P9-CCX-007

Examination of Orthopedic and Athletic Injuries

EDITION 3

Chad Starkey, PhD, LAT
Clinical Associate Professor
Coordinator, Division of Athletic Training
College of Health and Human Services
Ohio University
Athens, OH

Sara D. Brown, MS, ATC
Clinical Associate Professor
Director, Programs in Athletic Training
Sargent College of Health and Rehabilitation Sciences
Boston University
Boston, MA

Jeffrey L. Ryan, PT, MBA
Chief Clinical Operating Officer
Hahnemann Physician Practice Plan
Philadelphia, PA

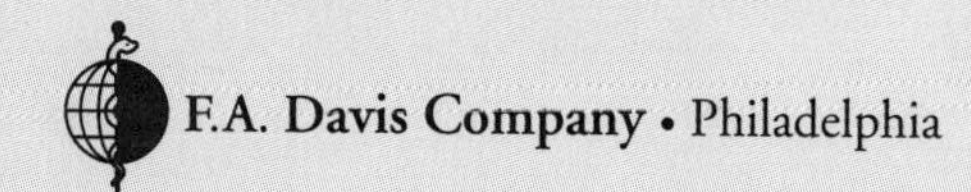

F.A. Davis Company
1915 Arch Street
Philadelphia, PA 19103
www.fadavis.com

Printed in the United States of America

Last digit indicates print number: 10 9 8 7 6 5 4 3 2 1

Senior Acquisitions Editor: Quincy McDonald
Manager of Content Development: George W. Lang
Developmental Editors: Molly Connors and Sarah Granlund
Art and Design Manager: Carolyn O'Brien

As new scientific information becomes available through basic and clinical research, recommended treatments and drug therapies undergo changes. The author(s) and publisher have done everything possible to make this book accurate, up to date, and in accord with accepted standards at the time of publication. The author(s), editors, and publisher are not responsible for errors or omissions or for consequences from application of the book, and make no warranty, expressed or implied, in regard to the contents of the book. Any practice described in this book should be applied by the reader in accordance with professional standards of care used in regard to the unique circumstances that may apply in each situation. The reader is advised always to check product information (package inserts) for changes and new information regarding dose and contraindications before administering any drug. Caution is especially urged when using new or infrequently ordered drugs.

Library of Congress Cataloging-in-Publication Data

Starkey, Chad, 1959-
Examination of orthopedic and athletic injuries / Chad Starkey, Sara D. Brown, Jeffrey L. Ryan. — Ed. 3.
p. ; cm.
Rev. ed. of: Evaluation of orthopedic and athletic injuries / Chad Starkey, Jeffrey L. Ryan. 2nd ed. c2002.
Includes bibliographical references and index.
ISBN-13: 978-0-8036-1720-9
ISBN-10: 0-8036-1720-8
1. Sports injuries. I. Brown, Sara D. II. Ryan, Jeffrey L., 1962- III. Starkey, Chad, 1959- Evaluation of orthopedic and athletic injuries. IV. Title.
[DNLM: 1. Athletic Injuries—diagnosis. 2. Orthopedic Procedures—methods. QT 261 S795e 2009]
RD97.S83 2009
617.1'027—dc22 2009022826

And everything that I thought fanciful and mocked as too extreme
Must be family entertainment here in the strange land of my dreams

C.A.S.

To Tom, Max, and Stephanie. You make everything seem right.

S.D.B.

To Dr. Chad Starkey for your foresight, direction, and, most of all, friendship. God knows that if it were not for the friendship we would have stopped this project after writing Chapter 1 of the first edition. And to Steve Bair, ATC, who gave me my most valuable professional life lesson: "J.R., always know what you don't know."

J.L.R.

RP
April 1986–May 2008

PREFACE

Much has changed since Jeff Ryan and I wrote the first edition of *Evaluation of Orthopedic and Athletic Injuries* in 1995. The words *outcomes* and *evidence* belonged more to the legal world than healthcare, and the focus of the diagnostic process was primarily on identifying the traumatized tissues rather than the effect the pathology had on an individual's lifestyle. The third edition of this text, now titled *Examination of Orthopedic and Athletic Injuries*, has four primary changes: organization of the chapters into two sections – Foundations of Examination, covering background concepts, and Regional Examination, focusing on specific anatomic areas; consideration of evidence-based practice (EBP); inclusion of the concept of disablement; and the addition of Sara D. Brown, MS, ATC, as a coauthor.

Chapter 3, Evidence-Based Practice in the Diagnostic Process, introduces the reader to the concepts and terminology used in EBP. In subsequent diagnostic chapters we present the current evidence (current at the time of the final editorial review) for clinical diagnostic procedures, focusing on the inter-rater reliability, intra-rater reliability, positive likelihood ratio, and negative likelihood ratio when this information is available in peer-reviewed journals. You will note that the usefulness of many popular orthopedic tests has not yet been determined. Although the absence of evidence does not necessarily mean that the procedure is invalid, it does indicate that research is still needed to confirm the test's efficacy. Interestingly, many of the most common orthopedic diagnostic tests lack peer-reviewed evidence.

Because of compelling evidence citing the lack of diagnostic accuracy, several special tests that were presented in the first and second editions of this text have been omitted from this edition. We have, however, included several procedures that have historically been taught and are commonly used in clinical practice but that do not pass scientific muster because they are either unreliable or provide little diagnostic value. We want to emphasize that instructors should *not* be compelled to teach students how to perform each procedure presented in *Examination of Orthopedic and Athletic Injuries*. Those with low diagnostic accuracy should be discussed as to why they are not clinically useful.

Most chapters include multiple "at a glance" practical evidence boxes that provide a concise summary of important or compelling findings in the diagnostic process. We present all the evidence with caution, knowing that much of the research is in its early stages and is subject to sudden and significant change. We will keep an updated list of evidence at http://davisplus.fadavis.com and we encourage both instructors and students to keep up-to-date with the current research.

We have divided Chapter 1 from the first edition into three chapters: The Injury Examination Process (Chapter 1), Examination and Management of Acute Pathologies (Chapter 2), and Musculoskeletal Diagnostic Techniques (Chapter 5). This division allows for more detail in the examination and management of acute (on-field) injuries and further explanation of musculoskeletal images. The examination and management concepts presented in Chapters 1 and 2 and the information presented in Injury Pathology Nomenclature (Chapter 4) provide the basis for the examination techniques presented in Section 2, Regional Examination. The Musculoskeletal Diagnostic Techniques chapter describes the usefulness of various forms of imaging, electromyography, and nerve conduction velocity testing, and provides basic instructions to prepare the patient for the procedure.

To make room for this new information, the relevant parts of the Cardiopulmonary Conditions and General Medical Conditions chapters from the second edition were merged into other chapters in the third.

As always, the most important component of this (or any text) is the instructors and students who use it. We invite your feedback and questions regarding this edition. Please feel free to email us at chadstarkey@aol.com or sara@bu.edu if we may be of any service to you.

Chad Starkey
Sara D. Brown
Jeffrey L. Ryan

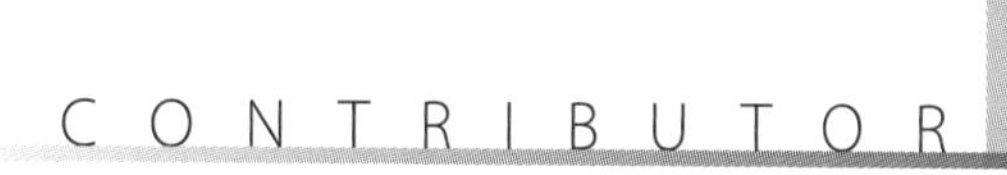

CONTRIBUTOR

Monique Mokha, PhD, ATC
Adjunct Faculty
Athletic Training Program
Nova Southeastern University
Boca Raton, FL

Diane Bartholomew, DHSc, ATC
Athletic Training Curriculum Administrator
Assistant Professor
Health and Movement Science Department
Graceland University
Lamoni, IA

Paul K. Canavan, PhD, ATC, PT, CSCS
Assistant Professor
Northeastern University
Athletic Training Education and Physical Therapy Department
Boston, MA

Laura E. Clark, MS, ATC
Athletic Training Clinical Instructor
Exercise Science, Health Promotion, and Recreation Department
Colorado State University – Pueblo
Pueblo, CO

Matthew J. Comeau, PhD, LAT, ATC, CSCS
Associate Professor and Program Director
Department of Health, Physical Education and Sport Sciences
Arkansas State University
Jonesboro, AR

Mike Dolan, MA, ATC, CSCS
Professor
Athletic Training Program
Department of Sports Medicine, Health and Human Performance
Canisius College
Buffalo, NY

Alana Eichman, MEd, LAT
Assistant Athletic Trainer
The University of Miami
Coral Gables, FL

Bradley M. Farrell, MS, ATC
Assistant Athletic Trainer
University of Louisville
Louisville, KY

Trenton E. Gould, PhD, ATC
Director, Athletic Training Education
School of Human Performance and Recreation
The University of Southern Mississippi
Hattiesburg, MS

Peter Koehneke, MS, ATC
Professor and Chair
Athletic Training Program Director
Department of Sports Medicine, Health and Human Performance
Canisius College
Buffalo, NY

Julie A. Rochester, MS, ATC
Director, Athletic Training Program
Associate Professor
Department of Health, Physical Education and Recreation
Northern Michigan University
Marquette, MI

Susan Rozzi, PhD, ATC, SCATA
Associate Professor
Department of Physical Education and Health
Program Director, Athletic Training
College of Charleston
Charleston, SC

Daniel R. Sedory, MS, ATC, NHLAT
Clinical Associate Professor and Program Director
Kinesiology Department
University of New Hampshire
Durham, NH

Brady L. Tripp, PhD, ATC
Clinical Assistant Professor
Director, Graduate Athletic Training Program
Department of Applied Physiology and Kinesiology
University of Florida
Gainesville, FL

Stacy Walker, PhD, ATC
Assistant Professor
Ball State University
School of Physical Education, Sport and Exercise Science
Muncie, IN

Kristi M. White, PhD, LAT
Assistant Professor
Department of Recreation and Sport Sciences
Ohio University
Athens, OH

Andrew P. Winterstein, PhD, LAT
Program Director
Athletic Training Education Program
Department of Kinesiology
University of Wisconsin
Madison, WI

ACKNOWLEDGMENTS

We thank the following individuals for their editorial and production assistance in the development of this manuscript: Christa Fratantoro, Senior Acquisitions Editor; Quincy McDonald, Senior Acquisitions Editor; George W. Lang, Manager of Content Development; Yvonne Gillam, Developmental Editor; Elizabeth Stepchin, Developmental Associate; Carolyn O'Brien, Art and Design Manager; David Orzechowski, Managing Editor; Sam Rondinelli, Production Manager; and Molly Connors and Sarah M. Granlund, Project Directors at Dovetail Content Solutions.

Thanks to Scott Gardner, MA, ATC, of Scott Gardner Photography (http://scottgardnerphotos.com). The quality of the photographs is a clear improvement over the first two editions. We also thank the following individuals who served as models for the new photographs: Ben Batchelder, Navdeep Boparari, John Bowman, Matt Broaddus, Garrett Chin, Jeff Doeringer, Erin Driscoll, Nadia Edwards, Alana Eichman, Brian Fairbrother, Carrie Gladwell, Aimee Gros, Marisa Hard, Trish Harris, Ellen Herman, Matt Hoch, Megan Hunt, Ashley Jones, B. Andrew Krause, Heather Lawrence, Brian McGivern, Paula Meszaros, Angela Michael, Kyle Montgomery, Claire Olson, Andy Palko, Jacqueline Schwieterman, Kayla Shinew, Chris Stephan, Jason White, and Colleen Whitkopp.

We would like to thank René Revis Shingles, PhD, ATC (Culturally Competent Care box in Chapter 1) and Monique Mokha, PhD, ATC, (Chapter 7, Evaluation of Gait) for their contribution to this text. This edition includes a comprehensive ancillary package. Much thanks goes to Erin M. Driscoll, MS, ATC, who revised the Instructor's Guide and developed the PowerPoint presentation. We appreciate the efforts of Laura E. Clark, MS, ATC, Matthew J. Comeau, PhD, LAT, ATC, CSCS, Jeremy Dicus, MS, ATC, LAT, and Eric J. Fuchs, ATC, NREMT-B, who developed the test bank. We also thank our reviewers, who are listed previously.

Lastly, Chad would like to thank Jeff Ryan for 10 years of coauthorship in the first two editions of this text. In addition to being a supportive and driven coauthor, he has been an unparalleled friend, and his contributions to my life and career cannot be repaid. I am fortunate that Sara Daniels Brown, MS, ATC, agreed to serve as the coauthor of this edition. Her perspective and knowledge of EBP provided the basis on which this third edition is founded.

CONTENTS

SECTION 1

Foundations of Examination

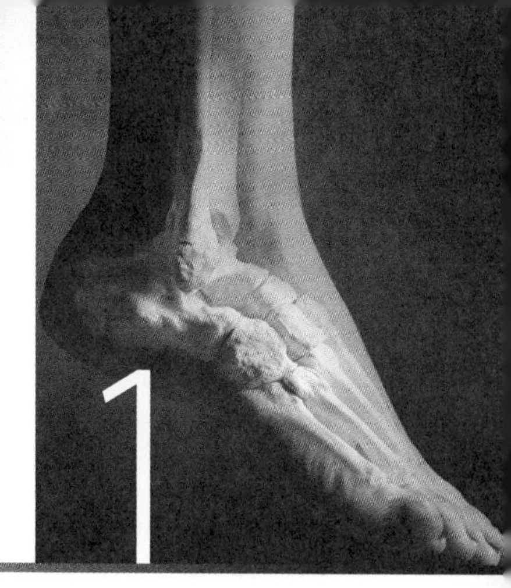

CHAPTER 1

The Injury Examination Process

Structure governs function. In the human body, anatomy is the structure and physiology and biomechanics are the functions. To perform a competent injury examination, a basic knowledge of the specific structure and function of the body part must be matched with an understanding of how these parts work together to produce normal movement (biomechanics). When injury occurs, **pathomechanics**, such as limping, may result. Conversely, an abnormal movement pattern, particularly one that is repeated thousands of times, such as a shortened stride length when running, can result in injury. The examination process consists of connecting the findings of dysfunctional anatomy, physiology, or biomechanics with the unique circumstances of the individual.

Successful management and rehabilitation of injuries depends on obtaining an accurate initial diagnosis of the injury; however, the process does not end there. The examination process is ongoing throughout all phases of recovery. The effectiveness of the treatment and rehabilitation protocol, and subsequent modification, is based on the ongoing reexamination of the patient's functional status.

Regardless of whether the examination is an initial **triage** of the injury or a reevaluation of an existing condition, a systematic and methodical evaluation model leads to efficiency, consistency, and accuracy in the evaluation process. The final determination of the patient's condition is derived through a **differential diagnosis** process in which pathologies that have similar **signs** and symptoms are progressively excluded based on examination findings. The clinical diagnosis may then be confirmed through imaging, laboratory tests, and other examination techniques.

Occasionally, a finding obtained during an examination will warrant immediate referral to a physician for medical diagnosis and management. The examination process should always attempt to rule in or rule out these conditions. Much of the exclusionary process is intuitive: a patient who is talking is obviously breathing. Findings such as bone angulation associated with an obvious fracture may become evident during the secondary survey. Other findings such as localized numbness may become apparent later in the clinical examination. If the patient's **disposition** is not clear, err on the side of caution and refer the patient for further medical examination.

Systematic Examination Technique

This chapter describes the examination model used in this text, one of many that are available. Any examination model must incorporate: (1) the justifiable inclusion or exclusion of each step and (2) adaptability to the specific needs of the situation.

Triage The process of determining the priority of treatment.

Sign An observable condition that indicates the existence of a disease or injury.

Disposition The immediate and long-term management of an injury or illness.

The examination should gather **objective data** to better organize, interpret, and monitor a patient's progress and develop treatment priorities. Baseline measurements such as pain scales obtained during the initial examination are recorded and referenced during subsequent reexaminations to document the patient's progress and identify the need for changes in the patient's treatment and rehabilitation protocol. The initial report serves as the baseline when planning the treatment and rehabilitation program. Through reevaluating the patient's condition and comparing it with the initial findings, the patient's progress may be monitored and subsequent adjustments made in the rehabilitation plan.

The findings of the initial and follow-up examinations and any subsequent referrals must be documented in the patient's medical record. Besides serving a legal purpose, medical records have an important practical purpose. Through the use of clear, concise terminology and objective findings, the medical record serves as a method of communicating the patient's current medical disposition to all who read it.

Description of the Examination Model

The model used in this text is divided into four primary components, each achieving a specific objective. The individual components, as well as the steps within each one, are presented sequentially, with one task completed before another is begun. In practice, the examination sequence and content vary based on the findings obtained, and more experienced clinicians will combine tasks such as inspecting the injured area while conducting the history. Sometimes, too, findings during the examination dictate that components be omitted entirely. For example, when a long bone fracture is suspected, range of motion (ROM) of the adjacent joints should be excluded.

One goal of the examination process is to obtain a clinical diagnosis. Another goal is to obtain sufficient information to determine a treatment plan that will improve the patient's quality of life. The **Nagi disablement model** provides a broader framework for the examination process, encouraging the clinician to consider the patient beyond the immediate examination findings. The principles associated with the Nagi model are applied in this text (Box 1-1). For example, identifying functional limitations by observing the patient performing the problematic tasks provides the foundation for the remainder of the examination. The clinical puzzle is to discover the underlying impairments that causes the functional limitation.

Although the physical aspect of the examination holds the immediate priority, the patient's psychological and emotional state must also be considered. People react differently to injury, with varying levels of pain tolerance, apprehension, fear, and desire to return to activity. The examination process may be adjusted based on the patient's psychological status. For instance, a patient who is apprehensive or fearful during the evaluation may relax if the examiner takes time to explain each step in the process in detail.

The Role of the Uninjured Paired Structure

The uninjured (opposite) body part provides an immediate reference point to determine the relative dysfunction of the injured segment. In the case of an injured extremity, the patient may use the uninjured limb to demonstrate the mechanism of injury or the movements that produce pain (Table 1-1). A portion of the history-taking process should be used to identify prior injury of the uninjured limb that could influence the bilateral comparison.

Although the role and importance of the uninjured body part is clear, where its examination fits into the evaluation process is not. One strategy is to perform each task on the uninjured body part before involving the injured side. The rationale for this technique is that the patient's apprehension will decrease if the evaluation is performed first on the uninjured side. The other school of thought suggests that testing the uninvolved limb first may increase the patient's apprehension and cause **muscle guarding**. This text assumes that the noninjured body part will be evaluated first; however, the urgency of some acute injuries such as joint dislocations makes comparison to the noninjured limb irrelevant.

Clinical Assessment

The term "assessment" describes the broad array of techniques used to obtain information regarding the patient's condition and the impact of the condition on the patient's life, including physical activity. Compared to acute evaluations, clinical assessments are performed in a relatively controlled environment. In the clinical setting, the clinician has luxuries that are not available at an athletic venue, including evaluation tools (e.g., tape measures, goniometers), medical records, and, perhaps most importantly, time.

An injury evaluation normally includes physical contact between the patient and the clinician. At times, the physical contact may involve areas of the patient's body—such as the pelvic region or the chest in female patients—that call for the utmost in discretion. Regardless of the area of physical contact or the gender of the patient and clinician, the patient must always give informed consent for the clinician to perform the evaluation. Patients who are younger than 18 years old or who have a cognitive impairment that would

Objective data Finite measures that are readily reproducible regardless of the individual collecting the information.

Muscle guarding Voluntarily or involuntarily assuming a posture to protect an injured body area, often through muscular spasm.

HISTORY

Past Medical History

- **Establish general information** (age, activities, occupation, limb dominance)
- **Establish prior history of injury to area**
  - When (in years, months or days)? Number of episodes?
  - Seen by physician or other health care provider?
  - Immobilization? If so, how long?
  - Surgery? Type?
  - Limitation in activity? Duration of?
  - Residual complaints? (Full recovery?)
  - Is this a similar injury? How is it different?
- **Establish general health status** (medications, mental status, chronic or acute diseases, etc.)

History of the Present Condition

- **Establish chief complaint**
  - What is the patient's disability? What can patient not do that is impacting life?
  - What is the primary problem and the impact on ADLs and/or sport?
  - What is the duration of current problem?
  - Self-initiated treatment
- **Establish pain information**
  - Pain location, type, and pattern. Does it change?
  - What increases and decreases pain?
  - Pattern relative to sports participation and/or occupation?
  - Pattern relative to specific sport demands
- **Establish changes in demands of activity and/or occupation**
  - Changes in activity?
  - New activity pattern?
  - New equipment?
  - Activities of daily living
- **Other relevant information**
  - Pain/other symptoms anywhere else? Altered sensations?
  - Crepitus, locking, or catching?

INSPECTION*

- **Obvious deformity**
- **Functional Assessment**
  - What functional limitations does the patient demonstrate?
  - What impairments cause the functional limitations? Which are most problematic?
- **Swelling and discoloration**
- **General posture**
- **Scars, open wounds, cuts, or abrasions**

PALPATION*

- **Areas of point tenderness**
- **Change in tissue density** (scarring, spasm, swelling, calcification)
- **Deformity**
- **Temperature change**
- **Texture**

JOINT AND MUSCLE FUNCTION ASSESSMENT

- **Active range of motion**
  - Evaluate for ease of movement, pain, available range (quantified via goniometry)
- **Manual muscle tests**
  - Evaluate for pain and weakness
- **Passive range of motion**
  - Evaluate for difference from active ROM, pain, end-feel, available range (quantified via goniometry)

JOINT STABILITY TESTS*

- **Stress Testing**
  - Evaluate for increased pain and/or increased or decreased laxity relative to opposite side
- **Joint Play**
  - Evaluate for increased pain and/or increased or decreased mobility relative to opposite side

SPECIAL TESTS*

- **Selective tissue testing**
  - Stress specific structures to identify laxity, tightness, instability, or pain.
- **Provocation/alleviation testing**
  - Identify positions or maneuvers that increase or decrease symptoms

NEUROLOGICAL ASSESSMENT*

- **Sensory**
  - Assess spinal nerve root and peripheral nerve sensory function
- **Motor**
  - Determine spinal nerve root and peripheral motor nerve function
- **Reflex**
  - Assess spinal level reflex function

VASCULAR ASSESSMENT*

- **Capillary refill**
  - Assess for adequate perfusion
- **Distal pulses**
  - Assess for adequate blood supply

CLINICAL DIAGNOSIS

- **Include all diagnoses that have not been excluded by the examination process**

DISPOSITION

- **Prognosis**
  - Predict probable short- and long-term outcome of the condition
- **Intervention**
  - Determine the patient's course of care
- **Return to activity**
  - Develop criteria for return to sport, work, and/or daily activity

* Compare bilaterally

Overview of the key elements of the examination model used throughout this text.

preclude an informed consent must have their needs represented by a guardian if at all possible.

Informed consent should include a statement that the patient understands that physical contact will occur and gives the clinician permission to proceed with the evaluation process. Furthermore, the patient understands that if he or she becomes uncomfortable with the physical contact during the evaluation, he or she can ask the examiner to stop. Informed consent may be established in the form of a signed written statement or, in the case of an on-field injury during athletics, it may be verbal in nature if a signed form is not already on file. A patient suffering a medical emergency may not be able to give consent for treatment. In this case, a clinician's duty to provide

Box 1-1
Nagi Model of Disablement

The Nagi Model of Disablement presents a framework to identify how the patient's pathology impacts body structure, operation, and psyche (impairments); how impairments influence function (functional limitations); and how these functional limitations impact the person's life (disability). Identified functional limitations are connected to impairments. One impairment may cause other impairments that further increase functional disability.[1] Traditional evaluation models focus on the patient's pathology and tend to neglect the impact of the injury or illness on the person's ability to function on a personal and societal level.

While the examination process in this book focuses on the identification of impairments and functional limitations, doing this in the absence of understanding the resulting disability leads to ineffective treatment. Likewise, not all impairments result in functional limitations. For example, a patient may have decreased ROM in a joint without any impact on the ability to perform daily activities. In this example, a treatment approach that focuses on impairment-level treatment (increasing the ROM) will have limited impact on the patient's quality of life.

The following illustrates the primary components of the Nagi model using a sprained knee ligament as an example

	Definition	Examples of Assessment Techniques	Measurement/Finding
Active Pathology	Interruption or interference of normal bodily processes or structure	Imaging Lab work	Ligament disruption
Impairment	Anatomical, physiological, mental or emotional abnormalities	History Pain questionnaires Instrumented testing Joint play Manual muscle tests Stress tests Special tests	Increased laxity with firm end feel Pain at rest = 3.0/10 Pain at worst = 7.5/10
Functional Limitation	Restriction of lack of ability to perform an action or activity in the manner or range considered normal (which results from impairment). How the impairment impacts the patient's ability to perform a task.	Observation during functional task such as walking or reaching.	Inability to walk normally
Disability	An inability or limitation in performing socially defined activities and roles expected of individuals within a social and physical environment.	Question patient regarding impact on life. What can the patient not do that he/she desires to?	Unable to participate in football practice.

Column 2 information from Nagi, SZ. Disability concepts revisited. In Pope, AM, Tarloy, AR (eds). *Prevention in Disability in America: Toward a National Agenda for* Prevention. Washington, DC: National Academy Press, 1991, p. 7.

emergency medical care overrides obtaining consent. Certain religions may limit the type of care rendered to the patient (see Box 1-2).

History

The most informative portion of an examination is the patient's history. Identifying the mechanism of injury, appreciating the influence of any underlying medical conditions, and understanding the impact of the condition on the patient's life are examples of information obtained in this component. The result of the patient's reported and documented medical history sets the tone and structure for the remaining physical examination.[2]

The remainder of the examination helps to refine the information derived from the history. The history provides information about the structures involved, the extent of the tissue damage, and the resulting disability. When examining acute conditions, identifying the mechanism of injury is vital to understanding the forces placed on certain structures. For chronic conditions, a determination of changes in training routines, equipment, or posture will help narrow the diagnostic possibilities and directly influence the intervention strategy.

Table 1-1 Role of the Noninjured Limb in the Examination Process

Segment	Relevance
History	**Past medical history:** Establishes preinjury health baseline and identifies conditions that can influence the current problem. **History of present condition:** Replicates the mechanism of injury, primary complaint(s), and functional limitations and disability.
Inspection	Functional assessment provides information regarding how the condition impacts the patient's ability to perform relevant tasks. Provides a reference for symmetry and color of the superficial tissues. Observation of function determines any limitation(s) between the extremities. Most meaningful when compared to baseline measures.
Palpation	Provides a reference for the comparison of bilateral symmetry of bones, alignment, tissue temperature, or other deformity as well as the presence of increased tenderness
Joint and Muscle Function Assessment	Provides a reference to identify impairments relating to available ROM, strength, and pain with movement.
Joint Stability Test	Provides a reference for end-feel, relative laxity or hypomobility, and pain
Special Tests	Provides a reference for pathology of individual ligaments, joint capsules, and musculotendinous units, and the body's organs.
Neurological Test	Provides a reference for bilateral sensory, reflex, and motor function
Vascular Screening	Determines blood circulation to and from involved extremity

Box 1-2

Culturally Competent Care

The information gained during a patient examination must be pertinent and accurate to arrive at the proper clinical diagnosis. Miscommunication or misinterpretation often can occur because of differing cultural conventions between the clinician and the patient, possibly leading to an incorrect diagnosis, inappropriate care, or patient noncompliance.[3,4] To minimize this risk clinicians should learn to:

- Involve patients in their own health care.
- Understand cultural groups' attitudes, beliefs, and values as related to issues of health and illness.
- Use cultural resources and knowledge to address health care problems.
- Develop care plans that are holistic and include patients' cultural needs.

"Culture" is the values, beliefs, and practices shared by a group and influences an individual's health beliefs, practices, and behaviors. Evaluating patients within a cultural context helps the clinician gain accurate information. It also conveys concern about the patient as a person, not as a body part or injury (e.g., "my ACL patient"). Therefore, using patient-first language, that is, addressing the patient rather than the condition is more appropriate (e.g., "my patient who has an ACL injury").

Remember that culture is present, operating, and influencing the interchange in every evaluation (whether the interaction is between members of different cultures or within the same culture). The following are some cultural aspects that must be considered during the evaluation process.

History

Clear communication between the clinician and patient is critical for taking an accurate history. Whether you are using verbal and/or nonverbal communication skills, it is important to understand the cultural context in which the exchange is occurring.

- Convey respect: Patients, particularly adult patients, are addressed formally (Miss, Mr., Mrs., Ms.) unless otherwise directed to do so by the patient.
- Language: Barriers can exist when English is spoken as a second language or if the patient does not speak English. Likewise, barriers can exist even when speaking the same language or dialect. Some communication interventions include:
- Determine the level of English fluency.
- Obtain the services of an interpreter, if needed.
- Recognize that dialects are acceptable.
- Avoid stereotyping because of language and speech patterns.
- Clarify slang terms.

Continued

Box 1-2
Culturally Competent Care—cont'd

- Use jargon-free language.
- Use pictures, models, or materials written in the patient's language.
- Speak more slowly, not more loudly.
- Ask about one symptom at a time.

To ensure that the patient understands your instructions, have him or her paraphrase your instructions. If you are working in a setting where other languages are spoken, consider learning the languages of the patient or obtain the services of an interpreter. If an interpreter is used, speak to, and make eye contact with, the patient, not the interpreter.

- **Verbal versus nonverbal communication**: The actions of the clinician can be just as important as what is said (or not said). If a person has difficulty understanding what you are saying, he or she will increase his or her reliance on secondary forms of communication such as body language and facial expressions. Likewise, the clinician should be familiar with assessing the patient's body language from a cultural perspective, including level of eye contact and use of silence.
- **Narrative sequence**: Clinicians often ask history questions and expect answers in a chronological order. However, not all patients describe the history chronologically. Some relay what happened episodically, indicating those "episodes" or "stories" deemed important to the injury. Allow the patient to respond to the question in the sequence he or she feels comfortable. Taking notes will help organize the pertinent information.
- **Religious considerations**: Some religions prohibit or limit the amount of medical intervention that can occur. Obtaining cultural information, including religious considerations, as part of the preparticipation medical examination history potentially minimizes the risk of providing unwanted or prohibited care. For example, if an acute injury situation arises where the patient is unconscious, knowledge about the patient's preferences will assist the clinician in providing care that is consistent with those preferences.
- **Family considerations**: Including immediate and extended family in the decision-making process is often important. Family members can assist with therapeutic regimens, thereby improving compliance.
- **Use of complementary and alternative medicine (CAM); traditional and folk medicines or practices**: Ask patients if they are using home remedies, traditional medicines or practices, herbal supplements, or other health care practices not considered a part of conventional medicine. As a clinician, you want to work cooperatively with patients, understanding and respecting their health care practices in order to provide the best possible care. In addition, some alternative medicines or treatments may negatively interact with mainstream medical care.

Inspection

When inspecting your patient, remember that differences in skin pigmentation and conditions must be considered.

- **Skin assessment** (coloration and discoloration): Skin pigmentation varies between and within cultural groups. Use enough lighting to differentiate changes in skin tone. When inspecting dark-pigmented skin for pallor, cyanosis, and jaundice, check the mucous membranes, lips, nail beds, palms of hands, and soles of feet to determine the problem.
- **Skin conditions**: Be aware that keloids, scars that form at the site of a wound and grow beyond its boundaries, are most common in African American and Asian patients (refer to Fig. 1-3). Ascertain if the patient is prone to keloids, particularly if surgery is indicated. There may be steps the physician can take to minimize the scarring.

Issues Regarding Physical Contact

When palpating the patient, care must be taken to touch in a manner that is culturally appropriate.

- **Religious considerations**: Permission must be granted before touching any patient. In some cultures and religions, the act of physically being touched or exposing body areas may carry with it certain moral and ethical issues.
- **Gender considerations**: The standard for the "appropriateness" of touching can be influenced by the gender of the patient and the clinician. Some patients may not feel comfortable being examined by an individual of the opposite gender. If a clinician is of the opposite gender of the patient, the process should be observed by a third party (e.g., another clinician, coach, parent/guardian, or family member).

Not all individuals in a given ethnic or racial group behave the same way. The levels of acculturation and socioeconomic status are just two factors that influence health care beliefs and practices. Therefore, use this information as a guide during the evaluation process. Further information may be obtained from the following sources:

Office of Minority Health, U.S. Department of Health and Human Services

Center for Cross-Cultural Health (A clearing house of information, training, and research)

National Center for Complementary and Alternative Medicine

Resources for Cross-Cultural Health Care

Obtaining a medical history relies on the ability to communicate with the patient. The quality, depth, and breadth of information gained from the patient's responses will correspond to the clinician's communication skills. Sociocultural differences between the clinician and patient may create an unrecognized communication barrier that can negatively influence the rest of the evaluation. An awareness of these differences can facilitate communication and improve patient care (Box 1-2).

Open-ended inquiries are useful during the history-taking process because they allow the patient to describe the nature of the complaint in detail. Asking questions that can be answered "yes" or "no" limits the amount of information that can be deduced from the patient's response. Consider the different responses to, "Does your shoulder hurt when you raise your arm?" versus, "Tell me about what makes your shoulder hurt." Occasionally, however, when time is critical such as the immediate examination of an acute, potentially **catastrophic** injury, closed-ended questions are necessary, for example, "Can you move your fingers?" (see Chapter 3).

Past medical history

For nonacute examinations, patients or their parents are usually asked to complete medical history forms that detail any underlying health conditions, prior injuries, factors that might predispose them to injury, and the course of the current condition. This information provides important baseline information that can serve as the foundation of the examination. Increasingly, clinicians are asking patients to complete disability questionnaires such as the Disabilities of the Arm, Shoulder and Hand (DASH). These questionnaires quantify the extent and nature of resulting disability and, when repeated, offer reliable information regarding the effectiveness of any intervention (Box 1-3).[5]

Box 1-3
Functional Outcome and Disability Questionnaires

Quantifying the extent of a patient's ROM tells us little about how the patient is actually doing with regard to functioning in everyday life. Initially, these outcome measures were used for research but their use has expanded where to the point that functional outcome measures and disability questionnaires are being completed on a routine basis so that the patient's progress with regard to impact of a condition on quality of life can be determined. Some of the measures are more global and others are condition-specific.

Global

Short Form 36 (SF-36): Thirty-six questions completed by the patient; yields a profile of functional health and well-being

Tegner Activity Scale: Numerical rating from 0 to 10 indicating the patient's ability to perform specific activities. A score of 10 indicates an ability to participate in competitive sports including soccer and football.

Low Back

Oswestry Disability Questionnaire: Ten-section questionnaire assesses the impact of low back pain on everyday life.

Roland-Morris Disability Questionnaire: Patient marks any of 18 statements that describe the impact of his or her back pain.

Knee

Lysholm Knee Scale: Reflects physical parameters such as ability to climb stairs and squat, episodes of giving way, swelling, and pain.

Activity Rating Scale: Used to measure the activity level of patients with knee pain based on straight-ahead running, cutting, decelerating, and pivoting.

Cincinnati Knee Rating System: Classifies disability based on six functional measures: walking, using stairs, squatting and kneeling, straight running, jumping and landing, and twists, cuts, and pivots.

Ankle

Foot and Ankle Outcome Score (FAOS): Self-report of foot or ankle pathology on pain, other symptoms, activities of daily living and ability to participate in sports and recreation

Upper Extremity

Disabilities of the Arm, Shoulder, and Hand (DASH): 30-item questionnaire completed by patient that measures physical function and symptoms

Catastrophic An injury that causes permanent disability or death.

For those working in the collegiate athletic setting, the National Collegiate Athletic Association (NCAA) has recommended specific components of the student-athlete's medical record (Box 1-4).[6]

The past medical history portion of the examination should include the items below. When possible, request documentation (e.g., operative and rehabilitation reports) that supplement the patient's explanation.

- **Previous history:** Is there a history of injury to the body area? Are there any possible sources of weakness from a previous injury? Is there is a history of injury to this body part on either side? If so, ask the patient to describe and compare this injury with the previous injury. Was the onset similar? Do the present symptoms duplicate the previous symptoms? Asking about injury to the entire extremity is important because injury to one structure, even though not currently symptomatic, can impact forces imposed on the adjacent, currently injured structure.

  A history of injury to the body area, prior medical conditions, and **congenital** conditions can predispose the person to further injury or influence the evaluation findings. If the injury appears to be a chronic condition or if previous injury to this body part has occurred, prior medical referral and subsequent treatment and rehabilitation protocol must be determined:
  - When did this episode occur? Has it reoccurred since the initial onset?
  - Who evaluated and treated this injury previously?
  - What diagnosis was made?
  - What diagnostic tests were performed? (e.g., radiographs, magnetic resonance imaging [MRI], blood work)
  - What was the course of treatment and rehabilitation?
  - Was surgery performed or medication prescribed?
  - Did the previous treatment plan change the symptoms?
  - Was there a successful return to the desired level of activity?

Understanding how similar prior injuries were managed and their subsequent outcome provides a baseline reference for future diagnostic procedures and rehabilitation planning.

- **General medical health:** What is the patient's general health status and what, if any, **comorbidities** are present? Athletes are often assumed to be in prime physical health. Unfortunately, this is not always correct. Current advances in medical treatment, including the

Box 1-4
NCAA Guideline 1B: Medical Evaluations, Immunizations, and Records

- History of injury, illness, pregnancy, and surgery of both athletic and nonathletic origin
- Physician referrals and subsequent feedback regarding treatment, rehabilitation, and disposition
- Preparticipation and preseason medical questionnaire detailing the following:
  - Acute and chronic illnesses
  - Acute and chronic injuries (athletic and nonathletic)
  - Surgery and hospitalization
  - Allergies
  - Medications taken on a regular basis
  - Conditioning status
- Concussions sustained
- Episodes involving the loss of consciousness, including **syncope**
- Exercised-induced asthma or bronchospasm
- Loss of paired organs
- Heat illness
- Cardiac conditions, including those involving the immediate family. Cardiovascular screening should be conducted every 2 years.
- **Sudden death** in a family member younger than age 50 years
- Family history of **Marfan syndrome**
- Immunization records:
  - Measles, mumps, rubella
  - Hepatitis B
  - Diphtheria, tetanus, meningitis
- Other documentation, signed by the athlete (and parent if the athlete is younger than age 18 years)
- Release of medical records
- Consent to treatment

use of medications, have allowed people to participate in athletics and exercise who previously would have been unable to. Prior physical examinations, including preparticipation and annual physical examinations, may reveal congenital abnormalities or diseases that could affect the evaluation and treatment of the injury.

The signs and symptoms of certain tumors and other systemic pathologies may masquerade as overuse injuries, strains, sprains, and other inflammatory conditions.[7] For example, testicular cancer may clinically appear to be a chronic adductor strain. Patients who present with apparent musculoskeletal injuries, but are lacking a relevant history to explain the symptoms or have symptoms that fail to resolve within a typical timeframe, must be promptly referred to a physician (Table 1-2).

- **Relevant illnesses and lab work**: Chronic, systemic illnesses or laboratory findings that can affect injury management and influence the healing process and should be noted at the time of examination. For example, people with diabetes often have associated sensory and vascular deficits that delay healing and alter pain perception.
- **Medications**: What prescription or over-the-counter medications, supplements, and/or herbal remedies is the individual taking? Certain medications impede tissue healing and may interact with any medications used to treat the current condition (Table 1-3).
- **Smoking**: Cigarette smoking as associated with a decreased tolerance for exercise, an increased risk for low back pain and musculoskeletal disorders, and an increased risk for cardiovascular disease. In addition, smoking may delay fracture and wound healing.[8]

History of the present condition

The following information should be obtained during the history-taking process:

- **Mechanism of the injury:** How did the injury occur? The description of the mechanism of injury helps to identify the involved structures and the forces placed on them. Was the trauma caused by a single traumatic force (macrotrauma), or was it the accumulation of repeated forces (microtrauma), resulting in an **insidious** onset of the symptoms? For example, "I got hit on the outside of my knee," describes a mechanism that produces compressive forces laterally and tensile forces medially.

For athletic injuries, practice and game videos can be used to help identify the mechanism of injury. These films may allow the medical team to actually view the mechanism and circumstances surrounding the injury.

- **Relevant sounds or sensations at the time of injury:** What sensations were experienced? Did the patient or bystanders hear any sounds, such as a "pop" that could be associated with a tearing ligament or a "crack" associated with bone fracturing? Determining the relationship between true physical dysfunction and the reported sensations is useful. For example, true "giving way" or instability would involve the subluxation of a joint (see Chapter 4). The physical sensation of a joint's giving way, but without true joint subluxation, indicates pain inhibition or weakness of the surrounding muscles.
- **Onset and duration of symptoms:** When did this problem begin? With acute macrotrauma, the signs and symptoms tend to present themselves immediately. The signs and symptoms associated with chronic or insidious microtrauma, such as **overuse syndromes**, tend to progressively worsen with time and continued stresses. The severity of overuse conditions may be graded based on the duration of time since the onset of symptoms and the amount of associated dysfunction. In the early stages, patients with overuse syndromes complain of pain associated with fatigue and after activity. As the condition progresses, pain is also described at the onset of activity and then progresses to pain of a constant nature.
- **Pain:** Because of changes in physiology following an injury, acute injuries often have a localized "stinging" type pain. A few hours later the pain becomes more diffuse and is may be described as "burning" or "aching." The location, type and severity of pain should be quantified whenever possible (Box 1-5).
    - **Location of pain**: Ask the patient to point to the area of pain. In many cases, the location of the pain correlates with the damaged tissue. Often following an acute injury the patient is able to use one finger to isolate the area of pain and is more likely to isolate the involved structure or structures. As time passes following the injury, pain becomes more diffuse and the patient tends to identify the painful area by sweeping the hand over a general area. Also ask the patient about any changes in the location, type, and duration of pain throughout the course of the day.

Congenital A condition existing at or before birth.

Syncope Fainting caused by a transient loss of oxygen supply to the brain.

Sudden death Unexpected and instantaneous death occurring within 1 hour of the onset of symptoms; most often used to describe death caused secondary to cardiac failure.

Marfan syndrome A hereditary condition of the connective tissue, bones, muscles, and ligaments. Over time, this condition results in degeneration of brain function, cardiac failure, and other visceral problems.

Comorbidity The presence of multiple unrelated disorders in the same person at the same time.

Insidious Of gradual onset; with respect to symptoms of an injury or disease having no apparent cause.

Overuse syndrome Injury caused by accumulated microtraumatic stress placed on a structure or body area.

Table 1-2 Referral Alerts

Finding	Possible Active Pathology or Condition
Chest pain Dizziness Shortness of breath Unexplained pain in the left arm Unexplained swelling of the ankle Unexplained weight gain	Congestive heart failure Myocardial infarction Splenic rupture
Unexplained weight loss Moles or other acute skin growths Slow to heal skin lesions Blood in the stool Unremitting night pain	Cancer
Blood in the urine Pain in the flank following the course of the ureter Low back pain associated with the above	Kidney stones Kidney/bladder infections
Loss of balance/coordination Loss of consciousness Bilateral hyperreflexia Acute hyporeflexia Inability to produce voluntary muscle contractions Unexplained general muscular weakness Bowel or bladder dysfunction	Neurological involvement
Unexplained pain Symptoms that fail to resolve in the expected time	Unknown, warrants medical examination
Fever, chills, and/or night sweats	Systemic disease or infection
Amenorrhea Severe dysmenorrhea	Pregnancy Ectopic pregnancy

Table 1-3 Potential Medication Effects on Musculoskeletal Healing

Medication (or medication family)	Generic Name (trade name) Example	Potential Negative Effect
Beta-blockers	Metoprolol (Lopressor) Propranolol (Inderal) Atenolol (Tenormin)	Decreased tolerance to exercise coupled with reduced perceived exertion.
Corticosteroid	Methylprednisolone (Medrol) Dexamethasone (Decadron)	Prolonged use: Muscle weakness, loss of muscle mass, tendon rupture, osteoporosis, aseptic necrosis of femoral and humeral heads, spontaneous fractures[9]
Cox-2 Inhibitors (type of NSAID)	Celecoxib (Celebrex)	Inhibit healing of soft-tissue and bone in animal models.[10]
Nonsteroidal Anti-Inflammatory Drugs	Ibuprofen (Motrin) Diclofenac (Voltaren)	Delayed fracture healing or nonunion of fracture,[11] delayed soft tissue healing in animal models[10,12]
Salicylates	Aspirin	Prolonged bleeding times
Anticoagulant	Warfarin (Coumadin)	Prolonged bleeding times

Box 1-5
Pain Rating Scales

Visual Analog Scale (VAS)

Pain as bad as it could be ▬▬▬▬▬▬▬▬▬▬ No pain

Using a 10-cm line, the patient is asked to mark the point that represents the current intensity of pain. The VAS value is then calculated by measuring the distance in centimeters from the right edge of the line.

Numeric Rating Scale (NRS)

No pain 0 1 2 3 4 5 6 7 8 9 10 Pain as bad as it could be

The patient is asked to circle the number from 0 (no pain) to 10 (worst pain imaginable) that best describes the current level of pain. Only whole numbers are used with this scale.

The VAS and NRS are common clinical techniques that are used to quantify the amount of pain that a patient is experiencing over time. They are also useful for measuring pain before and after treatment.

A. Where is your pain?

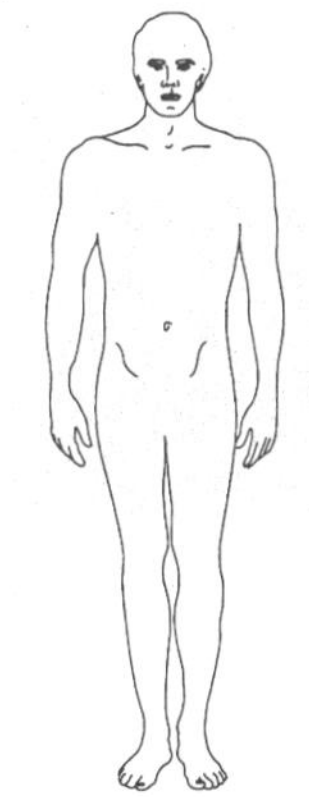

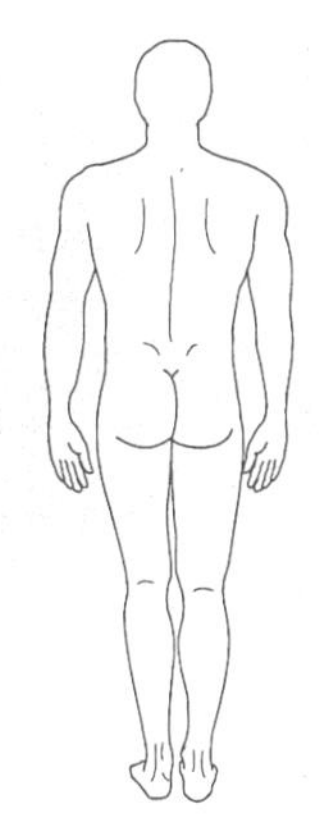

Using the above drawing, please mark the area(s) where you feel pain. Mark an "E" if the source of the pain is external or "I" if it is internal. If the source of the pain is both internal and external, please mark "B".

B. Pain rating index

Many different words can be used to describe pain. From the list below, please circle those words that best describe the pain you are currently experiencing. Use only one word from each category. You do not need to mark a word in every category -- **Only mark those words that most accurately describe your pain.**

1. Flickering, Quivering, Pulsing, Throbbing, Beating, Pounding

2. Jumping, Flashing, Shooting

3. Pricking, Boring, Drilling, Stabbing

4. Sharp, Cutting, Lacerating

5. Pinching, Pressing, Gnawing, Cramping, Crushing

6. Tugging, Pulling, Wrenching

7. Hot, Burning, Scalding, Searing

8. Tingling, Itchy, Smarting, Stinging

9. Dull, Sore, Hurting, Aching, Heavy

10. Tender, Taut, Rasping

11. Tiring, Exhausting

12. Sickening, Suffocating

13. Fearful, Frightful, Terrifying

14. Punishing, Grueling, Cruel, Vicious, Killing

15. Wretched, Blinding

16. Annoying, Troublesome, Miserable, Intense, Unbearable

17. Spreading, Radiating, Penetrating, Piercing

18. Tight, Numb, Drawing, Squeezing, Tearing

19. Cool, Cold, Freezing

20. Nagging, Nauseating, Agonizing, Dreadful, Torturing

McGill Pain Questionnaire

Pain assessment instruments such as the McGill Pain Questionnaire are often used for patients who have complex pain problems. In Part A of the questionnaire identifies the area(s) of pain and if the pain is deep or superficial. Part B provides descriptors that are used to determine the intensity and nature of the patient's pain. A visual analog or numeric rating scale is often included as a part of the questionnaire.

Figures from Starkey C. *Therapeutic Modalities,* (ed 3). Philadelphia: FA Davis 2004.

- **Type of pain**: When injured, different tissues may respond by producing different types of pain. Pain associated with fractures is often described as "sharp" due to the rich innervation of the periosteum. Nerve pathology can be described as "electricity," "lightening," or "pins and needles" extending from **proximal** to **distal** (or, in rare occasions, distal to proximal) in the extremity. Sharp, localized "stinging" pain is common immediately following acute injury; with time, the pain will transition to a "aching" or "throbbing" sensation.
- **Referred pain:** Referred pain, or pain at a site other than the actual location of trauma, can mislead the patient and the clinician as to the actual location of the pathology. Resulting when the central nervous system (CNS) misinterprets the location and source of the painful stimulus, referred pain patterns can indicate internal injury, such as when damage to the spleen results in left shoulder pain. Musculoskeletal injury can also cause referred pain, such as when rotator cuff involvement refers pain to the insertion of the deltoid muscle. Nerve trauma can produce radicular pain.
- **Radicular pain**: Radicular symptoms can result when a nerve root or peripheral nerve is compressed or otherwise damaged. Radicular pain occurs along relatively common distributions of innervation (dermatomes) and is discussed further in the appropriate chapters of this text.
- **Daily pain patterns:** When during the course of the day is the pain worse? Better? What is the pattern during activity? Pain that is worse in the morning and eases as the day progresses may be associated with **tissue creep** that occurs when tissues are shortened during the night (see Chapter 4). The opposite pattern, better in the morning and worse later in the day, can be associated with muscular fatigue or prolonged compressive forces, as in the case of a herniated disc.
- **Provocation and alleviation patterns:** What activities or positions relieve and worsen the pattern? The patient's description of a position that provokes the pain may direct the sequence of the examination and also helps identify what tissues may be stretched or compressed. For example, a patient may describe the functional limitation of increased shoulder pain with overhead movement, a provoking movement that can be replicated during the ROM portion and special testing portion of the examination. Patients with a cervical disc problem may describe certain positions that decrease pain, such as lateral bending, illustrating an alleviation pattern.

- **Other symptoms:** Does the patient describe other symptoms, such as weakness or **paresthesia**? Does the limb "give out"? Does the patient complain that the extremity feels "cold," indicating possible arterial involvement or "heavy," indicating possible venous or lymphatic involvement? Questioning the patient about the onset of symptoms such as **effusion** may help identify the involved structure.
- **Treatment to date:** Has the patient attempted any self-treatment or sought help from anyone else for this condition? A complete description of medications, alternative therapies, first aid procedures, and any other interventions such as prescription or over-the-counter foot orthotics is necessary to understand the full scope of the condition.
- **Affective traits:** Does the patient have any influences that would impede or exaggerate the desire to return to activity? Patients may understate the magnitude of their symptoms if an injury may prevent them from participating. Sometimes patients may overstate—or exaggerate—their symptoms either as a reason for poor performance or for possible financial gain.

  Depression is frequently associated with chronic pain, such as with nonspecific low back pain, and can negatively impact treatment outcomes. Questioning the patient specifically about recent feelings of depression and a decline in interest or pleasure in doing things can help identify those with depressive tendencies.[13] Fear-avoidance behaviors, where patients opt to not participate in a given activity due to fear of further injury or re-injury, and emotional distress are also associated with poor outcomes in patients with low back pain.[14]
- **Resulting functional limitations and disability:** What is the patient unable to accomplish and what activities are restricted? As described in Box 1-1 the concept of connecting identified impairments with functional limitations and resulting disabilities is key to developing an effective intervention strategy that works for the individual. For example, a runner who experiences pain at mile 20 may not have a disability if his goals can be met with runs of 10 miles.

At the conclusion of the initial history-taking process, a clear picture of the events causing the injury; predisposing conditions that may have led to its occurrence; and the activities, motions, and postures that increase or decrease the symptoms should be formed. The impact of the injury on the patient's life should be known. The remainder of the

Proximal Toward the midline of the body; the opposite of distal.

Distal Away from the midline of the body, moving toward the periphery; the opposite of proximal.

Tissue creep The gradual and progressive deformation of tissues to adapt to postural changes including immobilization or pathomechanics.

Paresthesia The sensation of numbness or tingling, often described as a "pins and needles" sensation, caused by compression of or a lesion to a peripheral nerve.

Effusion The accumulation of excess fluid within a joint space or joint cavity.

examination is used to expand on and further investigate the findings obtained during the history-taking process. Further information regarding the history of the injury is continued throughout the examination. Expand on the history during the remainder of the examination, backtracking or asking further questions as you follow leads to fully ascertain all the facts regarding the patient's condition.

Physical Examination

Next in the process is the physical examination, during which the clinician continues to pare down the differential diagnosis, determine a clinical diagnosis, and identify functional limitations and underlying impairments. The differential diagnosis includes all those possible diagnoses that have not been excluded by the examination findings. For example, with an acute ankle injury the initial differential diagnosis must include the possibility of a fracture that must be ruled in or out during the examination process.

Blood, synovial fluid, saliva, and other bodily fluids can potentially transmit bloodborne pathogens such as the **hepatitis B virus** (HBV) and the **human immunodeficiency virus** (HIV).[15] All bodily fluids must be treated as though they contain these viruses.[16] The treatment of acute injuries that involve bleeding, postsurgical wounds, and the handling of soiled dressings, instruments, or other blood or fluid-soiled object must be managed as if contaminated (Box 1-6).

Box 1-6
Standard Precautions Against Bloodborne Pathogens

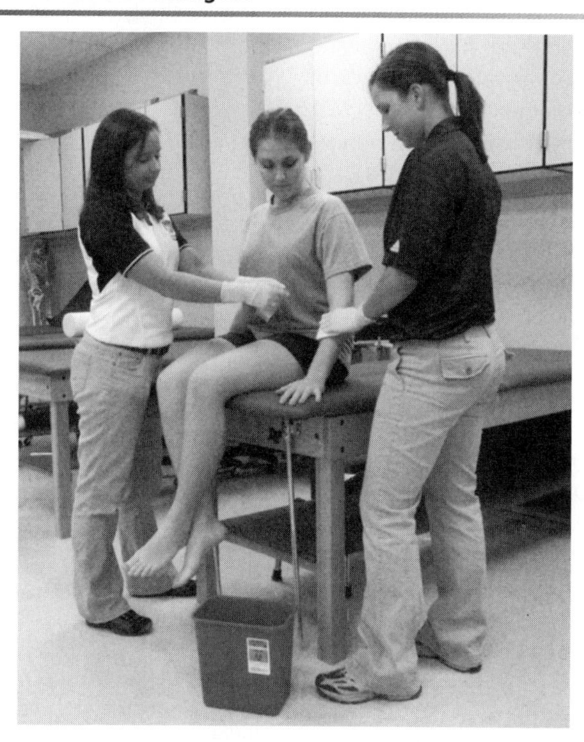

The use of standard precautions against bloodborne pathogens reduces the possibility of accidental exposure to biohazards, bloodborne substances such as hepatitis B or human immunodeficiency virus (HIV) that are potentially toxic to humans, animals, or the environment. Methods of protecting against accidental exposure include using gloves, biohazard disposal containers, and washing soiled towels, uniforms, and other material separately, according to the accepted guidelines. Approved disinfectants must be used to clean up blood and soiled dressings and instruments must be properly disposed of or cleaned.

Each health care facility should have established policies and procedures and conduct an annual training of the steps used in protecting employees from exposure to bloodborne pathogens while preventing possible transmission of disease between the clinician and patient.

- Protect skin and mucous membranes against exposure to blood and other fluids through the use of a barrier membrane, such as rubber gloves.
- Immediately wash skin coming into contact with a potential carrying agent with soap and water.
- Clean contaminated surfaces, such as tables and countertops, with a 1:10 mixture of household bleach and water.
- Dispose of all used needles, scalpels, and other sharp objects in a proper manner using a rigid biohazard container.
- Staff members with open, draining sores or skin lesions should not provide direct patient care until the condition clears.
- Bag soiled linen or uniforms and wash them separately from other items in hot water and detergent.
- Wash hands after removing protective gloves.

Inspection

The inspection is a continual process that begins as soon as the patient enters the facility. An initial observation of **gait**, posture, and function may provide information about the patient's compensatory postures and movement patterns. Any guarding or postures where the patient splints the body part in a protective position should be noted. Bilateral comparison of paired body parts such as the extremities or eyes must be performed when applicable, noting and exploring any deviation from the expected mirror image of the **contralateral** side.

Inspect the injured body part and compare the results with the opposite structure for:

- **Deformity:** Visual deviations from normal can be subtle, **gross**, or somewhere in between. Some fractures and joint dislocations result in gross deformity, with angulation or clear disruption of normal joint contour. Signs of joint displacement or bony fracture warrant ruling out any other significant trauma, appropriate splinting, and the immediate referral to a physician. This process is explained further in Chapter 2.

  Careful bilateral inspection may reveal differences in otherwise healthy-looking body parts (Fig. 1-1).
- **Swelling**: Any enlargement of a body part can be subtle or dramatic and occur rapidly or over time. The onset, look, and feel of a swollen body part can help identify the nature of injury. For example, an acute joint effusion resulting from a **hemarthrosis** is typically readily apparent. Joint swelling that forms over a number of hours is most likely the result of excess synovial fluid production. **Edema** resulting from a tibial stress fracture can be slight and localized. The amount of swelling can be measured in a quantifiable manner using girth measurements (Special Test Box 1-1) or volumetric measurements (Fig. 1-2). Girth measurements require less equipment and demonstrate high interrater reliability, and results closely represent the results of volumetric measurements.[17,18]

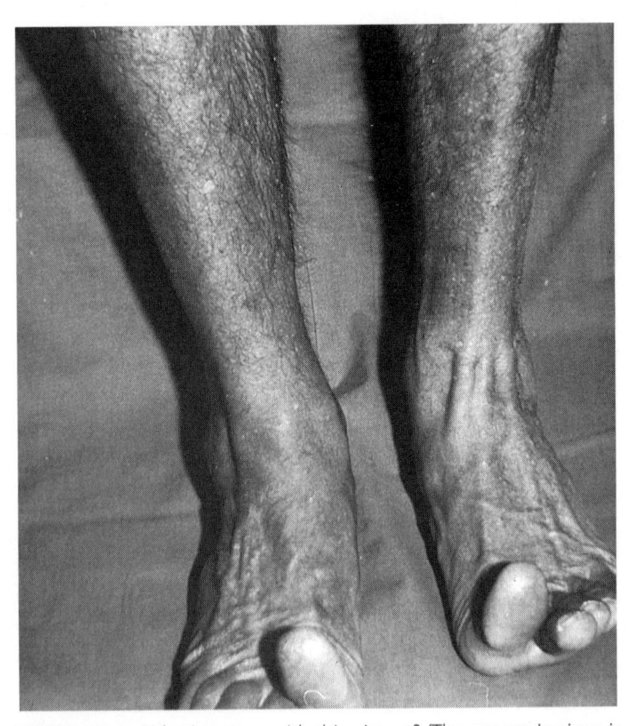

FIGURE 1-1 ■ What's wrong with this picture? (The answer is given in the legend of Figure 1-2.) The patient has few complaints other than decreased strength during dorsiflexion of the right ankle. There is no history of trauma to the body area. Carefully examine both ankles to determine the cause of these complaints.

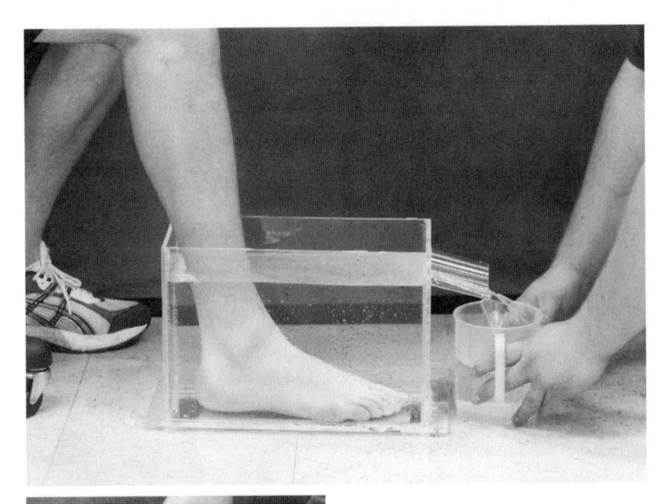

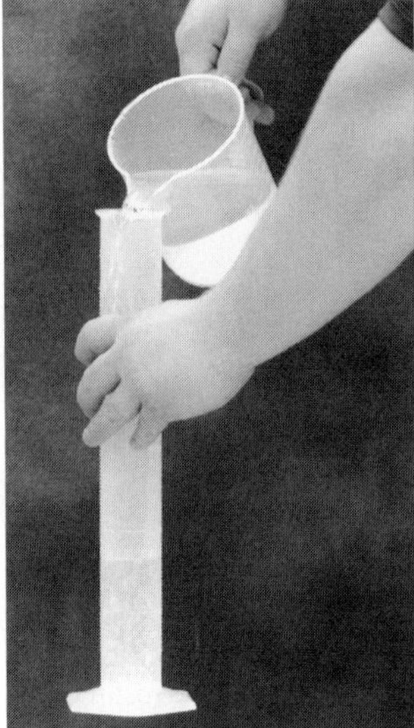

FIGURE 1-2 ■ Volumetric measurement. **(A)** The tank is filled with water up to the specified level and the limb is gently immersed. **(B)** The overflow water is collected and poured into a calibrated beaker to determine the mass (volume) of the limb. This measurement is obtained by either reading a graduate cylinder or, more accurately, by weighing the water expelled. Volumetric measurement of limb volume is most commonly used as a research tool, but can provide important clinical information. **Answer to Figure 1-1:** The right tibialis anterior tendon is ruptured. Note the absence of its tendon as it crosses the joint line.

Hepatitis B virus (HBV) A virus resulting in inflammation of the liver. After a 2- to 6-week incubation period, symptoms develop, including gastrointestinal and respiratory disturbances, jaundice, enlarged liver, muscle pain, and weight loss.

Human immunodeficiency virus (HIV) The virus that causes acquired immune deficiency syndrome (AIDS).

Gait The sequential movements of the spine, pelvis, knee, ankle, foot, and upper extremity when walking or running.

Contralateral Pertaining to the opposite side of the body or the opposite extremity.

Gross Visible or apparent to the unaided eye.

Hemarthrosis Bleeding into a joint cavity.

Edema The collection of fluids in the intercellular spaces.

Special Test 1-1
Girth Measurement

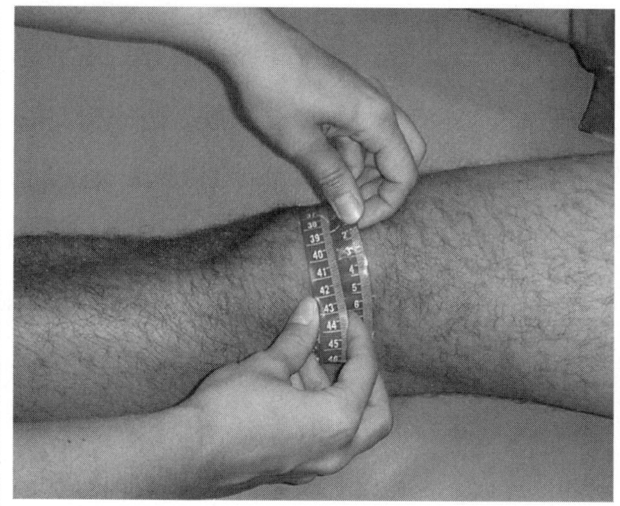

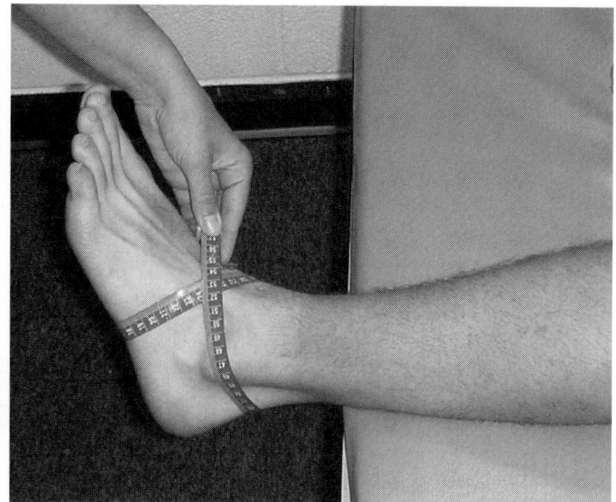

Girth measurements provide a quantifiable and reproducible measure of a limb's atrophy or hypertrophy. For a more precise measure, refer to Figure 1-2.

Patient Position	Supine
Position of Examiner	Standing to access the body part
Evaluative Procedure	**1.** To determine capsular swelling, identify the joint line using prominent bony landmarks. To determine muscular atrophy, make incremental marks (e.g., 2, 4, and 6 inches) from the joint line **(A)**. **2.** Do not use a measuring tape made of cloth (cloth tapes tend to stretch and cause the markings to fade). **3.** Lay the measuring tape symmetrically around the body part, being careful not to fold or twist the tape. **4.** To measure ankle girth use a figure-8 technique. Position the tape across the malleoli proximally and around the navicular and the base of the fifth metatarsal distally **(B)**. **5.** Pull the tape snugly and read the circumference in centimeters or inches. **6.** Take three measurements and record the average. **7.** Repeat these steps for the uninjured limb. **8.** Record the findings in the patient's medical file.
Positive Test	A significant difference in the girth between the two limbs based on factors such as lower or upper extremity, side dominance, and so on.
Implications	Increased girth across the joint line: Edema Increased girth across muscle mass: Hypertrophy or edema Decreased girth across muscle mass: Atrophy
Evidence	There is a strong positive correlation (0.90) between figure-8 and volumetric ankle measurements

*** Practical Evidence**

When used to determine muscle volume, most body composition methods, including girth measurements, tend to be more accurate on males than females because of the overlying adipose tissue layer in females.[19] Intra-rater and inter- rater reliability of girth measurement is significantly improved when landmarks are consistently identified and used. In the case of the ankle, the minimally detectable clinically relevant change is 9.6mm.[20]

- **Skin**: Does the area show redness that may be associated with inflammation? Is **ecchymosis** present, indicating a contusion or other **soft tissue** disruption? Is the ecchymosis located at or distal to the injured structure? Ecchymosis located distal to the site of injury indicates pooling of the blood secondary to the effects of gravity. Are there any open wounds that warrant referral or first aid? Are there signs of previous trauma, keloids, or surgical scars that have not been explained in the history (Fig. 1-3)?
- **Infection**: Does the body area show signs of infection (e.g., redness, swelling, pus, red streaks, swollen **lymph nodes**)? Infections can occur in both open and closed wounds. Red streaks that follow the lymphatic system necessitate immediate physician referral.

Functional assessment

Ask the patient to perform those functional tasks that were identified as problematic during the history-taking portion of the clinical examination. These limitations can occur during activities of daily living, such as reaching, or during more complex tasks such as throwing a baseball. Consider the underlying impairment that could lead to the functional limitations. For example, painful or limited knee flexion can cause a compensatory hip hike to sufficiently shorten the limb while climbing stairs. The results of the functional assessment form the framework for the remaining physical examination, where the impairments are identified and measured.

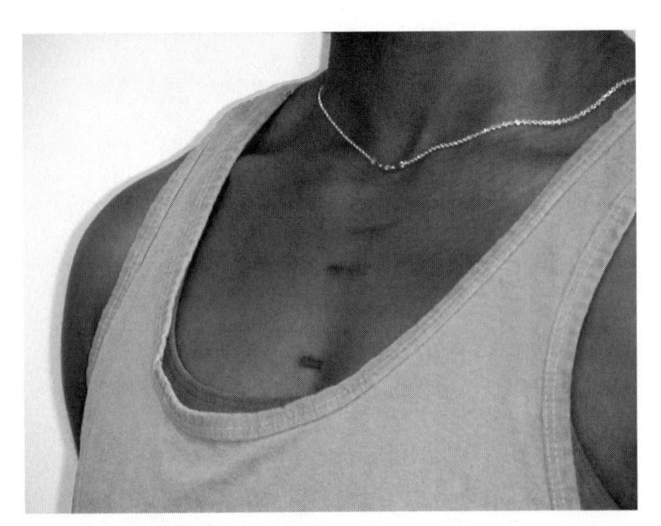

FIGURE 1-3 ■ Keloid formation. These firm, nodular masses represent the overdevelopment of collagen-rich scar tissue. Keloid formation is most prevalent among African Americans.

Standardized, reproducible functional tests are designed to assess how the body parts work together to produce functional activity (e.g., reaching, one leg hop for distance, ROM, strength, and balance). These assessments are then expanded to replicate the activity to be performed by the patient under the precise demands faced during real-life situations (e.g., running, jumping, stair climbing, stacking boxes on a pallet). Specific functional tests are described in Appendix B. Standardized functional assessment tools are often used to help determine outcome measures. By assessing a patient's functional status throughout the course of a condition, the relative effectiveness of an intervention can be determined.

Palpation

Palpation, the process of touching and feeling the tissues, allows the examiner to detect tissue damage or change by comparing the findings of one body part with those of the opposite one. It also helps to identify areas of point tenderness. Palpation is performed bilaterally and in a specific sequence, beginning with structures away from the site of pain and progressively moving toward the potentially damaged tissues. Thus, different potential sources of pain can be ruled out and possible involved secondary structures can be identified. While assessing pulse and sensation technically involve palpation, these are typically classified with other parts of the examination.

One method of sequencing is to palpate the bones and ligaments first and then palpate the muscles and tendons, and then, finally, locate any other areas such as pulses. The second form of sequencing is to palpate all structures (e.g., bones, muscles, ligaments) farthest from the suspected injury and then palpating progressing toward the injured site. Regardless of the palpation strategy used, a thorough knowledge of topical anatomy is crucial to ensure that the connection is made between the location of the finding and the associated structure. Some examination models delay the palpation process until the end of the evaluation because this is often the most painful aspect of the evaluation. Excess pain with palpation can produce apprehension, causing the patient to guard the area and alter the remainder of the evaluation.

Ecchymosis A blue or purple area of skin caused by blood escaping into the extravascular spaces under the skin.

Soft tissues Structures other than bone, including muscle, tendon, ligament, capsule, bursa, and skin.

Lymph nodes Nodules located in the cervical, axillary, and inguinal regions, producing white blood cells and filtering bacteria from the bloodstream. Lymph nodes become enlarged secondary to an infection.

During the palpation, make note of the following potential findings:

- **Point tenderness:** Palpate toward the injured area, beginning with gentle and progressively increasing pressure, visualizing the structures that lie beneath your fingers. Certain areas of the body (e.g., the anatomical snuff box, orbital rim, costochondral joints) are normally tender. To be a meaningful finding, palpation should elicit increased tenderness of the structure relative to the surrounding structures and the same structure on the opposite side of the body.
- **Trigger points**: A trigger point is a hypersensitive area located in a muscle belly that, when irritated as during palpation, refers pain to another body area. Trigger points feel like small nodules within the tissue. The cause-and-effect relationship between the symptoms and the patient's pathology should be determined.
- **Change in tissue density**: Determine any differences in the density or "feel" of the tissues, possibly indicating muscle spasm, hemorrhage, edema, scarring, myositis ossificans, or other conditions (Table 1-4).
- **Crepitus**: Note a crunching or crackling sensed with the rubbing of tissues. Termed crepitus, this may indicate a fracture when felt over bone or inflammation when felt over tendon, bursa, or joint capsule. **Crepitus** is sometimes audible such as when bony fracture sites grind against each other or when air enters the tissues such as after an orbital fracture or pneumothorax.
- **Tissue temperature**: Feel for an altered temperature of the injured area relative to the surrounding sites. An increased temperature is typical during an active inflammatory process such as occurs following an acute injury or in the presence of infection. A decreased temperature is associated with vascular insufficiency.

Table 1-4 Possible Causes of Changes in Tissue Density

Tissue Feel	Possible Cause
Spongy, boggy over a joint	Synovitis
Hard, warm	Blood accumulation
Dense thickening	Scar tissue formation
Dense/viscous	Pitting edema
Increased muscle tone	Muscle spasm, muscle hypertrophy
Hard	Bone or bony outgrowth (exostosis

Joint and Muscle Function Assessment

The results of active and passive ROM assessments and manual muscle testing begin to quantify the patient's current functional status. As with all evaluation tools, bilateral comparison is used and, when possible, results are compared against established **normative data**. The examination includes assessment of all available motions at the involved joint and the joints proximal and distal to the affected area. Pain and/or dysfunction proximal or distal to the involved structure can change the stress on that tissue and must be addressed for full recovery.

Common terminology such as flexion, extension, abduction, and adduction describes most joint motions. Some joint motions, such as ankle inversion, are unique to specific joints (Table 1-5). These specific motions are discussed in the individual chapters.

Table 1-5 Joint Motion Description by Body Area

Body Area	Common Descriptors	Atypical Descriptors
Cervical Spine	Flexion	Lateral or side bending (lateral flexion)
	Extension	Capital flexion
	Rotation	Capital extension
Shoulder Complex	Flexion	Horizontal abduction
	Extension	Horizontal adduction
	Abduction	Elevation
	Adduction	
	Internal rotation	
	External rotation	
Elbow/Forearm	Flexion	Pronation
	Extension	Supination

Continued

Crepitus Repeated crackling sensations or sound emanating from a joint or tissue.

Normative data Normal ranges of data collected for comparison during the evaluation of an athlete. On many measures, athletes have norms different from the general population.

Table 1-5 Joint Motion Description by Body Area—cont'd

Body Area	Common Descriptors	Atypical Descriptors
Wrist/Hand	Flexion Extension	Radial deviation Ulnar deviation
Fingers	Flexion Extension Abduction Adduction	Opposition Apposition
Thumb (CMC joint)	Flexion Extension Abduction Adduction	Opposition Apposition
Lumbar Spine	Flexion Extension Rotation	Lateral or side bending (lateral flexion)
Hip	Flexion Extension Abduction Adduction Internal rotation External rotation	
Knee	Flexion Extension Internal rotation External rotation	
Ankle/Foot		Plantarflexion Dorsiflexion Pronation Supination Inversion Eversion
Toes	Flexion Extension Abduction Adduction	

Abduction = Lateral movement of a body part away from the midline of the body. In the feet, the movement is in reference to the midline of the foot.
Adduction = Medial movement of a body part toward the midline of the body. In the feet, the movement is in reference to the midline of the foot.
Eversion = The movement of the plantar aspect of the calcaneus away from the midline of the body.
Extension = The act of straightening a joint and increasing its angle. Ankle extension is referred to as plantarflexion.
Flexion = Bending a joint and decreasing its angle. Ankle flexion is referred to as dorsiflexion
Inversion = The movement of the plantar aspect of the calcaneus toward the midline of the body.
Pronation = (1) The combined motion of eversion, abduction, and dorsiflexion of the foot and ankle. (2) Movement at the radioulnar joints allowing for the palm to be turned downward.
Supination = (1) The combined motion produced by inversion, adduction, and plantarflexion of the foot and ankle. (2) Movement at the radioulnar joints allowing for the palm to turn upward, as if holding a bowl of soup.

The evaluation of active and passive ROM may be made by gross observation or, more precisely, objectively measured with the use of a goniometer or inclinometer (Goniometry Box 1-1). The patient's age and gender influence ROM. In the high school and college-aged population, women have a greater ROM in all planes than do men. ROM decreases after age 20 for both genders, but this decrease occurs to a greater extent in women.[25,26]

Goniometry Box 1-1
Goniometer Use Guidelines

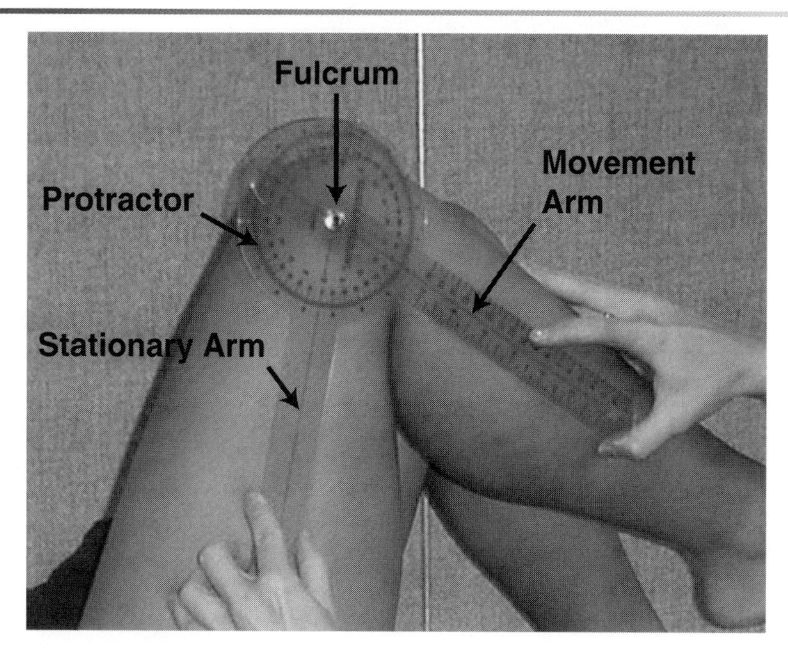

With proper training and practice goniometers can yield accurate and quantifiable measures of a patient's active and passive ROM. Each joint has different landmarks for the fulcrum, stationary arm, and movement arm.

Goniometer Segments

Protractor: Measures the arc of motion in degrees. Full-circle goniometers have a 360° protractor; half-circle goniometers have a 180° protractor.

Fulcrum: The center of the axis of rotation of the goniometer

Stationary arm: The portion of the goniometer that extends from, and is part of, the protractor

Movement arm: The portion of the goniometer that moves independently from the protractor around an arc formed by the fulcrum

Procedure

1. Select a goniometer of the appropriate size and shape for the joint being tested.
2. Position the joint in its starting position.
3. Identify the center of the joint's axis of motion.
4. Locate the proximal and distal landmarks running parallel to the joint's axis of motion.
5. Align the fulcrum of the goniometer over the joint axis.
6. Align the stationary arm along the proximal body segment and the movement arm along the distal segment.
7. Read and record the starting values from the goniometer.
8. Move the distal joint segment through its ROM.
9. Reapply the goniometer as described in Steps 5 and 6.
10. Read and record the ending values from the goniometer.

Recording Results

There are several different methods and documentation forms for recording goniometric data. Most systems use the neutral position as "0" and document the amount of motion from this point. For example, 10° of knee extension and 120° of knee flexion would be recorded as:

10° – 0° – 120°

In a case where the patient is unable to obtain the starting ("0") position, zero is the first number cited or is omitted. For example a limitation in the ROM, lacking 10° of knee extension would be recorded as:

0° – 10° – 120° or **10° – 120°**

Avoid the use of negative numbers.

Active range of motion

Joint movement occurs through physiological and accessory motions. Active range of motion (AROM), joint motion produced by the patient contracting the muscles, assesses physiological motion and osteokinematics. AROM is evaluated first unless it is **contraindicated** by immature fracture sites or recently repaired soft tissues. Accessory motions, or arthrokinematics, are those patterns that must occur for normal osteokinematic motion but are not under voluntary control. For example, to flex the glenohumeral joint (osteokinematics) the humeral head must slide inferiorly (arthrokinematics). Accessory motions are assessed using joint play (p. 24).

First evaluating the AROM determines the patient's willingness and ability to move the body part through any or all of the ROM. An unwillingness to move the extremity could signify extreme pain, neurological deficit, or possible **malingering**.

While the joint is actively moved through all the possible motions in the cardinal planes observe the ease with which the movement is made and the total ROM obtained (Fig. 1-4). Also note any compensation or abnormal movement in the surrounding structures. The patient may verbally or nonverbally describe a **painful arc** within the ROM.

Manual muscle testing

Manual muscle testing (MMT) is used to assess for strength and provocation of pain by relatively isolating muscles or groups of muscles. True isolation, where no other muscles are active, is not possible to achieve clinically, but EMG analysis can assess the positions in which muscles are most active. These positions are used for MMT. MMT can help identify the involved muscles or muscle group by ascertaining whether or not pain is present.

Resisted range of motion (RROM), alternatively, assesses gross strength of an entire muscle group throughout a cardinal plane of motion. Often, movements assessed during manual muscle testing are the same as those assessed with RROM. For example, strength of the quadriceps is assessed using knee extension. While RROM is used to assess the strength of muscle groups throughout the full ROM within the cardinal planes, its usefulness is relegated to determining a general weakness. MMTs are described throughout this text.

*** Practical Evidence**

Because of the relative lack of testosterone, girls are typically weaker than boys from the age of 9 and beyond.[27] Strength normally increases with age until 20 to 30 years. In the fifth or sixth decade of life the rate of muscle strength decay increases.[28]

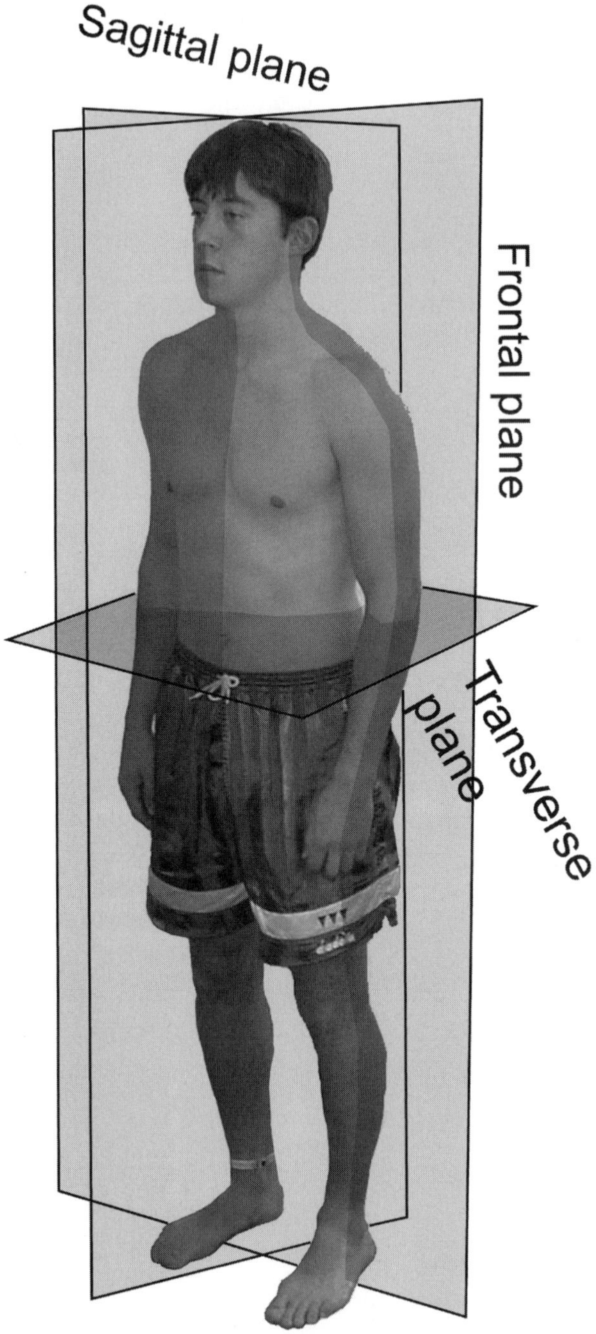

FIGURE 1-4 ■ The cardinal planes of the body. The sagittal plane divides the body into left and right sides. The transverse plane bisects the body into superior and inferior or proximal or distal segments. The frontal (coronal) plane divides the body into anterior and posterior segments. Movement in the frontal plane occurs around an anterior–posterior axis; movement in the sagittal plane occurs around a medial–lateral axis; movement in the transverse plane occurs around a vertical axis.

Contraindication Procedure that may prove harmful given the patient's current condition.

Malingering Faking or exaggerating the symptoms of an injury or illness.

Painful arc An area within a joint's range of motion that causes pain, representing compression, impingement, or abrasion of the underlying tissues.

Isometric MMT performed in the mid-range of the joint's ROM, also known as a **break test**, better differentiates between muscle pathology and injury of noncontractile tissues such as ligaments. Noncontractile tissues are less likely to be taut in a joint's midrange. MMT performed throughout the range may provide additional information about changes in strength with positioning, but the reliability and validity decrease due to potential input from other tissues. Instrumented testing such as a hand-held dynamometer allows the muscle force being generated to be quantitatively assessed.[29]

The ability to perform AROM serves as the foundation for grading manual muscle tests. As identified in Table 1-6, the ability to perform pain-free AROM against gravity would receive a minimum score of "Fair" or "3/5" as gravity is providing resistance to the motion. If the patient were unable to achieve a grade of Fair, the position would be changed to reduce the effects of gravity. If the patient is able to achieve a grade of Fair, then resistance is progressively added to determine the final grade. With the exception of identifying neurological involvement, the use of these grading scales to quantify strength in athletes and others involved in strenuous physical activity is rarely beneficial (Fig. 1-5). Multiple repetitions of a single test may be needed before symptoms are reproduced, particularly when the patient notes that symptoms are present only when fatigue is a contributing factor.

Manual muscle tests (MMT) are useful in determining the strength of muscles and muscle groups when administered by highly trained personnel, but are prone to low interrater and intrarater reliability measures, especially for grades 4 and 5 (Manual Muscle Test 1-1).[30,31] Procedural consistency using standardized positions and hand placements is important for maximum reliability and validity during MMT.

During manual resistance, the limb is stabilized proximally to prevent other motions from compensating for weakness of the involved muscle. Resistance is provided distally on the bone to which the muscle or muscle group attaches, not distal to a second joint. **Compensation** occurs when postural changes are used to substitute for a loss of motion or weakness, such as using shoulder girdle elevation to compensate for a loss of glenohumeral

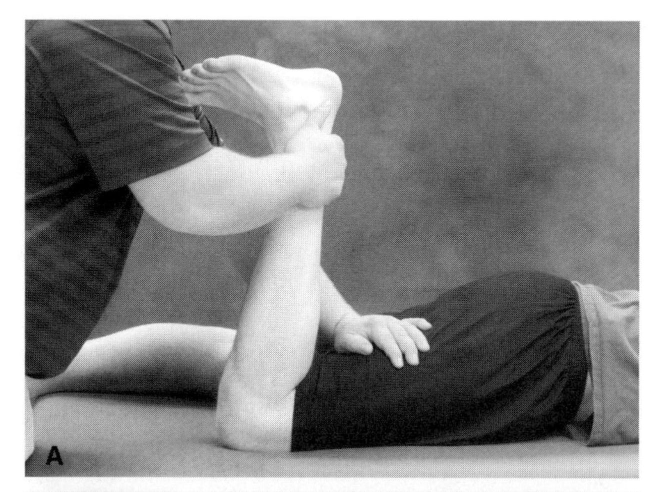

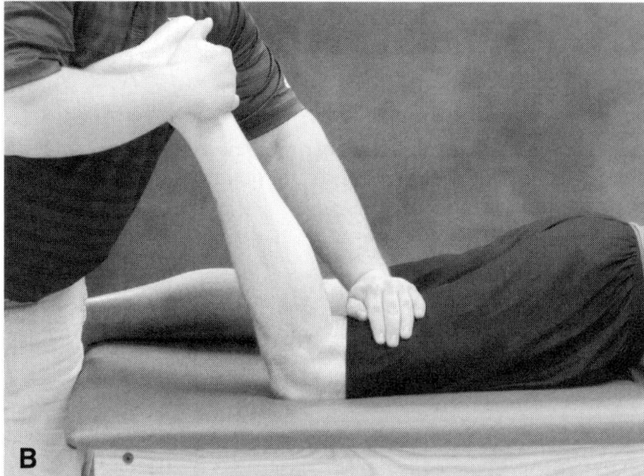

FIGURE 1-5 ■ Manual muscle test of the hamstring muscle group. **(A)** When the knee is flexed beyond 90° in the prone position gravity assists the motion of the hamstrings. **(B)** If the knee is flexed less than 90° the hamstring muscles must work to overcome both gravity and the examiner's manual resistance.

Table 1-6 Grading Systems for Manual Muscle Tests

Verbal	Numerical	Clinical Finding
Normal	5/5	The patient can resist against maximal pressure. The examiner is unable to break the patient's resistance.
Good	4/5	The patient can resist against moderate pressure.
Fair	3/5	The patient can move the body part against gravity through the full ROM.
Poor	2/5	The patient can move the body part in a gravity-eliminated position through the full ROM.
Trace	1/5	The patient cannot produce movement, but a muscle contraction is palpable.
Zero	0/5	No contraction is felt.

Break test An isometric contraction against manual resistance provided by the examiner; used to determine the patient's ability to generate a static force within a muscle or muscle group.

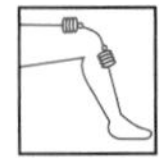

Manual Muscle Test 1-1
Muscle Testing Guidelines

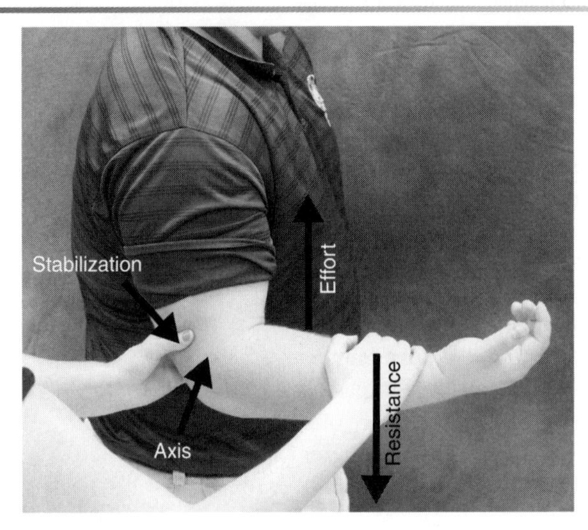

These procedures are used when attempting to isolate an individual muscle or muscle group (manual muscle test). Specific techniques are described in the appropriate chapters throughout this text.

Patient Position	Position the patient so that the muscle(s) tested must work against gravity.
Position of Examiner	As needed to stabilize proximal to the joint being tested and provide resistance distal to the joint.
Evaluative Procedure	**1.** Provide stabilization proximal to the joint to isolate the joint to the motion/muscle(s) being tested. Do not apply resistance at this point. **2.** Instruct the patient to perform the requested motion, such as elbow flexion with the forearm supinated. **3.** While the patient is attempting the motion, palpate the muscle(s) to ensure that it is contracting. **4.** If the patient is able to complete the ROM against gravity, a starting grade of "Fair" or "3" is assigned. **5.** Position the joint in the mid-ROM and apply resistance. Instruct the patient, "Don't let me move you." Gradually increase the resistance. **6.** Apply resistance as far away as possible from the target joint without crossing the distal joint. **7.** Ensure that the muscles distal to the joint being tested are relaxed. **8.** If the patient is unable to complete the ROM against gravity, reposition the body part to a gravity-eliminated position and request that the patient attempt to perform AROM again.
Positive Test	Weakness and/or pain compared to the contralateral side
Implications	See Table 1-6.

ROM = range of motion; AROM = active range of motion.

abduction. Compensation may also occur through muscular **substitution**, especially by more proximal muscle groups, as the patient attempts to overcome weaknesses of the muscle being tested by recruiting other muscles (e.g., upper trapezius recruitment during shoulder abduction to compensate for a torn supraspinatus tendon). When the patient uses compensatory motions, the amount of resistance used against the contraction should be reduced and the patient's MMT grade reduced accordingly.

*** Practical Evidence**

The clinical relevance (and interrater reliability) of manual muscle testing is improved when muscle strength is described as "normal" or "not normal" rather than ordinal grading systems such as 0 to 5.[32]

Passive range of motion

After muscle function is assessed, passive range of motion (PROM) where the clinician moves the joint through the

ROM is evaluated for the quantity of available movement as compared to AROM and changes in the pain pattern. **Overpressure** should be applied at the end of the ROM to identify the **end-feel** that indicates what type of structures are stressed at the terminal ROM. The different end-feels as established by Cyriax are listed in Table 1-7.[33] Certain movements have particular normal end-feels (e.g., elbow extension should have a hard or bony end-feel). Knowledge of these end-feels is necessary to identify pathological limits to ROM (Table 1-8).

A capsular pattern is the characteristic loss of motion caused by shortening or adhesions of the joint capsule. Each synovial joint has a unique capsular pattern. Full joint motion cannot occur if the capsular fibers are shortened. Noncapsular patterns occur when nonjoint capsular structures are involved. The capsular patterns for the major joints of the body are described in the relevant chapters of this text.

Useful information can be obtained by comparing the range of movement obtained for AROM with that obtained for PROM. Typically, PROM is greater than AROM. When AROM and PROM are equal and both fall short of the expected ROM, capsular adhesions or joint tightness may be restricting the motion. AROM that is less than PROM signifies a muscular weakness or a lesion within the active **contractile tissue** that is causing pain and inhibiting motion. Although data exist describing normal ROM, this information may not be helpful in determining whether or not a functionally sufficient amount of range is available for the individual. For example, consider a gymnast who must have 0 to 140 degrees of hip flexion (as opposed to the normal value of 0 to

Table 1-7 Physiological (Normal) End-Feels to PROM

End-Feels	Structure	Example
Soft	Soft tissue approximation	Knee flexion (contact between soft tissue of the posterior leg and posterior thigh)
Firm	Muscular stretch	Hip flexion with the knee extended (passive elastic tension of hamstring muscles)
	Capsular stretch	Extension of the metacarpophalangeal joints of the fingers (tension in the palmar capsule)
	Ligamentous stretch	Forearm supination (tension in the palmar radioulnar ligament of the inferior radioulnar joint, interosseous membrane, oblique cord)
Hard	Bone contacting bone	Elbow extension (contact between the olecranon process of the ulna and the olecranon fossa of the humerus)

Table 1-8 Pathological (Abnormal) End-Feels to PROM

End-Feels	Description	Example
Soft	Occurs sooner or later in the ROM than is usual or occurs in a joint that normally has a firm or hard end-feel; feels boggy	Soft tissue edema Synovitis
Firm	Occurs sooner or later in the ROM than is usual or occurs in a joint that normally has a soft or hard end-feel	Increased muscular tone, capsular, muscular, ligamentous shortening
Hard	Occurs sooner or later in the ROM than is usual or occurs in a joint that normally has a soft or firm end-feel; feels like a bony block	Osteoarthritis Loose bodies in joint Myositis ossificans Fracture
Spasm	Joint motion is stopped by involuntary or voluntary muscle contraction.	Inflammation Strain Joint instability
Empty	Has no real end-feel because end of ROM is never reached owing to pain; no resistance felt except for patient's protective muscle splinting or muscle spasm	Acute joint inflammation Bursitis Abscess Fracture Psychogenic origin

Contractile tissue Tissue that is capable of shortening and subsequently elongating; muscular tissue.

120 degrees) in order to execute a move. Even if the patient is able to complete full AROM, PROM should be performed with emphasis on the quality of the end-feel.

Joint stability tests

Joint stability is provided by contractile and noncontractile tissue, ligament, and capsule. The contribution of these noncontractile tissues to joint stability is assessed by stress testing and joint play. Stress testing isolates specific ligaments and/or portions of the joint capsule, while joint play assesses accessory motions, those motions that are essential for normal physiological movement. Not every joint stability test described in this text has to be performed in each and every case. Only those joint stability tests needed for the differential diagnosis should be performed.

Joints may either be **hypermobile**, having more laxity than the norm, or **hypomobile**, an amount of mobility that is considered below the normal limits. As described in Chapter 6, joints must have an appropriate amount of accessory motion for proper motion to occur. However, some adaptations may occur normally as the result of repeated activity. Athletes may demonstrate expected mobility patterns in some joints. For instance baseball pitchers tend to have an increased amount of external rotation and a decreased amount of internal rotation than the rest of the population.

Testing involves the application of a specific stress to a noncontractile tissue to assess its laxity. However, a distinction must be made between laxity and instability. Laxity is a clinical sign and instability is the symptom.[34] Laxity describes the amount of "give" within a joint's supportive tissue. A person may have congenital laxity throughout all joints as determined by generalized measures, such as having the patient attempt to pull the thumb to the forearm (Fig. 1-6). Instability is a joint's inability to function under the stresses encountered during functional activities. The amount of joint laxity does not always correlate with the degree of joint instability.[1] The case of laxity in the absence of reported instability illustrates an identified impairment without a functional limitation.

To limit the potential splinting effects of patient apprehension, joint stability tests should first be performed on the injured limb and then the uninjured extremity.[35]

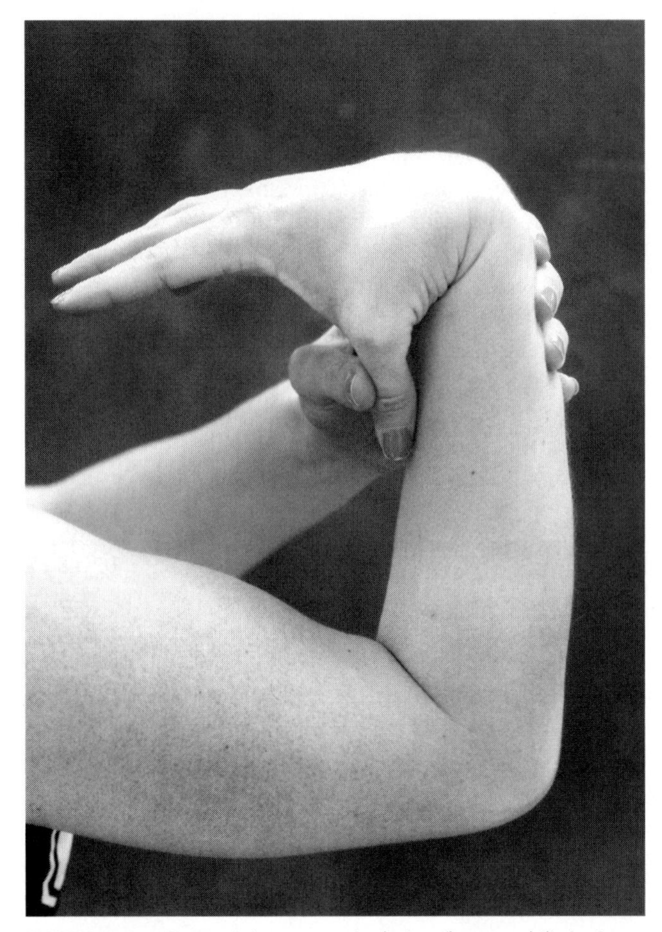

FIGURE 1-6 ■ Determining systemic laxity (hypermobility). Some patients may be naturally lax in all joints. A simple test to determine laxity is to have the patient attempt to pull the thumb to the forearm. If this can be accomplished it may be assumed that all of the patient's joints are lax.

Stress testing

Ligamentous stress testing is used to identify the presence of joint laxity. Sprains are graded on a three-degree scale that is based on the amount that the joint opens and the quality of the **end-point** relative to the opposite uninvolved, uninjured joint (Table 1-9).[36]

Joint play

Normal observable ROM cannot be achieved without sufficient accessory (arthrokinematic) motion. These accessory motions occur via rolling, spinning, or gliding of the joint

Table 1-9 Grading System for Ligamentous Laxity

Grade	Ligamentous End-Feel	Damage
I	Firm (normal)	Slight stretching of the ligament with little, if any, tearing of the fibers. Pain is present, but the degree of laxity roughly compares with that of the opposite extremity.
II	Soft	Partial tearing of the fibers. There is increased play of the joint surfaces upon one another or the joint line "opens up" significantly when compared with the opposite side.
III	Empty	Complete tearing of the ligament. The motion is excessive and becomes restricted by other joint structures, such as secondary restraints or tendons.

surfaces and are assessed using joint play. The concave–convex rule identifies the direction of accessory motions (Fig. 1-7).

Joint play is assessed with the patient relaxed and the joint in the loose-packed, or resting, position to minimize the influence of bony alignment (congruency). A gliding or distracting stress is then applied and the relative amount of movement assessed and compared bilaterally. The findings of joint play assessment can be rated as normal; hypermobile, such as following injury to a ligament; or hypomobile, such as following a period of immobilization. A six-point scale is typically used, with a score of 3 indicating normal mobility:

0 = **ankylosed**
1 = considerably decreased
2 = slightly decreased
3 = normal
4 = slightly increased
5 = considerably increased
6 = dramatically increased; pathological

All stress tests are evaluated bilaterally and, whenever possible, compared with baseline measures. The proper joint angle must be obtained to isolate specific tissues within the joint. Performing ligamentous tests with the joint in the incorrect position can yield false results.

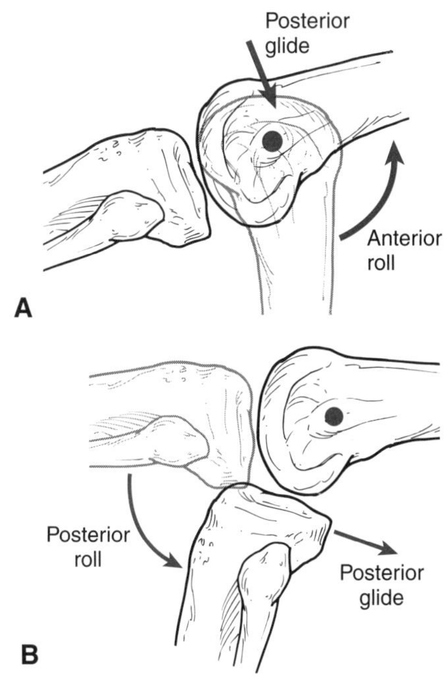

FIGURE 1-7 ■ The convex–concave rule. **(A)** Moving convex joint surface rolls and glides in opposite directions to offset natural translation. **(B)** A moving concave joint surface rolls and slides in the same direction.

End-point The quality and quantity at the end of motion for any stress applied to a tissue.

Ankylosed Fusion of a joint as the result of pathology or surgical design.

Special Tests

Special tests involve specific procedures applied to selected tissues. Therefore, these tests are unique to each structure, joint, or body part. Examples of special tests include the impingement test in the shoulder or the McMurray's test for a meniscal tear. Like all examination techniques, some special tests are more helpful to the diagnostic process than others, and the concepts introduced in Chapter 3 are used to determine whether or not tests should be included in the examination of the current injury.

Unlike stress testing, these tests are typically not graded but, rather, results are compared, either from side to side or as a provocation (causing pain or instability) or alleviation (reduce pain or other symptoms) test and are reported as "positive" or "negative."

Neurological Screening

Neurological assessments involve an upper and lower quarter screen of sensation, motor function, and deep tendon reflexes. Neurological tests are used to identify nerve root impingement, peripheral nerve damage or entrapment, central nervous system (CNS) trauma, or disease. Any neurological signs must be determined so that proper management techniques may be performed. Lower quarter screens are presented in Neurological Screening Box 1-1, and upper quarter screens are presented in Neurological Screening Box 1-2. Inter-rater reliability in identifying patterns associated with nerve root or peripheral nerve involvement is good between experienced examiners.[20]

During the clinical evaluation of orthopedic injuries, neurological examination is indicated when the patient complains of numbness, paresthesia, muscular weakness, pain of unexplained origin, or has sustained a cervical or lumbar spine injury.

Sensory testing

Each spinal nerve root innervates a discrete area of skin. These areas, known as dermatomes, have central autogenous zones that are supplied by only one nerve root with the peripheral areas being supplied by other nerve roots. When a single nerve root is compressed or otherwise inhibited, the skin in the autogenous zone will have reduced sensory function (paresthetic or anesthetic); the remaining portion of thedermatome will have decreased sensory function (hypoesthesia).

*** Practical Evidence**

Having the patient indicate areas of pain or unusual sensation on a drawing of the human body and then mapping the results to dermatome charts is a reliable in identifying pain of neurological origin.[37]

Sensory testing involves a bilateral comparison of light touch discrimination, using a light stroke within the central autogenous zone of the dermatome to avoid overlap of

Neurological Screening Box 1-1
Lower Quarter Neurologic Screen

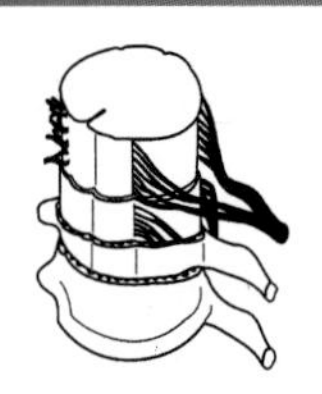 Nerve Root Level	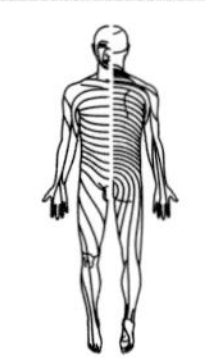 Sensory Testing	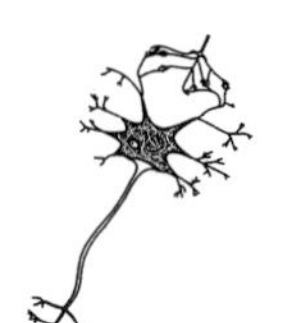 Motor Testing	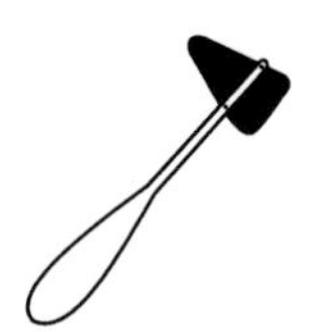 Reflex Testing
L1	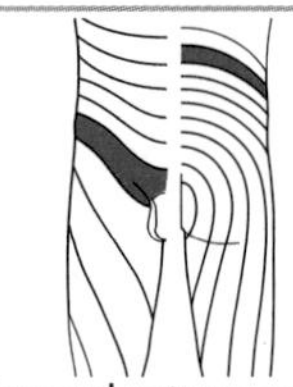 Femoral cutaneous n.	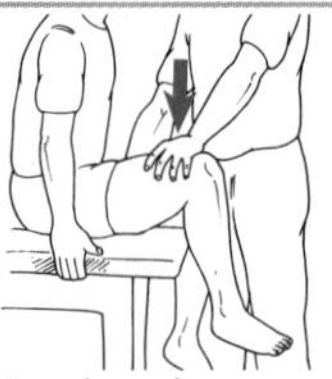 Lumbar plexus	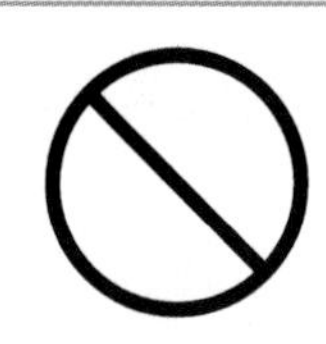 None
L2	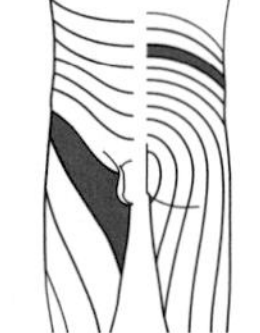 Femoral cutaneous n.	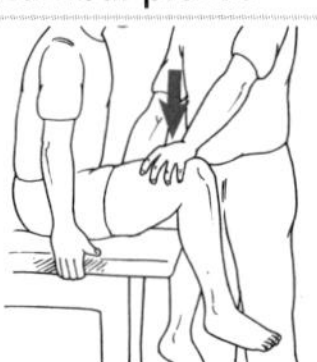 Lumbar plexus	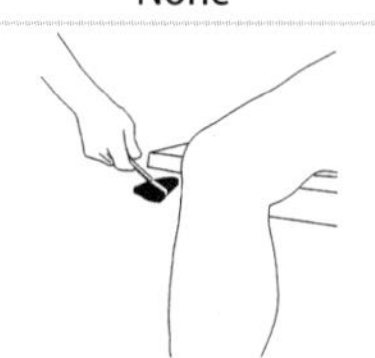 Femoral n. (partial)
L3	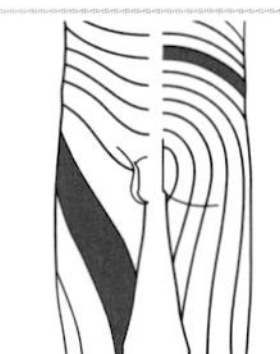 Femoral cutaneous n.	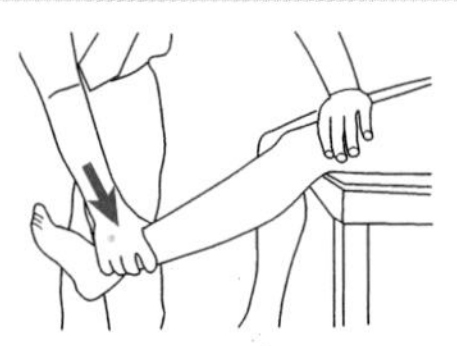 Femoral n.	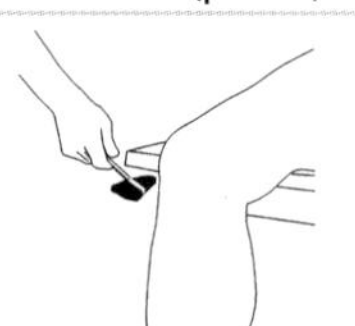 Femoral n. (partial)
L4	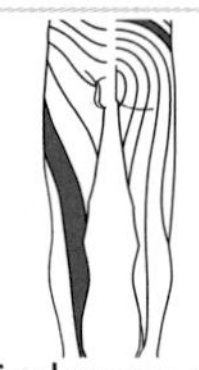 Saphenous n.	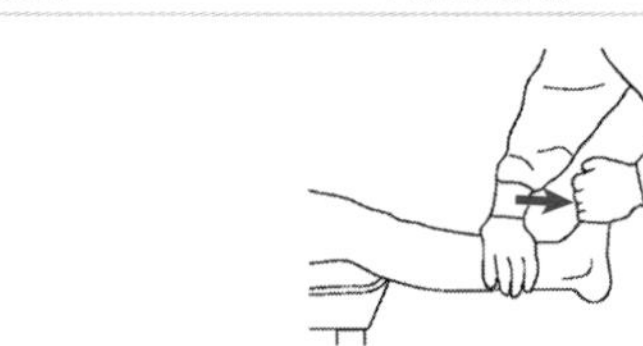 Deep peroneal n.	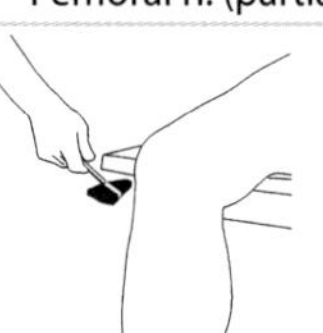 Femoral n. (partial)
L5	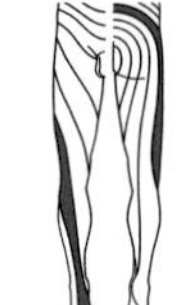 Superficial peroneal n.	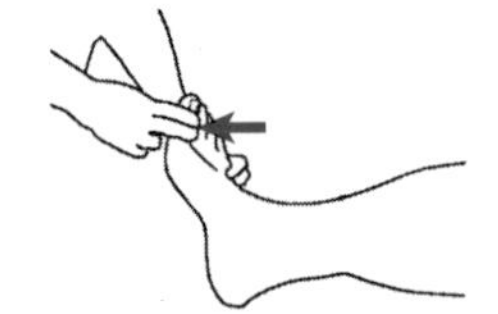 Deep peroneal n.	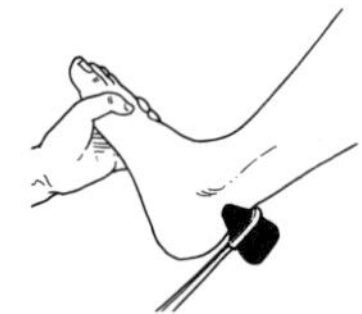 Tibial n.
S1	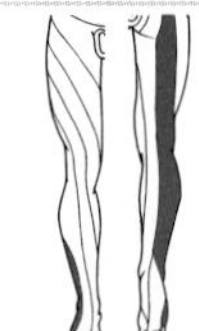 Posterior femoral cutaneous n. and sural n.	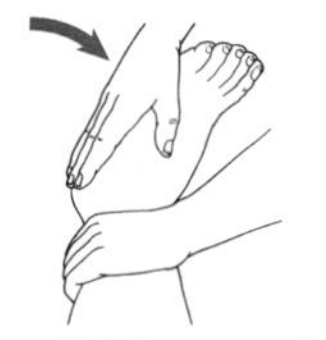 Superficial peroneal n.	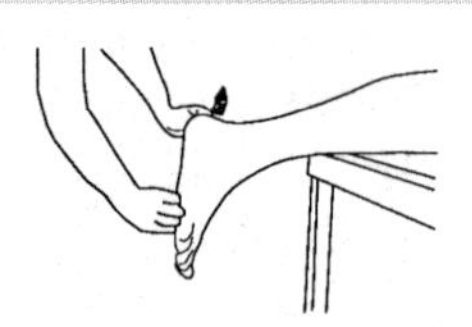 Tibial n.
S2	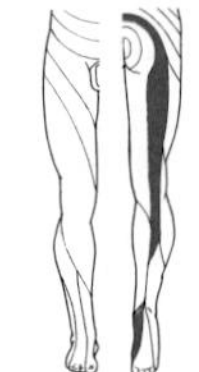 Posterior femoral cutaneous n.	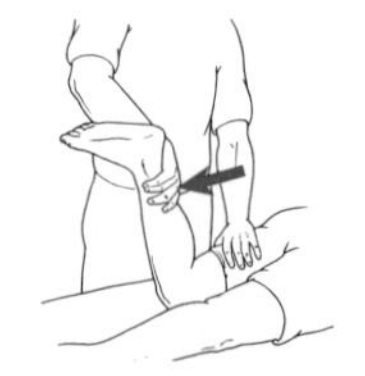 Tibial n. and common peroneal n.	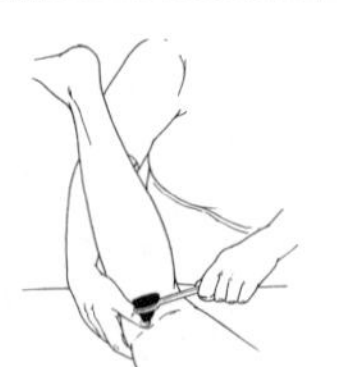 Tibial n.

Neurological Screening Box 1-2
Upper Quarter Neurologic Screen

Nerve Root Level	Sensory Testing	Motor Testing	Reflex Testing
C4	Supraclavicular n.	Shoulder shrug Dorsal scapular	None
C5	Proximal lateral brachial cutaneous n.	Axillary n.	Musculocutaneous n.
C6	Lateral antebrachial cutaneous n.	Musculocutaneous n. (C5 & C6)	Musculocutaneous n.
C7	Radial n.	Radial n.	Radial n.
C8	Ulnar n. (mixed)	Median n.	None
T1	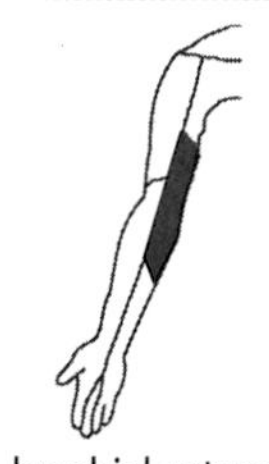 Med. brachial cutaneous n.	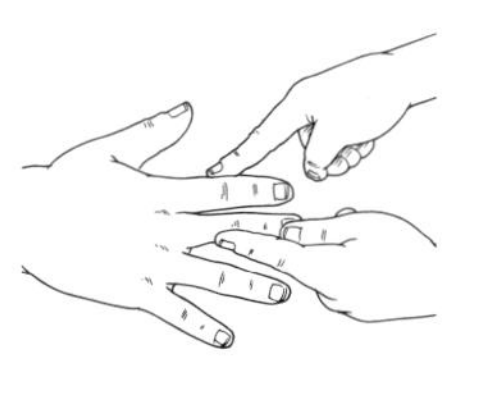 Med. brachial cutaneous n.	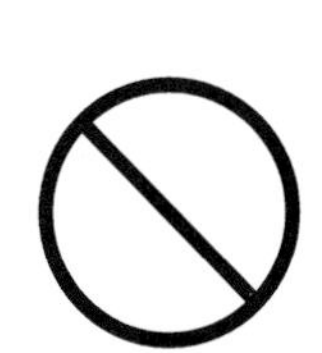 None

multiple nerve roots and more accurately identify the breadth of the involved area (Fig. 1-8). The stroke should be felt to an equal extent on each side. Sensory tests using sharp and dull discrimination and two-point discrimination may also be used to assess sensation in a more quantified manner. (Fig. 1-9).[38] Different types of sensory tests are used to assess to differentiate between types of nerves involved. All sensory testing begins with a thorough explanation of the test to the patient; however, actual testing should be conducted with the patient's eyes closed or head averted to avoid visual influence. The technique should first be tried on an area of normal sensation so that the patient has an accurate understanding of expected sensations.[39]

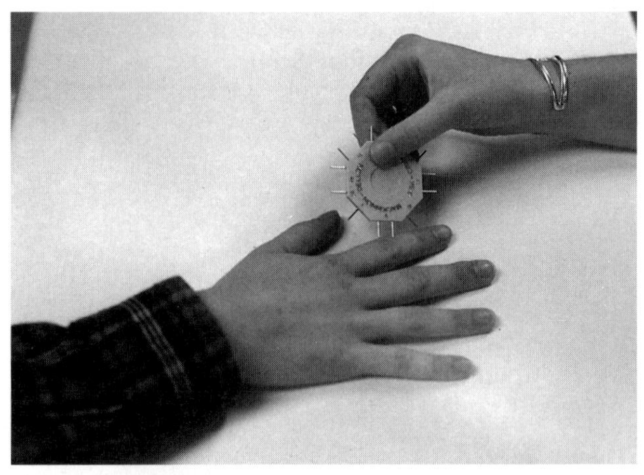

FIGURE 1-9 ■ Two-point discrimination test. This examination procedure is used to determine the amount of sensory loss. Normal results are that the patient can distinguish points that are at most 4 to 5 mm apart.

Motor Testing

Manual muscle tests using the procedures described in Manual Muscle Test Box 1-1 are used to test the motor nerves that are innervating the extremities (see Neurological Screening Boxes 1-1 and 1-2). Although innervation of all muscles tends to overlap, some muscles are more pure

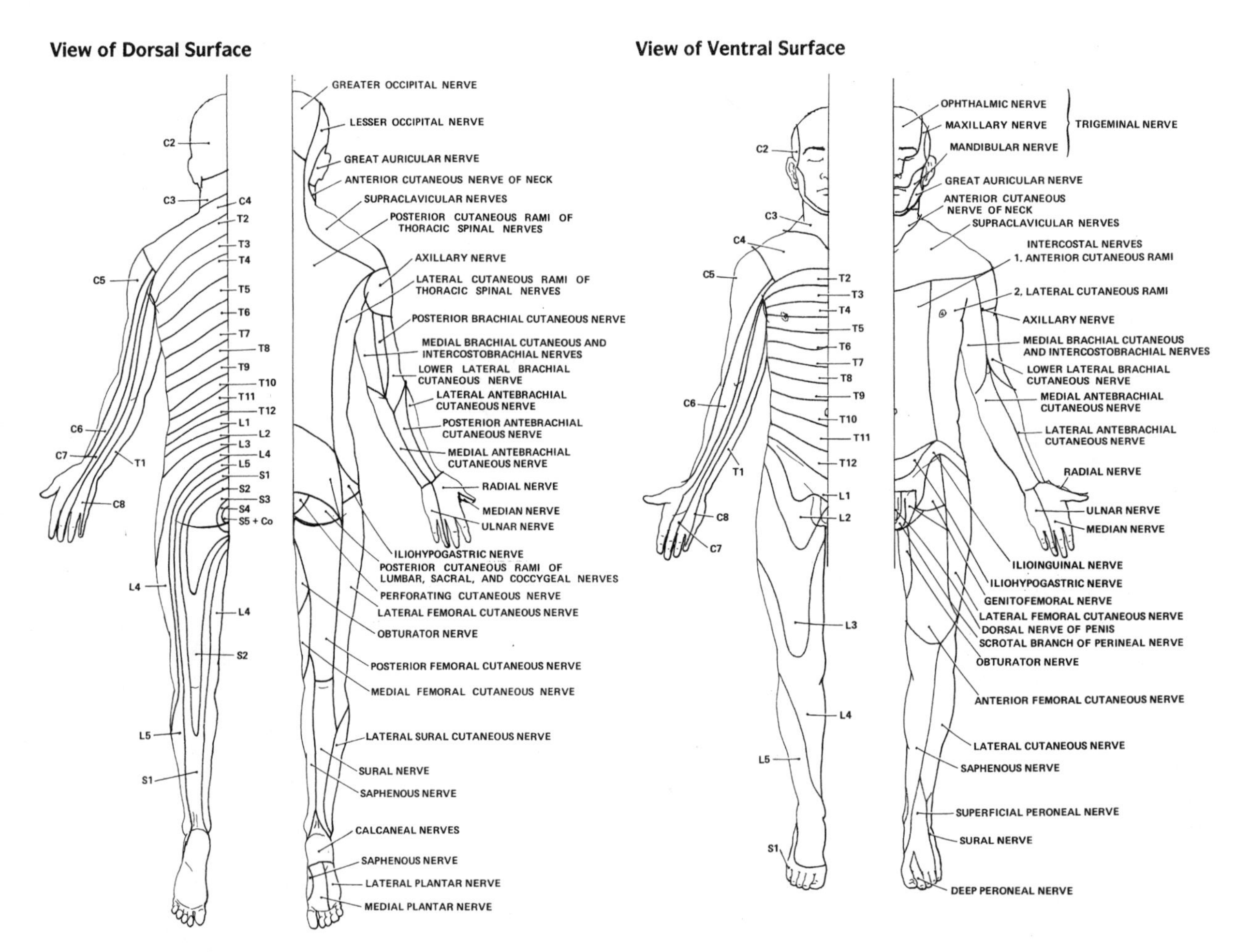

Cutaneous innervation of the back of the body. Dermatomes are on the left, and peripheral nerves are on the right.

Cutaneous innervation of the front of the body. Dermatomes are on the left, and peripheral nerves are on the right.

FIGURE 1-8 ■ The body's dermatomes. These charts describe the area of skin receiving sensory input from each of the nerve roots. Note that there are many different dermatome references. (From Rothstein, JM, Roy, SH, and Wolf, SL: *The Rehabilitation Specialist's Handbook*. ed 2. Philadelphia: FA Davis, 1998.)

than others with regard to their innervation and are initially tested. If weakness is detected in a neurological motor test screen that is innervated by a specific nerve root, identify another muscle that shares that innervation and perform a manual muscle test. If only one muscle is weak, pathology to the muscle or the peripheral nerve supplying it (if different from the second muscle) should be suspected. If both muscles are weak, then the nerve root or peripheral nerve supplying the muscles is implicated.

Reflex testing

Deep tendon reflexes (DTRs), myotatic reflexes, provide information about the integrity of the cervical and lumbar nerve roots and their afferent (toward the CNS) and efferent (from the CNS) pathways. The impact of the reflex hammer on the muscle tendon stretches the tendon, stimulating Golgi tendon organs and muscle spindles. These receptors send a signal to the spinal cord indicating that the muscle is being stretched. In turn, the spinal cord sends a motor impulse to the muscle instructing it to fire and therefore take the stretch off of the muscle.[39]

Reflex testing is limited because not all nerve roots have an associated DTR. A standard scale for grading DTRs is used (Table 1-10). Asymmetry in reflex testing is more remarkable than is bilaterally equal hyperreflexia and may still not be pathological. Because of natural variability, the results of reflex testing should be interpreted in light of other examination findings.[40] Increased response to a reflex test indicates an **upper motor neuron lesion**, while decreased responses could signify a **lower motor neuron lesion**.

DTRs are assessed with the target muscle/tendon on slight stretch and relaxed. The patient should be instructed to look away from the target site. The tendon should be struck briskly by the reflex hammer and the reaction noted. The reflex should be elicited multiple times with any change in response noted. In some patients, eliciting a reflexive response is difficult. For these individuals, the technique of having the patient contract a muscle away from the target area, the **Jendrassik maneuver,** may be helpful.[41] Nerve root level reflex testing for the upper and lower extremities is presented in Appendix A.

Vascular Screening

Clinical examination of the vascular system provides a gross assessment of the blood flow to and from the extremities. Decreased arterial blood flow can produce pain by depriving the tissues of oxygen; inhibition or failure of the vascular return network can produce pain secondary to edema (Table 1-11). Symptoms often worsen during and following activity.

Adequate arterial supply to the extremity is grossly determined by establishing the presence of a pulse. Lower extremity pulses are assessed at the femoral, posterior tibial, and dorsal pedal arteries. In the upper extremity, the brachial, radial, and ulnar arteries are frequently used. The carotid artery (supplying the brain) is used to determine a systemic pulse.

The capillary refill in the nail beds of the toes and fingers can provide some clinical evidence as to the status of the cardiovascular and respiratory systems (Special Test Box 1-2). If blood and/or oxygen supply to the extremities is diminished the nail beds often become cyanotic. Capillary refill should be assessed in digits that have a unique blood supply.

Table 1-10 Deep Tendon Reflex Grading

Grade	Response
0	No reflex elicited
1+	Hyporeflexia: Reflex elicited with reinforcement (precontracting the muscle)
2+	Normal response
3+	Hyperreflexia (brisk)
4+	Hyperactive with **clonus**

Table 1-11 Signs of Vascular Inhibition in the Extremities

Arterial Deficiency	Venous Inhibition
Decreased pulse	Edema in the distal extremity
Decreased capillary refill	Noticeable "pitting" after removing the socks
Cyanotic color	Dark discoloration

The Role of Evidence in the Examination Process

With more than 100 orthopedic tests available for the knee alone, it quickly becomes clear that not all of them can be performed during the examination of each patient. Using the results of the history and functional assessment conducted early in the process helps whittle down or modify the orthopedic tests to be used. If the patient is complaining of a condition with a gradual onset, examination techniques to help identify an acute fracture can be omitted.

Applying the best evidence allows us to pare the list still further. Incorporating tests and measures that change the probability (or likelihood) of a certain diagnosis and

---

Upper motor neuron lesion A lesion proximal to the anterior horn of the spinal cord that results in paralysis and loss of voluntary movement, spasticity, sensory loss, and pathological reflexes.

Lower motor neuron lesion A lesion of the anterior horn of the spinal cord, nerve roots, or peripheral nerves resulting in decreased reflexes, flaccid paralysis, and atrophy.

Clonus Neuromuscular activity in the skeletal muscle marked by rapidly alternating involuntary contraction followed by relaxation.

Special Test 1-2
Capillary Refill Testing

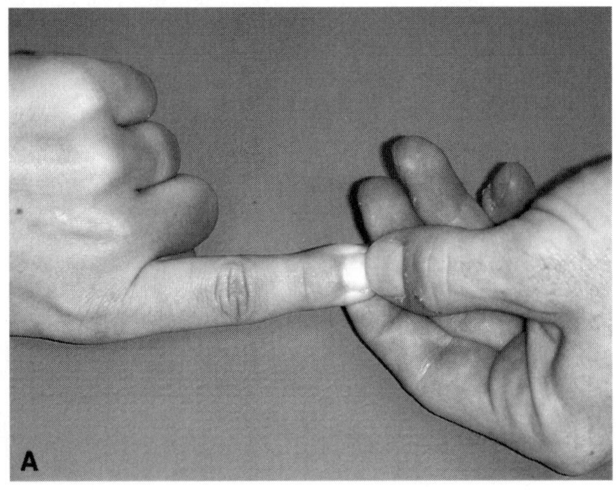

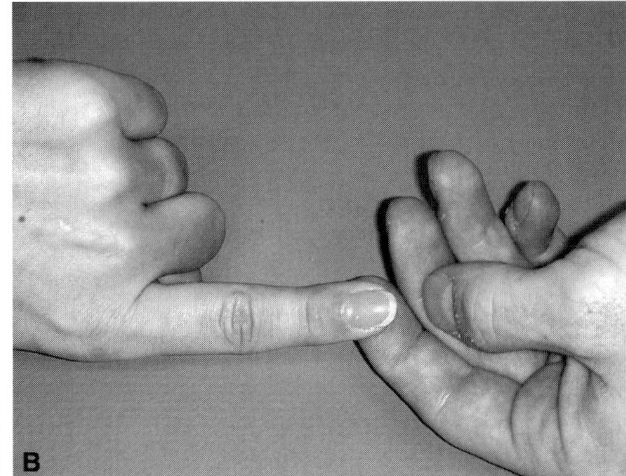

The capillary refill test provides gross information on the quality and quantity of blood flow to the extremities.

Patient Position	***Fingers***: Sitting or lying supine. The extremity is placed in a gravity-neutral position (horizontal). ***Toes***: Lying supine.
Position of Examiner	In front of or beside the patient.
Evaluative Procedure	Observe the color of the nail bed. Squeeze the fingernail so that the nail bed turns white or a lighter shade and hold for 5 sec. **(A)** Release the pressure and note the speed of the refill as indicated by the baseline color returns to the nail bed. **(B)** Repeat using the other fingers or toes and then perform on the opposite extremity.
Positive Test	Markedly slow or absent return of the nail's natural color.
Implications	***Unilateral:*** Occlusion of an artery or arteriole supplying the finger. ***Bilateral:*** Possible systemic cardiovascular compromise or disease.
Evidence	Absent or inconclusive in the literature.

eliminating those that do not help include or exclude diagnoses makes the examination still more refined, accurate and efficient. When clinical prediction rules, such as the Ottawa Ankle Rules, exist, they should be followed whenever possible. The role of evidence in the clinical examination process is described in Chapter 3.

REFERENCES

1. Ageberg, E, et al: Balance in single-limb stance in patients with anterior cruciate ligament injury: Relation to knee laxity, proprioception, muscle strength, and subjective function. *Am J Sports Med,* 33:1527, 2005.
2. Bertilson, BC, Brunnesjö, DN, and Strender L: Reliability of clinical tests in the assessment of patients with neck/shoulder problems – Impact of history. *Spine,* 28:2222, 2003.
3. McHenry, DM: A growing challenge: patient education in a diverse America. *J Nurses Staff Dev,* 23:83, 2007.
4. Spector, RE: *Cultural Diversity in Health and Illness* (ed 6). Stamford, CT: Appleton & Lange, 2003.
5. Michener, LA, and Leggin, BG: A review of self-report scales for the assessment of functional limitation and disability of the shoulder. *J Hand Ther,* 14: 68-76, 2001.
6. National Collegiate Athletics Association: Sports Medicine Handbook 2006–07 (ed 18). Retrieved from http://www.ncaa.org/library/sports_sciences/sports_med_handbook/2007-08/2007-08_sports_medicine_handbook.pdf (Accessed August 3, 2008).
7. Muscolo, DL, et al: Tumors about the knee misdiagnosed as athletic injuries. *J Bone Joint Surg,* 85(A):1209, 2003.
8. Warltier, DC: Perioperative abstinence from cigarettes. Physiologic and clinical consequences. *Anesthesiology,* 104: 356, 2006.
9. Roach, S: Hormones and related drugs. In *Pharmacology for Health Professionals.* Baltimore: Lippincott Williams & Wilkins, 2005, pp 355–356.
10. Cohen, DB, et al: Indomethacin and celecoxib impair rotator cuff tendon-to-bone healing. *Am J Sports Med,* 34:352, 2006.
11. Giannoudis, PV, et al: Nonunion of the femoral diaphysis: The influence of reaming and non-steroidal anti-inflammatory drugs. *J Bone Jt Surg [Am],* 82-B:655, 2000.

12. Warden, SJ, et al: Low-intensity pulsed ultrasound accelerates and a nonsteroidal anti-inflammatory drug delays knee ligament healing. *Am J Sports Med*, 34:1094, 2006.
13. Haggman, S, Maher, CG, and Refshauge, KM: Screening for symptoms of depression by physical therapists managing low back pain. *Phys Ther*, 84: 1157, 2004.
14. Grotle, M, Vøllestad, NK, and Brox, JI: Clinical course and impact of fear-avoidance beliefs in low back pain. Prospective cohort study of acute and chronic low back pain: II. *Spine*, 31: 1038, 2006.
15. Herring, SA, et al: Mass participation event management for the team physician: A consensus statement. *Med Sci Sports Exer*, 36:2004, 2004.
16. American Academy of Pediatrics Committee on Sports Medicine and Fitness: Human immunodeficiency virus and other blood-borne viral pathogens in the athletic setting. *Pediatrics*, 104:1400, 1999.
17. Mawdsley, RH, Hoy, DK, and Erwin, PM: Criterion-related validity of the figure-of-eight method of measuring ankle edema. *J Orthop Sport Phys Ther*, 30:149, 2000.
18. Peterson, EJ, et al: Reliability of water volumetry and the figure of eight method on subjects with ankle joint swelling. *J Orthop Sports Phys Ther*, 29:609, 1999.
19. Daniel, JA, Sizer, PS, and Latman, NS: Evaluation of body composition methods for accuracy. *Biomed Instrum Technol*, 39:397, 2005.
20. Rohner-Spengler, M, Mannion, AF, and Babst, R: Reliability and minimal detectable change for the figure-of-eight-20 method of measurement of ankle edema. *J Orthop Sports Phys Ther*, 37:199, 2007.
21. Petersen, EJ, et al: Reliability of water volumetry and the figure of eight method on subjects with ankle joint swelling. *J Orthop Sports Phys Ther*, 29:609, 1999.
22. Tatro-Adams, D, McGann, SF, and Carbone, W: Reliability of the figure-of-eight method of ankle measurement. *J Orthop Sports Phys Ther*, 22:161, 1995.
23. Dewey, WS, et al: The reliability and concurrent validity of the figure-of-eight method of measuring hand edema in patients with burns. *J Burn Care Res*, 28:157, 2007.
24. Leard, JS, et al: Reliability and concurrent validity of the figure-of-eight method of measuring hand size in patients with hand pathology. *J Orthop Sports Phys Ther*, 34:335, 2004.
25. Grimston, SK, et al: Differences in ankle joint complex range of motion as a function of age. *Foot and Ankle* 14:215, 1993.
26. Kendall, FP, et al: *Muscles: Testing and Function, with Posture and Pain*. Baltimore, Lippincott Williams & Wilkins, 2005, p. 18.
27. Round, JM, et al: Hormonal factors in the development of differences in strength between boys and girls during adolescence: a longitudinal study. *Ann Hum Biol*, 26:49, 1999.
28. Goodpaster, BH, et al: The loss of skeletal muscle strength, mass, and quality in older adults: the health, aging and body composition study. *J Gerontol A Biol Sci Med Sci*, 2006 61:1059, 2006.
29. Aitkens, S, et al: Relationship of manual testing to objective strength measurements. *Muscle Nerve*, 12:173, 1989.
30. Escolar, DM, et al: Clinical evaluator reliability for quantitative and manual muscle testing measures of strength in children. *Muscle Nerve*, 24:787, 2001.
31. Dvir, Z: Grade 4 in manual muscle testing: The problem with submaximal strength assessment. *Clin Rehabil*, 11:36, 1997.
32. Jepsen, JR, et al: Manual strength testing in 14 upper limb muscles. A study of inter-rater reliability. *Acta Orthop Scand*, 75:442, 2004.
33. Norkin, CC, and White, DJ: *Measurement of Joint Motion: A Guide to Goniometry* (ed 3). Philadelphia, FA Davis, 2003, p. 8.
34. Snyder-Mackler, L, et al: The relationship between passive joint laxity and functional outcome after anterior cruciate ligament surgery. *Am J Sports Med*, 25:191, 1997.
35. Smith, CC: Evaluating the painful knee: A hands-on approach to acute ligamentous and mensical injuries. *Adv Stud Med*, 4:362, 2004.
36. Stanitski, CL: Anterior cruciate ligament injury in the skeletally immature patient: Diagnosis and treatment. *J Am Acad Orthop Surg*, 3:146, 1995.
37. Bertilson, B, et al: Pain drawing in the assessment of neurogenic pain and dysfunction in the neck/shoulder region: Inter-examiner reliability and concordance with clinical examination. *Pain Med*, 8:134, 2007.
38. Gellman, H, et al: Carpal tunnel syndrome. An evaluation of the provocative diagnostic tests. *J Bone Joint Surg Am*, 68:735, 1986.
39. Reese, NB: Techniques of the sensory examination. In *Muscle and Sensory Testing* (ed. 2). St. Louis, MO: Elsevier Saunders, 2005, p 522.
40. Dick, JPR: The deep tendon and the abdominal reflexes. *J Neurol Neurosurg Psychiatry*, 74:150, 2003.
41. Delwaide, PJ, and Toulouse, P: The Jendrassik maneuver: quantitative analysis of reflex reinforcement by remote involuntary muscle contraction. In: Desmedt JE, et al. Motor *Control Mechanisms in Health and Disease*. New York, Raven Press, 1983, pp 661–669.

CHAPTER 2

Examination and Management of Acute Pathologies

The circumstances surrounding an acute orthopedic injury dramatically influence the nature and duration of an examination. Consider the ambulatory evaluation, characterized by the patient coming to you for care on the sidelines. In many cases, this examination process mimics that described in Chapter 1. An on-field examination, which occurs at athletic venues such as a court, rink, gymnasium, pool, or field, initially focuses on establishing the absence of severe injury and then progresses through a series of examination techniques designed first to identify gross pathology and concluding with establishing the patient's ability and willingness to move and bear weight.

This chapter focuses on the immediate management of orthopedic pathology. Other possible **emergent** conditions such as **anaphylaxis**, myocardial infarctions, and other medical conditions that may require emergency interventions are not presented in this chapter.

The first goal of the immediate examination is to determine if the condition requires emergency management to save the patient's life or extremity. In order of their importance, the immediate examination must rule out:

- Inhibition of the cardiovascular and respiratory systems (ABCs)
- Life-threatening trauma to the head or spinal column
- Profuse bleeding
- Fractures
- Joint dislocation
- Peripheral nerve injury
- Other soft tissue trauma

Based on the findings of this triage, the immediate **disposition** of the athlete must be determined. The on-field management of the injury, the safest method of removing the athlete from the field, and the urgency of referring the patient for further medical care are the focus of the decision-making process.

On-field examinations are best performed with two responders. In cases of head or spine trauma, one individual is responsible for stabilizing the cervical spine while the other performs the needed examination techniques. For noncatastrophic conditions, one responder conducts the examination while the other communicates with and calms the athlete and controls the surrounding scene (Fig. 2-1). In all cases the responders should ensure that play has stopped (or has been moved in the event of a practice-related injury) so that the responders and the victim are protected from further sports-related activity.

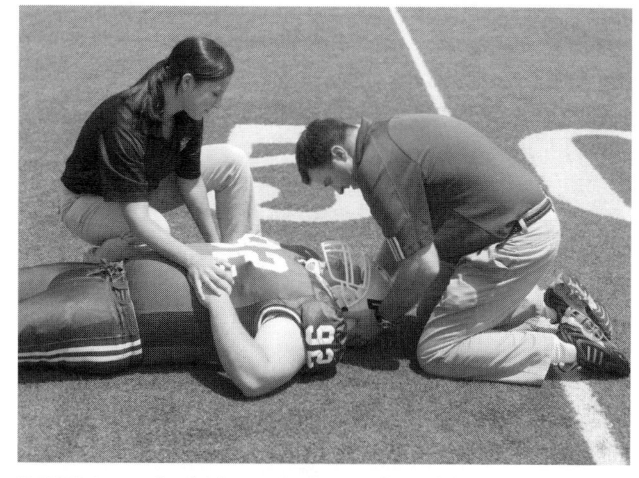

FIGURE 2-1 ■ On-field examination performed by two responders. One responder communicates with and calms the athlete while the second performs the examination. This method is optimal for handling on-field injuries, especially in emergency situations.

Emergent In need of prompt care; emergency.

Anaphylaxis A severe, potentially life-threatening allergic reaction.

When one responder is responsible for the on-field injury examination, a clear communication and evaluation protocol is needed so that relatively untrained people can assist (Fig. 2-2). The coaching staff and other personnel should receive regular training in cardiopulmonary resuscitation (CPR), including use of an automated external defibrillator (AED), and be prepared to provide assistance in the event of a catastrophic injury.

∗ Practical Evidence

Early defibrillation using an AED saves lives. Early defibrillation is the single most important intervention in improving survival following sudden cardiac arrest. For every minute that defibrillation is delayed the chance of surviving sudden cardiac arrest declines by 10%.[1,2]

Emergency Planning

The planning of medical coverage for events must take into account the worst case scenario: **catastrophic** conditions to athletes, spectators, and others at the venue. Each institution should have a written **Emergency Action Plan** (EAP) that identifies the personnel, equipment, lines of communication, and standard procedures should a potentially catastrophic event occur (Box 2-1).[3] When visiting an away site, communicate with the host institution to determine the EAP for that venue.

An on-field communication plan must be established for managing on-field injuries. The use of preestablished hand signals or walkie-talkies allows the individuals conducting the on-field evaluation to communicate with the sideline personnel. The need for emergency equipment, the team physician, other emergency personnel, and transport squad on the field can be relayed quickly.

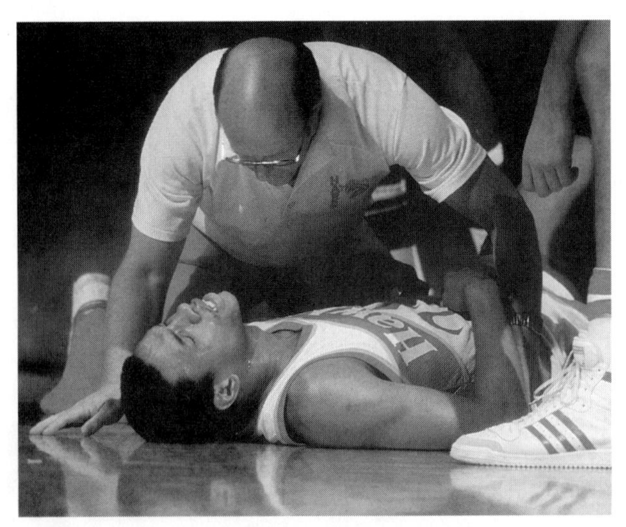

FIGURE 2-2 ■ One examiner responding to an on-field injury. This method requires that the individual perform the evaluation, communicate with the athlete, and, if necessary, summon emergency personnel.

Sport-Specific Rules

Each sport at each level of competition has rules governing the on-field evaluation of injuries during sanctioned competition. In most cases, the official must summon assistance onto the playing area and, in some sports such as wrestling, the examination must be completed and the disposition of the athlete determined within a limited period of time. Once the time period ends, the athlete is disqualified from competition regardless of ability to continue based on a medical evaluation.

Table 2-1 provides a general summary of sport-specific rules as they pertain to medical examination and care. These rules vary by governing organization, state, and venue. The medical staff is responsible for knowing the rules governing medical assistance. Before each contest, meet with the officials and other emergency personnel to clarify rules as they pertain to injury examination and protective equipment.

Critical Findings

During the examination of an acute injury, a finding may be so profound that no other information need be collected; management procedures are implemented and the athlete is immediately transported to an appropriate medical facility. Such findings include acute neurological symptoms (indicative of cervical spine or head pathology), signs of cardiovascular distress, bone angulations or deformity (associated with fractures or joint dislocations), gross joint instability, and vascular deficits. When the severity of the condition is uncertain, always err on the side of caution and refer the athlete for further medical attention.

If the initial examination cannot rule out a catastrophic condition, management of the condition becomes the first priority (Table 2-2). In addition to activating the EAP, injury management strategies must be implemented.

The On-Field Examination

When examining an on-field injury, obtaining a precise clinical diagnosis and identifying the functional limitations are less important than determining the extent of the injury and how to transport the athlete safely. Immediately after the injury, the examination focuses on determining if—and how—to splint the body part; how to remove the athlete from the playing area; and if the athlete should be transported to the sideline, sports medicine facility, or directly to the hospital. The examination must first rule out life- or limb-threatening conditions (including head and spinal cord trauma), followed by assessment for fractures/dislocations, peripheral nerve pathology, joint instability, and muscle trauma.

Box 2-1

Emergency Action Plan (EAP) Checklist*

The following elements are recommended in the development of a comprehensive EAP for sudden cardiac arrest (SCA) in athletics. Actual requirements and implementation may vary depending on the location, school, or institution.

I. Development of an EAP
- Establish a written EAP for each individual athletic venue.
- Coordinate the EAP with the local EMS agency, campus public safety officials, on-site first responders, administrators, athletic trainers, school nurses, and team and consulting physicians.
- Integrate the EAP into the local EMS response.
- Determine the venue-specific access to early defibrillation (less than 3 to 5 minutes from collapse to first shock recommended).

II. Emergency Communication
- Establish an efficient communication system to activate EMS at each athletic venue.
- Establish a communication system to alert on-site responders to the emergency and its location.
- Post the EAP at every venue and near telephones, including the role of the first responder, a listing of emergency numbers, and street address and directions to guide the EMS personnel.

III. Emergency Personnel
- Designate an EAP coordinator.
- Identify who will be responsible and trained to respond to a SCA (likely to be first responders include athletic trainers, coaches, school nurses, and team physicians).
- Train targeted responders in CPR and AED use.
- Determine who is responsible for personnel training and establish a means that training has occurred.
- Identify the medical coordinator for on-site AED programs.

IV. Emergency Equipment
- Use on-site or centrally located AED(s) if the collapse-to-shock time interval for conventional EMS is estimated to be more than 5 minutes.
- Notify EMS dispatch centers and agencies of the specific type of AED and the exact location of the AED on school grounds.
- Acquire pocket mask or barrier-shield device for rescue breathing.
- Acquire AED supplies (scissors, razor, towel, and consider an extra set of AED pads).
- Consider bag-valve masks, oxygen delivery systems, oral and nasopharyngeal airways, and advanced airways (e.g., endotracheal tube, Combitube, or laryngeal mask airway).
- Consult with physician regarding emergency cardiac medications (e.g., aspirin, nitroglycerin).
- Determine who is responsible for checking equipment readiness and how often and establish a means of documentation.

V. Emergency Transportation
- Determine transportation route for ambulances to enter and exit each venue.
- Facilitate access to SCA victim for arriving EMS personnel.
- Consider on-site ambulance coverage for high-risk events.
- Identify the receiving medical facility equipped in advanced cardiac care.
- Ensure that medical coverage is still provided at the athletic event if on-site medical staff accompany the athlete to the hospital.

VI. Practice and Review of Emergency Action Plan
- Rehearse the EAP at least annually with athletic trainers, athletic training students, team and consulting physicians, school nurses, coaches, campus public safety officials, and other targeted responders.
- Rehearse mock SCA scenarios.
- Establish an evaluation system for the EAP rehearsal, and modify the EAP if needed.

VII. Postevent Catastrophic Incident Guidelines
- Establish a contact list of individuals to be notified in case of a catastrophic event.
- Determine the procedures for release of information, aftercare services, and the postevent evaluation process.
- Identify local crisis services and counselors.
- Prepare an incident report form to be completed by all responders and the method for system improvement.

*EMS, emergency medical services; CPR, cardiopulmonary resuscitation; and AED, automated external defibrillator.
From: Drezner, JA, et al: Inter-association task force recommendations on emergency preparedness and management of sudden cardiac arrest in high school and college athletic programs. *J Athl Train*, 42:143, 2007.

Table 2-1 Rules Affecting Examination During Athletic Competition

Sport	Rule(s)
Baseball	Hard casts must be properly padded. Players are permitted to wear only one elbow pad that does not exceed 10 inches in length.[4]
Basketball	An injured player must temporarily leave the contest if the athletic trainer or other staff member comes onto the court requiring a stoppage in play.[5] Equipment deemed dangerous to others by the officiating crew is prohibited.[5] Pre-event approval of protective equipment is required.
Field Hockey	Protective equipment that increases the size of the goalkeeper is not allowed.[6]
Football	No equipment that would endanger others such as metal is allowed. Hard equipment must be covered with thick foam padding; therapeutic/ preventative knee braces must be covered or worn under clothing.[7] After an injury timeout, the injured player must leave for at least one down.[7]
Ice Hockey	Use of pads or protectors made of metal or any hard substance that could cause injury is prohibited.[8]
Soccer	Athletic trainers or other staff may not enter the field unless instructed by an official. Casts, knee braces, and other hard braces must be properly padded.[9]
Softball	Casts, braces, splints, and/or prostheses may be worn provided they are well-padded and not distracting.[10]
Tennis	Time-limited medical and bleeding timeouts may be used to treat the athlete.[11]
Wrestling	Two injury timeouts may be given for a cumulative maximum of 90 seconds for the entire match. A third nonbleeding injury will end the match. Bleeding timeouts do not count as an injury timeout, but the number and length of time allowed to treat the wound are left to the official's discretion. No more than two attendants may be allowed on the mat during these timeouts.[12]
All Sports	Athletes who have open wound must be removed from competition until the bleeding is controlled and the wound appropriately covered. Uniforms that are saturated with blood must be changed.

Refer to current national governing agencies and individual conference rules regarding competitor safety.

Table 2-2 Conditions Warranting Termination of the Evaluation

Segment	Findings that Warrant Immediate Physician Referral
History	Reports of the inability to feel or move one or more limbs (confirm with neurologic screen) Reports of significant chest pain Reports of difficulty breathing (e.g., anaphylaxis, pneumothorax)
Inspection	Obvious fracture Obvious joint dislocation Prolonged loss of consciousness Cyanosis Unequal chest expansion
Palpation	Disruption in the contour of bone, indicating a fracture or joint dislocation Malalignment of joint structures
Joint and Muscle Function Assessment	Inability of the muscle to produce torque
Joint Stability Tests	Gross joint instability
Neurologic Tests	Sensory dysfunction Motor dysfunction Pathologic changes in reflex Inability to maintain balance, loss of coordination, and other signs and symptoms of brain injury
Vascular Screening	Diminished or absent pulse Pooling of venous blood, suggesting inhibition of venous return

Because the purpose of the on-field examination differs from that of a clinical examination, the model used will also differ. Part of the inspection process begins before a history is taken, and only gross measures of joint range of motion, muscle function, and joint stability are assessed. Special tests are usually not performed at this point. In the event of possible vertebral fracture or dislocation, or spinal cord or nerve root trauma, neurological testing will assume increased importance, as will vascular screening if a fracture or dislocation of a major joint is present.

Another difference between clinical and on-field acute examinations is the less than ideal conditions in which the acute examination is conducted. The luxury of an examination table is replaced by the challenge of examining an athlete who is **prone** on the ground or sitting awkwardly on a bench. The examination may also be complicated by protective equipment and environmental conditions.

The best way to acclimate yourself to performing an on-field examination is to practice these skills with a person lying on the ground wearing football equipment or on the ice while wearing hockey equipment. The mechanics of the range of motion, stress, and special tests described in this text are more difficult when performed while kneeling. Other athletic venues such as swimming pools and gymnastics pits also present challenges to the acute examination process.

Equipment Considerations

Athletic equipment can hinder many components of the on-field examination. In most cases, clothing is not removed to conduct the on-field examination, but protective equipment such as ankle or knee braces can impede the immediate examination and must be removed or loosened to permit a complete evaluation. Methods to remove protective equipment safely are discussed in the on-field management sections in the applicable chapters of this text. Helmets, facemasks, and shoulder pads present a unique challenge to the on-field examination of suspected cervical spine trauma (see Chapter 21).

*** Practical Evidence**

Football face mask removal using a cordless screwdriver is easier than using tools that cut through the straps and results in less head movement.[13]

Primary Survey

The acute examination begins with the primary survey (Fig. 2-3). As you approach the athlete, observe for signs of movement. An athlete who is moving normally, holding an injured body part, or writhing in pain indicates consciousness, a functioning central nervous system (CNS), and cardiovascular function. Far more critical are athletes who show no signs of movement or who are seizing, indicating possible CNS trauma. All unconscious individuals should be managed as if they are suffering from cervical spine trauma (see Chapter 21).

Stabilize the head and cervical spine, unless this is clearly not indicated by the mechanism of injury (Fig. 2-4). Establish the level of consciousness by speaking to the athlete. Avoid shaking or the use of "smelling salts" (e.g., ammonia capsules) in an attempt to determine the athlete's level of consciousness or to revive the athlete.

If the athlete continues to be unresponsive, the EAP should be immediately activated so that advanced life support will arrive promptly. Do not move an unconscious athlete unless airway clearance, CPR, or AED use is indicated or accessing the athlete's airway is anticipated.

Next, determine whether or not the athlete has an open Airway, is Breathing, and has Circulation (ABCs). If the athlete is conscious, systemic circulation can be assumed. The conscious athlete may show signs of **apnea** or **dyspnea**, in which case an obstructed airway should be suspected. Possible causes of obstructed airways on the playing field include chewing tobacco, mouthpieces, dislodged teeth, and swelling of the esophagus secondary to anaphylaxis.

Secondary Survey

A secondary survey is performed when the athlete is unconscious, unable to move (or should not be moved), or unable to communicate with the responder. The purpose of the secondary survey is to identify other serious conditions that require immediate management or that will change how emergency care is implemented. For example, CPR cannot effectively be administered when there is bleeding from a large artery because chest compressions will cause more bleeding.

Observe and palpate the other body areas, noting for the presence of any bleeding, gross deformity, or other signs of trauma to other parts of the body. In cases in which the injury is apparent, such as an obvious fracture or dislocation, the history of the injury often becomes irrelevant. In these cases, rule out the possibility of head and/or spinal trauma, calm the athlete, and perform a secondary screen to rule out injury to other body areas while initiating appropriate management of the condition. When appropriate, treat for shock.

The results of the primary and secondary survey are used to make the next clinical decision. Options at this

---

Prone Lying face down.

Apnea The temporary cessation of breathing.

Dyspnea Air hunger marked by labored or difficult breathing; may be a normal occurrence after exertion or an abnormal occurrence indicating cardiac or respiratory distress.

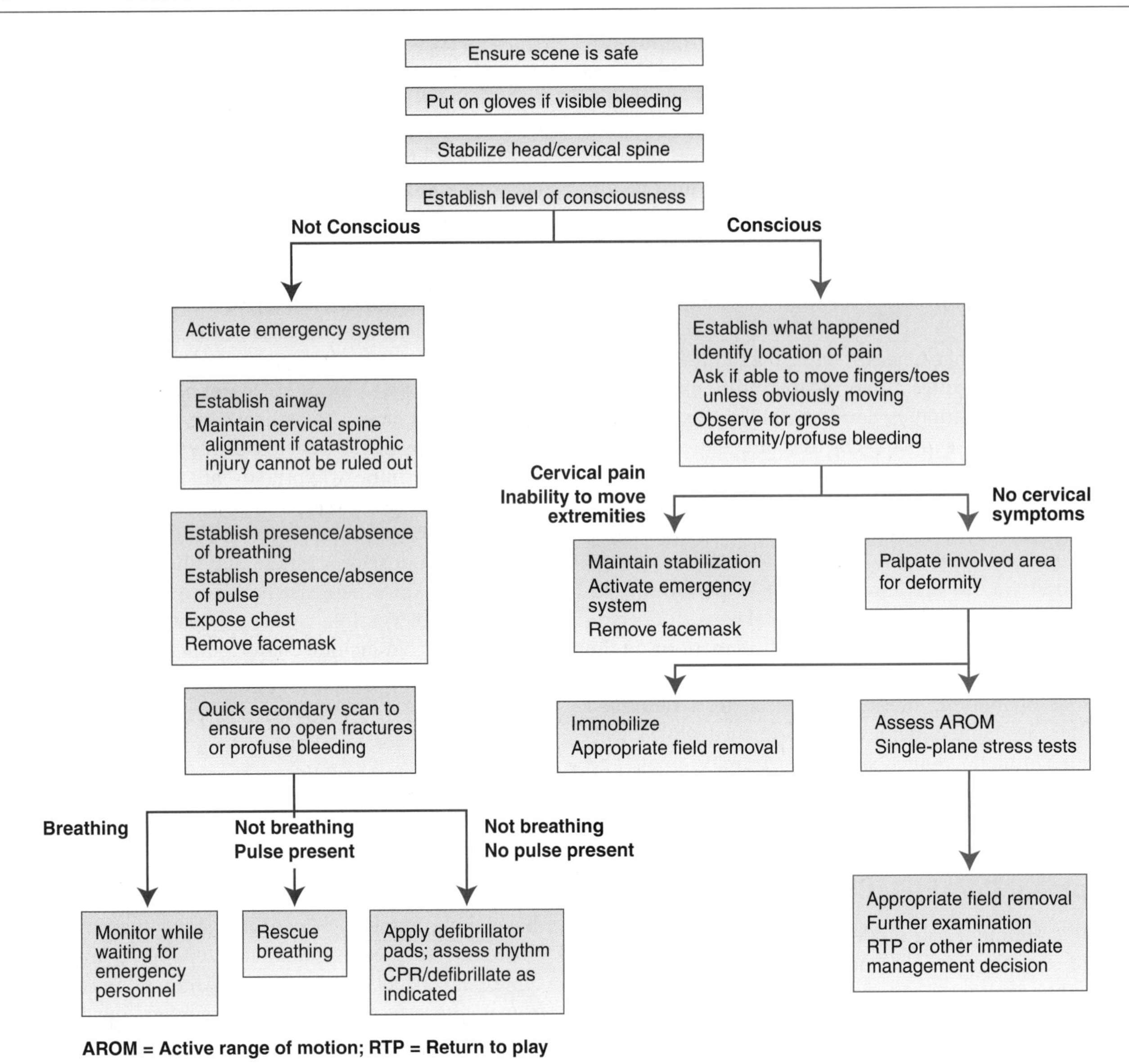

FIGURE 2-3 ■ Schematic representation of the on-field decision-making process.

point are: (1) activate the EAP and provide emergency intervention such as controlling bleeding, administering CPR or AED, or (2) continue with the examination process.

On-Field History

Once the presence of the athlete's airway and circulation has been established, the history taking process continues. If the athlete is unconscious or disoriented, as much information as possible is obtained from those who witnessed the episode. The history portion of the on-field evaluation is relatively brief compared with that associated with the clinical evaluation and tends to focus on the immediate events. The information to be identified includes:

- **Location of the pain:** Identify the site of pain as closely as possible. Although the athlete may be holding a particular area, do not assume that this is the only site of trauma because multiple injuries may have occurred. Ask the question, "Do you have pain anywhere else?"
- **Peripheral symptoms:** Question the athlete about the presence of pain or altered sensation that radiates into the distal extremities, suggesting spinal cord, nerve root, or peripheral nerve trauma.
- **Mechanism of the injury:** Identify the force that caused the injury (e.g., contact vs. noncontact injuries).
- **Associated sounds and symptoms:** Note any reports of a "snap" or "pop" at the time of injury that may indicate a tearing of ligaments or tendons or fracture.
- **History of injury:** Identify any relevant history of injury that may have been exacerbated by the current trauma or may influence the physical findings during the current evaluation.

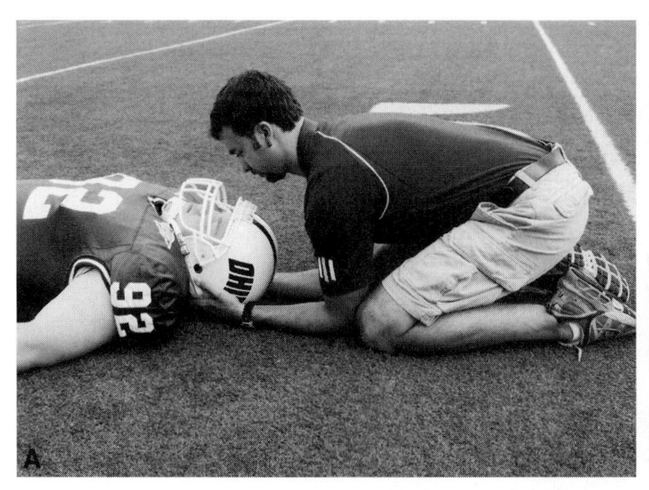

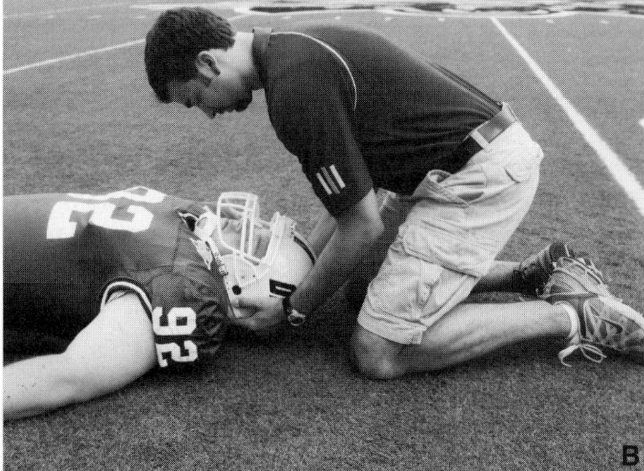

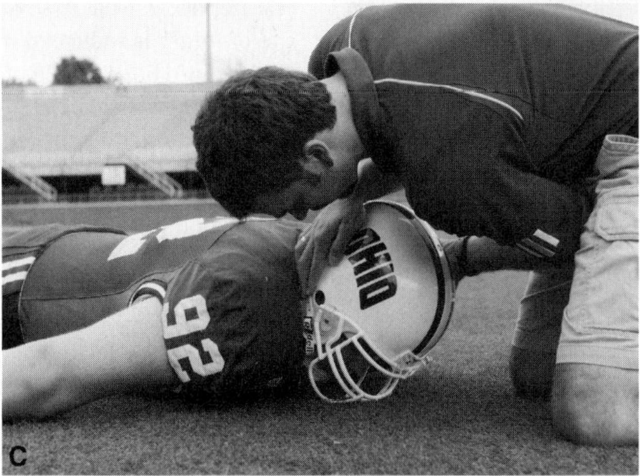

FIGURE 2-4 ■ Different c-spine stabilization techniques. **(A, B)** In-line stabilization and **(C)** prior to rolling the athlete supine.

On-Field Inspection

In an athlete-down situation, the observation process begins as soon as the athlete is in the responder's sight. As described in the Primary Survey section, observe for signs of movement and determine the level of consciousness first. Once the presence of the ABCs has been established, observe for the following:

- **Position of the athlete:** Is the athlete prone, **supine**, or side-lying? Is a body part in an awkward position? Is any gross deformity evident? These factors take on added importance if the athlete is unconscious and must be moved to begin CPR.
- **Inspection of the injured area:** This process is an abbreviated version of the steps presented during the clinical evaluation section, specifically observing for signs of a fracture (such as long bone angulation), joint dislocation (gross deformity), or edema.

On-Field Palpation

Two major areas to palpate are the bony structures and soft tissues. Findings of possible fractures, joint dislocations, or neurovascular pathology warrant terminating the evaluation and transporting the athlete to a medical facility.

Palpation of the bony structures

- **Bony alignment:** Palpate the length of the injured bone to identify any discontinuity. Although fractures of long bones are often accompanied by gross deformity, those of smaller bones may present no outward signs but are exquisitely tender during palpation.
- **Crepitus:** Note any crepitus, associated with fractures, swelling, inflammation, or air entering the subcutaneous tissues.
- **Joint alignment:** If the injury involves a joint, palpate along the joint line to determine whether the joint is aligned normally.

Palpation of the soft tissues

- **Swelling:** Swelling immediately after the injury is often associated with a major disruption of the tissues. Trauma to bursae tend to swell disproportionately to the severity of the injury. Tissues that have a rich blood

---

Supine Lying face up.

supply, such as the face, may present with a rapid formation of localized edema.

- **Painful areas:** Areas that are painful when palpated can indicate trauma to underlying tissue.
- **Deficit in the muscles or tendons:** Severe tearing of a muscle or tendon can result in a palpable defect. There is a "golden period" immediately after an injury that allows for defects to be palpated. After this period, edema and muscle spasm mask any underlying defect.

On-Field Joint and Muscle Function Assessment

While evaluating acute injuries on the field, range of motion (ROM) and functional testing provide information about the athlete's ability and willingness to move the involved extremity. AROM is the most important test to be performed while the athlete is still on the field, as this demonstrates willingness to move and an intact contractile structure. If the injury involves the lower extremity, expand functional testing to include the ability to bear weight.

Do not perform an on-field assessment of joint function when a fracture, dislocation, or muscle or tendon rupture is suspected. An approach to assessing the limb's function in a progressive manner includes:

- **Active range of motion:** The athlete is asked to move the limb through the ROM, while the quality and quantity of movement are noted.
- **Strength assessment:** If ROM test results are normal, break pressure can be used to determine the involved muscle group's ability to sustain a forceful contraction. Similar to PROM, the more specific manual muscle tests are delayed until a more detailed examination is performed.
- **Passive range of motion:** The decision to include PROM assessment is made on a case-by-case basis and is frequently delayed until the clinical evaluation. The degree of muscular and/or ligamentous damage and capsular disruption is assessed by placing the tissues on stretch. Do not perform PROM evaluations on the field if the athlete is unable to actively move the joint.
- **Weight-bearing status (lower extremity injuries):** If the athlete is able to complete the ROM tests, the athlete can be permitted to walk off the field, with assistance if necessary. If the athlete is unable to perform these tests or signs and symptoms of a potential fracture or dislocation exist, the athlete is removed from the field in a non–weight-bearing manner.

On-Field Joint Stability Tests

The purpose of on-field ligamentous testing is to gain an immediate impression of the integrity of the capsule and ligaments involved in the injury before muscle guarding or swelling masks the degree of instability. Often, on-field ligamentous testing involves only single-plane tests that are compared to the opposite side. Because these evaluations are performed on the playing surface, ligamentous testing is often conducted in less than ideal conditions.

On-Field Neurologic Testing

Neurologic testing becomes particularly important in the on-field evaluation of the athlete with a suspected head or spine injury. A thorough evaluation can ensure the proper management of these potentially catastrophic injuries. When responding to acute neurologic injuries, tests for cervical nerve root and cranial nerve involvement are needed (see Chapters 14 and 21).

Fractures or dislocations can impinge or lacerate peripheral nerves as well. Assessing motor function distal to the site of injury is indicated if it can be done without moving the involved bone or joint. For example, the athlete might be asked to move his or her fingers in the presence of an anterior glenohumeral joint dislocation. An assessment of distal sensation can also be included.

On-Field Vascular Assessment

After the dislocation of a major joint or the fracture of a large bone, the integrity of the distal vascular structures must also be determined. As with nerves, bony displacement may impinge on or lacerate the arteries and veins supplying the distal portion of the extremity. An athlete with damaged arteries may still present with an intact distal pulse, so further diagnostic testing is indicated post joint dislocation and reduction. Capillary refill should be assessed and formation of edema distal to the injured area, possibly signifying blockage of the venous return system, should be noted.[14] The specific processes for identifying these deficits are described in the appropriate chapters of this text.

*** Practical Evidence**

Identifying a distal pulse after knee dislocation does not rule out vascular damage. Following a dislocation angiography is recommended even with normal pulse and well-perfused limb. Angiography is not recommended if vascular injury is obvious (diminished pulse; signs of ischemia) because any delay in surgery worsens the outcome.[15]

Immediate Management

On completion of the on-field examination, a determination must be made regarding how to manage the athlete. Possible conclusions are:

- No splinting is needed: The athlete walks off under his or her own power.
- No splinting is needed: The athlete is assisted off the field.
- No splinting is needed: The athlete is transported directly to the hospital.

- Splinting is needed: The athlete walks off the field (upper extremity injury).
- Splinting is needed: The athlete is assisted off the field (lower extremity injury).
- Splinting is needed: The athlete is transported directly to the hospital.

The decision-making model will change according to physician availability and institutional protocol. Refer to Chapter 21 regarding the on-field management of head and spine injuries. On-field management strategies for upper and lower extremity injuries are presented in the corresponding chapters.

Splinting

Most fractures, dislocations, and significant joint sprains will need to be immobilized before removing the athlete from the field. A variety of splints are available for use, but vacuum splints are arguably the most widely used. The basic principles of immobilization are the same regardless of the type of splint used (Box 2-2).

Transportation

A decision must be made regarding how and when to transport the athlete from the playing area in the safest manner possible. If a fracture, dislocation, gross joint instability, or other significant musculoskeletal trauma is suspected, the involved body part must be splinted as described in the previous section before moving the athlete.

Based on the severity and type of injury being managed one of several methods may be used to remove the athlete from the field (Fig. 2-5). In the case of most upper extremity injuries, immobilize the body part and walk the athlete off the field. In cases of lower extremity injuries in which the athlete is unable to bear weight or upright posturing is contraindicated, several types of stretchers may be used; avoid carrying the athlete if possible. Injury to the spine requires the use of a spine board and rigid cervical collar.

Injured athletes who are lying on the field should first be moved to a sitting position, where they are again monitored for dizziness and lightheadedness. If sitting is achieved without a problem, the athlete is assisted to a standing position. Finally, give instructions regarding the extent of weight-bearing. If non–weight bearing on the injured limb, provide two human "crutches" of similar size.

Disposition

After removing the athlete from the field, a more detailed examination process ensues. The goals of this examination are to obtain enough information to formulate a return-to-play decision, to determine a diagnosis, and to decide on an immediate plan of care. This plan of care could include immediate referral for more advanced medical care or application of first aid measures such as

Box 2-2
Principles of Splinting and Immobilization

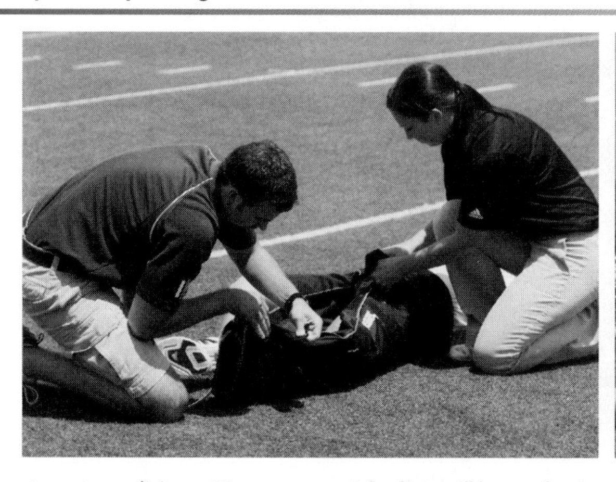

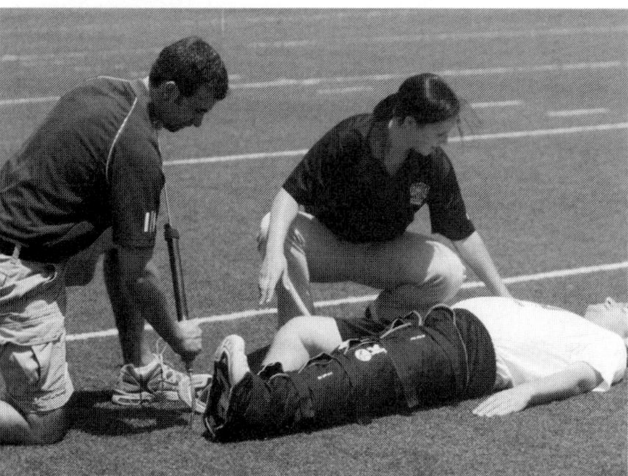

In most sports medicine settings commercial splints will be used to immobilize the body part, although upper extremity injuries can often be splinted against the torso. Regardless of the type of splint used, the splinting technique should limit motion of the involved joint and/or bone in three dimensions.

1. Unless otherwise directed by a physician, splint the extremity in the position in which it was found.
2. Establish a baseline level of sensation and skin temperature so that any changes can be noted.
3. Immobilize the joint(s) proximal and distal to the injured site.
4. Edema will most likely form soon after the injury. The splint should allow for edema and be regularly readjusted to account for swelling.[16]
5. To allow capillary refill to be checked, leave the fingers or toes uncovered when possible. Regularly assess capillary refill.
6. After immobilization, periodically question the athlete about increased pain, diminished or altered sensation, and changes in skin temperature.

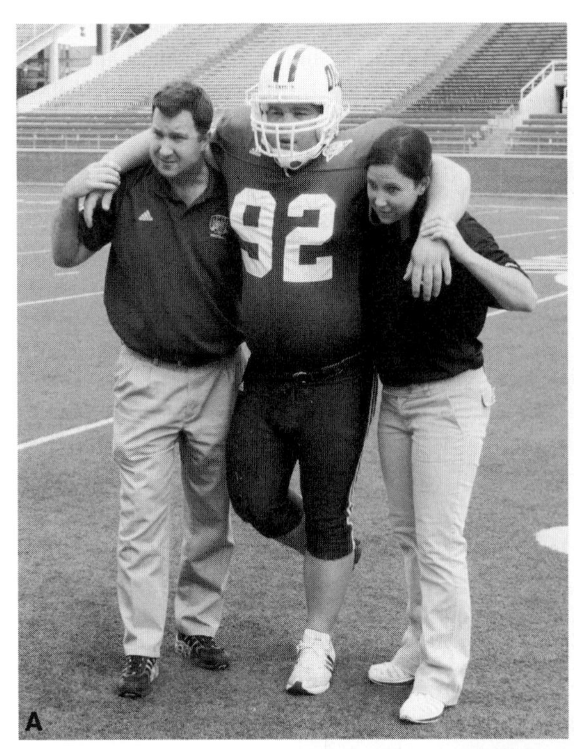

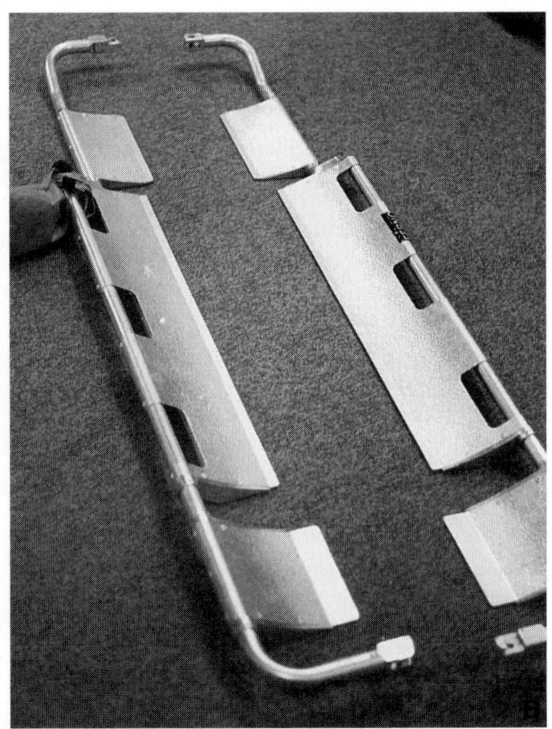

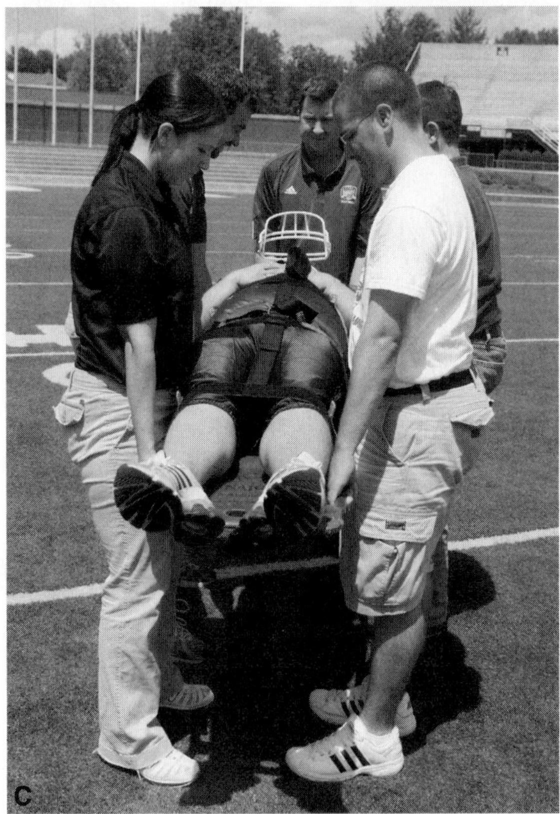

FIGURE 2-5 ■ Various athlete extraction techniques. (A) Assisted walking; (B) scoop stretcher; and (C) full spine board.

cold and compression with home instructions for continued monitoring.

Return to Activity Decision Making

Following the acute examination there will be instances in which the athlete obviously cannot continue to participate and other cases in which the trauma was obviously minor and the athlete's ability to play is evident. The challenging decision is for a case that lies in between these two situations. A physician may need to be consulted when making the return-to-play decision.

The return to play decision should be based on the relative risk of reinjury and the athlete's functional ability. The athlete's age and level of competition also factor into the decision-making process. Younger individuals are generally managed more conservatively than older athletes; for example, an injury that would not disqualify a professional athlete may disqualify a child from participating in a recreational league.

This decision is often made in an environment that is not conducive to obtaining objective measures (i.e., the sideline). The final determination is based on the assessment of function:

- **Strength and Range of Motion:** The athlete's strength and ROM should be approximately equal bilaterally and sufficient to protect both the injured area—and the athlete in general—from further injury.
- **Pain:** The athlete should report tolerable pain during exertional activities that does not result in noticeable change in function or worsen the condition.
- **Proprioception:** The athlete's involved extremity should demonstrate proprioceptive ability sufficient to protect the body part from further injury.
- **Functional activity progression:** Gradually increase the demands of the activity by introducing progressively more challenging tasks. For example, a soccer player with a lower extremity injury the functional progression would include demonstrating the ability to walk, jog, run straight ahead, change direction when jogging, and then change direction at high speed. Sport-specific skills such as dribbling are added once the athlete can complete this progression.

REFERENCES

1. Marenco, JP, et al: Improving survival from sudden cardiac arrest. The role of the automated external defibrillator. *JAMA*, 285:1193, 2001.
2. Zipes, DP, et al: ACC/AHA/ESC 2006 guidelines for management of patients with ventricular arrhythmias and the prevention of sudden cardiac death—executive summary. A report of the American College of Cardiology/American Heart Association Task Force and the European Society of Cardiology Committee for Practice Guidelines. *J Am Coll Cardiol*, 48:1064, 2006.
3. Andersen, JC, et al: National Athletic Trainers' Association Position Statement: Emergency planning in athletics. *J Athl Train*, 37:99, 2002.
4. 2005 Baseball Rules: Indianapolis: The National Collegiate Athletic Association, 2005.
5. Bilk, E, and Jacob, B, prep: 2004 Basketball Men's and Women's Rules and Interpretations. Indianapolis, The National Collegiate Athletic Association, 2003.
6. The International Hockey Federation: Rules of Hockey-Including Explanations. Lausanne, Switzerland, The International Hockey Federation, 2006.
7. Adams, JR, prep: 2005 Football Rules and Interpretations. Indianapolis, The National Collegiate Athletic Association, 2005.
8. Duffy, PJ, prep: 2004 Ice Hockey Rules and Interpretations. Indianapolis, The National Collegiate Athletic Association, 2003.
9. McCrath, CC, prep: 2004 Men's and Women's Soccer Rules. Indianapolis, The National Collegiate Athletic Association, 2004.
10. Abrahamson, D, prep: 2005 Softball Rules. Indianapolis, The National Collegiate Athletic Association, 2004.
11. USTA Regulations: Part 3, Section W. 2005.
12. Bubb, RG, prep: 2005 Wrestling Rules and Interpretations. Indianapolis, The National Collegiate Athletic Association, 2004.
13. Jenkins, HL, et al: Removal tools are faster and produce less force and torque on the helmet than cutting tools during face-mask retraction. *J Athl Train*, 37:236, 2002.
14. Miranda, FE, et al: Confirmation of the safety and accuracy of physical examination in the evaluation of knee dislocation for injury of the popliteal artery: A prospective study. *J Traum Inj Infect Crit Care*, 52:247, 2002.
15. Barnes, CJ, Pietrobon, R, and Higgins, LD: Does the pulse examination in patients with traumatic knee dislocation predict a surgical arterial injury? A meta-analysis. *J Trauma*, 53:1109, 2002.
16. Spain, D: Casting acute fractures. Part 1—Commonly asked questions. *Aust Fam Physician*, 29:853, 2000.

CHAPTER 3

Evidence-Based Practice in the Diagnostic Process

Evidence-based practice (EBP) in health care is an old concept with a new name, with the principles imbedded in everyday life. Much like making a purchase, EBP requires integration of current, best research results, clinical expertise, and the unique needs of the patient.[1] Consider helping a friend buy a new computer. First, you would **research** the various brands and models that are on the market; some are better than others. For a few more dollars you may be able to purchase a computer with more features, but are they worth it? During this process you would call on the second element, your **personal experience and expertise**. What brands have worked well in the past? Finally, you must consider the **needs** of your friend. Which features are important? Is cost or portability more significant? Failure to recognize these personal needs and values could lead to inaccurate results (unless you guessed correctly). If your friend simply does not want a laptop computer, no amount of research will make the laptop a wise purchase.

*** Practical Evidence**

Evidence-based practice, a foundation of best practice, is the incorporation of three elements into the decision-making process of patient care: (1) best available research, (2) clinical expertise, and (3) the needs and values of the individual patient.

EBP has come into focus as the result of rising medical costs, including surgery and rehabilitation, that were being paid by insurance companies. As a result of the high costs of the surgical techniques and rehabilitation devices used, insurance companies began to question their **efficacy**. Research indicated that some techniques did not provide significant improvement in the patient's condition. Other procedures required prolonged follow-up care or repeat surgeries, provided no additional benefit to the patient, or were less efficient and more expensive than other techniques.[2] To receive payment, insurance companies began to require that clinicians prove the procedures they were using actually helped patients improve in a timely, efficient manner. Thus began the modern movement toward evidence-based practice.

Applying EBP to patient care assists in making informed decisions about the most effective approaches to prevention, **diagnosis**, and management of a particular condition. Clinically there are multiple versions of how to perform a special test and multiple theories on the "best" approach to rehabilitate a patient who has just had anterior cruciate ligament (ACL) surgery. Are each of these approaches equally effective, are some better than the others, and are some just wrong?

EBP is a process rather than a technique.[3] Information—evidence—is gathered from non-biased sources such as peer-reviewed journals that address the clinical problem. Box 3-1 identifies the levels of evidence. Some types of information are more compelling than others. For example, **meta-analysis** collectively examines a body of research on a specific topic. Combined with **randomized clinical trials**, these types of research provide the strongest arguments for the inclusion or exclusion of a particular technique for a specified population. The weakest level of evidence, although not always "bad" or unusable, is often

Efficacy The ability of a protocol to produce the intended effects.

Diagnosis A conclusion reached by identifying and classifying the signs, symptoms, and clinical, radiographic, or laboratory procedures.

Meta-analysis A research technique that combines the results of multiple studies that have similar research hypotheses.

Randomized clinical trial A study in which subjects are randomly assigned to a control group or a treatment group.

Box 3-1
Puzzlin' Evidence

Not all evidence is created equally. The data and methods used to derive conclusions are varied, some stemming from well constructed research designs to those that do not pass muster with the scientific community. Certainly the findings of double-blind, randomized control studies are (or should be) more meaningful than an advertisement claiming that "4 out of 5 doctors recommend…"

The Centre of Evidence-Based Medicine has developed criteria to evaluate the quality of research. Termed "Levels of Evidence," it describes hierarchy of the different sources of data from which clinical decisions are made. Those at the top of the hierarchy carry more weight than the ones ranked lower:

Meta-analysis: Technique that combines the results of similar high-quality research studies and draws a conclusion based on statistical results.

Systematic review: A literature review that critiques and synthesizes high-quality research relating to a specific, focused question.

Randomized clinical trials: A research technique in which subjects are randomly assigned to an experimental or control group. The experimental group receives the treatment. The control group does not. The results for each group are statistically compared to identify any differences.

Cohort studies: Two groups, one that receives the treatment and one that does not, are studied forward over time to determine the impact of the treatment.

Case-control studies: Similar to a cohort study, but groups are studied from a historical perspective (backwards in time). Differences between groups of patients with (the case group) and without the a specified condition (the control group) are identified.

Case series: Report on a series of patients with a particular condition; no control group is used

Case reports: A precise description and analysis of one or more clinical cases.

Expert opinion: Opinion based on general principles, animal or human-based laboratory research, physiology, and clinical experience.

Often two sources may be contradictory regarding the usefulness of clinical techniques. In this case it is important to factor in the strength of the source (based on the hierarchy above) and the weight of the recommendations. The recommendations derived from a randomized clinical trial must be given more consideration than those from a case report.

Much of what we learn, practice, and teach has either not been critically analyzed or is still used despite the fact that the evidence does not support its inclusion in the diagnostic process.

the most prevalent and from the most surprising source: expert opinion (including textbooks).

Your clinical expertise and the input from others also contribute to **best practice**. Quality published research on the clinical signs and symptoms, examination techniques, and management of many conditions may simply not exist. In other cases the research may not be applicable to your patient.[4] For example, research on the diagnosis of shoulder conditions in the elderly may not be applicable to the diagnosis of shoulder conditions in the younger population. Likewise, recent research on the clinical diagnostic techniques of relatively rare conditions may not exist. In these instances your clinical judgment, based on your knowledge of anatomy, biomechanics, orthopedic examination techniques, and past experiences, serves as the best available evidence.

The process from the initial diagnosis through management and rehabilitation must be **patient-centered**, accounting for the patient's needs, values, and long-term goals. A patient who has no desire to return to competitive athletics after an injury would be managed much differently than a patient who does. At times, the patient's family should be involved in the decision-making process to ensure agreement and compliance with the recommended course of care. Failure to personalize care, regardless of the research findings for the condition being managed, may alienate the patient and detract from the final outcome. Refer to Box 1-2, Culturally Competent Care, for more information about interpersonal aspects of the examination process.

Evidence-based practice, including best available research, clinical expertise, and the patient's needs and values, serves as the foundation for best health care practice. Adopting this approach provides a systematic method for structuring the clinical diagnostic approach and determining management strategies. This chapter details the components of EBP only as it relates to clinical diagnostic techniques and describes how these components are incorporated into the remainder of this text. Many excellent resources describe the process of researching and interpreting the literature and present a broader picture of the evidence-based process.

Best practice Methods or procedures that through research and experience have demonstrated the optimal, most expedient results.

The Role of Evidence-Based Practice in Orthopedic Examination and Diagnosis

Hundreds, if not thousands, of orthopedic examination techniques are described in the literature. Which ones are best suited for which patient? Does every known orthopedic test need to be performed on each patient? EBP principles are used as a framework to improve the precision and efficiency of the diagnostic process. Let us assume that there are 50 special tests for the glenohumeral joint. Even if time allowed, do all of the 50 special tests have to be performed for each patient complaining of shoulder pain you examine? Identifying the tests that are most appropriate and accurate for the **symptoms** obtained during the history-taking process reduces the number of special tests that must be performed. When we weigh the evidence of how useful these tests are in identifying **pathology** we could potentially pare their number down to three or four (Fig. 3-1).

Understanding the principles that assess the relative usefulness of the examination features is needed to interpret and incorporate research findings. The components of clinical examination should be supported by evidence that confirms their usefulness in ruling in or ruling out a diagnosis.[5]

Fundamentals of Interpreting Research

EBP requires thoughtful interpretation and integration of published research. This section introduces the EBP concepts used throughout this text by describing the basic interpretation and clinical application of research findings. We will use a hypothetical example to illustrate these points. For our example we will walk through the process of determining the usefulness of the McManus test, a new (and fictitious) stress test that is intended to identify damage to the ACL (Fig. 3-2). To determine if we should include the McManus test as a part of our ACL examination procedure we must consult the literature to determine the test's reliability and its ability to rule in or rule out ACL tears.

Reliability

Before the **diagnostic accuracy** of a test can be established, its reliability, how often the same results are obtained, must be determined.[6] A test cannot be diagnostically accurate without acceptable reliability. Clinically, there are two types of reliability: Intra-rater reliability and inter-rater reliability.

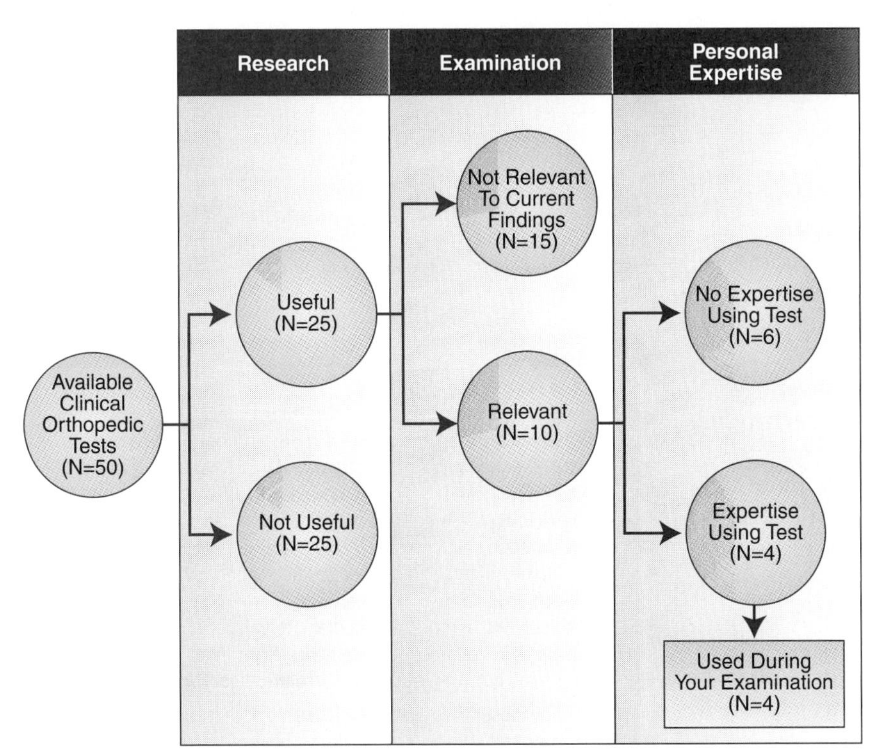

Figure 3-1 ■ Paring down the number of clinical tests to use in an examination. Consider a pool of 50 orthopedic diagnostic tests for a particular body area. After researching the various tests (hopefully found in one or two journal articles), we find that 25 of them are clinically useful and 25 are not. Based on the patient's history and clinical signs and symptoms, 15 are not needed for the differential diagnosis, leaving 10 in the pool. Of these 10, there are 6 procedures that you are not versed in. Assuming that the remaining 4 tests are accurate (which we deduced from the research phase), we can be assured that we will reach a correct diagnosis by including these 4 tests in our overall examination of this patient.

Symptom A condition not visually apparent to the examiner, indicating the existence of a disease or injury. Symptoms are usually obtained during the history-taking process.

Pathology A condition produced by an injury or disease.

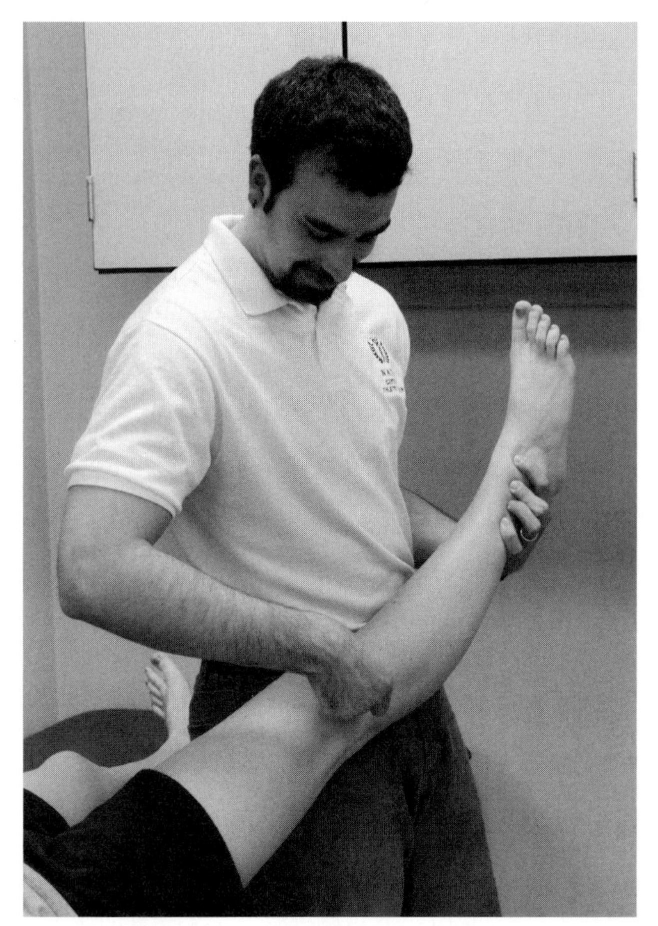

Figure 3-2 ■ The McManus test, a fictitious test used to identify ACL pathology as an illustration of EBP concepts.

Intra-rater (intra-examiner) reliability describes the extent to which the same examiner obtains the same results on the same patient. If the same examiner performs the McManus test on the same patient multiple times, how consistently will the same result (positive or negative) be obtained?

Inter-rater (inter-examiner) reliability describes the extent to which different examiners obtain the same results for the same patient. If the different examiners perform the McManus test on the same patient multiple times, how consistently will they obtain the same findings?

Depending on the type of test, statisticians report reliability using the kappa coefficient or intraclass correlation coefficient (ICC) (Box 3-2). Clinically, however, the most important aspect of these statistical measures is the interpretation of their relative usefulness. Remember that the closer the reliability measure is to 1.0, the better it is and the closer to 0.0, the less reliable it is:

If the reliability measure falls within this range...	...then the clinical usefulness is
Less than 0.5	Poor
0.5–0.75	Moderate
Greater than 0.75	Good

Not Reliable — Very Reliable

Poor | Moderate | Good

0 0.1 0.2 0.3 0.4 0.5 0.6 0.7 0.8 0.9 1.0

The first step in establishing the usefulness of the McManus test is determining its reliability. To establish **intra-rater reliability** we would ask the same clinician to perform the McManus test on multiple patients on at least two different occasions. The sample would consist of some patients who were ACL-deficient and some who were not. The clinician would not know (be "blinded" to) the patient's history or condition when performing the test. We would then compare the examiner's result for consistency using the kappa coefficient. To what extent does the examiner reach the same finding on each patient each time?

To establish **inter-rater reliability**, we would have multiple clinicians perform the McManus test on the same group of patients. Again, blinding is important. We would then measure the extent of agreement in the examiners' determination of positive and negative results. Fortunately, the McManus test performed well, yielding an inter-rater reliability of 0.76 and an intra-rater reliability of 0.86.

*** Practical Evidence**

When a task is correctly repeated multiple times by a trained practictioner using the same technique, and the same scale is applied to interpret the results, intra-rater reliability improves.

Diagnostic Accuracy

After determining that the McManus test is reliable, the test is then assessed for its diagnostic accuracy. How often do the results correctly identify whether or not the pathology is present?

Box 3-2
Measures of Reliability

When a statistician determines the percentage agreement of positive or negative findings for procedures that produce a "yes/no" or "true/false" result (nominal data), the **kappa coefficient** (κ) is used. This statistic accounts for differences attributed to chance alone. Most special tests yield this type of result, meaning that it is either positive or negative, rather than graded on a scale (such as seen with ligamentous tests). Reliability between two or more repeated of interval measurements (e.g., temperature) or ratio measurements (e.g., range of motion) are expressed using an **intraclass correlation coefficient** (ICC).

The closer the reliability measures (κ or ICC) are to 1.0, the more reliable are the findings; the closer to 0.0, the more unreliable they are. The diagnostic accuracy of a test is suspect in the presence of low reliability.[1]

Reliability is influenced by factors such as consistency in performing a skill, how the results are interpreted, the experience and training of the examiner, and the equipment used.

To assess diagnostic accuracy, we first identify a population of individuals on whom the test might be conducted. In this example, our population would be individuals presenting to us with knee pain. We know that a certain number of these individuals have sustained an ACL injury (the **prevalence** of a condition) and are trying to determine how effective our test is at correctly categorizing those people who have an ACL tear and those who do not.

Prevalence, the extent to which a condition is present in a specific population, is an important consideration for diagnostic statistics. The prevalence of any condition can change based on the group being studied. For example, prevalence of ACL **sprains** for everyone in the United States would be much different than the prevalence in a population who reports to an orthopedic clinic because of acute knee pain. In your group of friends, there is a slight chance that one or more has an ACL-deficient knee. In an orthopedic clinic the chances of finding someone who has ACL pathology is much greater simply because of the type of patients seen at the facility. Prevalence information is helpful to establish the **pretest probability** that a condition exists in a given population.

*** Practical Evidence**

Simply because of random chance, changes in the prevalence of a condition affect the ability to identify the pathology. If 1 in 100 patients has a torn ACL, then there is a 1% chance of simply guessing (or pulling the name out of a hat) the person who is injured, and a 99% chance that you can correctly identify people who have intact ACLs. If 50 in 100 patients have a torn ACL, there is a 50% chance of randomly identifying those with ACL deficiency.

Diagnostic Gold Standard

Our test results are compared to a **diagnostic gold standard** (also known as the reference standard). Gold standards have the highest diagnostic accuracy but are generally more expensive, less accessible, slower, invasive, and/or require additional personnel as compared to the clinical test. **Arthroscopy** is the gold standard for diagnosing ACL tears.[7,8] The clinical results of the McManus test will be compared to those obtained during arthroscopy.

The clinical diagnostic results are compared to the gold standard via a table consisting of two columns and two rows (a 2 × 2 contingency table). One of four outcomes can occur:

	Gold Standard	
	Positive	Negative
Clinical test positive	True positive (TP)	False positive (FP)
Clinical test negative	False negative (FN)	True negative (TN)

- **True positive:** The clinical test and the gold standard are both positive, and the condition is correctly identified. The McManus test and arthroscopy both indicate ACL pathology.
- **False positive:** The clinical test incorrectly identifies a condition as present when, in fact, there is no pathology. The McManus test indicates ACL pathology, but the ACL is shown to be intact during arthroscopy.
- **True negative:** The clinical test and the gold standard are both negative. The absence of the pathology is correctly identified. The McManus test indicates no ACL pathology and the ACL is shown to be intact during arthroscopy.
- **False negative:** The clinical procedure identifies a condition as not present when, in fact, it is present. The McManus test indicates no ACL pathology, but the arthroscopy shows the ACL as torn.

The best diagnostic accuracy is achieved with a high rate of true positives and true negatives. Following a trial involving 40 patients with knee pain, the results of the McManus test are classified as positive or negative and are grouped by arthroscopic findings of the intactness of the ACL. In this case, the comparison of the McManus test to the reference standard of arthroscopy results in the 2 × 2 table below:

	Arthroscopy	
	Arthroscopy Positive for ACL Pathology	Arthroscopy Negative for ACL Pathology
McManus test positive	17 (TP)	3 (FP)
McManus test negative	6 (FN)	14 (TN)

FN = false negative; FP = false positive; TN = true negative; TP true positive.

Diagnostic Predictive Value

The **accuracy** of a test is determined by comparing the number of correctly classified patients (True Positives + True Negatives) to the total number of patients examined. A test that is 100% accurate correctly classifies every single patient; however, this level of accuracy is highly unlikely. Relying on accuracy to determine a test's usefulness can be deceptive because it is impacted by the prevalence of a condition.[6]

Research on the usefulness of diagnostic techniques may report the **positive predictive value** and **negative predictive value**. By comparing the True Positive rate to the

Sprain The stretching or tearing of ligamentous or capsular tissue.

Pretest probability The likelihood that a specific condition is present before the diagnostic test results are known.

Arthroscopy A minimally invasive procedure in which a tube-like instrument is inserted though the skin to visualize and repair underlying tissues.

overall positive rate (or True Positive/True Positive + False Positive), positive predictive values depict how often a positive finding is correct. Conversely, negative predictive values identify how often a negative finding is correct (True Negative/True Negative + False Negative).

Although useful, predictive values are less valuable than likelihood ratios because a low prevalence of a condition in a given population deflates the positive predictive value and inflates the negative predictive value. In other words, when the number of those who will test negative is large simply because of the low prevalence, the true positives will be much more difficult to find without including more false positives in the process.[9] Failing to consider prevalence rates when comparing predictive values from two different studies can lead to false conclusions. Because of the wide spectrum of prevalence rates and the resulting difficulty in making comparisons, predictive values are not reported in this text. See Box 3-3 for a further description of the influence of prevalence on predictive values.

Sensitivity and Specificity

Sensitivity and specificity describe how often the technique identifies the true positive and true negative results. **Sensitivity** describes the test's ability to detect those

Box 3-3
Relationship Between Prevalence and Predictive Value

Prevalence is the number of people affected by a condition. Depending on the group of people studied, the prevalence of a condition will change. Because of the differences in the physical demands of the sport, it is more likely that more cases of patellar tendinopathy would be identified in a group of 100 professional basketball players (say 25 out of 100) than in a group of 100 golfers (say 5 out of 100).

Prevalence affects the positive and negative predictive values. In our example of basketball players and golfers, random chance gives us a greater probability of finding a basketball player with patellar tendinopathy than a golfer. Differences in the prevalence of a condition make comparison of positive predictive values (PPV) and negative predictive values (NPV) between two different studies problematic.

The tables below illustrate the effect of two different prevalences on the PPV and NPV for the McManus test. Remember that we already know the test's ability to identify correctly those with and without the pathology (sensitivity and specificity).

Group I assumes that the prevalence of ACL pathology in the entire adult population of the United States is 0.02%, or 20 out of every 100,000 individuals. Because the number of those without the pathology is so overwhelmingly high, it makes sense that the negative predictive value will be very high: almost everyone is already negative. Because so few individuals have the pathology, the rate of false positives will also be high, and the PPV will be decreased.

The prevalence of ACL pathology changes in a sports medicine facility (Group II). First, our target population are those exclusively complaining of acute knee pain. In this population, a much higher proportion will have sustained damage to the ACL. Let us assume a prevalence of 20%, or 20,000 out of 100,000 patients have injured their ACL. Now, we can expect a slightly lower negative predictive value and a largely increased positive predictive value. There are fewer false positives simply because there are more people with ACL trauma.

Using the 2 × 2 tables below, compare the positive and negative predictive values for Groups I and II. Although the rate of detection for the McManus test is the same, the predictive values change based on the prevalence of ACL trauma in the two groups. The increased proportion of ACL-deficient people most significantly affects the positive predictive value. When examining the predictive values, the population used must be considered before making a determination of a test's usefulness.

Group I Prevalence = 20/100,000 (0.02%)

	Arthroscopy		
	Positive ACL Pathology	Negative ACL Pathology	Predictive Value
McManus test positive	15	18,000	PPV = 15/18,015 = 0.08
McManus test negative	5	82,000	NPV = 82,000/82,005 = 99.99

Group II Prevalence = 20,000/100,000 (20.0%)

	Arthroscopy		
	Positive ACL Pathology	Negative ACL Pathology	Predictive Value
McManus test positive	15,000	14,400	PPV = 15,000/29,400 = 51.02
McManus test negative	5000	65,600	NPV = 65,600/70,600 = 92.92

patients who actually have the disorder relative to the gold standard.[9] Also known as the *true positive rate*, sensitivity describes the proportion of positive results a technique identifies relative to the actual number of positives. Sensitivity is calculated as: True Positives/(True Positives + False Negatives). Compared to arthroscopy, the McManus test correctly identified 17 out of 23 individuals who have ACL pathology, yielding a sensitivity of 0.74.

	Arthroscopy	
	Arthroscopy Positive for ACL Pathology	Arthroscopy Negative for ACL Pathology
McManus test positive	17 (TP)	3 (FP)
McManus test negative	6 (FN)	14 (TN)
	Sensitivity = TP/(TP+FN) = 17/(17 + 6) – 0.74	

TP = true positive; FP = false positive; TN = true negative; FN = false negative.

Tests with high sensitivity accurately identify all or most patients with a given condition. The sensitivity value alone, however, can be misleading. While all True Positives are likely to be identified, the number of False Positives obtained along the way can also be high. To gain a better understanding of a test's overall usefulness, specificity must also be considered.

Specificity, the *true negative rate*, describes the test's ability to detect patients who do not have the disorder. The specificity of a diagnostic technique identifies the proportion of True Negatives the technique detects compared to the actual number of negatives in a given population. Specificity is calculated as: True Negatives/(True Negatives + False Positives). With a specificity of 0.82, the McManus test correctly identified those without ACL damage by yielding a negative result 82% of the time.

	Arthroscopy	
	Arthroscopy Positive for ACL Pathology	Arthroscopy Negative for ACL Pathology
McManus test positive	17 (TP)	3 (FP)
McManus test negative	6 (FN)	14 (TN)
	Sensitivity = TP/(TP + FN) = 17/(17 + 6) = 0.74	Specificity = TN/(TN + FP) = 14/(14 + 3) = 0.82

TP = true positive; FP = false positive; TN = true negative; FN = false negative.

A high sensitivity tells us that in most cases this test will identify ACL tears. Because of this negative tests results strongly rule out the presence of an ACL tear. **SnNout** is a useful reminder: In tests with a high sensitivity (Sn), a negative finding (N) effectively rules *out* the condition. Alternatively, a high specificity, where most of those without the condition are identified, makes positive results more convincing. The reminder **SpPin** is used: In tests with a high specificity (Sp), a positive finding (P) convincingly rules *in* the condition.[1]

The meaningfulness of sensitivity and specificity values changes relative to the condition being studied. When the failure to identify some conditions could produce catastrophic results, a high sensitivity is required and can come at the expense of specificity. Using our SnNout acronym, we would need to use a test with a high sensitivity in which a negative result is truly negative. For example, when examining a "high stakes" orthopedic condition such as a cervical spine fracture or joint dislocation the test with the highest sensitivity is used first to identify all potentially positive cases.

*** Practical Evidence**

Failure to detect arterial insufficiency could result in the loss of the distal extremity. Because palpation of a distal pulse (e.g., the dorsalis pedal pulse) is not highly sensitive in detecting damage to the proximal artery, a more definitive (sensitive) technique such as Doppler ultrasound should be used to determine if there is arterial damage.[10]

As with sensitivity, using only the specificity values is misleading in determining the usefulness of a diagnostic test. Detecting all of the True Negatives may also be at the expense of misclassifying those who actually do have the condition as False Negatives. Sensitivity and specificity determine how well a test detects true positives and true negatives. Yet, taken alone, these measures may not be sufficiently useful. Unless both the sensitivity and specificity values are high, determining the procedure's clinical usefulness is difficult (and often inconclusive). To avoid these pitfalls, sensitivity and specificity values are considered together and are expressed as likelihood ratios.

Likelihood Ratios

Likelihood ratios provide quick summaries of how positive and negative findings on a particular test determine a test's diagnostic usefulness. Likelihood ratios incorporate a test's sensitivity and specificity and are not influenced by the prevalence of a condition (see Box 3-3).

Likelihood ratios explain the shift in the pretest probability that a patient has a condition after a test result is obtained. Pretest probabilities are population-specific and derived from prevalence data from regional or national databases, practice databases, published research findings, or clinical experience.[6] Often, pretest probabilities must be estimated based on clinical experience because specific data are not available.

A likelihood ratio that is near or at 1 indicates that there is little to no shift in the pretest probability that a condition is present after the results—either positive or negative—of the test are considered. A likelihood ratio that is greater than 1 increases the probability that the condition exists, and an LR of less than 1 decreases the probability that the condition exists.[11] Consideration of likelihood ratio results can lead to one of three clinical decision options: [1]

- The post-test probability is so high that there is acceptable certainty that the pathology is present.
- The shift in post-test probability is inconclusive. A stronger test or tests, if available, are needed to rule in or rule out the pathology.
- The post-test probability is so low that there is acceptable certainty that the pathology is not present. Other diagnoses must be considered.

Following a positive or negative test result, how sure are we that the patient has the condition in question? A positive likelihood ratio describes the shift in the pretest probability that the condition is present based on a positive test result. A negative likelihood ratio describes the change in the pretest probability that a condition exists based on a negative test result.

Positive Likelihood Ratio

The positive likelihood ratio (LR+) expresses the change in our confidence that a condition is present when the test is positive. The higher the LR+, the more a positive test enhances the probability that the pathology is present.

A LR+ is calculated as:

$$\text{sensitivity}/(1 - \text{specificity})$$

Using our sensitivity and specificity information for the McManus test presented earlier, the likelihood ratio can be calculated:

	Arthroscopy	
	Arthroscopy Positive for ACL Pathology	Arthroscopy Negative for ACL Pathology
McManus test positive	17 (TP)	3 (FP)
McManus test negative	6 (FN)	14 (TN)
	Sensitivity = 0.74 LR+ = Sensitivity / (1 − specificity) = 0.74 /(1 − 0.82) = 4.11	Specificity = 0.82

TP = true positive; FP = false positive; TN = true negative; FN = false negative.

A positive result using the McManus test is about four times more likely to be seen in a patient with our target condition.

Negative Likelihood Ratio

The negative likelihood ratio (LR−) expresses the probability that the pathology is still present even though the test was negative. How convincing is a negative test in diminishing the likelihood that the patient has the pathology? The closer the LR− is to 1, the less significant is the change in pretest probability. The lower the LR− is, the lower is the probability that the condition exists.

The LR− is calculated as:

$$(1 - \text{sensitivity})/\text{specificity}$$

A high sensitivity (or true positive rate), will deflate the LR−. A negative McManus test would not convincingly rule out the possibility of an ACL tear because there is only a small shift in the pretest probability.

	Arthroscopy	
	Arthroscopy Positive for ACL Pathology	Arthroscopy Negative for ACL Pathology
McManus test positive	17 (TP)	3 (FP)
McManus test negative	6 (FN)	14 (TN)
	Sensitivity = 0.74 LR+ = 4.11 LR− = (1 − Sensitivity)/ Specificity = (1 − 0.74)/0.82 = 0.32	Specificity = 0.82

TP = true positive; FP = false positive; TN = true negative; FN = false negative.

Interpreting Likelihood Ratios

Likelihood ratios tell us the extent to which the outcome of our test changes the probability that the patient has the suspected condition. This change in probability can be interpreted using a likelihood ratio nomogram (Fig. 3-3) or general guidelines. The general guidelines for interpretation of likelihood ratios are presented in Table 3-1.[12,13]

To use the nomogram, the pretest probability that the patient has the condition must be known or estimated. Remember that the pretest probabilities are based on a specific group of people (e.g., athletes, construction workers, the elderly) and are derived from the results of on-going research.[6] Often, pretest probabilities must be estimated based on clinical experience because specific data is not available.

If the pretest probability that a specific pathology exists is already high, then only a test having a large LR+ will help confirm the diagnosis. If the pretest probability that a specific pathology exists is low, then only a test with a very small LR− will lower that probability even more. Tests with LR+ or LR− values that approach 1.0 have little clinical usefulness and can be omitted from the clinical diagnostic procedure.

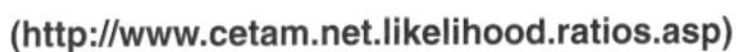

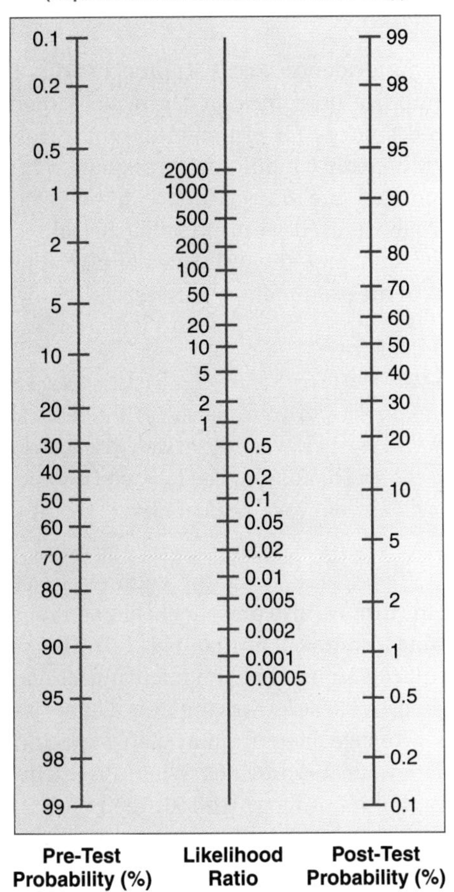

Figure 3-3 ■ Nomogram. The pretest probability is identified on the left side of the nomogram, the positive or negative likelihood ratio is plotted on the middle column, and a line connecting the two points is continued through the third column. The intersection in the third column indicates the change in probability that the condition exists given the results of the test.

Table 3-1 Interpretation of Likelihood Ratios

Positive Likelihood Ratio	Negative Likelihood Ratio	Shift in Probability Condition is Present
>10	<0.1	Large, often conclusive
5–10	0.1–0.2	Moderate but usually important
2–5	0.2–0.5	Small, sometimes important
1–2	0.5–1	Very small, usually unimportant

Ample data exist on knee injuries and the incidence of injury to the ACL. In an early study of knee injury in women's college basketball, 26% of those who sustained an acute knee injury sustained damaged to their ACL.[14] Risk factors or reported history also help in generating a pretest probability hypothesis. For example, women who play basketball or soccer are two to four times more likely to sustain an ACL injury as compared to their male counterparts.[14,15] Athletes between 15 and 25 years of age sustain more than 50% of all ACL injuries.[15] The majority of non-contact ACL injuries occur from planting and pivoting.[14,15]

Using our example, consider a 20-year-old woman who comes in seeking evaluation for an acute knee injury that occurred yesterday while she was playing basketball. Our initial differential diagnosis includes about a 25% probability that she has sustained injury to her ACL. In this case, the McManus test is positive and we know its LR+ is 4.11. Using a nomogram to plot our results, we find that the post-test probability that she has injured her ACL is approximately 50% (Fig. 3-4). Had we obtained a negative result with the McManus test, the post-test probability that has injured her ACL would be between 5% and 10%, using the known LR− of 0.32. Using the interpretation guidelines, we have obtained a small but potentially useful shift in probability that she has injured her ACL.

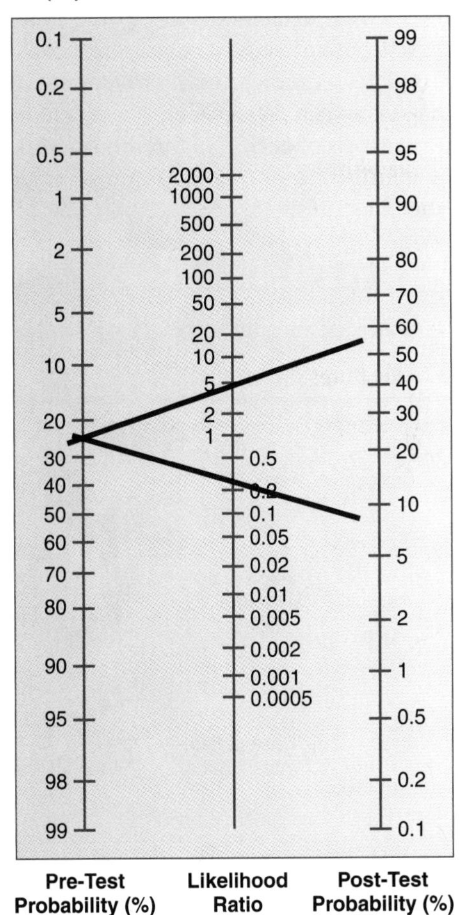

Figure 3-4 ■ Nomogram for the McManus test. These lines show the changes in pretest probability of a patient having an ACL sprain with a positive or negative McManus test result. Use the nomogram in Figure 3-2 to plot the changes in post-test probability for a condition that has a low pretest probability that is diagnosed using a test with a high LR+.

Clinical Decision Rules

Clinical decision rules (CDRs), also known as clinical prediction rules, are groups of findings that, when considered collectively, improve decision making, decrease costs, and ultimately improve patient outcomes. CDRs are developed by identifying the clinical signs and symptoms that most significantly predict the presence of the pathology. Data from this collection of validated, reliable items are analyzed to identify the items that contribute most to making an accurate clinical decision, providing the basis of the CDR. These rules must then be tested in various groups to ensure that they should, in fact, be included. Finally, the impact of the CDR on cost, patient satisfaction, and/or outcome is evaluated.[16]

For example, the Ottawa Ankle Rules were developed to reduce unnecessary radiographs for patients presenting to emergency rooms after traumatic foot and ankle injuries (Box 3-4; also see Chapter 9). Using only the clinical findings of the ability to bear weight and areas of point tenderness, this simple diagnostic protocol results in fewer radiographs, lower costs, decreased time in the emergency room, increased patient satisfaction, and (most importantly) no undetected fractures (100% sensitivity).[17,18] Common diagnostic clinical decision rules include those used for the diagnosis of deep vein thrombosis, mild traumatic brain injuries, cervical spine injuries, ankle fractures, and knee fractures.[14,19]

Use of Evidence in this Text

Developing an evidence-based approach will increase efficiency, improve outcomes, and provide a thoughtful, individualized strategy for examination and diagnosis of those with orthopedic conditions. Throughout this text we have incorporated the best evidence as it is currently available. While we used an orthopedic special test as an example in this chapter, the principles of EBP apply to all components of the examination process.

*** Practical Evidence**

Remaining current with *all* the literature is impossible. Use clinical questions that relate to your patient as the foundation for evidence-based practice. When faced with a clinical challenge, refer to the current literature on that topic and incorporate the published findings into your decision-making process.

Reliability data of specific procedures is reported throughout the text. We also present likelihood ratios, when available, using a graphical format (Fig. 3-5). This provides you with a quick summary of the relative usefulness of a positive or negative test in arriving at a diagnosis. Likelihood ratios were calculated from available specificity and sensitivity data when not provided. When specificity equals 1 (indicating that all of those without the condition were correctly identified), we did not calculate the positive likelihood ratio because the denominator will be 0. In this case,

Box 3-4
Ottawa Ankle Rules

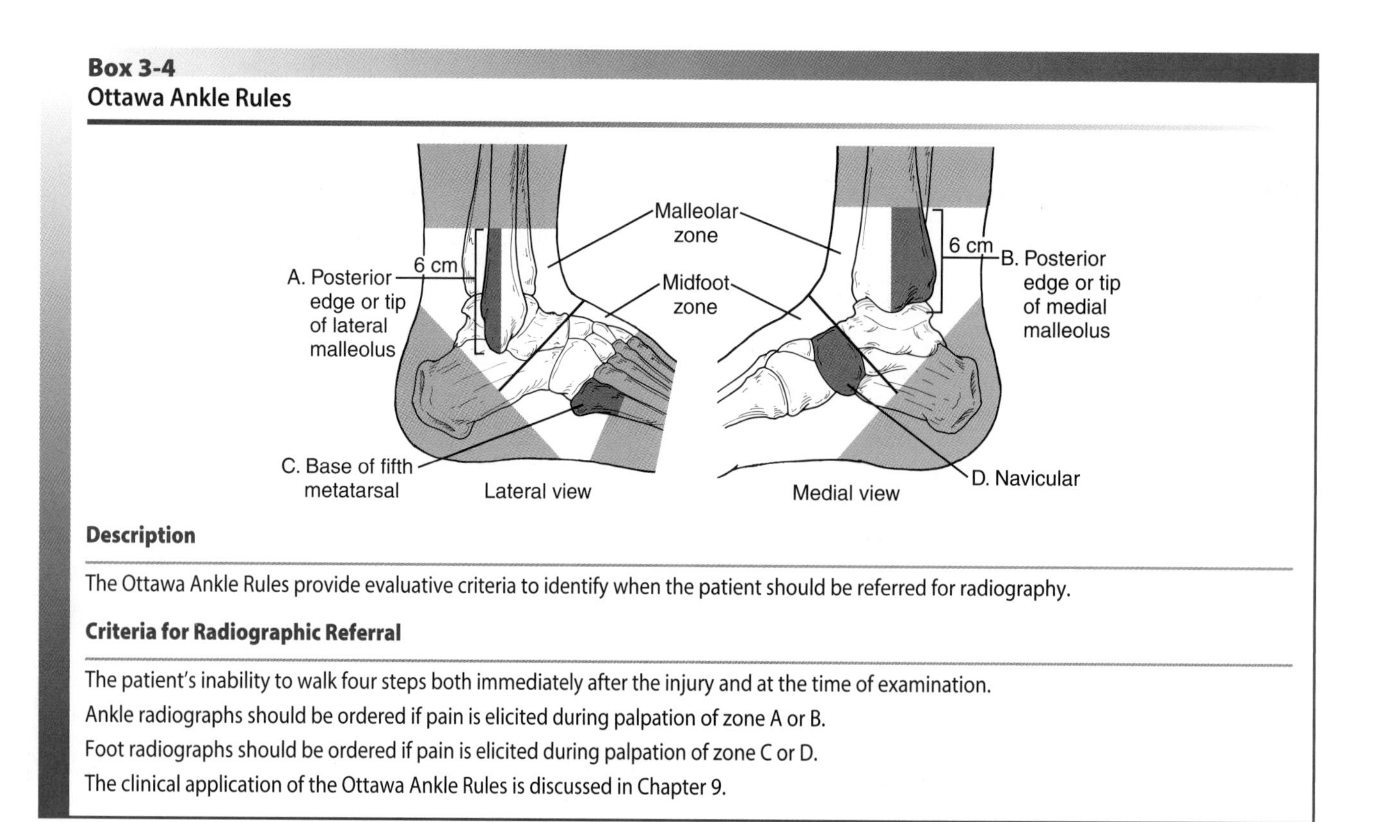

Description

The Ottawa Ankle Rules provide evaluative criteria to identify when the patient should be referred for radiography.

Criteria for Radiographic Referral

The patient's inability to walk four steps both immediately after the injury and at the time of examination.

Ankle radiographs should be ordered if pain is elicited during palpation of zone A or B.

Foot radiographs should be ordered if pain is elicited during palpation of zone C or D.

The clinical application of the Ottawa Ankle Rules is discussed in Chapter 9.

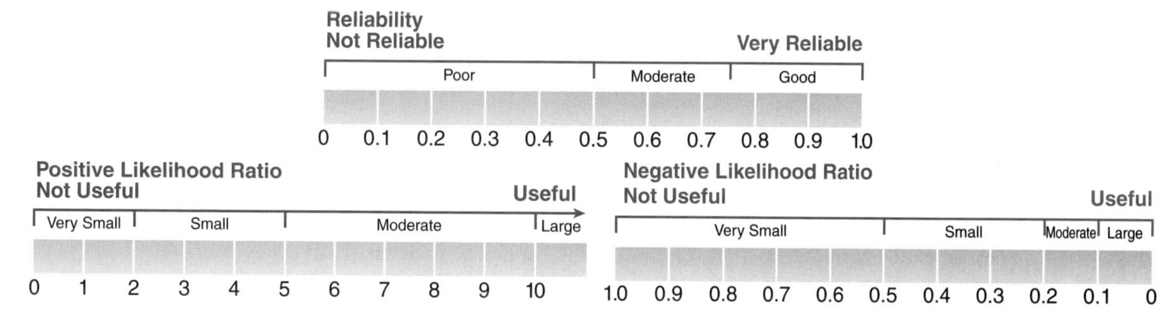

Figure 3-5 ■ Presentation of reliability and positive and negative likelihood ratio values used in this text.

you can assume that a positive finding generates a large shift in the post-test probability that the condition exists.[6] Sensitivity and specificity values for many orthopedic diagnostic techniques are reported in Appendix A.

Incorporating Evidence-Based Practice into Clinical Diagnosis

A clinical diagnostic technique is useful—and should be included in the examination process—if it meaningfully assists in identifying the presence (or absence) of the pathology. Many of the clinical techniques are used more because of tradition than science, with a positive or negative finding adding little to the diagnostic picture. Other techniques have been examined only by the individual(s) who developed the procedure, adding a bias to the outcome (who would publish a paper declaring "I invented this test, but it does not work"?). Lastly, a large percentage of the orthopedic clinical techniques used have not been the subject of rigorous study.

To be determined as useful, a clinical technique must be reliable and it must increase or decrease the probability that the condition is present. If a procedure has low intra- or inter-rater reliability, then the usefulness is limited because the technique is not accurately reproducible and the findings will vary from attempt to attempt (intra-rater reliability) or from clinician to clinician (inter-rater reliability). To be clinically useful, a procedure must demonstrate moderate (>0.5) to good (>0.75) reliability. Of course, the closer the reliability is to 1.0, the more comfortable we are with the reproducibility of the results.

Likelihood ratios combine the influences of sensitivity and specificity to determine the impact that a positive or negative test finding has on the probability that given condition exists. A positive test result must have a minimum LR+ value of 2.0 (small) to significantly add to the pretest probability that the condition is present. A LR− value of 0.2 or less meaningfully lowers the probability that the condition is present.

Our hypothetical McManus test passed the first criteria of intra- and inter-rater reliability, yielding a 0.76 inter-rater reliability and 0.86 intra-rater reliability values. This means that the test is reproducible and we can accept the findings of the same person over time and the results of two different clinicians. The likelihood ratios, although not as strong as we would like, did generate a meaningful shift in post-test probability. The McManus test has a 4.11 LR+, meaning that a positive finding increases the chance that ACL damage is present. The LR− value of 0.32 means that a negative test finding decreases the chance that the ACL has been torn.

Given that other tests, such as the Lachman or pivot-shift test, have higher LR+ and lower LR− values, it is unlikely that the McManus test will significantly contribute to making a clinical diagnosis. As such, we should use the Lachman and/or pivot-shift test rather than the McManus test. We can efficiently examine a knee for ACL pathology and accurately conclude that the ACL is torn without performing the McManus test. Likewise, since the Lachman test has a higher LR+ value >10, if it was positive there would be no need to perform other orthopedic tests such as the pivot-shift or McManus to confirm the presence of an ACL tear.

Adopting an evidence-based approach to patient care requires a commitment to asking well-formed clinical questions and seeking answers from contemporary resources. As is the nature of research, much of the EBP information presented in this text will change with time. The reader is advised to supplement the information provided in this text with that found in current peer-reviewed journals.

REFERENCES

1. Straus, SE, et al: *Evidence-based Medicine*, ed 3. Philadelphia, Elsevier Churchill Livingstone, 2005.
2. Bourne, RB, Maloney, WJ, and Wright, JG: The Orthopaedic Forum. An AOA critical Issue: The outcome of the outcomes movement. *J Bone Joint Surg* 86A:633, 2004.
3. Steves, R, and Hootman, JM: Evidence-based medicine: What is it and how does it apply to athletic training? *J Athl Train*, 39:83, 2004.
4. Cook, DJ, and Levy, MM: Evidence-based medicine. A tool for enhancing critical care practice. *Evidence-based Crit Care Med*, 14:353, 1998.
5. Davidoff, F, et al: Evidence based medicine (Editorial), *Br J Med*, 310:1085, 1995.
6. Cleland, J: *Orthopedic Clinical Examination: An Evidence-Based Approach for Physical Therapists*. Carlstadt, NJ, Icon Learning Systems, 2005.

7. Scholten, RJ, et al: Accuracy of physical diagnostic tests for assessing ruptures of the anterior cruciate ligament: a meta-analysis. *J Fam Pract*, 52:689, 2003.
8. Moore, SL: Imaging the anterior cruciate ligament. *Orthop Clin North Am*, 33:663, 2002.
9. Loong, T-W: Understanding sensitivity and specificity with the right side of the brain. *BMJ*, 327:716, 2003.
10. Barnes, CJ, Pietrobon, R, and Higgins, LD: Does the pulse examination in patients with traumatic knee dislocation predict a surgical arterial injury? A meta-analysis. *J Trauma*, 53:1109, 2002.
11. Fritz, JM, and Wainner, RS: Examining diagnostic tests: An evidence-based perspective. *Phys Ther*, 81:1546, 2001.
12. Denegar, CR, and Fraser, M: How useful are physical examination procedures? Understanding and applying likelihood ratios. *J Athl Train*, 41:201, 2006.
13. Jaeschke, R, Guyatt, JH, and Sacket, DL: User's guide to the medical literature, III: how to use an article about a diagnostic test. B: What are the results and how will they help me in caring for my patients? The Evidence-Based Medicine Working Group. *JAMA*. 271:703, 1994.
14. Arendt, EA, Agel, J, and Dick, R: Anterior cruciate ligament injury patterns among collegiate men and women. *J Athl Train*, 34:86, 1999.
15. Griffin, LA, et al: Understanding and preventing noncontact anterior cruciate ligament injuries. A review of the Hunt Valley II meeting, January 2005. *AJSM*, 34:1512, 2006.
16. Childs, JD, and Cleland, JA: Development and application of clinical prediction rules to improve decision making in physical therapist practice. *Phys Ther*, 86:122, 2006.
17. Stiell, IG, et al: A study to develop clinical decision rules for the use of radiography in acute ankle injuries. *Ann Emerg Med*, 21:384, 1992.
18. Nugent, PJ: Ottawa Ankle Rules accurately assess injuries and reduce reliance on radiographs. *J Fam Pract*, 53:785, 2004.
19. Perry, JJ, and Stiell, IG: Impact of clinical decision rules on clinical care of traumatic injuries to the foot and ankle, knee, cervical spine, and head. *Injury*, 37:1157, 2006.

CHAPTER 4

Injury Pathology Nomenclature

A standard approach to describing mechanisms of injury and the resulting pathology is required to make an accurate diagnosis and to communicate among health care providers. A diagnosis of "sprain" must mean the same to each person so that the correct tissue is targeted during the treatment process. Interestingly, even terminology changes as more and more is known about the body. For example, until recently "tendinitis" was used to describe most nonacute tendon pathologies. We now know that many tendon conditions are not inflammatory in nature, as the "itis" suffix implies. Instead, tendon pathology often results from degenerative changes, and the term "tendinosis" is more appropriate. It is easy to see how the nomenclature might influence the treatment. A patient with an "itis" might effectively be treated with agents designed to reduce inflammation. Treatment of a patient with an "osis" would likely take a different path. In addition to a common labeling approach, a common understanding of how different tissues respond to different types of stress is critical to understanding how various mechanisms result in injury.

Tissue Response to Stress

The tissues that form the human body react to the forces—stress—placed on them in a meaningful and predictable manner, as described by the **Physical Stress Theory** (Fig. 4-1).[1] The term "stress" is broad and encompassing enough to describe physical forces applied to the body as well as psychological, social, and emotional factors. This chapter focuses on the physical forces applied to human tissues. Stress can also affect the body systemically, such as cardiovascular and muscular enhancements when running, or regionally, such as when performing a one-armed biceps curl.

Some stress is needed for soft tissue and bone to maintain homeostasis (maintenance level). This level of activity varies from person to person but so long as the stressors applied to the body stay within this range, no physiological changes occur. When the relative level of applied stress falls below the maintenance level, the tissues **atrophy**. This can be seen after long-term immobilization of an arm or leg: when the cast or brace is removed the girth of the muscles of the immobilized portion of the limb is significantly less than the healthy limb.

Hypertrophy occurs when the duration and magnitude of the stress applied to the body are progressively increased at a rate that allows the tissues to accommodate their cellular structure and composition to meet the imposed demands.[1] Examples of the beneficial changes in this stage include increased muscle girth and increased bone mineral density and strength. If the body cannot adapt to these forces, tissue **injury** or **cell death** occurs.[1]

Stress–Strain Relationships

Stress–strain curves (Fig. 4-2) describe the amount of tensile load specific tissues can tolerate before damage results. During the early stages of tension development, called the

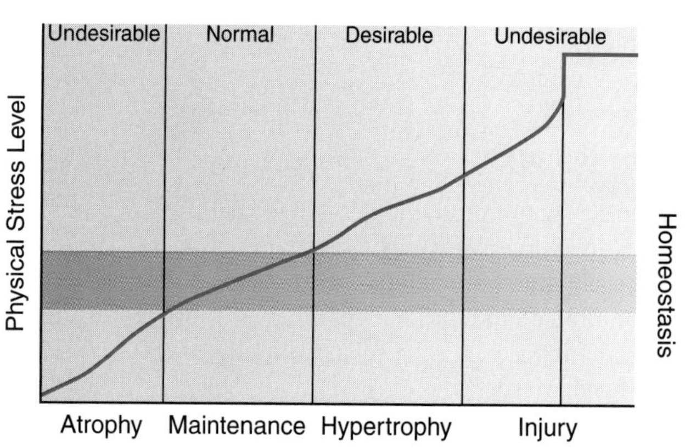

Figure 4-1 ■ The Physical Stress Theory. The body and specific tissues respond in a predictable manner to stresses placed upon them.

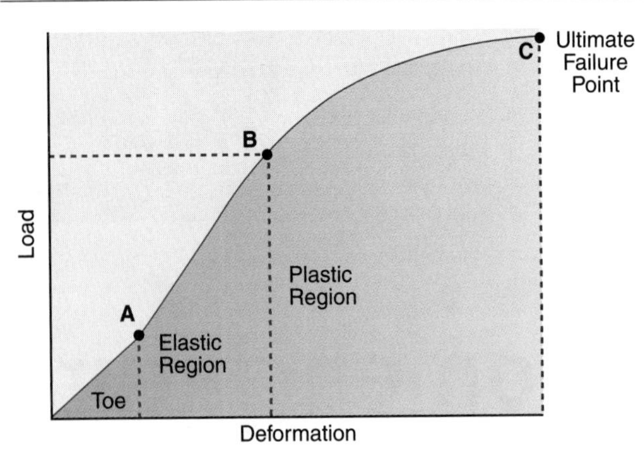

FIGURE 4-2 ■ Load-deformation curve for a connective tissue tested in tension. Initially, the crimp straightens with little force (toe region). Then, collagen fibers are stretched as the elastic region begins at **A**. After the elastic region ends **(B)**, further force application causes a residual change in tissue structure (plastic region). Continuation of load may case the tissue to rupture at its ultimate failure point **(C)**. (From Butler, DL, et al: Biomechanics of ligaments and tendons. *Excer Sport Sci Rev*, 6:144, 1978, with permission from Lippincott Williams & Wilkins.)

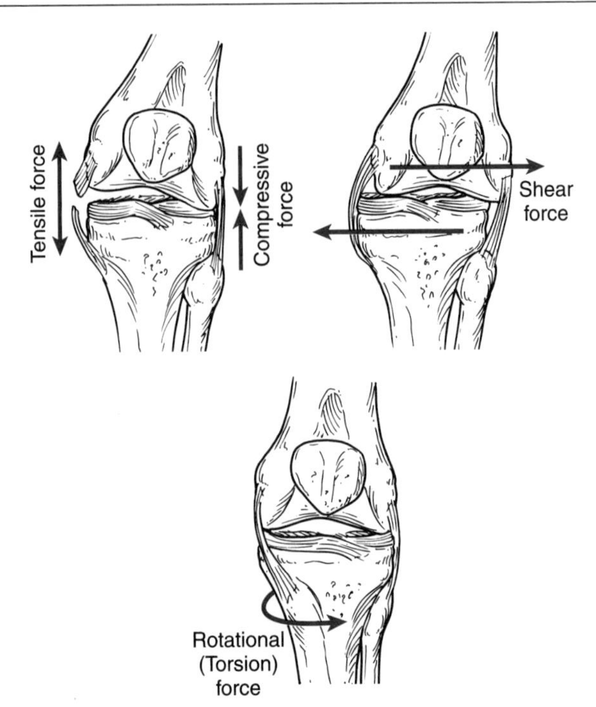

FIGURE 4-3 ■ Forces placed on a joint. **Tensile forces** "tear" the structure by stretching the tissue. **Compressive forces** place opposing forces on the structure. Note that tensile forces and compressive forces may occur on opposite sides of the joint. **Shear forces** place a stress perpendicular to the tissues. **Rotational forces** (torsion) place an angular stress on the tissues.

toe region, the tissue slack is being taken up and there is relatively little change in strength. When no more slack remains, elongation continues and stiffness increases. At some point, maximum stiffness occurs and any further stress results in tissue failure. Tissue stiffness increases with aging, a predisposing factor in many soft tissue injuries.

Mechanisms of Injury

Identifying the mechanism of injury is one of the goals of the history-taking process. In response to questions, the patient tends to describe what happened: "I fell with my arm outstretched and landed on my hand" or "It started hurting when I started running outside." **Macrotrauma** occurs when a single force exceeds the tissue's failure point. **Microtrauma** occurs when the body receives repeated submaximal forces over time, and the tissue is unable to adapt.

The most common forms of acute musculoskeletal trauma are the result of tensile, compression, shear, or torsion forces (Fig. 4-3). Certain parts of the body have unique descriptors of the forces leading to injury. For example, whiplash describes a rapid flexion–extension injury to the cervical spine.

Tensile Forces

A tensile force exerts a longitudinal "tearing" stress on the structure, such as a weight suspended by a rope. Tissues, especially muscles and tendons, are better able to adapt and accommodate to tensile forces when they are gradually applied than those that all received abruptly (see Stress/Strain).

Muscle tissue (including tendons), ligaments, and fascia are most prone to injury as the result of tensile forces. Motion that stretches these structures beyond their normal limits and exceeds the tissues' tensile strength results in tearing of the structure. In ligaments, tensile forces are caused by an overstretching of the structure, such as a valgus force stressing the medial collateral ligament of the knee. In muscles and tendons, tensile injury occurs when the joint's normal range is exceeded. A muscle that crosses two joints, for example, the rectus femoris, is more apt to be injured as the result of overstretching than a one-joint muscle such as the vastus lateralis. More commonly, musculotendinous strains are the result of **dynamic overload** where the muscle is contracting eccentrically while an **antagonistic** force attempts to elongate the muscle. For instance, strains of the hamstring group often occur while the muscle is eccentrically contracting to slow knee extension during running.

Compression Forces

Compression forces result when stresses are applied at each end of a structure. Compressive injuries can result from an acute mechanism, such as a distal radius fracture after falling on an outstretched arm or from chronic overload, such as vertebral disc failure from repetitive forces in diving.

Shear Forces

Shear forces occur perpendicularly across the long axis of a structure. When a shear force of sufficient magnitude is applied across a bone, a transverse fracture may occur (see p. 79). When a shear force of sufficient magnitude is applied across a joint, dislocation is imminent.

Torsion Forces

Torsion forces occur with twisting, such as when the foot is fixed and the knee rotates during a change of direction. Torsion forces are magnified by shoewear that fixes the foot more firmly to the ground and may result in fractures and sprains.

Direct Blow

The term describes exactly what occurs: a blow directly to the body part. Resulting in contusions, fractures, and possibly dislocations, direct blows are easily described by the patient.

Soft Tissue Pathology

Soft tissue pathology, the most common form of orthopedic injury, includes damage to the muscles and their tendons, skin, joint capsules, ligaments, nerves, and bursae. These injuries hinder motion at one or more joints, decrease the ability of the muscle to produce force, create joint instability, make volitional control difficult or impossible, or mechanically limit the amount of motion available.

Musculotendinous Injuries

Injuries to a muscle belly or tendon adversely affect the muscle's ability to generate and sustain tension within the muscle because of mechanical insufficiency or pain. If the **musculotendinous unit** has been mechanically altered through partial or complete tears, the muscle can no longer produce the forces required to perform simple movements or meet the demands required by athletic or work activity. Partial muscle or tendon tears cause decreased force production secondary to pain elicited during the contraction. Complete tears of the unit result in the muscle's mechanical inability to produce force.

Strains

Strains are noncontact injuries of the musculotendinous unit caused by excessive tension within its fibers. Several fibers, myofibers, are bound together to form muscle bundles.[2] Excessive **tensile forces** are produced when the muscle is stretched beyond its normal range of motion (ROM), causing the fibers to fail. Muscle fibers can also be traumatized by **dynamic overload,** occurring when the muscle generates more force than its fibers can withstand. The amount of tension produced during dynamic overload, such as during an **eccentric muscle contraction**, is an elongating force exerted on the body distal to a muscle's attachment. Muscles that cross two joints are more prone to strains because of increased eccentric tension.[3] Although muscle strains are frequently associated with decreased flexibility, most occur secondary a strength imbalance between the agonist and antagonist muscles. No convincing evidence exists that stretching reduces injury risk.[4]

The severity of a strain is based on the number and extent of the fibers that have been traumatized. A three-degree scale is used (Examination Findings 4-1):

- **First-degree strains** involve stretching of the fibers and/or damage to the myofibrils, traumatizing less than 5% of the musculotendinous unit.[2] Pain increases as the muscle contracts, especially against resistance, and the site of injury is point tender. Swelling may also be present.
- **Second-degree strains** involve the actual tearing of some of the muscle fibers, extracellular matrix, and fascia.[2] The inflammatory response is more pronounced than in first-degree strains. These injuries present with the same findings as first-degree strains but are more severe and ecchymosis may be present.
- **Third-degree strains** involve the complete rupture of the muscle and blood vessels, resulting in a total loss of function and a palpable defect in the muscle that is rapidly obscured by swelling. The tissues become ischemic, causing further muscle damage and edema formation. Pain, swelling, and ecchymosis are also present.

Muscle strains tend to occur at the junction between the muscle's belly and its tendon, the musculotendinous junction, regardless of the type of muscle.[2,5] With first- and second-degree strains, local tenderness is present over the site of the injury (i.e., pain is elicited at the injury site when the muscle is either actively shortened or passively elongated). Manual muscle testing results in decreased strength secondary to pain or the muscle's mechanical inability to produce force. In third-degree strains, the muscle is incapable of producing force, but the patient may be able to move the joint through muscular substitution or compensation. No tension within the involved muscle is felt with passive elongation and, after the initial pain has subsided, pain may be minimal to nonexistent.

Depending on the depth of the muscle relative to the skin, swelling and ecchymosis may be visible. The force of gravity can cause these fluids to accumulate distal to the actual site of the injury (Fig. 4-4). The muscular defect, often palpable in second-degree strains, may be visible as well as palpable in third-degree strains. Strains that involve more than half of the cross-sectional area or tears deep within the muscles, and/or that result in edema have longer recovery times than strains lacking these characteristics.[3]

The same mechanism that produces a strain in a skeletally mature individual may result in an avulsion of the

---

Antagonistic In the opposite direction of movement (e.g., the antagonistic motion of extension is flexion).

Musculotendinous unit The group formed by a muscle and its tendons.

Eccentric muscle contraction A contraction in which the elongation of the muscle is voluntarily controlled. Lowering a weight is an example of an eccentric contraction.

Examination Findings 4-1
Muscle Strains

Examination Segment	Clinical Findings
History	***Onset:*** Acute. ***Pain characteristics:*** Pain is initially located at the site of the injury, which tends to be at or near the junction between the muscle belly and tendon. After a few days, pain becomes more diffuse and difficult to localize. The distal musculotendinous junction is most often involved. ***Mechanism:*** Strains usually result from a single episode of overstretching or overloading of the muscle but are more likely to result from eccentric loading.[2] ***Predisposing conditions:*** Imbalance in the strength of the agonist/antagonist muscle groups. History of strain to the involved muscle. Muscle tightness and improper warm-up before activity.
Inspection	Ecchymosis is evident in cases of severe muscle strains. Gravity causes the blood to pool distal to the site of trauma. Swelling may be present over or distal to the involved area. In severe acute cases or in a chronic condition a defect may be visible in the muscle or tendon. If the strain involves a muscle of the lower extremity, the patient may walk with a limp.
Palpation	Point tenderness and increased tissue density associated with spasm exists over the site of the injury, with the degree of pain increasing with the severity of the injury. A defect may be palpable at the injury site.
Joint and Muscle Function Assessment	***AROM:*** Pain is elicited at the injury site. In the case of second- or third-degree strains, the patient may be unable to complete the movement. ***MMT:*** Muscle strength is reduced. Pain increases as the amount of resistance is increased. Third-degree strains result in total a loss of function of the involved muscle. ***PROM:*** Pain is elicited at the injury site during passive motion in the direction opposite that of the muscle, placing it on stretch. Active contraction of the antagonistic muscle can also produce pain by stretching of the involved muscle.
Joint Stability Tests	***Stress tests:*** Stress tests of the ligaments crossing the joint(s) serviced by the muscle should be performed. Strains may occur as the body attempts to protect against ligament injury. ***Joint play:*** Rule out hypermobility
Neurologic Screening	Use to rule out nerve entrapment that clinically appears as a strain. Tearing of muscle may also damage peripheral nerves.
Vascular Screening	Within normal limits
Functional Assessment	Limping will be observed if the lower extremity is involved. Increased symptoms with activities requiring eccentric control.
Imaging Techniques	MRI can be used to identify tears in the muscle and/or tendon. Diagnostic ultrasound
Differential Diagnosis	Tendinopathy, underlying joint instability, stress fracture, nerve entrapment, avulsion fracture
Comments	Strains more frequently occur in muscles that span two joints than one-joint muscles. In the presence of a complete muscle tear (rupture), trauma to the associated joint structures should be ruled out. Active range of motion does not rule out a complete tear of the muscle belly or rupture of the tendon. Other intact muscles— including secondary movers—may still produce active motion.

AROM = active range of motion; MMT = manual muscle test; PROM = passive range of motion.

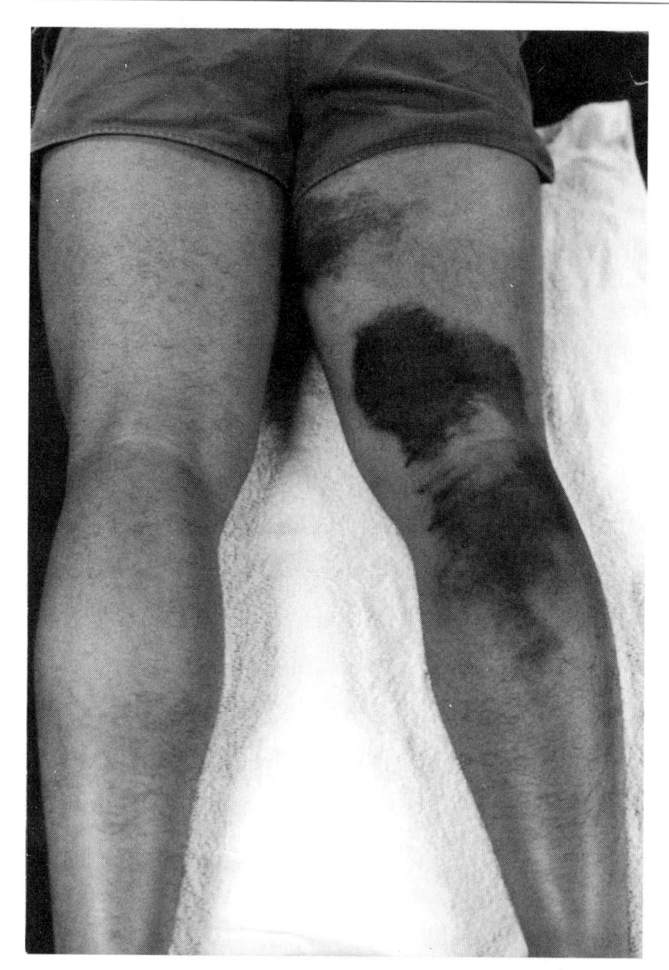

FIGURE 4-4 ■ Ecchymosis associated with a muscular strain. Gravity causes blood that has seeped into the tissues to drift inferiorly.

muscle's origin or insertion in skeletally immature individuals. These apophyseal avulsions should be ruled out via radiographs or magnetic resonance imaging (MRI).

Tendinopathy

The generic term "tendinopathy" is used to describe any tendon pathology. Differentiating between tendinitis, an inflammation of the tendon, and tendinosis, a degenerative condition, is difficult without a histologic exam. Often, both conditions are present simultaneously, although tendinosis is far more prevalent than tendinitis.[6]

As indicated by the "-itis" suffix, tendinitis is the inflammation of the structures encased within the tendon's outer layering.[7] The tendon is surrounded by a highly vascular paratenon that is susceptible to inflammation, most commonly at the tendon's bony attachment.[6] Because of the relative lack of blood supply many tendons lack a direct inflammatory response and degenerative changes, or tendinosis, tends to result. Tendinosis is characterized by degeneration of collagen and little evidence of healing.

Tendons are injured acutely, as in the case of a rupture, or as the result of repetitive stresses (Table 4-1). Repeated loading of the tendon results in decreased blood flow which, in turn, limits tissue viability. Once exposed to this repetitive loading, the tendon responds by either inflammation of the sheath (tendinitis), degeneration of the tendon itself (tendinosis), or a combination of both.[8] With chronic irritation, the tendon thickens and becomes more susceptible to partial- or full-thickness rupture (Examination Findings 4-2).

Table 4-1 Mechanisms Leading to Tendinopathy

Mechanism	Implications
Microtrauma	Repetitive tensile loading, compression, and abrasion of the working tendons. Insufficient rest periods allow for the accumulation of the microtrauma, possibly leading to tendon failure.
Macrotrauma	A single force placed on the muscle, causing discrete tearing within the tendon or at the musculotendinous junction. This area becomes the weak link when the forces of otherwise normal activity are sufficient to cause further inflammation.
Biomechanical Alteration	The alteration of otherwise normal motion with redistribution of the forces around a joint, resulting in new tensile loads, compressive forces, or wearing of the tendons. Examples of this include running on uneven terrain or using poor technique with sporting equipment such as a tennis racquet.

Tenosynovitis, an inflammation of the synovial sheath surrounding a tendon, is more common in the hands and feet because of the relatively small size of the tendons located there. Over time, adhesions can develop, causing restricted movement of the tendon within its sheath. Not all tendons are encased by a synovial sheath. Some are encased by a peritendinous layer of thick tissue. Such inflammation is termed **peritendinitis.**[9] The signs and symptoms of tenosynovitis are similar to those of tendinitis, except that the pain tends to be more localized and crepitus is more pronounced.

The clinical grading of tendinopathy is based on when symptoms occur:

- **First-degree tendinopathy** is marked by pain and slight dysfunction during activity.
- **Second-degree tendinopathy** results in decreased function and pain during and after activity.
- **Third-degree tendinopathy** is characterized by constant pain that prohibits activity.

Prolonged tendinopathy or a single traumatic force can result in a partial (part of the tendon is disrupted) or full (the tendon is completely disrupted) tearing of a tendon. An exception is in the rotator cuff tendons of the glenohumeral joint. These types of tears are termed partial-thickness or full-thickness tears, referring to the depth of the tear rather than to how much of the tendon is torn. Therefore, although a full-thickness tear penetrates

Examination Findings 4-2
Tendinopathy

Examination Segment	Clinical Findings
History	***Onset:*** Insidious. An acute inflammation may occur following a rapid increase in activity, such as running a marathon. ***Pain characteristics:*** Pain in tendon, often near the bony insertion, that increases or decreases with the level of activity. ***Mechanism:*** Results from microtraumatic forces applied to the tendon ***Predisposing conditions:*** History of muscle tightness, poor conditioning, increase in the frequency, duration, and/or intensity of activity, changes in footwear or surfaces
Inspection	Swelling may be noted, but joint effusion is rare.[6] If a tendon of the lower extremity is involved, the patient may walk with a limp or demonstrate some other compensatory gait. In chronic cases, atrophy of the involved muscle may be noted. A guarding posture may be noted where the patient avoids placing stressing the tendon.
Palpation	The tendon is tender to the touch. Crepitus or thickening of the tendon may be noted.
Joint and Muscle Function Assessment	***AROM:*** Pain throughout the range of motion as force is generated within the tendon. ***MMT:*** Strength is decreased secondary to pain. ***PROM:*** Pain is elicited during the extremes of the range of motion as the tendon is stretched. Pain can be elicited earlier in the ROM in more severe cases.
Joint Stability Tests	***Stress tests:*** Rule out underlying joint instability. ***Joint play:*** Rule out underlying joint hypomobility or hypermobility.
Special Tests	Specific to the involved joint
Neurologic Screening	Used to rule out neuropathy
Vascular Screening	Within normal limits
Functional Assessment	Activities that load or stretch the involved tendon(s) increase the symptoms. The patient may use compensatory motions to avoid stressing the involved tendon. Patient describes increased symptoms with movements that load the tendon eccentrically.
Imaging Techniques	Radiographs may be used for exclusion in the differential diagnosis. MR and/or ultrasonic images may be used to detect tendinosis, but these findings are poorly correlated to clinical findings.[6]
Differential Diagnosis	Loose bodies, osteoarthritis, bursitis, sprain, synovitis, fat pad impingement, nerve entrapment
Comments	Differentiating between an acute tendinitis and chronic tendinosis is necessary for appropriate intervention. Owing to the relative avascularity of the major tendons, tendinosis is more common that an actual tendinitis.

AROM = active range of motion; MMT = manual muscle test; PROM = passive range of motion.

through the depth of the tissue, part of the tendon may still be intact. Tendon tears are more common after corticosteroid injections or in persons who abuse anabolic steroids, as these chemicals weaken the tendon tissue.

Calcium formation within the tendon, **calcific tendinitis** (calcific tendinopathy), may also develop with long-term tendinopathy. The calcium buildup within the substance of the tendon causes pain with active contraction. Over time, it may lead to decreased ROM and decreased strength.

With all tendinopathies, active ROM may produce pain at the end of the range of motion, especially if the tendon meets a bony structure. Passive motion in the muscle's antagonistic direction results in pain as the tendon is stretched. The dynamic tension produced during resisted range of motion results in pain, decreasing the amount of force produced. MRI can identify the presence of tendinopathy.[6,10]

Treatment of tendon pathology involves avoiding the aggravating activity, correcting any imbalances that might be overstressing the tendon, and a gradual return to activity to allow the tissue to accommodate to new stresses.

Contusions

Contusions are soft tissue injuries resulting from direct blows that range in severity from mildly annoying to incapacitating. Capillary bleeding and the breakdown of hemoglobin provide the characteristic initial redness that gradually deepens to dark purple and blue, finally fading to yellow as the region heals.

Contusions to superficial bone are exquisitely painful, as the periosteum is richly innervated. (Think of unwittingly hitting your shin on a table corner.) Pain associated with contusions to muscle is initially localized and then becomes diffuse, as the bleeding pools according to the laws of gravity and the surrounding muscle protectively spasms. Evaluation of contusions should include eliminating other underlying injuries, such as fractures or superficial nerve damage. MRI and diagnostic ultrasound are highly sensitive in detecting edema and hemorrhage associated with contusions.[11]

The treatment of contusions consists of ice, gentle stretching, and padding to protect against further injury. Heterotopic ossification can occur after a severe contusion to a large muscle such as the quadriceps or deltoid.

Heterotopic ossification

Heterotopic ossification (HO), previously known as myositis ossificans, is the formation of bone within a muscle belly's fascia and other soft tissues. Heterotopic means "in the wrong place." Because it is not necessarily association with muscle inflammation nor is muscle the only involved tissue, the term "myositis" is no longer preferred (Fig. 4-5). The **etiology** of HO can be traced to the genetic formation of abnormal tissue, neurologic disease such as traumatic brain injury, or trauma.[12] This text addresses only HO resulting from trauma (Examination Findings 4-3).

Heterotopic ossificans occurs secondary to a traumatic injury such as a deep contusion, multiple contusions, or, less frequently, a muscle strain. An MRI can be used to identify the size and location of an intramuscular hematoma. If indicated, the **hematoma** may be **aspirated** to restore function and decrease the chance of heterotopic ossification.[4]

The quadriceps femoris, hip adductor group, or biceps brachii muscles are most commonly involved. The ossification area can be traced to an error in the body's healing process and a delay in the proper treatment of the initial trauma. After the injury, various factors stimulate **stem cells** to differentiate into **osteoblasts**, giving rise to the formation of immature bone.[12] A hematoma or heterotopic ossification within a fascial compartment can lead to a **compartment syndrome** (Box 4-1).

Calcification appears on radiographic examination approximately 3 weeks after the injury. As the size of the mass continues to expand, it becomes palpable. The

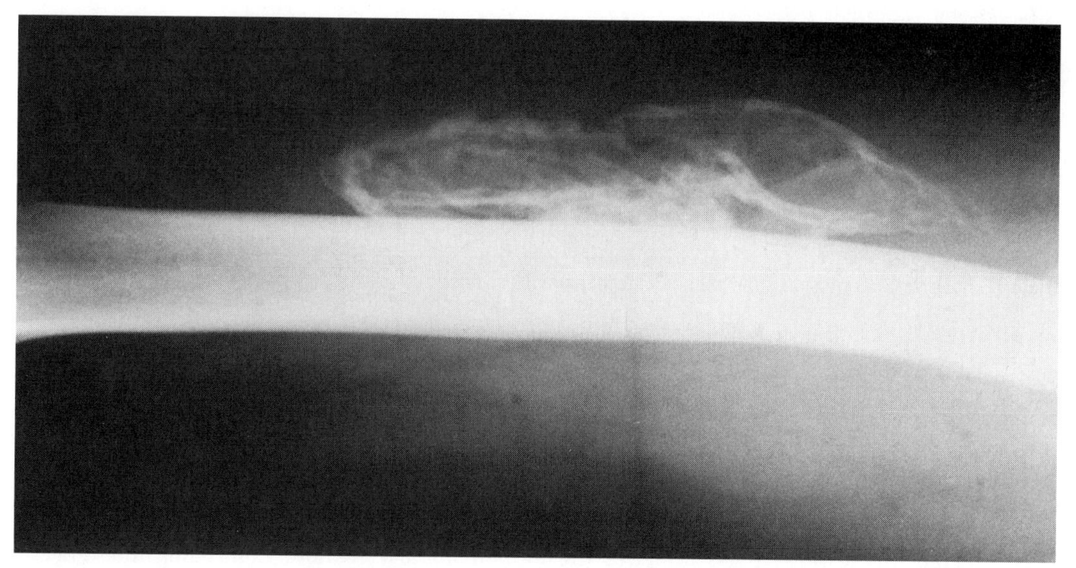

FIGURE 4-5 ■ Radiograph of heterotopic ossification. This calcification has occurred in the biceps brachii of a football lineman who sustained multiple blows to the muscle during the act of blocking.

Etiology The cause of a disease (also the study of the causes of disease).

Hematoma A collection of clotted blood within a confined space (hemat blood; oma tumor).

Aspirate The removal of fluid from the body using a needle and syringe.

Stem cells Generic cell types that can develop into specialized cells.

Osteoblasts Cells responsible for the formation of new bone.

Examination Findings 4-3
Heterotopic Ossification

Examination Segment	Clinical Findings
History	***Onset:*** The initial trauma is a hematoma caused by a single acute or repeated blows to the muscle. The ossification occurs gradually. ***Pain characteristics:*** Pain occurs at the site of ossification, usually the site of a large muscle mass that is exposed to blows (e.g., the quadriceps femoris or biceps brachii muscles). ***Other symptoms:*** A fever may develop. ***Mechanism:*** Calcium within the muscle fascia secondary to an abnormality in the healing process ***Predisposing conditions:*** History of heterotopic ossification
Inspection	A superficial bruise may be noted. Edema of the distal joint closest to the site injury occurs. Ecchymosis may be present.
Palpation	Acutely, the muscle is tender. As the ossification develops, it may become palpable within the muscle mass. Swelling and warmth may be felt at the site of injury.
Joint and Muscle Function Assessment	***AROM:*** As the ossification grows, the number of contractile units available to the muscle decreases. Antagonist motion is painful secondary to decreased flexibility within the affected muscle mass. ***MMT:*** Decreased secondary to pain; the ossification does not allow the muscle to contract normally ***PROM:*** Decreased secondary to pain and adhesions within the muscle
Joint Stability Tests	***Stress tests:*** None ***Joint play:*** None
Special Tests	None
Neurologic Screening	Within normal limits
Vascular Screening	Within normal limits
Functional Assessment	Compensatory motions to avoid using the muscle containing the ossification.
Imaging Techniques	Radiographic examination shows the ossification as it matures. A bone scan may be positive in the earlier stages. CT scans or, less preferably, MR images are used for comprehensive examination and to differentiate from other forms of tumors.
Differential Diagnosis	Contusion, strain, tumor (osteosarcoma), exostosis
Comments	Early stretching and ROM following a muscle contusion may limit the formation of HO.

AROM = active range of motion; CT = computed tomography; HO = heterotopic ossification; MMT = manual muscle test; MR = magnetic resonance; PROM = passive range of motion; ROM = range of motion.

joint's ROM is affected as the bony mass impedes the muscle's ability to actively contract or passively lengthen. For this reason, a differential diagnosis must be made between muscle strains and contusions to predict the possible ossification.

Immediate sustained stretching with the knee maintained in 120 degrees of flexion may be helpful in reducing the incidence of heterotopic ossificans and the time lost from activity due to quadriceps contusions.[13] Nonsteroidal anti-inflammatory medications may help prevent hematoma formation.[4] Controlling inflammation, protecting the injured tissues, and ROM exercises can help prevent the formation of HO and lead to its resolution. In rare cases, the mass may require surgical excision once it is fully matured.

Bursitis

Bursae are fluid-filled sacs that serve to buffer muscles, tendons, and ligaments from other friction-causing structures and facilitate smooth motion. Although common sites of bursa formation do exist, such as over the patella

Box 4-1
Compartment Syndromes

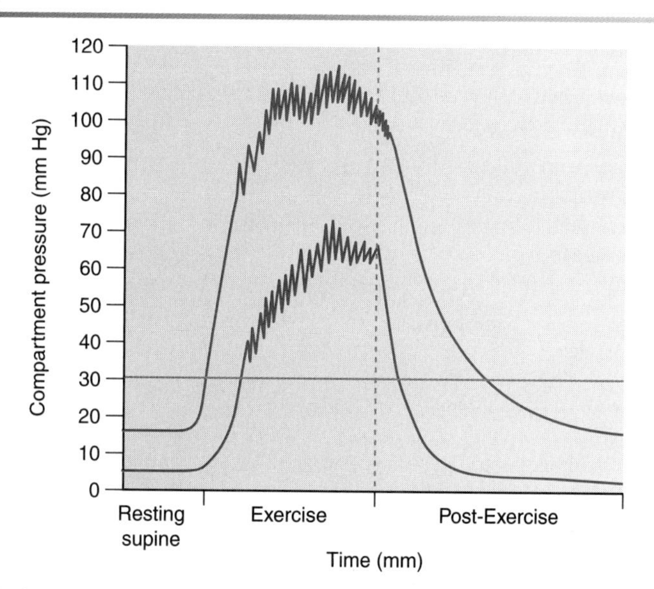

"Compartments" are areas within the extremities defined by relatively unyielding borders such as dense fascia and bone. An increase in pressure, caused by increased blood volume, excess fluid, or muscle hypertrophy can result in a disruption of distal arterial, vascular, and nerve function. Blood supply to the structures within the compartment is also compromised.

Acute compartment syndromes result from trauma such as contusions and fractures. Chronic compartment syndromes (also referred to as exertional or recurrent compartment syndromes) occur during exercise as muscles enlarge but the compartment cannot expand to accommodate the increased volume. The anatomical compartments most disposed to this condition are located in the leg and forearm.

Patients will complain of pain, numbness, and/or paresthesia in the distal extremity. The classic signs—The "five P's"—pain, pallor (redness), pulselessness, paresthesia, and paralysis, are indicative of late-stage of compartment syndrome. Acute compartment syndromes are medical emergencies. If a pulse is absent, the extremity is in immediate danger. Refer to Compartment Syndromes in Chapter 9 for more information.

and olecranon process, bursae develop over areas where they are needed to reduce friction. Bursae cannot be specifically palpated unless they are inflamed. The triggering event causing bursitis is irritation of the bursal sac secondary to a disease state, increased stress, friction, or a single traumatic force that activates the inflammatory process (Examination Findings 4-4).

The clinical findings of bursitis depend on the location of the involved structure. Bursae that are immediately subcutaneous can enlarge greatly. However, the swelling remains localized within the sac. Often the underlying joint can be moved without causing pain. Bursae separating tendinous, bony, or ligamentous tissues often cause exquisite pain during all forms of joint movement, possibly limiting joint motion.

Bursal inflammation can also be the result of local or systemic infection. Lacerations, abrasions, or puncture wounds entering a bursa can introduce an infectious agent, resulting in the subsequent enlargement of the bursa. A **staphylococcal infection** can localize within a bursa, producing symptoms resembling those of an overuse syndrome. Bursal infections may be accompanied by red streaks along the extremity and enlarged proximal lymph nodes. An analysis of the bursal fluid is required to determine the cause of the bursitis.[14]

Joint Structure Pathology

The most prevalent soft tissue injuries involving the joint structures are those involving the capsular and ligamentous tissues and are prevalent at the ankle, knee, and shoulder.[15] These injuries directly affect the joint's stability during movement.

Sprains

Sprains occur when a joint is forced beyond its normal anatomical limits, resulting in the stretching or tearing of the ligaments, joint capsule, or both. Although ligaments are commonly thought of and presented as discrete structures, they are often thickened areas within the joint capsule. When damaged, the ligaments that are within the joint capsule or part of the joint capsule produce more swelling than the ligaments that are **extracapsular** because of the associated disruption of the capsule (Examination Findings 4-5).

Staphylococcal infection An infection caused by *Staphylococcus* bacteria.

Extracapsular Outside of the joint capsule.

Examination Findings 4-4
Bursitis

Examination Segment	Clinical Findings
History	***Onset:*** Acute in the case of direct trauma to the bursa; insidious in the case of overuse or infection ***Pain characteristics:*** Pain occurring at the site of the bursal sac ***Mechanism:*** Chemical: Calcium or other chemical deposits within the bursa activating the inflammatory response. Mechanical: Repetitive rubbing of the soft tissue over a bony prominence or a direct blow, possibly related to improper biomechanics. Septic: Viral or bacterial invasion of the bursa. ***Predisposing conditions:*** Improper biomechanics, poor padding of at-risk bursae (e.g., suprapatellar bursa, olecranon bursa).
Inspection	Local swelling of bursae can be very pronounced, especially those located over the olecranon process and patella. Chronic or septic bursitis may appear red with accompanying lymphatic streaking.
Palpation	Point tenderness is noted over the site of the bursa. Localized heat and swelling may be noted.
Joint and Muscle Function Assessment	***AROM:*** Pain may be noted. ***MMT:*** Strength limited secondary to pain. As the muscle contracts, it compresses the bursal sac. ***PROM:*** Pain is produced if the motion causes the tendon or other structure to rub across or compress the inflamed bursa.
Joint Stability Tests	***Stress tests:*** Rule out underlying instability. ***Joint play:*** Rule out underlying hypermobility.
Special Tests	None
Neurologic Screening	Within normal limits
Vascular Screening	Within normal limits
Functional Assessment	Increased pain and/or weakness with tasks that require strength of involved muscles
Imaging Techniques	T2-weighted MRI with fat suppression are used to image bursae.
Differential Diagnosis	Contusion, tendinopathy, septic joint, synovitis
Comments	Signs and symptoms of an infected bursa warrant immediate referral to a physician. Chronic bursal irritation is often associated with tendon pathology.

AROM = active range of motion; MMT = manual muscle test; MRI = magnetic resonance imaging; PROM = passive range of motion.

The three degrees of sprains, based on the amount of laxity produced by the injury relative to the opposite limb, are as follows (see also Table 1-9):

- **First-degree sprain:** The ligament is stretched with little or no tearing of its fibers. No abnormal motion is produced when the joint is stressed, and a normal, firm **end-point** is felt. Local pain, mild point tenderness, and slight swelling of the joint are present.
- **Second-degree sprain:** Partial tearing of the ligament's fibers has occurred, resulting in joint laxity when the ligament is stressed. A soft but definite end-point is present. Moderate pain and swelling occur and a loss of the joint's function is noted.
- **Third-degree sprain:** The ligament has been completely ruptured, causing gross joint laxity, possible instability, and an empty or absent end-point. Swelling is marked, but pain may be limited secondary to tearing of the local nerves. A complete loss of function of the joint is usually noted.

Joint dislocation

Dislocations involve the disassociation of the joint's articulating surfaces caused by forces that rupture many of the joint's soft tissue restraints. Frank joint dislocations result in obvious deformity and therefore normally do not require any evaluative tests beyond assessing distal vascular and nerve supply (Fig. 4-6). In some instances, the dislocation

Examination Findings 4-5
Sprains

Examination Segment	Clinical Findings
History	***Onset:*** Acute ***Pain characteristics:*** Pain is localized to the site of injury with first-degree sprains. As the severity of the sprain increases, the pain radiates throughout the joint. ***Other symptoms:*** A "popping" sensation or sound may be reported by the patient. ***Mechanism:*** Sprains result from tensile forces caused by the stretching of the ligament. ***Predisposing conditions:*** A history of a sprain can predispose the ligament to further injury. Shoe wear that increases the friction between the shoe–surface interface may increase the chance of lower extremity sprains. Women have a greater risk of some knee ligament sprains, but the exact cause has not been determined.
Inspection	Acutely, localized swelling is evident with injury to superficial structures. Effusion may be visible. Ecchymosis may form at and distal to the site of injury.
Palpation	Point tenderness is noted over the ligament. The entire joint may be tender. Palpable effusion may be noted
Joint and Muscle Function Assessment	***AROM:*** Limited by pain in the direction that stresses the involved ligament (or ligaments) ***MMT:*** Resisting through the range may be painful, especially at the end range. Isometric contractions may not produce as intense pain. ***PROM:*** Limited by pain, especially in the direction that stresses the involved ligament (or ligaments)
Joint Stability Tests	***Stress tests:*** The ligament can be stressed by producing a force through the joint that causes the ligament to stretch. The examiner should note the amount of increased laxity compared with the opposite side, as well as the quality of the end-point. The end-point should be distinct and crisp. A soft, "mushy," or absent end-point is a sign of ligamentous damage. ***Joint play:*** Hypermobility of the involved joint
Special Tests	Based on the joint being examined
Neurologic Screening	Within normal limits
Vascular Screening	Within normal limits
Functional Assessment	Depending on severity of sprain, instability during functional movements may be present.
Imaging Techniques	Radiographs and/or CT scans to rule out fracture; stress radiographs to identify laxity Some ligaments, such as the anterior cruciate ligament, can be visualized via MR images.
Differential Diagnosis	Strain, epiphyseal fracture, osteochondral fracture, joint subluxation/dislocation
Comments	Strains can occur simultaneously with sprains, as the muscles attempt to protect the joint.

AROM = active range of motion; MMT = manual muscle test; PROM = passive range of motion.

may cause the joint surfaces to protrude through the skin, an open dislocation (Fig. 4-7).

Because of the inherent risk of injury to bony, vascular, neurologic, and other soft tissue structures, joint reduction should be performed in the most expedient and safest manner by individuals who are trained to do so. When a major joint (e.g., the shoulder, knee, ankle) is dislocated, the presence of the distal pulse and the normal sensory distribution of the involved extremity must be established (Examination Findings 4-6). Dislocations of major joints are medical emergencies. The possible involvement of the neurovascular structures increases the urgency for prompt medical treatment.

Joint subluxation

Subluxation is a vague term with many definitions ranging from a subtle, chronic instability, to joint surfaces that partially separate, to a joint that dislocates and spontaneously reduces. For this text we will define a subluxation as a partial or complete disassociation of the joint's articulating surfaces

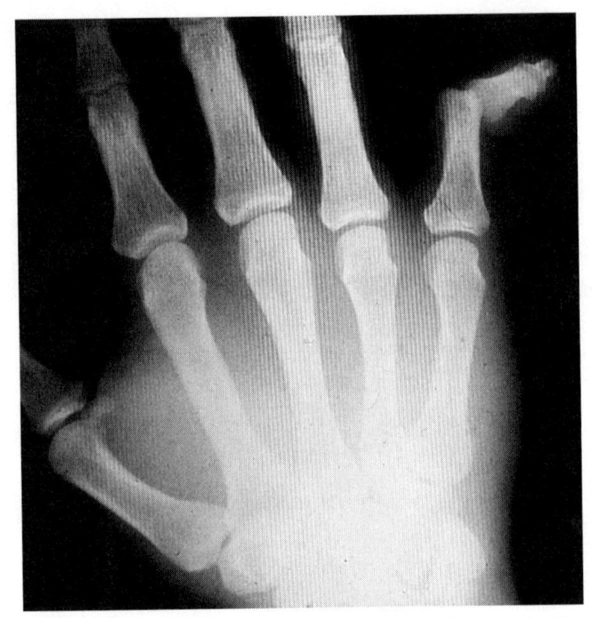

FIGURE 4-6 ■ Radiograph of a dislocation of the fifth proximal interphalangeal joint (PIP joint).

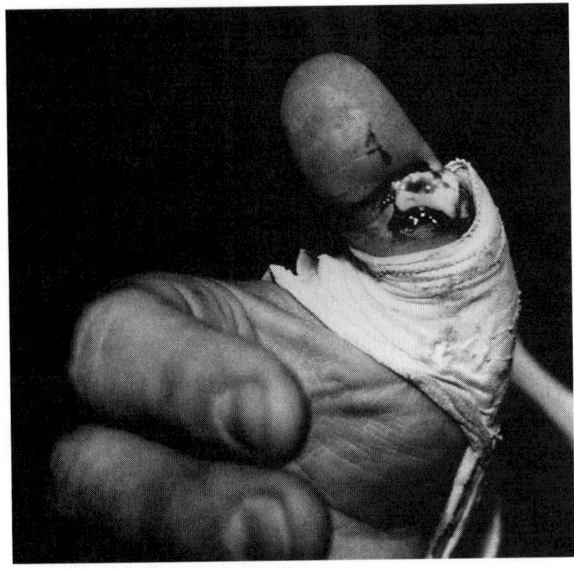

FIGURE 4-7 ■ Open dislocation of the thumb's interphalangeal joint. Note the glossy appearance of the proximal articular surface. There appears to be a defect of the hyaline cartilage on the ulnar side of the bone.

Examination Findings 4-6
Joint Dislocations

Examination Segment	Clinical Findings
History	***Onset:*** Acute ***Pain characteristics:*** At the involved joint ***Mechanism:*** Dislocation caused by a stress that forces the joint beyond its normal anatomical limits ***Predisposing conditions:*** Repeated dislocation as the joint's supportive structures are progressively stretched
Inspection	Gross joint deformity may be present and swelling is observed.
Palpation	Pain is elicited throughout the joint. Malalignment of the joint surfaces may be felt.
Joint and Muscle Function Assessment	***AROM:*** ROM is not possible because of the disruption of the joint's alignment. ***MMT:*** Contraindicated in the presence of an obvious dislocation ***PROM:*** Contraindicated in the presence of an obvious dislocation
Joint Stability Tests	***Stress tests:*** Contraindicated in the presence of an obvious dislocation ***Joint play:*** Contraindicated in the presence of an obvious dislocation
Special Tests	Contraindicated when the joint is dislocated.
Neurologic Screening	Sensory distribution distal to the dislocated joint must be established.
Vascular Screening	The presence of the distal pulse must be established. A lack of circulation to the distal extremity threatens the viability of the body part.
Functional Assessment	Contraindicated when the joint is dislocated
Imaging Techniques	Radiographs and/or MRI are obtained to confirm and quantify the magnitude of joint disruption. Imaging may be obtained post-reduction to evaluate the integrity of joint surfaces.
Differential Diagnosis	Fracture, sprain, subluxation, tendon rupture
Comments	Dislocations of the major joints represent medical emergencies.

AROM = active range of motion; MMT = manual muscle test; MRI = magnetic resonance imaging; PROM = passive range of motion.

that spontaneously return to their normal alignments. The amount of force required to displace the bones is often sufficient to cause soft tissue or bony injury. Stretching and tearing of the joint capsule and ligaments and bony fractures must be suspected after a subluxation.

Subluxating joints are a progressive condition in which each subluxation predisposes the joint to subsequent episodes resulting from stretching of the supporting soft-tissue structures. All first-time subluxations should be examined by a physician and a determination made on how to manage subsequent subluxations of the joint.

Clinically, joint subluxations are often identified by a reported history of the "joint's going out and then popping back in." The joint's range of motion is limited by pain, instability, and apprehension. Chronically, the joint displays instability during ligamentous and capsular testing and joint play assessment. Functionally, the patient describes avoiding maneuvers, such as cutting, that might produce instability. These tests may produce an **apprehension response,** meaning that the patient displays anxiety and/or muscle guarding that a specific test or functional demand will cause the joint to again subluxate (Examination Findings 4-7).

Examination Findings 4-7
Joint Subluxations

Examination Segment	Clinical Findings
History	***Onset:*** Acute or chronic. Chronic subluxation can occur as the joint's supportive structures are progressively stretched. ***Pain characteristics:*** Pain occurs throughout the involved joint. Associated muscle spasm may involve the muscles proximal and distal to the joint. ***Other symptoms:*** Patients may not realize that their joint is actually subluxating and may report other symptoms such as pain, apprehension, or the joint "giving way." ***Mechanism:*** Joint subluxation results from a stress that takes the joint beyond its normal anatomical limits. ***Predisposing conditions:*** History of joint subluxation or dislocation; congenital hyperlaxity
Inspection	Swelling may be present. No gross bony deformity is noted because the joint relocates.
Palpation	Pain elicited along the tissues that have been stretched or compressed
Joint and Muscle Function Assessment	***AROM:*** Limited to pain and instability The patient is unwilling or unable to move joint to the end range. ***MMT:*** Muscular strength is decreased secondary to pain and joint instability. ***PROM:*** Limited secondary to pain and possible instability
Joint Stability Tests	***Stress tests:*** Pain is elicited during stress testing of the involved ligament (or ligaments). Laxity of the tissues is present, particularly post-acutely. The patient may note instability and react to guard against this by contracting the surrounding musculature or pulling away, an apprehension response. ***Joint play:*** Hypermobility
Special Tests	Based on the body part being examined
Neurologic Screening	Transient paresthesia of the nerves crossing the joint may be present
Vascular Screening	Repeated subluxations may result in occlusion of the vessels crossing the joint. Assess distal capillary refill and note for venous pooling in the distal extremity.
Functional Assessment	May describe sensation of instability with motions that stress the joint. Observation may reveal avoidance of those positions secondary to this apprehension.
Imaging Techniques	Radiographs; MR may be used to rule out bony or soft tissue injury.
Differential Diagnosis	Sprain or damage to other supportive structures (e.g., labrum), nerve pathology
Comments	Not applicable

AROM = active range of motion; MMT = manual muscle test; MR = magnetic resonance; PROM = passive range of motion.

Synovitis

The inflammation of a joint's capsule often occurs secondary to the presence of existing inflammation in or around the joint that spreads to the **synovial membrane** (Fig. 4-8). The patient complains of "bogginess" within the joint and tends to hold it in a position that applies the least amount of stress on the capsule's fibers (usually a position between the extremes of the joint's ROM) (Examination Findings 4-8).

Cellulitis

Cellulitis is the result of bacterial infection of the skin's connective tissue that is marked by edema, redness, and tightening of the skin. No outward leakage of pus and no sign of a **furuncles** or pustules are noted. One or more veins on the proximal side of the infection may turn red, representing **lymphangitis**. If the infection spreads, the patient may display a fever and complain of chills, fatigue, and an overall feeling of malaise.

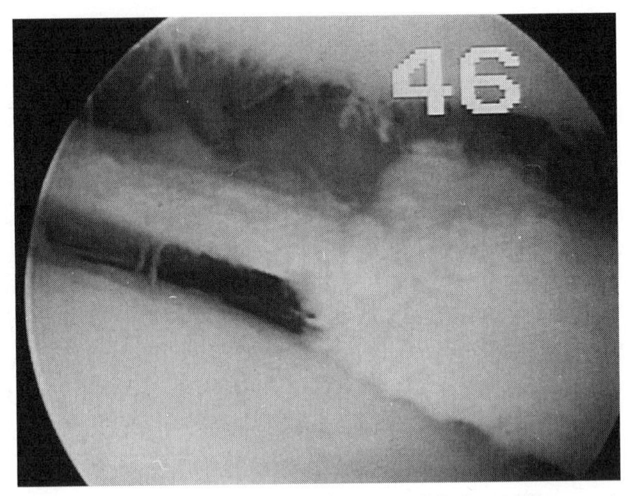

FIGURE 4-8 ■ Arthroscopic view of synovitis of the knee joint capsule. The hairlike strands emerging from the top border of the joint represent inflammation of the synovial capsule.

Examination Findings 4-8
Synovitis

Examination Segment	Clinical Findings
History	***Onset:*** Insidious; often subsequent to a previous injury to the joint ***Pain characteristics:*** Pain occurring throughout the entire joint, causing aching at rest and increased pain with activity ***Other symptoms:*** Not applicable ***Mechanism:*** Synovitis often begins after an injury to a joint. The resulting inflammatory reaction triggers inflammation within the synovium. ***Predisposing conditions:*** Underlying pathology within the joint
Inspection	The joint may appear swollen. The patient may move the joint in a guarded manner. Joints affected by synovitis do not appear red. Persistent synovitis can result in muscle atrophy secondary to pain and decreased joint ROM.
Palpation	Warmth may be felt. A "boggy" swelling is present. Diffuse soreness is usually present.
Joint and Muscle Function Assessment	***AROM:*** Limitations exist within the capsular pattern of the joint. ***MMT:*** Weakness secondary to muscle guarding ***PROM:*** Normally, this is greater than AROM but is still limited by pain.
Joint Stability Tests	***Stress tests:*** Not applicable ***Joint play:*** In the absence of underlying pathology to the capsule, joint play is normal.
Special Tests	None
Neurologic Screening	Within normal limits
Vascular Screening	Within normal limits
Functional Assessment	Avoid maneuvers that increase stress on the joint. **Antalgic** gait present with lower extremity joint involvement.
Imaging Techniques	In most cases, the diagnosis of synovitis is made without the need for imaging studies.
Differential Diagnosis	Joint **sepsis**, sprain, osteochondral fracture
Comments	The signs and symptoms of synovitis may mimic those of an infected joint.

AROM = active range of motion; MMT = manual muscle test; PROM = passive range of motion.

Individuals suspected of suffering from cellulitis must be immediately referred to a physician. The treatment approach consists of the oral, injected, or intravenous administration of antibiotics. Hospitalization may be required. If a patient with cellulitis remains untreated, gangrene, meningitis, widespread lymphangitis, or a generalized body-wide infection may develop.

Although cellulitis is not communicable, patients are withheld from activity because of the presence of an underlying infection. With treatment, most bouts of cellulitis resolve in 7 to 10 days.

Articular Surface Pathology

The articular or **hyaline cartilage** lining a bone's joint surface may be acutely injured or damaged as the result of degenerative changes caused by aging. Most of these injuries are irreversible and result in chronic joint pain, dysfunction, or both.

Osteochondral defects

Osteochondral defects (OCDs) can result from trauma or from gradual softening of the underlying bone. Including the articular cartilage and underlying cortical bone, OCDs present a diagnostic and treatment challenge, particularly if the involved surface is weight-bearing. The severity of an OCD is based on the depth of the defect and the proportion of the articular surface that is involved. **Partial-thickness** OCDs involve the outer layering of the articular cartilage. **Full-thickness** OCDs expose the underlying bone and are almost always symptomatic (Fig. 4-9).

Osteochondral defects are categorized into two groups based on the age at onset. **Juvenile osteochondritis** affects patients younger than age 15 years, and **adult osteochondritis** affects patients age 15 years or older.[16] Osteochondral defects can affect most joints, but the talus, femur, patella, capitellum, and humeral head are most frequently affected.

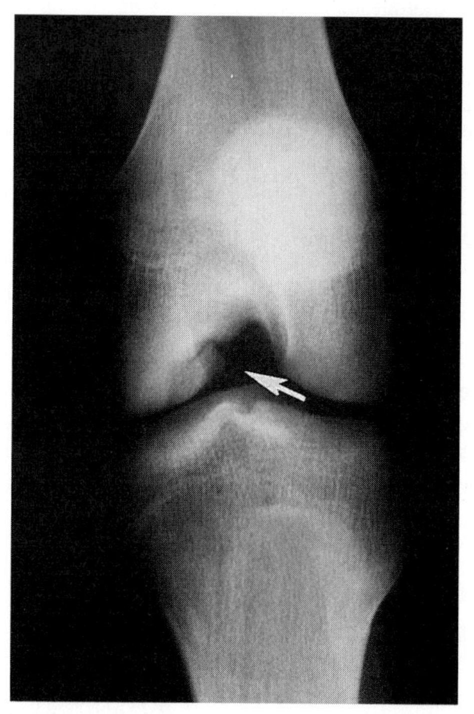

FIGURE 4-9 ■ Radiograph of an osteochondral defect. Note the small fracture line on the medial portion of the trochanteric groove.

The bony fragment may be stable within the joint or free floating within the joint space, **osteochondritis dissecans,** where it can cause greater problems of pain, loss of range of motion, and decreased joint function (Fig. 4-10). The underlying cause resulting in the destruction of bone has been proposed to be **ischemia**, trauma, and degenerative changes.[17] As the depth of the defect increases, the stresses applied to the underlying bone are increased, resulting in pain during activity. The amount of disability occurring after an OCD also depends on the location of the defect on the articular surface. If the defect is located in an area of high joint forces, the disability secondary to pain is increased.

The chief complaints include increasing pain, episodes of the joint "locking," and an inability to function. The onset is usually not related to any specific trauma. The complaints of pain are usually specific to the area of the affected joint and the stage of injury (Table 4-2). As the condition

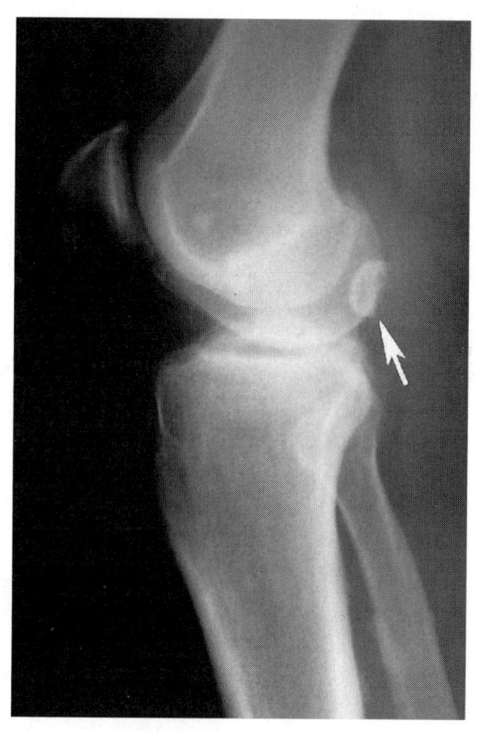

FIGURE 4-10 ■ Radiograph of a free-floating body, osteochondritis dissecans, in the joint space.

Synovial membrane The membrane lining a fluid-filled joint.

Furuncles A boil characterized by redness, leakage of pus, and necrosis of the involved tissue.

Antalgic Having a pain-relieving quality; analgesic.

Sepsis Infection.

Hyaline cartilage Cartilage located on the articular surface of bones, especially suited to withstand compressive and shearing forces.

Ischemia Local and temporary deficiency of blood supply caused by the obstruction of blood flow to a body area.

Table 4-2 Progressive Stages of Osteochondral Defects

Stage	Description
I	Soft tissue swelling Mild osteoporosis Frank fracture resulting from acute trauma
II	Microfractures begin to develop Irregular contour of the articular surface Subcortical bone begins to thin and defragment
III	Necrotic tissue is replaced by granulation tissue Structural weakness of the underlying bone alters the shape of the articular surface

progresses, the joint's ROM decreases and the patient's ability to produce forceful contractions of the surrounding muscles declines (Examination Findings 4-9).

Treatment of osteochondral defects varies widely in technique and outcomes. In general, osteochondral fractures on weight-bearing surfaces are difficult to treat. Débridement, **mosiacplasty**, autografts, allografts, and chondrocyte implantation are all used.

Arthritis

Although there are several causes for arthritis, the degeneration of a joint's articular surface, the most common type found in athletes, is **osteoarthritis**. This chronic condition most often affects the body's weight-bearing joints, especially the knees. With time, the articular surfaces begin to degenerate, and the regenerative process causes bony outgrowths on what should be an otherwise smooth surface (Fig. 4-11). This degeneration of the articular cartilage can eventually lead to the complete destruction of the cartilage and exposure of the subchondral bone. Flaking pieces of bone can result in loose bodies and chronic synovitis.

The outward signs and symptoms of osteoarthritis depend on the duration of the condition. Acute cases present with minimal swelling and redness. Typically, the chief complaint is pain during joint motion while the joint surfaces are compressed. When the problem becomes chronic, the patient suffers from unremitting pain and inability to function. The affected area may be marked by obvious deformity (Examination Findings 4-10).

Rheumatoid arthritis is a systemic autoimmune condition that affects the articular cartilages of multiple joints. As the condition worsens, the joints appear to be hard and nodular, with even simple movement resulting in profound pain. The patient often has a family history of rheumatoid arthritis and his or her hand and multiple other joints are affected. In addition, the patient may experience associated medical complications such as inflammation of the lungs, blood vessels, and other organs.

Juvenile rheumatoid arthritis most commonly affects children age 6 months to 16 years, typically presenting as unexplained joint pain and swelling. The disease may progress to include intermittent rashes and high fever.

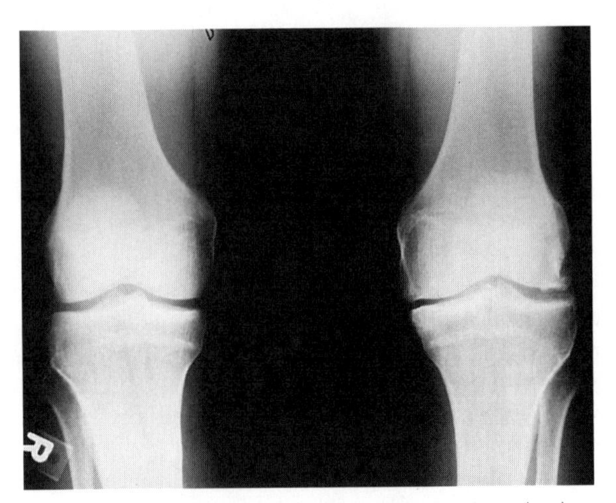

FIGURE 4-11 ■ Radiograph of an arthritic joint. Note the loss of definition in the joint space of the left knee (on the right above).

Lyme Disease

Lyme disease is a complex illness that affects multiple systems within the body. Caused by the *Borrelia burgdorferi* virus, it is transmitted to humans via a deer tick bite. If treated in its early stages, it can usually be well managed with limited progression of symptoms.

Not all tick bites transmit the disease. Imbedded ticks should be removed promptly because the tick may need to be attached for longer than 24 hours to transmit the infection. Individuals who are at risk of exposure should check for ticks routinely. After the tick is removed, the area should be observed carefully and medical attention should be sought if local symptoms appear.

An early manifestation of the disease is the development of an erythematous macule or papule at the site of the bite. Over a period of days, the infection spreads over the skin to create an erythematous migrans. Over time, the infection may spread via the blood. Secondary symptoms include fever, chills, headache, **arthralgias**, myalgias, and secondary skin site lesions. The disease can spread to the heart, creating carditis; the nervous system in the form of meningitis or cranial nerve palsy; and, very commonly, the joints in the form of unexplained pain and inflammation that is often confused with arthritis.[18] The knee is most commonly affected.

The diagnosis of Lyme disease is made primarily through clinical examination and serologic testing. Lyme disease progresses through three stages, but the symptoms may overlap among them (Table 4-3).[18]

In the early stages of the disease, blood tests may reveal that the patient has not become seropositive. After diagnosis, the treatment revolves around antibiotic therapy

---

Mosiacplasty A procedure used to encourage the growth of articular cartilage where small holes are bored into the epiphysis.

Arthralgia Painful joints.

Examination Findings 4-9
Osteochondral Defects

Examination Segment	Clinical Findings
History	***Onset:*** Acute or insidious ***Pain characteristics:*** Complaints of pain in the joint during weight-bearing activities. Depending on the site of the defect, the entire joint may be painful secondary to a synovial reaction (see Synovitis). Pain may be absent at rest. ***Other symptoms:*** Dislodged bony fragments may cause joint locking. ***Mechanism:*** ***Acute:*** A rotational or **axial load** placed on two opposing joint surfaces. The resulting friction results in a tearing away of the cartilage. ***Chronic:*** A progressive degeneration of the articular cartilage. ***Predisposing conditions:*** Joint trauma
Inspection	Effusion is present. The patient tends to hold the joint in a pain-free position.
Palpation	The joint line may be tender from the defect, but the defect itself is usually not palpable. Joint effusion Tenderness may also be caused by synovitis.
Joint and Muscle Function Assessment	***AROM:*** Limited due to pain and swelling ***MMT:*** Strength is decreased secondary to pain, if the joint is compressing the defect (position-dependent). ***PROM:*** Increased relative to the AROM but still limited by pain and swelling
Joint Stability Tests	***Stress tests:*** Underlying instability may be a causative factor. ***Joint play:*** Hypermobility may be present.
Special Tests	Specific to the involved joint.
Neurologic Screening	Within normal limits
Vascular Screening	Within normal limits
Functional Assessment	Patient describes avoiding weight-bearing maneuvers that increase pressure on the defect. AROM, PROM, and MMT may be reduced secondary to a loose body lodging between the joint surfaces, creating a mechanical block against movement.
Imaging Techniques	The defect may be present on standard radiographic examination. Better imaging is obtained through the use of MRI. The definitive diagnosis is based on MR images.
Differential Diagnosis	Sprain, synovitis
Comments	Osteochondral fractures are associated with a rapid-onset hemarthrosis.

AROM = active range of motion; MMT = manual muscle test; MRI = magnetic resonance imaging; PROM = passive range of motion.

usually completed over a 2- to 3-week period. Although a Lyme disease vaccine is available, indications for its prescription have not been established. Individuals with a high risk of exposure to deer ticks should be vaccinated against Lyme disease.

Bony Pathology

Acute fracture tend to require more force than soft tissue injuries. In cases of acute fractures to the **long bones**, the ribs, and the spine, proper initial management of the injury

Axial load A force applied through the long axis of a bone or series of bones.

Long bones A bone possessing a base, shaft, and head.

Examination Findings 4-10
Osteoarthritis

Examination Segment	Clinical Findings
History	***Onset:*** Insidious ***Pain characteristics:*** Pain occurs throughout the involved joint. ***Other symptoms:*** Not applicable ***Mechanism:*** Osteoarthritis develops secondary to trauma and irregular biomechanical stresses being placed across the joint. Rheumatoid arthritis is caused by a systemic disorder that activates an inflammatory response in the body's joints. ***Predisposing conditions:*** For osteoarthritis, previous trauma to the joint has occurred. Rheumatoid arthritis is associated with a family history of the disorder. Certain occupations and obesity may overload the joints, causing increased forces over time.
Inspection	In chronic cases, gross deformity of the joint is noticed. Individuals with cases of shorter duration present with swelling.
Palpation	Warmth and swelling are identified in the affected joint. The articular surfaces, when and where palpable, are tender to the touch.
Joint and Muscle Function Assessment	***AROM:*** May be limited by pain, often becoming **contractured** as the condition progresses. ***MMT:*** Decreased secondary to pain. ***PROM:*** Pain is decreased relative to AROM.
Joint Stability Tests	***Stress tests:*** Test results may be positive if a deformity has developed, causing the stressed capsule and ligaments to elongate over time. ***Joint play:*** Distraction of the joint surfaces will reduce the pain associated with joint motion.
Special Tests	Specific to the involved joint.
Neurologic Screening	Within normal limits
Vascular Screening	Within normal limits
Functional Assessment	The patient demonstrates compensations to avoid using the involved body part. When arthritis affects the joints of the lower extremity, an antalgic gait is produced.
Imaging Techniques	AP, PA, lateral, and oblique radiographs In the lower extremity, weight-bearing views to identify decreased joint spaces will be obtained.
Differential Diagnosis	Lyme disease, juvenile rheumatoid arthritis, infection
Comments	The differential diagnosis of RA is made using blood markers.

AP = anteroposterior; AROM = active range of motion; MMT = manual muscle test; PA = posteroanterior; PROM = passive range of motion.

is essential to minimize the chance of a permanent disability or possibly death.

Injuries to bones of the pediatric and adolescent populations bring a unique set of challenges to the evaluation. The presence of **growth plates** as a weak link in the skeletal system increases the risk of traumatic fractures and overuse injuries and creates the possibility of long-term consequences of injury in skeletally immature individuals. Growth plate injuries are categorized using the Salter–Harris system (Box 4-2).[19]

Exostosis

Wolff's law states that a bone remodels itself in response to forces placed on it, a naturally occurring phenomenon that allows bones to adapt and become stronger.[20] Growth of

Contracture A pathological shortening of tissues causing a decrease in available motion.

Growth plates The area of bone growth in skeletally immature individuals; the epiphyseal plate.

Table 4-3 Stages of Lyme Disease

Stage	Onset After Exposure	Symptoms
1	3–30 days	A rash at the site of the bite (erythema migrans) Fever Headache Myalgias Arthralgias
2	Weeks to months	Increasing severity of illness with an increase in symptoms from stage 1 Malaise Neurologic symptoms (headache, cranial nerve palsies [especially Bell's palsy], lymphocytic meningitis with or without radiculopathy) Cardiovascular symptoms (carditis characterized by atrioventricular conduction abnormalities)
3	Months to years	Synovial involvement Nervous system involvement (chronic neurologic Lyme disease, subtle encephalopathy, peripheral neuropathy, cognitive impairment most likely affecting short-term memory, paresthesias in a stocking or stocking/glove distribution) Systemic skin rashes Arthritis

extraneous bone, exostosis, can occur as a stress reaction from injury or from irregular forces placed on the bone (Fig. 4-12). The bone develops an exostosis at the site of the stress that may become painful and, in some cases, forms a mechanical block against movement (Examination Findings 4-11).

Apophysitis

Sometimes termed "growing pains," apophysitis is an inflammatory condition involving a bone's growth plate. In adolescents, the growth plate represents the weak link along the bone. Some of these growth areas serve as, or are close to, the attachment sites for the larger, stronger muscle groups in the body. Tightness of these muscles or repetitive forces applied to the bone by these muscles can result in inflammation and the eventual separation of these areas away from the rest of the bone (Fig. 4-13).

Apophysitis often includes a history of recent rapid growth. As the skeleton rapidly matures, the muscular tissues do not fully adapt to the new bone length and apply increased stress to the growth plate. Lack of flexibility may be a contributing cause, but after apophysitis has occurred, the flexibility of the muscle group attaching to the site decreases further. Resistance exercises (e.g., weight lifting) result in pain as the forces generated are transmitted to the affected area.

Fractures

Classification schemes of bony fractures are based on the location of the fracture relative to the rest of the bone (Inspection Findings Box 4-1); the magnitude of the

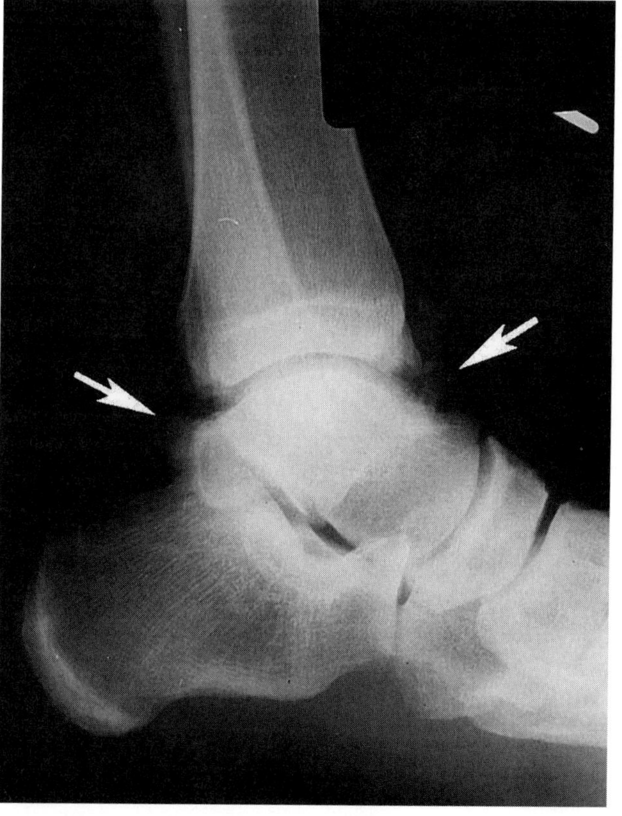

FIGURE 4-12 ■ Radiograph of exostosis of the subtalar joint. Note the bony outgrowths indicated by the arrows.

Box 4-2
Salter–Harris Classification of Epiphyseal Injuries

Fracture Configuration	Type
	I: Fracture extends through the physis, separating the two segments. Common in infants.
	II: Fracture starts through the physis and ends on the shaft, creating a displaced wedge.
	III: The fracture line extends perpendicularly through the joint surface and then transversely across the physis, resulting in partial displacement of the segment. Growth of the involved physis may be compromised.
	IV: Similar to a type III fracture, but the transverse fracture line extends across the physis into the shaft. Surgical fixation is often required and physeal growth may be affected.
	V: A crushing injury that compresses the physis. If undetected, **avascular necrosis** may occur and growth may be inhibited.

fracture line or lines (Inspection Findings Box 4-2); and the shape and direction of the fracture (Inspection Findings Box 4-3). Although it is common practice, the use of relatively nondescriptive terms (e.g., boxer's fracture: fracture of the fourth or fifth metacarpal) or the identification of a fracture type by an individual's name (e.g., Colles' fracture: fracture of the distal radius that is displaced dorsally) tends to become corrupted over time and may be less accurate.

Fractures that fail to heal within 9 months of the expected time required (for example, a fracture that is expected to heal in 2 months that has not yet healed in 11 months) are termed **nonunion fractures**. Healed fractures that leave the bone in a functionally unacceptable position are described as **malunion fractures**.

Avascular necrosis Death of cells secondary to lack of an adequate blood supply.

Examination Findings 4-11
Exostosis

Examination Segment	Clinical Findings
History	***Onset:*** Insidious ***Pain characteristics:*** Exostosis involving the extremities most often results in the localization of pain and other symptoms. Spinal exostosis can result in pain being referred along the distribution of affected nerve roots. ***Mechanism:*** Exostosis is the result of repeated strain placed on a bone or the bony insertion of a tendon. May also result from repeated compressive forces. ***Predisposing conditions:*** Previous trauma to the area, osteoarthritis
Inspection	Deformity may be noted over the site of pain.
Palpation	Point tenderness is present. A large bony outgrowth may be palpable.
Joint and Muscle Function Assessment	***AROM:*** Limited secondary to pain and/or bony block ***MMT:*** Dependent on joint position ***PROM:*** Equal to AROM
Joint Stability Tests	***Stress tests:*** Within normal limits ***Joint play:*** May be restricted in direction of exostosis.
Special Tests	Not applicable
Neurologic Screening	Within normal limits
Vascular Screening	Within normal limits
Functional Assessment	Patient demonstrates avoidance of movements that add tensile stress or compress the exostosis.
Imaging Techniques	Radiograph
Differential Diagnosis	Tumor, apophysitis (e.g., Osgood Schlatter's disease)

AROM = active range of motion; MMT = manual muscle test; PROM = passive range of motion.

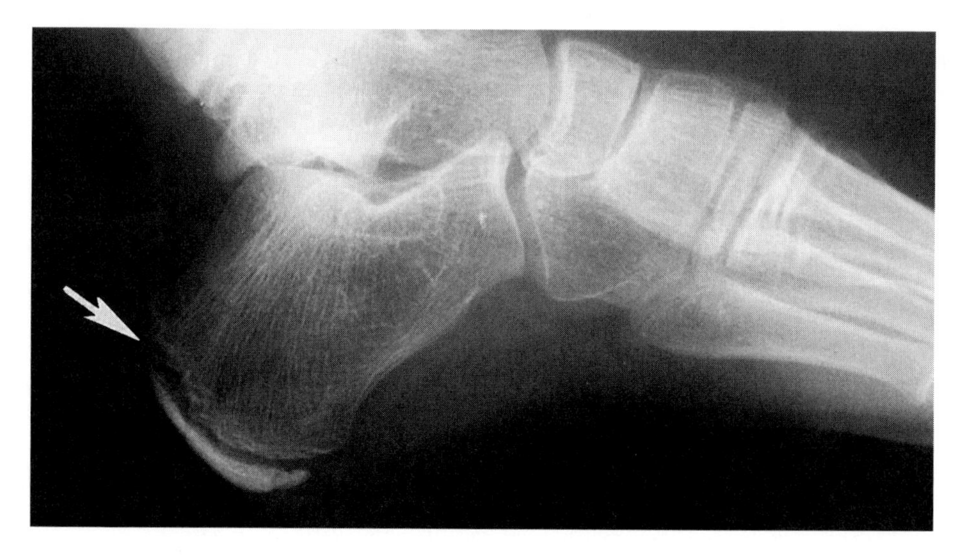

FIGURE 4-13 ■ Radiograph of calcaneal apophysitis.

Inspection Findings 4-1
Terminology Used to Describe the Fracture Location

Fracture	Description
	Diaphyseal fractures involve only the bone's **diaphysis** and are associated with a good prognosis for recovery.
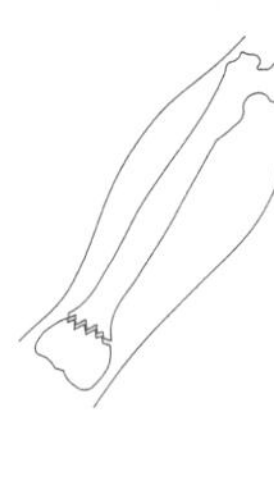	**Epiphyseal fractures** involve the fracture line crossing the bone's unsealed **epiphyseal line** and can have long-term consequences by disrupting the bone's normal growth. Epiphyseal fractures may mimic soft tissue injuries by resembling joint laxity during stress testing.
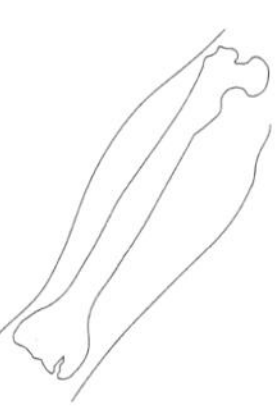	**Articular fractures** disrupt the joint's articular cartilage, which, if improperly healed, results in pain and decreased range of motion and can lead to arthritis of the joint.

Inspection Findings 4-2
Terminology Used to Describe the Relative Severity of the Fracture Line

Fracture	Description
	Incomplete fracture: Fracture line does not completely disassociate the proximal end of the bone from its distal end.
	Undisplaced fracture: Fracture line completely disassociates the two ends of the bone, but the two ends of the bone maintain their relative alignment to each other.
	Displaced fracture: Bony alignment is lost between the two segments; the surrounding tissues may be jeopardized.
	Open fracture: A bony segment of a displaced fracture exits the skin.

Inspection Findings 4-3
Terminology Used to Describe the Fracture Line

Fracture	Description
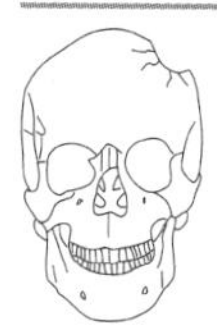	***Depressed fracture:*** Results from direct trauma to flat bones, causing the bone to fracture and depress.
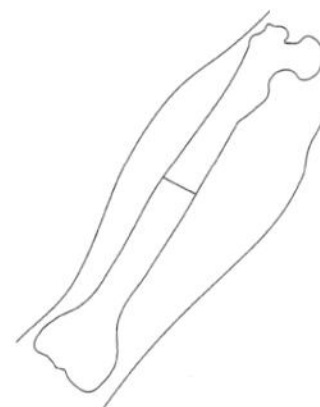	***Transverse fracture:*** Caused by a direct blow, shear force, or tensile force being applied to the shaft of a long bone and results in a fracture line that crosses the bone's long axis.
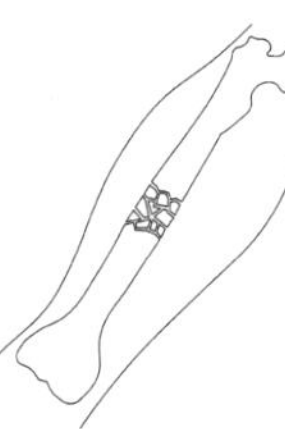	***Comminuted fracture:*** Result of extremely high-velocity impact forces that cause the bone to shatter into multiple pieces. This type of fracture often requires surgical correction.
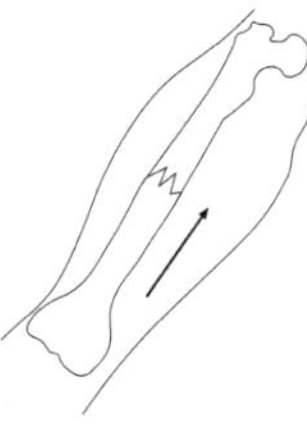	***Compacted fracture:*** Results from compressive forces applied through the long axis of the bone. One end of a fractured segment is driven into the opposite piece of the fracture, leading to a shortening of the involved bone.
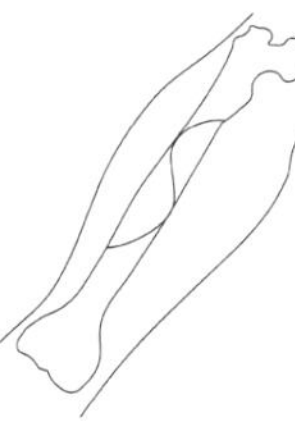	***Spiral fracture:*** The result of a rotational force placed on the shaft of a long bone, such as twisting the tibia while the foot remains fixated. The fracture line assumes a three-dimensional S-shape along the length of the bone.
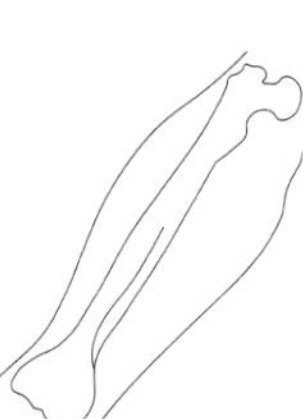	***Longitudinal fracture:*** Most commonly occur as the result of a fall and have a fracture line that runs parallel to the bone's long axis.
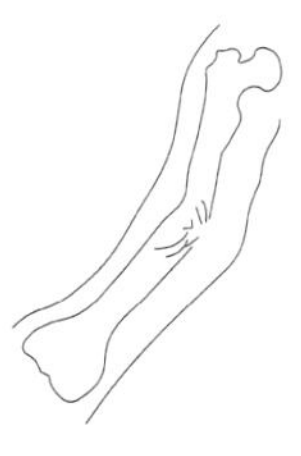	***Greenstick fracture:*** Generally specific to the pediatric and adolescent population, involve a displaced fracture on one side of the bone and a compacted fracture on the opposite side. The name is derived from an analogy to an immature tree branch that has been snapped.

Diaphysis The shaft of a long bone.

Epiphyseal line The area of growth found between the diaphysis and epiphysis in immature long bones.

Avulsion fractures

Avulsion fractures involve the tearing away of a ligament's or tendon's bony attachment (Fig. 4-14). Except for the case of large tendons (e.g., the patellar tendon), this injury may be missed easily because of the relatively small fracture site and the similarity to sprains or strains and their mechanisms. Tendon avulsions can also occur if a muscle is forcefully contracted and the attachment site is pulled away from the rest of the bone. When large tendons are involved, obvious deformity results as the tendon recoils from the fracture site. With smaller tendons or ligaments, pain is described at the fracture site and point tenderness is elicited. The stress testing of the joint may display the signs and symptoms of a third-degree sprain.

Stress fractures

A stress fracture is classified as a fatigue fracture or insufficiency fracture. **Fatigue fractures** occur when normal bone is subjected to abnormally high, repeated submaximal stresses and is linked to sudden changes in the frequency, intensity, or duration of activity beyond which the bone is accustomed. **Insufficiency fractures** occur when abnormally weak bones are subjected to normal forces.[21]

Although stress fractures most commonly occur in the lower extremities, this condition can be found in any bone that absorbs repetitive stress.[22,23] Stress fractures present as a complex injury because of their nondescript initial findings and their tendency to mimic the signs and symptoms of soft tissue injuries. Stress fractures occur when the bone's osteoclastic activity outweighs osteoblastic activity, causing a weakened area along the line of stress. If the external stress is not reduced (e.g., the patient continues running), the bone eventually fails.

The history reveals a chronic condition caused by repetitive stresses to the involved area. There may have been a recent change in the patient's workout routine, including changes in equipment, playing surfaces, frequency, duration, or intensity. Because of the related reduction in levels of estrogen and progesterone, **amenorrheic** women may be predisposed to developing stress fractures. With specific palpation, an area of exact tenderness can be discerned along any bony surface. Compression of long bones may result in increased pain (Examination Findings 4-12).

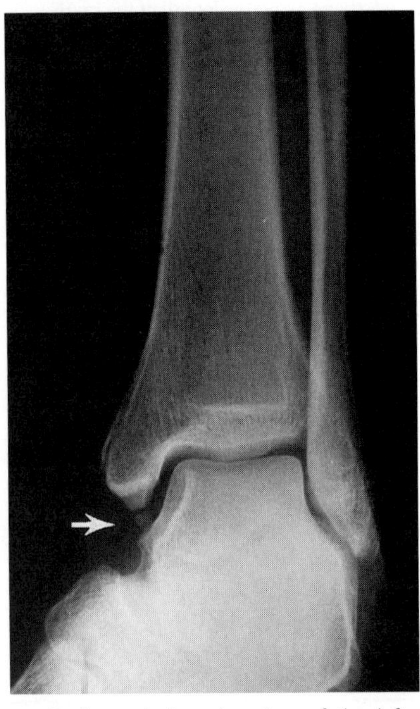

FIGURE 4-14 ■ Radiograph (anterior view of the left ankle) of an avulsion fracture of the attachment of the deltoid ligament (*arrow*).

Neurovascular Pathologies

Trauma to the neurovascular structures (i.e., nerves, arteries, and veins) is often a consequence of joint dislocation, bony displacement, concussive forces, or compartment syndromes (see Box 4-1). If untreated, vascular disruption can lead to the loss of the affected body part. Neurologic inhibition can lead to the loss of function in the involved part.

Peripheral Nerve Injury

Entrapment injuries to the peripheral nerves are common at the ankle, elbow, wrist, and cervical spine. Peripheral nerves located more distally from the spinal column have a greater probability of regeneration than a lesion that occurs more proximal to the CNS.

In some cases, nonneurologic tissue or swelling entraps the nerve, causing dysfunction in the form of paresthesia and muscular weakness. This condition is most commonly seen at the ulnar tunnel, pronator teres muscle, carpal tunnel, and tarsal tunnel. In each case, the complaints are of specific pain patterns and paresthesia. With careful manual muscle testing, muscle weakness may be elicited. Although these syndromes may be suspected on evaluation, they are confirmed via electrodiagnostic testing.

Stretch injuries to peripheral nerves may be divided into three categories based on the pathology and the prognosis for recovery. **Neurapraxia** is the mildest form of peripheral nerve stretch injury. The nerve, **epineurium**, and **myelin sheath** are stretched but remain intact. Symptoms are usually transient and include burning, pain, numbness, and temporary weakness on clinical evaluation.

Amenorrheic (amenorrhea) The absence of menstruation.

Neurapraxia A stretch injury to a nerve resulting in transient symptoms of paraesthesia and weakness.

Epineurium Connective tissue containing blood vessels surrounding the trunk of a nerve, binding it together.

Myelin sheath A fatty-based lining of the axon of myelinated nerve fibers.

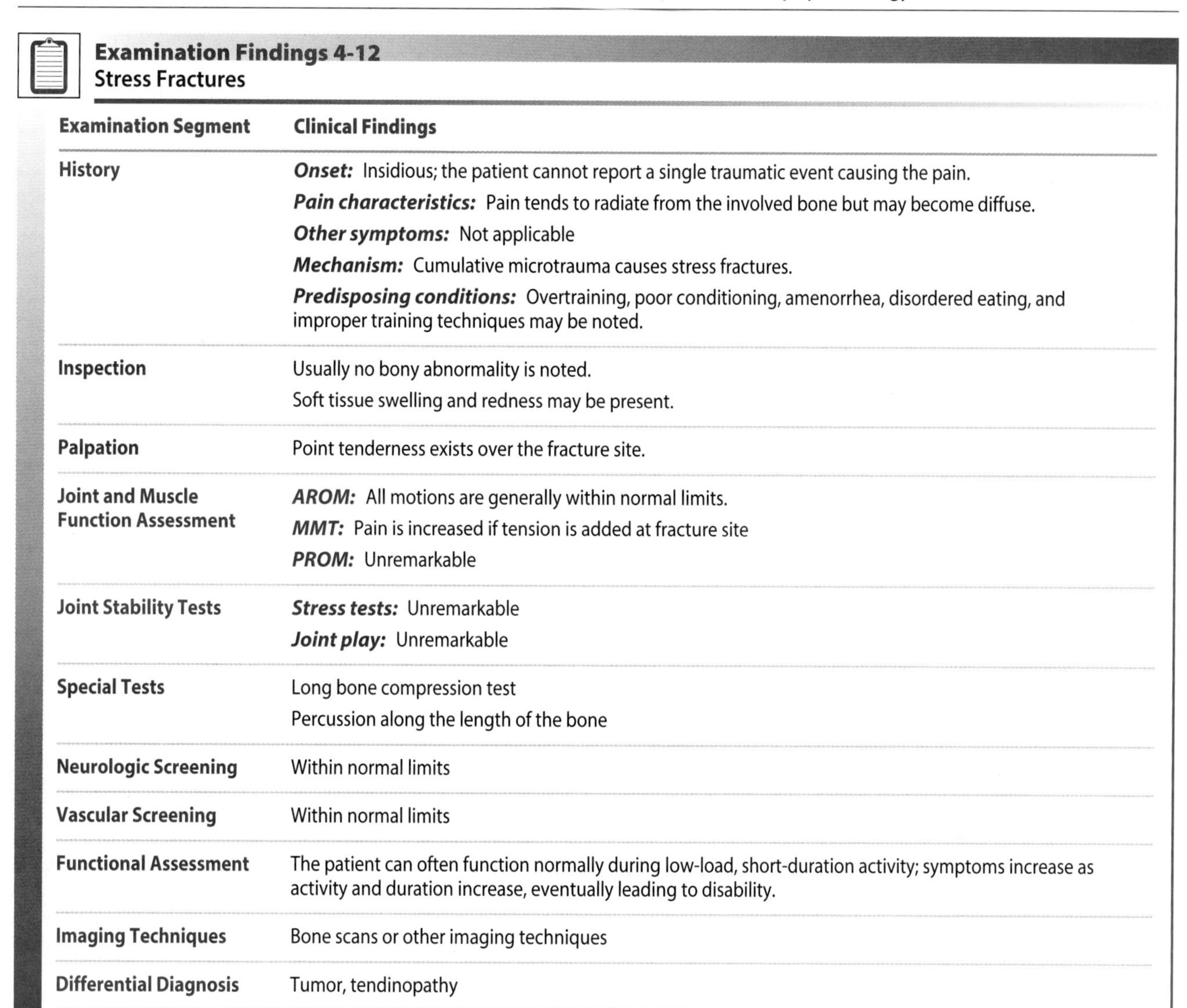

Examination Findings 4-12
Stress Fractures

Examination Segment	Clinical Findings
History	***Onset:*** Insidious; the patient cannot report a single traumatic event causing the pain. ***Pain characteristics:*** Pain tends to radiate from the involved bone but may become diffuse. ***Other symptoms:*** Not applicable ***Mechanism:*** Cumulative microtrauma causes stress fractures. ***Predisposing conditions:*** Overtraining, poor conditioning, amenorrhea, disordered eating, and improper training techniques may be noted.
Inspection	Usually no bony abnormality is noted. Soft tissue swelling and redness may be present.
Palpation	Point tenderness exists over the fracture site.
Joint and Muscle Function Assessment	***AROM:*** All motions are generally within normal limits. ***MMT:*** Pain is increased if tension is added at fracture site ***PROM:*** Unremarkable
Joint Stability Tests	***Stress tests:*** Unremarkable ***Joint play:*** Unremarkable
Special Tests	Long bone compression test Percussion along the length of the bone
Neurologic Screening	Within normal limits
Vascular Screening	Within normal limits
Functional Assessment	The patient can often function normally during low-load, short-duration activity; symptoms increase as activity and duration increase, eventually leading to disability.
Imaging Techniques	Bone scans or other imaging techniques
Differential Diagnosis	Tumor, tendinopathy
Comments	Repetitive stress fractures: seek underlying cause.

AROM = active range of motion; MMT = manual muscle test; PROM = passive range of motion.

Axonotmesis involves a disruption of the axon and the myelin sheath, but the epineurium remains intact. The signs and symptoms are the same as for neurapraxia, but those associated with axonotmesis have a longer duration. Because the axon undergoes **wallerian degeneration**, the return of normal innervation is unpredictable and sustained weakness may be experienced.

Neurotmesis, a complete disruption of the nerve, is the most severe form of peripheral nerve injury. The prognosis for the return of normal innervation is poor. This injury occurs under extremely high forces and usually entails concurrent injury to bones, ligaments, and tendons. Many times a nerve **graft** or tendon transfer is required to return function to the extremity. These procedures meet with limited success and are not conducive to the return to competitive athletics.

Complex Regional Pain Syndrome

Complex regional pain syndrome (CRPS), also known as reflex sympathetic **dystrophy** (RSD), is an exaggerated, generalized pain response after injury. CRPS is characterized

Wallerian degeneration Degeneration of a nerve's axon that has been severed from the body of the nerve.

Neurotmesis Complete loss of nerve function with little apparent anatomic damage to the nerve itself.

Graft An organ or tissue used for transplantation. An allograft is a donor tissue transplanted from the same species. An autograft tissue is transplanted from within the same individual.

Dystrophy The progressive deterioration of tissue.

by intense or unduly prolonged pain that is out of proportion to the severity of the injury, **vasomotor** disturbances, delayed functional recovery, and various associated **trophic** changes.[24] In type I CRPS there is no overt nerve damage. Type II CRPS involves damage to the peripheral nerves.

Patient complaints of CPRS include:

- Pain that is disproportionately increased relative to the severity of the injury
- Superficial hypersensitive areas (e.g., pain when clothing touches the skin)
- Edema
- Decreased motor function, leading to dystrophy
- Muscle spasm
- Dermatologic alterations, including the integrity of the skin, skin temperature changes, hair loss, and changes in the nail bed
- Vasomotor instability: **Raynaud's phenomenon, vasoconstriction, vasodilation, hyperhydrosis**
- Skeletal changes, including osteoporosis

The prognosis for patients with CRPS is extremely variable, but early intervention appears to improve the probability of a favorable outcome, making early recognition and referral a priority. Intervention includes rehabilitation with modalities and therapeutic exercise.[25] Symptomatic relief can be obtained through the use of various medications, including narcotics, central nervous system depressants, epidural injections, and muscle relaxants to reduce sympathetic activity.[24,26] In unyielding cases, surgical dissection of the nerve may be required to prevent the pain causing nerve transmission.[26]

REFERENCES

1. Mueller, MJ, and Maluf, KS: Tissue adaptation to physical stress: A proposed "Physical Stress Theory" to guide physical therapist practice, education, and research. *Phys Ther,* 82:383, 2002.
2. Clanion, TO, and Coupe, KJ: Hamstrings strains in athletes: Diagnosis and treatment. *J Am Acad Orthop Surg,* 6:237, 1998.
3. Anderson, K, Strickland, SM, and Warren, R: Hip and groin injuries in athletes. *Am J Sports Med,* 29:521, 2001.
4. Thacker, SB, et al: The impact of stretching on sports injury risk: A systematic review of the literature. *Med Sci Sport Exer,* 36: 371, 2004.
5. Almekinders, LC, Garrett, WE, and Seaber, AV: Histopathology of muscle tears in stretching injuries. *Trans Orthop Res Soc,* 9: 306, 1984.
6. Wilson, JJ, and Best, TM: Common overuse tendon problems: A review and recommendations for treatment. *Am Fam Phys,* 72:811, 2005.
7. Gross, MT: Chronic tendinitis: Pathomechanics of injury, factors affecting the healing response, and treatment. *J Orthop Sports Phys Ther,* 16:248, 1992.
8. Sharma, P, and Maffulli, N: Tendon injury and tendinopathy: Healing and repair. *J Bone Jt Surg,* 87-A:187, 2005.
9. Frey, CC, and Shereff, MJ: Tendon injuries about the ankle in athletes. *Clin Sports Med,* 7:103, 1988.
10. Kijowski, R, De Smet, A, and Mukharjee, R: Magnetic resonance imaging findings in patients with peroneal tendinopathy and peroneal tenosynovitis. *Skelet Radiol,* 36:105, 2007.
11. Alonso, A, Hekeik, P, and Adams, R: Predicting recovery time from the initial assessment of a quadriceps contusion injury. *Austral J Physiother,* 46:167, 2000.
12. Pape, HC, et al: Current concepts in the development of heterotopic ossification. *J Bone Joint Surg,* 86 (B):783, 2004.
13. Aronen, JG, et al: Quadriceps contusions: Clinical results of immediate immobilization in 120 degrees of knee flexion. *Clin J Sport Med,* 16:383, 2006.
14. It's bursitis, but which type? *Emerg Med* 21:71, 1989.
15. Starkey, C: Injuries and illnesses in the National Basketball Association: A 10-year perspective. *J Athl Train,* 35:161, 2000.
16. Sailors, ME: Recognition and treatment of osteochondritis dissecans of the femoral condyle. *J Athl Train,* 29:302, 1994.
17. Lindholm, TS, Osterman, K, and Vankkae, E: Osteochondritis dissecans of the elbow, ankle, and hip. *Clin Orthop,* 148: 245, 1980.
18. Jouben, LM, Steele, RJ, and Bono, JV: Orthopaedic manifestations of Lyme disease. *Orthop Rev,* 23:395, 1994.
19. McKinnis, LN: Radiologic evaluation of fracture. In McKinnis, LN: *Fundamentals of Musculoskeletal Imaging,* ed 2. Philadelphia, FA Davis, p 94, 2005.
20. Starkey, C: The injury response process. In Starkey, C: *Therapeutic Modalities,* ed 3. Philadelphia, FA Davis, 2004.
21. Shin, AY, and Gillingham, BL: Fatigue fractures of the femoral neck in athletes. *J Am Acad Orthop Surg,* 4:293, 1997.
22. Ward, WG, Bergfeld, JA, and Carson, WG: Stress fracture of the base of the acromial process. *Am J Sports Med,* 22: 146, 1994.
23. Yasuda, T, et al: Stress fracture of the right distal femur following bilateral fractures of the proximal fibulas. A case report. *Am J Sports Med,* 20:771, 1992.
24. Muizelaar, JP, et al: Complex regional pain syndrome (reflex sympathetic dystrophy and causalgia): Management with the calcium channel blocker nifedipine and/or the alpha-sympathetic blocker phenoxybenzamine in 59 patients. *Clin Neurol Neurosurg,* 99:26, 1997.
25. Sherry, DD: Short- and long-term outcomes of children with complex regional pain syndrome type I treated with exercise therapy. *Clin J Pain,* 15:218, 1999.
26. Kurvers, HA: Reflex sympathetic dystrophy: Facts and hypotheses. *Vasc Med,* 3:207, 1998.

Vasomotor Pertaining to nerves controlling the muscles within the walls of blood vessels.

Trophic Pertaining to efferent nerves controlling the nourishment of the area they innervate.

Raynaud's phenomenon A reaction to cold consisting of bouts of pallor and cyanosis, causing exaggerated vasomotor responses.

Vasoconstriction A decrease in a vessel's diameter.

Vasodilation An increase in a vessel's diameter.

Hyperhydrosis Excessive or profuse sweating.

CHAPTER 5

Musculoskeletal Diagnostic Techniques

Several hospital or laboratory-based neuromuscular diagnostic techniques are referenced throughout this text. Although a physician typically orders these procedures and interprets the results, knowledge of when these techniques are indicated, what conditions they identify, and basic interpretation techniques are valuable clinical skills. Table 5-1 presents an overview of the techniques discussed in this chapter and their most advantageous uses.

Table 5-1 Selected Diagnostic Techniques and Their Use

Technique	Best Use
Radiography	**Standard:** Bone lesions, joint surfaces, and joint spaces **Arthrogram:** Capsular tissue tears and articular cartilage lesions **Angiogram:** Blood vessel **Myelogram:** Pathologies within the spinal canal
Computed Tomography (CT)	Bony or articular cartilage lesions and some soft tissue lesions Quantify detailed bony lesions (e.g., size and location) Identify tendinous and ligamentous injuries in varying joint positions **Angiography:** Artery and/or vein pathology, including stenosis, aneurysms, and thrombi (clots)
Magnetic Resonance Imaging (MRI)	Visualize soft tissue structures, especially ligamentous and meniscal injuries **Magnetic resonance arthrography (MRA):** Used to image blood vessels. **Functional magnetic resonance imaging (fMRI):** Assess metabolic activity associated with brain function.
Nuclear Medicine	**Bone scan:** Identifies increased metabolic activity but may yield false-positive findings, especially in endurance athletes. **Positron emission tomography (PET):** Creates a three-dimensional image of physiological function in the body. **Single photon emission computed tomography (SPECT):** Produces three-dimensional images of internal structures.
Ultrasonic Imaging	Images tendon and other soft tissue imaging
Electromyography	Evaluates muscle physiology at rest and with activity. Identifies pathology of muscle secondary to nerve supply dysfunction or change in the muscle itself. Used in conjunction with nerve conduction study.
Nerve Conduction Study	Assesses function of motor and sensory nerves to detect nerve pathology, including axonal degeneration and neurotmesis.

Imaging Techniques

Radiographs, magnetic resonance images (MRI), computed tomography (CT), bone scans, and diagnostic ultrasound, collectively referred to as **diagnostic imaging**, are obtained by exposing the body to electromagnetic energy, or in the case of diagnostic ultrasound, acoustical energy, and determining how much energy is absorbed by the body, is reflected, or passes through the tissues. Most imaging technique is composed of a source (generator) that transmits the energy to the body and a collector that captures energy that has not been absorbed or scattered. From this, two- or three-dimensional images are constructed.

To obtain the clearest images of the involved structure(s), the diagnostic energy must strike the body from a specific direction and angle. Energy may pass from the anterior through the posterior tissues (anteroposterior [AP]), posterior to anterior (posteroanterior [PA]), or from a left or right lateral projection. The patient and generator may be aligned so that the energy strikes the body at a right angle, or images may be obtained using an oblique or acute angle (Fig. 5-1).

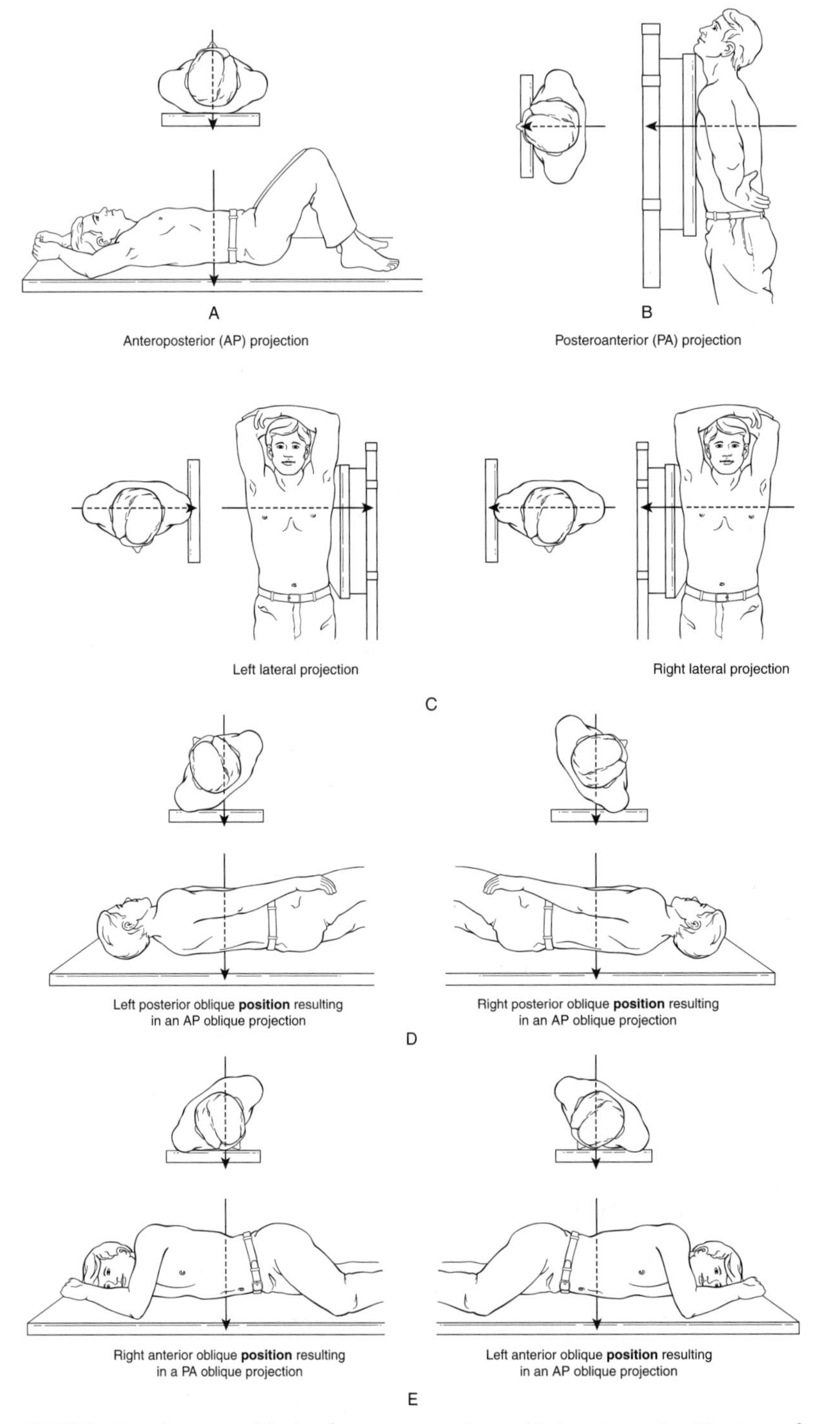

FIGURE 5-1 ■ Patient positioning for common radiographic imaging series. (Courtesy of McKinnis, L. *Fundamentals of Musculoskeletal Imaging*, 2nd ed. Philadelphia, FA Davis, 2005, p 18.)

Cost, accuracy, risk to the patient, and availability are factors in selecting which diagnostic technique is used. Because of its low cost and availability, radiography is a frequent first step to determine if there is bony pathology. For some suspected pathologies, other imaging techniques are quickly ordered in the presence of a negative radiograph and persistent symptoms.

Radiography

Radiographs are the most common imaging technique used in the diagnosis of orthopedic injuries. Discovered in 1895, the use of x-rays marked the first time that the internal structures could be viewed without invasive techniques.[1] Before this, the only method of viewing the internal structures was to actually cut the individual open. Note that "x-ray" describes the form of electromagnetic energy that is used; radiography describes the process of acquiring images (Fig. 5-2).

Although radiographs have limited utility beyond identification of fractures, because of their relatively low cost they are often obtained before MRI or CT scans. For example, in patients with suspected scaphoid fractures (see Chapter 18), radiographs lack the sensitivity of bone scans in detecting a fracture line.[2,3] The typical diagnostic approach includes initial radiographs and, if these are negative, a follow-up bone scan with 3 to 7 days of continued symptoms. Radiography has little utility in the early detection of stress fractures. Because of its improved sensitivity, MRI is replacing scintigraphy (bone scan) as the imaging of choice in detecting stress fractures early in the pathological process.[4]

Radiographic examination uses **ionizing radiation** to penetrate the body. Depending on the density of the underlying tissues, the radiation is absorbed or dispersed in varying degrees. High-density tissues such as bone absorb more radiation and are therefore more difficult to penetrate than less-dense tissue. The exposure to radiation leaves an imprint on special x-ray film (radiographic plate), producing the familiar radiographic image. Overexposure to ionizing radiation is hazardous, and care must be taken to protect the reproductive organs through the use of a lead apron.

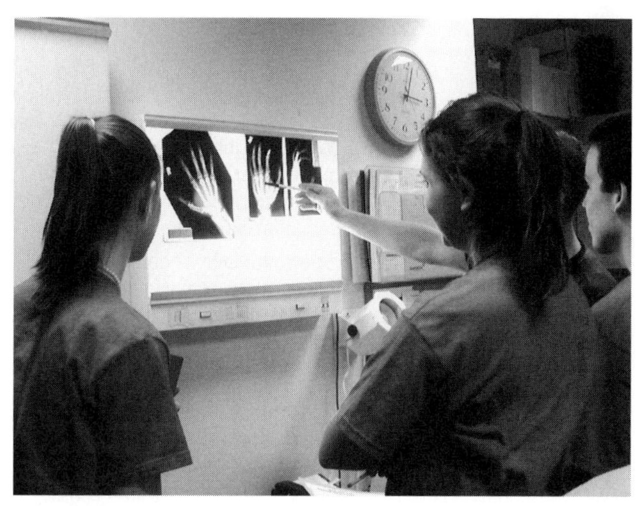

FIGURE 5-2 ■ Interpretation of radiographs is performed using the ABCS method: Alignment, Bones, Cartilage, and Soft tissue.

The interpretation of radiographic images can be based on the ABCS method:[5]

A—Alignment: The clinician observes for the normal continuity of the bones and joint surfaces and the alignment of one bone to another.

B—Bones: Bones should have normal density patterns, presenting with uniform color throughout the bone as compared bilaterally. Areas of decreased density appear as darkened areas within the bone. Fractures and abnormal bony outgrowths such as exostoses can also be visualized.

C—Cartilage: Although cartilage itself does not produce a radiographic image, the cartilage and ligamentous structures are inspected for what does not appear. The joint spaces should be smooth and uniform.

S—Soft tissue: Although soft tissue cannot be imaged, swelling within the confines of the soft tissue or between the soft tissue and the bones can be determined. In addition, the outline of soft tissues and even pockets of edema within soft tissue can be identified with adjusted exposure techniques.

Each body area has a standard series of radiographic views that are obtained to rule in or rule out a diagnosis (Table 5-2). The views ordered may be expanded based on

Table 5-2 Routine Radiologic Series by Body Area

Body Area	Views
Foot	AP, lateral, oblique
Ankle	AP, AP mortise, lateral, oblique
Knee	AP, lateral, intercondylar fossa
Patellofemoral	AP, lateral, merchant
Hip	AP, lateral
Lumbar spine	AP, lateral, oblique (right and left)
Thoracic spine	AP, lateral
Cervical spine	AP, lateral, oblique (right and left), open mouth
Shoulder	AP (internally rotated), AP (externally rotated)
Elbow	AP, lateral, oblique (internal and external),
Wrist, hand, and fingers	PA, lateral, oblique

AP = anteroposterior, PA = posteroanterior.

Ionizing radiation Electromagnetic energy that causes the release of an atom's protons, electrons, or neutrons. Ionizing radiation is potentially hazardous to human tissue.

the differential diagnosis, the patient's symptoms, or findings of earlier imaging series.

Assessment of a joint's ligamentous integrity often requires the use of imaging techniques, during which stress is applied to a joint to measure the amount of laxity, a stress radiograph (Figs. 5-3 and 5-4). This requires application of a force that stretches the ligament during the x-ray exposure, allowing for the measurement of excessive motion, determining a third-degree ligament injury, or ascertaining the amount of overall joint laxity.

Other forms of radiographic screening involve the use of radio-opaque dyes that are absorbed by the tissues, allowing visualization by radiographic examination. Collectively known as **contrast imaging,** arthrograms, myelograms, and angiograms have various applications to specific body systems. With the availability of MRI techniques, these types of studies are less frequently used in the diagnosis of orthopedic injuries.

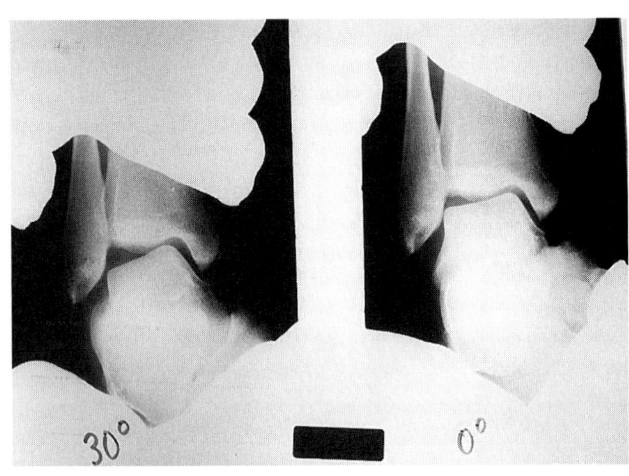

FIGURE 5-3 ■ Stress radiograph for inversion of the ankle.

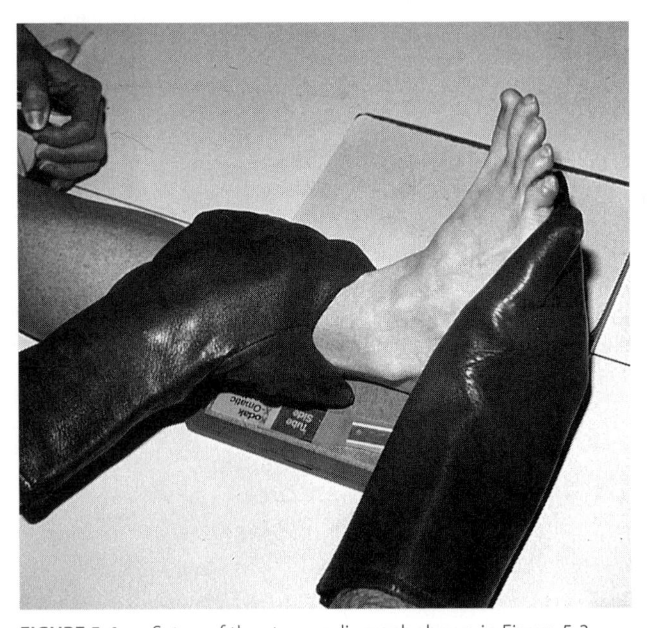

FIGURE 5-4 ■ Setup of the stress radiograph shown in Figure 5-3.

Computed Tomography Scan

CT scan uses many of the same principles and technology as radiography but is used to determine and quantify the presence of a specific pathology rather than as a general screening tool. In the case of CT scans, the x-ray source and x-ray detectors rotate around the body (Fig. 5-5). Instead of the image's being produced on film, a computer determines the density of the underlying tissues based on the absorption of x-rays by the body, allowing for more precision in viewing soft tissue. This information is then used to create a two-dimensional image, or slice, of the body.[1] These slices can be obtained at varying positions and thicknesses, allowing physicians to study the area and its surrounding anatomical relationships (Fig. 5-6).

In traditional CT imaging, the x-ray source rotates 360 degrees around the body to obtain one slice. In spiral,

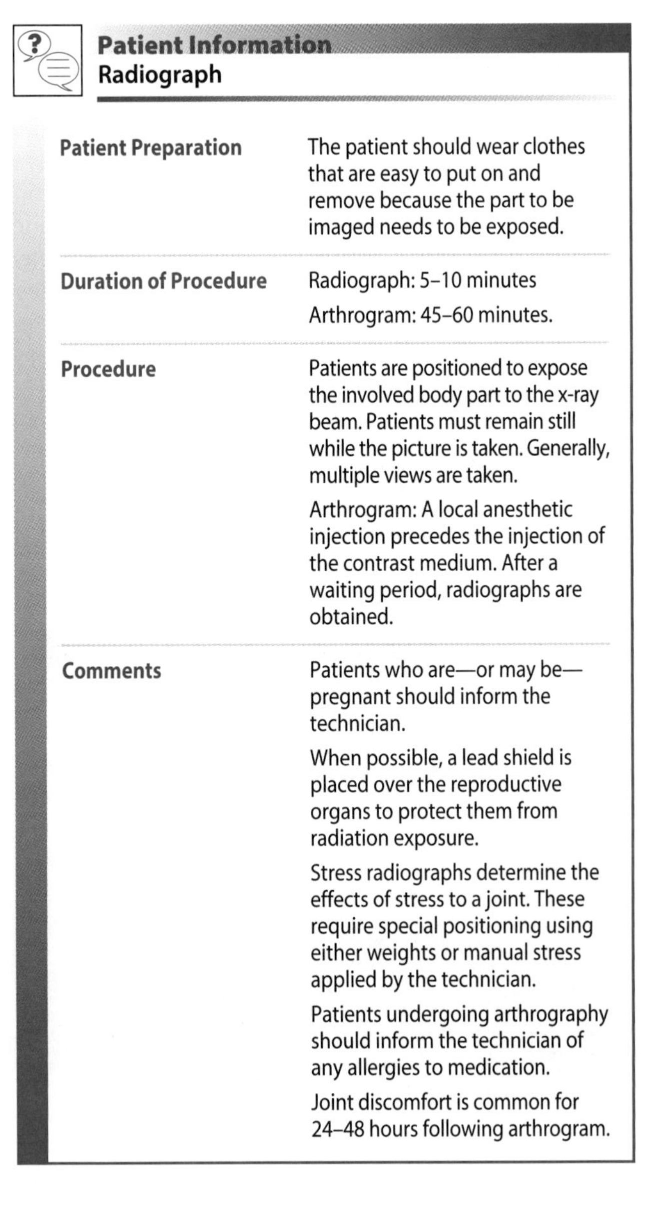

Patient Information
Radiograph

Patient Preparation	The patient should wear clothes that are easy to put on and remove because the part to be imaged needs to be exposed.
Duration of Procedure	Radiograph: 5–10 minutes Arthrogram: 45–60 minutes.
Procedure	Patients are positioned to expose the involved body part to the x-ray beam. Patients must remain still while the picture is taken. Generally, multiple views are taken. Arthrogram: A local anesthetic injection precedes the injection of the contrast medium. After a waiting period, radiographs are obtained.
Comments	Patients who are—or may be—pregnant should inform the technician. When possible, a lead shield is placed over the reproductive organs to protect them from radiation exposure. Stress radiographs determine the effects of stress to a joint. These require special positioning using either weights or manual stress applied by the technician. Patients undergoing arthrography should inform the technician of any allergies to medication. Joint discomfort is common for 24–48 hours following arthrogram.

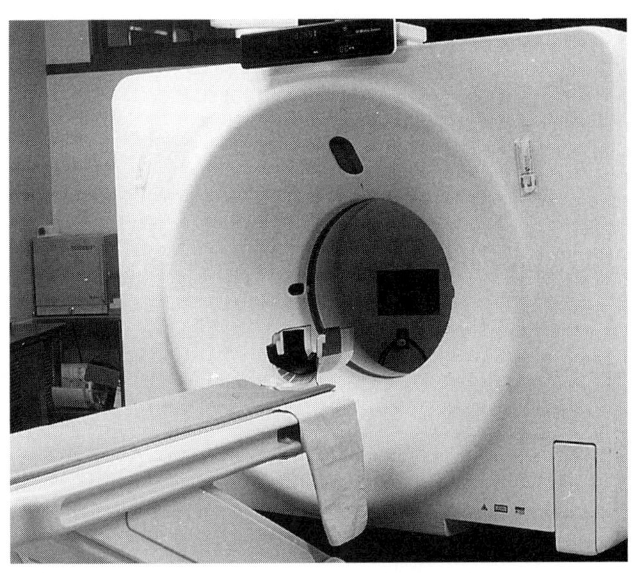

FIGURE 5-5 ■ CT scan device.

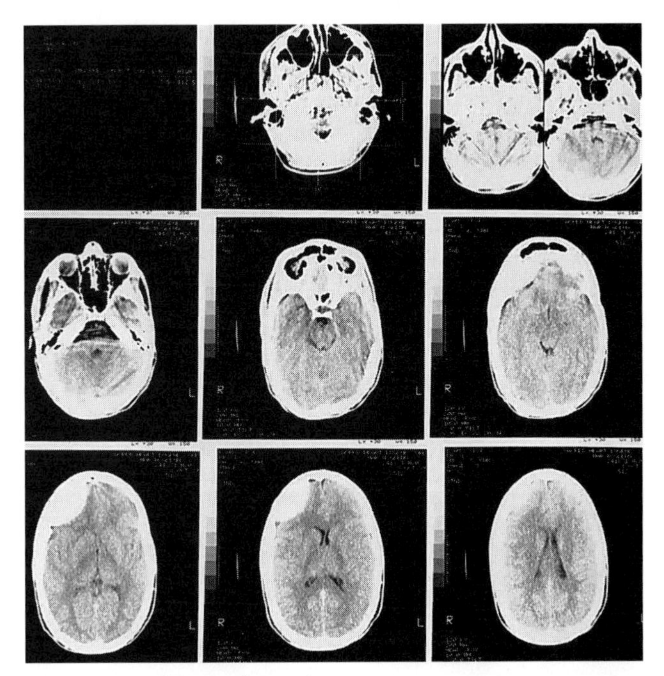

FIGURE 5-6 ■ CT scan of a cranium.

or helical, CT, the x-ray source scans in a continuous arc around the body (Fig. 5-7). The speed and number of slices acquired depends on the number of detectors. Spiral CT has improved accuracy, requires less radiation exposure, and has a faster acquisition time than traditional CT.

Optimal visualization of certain tissues requires injection or swallowing of a contrast medium prior to the scan. **CT angiography**, which involves use of a contrast medium injected into a vein, is often used to visualize blood vessels. **Single photon emission computed tomography** (SPECT) merges multiple two-dimensional images obtained from different angles and assembles them to form a three-dimensional image.

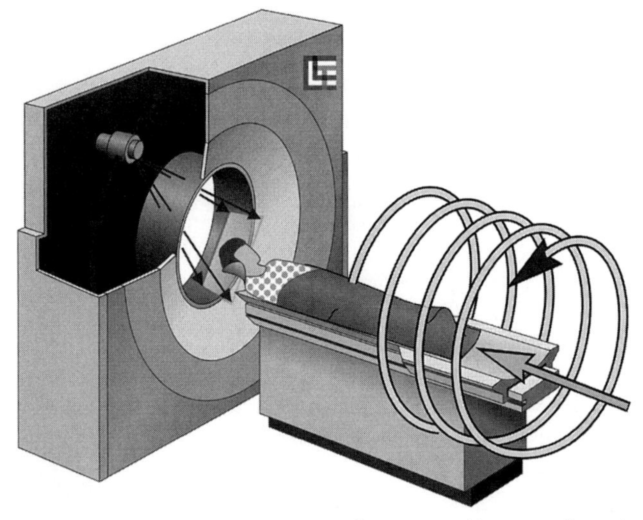

FIGURE 5-7 ■ Spiral (helical) CT scan. The patient table moves through the generator as the x-ray source rotates around the body, allowing the scan to be performed in a continuous arc. (Courtesy of McKinnis, L. *Fundamentals of Musculoskeletal Imaging*, 2nd ed. Philadelphia, FA Davis, 2005, p 119.)

Patient Information
CT Scan

Patient Preparation	The patient should wear loose-fitting clothing without zippers or snaps, as metal can distort the image. Patients may be asked to remove jewelry, hearing aids, dentures, or glasses, depending on the body part to be scanned. For CT angiography, patient may be asked to consume only clear liquids 12–24 hours before the procedure.
Duration of Procedure	5–30 minutes; faster if spiral CT is used.
Procedure	The patient lies still on a movable table that positions the target body part in the circle containing the scanning equipment. For CT angiography, the contrast medium is injected into a blood vessel prior to the scanning procedure.
Comments	Patients who are—or may be—pregnant should inform the technician. For CT angiography, patients should inform the technician of any allergies to medication.

Magnetic Resonance Imaging

Perhaps the greatest innovation in the noninvasive diagnosis of subcutaneous pathology, MRI acquires a detailed picture of the body's soft tissues (Fig. 5-8). Similar to a CT scan, MRI

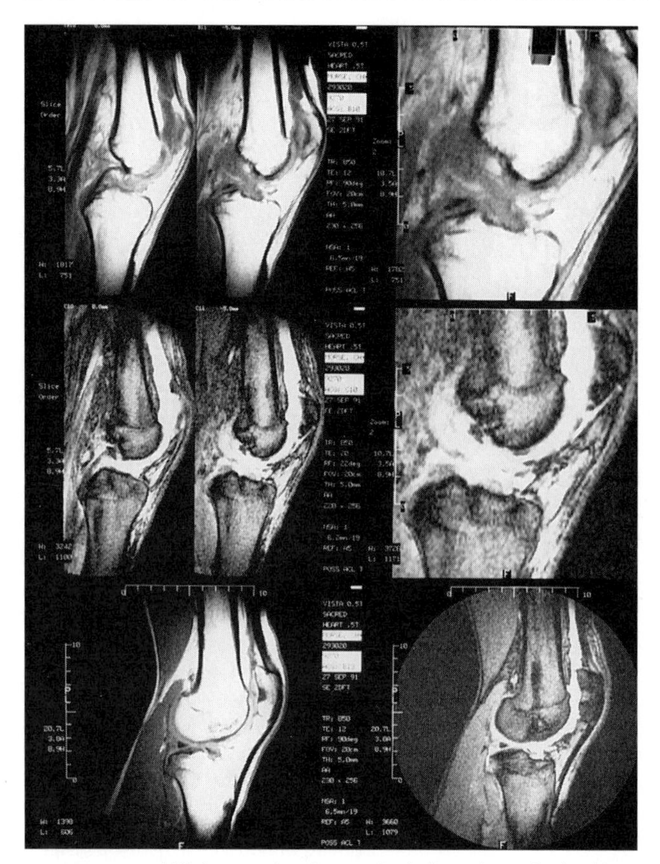

FIGURE 5-8 ■ MRI image showing sagittal slices through the knee. (Courtesy of Rothstein, JM, Roy, SH, and Wolf, SL: *The Rehabilitation Specialist's Handbook*. Philadelphia, FA Davis, 1991.)

is generally used to identify specific pathology or visualize a soft tissue structure (e.g., an anterior cruciate ligament sprain) rather than being used as a general screening tool. Compared with other imaging techniques, MRI offers superior visualization of the body's soft tissues.

These images are obtained by placing the patient in an MRI tube that produces a magnetic field, causing the body's hydrogen nuclei to align with the magnetic axis (Fig. 5-9). The tissues are then bombarded by electromagnetic waves, causing the nuclei to resonate as they absorb the energy. When the energy to the tissues ceases, the nuclei return to their state of equilibrium by releasing energy, which is then detected by the MRI unit and transformed by a computer into images.[1]

Similar to adjusting the contrast on your television screen or computer monitor, the contrast of the MR image can be "weighted" to better identify specific types of tissues (Box 5-1).[6] Contrast imaging media may be introduced into the tissues to delineate the structures further.

Unlike the ionizing radiation associated with radiographs and CT scans, the energy used during the MRI process produces no known potentially harmful effects. The only known limitations to the administration of this procedure lie with individuals who suffer from claustrophobia (who are fearful of entering the imaging tube) or those who have some types of implanted metal. MRI can often be safely used even if the

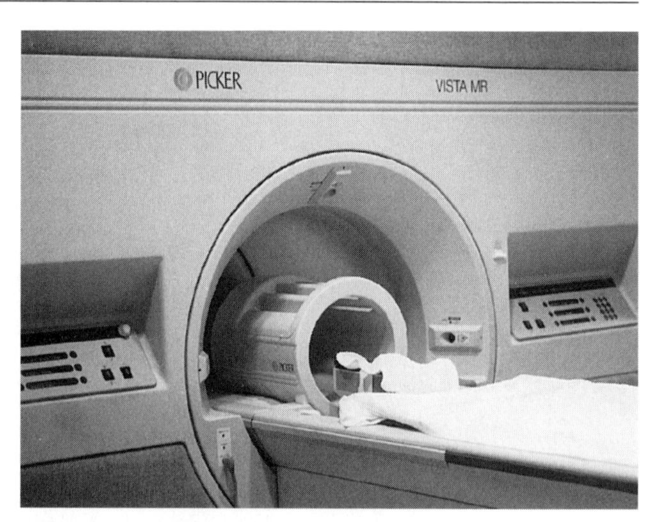

FIGURE 5-9 ■ MRI generator.

patient has implanted metal such as surgical staples, pins, plates and screws, as long as it has been in place for longer than 4 to 6 weeks. The open MRI eliminates or reduces claustrophobia by minimizing the immersion in the imaging tube and reducing the level of magnetism required to produce images.

Functional MRIs (fMRIs) are used to detect metabolic changes in the brain. fMRIs are useful in tracking changes in brain activity following stroke, traumatic brain injury, or tumor.

Magnetic resonance angiography (MRA) uses MRI to study blood vessels and its lack of invasiveness makes it preferable to a catheter study. Contrast material is sometimes injected into the bloodstream to better visualize the vessels (Fig. 5-10).

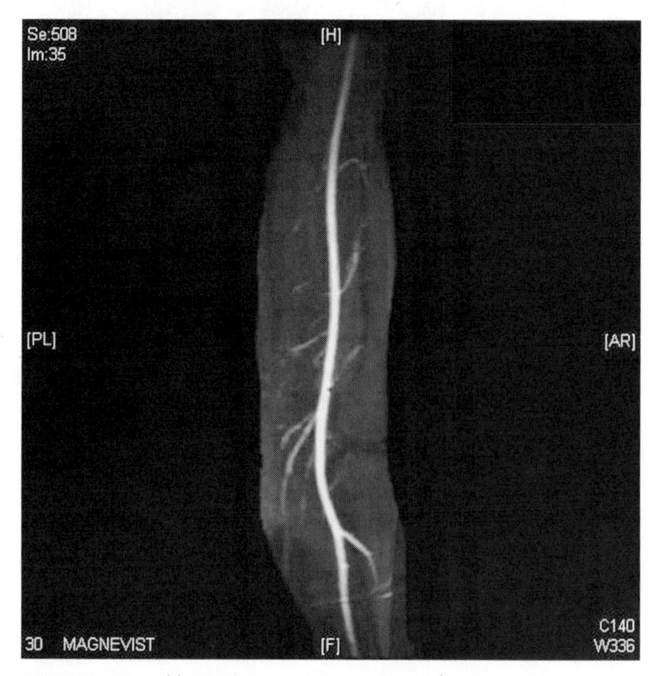

FIGURE 5-10 ■ Magnetic resonance angiography.

Box 5-1

Relative Signal Intensities of Selected Structures on Spin Echo in Musculoskeletal Magnetic Resonance Imaging

Structure	Sequence		
	T1-Weighted	Proton Density	T2-Weighted
Fat*	Bright	Bright	Intermediate
Fluid**	Dark	Intermediate	Bright
Fibrocartilage***	Dark	Dark	Dark
Ligaments, Tendon****	Dark	Dark	Dark
Muscle	Intermediate	Intermediate	Dark
Bone Marrow	Bright	Intermediate	Dark
Nerve	Intermediate	Intermediate	Intermediate

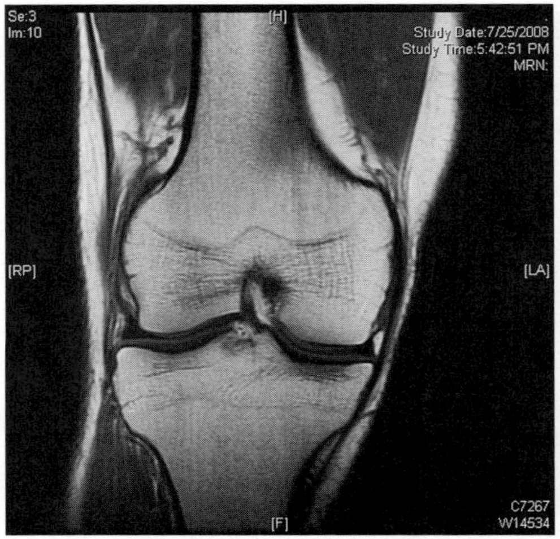

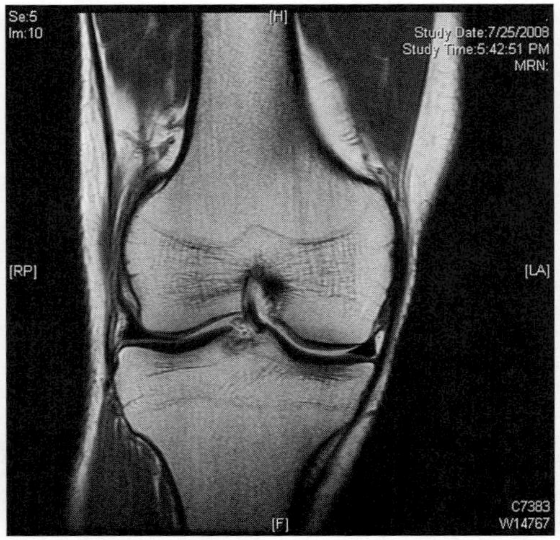

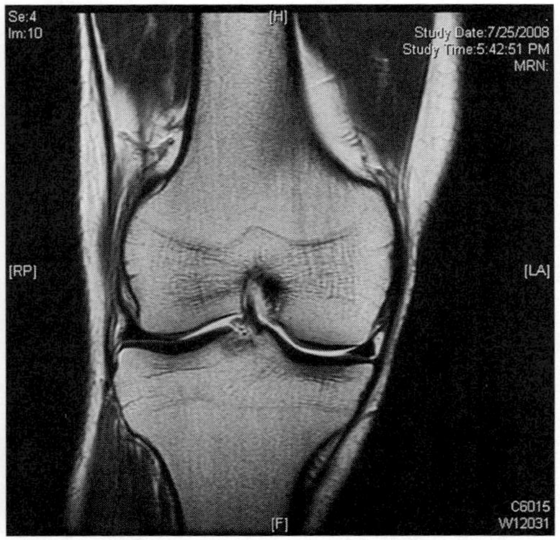

*Includes bone marrow.
**Includes edema, most tears, and most cysts.
***Includes labrum, menisci, triangular fibrocartilage.
****Signal may be increased because of artifacts.

MRI images are referenced from the frontal, sagittal, and transverse planes. They are read using a legend that numbers the slices as they progress through the body part. Each image can be referenced back to the legend image to determine where the slice is located. Sprains or other connective tissue damage involving loss of tissue continuity, fluid accumulation, or nerve entrapment are common pathologies that can be discovered via MRI (Fig. 5-11).

Bone Scan

Bone scans are a form of nuclear medicine used to detect bony abnormalities that are not normally visible on a standard radiograph. The patient receives an injection of a **radionuclide**, technetium-99m (Tc-99m), a **tracer element** that is absorbed by areas of bone undergoing excessive remodeling, or hotspots. These areas appear as darkened spots on the image and must be correlated with clinical signs and symptoms (Fig. 5-12). Bone scans can identify common pathologies, including degenerative disease, bone tumors, and stress fractures of the long bones and the vertebrae.[7]

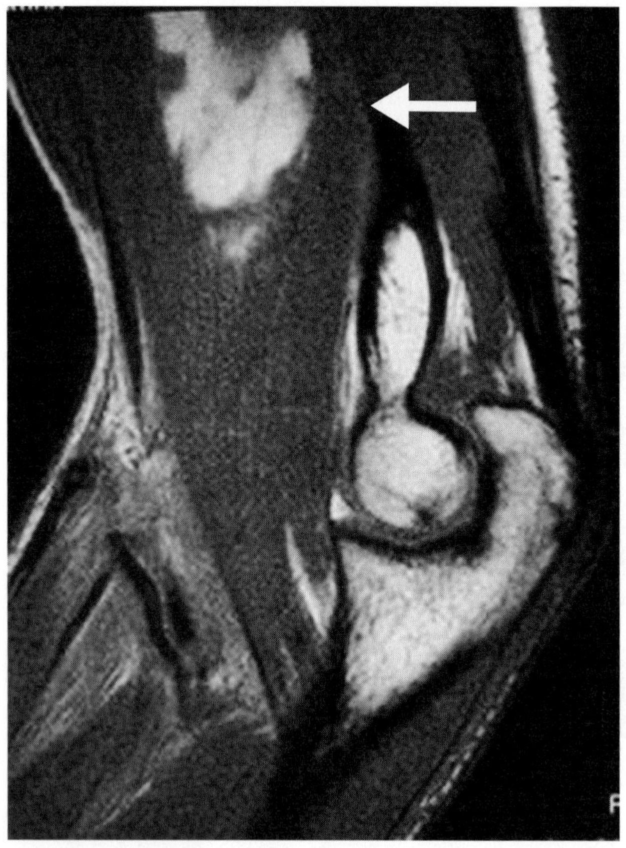

FIGURE 5-11 ■ MRI of a soft tissue injury. The arrow is indicating a hematoma in the right brachialis muscle (medial view).

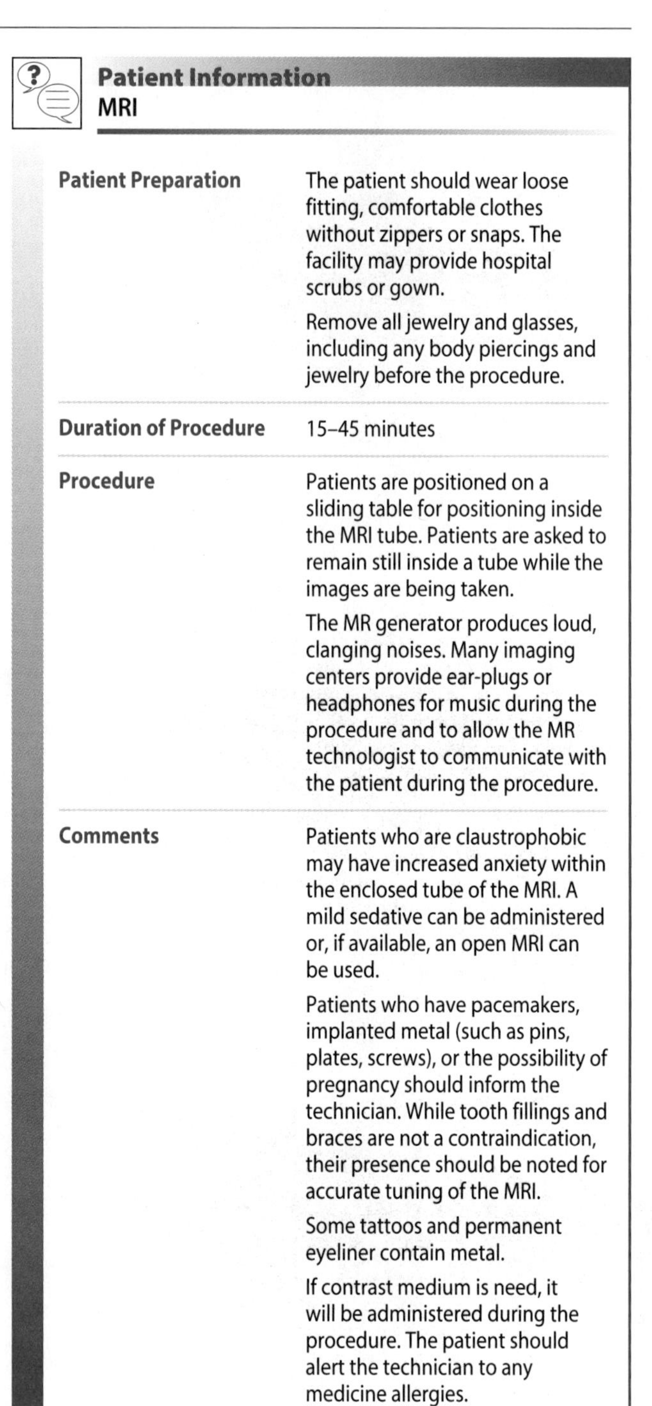

Patient Information
MRI

Patient Preparation	The patient should wear loose fitting, comfortable clothes without zippers or snaps. The facility may provide hospital scrubs or gown. Remove all jewelry and glasses, including any body piercings and jewelry before the procedure.
Duration of Procedure	15–45 minutes
Procedure	Patients are positioned on a sliding table for positioning inside the MRI tube. Patients are asked to remain still inside a tube while the images are being taken. The MR generator produces loud, clanging noises. Many imaging centers provide ear-plugs or headphones for music during the procedure and to allow the MR technologist to communicate with the patient during the procedure.
Comments	Patients who are claustrophobic may have increased anxiety within the enclosed tube of the MRI. A mild sedative can be administered or, if available, an open MRI can be used. Patients who have pacemakers, implanted metal (such as pins, plates, screws), or the possibility of pregnancy should inform the technician. While tooth fillings and braces are not a contraindication, their presence should be noted for accurate tuning of the MRI. Some tattoos and permanent eyeliner contain metal. If contrast medium is need, it will be administered during the procedure. The patient should alert the technician to any medicine allergies.

Diagnostic Ultrasound

Defects in soft tissue structures, primarily superficial muscle, the Achilles tendon, patellar tendon, and rotator cuff can be identified using diagnostic ultrasound (sonograms). Some internal organs, the testes, breasts, and fetus can also be viewed using sonograms. Diagnostic ultrasound uses sound waves having a frequency between

Radionuclide An atom undergoing disintegration, emitting electromagnetic radiation.

Tracer element A substance that is introduced into the tissues to follow or trace an otherwise unidentifiable substance or event.

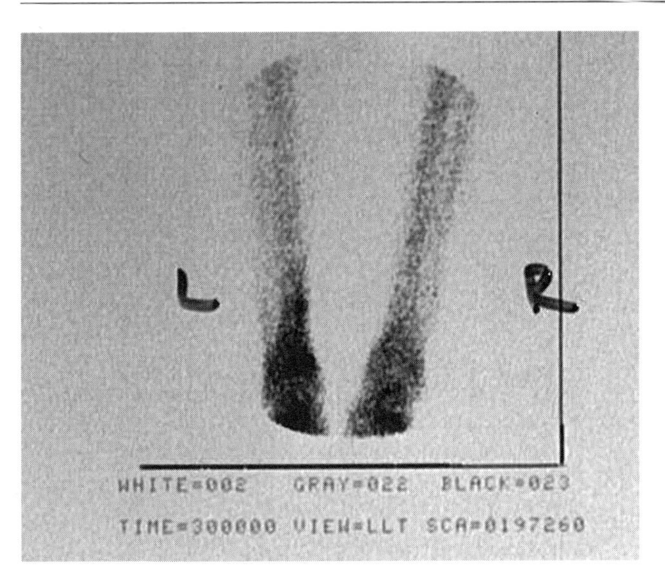

FIGURE 5-12 ■ Bone scan of the lower extremity. The darkened areas indicate "hot spots" of high uptake of the tracer element.

Patient Information
Bone Scan

Patient Preparation	The patient should wear comfortable clothing.
Duration of Procedure	Depends on type of scan and the time it takes for radioactive tracer to reach the target tissue. The imaging procedure itself takes 20–45 minutes.
Procedure	The radioactive agent is delivered into a vein. After waiting the proscribed period, the patient is asked to lie still on a table while the detector obtains and records the data.
Comments	Patients who are—or may be—pregnant should inform the technician. Patients should inform the technician of any allergies to medications.

1 and 15 **megahertz** (MHz) depending on the depth and type of tissues being imaged.

The frequency of the ultrasonic energy used is inversely proportional to the depth of the target tissue. Superficial structures such as muscle and tendon require energy with a higher frequency, normally in the range of 7 to 15 MHz. Imaging of deep internal organs require energy with a lower frequency.

A piezoelectric transducer delivers a brief pulse of ultrasonic energy into the tissues, then "listens" for a return echo. A computer interprets the strength of the returning sound wave and converts this information to display the type and depth of each structure (Fig. 5-13). The resulting image presents the tissues in cross section. Advanced units can generate color and three-dimensional images of the tissues.

Sonograms are relatively inexpensive and easy to obtain, but the quality of the resulting image is significantly influenced by the skill of the individual operating the unit. In some cases, the quality of images obtained from obese

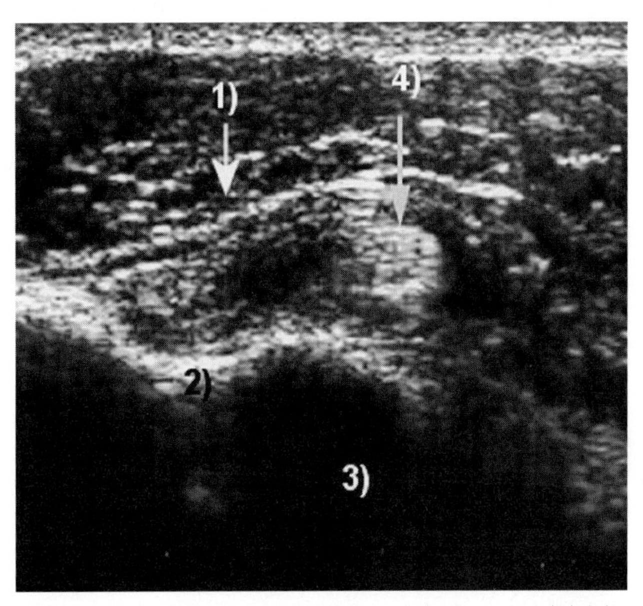

FIGURE 5-13 ■ Ultrasonic image (sonogram) showing a medial dislocation of the long head of the biceps brachii tendon. (1) pectoralis major tendon; (2) empty bicipital groove; (3) humerus; (4) displaced long head of the biceps tendon. (Courtesy of McKinnis, L. *Fundamentals of Musculoskeletal Imaging*, 2nd ed. Philadelphia, FA Davis, 2005, Figure 4-25, p 134.)

Patient Information
Diagnostic Ultrasound

Patient Preparation	The body part to be examined must be exposed. The patient should wear clothing that is easy to remove and put on.
Duration of Procedure	15–45 minutes
Procedure	The patient lies on a table. Gel, a coupling medium, is applied to the skin over the target and the technician runs the transducer head over the target area, capturing specific images on the computer.
Comments	Diagnostic ultrasound should not be confused with therapeutic ultrasound.

Megahertz One million cycles per second.

patients may be degraded as the result of scattering of the ultrasonic energy as it passes through dense pockets of adipose tissue. An equal level of skill is required to interpret the resulting image.

Nerve Conduction Study/ Electromyography

Nerve conduction studies (NCS) and electromyography (EMG) are diagnostic techniques used to detect pathology in peripheral nerves and the muscles they innervate. The techniques are performed by a trained health practitioner, often a neurologist or **physiatrist**. Peripheral nerve entrapments (such as carpal tunnel syndrome, tarsal tunnel syndrome), neurotmesis, nerve root injury, or muscle diseases such as **muscular dystrophy** and **myasthenia gravis** can be detected via NCS/EMG.

A motor NCS is used to examine motor peripheral nerve function and detect pathology along its path. In this procedure, the peripheral nerve is stimulated with an electrical current and activity from a muscle innervated by the nerve is identified and recorded. Two primary measurements are obtained: (1) **latency,** the time it takes for the impulse to travel to the target muscle and (2) **amplitude**, the magnitude of the nerve's response (Fig. 5-14). Comparing the amplitude of the muscle's electrical activity to the initial current strength provides a measure of the nerve's health. By stimulating different points along a peripheral nerve, NCS can detect the location of entrapments and isolate the location of specific pathology. A NCS is usually conducted in conjunction with an electromyographic (EMG) study.

An EMG study is an invasive procedure that involves inserting a thin detecting needle electrode into the muscle. The initial electrical activity with insertion of the electrode, which follows a characteristic pattern in a healthy muscle, is noted. The electrical activity of the resting muscle is then assessed. In normal muscle, the muscle should be electrically inactive. Spontaneous activity, or depolarizations, at rest could be indicative of muscle pathology. Finally, the patient is then asked to contract the muscle. The shape, size, and frequency of motor unit action potentials are noted.

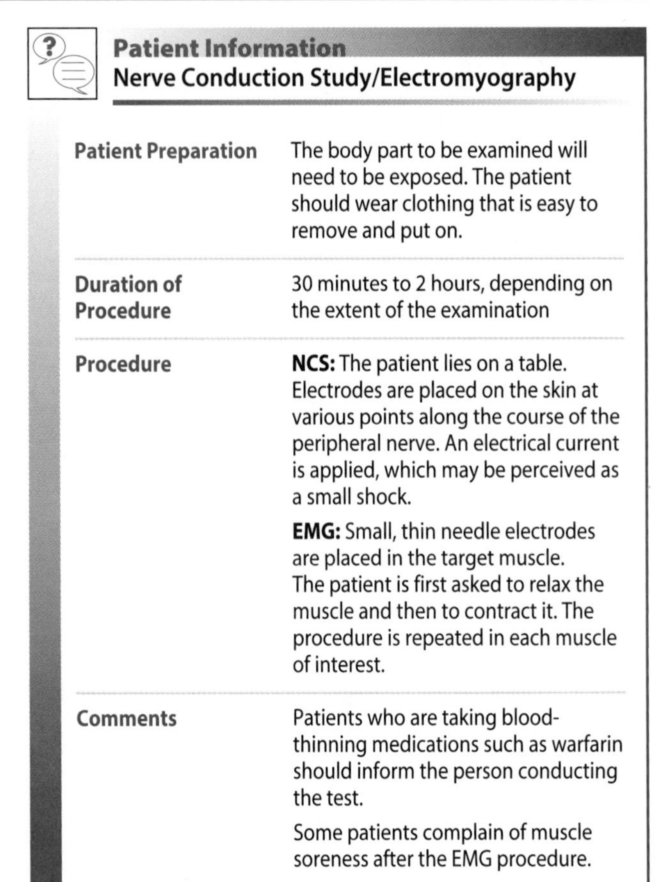

Patient Information
Nerve Conduction Study/Electromyography

Patient Preparation	The body part to be examined will need to be exposed. The patient should wear clothing that is easy to remove and put on.
Duration of Procedure	30 minutes to 2 hours, depending on the extent of the examination
Procedure	**NCS:** The patient lies on a table. Electrodes are placed on the skin at various points along the course of the peripheral nerve. An electrical current is applied, which may be perceived as a small shock. **EMG:** Small, thin needle electrodes are placed in the target muscle. The patient is first asked to relax the muscle and then to contract it. The procedure is repeated in each muscle of interest.
Comments	Patients who are taking blood-thinning medications such as warfarin should inform the person conducting the test. Some patients complain of muscle soreness after the EMG procedure.

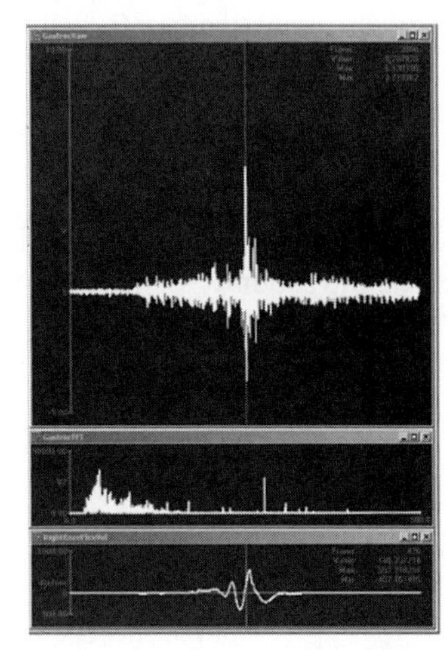

FIGURE 5-14 ■ EMG of a muscle innervated by the stimulated nerve.

Physiatrist A physician who specializes in physical medicine and rehabilitation.

Muscular dystrophy An inherited disease of the muscles causing progressive atrophy and weakness.

Myasthenia gravis A disease caused by a malfunction of the body's immune system, interrupting communication with motor nerves and causing weakness and fatigue.

REFERENCES

1. D'Orsi, CJ: Radiology and magnetic resonance imaging. In Greene, HL, Glassock, RJ, and Kelley, MA: *Introduction to Clinical Medicine*. Philadelphia, BC Decker, 1991, p 91.
2. Chakravarty, D, Sloan, J, and Brenchley, J: Risk reduction through skeletal scintigraphy as a screening tool in suspected scaphoid fracture: A literature review. *Emerg Med J*, 19:507, 2002.
3. Chakravarty, D, Sloan, J, and Brenchley, J: Risk reduction through skeletal scintigraphy as a screening tool in suspected scaphoid fracture: A literature review. *Emerg Med J*, 19:507, 2002.

4. Gaeta, M, et al: CT and MR imaging findings in athletes with early tibial stress injuries: Comparison with bone scintigraphy findings and emphasis on cortical abnormalities. *Radiology*, 235:553, 2005.
5. Schuerger, SR: Introduction to critical review of roentgengrams. *Phys Ther*, 68:1114, 1988.
6. Johnson, TR, and Steinbach, LS (eds): *Essentials of Musculoskeletal Imaging*. Rosemont, IL, American Academy of Orthopaedic Surgery, 2004, p 12.
7. Patton, DO, and Doherty, PN: Nuclear medicine studies. In Greene, HL, Glassock, RJ, and Kelley, MA: *Introduction to Clinical Medicine*. Philadelphia, BC Decker, 1991, p 81.

CHAPTER 6

Assessment of Posture

The term *posture* is used to describe the position of the body at a given point in time. Ideal posture is characterized by specific landmarks being aligned with the force of gravity, minimizing energy expenditure and maximizing function.[1] Proper posture requires the least amount of muscular effort, resulting in reduced stress on the joints and surrounding structures. Correct posture can improve performance, decrease abnormal stresses, and reduce the development of pathological conditions. Poor posture in and of itself usually does not prompt people to seek medical attention.

Faulty posture produces an increased amount of muscular activity and places increased stress on the joints and surrounding soft tissues.[2] Clinically, it is difficult to determine if the faulty posture is the result of muscle imbalances, caused by overuse of certain muscles during the **activities of daily living** (ADLs), or if these imbalances are the result of faulty posture. Restrictions in normal movement patterns may cause the body to acquire compensatory postures that still allow a functional motion to occur. Over time, these postures can result in adaptive changes and soft tissue dysfunction.[3]

Postural assessment is used to identify postural deviations that may be contributing to the patient's pain or dysfunction. The postural examination begins with the patient in a standing or sitting position, but can progress to include the dynamic postures of walking and running (see Chapter 7).[4] Static positions assessed in a medical facility may not replicate the postures that the patient normally assumes during athletic, school, home, or work activities.

This chapter presents the relationship between correct posture, common postural deviations, and associated pain and dysfunction. The cause-and-effect relationship between faulty posture, common compensatory motions, and associated musculoskeletal dysfunctions is also discussed.

Activities of daily living (ADLs) The skills and motions required for the day-to-day activities of life.

Clinical Anatomy

Before understanding how deviations in one region of the body affect another region, a review of basic anatomical and biomechanical concepts is needed. The musculoskeletal system is designed to function in a mechanically and physiologically efficient manner to use the least possible amount of energy. The change in position of one joint results in a predictable change in position of the other interrelated joints.[5] When a postural deviation or skeletal malalignment occurs, other joints in the kinetic chain undergo compensatory motions or postures to allow the body to continue to function as efficiently as possible. For example, a forward shoulder posture can result from tightness of the pectoralis minor. This, in turn, changes the functional positions of the scapula and may predispose the patient to chronic shoulder pain.[6,7]

The Kinetic Chain

The musculoskeletal system is a series of kinetic chains in which different joints are directly or indirectly linked to each other (Fig. 6-1). In a kinetic chain, movement occurring at one joint causes motion at an adjacent joint, creating a "chain reaction" of movements up or down the associated kinetic chain. Kinetic chains are classified as **open chain** (non–weight-bearing) or **closed chain** (weight-bearing). Because the definition of open- and closed kinetic chain motions become blurred, the terms "weight-bearing" and "non–weight-bearing" are often used instead. The lower extremity-pelvis-lumbar complex functions primarily in a closed kinetic chain; the upper extremity, scapulothoracic, and cervical spine function primarily in an open kinetic chain.[7,8]

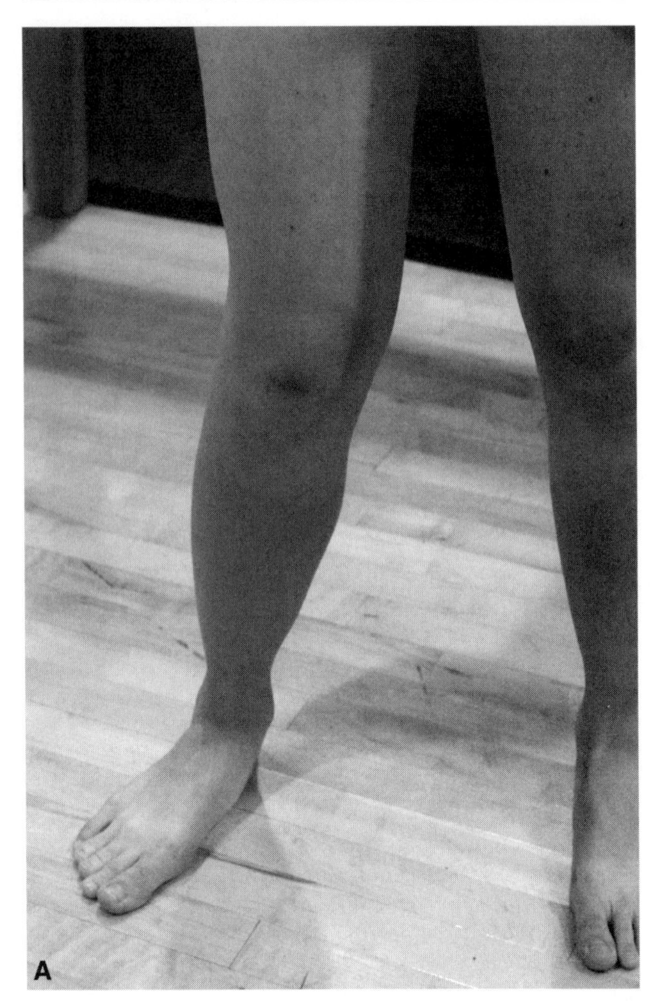

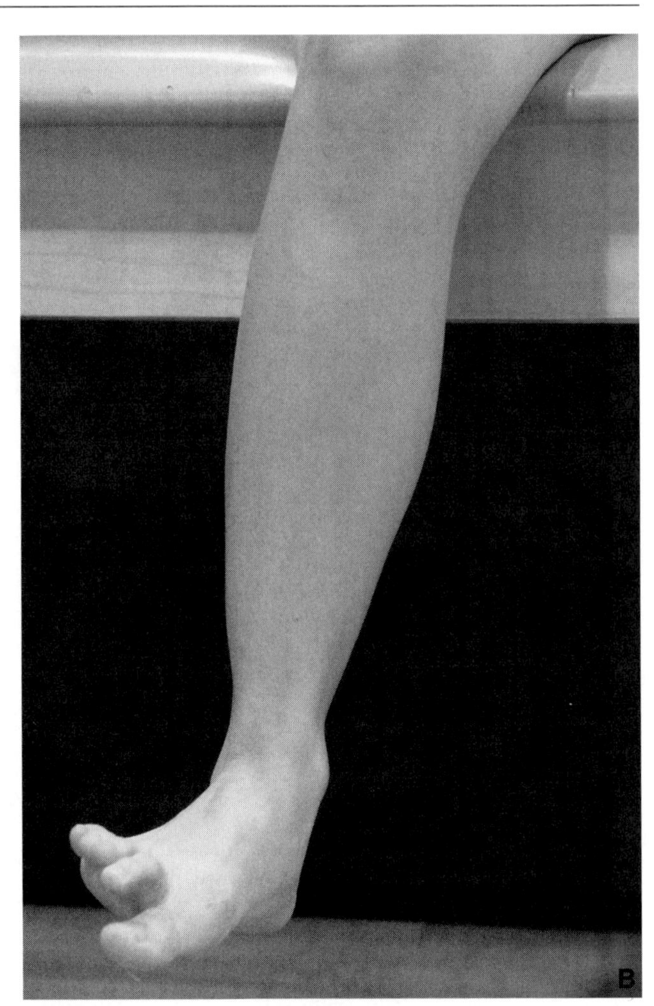

FIGURE 6-1 ■ **(A)** Weight-bearing and **(B)** non-weight-bearing examples of kinetic chains in the musculoskeletal system.

A closed kinetic chain is formed when the distal segment meets sufficient resistance or is fixated, such as the weight-bearing limb during walking or the upper extremity during push-ups or weight lifting. Because of the interdependency of each joint within a closed chain, the associated joints undergo predictable changes in position in response to a change in position of another joint along the chain. This can be demonstrated by standing up and "rolling" the foot inward. When maximum pronation is reached, the ankle naturally dorsiflexes, the tibia internally rotates, the knee flexes, and the hip internally rotates and flexes (see Fig. 6-1A). In an open kinetic chain the distal portion of the chain (the distal extremity) moves freely in space. When the inward rolling of the foot used in the closed kinetic chain is repeated with the foot non–weight-bearing, only the foot pronates and motion does not occur at the joints proximal to the foot and ankle (see Fig. 6-1B).

Kinetic chains are the underlying principle in determining the cause of postural deviations. Soft tissue dysfunction or bony anomaly occurring in one part of the kinetic chain can affect the proximal or distal joints and soft tissues along the chain, causing a specific postural deviation (Table 6-1).[8] The body attempts to compensate for these deviations to maintain efficient movement. An example of this compensatory strategy involves a structural condition of the foot called **forefoot varus**. If the body were unable to compensate for the abnormal position of the forefoot, a person would walk on the outside of the foot, not a very functional or efficient motion. To maximize propulsion and reduce the effect on gait, the foot compensates to forefoot varus by excessively pronating at the subtalar joint (STJ) and midtarsal joints to reach a foot-flat position (Fig. 6-2).

Compensatory postures can produce symptoms when joint range of motion (ROM) is excessive and produces joint stress; is excessive in its duration; or occurs at, or within, an inappropriate time.[5,9] If one motion is restricted, other joints in the area must compensate to allow for greater efficiency of movement.[10]

Adhesive capsulitis is another example of a soft tissue pathology that can alter the kinetic chain. In adhesive capsulitis, the **arthrokinematic** motions of the glenohumeral (GH) joint are decreased, prohibiting normal humeral elevation. Because the scapulothoracic articulation is included in the upper extremity kinetic chain, it compensates

Table 6-1 Examples of Compensatory Strategies of the Body

Compensatory Strategies				
Skeletal Malalignment	**Subtalar Joint**	**Tibiofemoral Joint**	**Hip Joint**	**Pelvis and Lumbar Spine**
Forefoot or Rearfoot Varus	Excessive and/or prolonged Pronation	Flexion Internal tibial rotation	Flexion Internal femoral rotation	Anterior rotation and excessive lumbar extension
Forefoot or Rearfoot Valgus	Early supination	Extension External tibial rotation	Extension External femoral rotation	Posterior rotation and excessive flexion

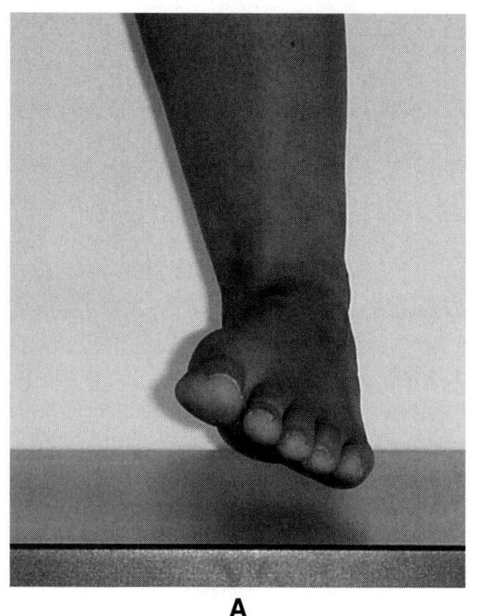
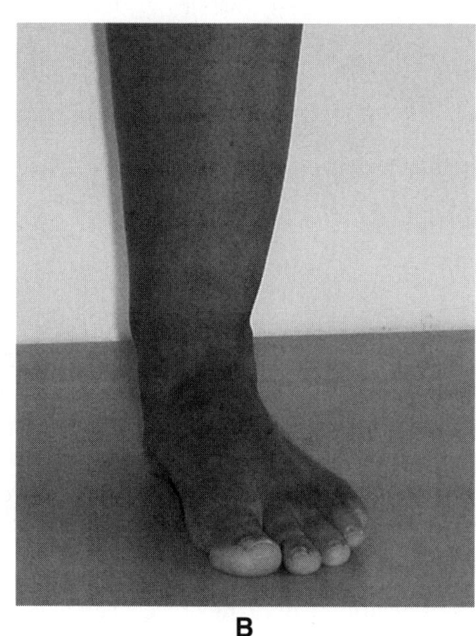

FIGURE 6-2 ■ **(A)** Uncompensated (STJ neutral) and **(B)** Compensated forefoot varus.

for the hypomobility of the GH joint by allowing excessive upward scapular rotation to permit functional humeral elevation (Fig. 6-3). When compensatory movement patterns or postures occur over a prolonged period they become "learned" and the body interprets them as being correct.[10]

Not all compensatory postures are detrimental. Some allow the body to function more efficiently, with less discomfort, or both. Such is the case for someone with **stenosis** in the lumbar spine. The individual assumes a flexed posture in the lumbar spine (decreased lumbar **lordosis**) to increase the otherwise narrowed space in the vertebral canal caused by stenosis. All the findings obtained during a postural evaluation must be interpreted before attempting to correct a compensatory postural deviation.

Muscular Function

Muscle contractions produce joint motion and provide dynamic **joint stability**. To perform these tasks properly, the muscles must have an optimal length–tension relationship. Muscles that are functionally too short or too long can produce adverse stress on the joints, work inefficiently, or create the need for compensatory motions during activity (Table 6-2). Different abnormal postures provide clues as to which muscles might be problematically shortened or lengthened. For example, increased lordosis is commonly associated with lengthened abdominal muscles. A passive insufficiency is created, making the abdominals less capable of working effectively.

Muscular Length–Tension Relationships

The **muscular length–tension relationship** describes the effect of muscle length and the amount of tension (force) produced. The tension-developing capacity of a muscle

Arthrokinematic Action and reaction of articular surfaces as a joint travels through its range of motion.

Stenosis (spinal) A narrowing of the vertebral foramen through which the spinal cord or spinal nerve root pass.

Lordosis Anterior curvature of the spine.

Joint stability The integrity of a joint when it is placed under a functional load.

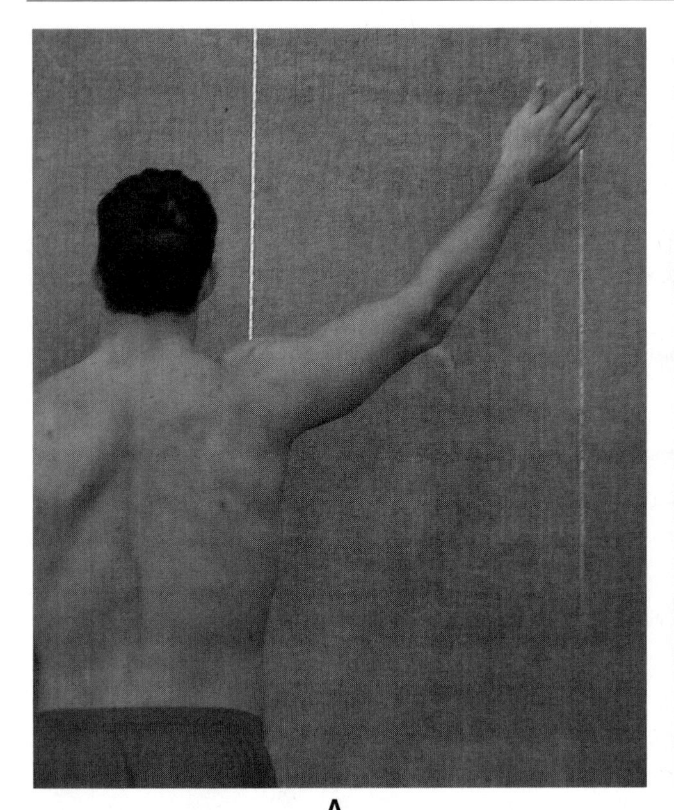

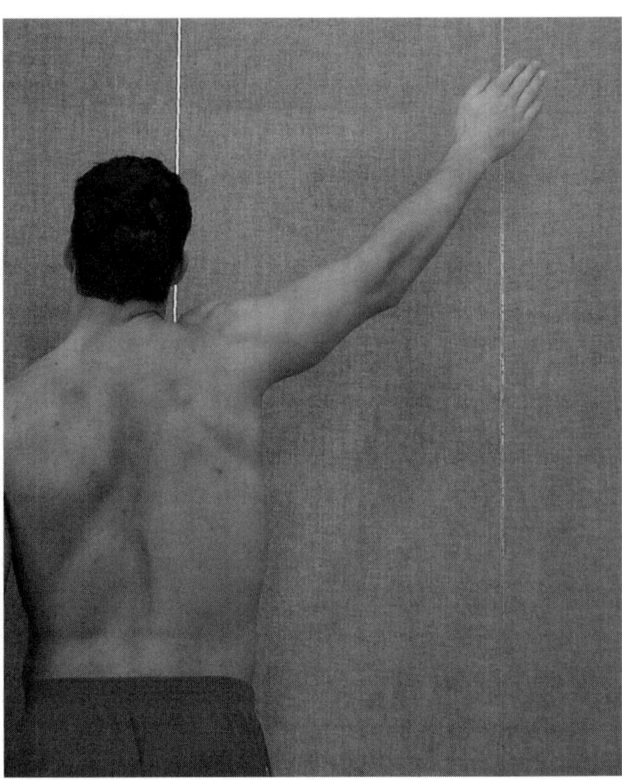

FIGURE 6-3 ■ **(A)** Normal scapulohumeral elevation. **(B)** Scapulohumeral elevation compensated with increased upper trapezius activity.

occurs within the **sarcomere** unit at the crossbridges formed between **actin** and **myosin** myofilaments. The optimal relationship between length and tension is the joint position where the muscle can generate the greatest amount of tension with the least amount of effort. At this length, the crossbridges between actin and myosin filaments within the sarcomere are at their most efficient position.

If a muscle is shortened or lengthened the interaction of crossbridges between actin and myosin filaments is reduced because there is either too much or too little overlap (Fig. 6-4). **Active insufficiency** occurs when a muscle is shortened and the actin and myosin myofilaments are overlapped to the point where maximum tension cannot be produced. **Passive insufficiency** occurs when the muscle is lengthened and the actin and myosin myofilaments lack sufficient overlap to generate force. In passive insufficiency, the muscle cannot generate sufficient tension to be effective in providing proper movement or stability.[10]

Table 6-2 Muscle Length and the Ability to Perform Function

Muscle Length	Ability to Provide Mobility	Ability to Provide Stability
Normal	Efficient	Efficient
Shortened	Inefficient	Efficient
Elongated	Efficient	Inefficient

Agonist and Antagonist Relationships

A muscle that contracts to perform the primary movement of a joint is termed the **agonist muscle**. The **antagonist muscle** performs the opposite movement of the agonist muscle and must reflexively relax to allow the agonist's motion to occur. This reflexive response is termed **reciprocal inhibition**. The biceps brachii and triceps brachii muscles are an example of agonist and antagonist muscles. During elbow flexion, the biceps brachii is the agonist performing the action of elbow flexion. The antagonist is the triceps brachii because it performs the opposite motion of elbow extension. The triceps brachii must reflexively relax and elongate while the biceps brachii contracts to allow normal, smooth elbow flexion. If an antagonist muscle did not receive an inhibitory impulse to relax, but instead received an excitatory stimulus of the same magnitude as the agonist, the joint would not move because both sets of muscles would be equally contracting.

The concurrent contraction of the agonist and antagonist muscles, **co-contraction**, is a technique often used

---

Sarcomere A portion of striated muscle fiber lying between two membranes.

Actin A contractile muscle protein.

Myosin A contractile muscle protein.

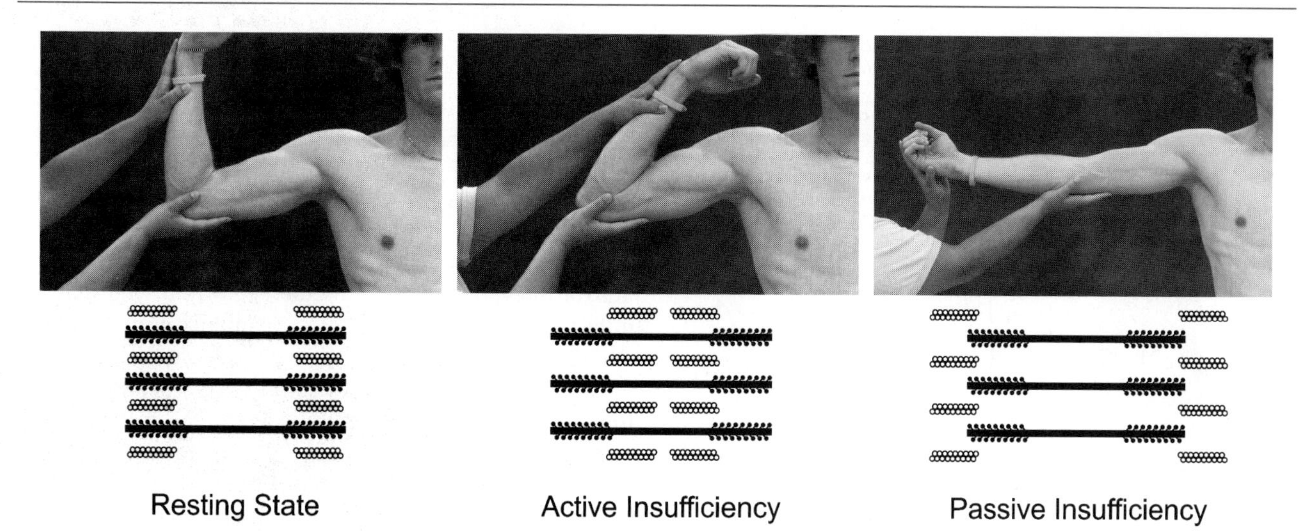

FIGURE 6-4 ■ Relationship of actin and myosin cross bridges. When the muscle is in its resting state, there is full communication between the actin and myosin, allowing for a strong contraction. Active insufficiency is created when the muscle has maximally shortened to its fullest point and the filaments can no longer slide. When the muscle is fully elongated, passive insufficiency, there is decreased communication between the actin and myosin, decreasing the strength the muscle can generate.

when restoring the dynamic stability of a joint. The smooth, deliberate movements of the body during normal ADLs are allowed to occur because of this excitatory/inhibitory reflex loop between the agonist and antagonist muscle groups. Proper balance between the lengths of the agonist and antagonist muscle groups is also necessary to maintain correct posture and avoid undue stress on the involved joints.

Muscle Imbalances

Length–tension relationships and agonist versus antagonist muscles allow us to better understand the implications of muscle imbalance. Muscle imbalances are characterized by an impaired relationship between a muscle that is overactivated, subsequently shortened and tightened and another that is inhibited and weakened.[11] Table 6-3 lists some of the common causes of muscle imbalances.

Different muscle types exhibit different patterns of activity in response to pain, postural deviations, or soft tissue dysfunction.[10,11] Skeletal muscles are classified as either postural (also referred to as tonic) or phasic (Table 6-4). Postural muscles primarily function to support the body against the forces of gravity. They are composed of a higher percentage of slow twitch muscle fibers, are slower to fatigue, and do not respond as quickly when activated.[11] Postural muscles have a greater tendency to become overactivated and shortened in response to stresses or pain (Fig. 6-5). **Trigger points** are hypersensitive soft tissue manifestations commonly seen in postural muscles undergoing stresses.[11]

Phasic muscles are primarily responsible for movement of the body. With a higher proportion of fast twitch muscle fibers than postural muscles, phasic muscles contract more quickly and generate a greater amount of force. Phasic muscles tend to rapidly fatigue because of the higher percentage

Table 6-3 Causes of Muscle Imbalances

Cause	Result
Nerve Pathology	Paralysis, muscle weakness, or muscle spindle inhibition
Pain	Inhibition or muscle spasm
Joint Effusion	Reflexive inhibition of muscle
Poor Posture	Alteration in muscle length–tension relationship
Repetitive Activity of One Muscle Group	Adaptive shortening and increased recruitment

Table 6-4 Postural versus Phasic Muscles

Characteristic	Postural Muscles	Phasic Muscles
Function	Support body against forces of gravity	Movement of the body
Muscle Fiber Type	Higher percentage of slow-twitch fibers	Higher percentage of fast-twitch fibers
Response to Dysfunction	Become overactivated and tightened or shortened	Become inhibited and weakened
Common Soft Tissue Dysfunction	Prone to trigger points	Prone to strains and tendinopathies

Trigger point A pathological condition characterized by a small, hypersensitive area located within muscles and fasciae.

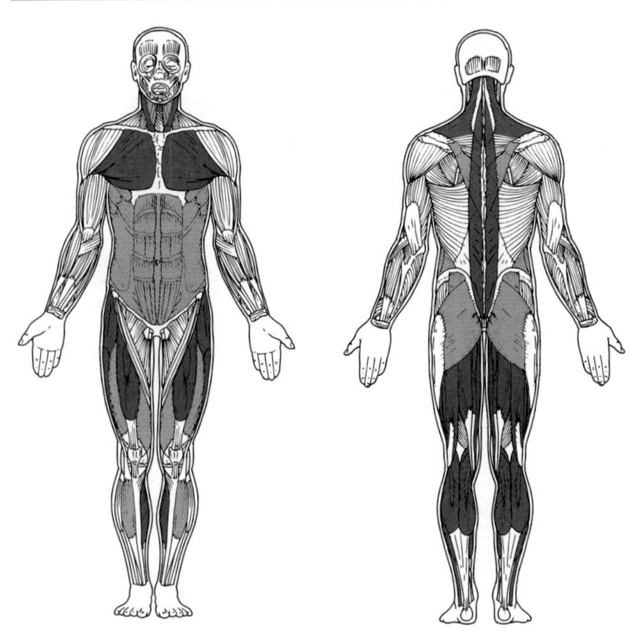

FIGURE 6-5 ■ Postural and phasic muscles. Red = Postural; Tan = Phasic

Common Postural Muscles	Common Phasic Muscles
Sternocleidomastoid	Scalenes
Pectoralis major	Subscapularis
Upper trapezius	Lower trapezius
Levator scapula	Rhomboids
Quadratus lumborum	Serratus anterior
Iliopsoas	Rectus abdominis
Tensor fascia latae	Internal obliques
Rectus femoris	External obliques
Piriformis	Gluteus minimus
Hamstring group	Gluteus maximus
Short hip adductors	Gluteus medius
Gastrocnemius	Vastus medialis
Soleus	Vastus lateralis
Erector spinae	Tibialis anterior
Longissimus thoracic	Peroneals
Multifidus or rotatores	
Tibialis posterior	

of fast twitch fibers and have a greater tendency to become weak and inhibited in response to pain.[11] Muscle strains and tendinopathies are common soft tissue dysfunctions seen in phasic muscles.

When a muscle becomes overactivated and shortened and its antagonist is weakened, the muscular balance around the joint changes. The overactivated muscle influence the manner that the underlying joint (or joints) move and alter the compressive or tensile forced placed on the joint.[10] Muscle imbalances expend more energy and create inefficient and stressful movement patterns and postures for the body.[11,12]

When designing a rehabilitation program to correct a muscle imbalance, the initial emphasis is on elongating the shortened, overactivated muscle group before strengthening the inhibited and weakened group. An inhibited, weakened muscle cannot sufficiently gain strength until the antagonist muscle is closely restored to its normal muscle length.[11]

Noncontractile Soft Tissue Influences

Muscle imbalances can also lead to abnormal compressive and/or shear forces being produced within the joint. A joint's capsule and surrounding ligaments undergo adaptive changes (i.e., remodeling) from prolonged overstressing or understressing. Faulty posture and associated muscle imbalances can alter the joint position, causing increased stress on different portions of the joint capsule and surrounding ligaments. While areas of a joint capsule that are continually stressed may elongate, areas that are slack and not stressed (usually on the opposite side of the tensile forces) may undergo adaptive shortening. The shoulder provides an example of a common noncontractile soft tissue imbalance. A person who has acquired pronounced rounded, forward shoulders can experience adaptive shortening of the posterior portion of the GH capsule and elongation of the anterior portion of the GH capsule. To compensate for forward shoulder posture, the humeral head externally rotates to allow the hands to assume a more functional posture. This reduces normal stresses on the posterior capsule, which, in turn, adaptively shortens. This position is further exaggerated as the anterior chest muscles adaptively shorten to maintain the posture while the posterior muscles—the middle and lower trapezius and serratus anterior—elongate.

Clinical Examination of Posture

Posture plays both direct and indirect roles in the onset of overuse injuries. Overuse injuries are characterized by pain with an insidious onset, usually brought on by repetitive tasks performed in specific postures.[13] When evaluating a musculoskeletal injury, general observation of posture must occur early in the examination process.

The clinical examination of posture is not an exact science.[14–16] Although the use of radiographs, photographs, and computer analyses are the most objective and accurate methods for determining skeletal postural deviations,[17,18] clinical tools such as **plumb lines**, goniometers, flexible rulers, and inclinometers can increase the validity and reliability of the inspection process (Fig. 6-6).[18]

Clinically, posture can be described by the terms normal, mild (25% deviation from normal), moderate (50% deviation), and severe (75% deviation).[18] This subjective method for quantifying postural deviations demonstrates fair to poor inter-tester reliability.[18] Whenever possible, use measurements to further quantify the skeletal malalignments

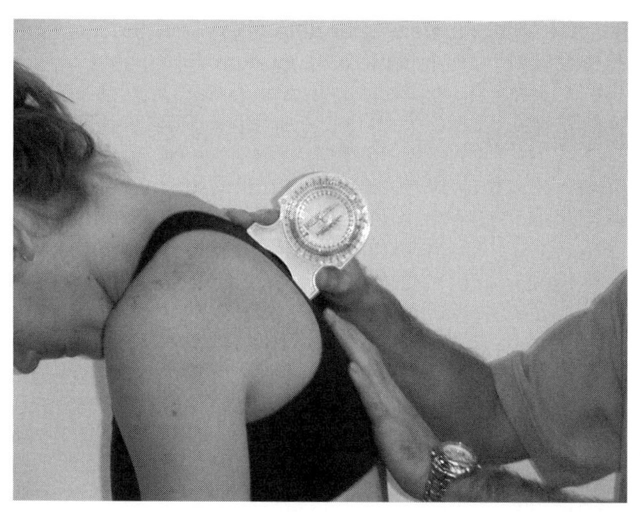

FIGURE 6-6 ■ An inclinometer can also be used to the measure range of motion.

causing postural deviations. Objective, quantifiable measurements can also assist in determining whether the current treatment plan is effective and if the patient's posture is improving.

The use of inspection and palpation in the assessment of posture varies from that during the examination of specific body areas. Although inspection and palpation are described as separate entities in this chapter, in practice these two segments occur simultaneously, each validating or refuting the findings of the other. As posture is being observed, the clinician simultaneously palpates to determine specific positions of joints and structures. The use of palpation to identify painful areas is not emphasized during the assessment of posture.

Posture is commonly assessed in two positions: standing and sitting. In addition, assessing posture in any other static or dynamic positions that produce the patient's symptoms should also be performed, including postures assumed by the patient for prolonged periods during the day or during normal ADLs. Certain movements can be performed before assessing a person's posture to assist in reinforcing that a natural, habitual posture is being assumed. The patient can be instructed to perform a sequence of movements referred to as the **orthoposition** and self-balancing position to obtain a relatively natural posture. Ask the patient to[19,20]:

1. March in place 10 times.
2. Roll the shoulders forward and backward three times.
3. Nod the head and neck forward and backward five times.
4. Inhale and exhale deeply.

Plumb line A string and pendulum that hangs perpendicular to surface.

Orthoposition Normal or properly aligned posture.

History

A thorough history assists in determining whether postural dysfunction is contributing to the patient's pathology and symptoms (Table 6-5). Repetitive tasks while maintaining a certain posture can lead to overuse injuries as well, so the history needs to identify any repetitive motions that are routinely performed.

If the mechanism of injury (MOI) for a particular injury has an insidious onset and symptoms have gradually increased over time, then the history needs to investigate further the person's day-to-day tasks and postures. If the MOI can be traced to a specific force at a particular time, the history determines the factors that might have predisposed the patient to the injury. However, in this case, improper posture may have contributed to the present symptoms.

The following information should be obtained to determine whether posture is contributing to the current pathology.

*** Practical Evidence**

As the weight of a book backpack increases, there is a proportional increase in the risk of onset of low back pain in adolescents.[21]

Mechanism of injury

Many overuse injuries associated with postural faults have an insidious onset with no specific cause of the pain. A nonspecific mechanism or time of injury may indicate that

Table 6-5 Factors Influencing Posture

Factor	Example
Neurologic Pathology	Winging of the scapula secondary to inhibition of the long thoracic nerve
Muscle Imbalances	Increased pelvic angles secondary to weak abdominal muscles
Hypermobile Joints	Genu recurvatum
Hypomobile Joints	Flexion contracture
Decreased Muscle Extensibility	Decreased pelvic angles secondary to tightness of the hamstring muscles
Bony Abnormalities	Toe in or toe out posture secondary to internal or external tibial torsion
Leg Length Discrepancies	Functional scoliosis
Pain	Antalgic posture (e.g., side bending cervical spine to decrease compression on a nerve root)
Lack of Postural Awareness	Acquired bad habits (e.g., slouching in chair)

the injury is possibly caused by poor posture. Common responses pointing toward possible postural involvement in an injury include:

- An insidious onset of pain
- Pain worsening as the day progresses
- Description of pain associated with specific posture
- Complaints of intermittent pain
- Vague or generalized pain descriptions
- Initially starting as an ache that has progressively worsened over time.

Type, location, and severity of symptoms

Are the symptoms constant or intermittent? Are they worse during a certain time of the day (i.e., morning, afternoon, evening)? Many postural dysfunctions are worse, or produce more symptoms, in the evening after the individual has maintained the posture all day. Which positions or postures increase or decrease the symptoms? Some activities, such as gymnastics, regularly require unusual postures. If the symptom is primarily pain, then what type of pain is it: burning, sharp, aching, pulsating? Is the patient experiencing paresthesia? If so, is it constant or intermittent?

Side dominance

Is the patient right or left side dominant? If one side is used for most, if not all tasks, then bilateral imbalances are likely to occur, exposing the patient to overuse injuries.

Activities of daily living

What is the patient's usual day like? Many people have repetitive daily schedules. Which types of activities does the patient perform and for what duration and frequency? To better understand the motions associated with specific pain-producing tasks, it is helpful to have the patient demonstrate specific motions as they are being described (Table 6-6).

Driving, sitting, and sleeping postures

Has anything been changed in the person's daily routine over the past few months (Table 6-7)? Changes in a routine often provide information about the instigating factor. For example, a change in mattress could provoke or decrease symptoms.

*** Practical Evidence**

A medium-firm mattress is associated with decreased pain and disability for individuals with low back pain.[23]

Level and intensity of exercise

Is exercise performed on a regular or sporadic basis or not at all? Has the exercise routine changed in any way? A rapid change in exercise duration or intensity may make a previously benign postural fault problematic.

Medical history

Has this problem occurred before? If so, was medical attention sought and what treatments were rendered? Are there any medical problems that should be identified? A general health questionnaire may be helpful to use before the evaluation to uncover any medical conditions.

Inspection

Ensure that the area used for postural assessment is private to protect the modesty of the patient and is at a comfortable temperature. When possible, males should wear only shorts that expose the majority of the legs. Females also wear shorts that expose most of their legs and a halter-type top that exposes the whole back. To allow observation of foot positions, shoes should not be worn. Do not alert the patient that posture is being assessed at this time. Patients who are aware that posture is being assessed will become conscious about their posture and may stand more erect than usual.

Use a systematic approach when assessing posture to avoid overlooking a specific region. The evaluation process may start at the foot and work superiorly or vice versa. This chapter describes posture starting at the feet and working superiorly. Whenever comparing bilaterally for symmetry, place your eyes at the same level as the region you are observing.

Overall impression

The first component of a postural assessment is the determination of the patient's general body type: ectomorph, mesomorph, or endomorph (Box 6-1). A person's body type is largely inherited and can influence the types of activity in which he or she may engage. For example, an ectomorph is more apt to be a distance runner than an endomorph. The Body Mass Index (BMI) is used describe the person's relative mass based on height and weight (Box 6-2).

Views of Postural Inspection

Posture is inspected from all views or planes with the body in orthoposition: lateral (sagittal plane), anterior (frontal plane), and posterior (frontal plane). A plumb line may be used to assist in identifying postural deviations. When using a plumb line, align the patient using the feet as the permanent landmark. Position the plumb line slightly anterior to the lateral malleolus from the lateral view and equidistant from both feet from the anterior and posterior views. Inspection Findings 6-1 presents ideal posture in each of the three planes.

Lateral view

Observation of posture from the lateral view involves making determinations of the anterior and posterior alignment relative to the frontal plane (see Inspection Box 6-1). Table 6-8 lists common postural deviations noted from the lateral view.

Anterior view

For the anterior view, the plumb line bisects the midline of the body in the sagittal plane. The major regions of the body are observed from this view and symmetry is compared

Table 6-6 Examples of Daily Stresses and Their Possible Resulting Pathologies

Activity	Associated Tasks	Possible Postural Deviations	Possible Soft Tissue Dysfunctions	Corrections
Desk Job	Computer use: Is the station ergonomically correct? Is it a multiuse station?	FHP, FSP, general postural faults caused by muscle fatigue or poor postural sense throughout trunk and upper quadrant	Soft tissue syndromes of the cervical, thoracic, and shoulder regions, including, myofascial syndromes, muscle imbalances, muscle strains, thoracic outlet syndrome, carpal tunnel syndrome, or other nerve entrapment syndromes throughout the upper extremity	1. Proper ergonomic design of work station 2. Frequent breaks with performance of postural exercises and stretches 3. Maintenance of proper sitting posture at work
	Telephone use: How is the phone held? Is the phone cradled between the ear and shoulder? Is the same side used?	Prolonged cervical lateral flexion, shoulder elevation	Adaptive shortening of cervical lateral flexors, lengthening of contralateral muscles, myofascial syndromes in all the above areas mentioned, joint or nerve root related problems in the cervical spine caused by compression of one side (narrowing of intervertebral foramen and compression of the ipsilateral facet joints)	Use of a telephone headset to maintain the head in the neutral position and leave the hands free to perform other tasks with minimal strain
	What type of chair is used? Is it ergonomically correct?	Inadequate lumbar support: Leads to "slouched" posture and flexed lumbar, thoracic spine, FSP, and FHP Inadequate arm rests: Leads to increased upper extremity work causing fatigue of shoulder girdle muscles	Muscle imbalances throughout trunk, shoulder girdle region, upper extremities; myofascial syndromes; TOS at any of three entrapment sites (anterior or mid scalenes, first rib and clavicle, pectoralis minor and rib cage); other nerve entrapment syndromes	1. Ergonomically correct chair with adequate lumbar support and arm rests at correct height 2. The chair placed correctly in front of the computer and not angled to perform computer work and other tasks at the same time. 3. Frequent breaks from computer work to perform postural exercises or stretches 4. Maintenance of proper sitting posture at work.
	Are bifocals worn? Are regular glasses worn and is the prescription up-to-date? Is there glare on the computer screen?	FHP, FSP from straining to read the screen	TMJ dysfunctions; myofascial syndromes; joint and nerve dysfunctions; muscle imbalances; headaches	1. Change of computer screen angle or height 2. Change of glasses as needed 3. Use of anti-glare screens and shields; decrease in glare from overhead fluorescent lighting

Continued

Table 6-6 Examples of Daily Stresses and Their Possible Resulting Pathologies—cont'd

Activity	Associated Tasks	Possible Postural Deviations	Possible Soft Tissue Dysfunctions	Corrections
Manual Labor	Frequency of bending, lifting, repetitive motions? (If possible, the patient should demonstrate the actual positions assumed and motions performed.)	Improper bending encompassing flexed lumbar spine; decreased use of leg muscles or increased use of back muscles; flexed thoracic and cervical spine with increased stress of soft tissue structures of back; combined motions of lumbar spine flexion and rotation	Muscle imbalance; myofascial syndrome; muscle strains or ligamentous sprains; joint or disc pathology	1. Teach proper lifting technique: maintenance of neutral spine; flexing at hips; use of legs rather than back muscles; maintenance of cervical lordosis or thoracic kyphosis; use of pivoting with feet versus rotation of spine when turning 2. Perform extension exercises throughout day to counteract flexion 3. Use assistive devices to lift heavy objects; use more trips with less weight per trip; and use partner to lift heavy and bulky objects
	Repetitive overhead tasks?	Cervical spine in prolonged extension	Muscle imbalances; cervical spine facet joint or nerve compression; myofascial syndromes; with the presence of a FSP, patients are more prone to shoulder impingement syndromes	1. Frequent breaks from overhead activities 2. Use of stool or device to attempt to keep work at eye level
	Is any specific equipment used repetitively?	Repetitive motions with use of specific tool increasing stress on certain tissues	Muscle imbalances; tendinopathy; strains; nerve entrapment syndromes	1. Stretching of muscles used during operation of tools 2. Ergonomically correct tools
Student	Is a backpack used? How heavy is the backpack?	FHP; FSP; flexed trunk and lumbar spine	Myofascial syndromes; TOS; facet or disc pathology; muscle imbalances	1. Use of both shoulder straps while wearing backpack to avoid carrying the weight over one shoulder 2. Limiting the weight of the backpack to 10 to 15 percent of body weight for adolescents.[22]
Athletics	Sports and position? Frequency, duration and intensity of involvement?	Possible overuse injuries or overtraining techniques based on the sport and position played; identification of relationship between changes in the pattern of participation and the onset of symptoms (e.g., surfaces, direction)	Myofascial syndrome; muscle strains or ligamentous sprains; muscle imbalances	1. Conditioning to prepare specific tissues for the rigors of the sport and position. Proper stretching before and after participation 2. Change in training regimen as necessary 3. Change of position 4. Increased awareness of stresses

FHP = forward head posture; FSP = forward shoulder posture; TMJ = temporomandibular joint; TOS = thoracic outlet syndrome.

Table 6-7 Driving, Sitting, and Sleeping Postures

ADL	Posture	Possible Postural Deviations	Postural Correction
Driving	Inadequate lumbar support?	Flexion of lumbar spine and thoracic spine, FSP, and FHP	Use lumbar support cushion
	Reclined seat angle—hips flexed less than 90°?	Flexion of lumbar and thoracic spine; increased scapula protraction; excessive arm elevation to reach steering wheel; FSP; FHP	Adjust seat angle so hips are at 90° of flexion
	Seat distance too far from steering wheel and pedals?	Flexion of lumbar and thoracic spine; protraction of scapula; FSP; FHP; increased pelvis and leg activity to reach for pedals	Adjust seat distance so elbows and knees are flexed approximately 30°–45°; the hands should reach the steering wheel and the thoracic spine and scapula should maintain contact with the seatback
	Frequency, length of time spent driving?	Muscle imbalances and overuse syndromes when incorrectly postured with prolonged sitting position	1. Use correct posture while driving 2. Take frequent rest stops and perform stretching exercises (e.g., trunk extension, hamstring stretches)
Sitting	Although some sitting postures are covered in Table 6-6, it is important to identify all different types of sitting postures assumed throughout the day	See Table 6-6 for description of postural deviations while sitting.	Use proper sitting posture that incorporates the following: body weight slightly anterior to ischial tuberosities; maintenance of normal lumbar lordosis; hips slightly higher than knees; feet flat on floor; shoulder maintained in a "back and down" position (retracted and depressed); arms supported at the proper height to maintain good shoulder position; head retracted and in a neutral position Postures may vary from the above description; the key is to understand what correct posture entails for that individual and to work from that position, changing various amounts of each movement to find a more "correct or functional" position for each individual
Sleeping	Mattress support (firm or soft)? Recent change in mattress?	A soft mattress may not provide adequate support; firm mattresses may be too rigid to conform to the natural curves of the body	Change mattress according to desired support.
	Number of pillows used? Type of pillow used?	Using too many pillows places the head and neck in excessive lateral flexion toward the opposite side during sleeping; may cause prolonged compression and distraction at the neck on the weight-bearing side	Use an adequate number (and size) of pillows to maintain the head in the neutral position while sleeping
	Sleep posture?	Different positions place abnormal stresses on the soft tissues or may perpetuate postural changes	Use positions that are not at the extremes of motion (i.e., too much flexion or extension, use pillows between the legs when sidelying)

FHP = forward head posture; FSP = forward shoulder posture.

Box 6-1
Classifications of Body Types

	Ectomorph	Mesomorph	Endomorph
	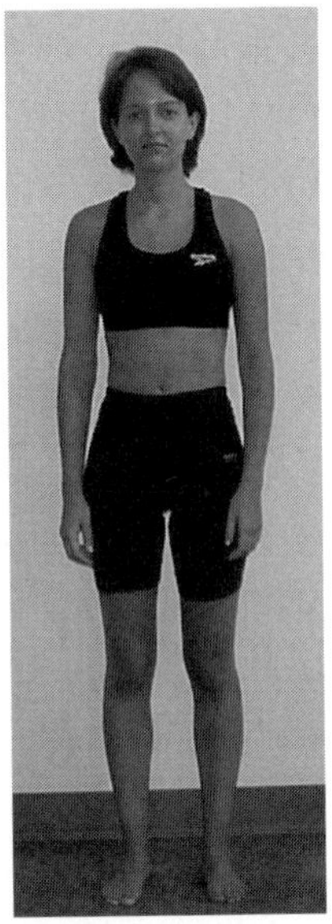	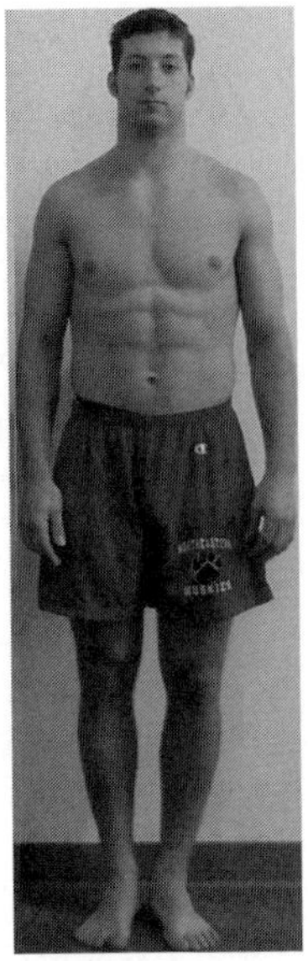	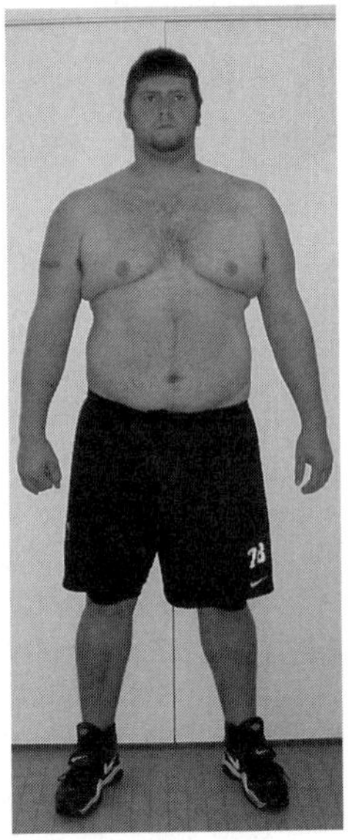
Description	Slender, thin build; relatively low body mass index	Medium, athletic build, relatively average body mass index	Stocky build; relatively high body mass index
Joint Shape	Small, flat joint surfaces	Medium joint surfaces	Large, concave-convex joint surfaces
Muscle Mass	Minimal muscle bulk, thin muscles	Medium muscle build	Thick muscle mass
Joint Mobility	Increased	Within normal limits	Decreased
Joint Stability	Decreased	Within normal limits	Increased

Box 6-2
Body Mass Index

Historically, the medical determination of obesity was made based on the percentage of body fat or total body weight. Depending on the measure being used, obesity is used to describe a person who is 20 to 30 percent over the average weight based on gender, age, and height. Body mass index (BMI) is an indirect estimation of the percentage of body fat.[24] The BMI, based on height and weight, is calculated by:

$$(\text{Weight [lbs.]} \times (705)/(\text{height [in.]} \times (\text{height [in.]})$$

or

$$\text{Weight (kg)}/(\text{height [m]} \times (\text{height [m]})$$

A BMI of 27.0 is the most commonly used threshold to define obesity. The National Center for Health Statistics proposes the following classification scheme for adult BMI. Note that there are specific formulas for children and teenagers:[24]

Underweight: <18.5

Normal: 18.5–24.9

Overweight: ≥ 25.0

Pre-obese: 25.0–29.9

Class I obesity: 30.0–34.9

Class II obesity: 35.0–39.9

Class III obesity: ≥ 40.0

BMI does not accurately describe the amount of body fat for certain groups of people, especially athletes.[25] For example, a 6 feet tall (1.83 m) muscular basketball player who weighs 200 lbs (90.7 kg) would have a BMI of 27.1 (90.7 kg/[1.83 m × 1.83 m]). This individual would fall into the pre-obese classification, even though he or she may have a low percentage of body fat. Therefore, obesity should be determined on a case-by-case basis taking the individual's gender, height, weight, age, BMI, percent body fat, and level of activity into consideration.

Inspection Findings 6-1
Assessment of Ideal Posture

Lateral	Anterior	Posterior
	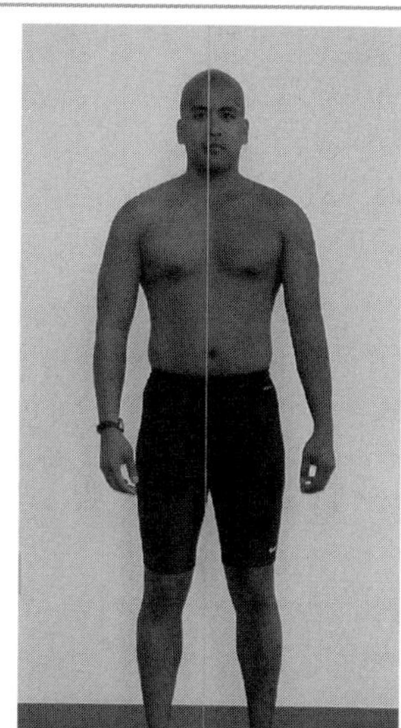	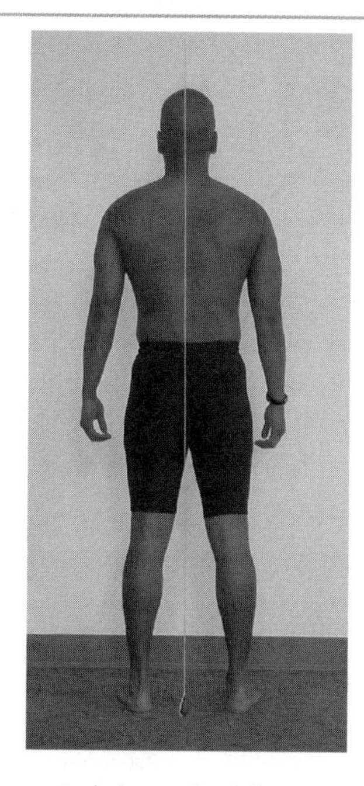
Alignment relative to plumb line: Lower extremity • Lateral malleolus: Slightly posterior • The tibia should be parallel to the plumb line and the foot should be at a 90° angle to the tibia • Lateral femoral epicondyle: Slightly anterior • Greater trochanter: Plumb line bisects	Alignment relative to plumb line: Lower extremity • Feet: Evenly spaced from plumb line • Tibial crests: Slight external rotation • Knees: Evenly spaced from plumb line • Patella: Facing anteriorly • Consistent angulation from joint-to-joint • The lateral malleoli, fibular head, and iliac crests should be bilaterally equal	Alignment relative to plumb line: Lower extremity • Feet evenly spaced from plumb line • Feet in slight lateral rotation: Lateral 2 toes are visible • Knees evenly spaced from plumb line • Consistent angulation from joint-to-joint
Torso		
• Midthoracic region: Plumb line bisects	• Umbilicus: Plumb line bisects, although surgical procedures may alter the alignment. • Sternum: Plumb line bisects • Jugular notch: Plumb line bisects	• Median sacral crests: Plumb line bisects • Spinous processes: Plumb line bisects • Paraspinals musculature bilaterally symmetrical
Shoulder		
• Acromion process: Plumb line bisects	• Acromion processes: Evenly spaced from plumb line • Shoulder heights equal or dominant side slightly lower • Deltoid, anterior chest musculature bilaterally symmetrical and defined	• Scapular borders: Evenly spaced from plumb line • Acromion processes: Evenly spaced from plumb line • Deltoid, posterior musculature bilaterally symmetrical • Shoulder heights equal or dominant side slightly lower
Head and Neck		
• Cervical bodies: Plumb line bisects • Auditory meatus: Plumb line bisects	• Head is bisected by plumb line • Nasal bridge: Plumb line bisects • Frontal bone: Plumb line bisects	• Cervical spinous processes: Plumb line bisects • Occipital protuberance: Plumb line bisects

Table 6-8 Deviations Noted from the Lateral View

Body Region	Deviation from Ideal Posture	Structural Relationships
Talocrural Joint	Dorsiflexed	Knee flexed, hip flexed
	Plantarflexed	Genu recurvatum, hip extended
Knee Joint	Lateral epicondyle posterior to plumb line	Genu recurvatum, ankle plantarflexed, hip extended
	Lateral epicondyle anterior to plumb line	Knee flexed, hip flexed, and ankle dorsiflexed
Hip Joint	Greater trochanter posterior to plumb line	Hip flexed, anterior pelvic tilt, increased lumbar lordosis
	Greater trochanter anterior to plumb line	Hip extended, posterior pelvic tilt, decreased lumbar lordosis
Pelvic Position	Angle between ASIS, PSIS, and a horizontal line greater than 10°: Anterior pelvic tilt (see Goniometry Box 6-1)	Increased lumbar lordosis, hip flexed
	Angle between ASIS and ipsilateral PSIS less than 8°: Posterior pelvic tilt	Decreased lumbar lordosis, hip extended
Lumbar Spine	Lumbar vertebral bodies anterior to plumb line: Increased lumbar lordosis	Anterior pelvic tilt, hip flexed
	Lumbar vertebral bodies posterior to plumb line: Decreased lumbar lordosis	Posterior pelvic tilt, hip extended
Thoracic Spine	Mid-thorax posterior to plumb line: Increased thoracic kyphosis	Forward head posture, forward shoulder posture, shortened anterior chest musculature
	Midthorax anterior to plumb line: Decreased thoracic kyphosis	Inability to flex through thoracic spine, possible shortened thoracic paraspinal muscles
Shoulder Joint	Acromion process posterior to plumb line: Retracted shoulders or scapulae	Decreased thoracic kyphosis
	Acromion process anterior to plumb line: Rounded shoulder or protracted scapulae	Forward head posture, increased thoracic kyphosis, shortened anterior chest musculature, poor postural control of the scapula
Cervical Spine	Lower cervical vertebral bodies posterior to plumb line: Decreased cervical lordosis	Decreased cervical lordosis
	Lower cervical vertebral bodies anterior to plumb line: Increased cervical lordosis	Forward head posture, forward shoulder posture
Head Position	External auditory meatus posterior to plumb line: Head retraction	Decreased cervical lordosis
	External auditory meatus anterior to plumb line: Forward head posture	Forward shoulder posture, suboccipital restrictions

ASIS = anterior superior iliac spine; PSIS = posterior superior iliac spine.

bilaterally (see Inspection Findings 6-1). Table 6-9 presents common postural deviations that may be observed from the anterior view.

Posterior view

Many observations found in the posterior view help to confirm the findings from the anterior view (see Inspection Box 6-1). The plumb line should be of equal distance from both feet, bisecting the spinal column or trunk and head. From the posterior view, observe for bilateral symmetry of the major regions of the body. Table 6-10 presents postural deviations that may be observed from the posterior view.

Inspection of leg length discrepancy

A leg length discrepancy (LLD) can contribute to lower limb and back pathology.[26] Hip osteoarthritis and lower extremity stress fractures are more frequent on the longer limb.[27] The amount of LLD that results in pathology is debatable. In general, those who develop LLD early in life tolerate more difference, while those who are athletic, stand on their feet frequently, or develop LLD later in life tolerate less difference.[27]

The two categories of LLDs are structural (true) and functional (apparent) (Table 6-11).[26,28,29] Although the most accurate methods for determining unequal leg lengths are by radiograph and CT evaluation, several methods can be used clinically.[27,30,31]

The most clinically reliable and valid way of determining an LLD is the premeasured block method (Special Test 6-1).[32] The most common, yet least reliable, method of determining am LLD is measuring the distance between the **anterior superior iliac spine** (ASIS) and medial malleolus to determine a structural leg length difference and from the navel to the

Table 6-9 Postural Deviations Observed from the Anterior View

Body Region	Deviation from Ideal Posture	Structural Relationships
Feet	Internally rotated feet (pigeon toed)	Internally rotated tibia, femoral anteversion, or STJ pronation
	Externally rotated feet (duck feet)	Externally rotated of tibia, femoral retroversion, or STJ supination
	Flattened medial arch	Excessive STJ and midtarsal pronation, internal tibial rotation
	High medial arch	Excessive STJ and midtarsal supination, external tibial rotation
Tibial Position	External tibial rotation: Tibial crests positioned lateral to midline	Femoral retroversion, supinated STJ, laterally positioned patella
	Internal tibial rotation: Tibial crests positioned medial to midline	Femoral anteversion, pronated STJ, laterally positioned patella
Patellar Position	Squinting patellae	Internally rotated tibia, femoral anteversion, pronated STJ
	Frog-eyed patellae	Externally rotated tibia, femoral retroversion, supinated STJ
Leg Positions	Genu varum	Increased angle of inclination of femur, femoral retroversion, supinated STJ
	Genu valgum	Decreased angle of inclination of femur, femoral anteversion, pronated STJ
	Tibial varum	Structural deformity of the tibias causing excessive STJ pronation
Pelvic Position	Asymmetrical iliac crest height	Leg length discrepancy, scoliosis
	Asymmetrical ASIS height	One ilium is rotated either anteriorly or posteriorly, leg length discrepancy, or congenital anomaly
Chest Region	Pectus carinatum: Outward protrusion of the chest and sternum	Not applicable
	Pectus excavatum: Inward position of the chest and sternum	Not applicable
Shoulder Region	Asymmetrical shoulder heights	Scoliosis
		Side dominance
Head and Cervical Spine	The head side bent or rotated; asymmetrical muscle mass of neck	Poor postural sense, overuse of one side, torticollis (congenital deformation or acute spasm of the sternocleidomastoid muscle)

ASIS = anterior superior iliac spine; STJ = subtalar joint.

medial malleolus to identify a functional leg length difference (Fig. 6-7). The tape measure method lacks validity as compared to the block method in that it does not account for possible contributions from the foot.[27] If a functional leg length discrepancy is suspected, further testing of soft tissue lengths and joint ROM must be used to determined the source (or consequence) of the difference.

An actual difference in lengths of the femurs or tibias can be grossly assessed in the supine position with the feet placed flat and in equal positions on the examining table with the knees flexed to 90 degrees. Observing the height of the knees from the anterior view will determine whether one tibia is longer than the other. Observing the length of the knees from the lateral view can be used to determine if one femur is longer than the other, but does not rule out apparent leg length discrepancies caused by the shape and position of the pelvis (Fig. 6-8).[34] During weight bearing, the position of the feet can also provide evidence of an LLD. The foot on the shorter leg supinates and the foot on the longer leg pronates in an attempt to compensate for the discrepancy in length (Fig. 6-9).

Palpation

When assessing posture, accurate palpation of key landmarks assists in identifying various postural deviations.

Lateral aspect

- **Pelvic position:** Palpate the ASIS and posterior superior iliac spine (PSIS) on the same side, placing marks on these landmarks to improve consistency. The relationship between the ASIS and PSIS, normally 9° to 10° from a line horizontal to the ground, indicates if the innominate bone is properly positioned or is rotated anteriorly or posteriorly (Goniometry Box 6-1). Compare right to left. Side-to-side pelvic asymmetry in the sagittal plane is common in asymptomatic individuals[35] and does not appear to be associated with low back pain.[36]

Table 6-10 Postural Deviations Observed from the Posterior View

Body Region	Deviation from Ideal Posture	Structural Relationships
Calcaneal Position	Calcaneal varum	STJ and midtarsal joints in a supinated position
	Calcaneal valgum	STJ and midtarsal joints in a pronated position
Posterior Leg Musculature	Asymmetry in girth or definition of musculature	Leg side dominance Atrophy caused by injury or immobilization of one side
Iliac Crest Heights	Asymmetry of iliac crest heights	Possible leg length discrepancy Scoliosis
Back Musculature	Asymmetry between mass or definition of erector spinae musculature	Side dominance or overuse of one side of the musculature (e.g., rowing) Scoliosis
Spinal Alignment	The spinous processes not in vertical alignment	Structural or functional scoliosis Asymmetry of scapula Asymmetry of spinal musculature Asymmetry of rib cage Side dominance
Scapular Position	Unequal height	Scoliosis Muscle imbalance caused by paralysis or weakness of musculature
	Excessively protracted or asymmetrically protracted	Muscle imbalance Poor posture Scoliosis Forward shoulder posture Forward head posture
	Asymmetrically rotated	Muscle imbalance Side dominance Forward shoulder posture Forward head posture
	Winging scapula	Poor posture Muscle imbalance Muscular weakness
Shoulder Heights	Shoulder heights unequal	Scoliosis Dominant side Scapula positioning
Neck Musculature	The upper trapezius hypertrophied in relation to other periscapular muscles	Overused in normal upper extremity activities or overemphasized in weight lifting Side dominance
Head Position	The head not sitting in a vertical position in relation to the neck Side bend, rotated	Caused by muscle imbalance Poor postural, proprioceptive sense Compensation for scoliosis Torticollis (acquired or congenital)

STJ = subtalar joint.

Table 6-11 Leg Length Differences

Category Type	Description	Possible Causes
Functional or Apparent Leg Length	Leg length difference that is attributed to something other than the length of the tibia and/or femur.	Tightness of muscle or joint structures or muscular weakness in the lower extremity or spine. Examples include knee hyperextension, scoliosis, or pelvic muscle imbalances.
Structural or True Leg Length	An actual difference in the length of the femur or the tibia of one leg compared with the other	Possibly from disruption in the growth plate of one of the long bones or a congenital anomaly

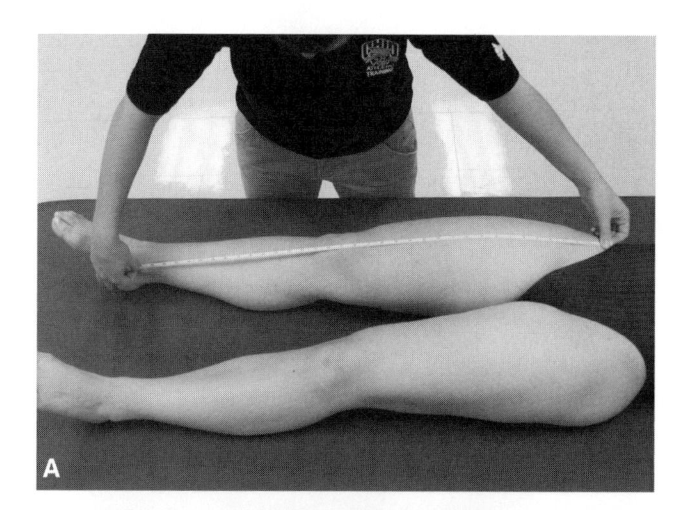

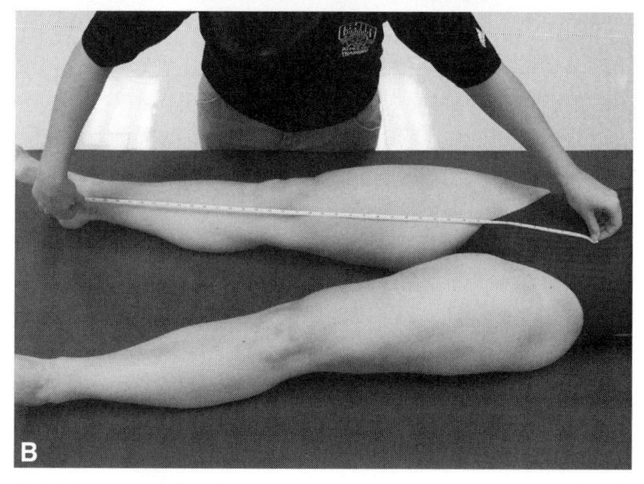

FIGURE 6-7 ■ **(A)** Test for the presence of a structural (true) leg length discrepancy. Measurements are taken from the anterior superior iliac spine to the medial malleolus. Bilateral discrepancies of greater than 10–20 mm are considered significant. **(B)** Test for the presence of an functional (apparent) leg length discrepancy. Measurements are taken from each medical malleolus to the umbilicus. This test is meaningful only if the test for a true leg length difference is negative.

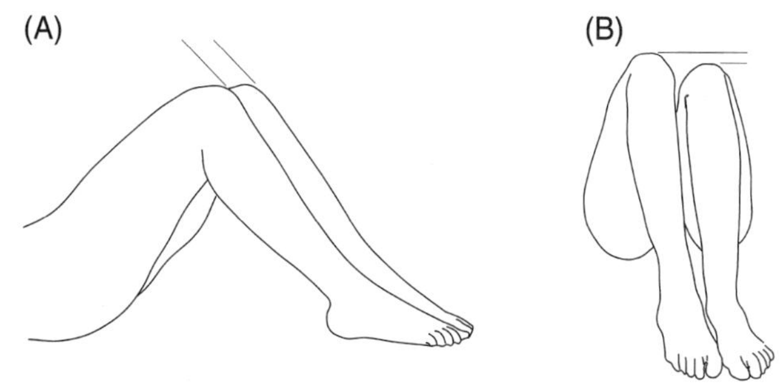

FIGURE 6-8 ■ Clinical discrimination between femoral and tibial leg length differences. **(A)** When viewing the patient from the lateral side, an increased anterior position of one knee indicates a discrepancy in the lengths of the femurs. **(B)** When viewing the knees from the front, a difference in height indicates a discrepancy in the lengths of the tibias. (Courtesy of Rothstein, JM, Roy, SH, and Wolf, SL: *The Rehabilitation Specialist's Handbook*. Philadelphia, FA Davis, 1991.)

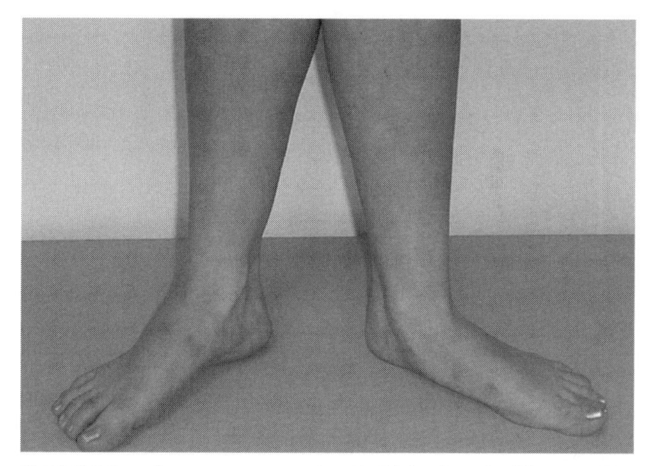

FIGURE 6-9 ■ Foot posture associated with leg length difference. The foot on the long-leg side (the patient's left foot) is pronated while the foot on the short-leg side is supinated.

Special Test 6-1
Measured Block Method of Determining Leg Length Discrepancies

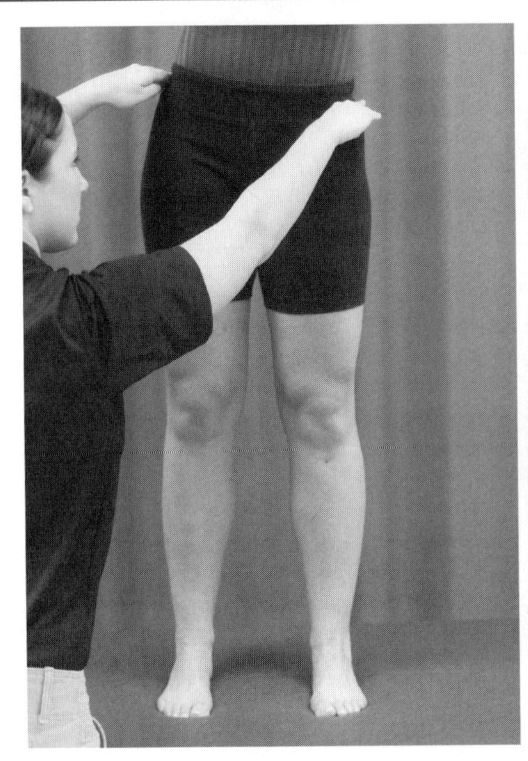

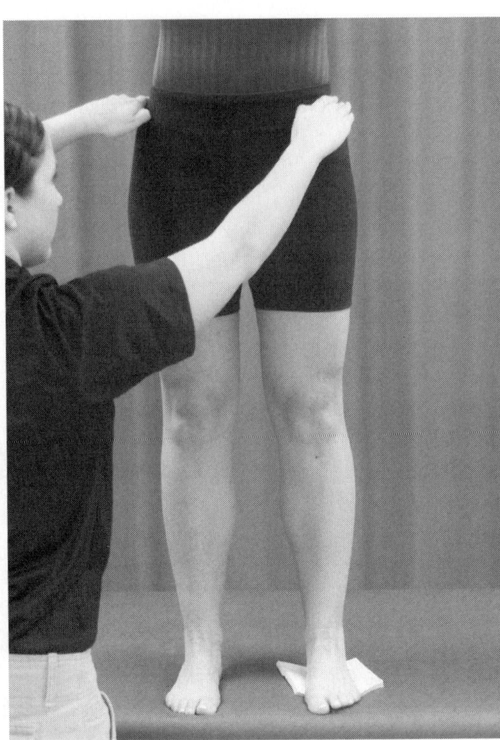

The block method of determining a leg length difference. Blocks of a known thickness are placed under the shorter extremity.

Patient Position	Standing on a firm surface with the feet shoulder-width apart and the weight evenly distributed
Position of Examiner	Standing in front of the patient
Evaluative Procedure	The starting levels of the iliac crests are noted. If heights are determined to be unequal, blocks of known thickness (measured in millimeters) are placed under the shorter leg until the iliac crests are of equal height. The leg length difference is calculated by totaling the sum of the heights of the individual blocks.
Positive Test	A leg length difference of 10–20 mm is frequently cited as the level at which treatment is considered. Patients who acquire the LLD at an early age may tolerate more difference. Patients who are athletic or must stand for much of the day may tolerate less.[27,33]
Comment	When the iliac crests are level, observe the heights of the ASIS. If the ASIS are not an equal height, then the patient has asymmetrical innominate bones.
Evidence	***Intra-rater reliability***

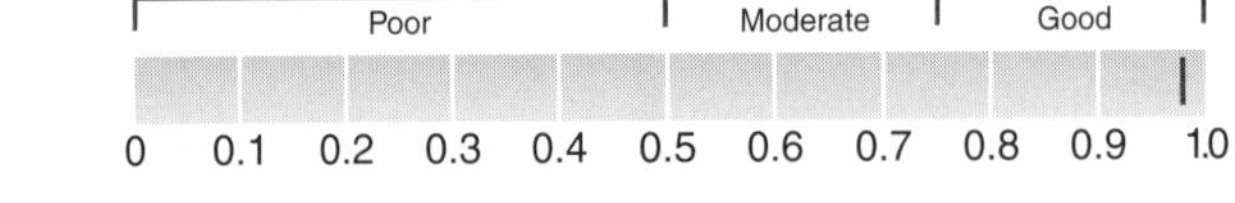

Inter-rater reliability

Not Reliable | Very Reliable
Poor | Moderate | Good
0 0.1 0.2 0.3 0.4 0.5 0.6 0.7 0.8 0.9 1.0

ASIS = anterior superior iliac spine; LLD = leg length discrepancy

Goniometry Box 6-1
Assessment of Pelvic Position

Neutral	Anterior Pelvic Tilt	Posterior Pelvic Tilt
8–10° angle between the ASIS and PSIS relative to horizontal	More than a 10° angle between the ASIS and PSIS relative to horizontal	Less than an 8° angle between the ASIS and relative to horizontal

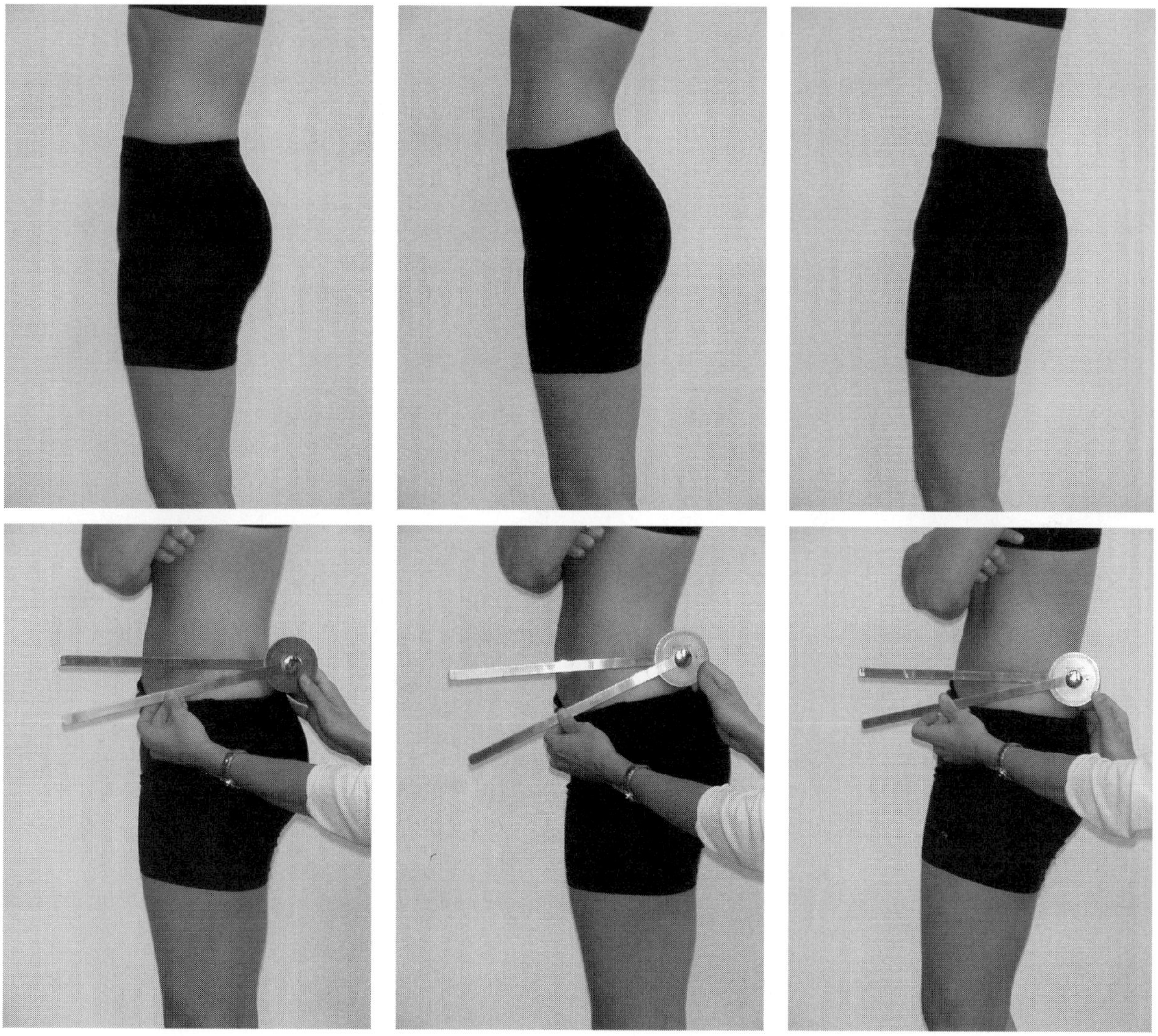

ASIS = anterior superior iliac spine; PSIS = posterior superior iliac spine.

Anterior aspect

- **Patellar position:** Before palpating for patellar position, ensure that the patient is standing comfortably with the feet symmetrically rotated and in an equal stance. Patellar position is observed while the patient is standing, lying supine, long sitting, and during dynamic moment. To assist in determining patellar position, place the thumbs on the medial borders of the patellae and the index fingers on the lateral borders. Further information regarding patellar position is provided in Chapter 11.
- **Iliac crest heights:** Palpate the lateral portions of both ilia moving superiorly until reaching the most superior aspect of the iliac crests. Place the palmar aspects of the index and middle fingers on top of the iliac crests as if forming two "table tops." When you have located the landmarks, determine if your hands are level and that the iliac crest heights are equal (Fig. 6-10). If one hand is higher than the other, then the iliac crests are unequal. Causes of unequal iliac crest height include true length discrepancy or functional LLD resulting from soft-tissue changes or excessive or restricted joint motion (Box 6-3).

Box 6-3
Resting Scapular Postures

Vertical Scapular Position

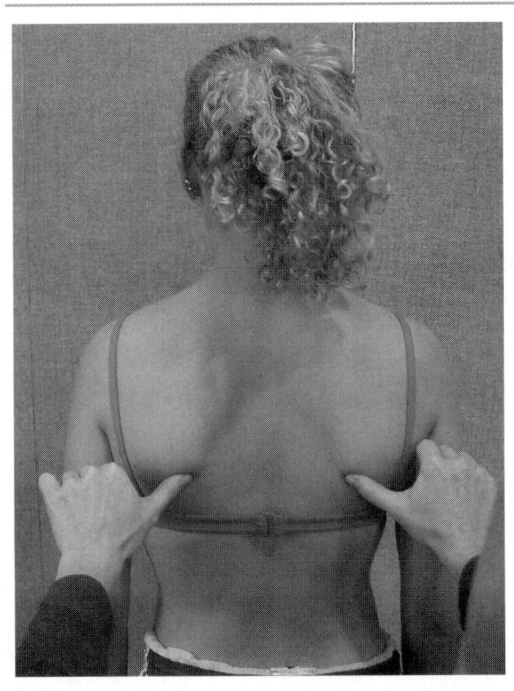

The vertical alignment of the scapulae are compared using the inferior angle as a landmark. The normal height correlates to thoracic vertebrae 7–9.[37]

Horizontal Scapular Position

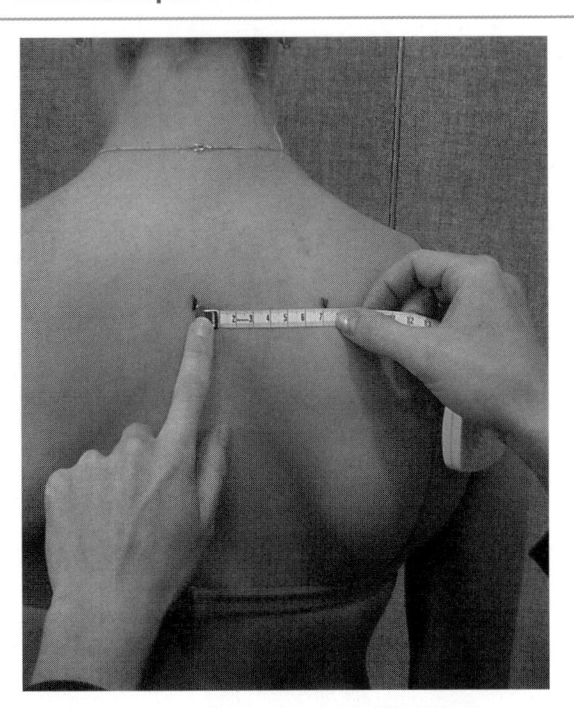

The distance from the T3 spinous process to the medial border of the scapula is measured with the patient standing. The normal value is 5–7 cm. An increased distance represents a protracted scapular position, a decreased distance, a retracted scapula.

Scapular Rotation

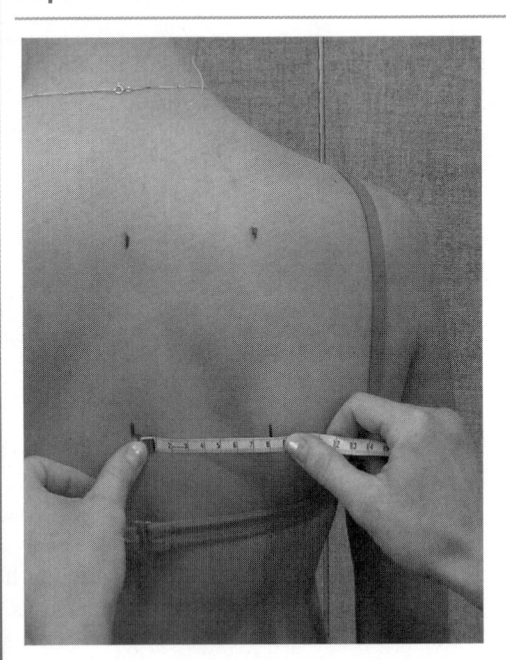

The distance from the T7 vertebrae to the inferior angle of each scapula is measured. An increased distance indicates an upwardly rotated scapula.

Scapular Winging

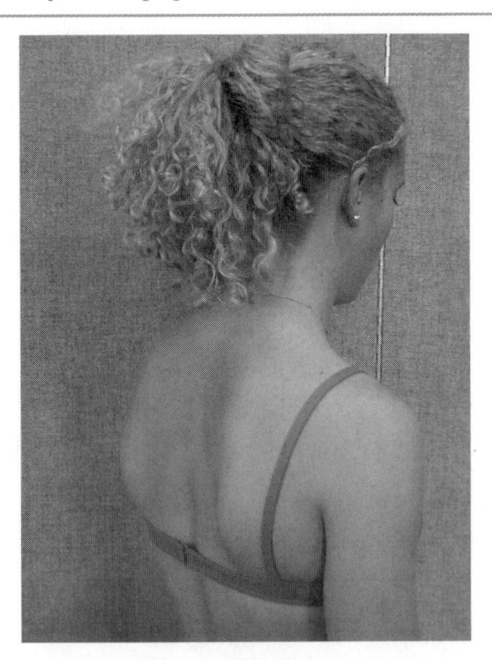

Protrusion of the medial border of scapula.

"Pseudowinging" is apparent when the inferior angle (not the entire medial border) is prominent and is associated with increased anterior tipping of the scapula.

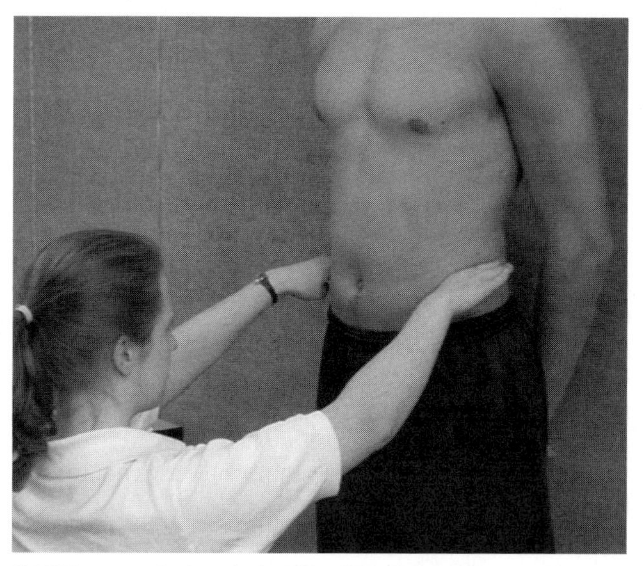

FIGURE 6-10 ■ Finding the heights of the iliac crests.

- **Anterior superior iliac spine (ASIS) heights:** Trace your thumbs down the anterior portion of both iliac crests until coming to the ASIS protuberance. Hook the thumbs on the most inferior ridges of the ASIS to ensure that the same aspect of the ASIS is being palpated on both sides. Determine whether your thumbs are level and the ASIS are of equal height (Fig. 6-11).
- **Lateral malleolus and fibula head heights:** Bilaterally palpate the most prominent projections of the lateral malleolus to determine if each is of equal height. Repeat this process for the fibular heads.
- **Shoulder heights:** Place the palmar aspect of the index and middle fingers on the superior surface of the acromion processes. The fingers should sit flatly on both acromion processes and be parallel to the ground (Fig. 6-12).

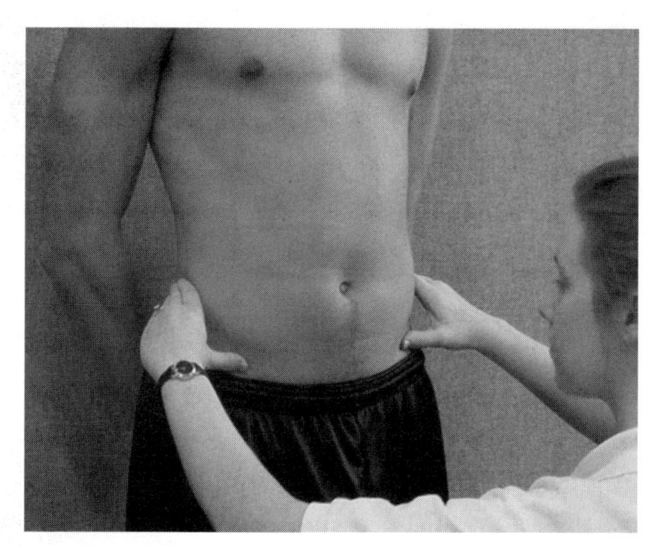

FIGURE 6-11 ■ Identifying the anterior superior iliac spine.

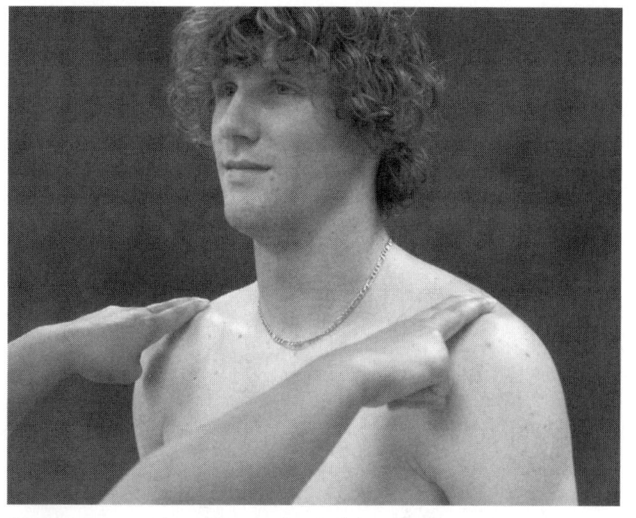

FIGURE 6-12 ■ Identifying the level of the shoulders.

Posterior aspect

Many of the same landmarks used for the anterior view are also used in the posterior view. This section discusses only landmarks that are specific to the posterior view.

- **PSIS positions:** Keeping the index and middle fingers in the position for measuring iliac crest heights, angle the thumbs 45 degrees downward and medially. Palpate for the PSIS, a relatively large, round protuberance, and hook your thumbs under the inferior margins of the PSIS. Determine if your thumbs are at equal heights (Fig. 6-13).
- **Spinal alignment:** Starting from the cervical vertebrae, trace your finger down each spinous process to the sacrum. A lateral deviation where more than one spinous process is not aligned vertically may reflect scoliosis. Refer to the section of this chapter on the spine for definitions of functional versus structural scoliosis.
- **Scapular position:** With the patient standing and relaxed, evaluate the scapula's resting position and note bilateral or unilateral elevation or depression, **protraction** or **retraction**, rotation, and **winging** (Box 6-3). Normally, the scapula on the dominant side is slightly more protracted than the nondominant shoulder. In normal posture, the scapula is angled 30 degrees relative to the frontal plane (the plane of the scapula) with the medial (vertebral) border parallel

Protraction (scapular) Movement of the vertebral borders of the scapula away from the spinal column.

Retraction (scapular) Movement of the scapular vertebral borders toward the spinal column.

Winging (scapular) The medial border of the scapula lifting away from the thorax.

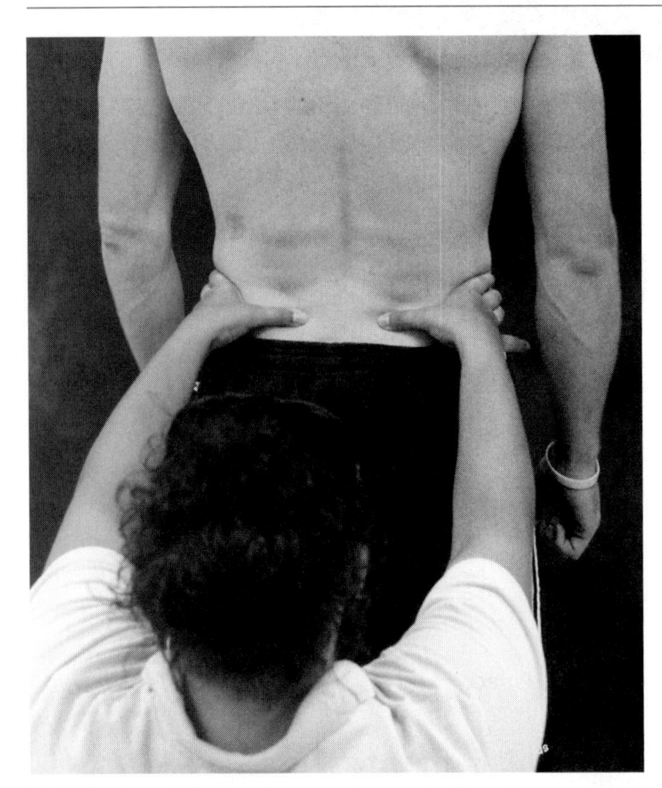

FIGURE 6-13 ■ Palpating the posterior superior iliac spines.

to the spine. The spine of the scapula is located at about the level of the second or third thoracic vertebrae while the inferior angle is at the level of the seventh to ninth thoracic vertebra. The scapula should rest flat against the thoracic wall.[37]

Muscle Length Assessment

Muscle length assessment objectively measures if specific muscles are shortened or elongated, contributing to postural abnormality. If a muscle crossing a specific joint is shortened, abnormal stresses may be placed on the joint over which the muscle crosses or the necessary mobility required for normal function may be lacking. If a muscle crossing a specific joint is in an abnormally elongated position, the joint may be affected by abnormal stresses or may lack the stability required for normal function. Consider a patient with low back pain who has increased anterior pelvic tilt (see Goniometry Box 6-1). The next task is to identify the underlying impairments and whether or not these contribute to functional limitations. The anterior tilt may be caused by a tight rectus femoris or iliopsoas muscles or lengthened hamstrings, but this assumption must be confirmed using, objective, measurable tests. As with all aspects of a clinical examination, muscle length assessment must use standard measures and be as objective as possible. However, for some muscle groups it is difficult to objectively measure the length. In these cases, a general estimate and comparison to the contralateral side or normative values is sufficient.

Before assessing the length of a muscle, rule out any bony or soft tissue restrictions that could be involved in the joint or joints that the muscle crosses.[11] Muscles that cross more than one joint (two-joint muscles) have a greater tendency to become shortened during normal ADLs than do muscles crossing only one joint. Specific, measurable tests are available for many of the **two-joint muscles** that commonly create postural problems as they become shortened in length. When assessing muscle length for most of the **one-joint muscles**, the normal ranges (measurements) for passive joint range of motion are used. One-joint muscles are less likely to become shortened. A goniometer used to measure joint angles assists in the objectivity of muscle length assessment.

Assessing for Shortness of the Lower Extremity Muscles

When muscle shortening occurs, various postural deviations may result. These are highlighted in Table 6-12. The specific procedures for assessing muscle length in selected lower extremity muscles are described in Muscle Length Boxes 6-1 through 6-3. The Ober test (see Special Test 10-19) and the Thomas test (see Special Test 12-3) are two additional tests for muscle length.

Assessing for Shortness of the Upper Extremity Muscles

When shortening occurs in upper extremity muscles, various postural deviations may result. These are highlighted in Table 6-13. The specific procedures for assessing muscle length in selected upper extremity muscles are described in Muscle Length Boxes 6-4 through 6-6.

Common Postural Deviations

Many people have less than ideal posture. However, not all postural deviations cause pathology. Clinicians must be able to identify normal posture, **asymptomatic** deviations, and postural deviations possibly causing soft tissue dysfunction and pain. When evaluating postural deviations, keep in mind that any potential muscle imbalances can either cause the poor posture or be a result of the poor posture. Postural deviations also can be a result of skeletal malalignment, anomalies, or a combination thereof. The next section discusses some common postural deviations observed for each joint.

Two-joint muscles A muscle that exerts its force across two different joints and whose strength depends on the position of those joints.

One-joint muscles A muscle that only exerts force across one joint.

Asymptomatic Without symptoms.

Table 6-12 Postural Deviations of the Lower Extremity as the Result of Muscle Shortness or Contracture

Muscle	Posture (resting position except where noted)
Foot and Toes	
Abductor hallucis	Forefoot varus
	Extended of the first MTP joint
Adductor hallucis	Hallux valgus
Flexor hallucis brevis	Flexed first MTP joint
Flexor hallucis longus	Flexed IP joint of the first toe
Flexor digitorum longus	Flexed DIP joints of the lateral four toes
Extensor digitorum longus	Extended lateral four MTP joints
Extensor hallucis longus and brevis	Extended first MTP joint
	Depressed head of the first MT
Ankle	
Tibialis anterior	Dorsiflexed talocrural joint; calcaneovarus
Tibialis posterior	Calcaneovarus, rearfoot supinates
Peroneus longus and brevis	Calcaneovalgus
Gastrocnemius and soleus	Plantarflexed talocrural joint
Knee	
Gastrocnemius	Flexed knee
Biceps femoris	Externally rotated tibia
Semimembranosus and Semitendinosus	Internally rotated tibia
Popliteus	Internally rotated tibia
Hamstring group	Flexed knee
	Posterior pelvic tilt
	Loss of normal lumbar lordosis
	Pelvic tilt (unilateral contracture of the hamstrings)
Quadriceps group	Knee extended
Hip	
Iliopsoas	Hip flexed, hip adducted
	Increased lumbar lordosis
	Anterior pelvic tilt
Gluteus minimus	Internally rotated femur, hip abduction
	When standing, pelvic tilt toward the side of the shortness (low side)
Gluteus medius	Abducted hip
	When standing, pelvic tilt toward the side of the shortness (low side)
Hip internal rotators	Internally rotated hip
Hip external rotators	Externally rotated hip
Adductor group	Adduction deformity
	When standing, pelvic tilt away from the side of the shortness (high side)
Sartorius	Hip flexed, abducted, and externally rotated
	Flexed knee.

DIP = distal interphalangeal; IP = interphalangeal; MT = metatarsal; MTP = metatarsophalangeal; MMT = manual muscle test.

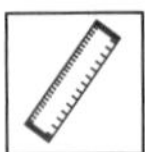

Muscle Length Box 6-1
Muscle Length Assessment for the Gastrocnemius

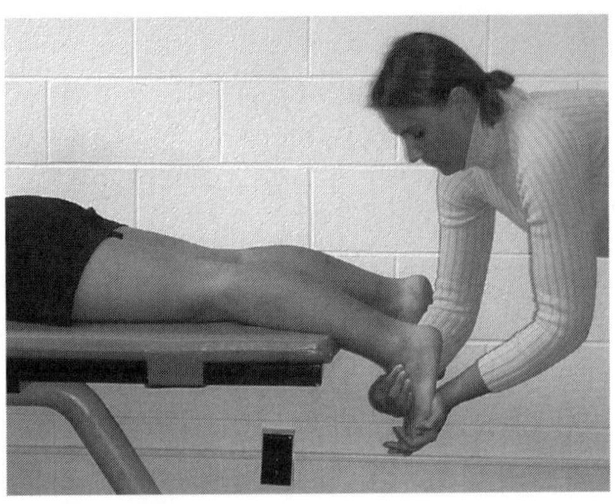

Patient Position	Prone with the foot off the edge of the table with the knee extended
Position of Examiner	One hand palpating the subtalar joint The other hand grasping the foot
Evaluative Procedure	While maintaining the subtalar joint in the neutral position, the foot is taken into dorsiflexion. ROM can be measured goniometrically by placing the axis over the lateral malleolus, the distal arm aligned parallel to the bottom of the foot, and the proximal arm aligned with the fibula.
Positive Test	Less than 10° of dorsiflexion may affect normal walking gait; less than 15° of dorsiflexion may affect normal running gait.
Implications	Tightness of the gastrocnemius can create overuse pathology at the foot, ankle, and knee.
Possible Pathologies	Plantar fasciitis, Sever's disease, Achilles tendinopathy, calcaneal bursitis, patellofemoral pathology.
Comment	The length of the soleus is assessed using dorsiflexion range of motion with the knee flexed to at least 60°.
Evidence	***Inter-rater reliability*** Not Reliable — Very Reliable Poor / Moderate / Good 0 0.1 0.2 0.3 0.4 0.5 0.6 0.7 0.8 0.9 1.0

ROM = range of motion.

Foot and Ankle

Pronated foot

A pes planus foot, or a flattened medial longitudinal arch is characteristic of excessively pronated subtalar and midtarsal joints. Excessive pronation is characterized by adduction and plantarflexion of the talus and eversion of the calcaneus when the foot is weight bearing (refer to Table 8-1 for a description of foot pronation and supination while weight bearing and non–weight bearing).

Two weight-bearing methods used to measure foot posture are the Feiss line and navicular drop tests (see Chapter 8, Special Tests 8-1 and 8-4). The subtalar neutral position is commonly used to determine non–weight-bearing foot position. In this position, the clinician is observing for static foot positions such as forefoot or rearfoot varus, which contribute to compensatory prolonged or hyperpronation and the resulting compensations up the kinetic chain (Fig. 6-14).

Supinated foot

Excessive weight-bearing supination is characterized by abduction and dorsiflexion of the talus and inversion of the calcaneus. A heightened medial longitudinal arch is also commonly observed. Forefoot or rearfoot valgus in the subtalar neutral position during non–weight bearing can be structural causes for excessive supination. A supinated or cavus foot has less shock-absorbing capacity, predisposing the foot to a number of stress-related conditions.

Foot posture index

The Foot Posture Index (FPI) was designed to improve the reliability and validity of classification of foot postures as supinated, neutral, or pronated and may be useful in

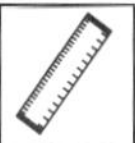

Muscle Length Box 6-2
Muscle Length Assessment for the Hamstring Group

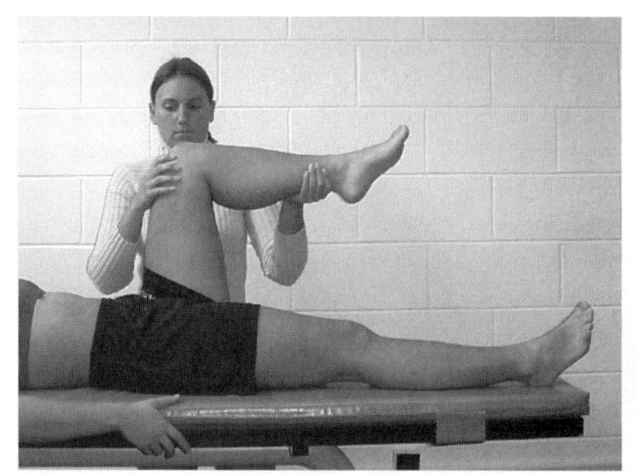

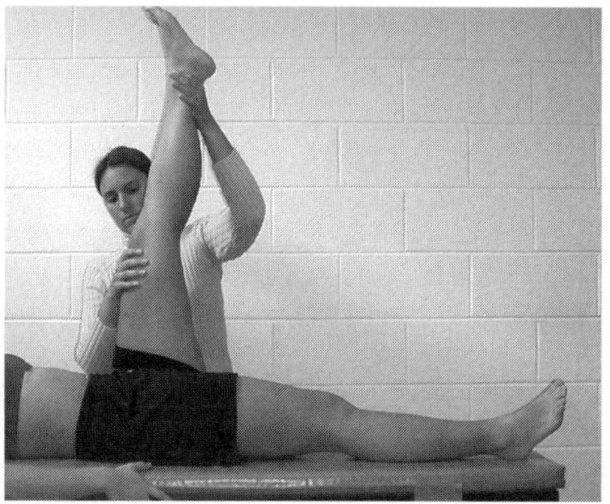

Patient Position	Supine
Position of Examiner	Standing at the side of the patient; the leg being assessed is placed in 90° of hip flexion and 90° of knee flexion (90/90 position)
Evaluative Procedure	The upper leg is stabilized in 90° of hip flexion and the lower leg is extended at the knee.
Positive Test	Lacking more than 20° of full knee extension.
Implications	Tightness of the hamstrings may affect the knee, thigh, hip, and spine.
Possible Pathologies	Muscle strains, patellofemoral dysfunction, ischial tuberosity inflammation, low back dysfunction
Evidence	***Inter-rater reliability***

Not Reliable — Very Reliable

Poor | Moderate | Good

0 0.1 0.2 0.3 0.4 0.5 0.6 0.7 0.8 0.9 1.0

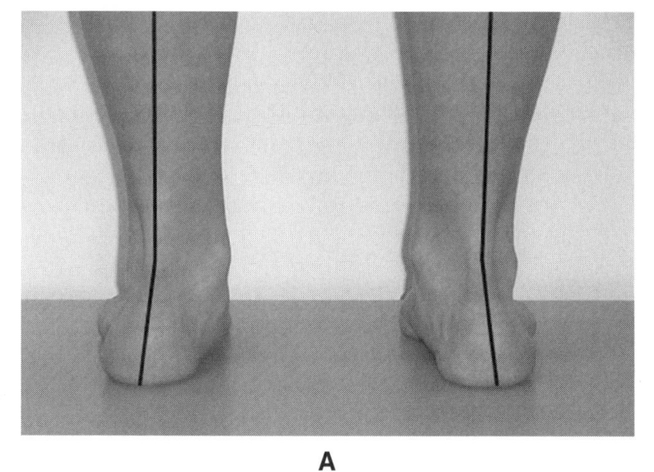

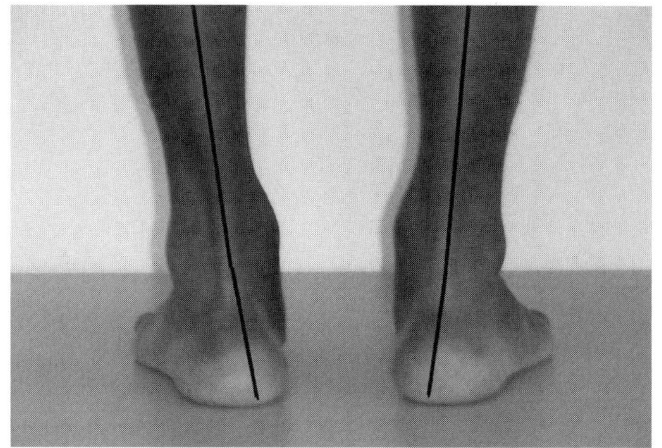

A B

FIGURE 6-14 ■ Alignment of the calcaneus and tibia. **(A)** Calcaneal eversion (calcaneovalgus). **(B)** Calcaneal inversion (calcaneovarus).

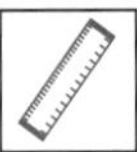

Muscle Length Box 6-3
Muscle Length Assessment of the Rectus Femoris

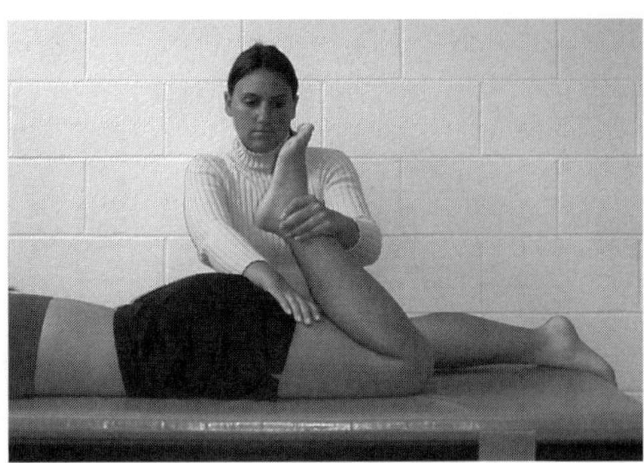

Patient Position	Prone
Position of Examiner	At the side of the patient
Evaluative Procedure	The knee is flexed. ROM can be measured using a goniometer with the axis placed over the lateral epicondyle, the distal arm aligned with the lateral malleolus, and the proximal arm aligned with the greater trochanter.
Positive Test	10° or greater difference as compared with the nonaffected side.
Implications	Tightness of the quadriceps may affect the knee, thigh, hip, and spine.
Possible Pathologies	Muscle strains, patellofemoral dysfunction, low back dysfunction
Evidence	***Intra-rater reliability*** Not Reliable — Very Reliable Poor / Moderate / Good 0 0.1 0.2 0.3 0.4 0.5 0.6 0.7 0.8 0.9 1.0

ROM = range of motion.

predicting injury risk.[38,39] Using simple palpation and inspection metrics with the patient in a relaxed stance, the FPI uses a 5-point Likert scale to assess six aspects of foot position:

1. Talar head palpation
2. Curves above and below the lateral malleoli
3. Inversion or eversion of the calcaneus
4. Bulge in the region of the talonavicular joint
5. Congruence of the medial longitudinal arch
6. Abduction or adduction of the forefoot on the rear foot

Each feature is assigned a rating from −2 to +2. Negative values reflect more supinated positioning and positive values reflect pronated positioning (Fig. 6-15). The scores are added with a composite score being used. A more pronated foot type as identified by the FPI is associated with an increased risk of medial tibial stress syndrome.[40]

The Knee

Alignment of the knee changes with age. Young children display a greater tibiofemoral angle than adults. The stressors introduced as the toddler transitions to walking change the knee from a varus alignment to a vertical alignment to a valgus alignment, gradually leading to a valgus alignment of less than 6 degrees by early adolescence.[40] Excessive valgus alignment in adolescence and beyond leads to potential pathology due to greater lateral compressive forces and tensile forces on the medial structures.[41]

Genu Recurvatum

This postural deviation is noted when the knee's axis of motion is significantly posterior relative to the plumb line, the person has greater than 5 degrees of knee hyperextension as measured with a goniometer, or the hyperextension is asymmetrical. A person with genu recurvatum

Table 6-13 Postural Deviations of the Upper Extremity as the Result of Muscle Shortness or Contracture

Muscle	Posture (resting position except where noted)
Fingers and Thumb	
Adductor pollicis	Adduction contracture of the thumb
Flexor pollicis longus	Flexed IP joint of the thumb
Flexor pollicis brevis	Flexed first MCP joint
Abductor pollicis longus	Extended first MC
	Slight radial deviation of wrist
Dorsal interossei	Abduction of the fingers relative to the third MC
Palmar interossei	Adduction of the fingers relative to the third MC
Lumbricales and Interossei	Flexed MCP joints
	Extended IP joints
Extensor digitorum	Hyperextended MCP joints (contracture).
	Hyperextended MCP joints during wrist flexion; extension of the wrist if the MCP joints are flexed (shortness).
Flexor digitorum superficialis	Flexed PIP joints (contracture)
	Flexed PIP joints if the wrist is extended; flexion of the wrist if the fingers are extended (shortness)
Flexor digitorum profundus	Flexed DIP joints (contracture)
	Flexed finger if the wrist is extended; wrist flexion if the fingers are extended (shortness)
Wrist and Hand	
Flexor carpi radialis	Radially deviated wrist
Flexor carpi ulnaris	Ulnarly deviated wrist
Extensor carpi radialis longus and brevis	Wrist extended, radial deviation
Extensor carpi ulnaris	Wrist extended, ulnar deviation
Elbow and Forearm	
Biceps brachii/brachialis	Flexed elbow and supinated forearm
Triceps brachii	Extended elbow
Shoulder	
Latissimus dorsi	Depressed shoulder girdle; limited humeral elevation
	Kyphosis of the thoracic spine
Pectoralis major	Humerus internally rotated and adducted; protracted scapula (clavicular portion of pectoralis major)
	Forward shoulder posture and/or depression of the shoulder girdle (sternal portion)
Pectoralis minor	Forward shoulder posture
Teres major	Premature rotation of the scapula during glenohumeral abduction
Rhomboid major and minor	Retracted scapulae
Trapezius (upper fibers)	Unilateral bending of the cervical spine

DIP = distal interphalangeal; IP = interphalangeal; MC = metacarpal; MCP = metacarpophalangeal; PIP = proximal interphalangeal.

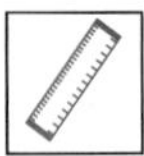

Muscle Length Box 6-4
Muscle Length Assessment of the Shoulder Adductors

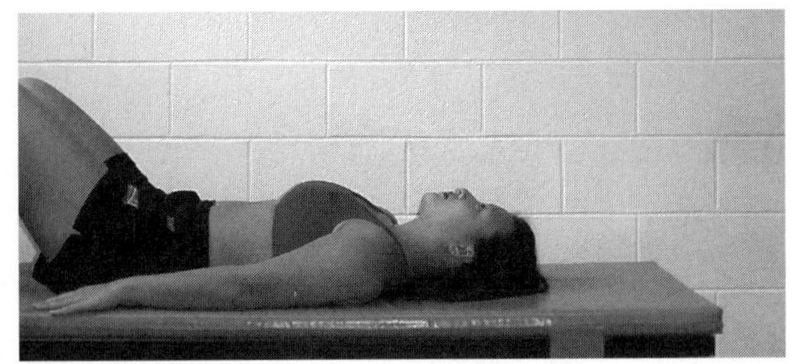

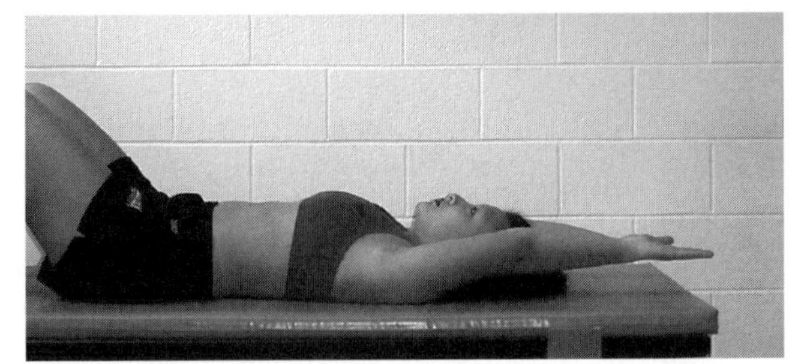

Starting Position	Ending Position
Patient Position	In the hook-lying position with the arms at the side
Position of Examiner	At the side of the patient
Evaluative Procedure	The patient flexes the shoulders above the head and attempts to place the arms on the table.
Positive Test	The patient cannot flex the arms above the head or the lumbar spine lifts off the table.
Implications	Shortness of the latissimus dorsi and teres major muscles
Evidence	Absent or inconclusive in the literature

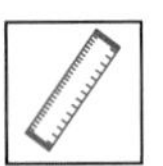

Muscle Length Box 6-5
Muscle Length Assessment of the Pectoralis Major Muscles

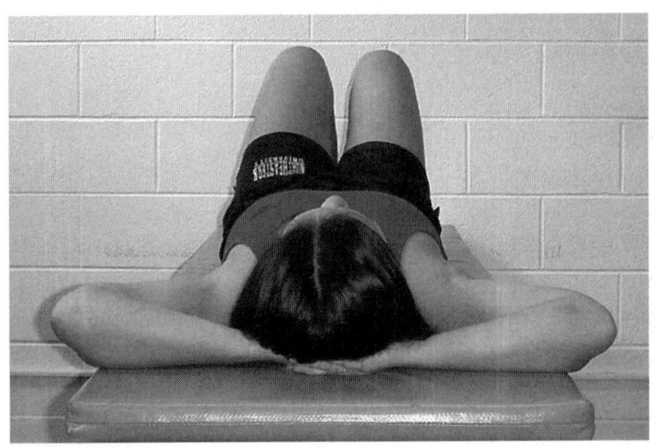

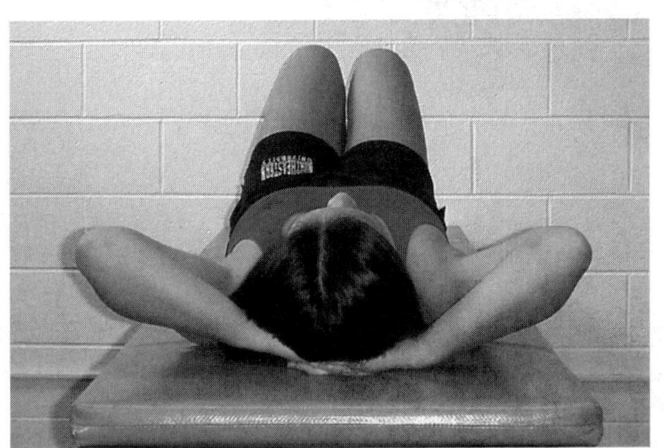

Normal Findings	Positive Findings
Patient Position	In the hook-lying position with the arms abducted, externally rotated, with the elbows flexed and the hands locked behind the head
Position of Examiner	At the head of the patient
Evaluative Procedure	The patient attempts to position the elbows flat on the table.
Positive Test	The elbows do not rest on the table. To establish an objective baseline, measure (in centimeters) the distance from the posterior aspect of the acromion process to the tabletop.
Implications	Tight pectoralis major muscles may create rounded shoulders and subsequent forward head posture, although shortness of the pectoralis minor is most commonly implicated.

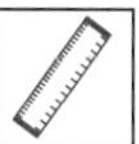

Muscle Length Box 6–6
Muscle Length Assessment of the Pectoralis Minor Muscles

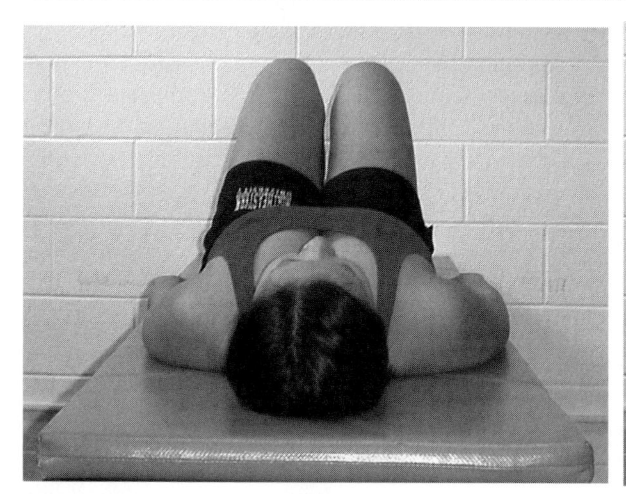

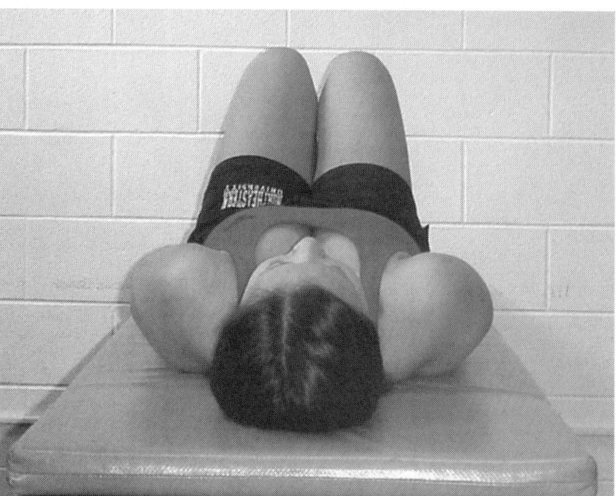

Normal Findings	Positive Findings
Patient Position	Supine with the arms at the side
Position of Examiner	At the head of the patient
Evaluative Procedure	Observe the position of the shoulders in reference to the table.
Positive Test	The posterior shoulder does not rest on the table. To establish an objective baseline, measure (in centimeters) the distance from the posterior aspect of the acromion process to the tabletop.
Implications	Tight pectoralis minor muscles may create rounded shoulders and subsequent forward head posture.
Modifications	**1.** Repeat the above test, but with the patient standing to avoid falsely positioning the scapula.[37] **2.** Measure from the sternoclavicular joint to the coracoid process.
Evidence	Tabletop measurement poorly correlated with more direct measurements of muscle length because of the supine positioning.[6]

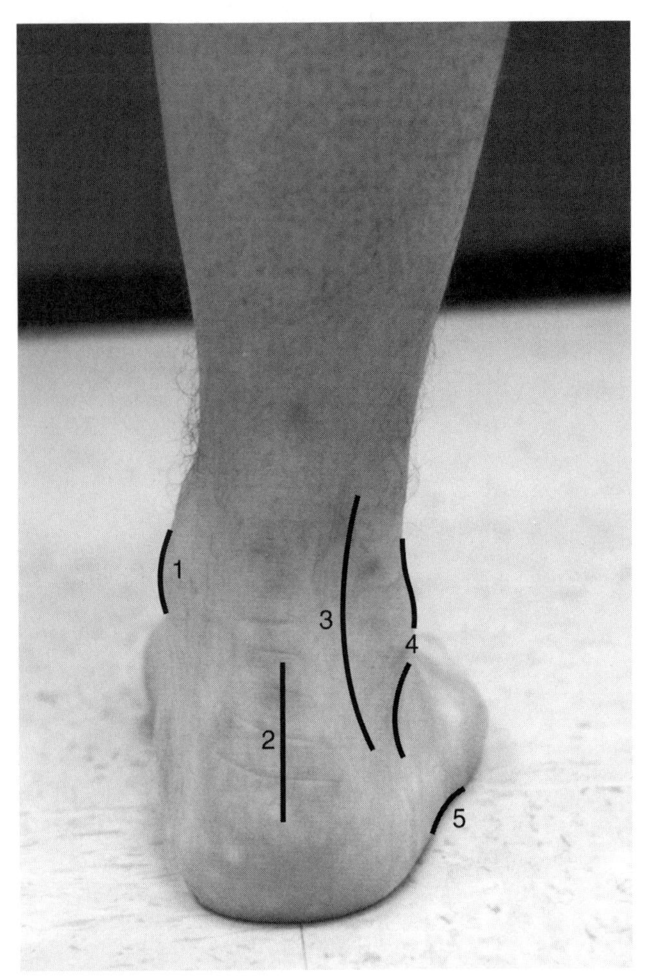

FIGURE 6-15 ■ Posterior view of a pronated foot as defined by the foot posture index. 1, talar navicular prominence; 2, calcaneal frontal plane position; 3, Helbing's sign; 4, inferior and superior lateral malleolar curves; 5, congruence of the lateral border.

often stands with the knee(s) "locked" in an extreme extended position (Inspection Findings 6-2). Genu recurvatum may be congenital or may be caused by pathology such as a combined tear of the anterior and posterior cruciate ligaments.

Genu valgum

Genu valgum is a medial angulation of the femur and tibia occurring at the knee. Normally, a slight medial angulation at the knee is present. However, with excessive genu valgum ("knock-kneed"), the knees are visibly closer together than the ankles during stance. Objectively measuring a person's Q angle determines if excessive genu valgum is present (see Chapter 10).

Genu valgum occurs because of structural anomalies at the hip, contributing muscular weaknesses occurring at the hip, or secondary to hyperpronation of the feet. Genu valgum can lead to or result from a number of different postural deviations in the lower extremity, such as increased foot pronation, internal tibial rotation, medial patellar positioning, and internal femoral rotation.

Genu varum

Genu varum ("bow-legged") is a lateral angulation of the femur and tibia occurring at the knee. The knees are further apart than the ankles while a person with genu varum is standing. Genu varum occurs because of structural anomalies at the hip or from excessive supination of the feet. A number of different postural deviations in the lower extremity can occur because of genu varum; these include foot supination, external tibial rotation, lateral patellar positioning, and external femoral rotation. See Inspection Findings 10-1 for photographs of genu varum and genu valgum.

Spinal Column

Hyperlordotic posture

This postural deviation entails an increase in the lumbar lordosis without compensation in the thoracic or cervical spines (Inspection Findings 6-3). Increased lower lumbar lordosis (anterior convexity) may have been acquired secondary to adaptive shortening of the hip flexors, rotating the ilia anteriorly and pulling the lumbar spine anteriorly. A large anterior abdominal mass, including during pregnancy, obesity, poor postural awareness, ligamentous laxity, and muscle weakness may also increase lumbar lordosis.

Kypholordotic posture

Kypholordotic posture is similar to hyperlordotic posture in that the patient has an increased lumbar lordosis; however, there is also a compensatory increase in thoracic **kyphosis** as an attempt to maintain the spine in a position of equilibrium (Inspection Findings 6-4). Kypholordotic posture increases the normal curvature in both the lumbar and thoracic spines. The lordosis cervical spine also increases and a forward head posture (FHP) is assumed in an attempt to compensate for the other regions of the spinal column. With this posture, adaptive changes in the lengths of the muscles can be observed throughout the entire trunk.

Swayback posture

Swayback posture is marked by increased lumbar lordosis and thoracic kyphosis that cause the hips to extend. This creates a position of instability because the spinal column relies on ligaments rather than muscles for support (Inspection Findings 6-5). Swayback posture commonly is commonly associated with an ectomorph or a lax ligamentous mesomorph body type. The joints are usually at the ends of their ranges, placing excessive strain on the surrounding ligamentous structures. In ideal posture, stability occurs because of a balance of static support from the ligamentous structures and dynamic support from surrounding muscles.

Flat back posture

An individual displaying a flat back posture has lost the normal "S" shaped curvature of the spine in the sagittal plane (Inspection Findings 6-6). The thoracic and lumbar curvatures are decreased and the spine is relatively straight. Often an associated FHP occurs to counteract the posterior

Inspection Findings 6-2
Genu Recurvatum

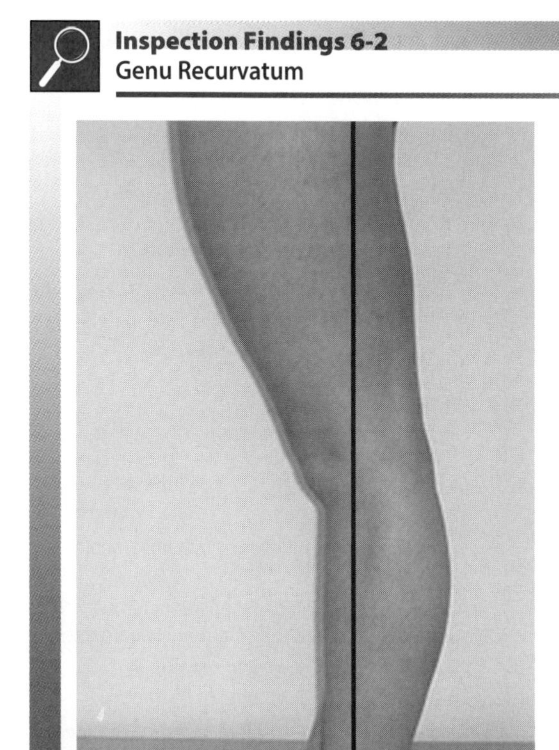

Potential Causes	Hypermobility of joints/lax ligaments (commonly seen in ectomorph body type) Combined posterior cruciate ligament and anterior cruciate ligament laxity[42] Poor postural sense
Resulting Effects	Increased stress on the ACL Increased tension on the posterior and posterolateral soft tissue structures Compressive forces on the anterior and medial compartments of the tibiofemoral joint

ACL= anterior cruciate ligament.

displacement of the thoracic and lumbar spines. A decreased lumbar lordosis is associated with a posterior pelvic tilt.

Scoliosis

Scoliosis involves the presence of lateral curvature of the spinal column (Inspection Findings 6-7). Scoliosis is named for the side of convexity and the region of the spine in which it is observed. There are two types of scoliosis: functional and structural. Functional scoliosis occurs as the spine attempts to compensate to maintain the head in a neutral position and keep the eyes level. It is usually caused by a muscle imbalance, muscle guarding, or a limb length discrepancy. A structural scoliosis is caused by a defect or congenital bony anomaly of the vertebrae. A subcategory of structural scoliosis is **idiopathic** scoliosis. Idiopathic scoliosis affects up 2 to 4 percent of the population, and females more often than males.[43,44] Idiopathic scoliosis is structural in nature but does not involve bony abnormalities of the vertebral body. The exact cause of idiopathic scoliosis is not clear. However, it seems to be caused by heredity, musculoskeletal, and neurologic factors.[43]

To determine if a scoliosis is structural or functional, observe the patient's spine during erect posture and then during a forward flexed (trunk) posture (Adam's forward bend test; see Special Test 13-2). A structural scoliosis is present in both positions. In contrast, functional scoliosis is demonstrated only while the individual stands erect and disappears during spinal flexion. Patients with functional scoliosis must be further examined to determine the underlying cause. School screening for scoliosis in childhood is no longer recommended.[45] Referrals for school-detected scoliosis result in unnecessary radiographs and bracing, which has negative psychosocial consequences. The long-term consequences of most cases of untreated idiopathic scoliosis are minimal.[44,45]

Shoulder and Scapula

Forward shoulder posture

Forward shoulder posture (FSP) is characterized by protraction and elevation of the scapulae and a forward, rounded position of the shoulders that may also involve scapula winging and internal humeral rotation (Inspection

Kyphosis Posterior curvature of the spine.
Idiopathic Of unknown origin.

Inspection Findings 6-3
Hyperlordotic Posture

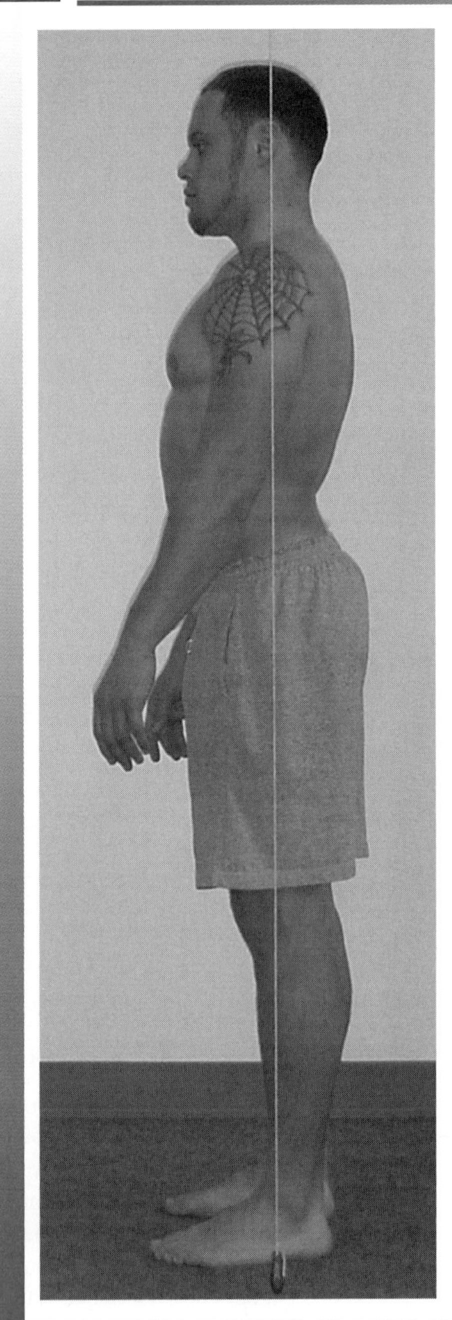

Joints Involved	Lumbar spine, pelvis, hip
Potential Cause	Tightened or shortened hip flexor muscles or back extensors Weakened or elongated hip extensors or abdominals Poor postural sense
Resulting Effects	Increased lumbar lordosis Anterior pelvic tilt Hip assuming a flexed position
Potential Associated Compressive or Distractive Forces and Pathological Conditions	Increased shear forces placed on lumbar vertebral bodies secondary to psoas tightness Increased compressive forces on lumbar facet joints Adaptive shortening of the posterior lumbar spine ligaments and the anterior hip ligaments Elongation of the anterior lumbar spine ligaments and the posterior hip ligaments Narrowing of the lumbar intervertebral foramen

Findings 6-8).[1,3,46] FSP often occurs concurrently with forward head posture.

When observed from the lateral view, forward shoulder posture is associated with an anterior displacement of the acromion process in relation to the plumb line. Common causes of FSP include poor postural sense (i.e., a person assuming a "slouched" posture); adaptively shortened anterior chest muscles (particularly the pectoralis minor), associated elongation of the posterior interscapular muscles (lower and middle trapezius, rhomboids); and abnormal cervical and thoracic spine sagittal plane curvatures, altering the resting position of the scapula.[1,6,47]

✱ Practical Evidence

In a patient with chronic shoulder pain, evaluate for pectoralis minor tightness. Pectoralis minor tightness is associated with increased scapular internal rotation and decreased scapular posterior tilting during shoulder elevation. Both of these mechanical changes decrease the subacromial space and predispose the patient to subacromial impingement.[6]

Inspection Findings 6-4
Kypholordotic Posture

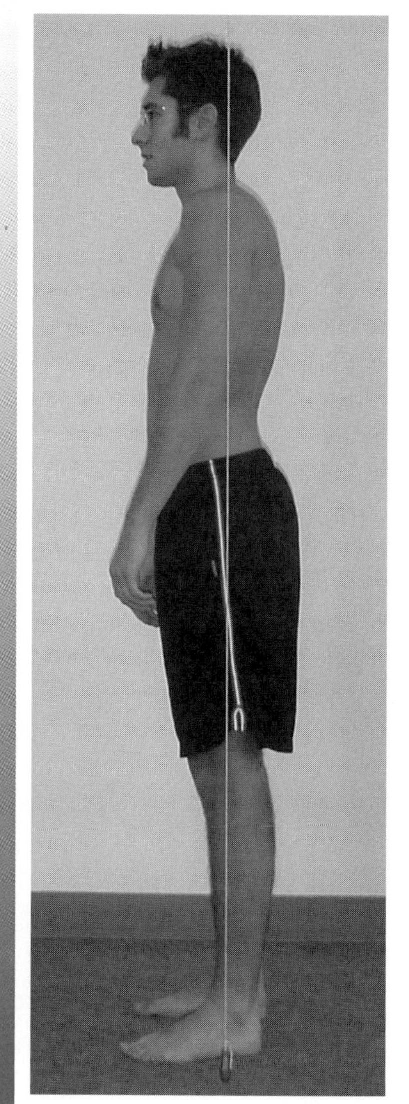

Joints Involved	Pelvis, hip joint, lumbar spine, thoracic spine, cervical spine
Potential Cause	Poor postural sense Muscle imbalance: Tightened or shortened hip flexors or back extensors Weakened or elongated hip extensors or trunk flexors
Resulting Effects	Anterior pelvic tilt Flexed hip joint Increased lumbar lordosis Increased thoracic kyphosis
Potential Associated Compressive or Distractive Forces and Pathological Conditions	Adaptive shortening of anterior chest musculature Elongation of thoracic paraspinal musculature Increased tensile forces on ligamentous structures in posterior aspect of thoracic spine and anterior aspect of lumbar spine Increased compression of lumbar facet joints Increased compression of thoracic anterior vertebral bodies Forward head posture Forward shoulder posture

Several consequences result from the presence of prolonged FSP. Biomechanical changes in the shoulder girdle can cause any number of the following soft tissue dysfunctions: degeneration of the acromioclavicular joint; bicipital or rotator cuff tendinopathy or impingement; muscular weakness; **myofascial** pain and trigger points; posterior capsular tightness; abnormal scapulohumeral rhythm; and can be attributed to excessive and habitual flexion of the back.[48–52] Adaptive shortening of the pectoralis minor or the anterior and middle scalene muscles can compress the subclavian artery, vein, and medial cord of the brachial plexus, resulting in **thoracic outlet syndrome** (Chapter 16).[51,53,54] An FSP can also be associated with traction placed on the brachial plexus at the origin of the suprascapular and dorsal scapular nerves, causing associated pain and muscle weakness of the supraspinatus, infraspinatus, and rhomboids in which they innervate.[54]

Scapula winging

Scapula winging, where the medial border projects posteriorly, can occur because of weakness of the periscapular muscles, especially the serratus anterior and middle and lower trapezius, and often occurs secondary to trauma to the long thoracic nerve. Winging is often more apparent with overhead movements. Scapula stabilization is essential for allowing normal arm mobility and biomechanics of the shoulder joint.

Myofascial A muscle and its associated fascia.

Inspection Findings 6-5
Swayback Posture

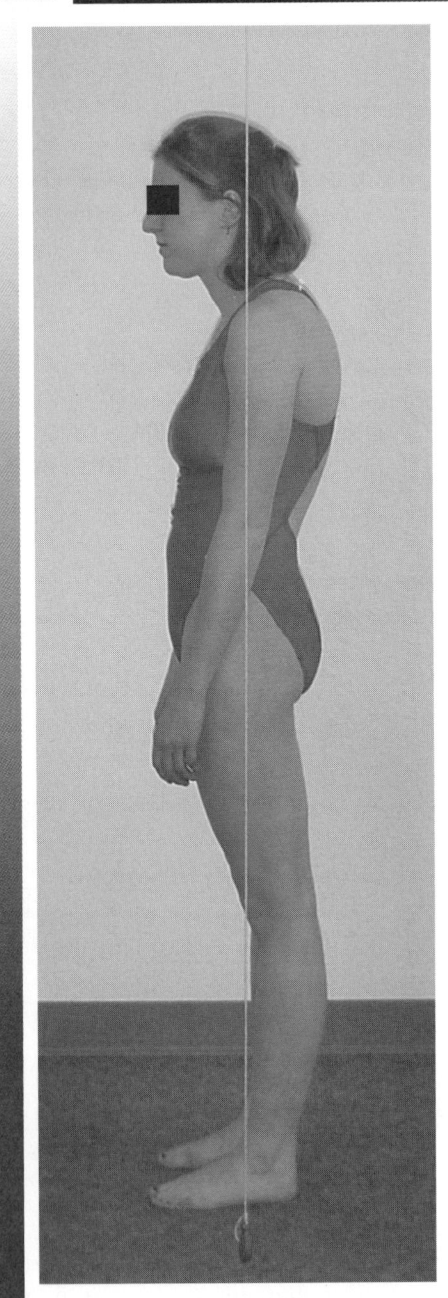

Joints Involved	Knee joint, hip joint, lumbar spine, lower thoracic spine, cervical spine
Potential Cause	Poor postural sense Tightened or shortened hip extensors Weakened or elongated hip flexors or lower abdominals Decreased general muscular strength
Resulting Effects	Genu recurvatum Extended hip joint Posterior pelvic tilt Anterior shift of the lumbosacral region Lumbar spine in neutral or minimal flexed position Increase in lower thoracic, thoracolumbar curvature (increase in lower thoracic kyphosis to cause posterior shift of trunk to compensate for anterior
Potential Associated Compressive or Distractive Forces and Pathological Conditions	Elongation or increased tensile forces on the ligamentous structures at the anterior hip joint and posterior aspect of the lower thoracic spine Adaptively shortened or increased compressive forces on the posterior ligamentous structures at the hip joint and anterior aspect of the lower thoracic spine Increased tensile forces on the soft tissue structures of the posterior knee; compressive forces on anterior knee Increased shearing forces L5/S1 Forward head posture Forward shoulder posture

Head and Cervical Spine

Forward head posture

Forward head posture (FHP), the anterior displacement of the head relative to the thorax, is a common postural deviation.[55] Observed from the lateral view, FHP is characterized by the external auditory meatus aligning anterior to the plumb line and anterior to the acromion process (Inspection Findings 6-9). This posture results in flexion of the lower cervical spine, flattening or flexion of the mid-cervical spine, and extension of the upper cervical spine (suboccipital region).

Causes of FHP include poor postural sense, use of bifocal lenses, muscle fatigue, FSP, and the need for glasses.[56] Several possible dysfunctions of the cervical spine, shoulder, temporomandibular joint, and general upper quadrant can occur as a result of FHP.[15,56] The head weighs approximately 13 lbs. Displacing this weight anteriorly on the cervical spine increases the amount of muscular activity in the posterior neck muscles and upper shoulder girdle muscles.[51]

Inspection Findings 6-6
Flat Back Posture

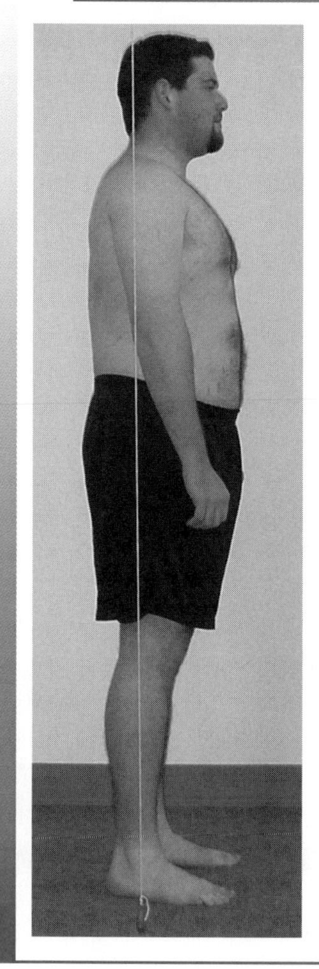

Joints Involved	Hip joint, lumbar spine, thoracic spine, cervical spine
Potential Causes	Shortened or tightened hip extensors, abdominal musculature Weakened/elongated hip flexors, back extensors Poor postural sense
Resulting Effects	Extended hip joint Posterior pelvic tilt Decreased lumbar lordosis Decreased thoracic kyphosis Flexed middle and lower cervical spine, extended upper cervical spine (FSP)
Potential Associated Compressive or Distractive Forces and Pathological Conditions	Adaptive shortening of soft tissue, compressive forces in posterior hip joint, anterior lumbar and mid-low cervical spines, posterior thoracic and upper cervical spines Elongation of soft tissue, tensile forces on the anterior hip joint, posterior lumbar and middle and lower cervical spines, anterior thoracic and upper cervical spines FHP resulting as compensation for the posterior displacement of the spine Knee flexion possibly occurring for the same reason

FHP = forward head posture; FSP = forward shoulder posture.

Forward head posture can also affect normal shoulder elevation. Elevation of the upper extremity requires cervical spine extension. If the mid and lower cervical spine remains in a flexed position, then full shoulder elevation cannot occur.[57] Certain muscle imbalances also result when FHP occurs concurrently with FSP (Table 6-14). Normally, the external auditory meatus aligns with the acromion process of the shoulder. If the AC joint and external auditory meatus are in alignment, but both landmarks are forward of the plumb line, then both FSP and FHP are present.

Table 6-14 Combination of Forward Head Posture and Forward Shoulder Posture

Muscles that Become Overactivated and Tightened	Muscles that Become Inhibited and Weakened
Pectoralis minor	Lower trapezius
Pectoralis minor	Middle trapezius
Upper trapezius	Serratus anterior
Upper rhomboids	
Levator scapulae	

Interrelationship Between Regions

Because each body part is closely linked to corresponding body parts, it is difficult to determine whether poor postural habits cause muscle imbalances, soft tissue dysfunctions, or pain or whether these conditions were the cause and poor posture was the result (Table 6-15). It is more important to understand the relationship and importance of correcting these factors because it is impossible to determine which was the cause or the effect after the fact.

Postural assessment is an important part of the evaluation process. Recognizing postural faults that are contributing to

Inspection Findings 6-7
Scoliosis

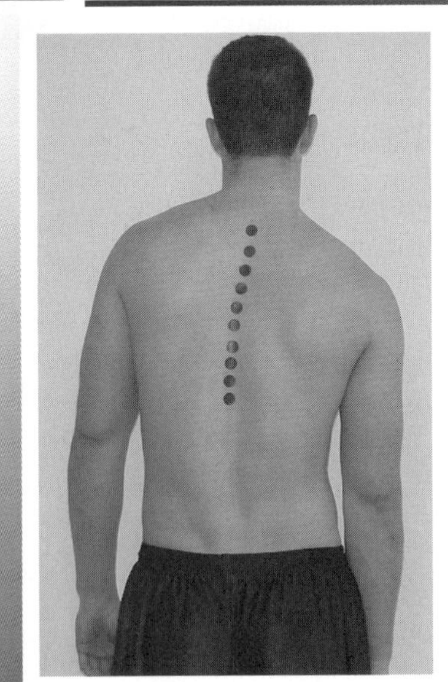

Left thoracic curve. Note the resulting asymmetrical scapular position.	
Structures Involved	Thoracic and lumbar vertebrae
Potential Causes	Structural scoliosis: Anomaly of vertebrae Functional scoliosis: Muscle imbalance, leg length discrepancy
Resulting Effects	Rotation of one or more vertebrae Compression of one facet joint; distraction of the opposite facet joint Shortened or tightened trunk muscles on concave side of the curvature Weakened or elongated trunk muscles on convex side of the curvature
Potential Associated Compressive or Distractive Forces and Pathological Conditions	Disc pathology Soft tissue pathology as the body attempts to compensate and maintain head posture Sacroiliac joint dysfunction Decreased mobility of spine and chest cage Asymmetry in chest expansion with deep breathing Decreased pulmonary function (if excessive in thoracic region) If caused by limb length inequality: Degenerative changes in lumbar spine, hip, knee joints in longer limb Muscle overuse on longer limb caused by increased muscle activity SI joint dysfunction Excessive pronation of longer limb with dysfunctions associated with pronation Alteration of pattern of mechanical stresses on joint involved—structural

SI = sacroiliac.

Inspection Findings 6-8
Forward Shoulder Posture

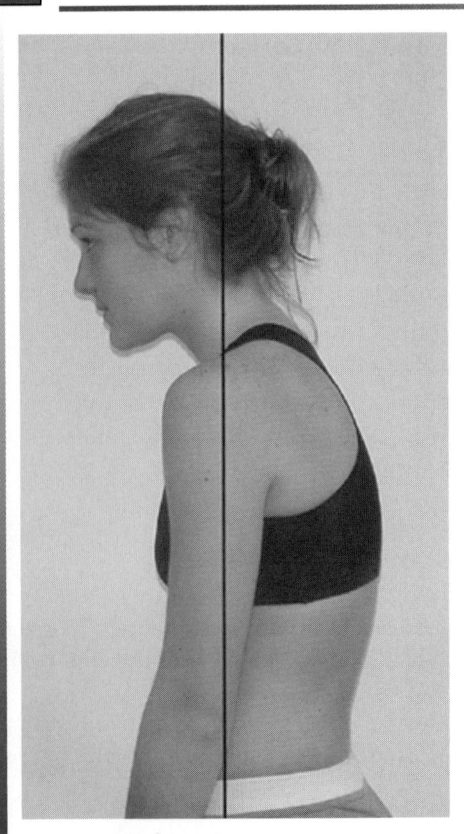

Structures Involved	Scapulothoracic articulation Glenohumeral joint Thoracic spine Cervical spine
Potential Causes	Shortened or overdeveloped anterior shoulder girdle muscles (pectoralis major, pectoralis minor) Weakened or elongated interscapular muscles (mid trap, rhomboid, lower trap) Poor postural awareness Abnormal cervical and thoracic spine sagittal plane alignments[47] Postural muscle fatigue Large breast development Repetitive occupational and sporting positions
Resulting Effects	Humeral head is displaced anteriorly; decreased posterior glide Forward head posture
Potential Associated Compressive or Distractive Forces and Pathological Conditions	Thoracic outlet syndrome Abnormal scapulohumeral rhythm and scapula stability Acromioclavicular joint degeneration Bicipital tendinopathy Impingement syndrome Trigger points, myofascial pain in periscapular muscles Abnormal biomechanics of GH joint

GH = glenohumeral.

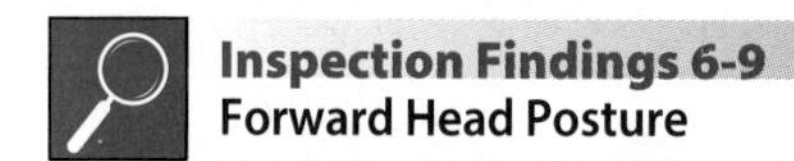

Inspection Findings 6-9
Forward Head Posture

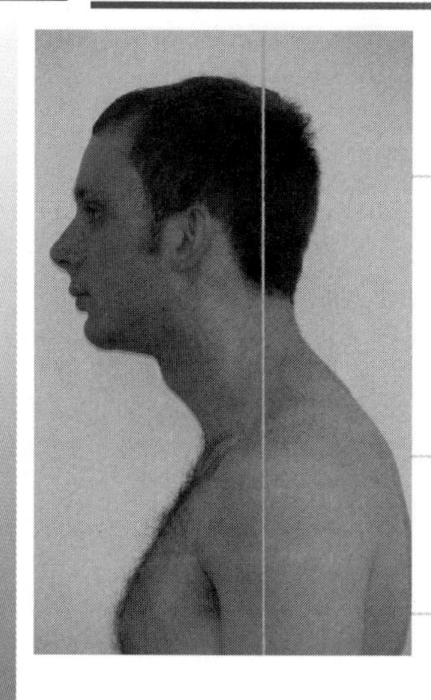

Structures Involved	Cervical spine GH joint Thoracic spine
Potential Causes	Wearing of bifocals Poor eyesight and need for glasses Muscle fatigue and weakness Poor postural sense Compensatory mechanism for other postural deviations (occupational activities and ADLs)
Resulting Effects	Flexed of lower cervical spine Flattening or flexion of mid-cervical spine Extended upper cervical spine
Potential Associated Compressive or Distractive Forces and Pathological Conditions	Adaptively shortened suboccipital muscles (capital extensors), scalenes, upper trapezius, and levator scapula Elongated and weakened anterior cervical flexors and scapular depressors Hypomobile upper cervical region with compensatory hypermobility of the mid-cervical spine Abnormal shoulder (GH joint) biomechanics; decrease in shoulder elevation Temporomandibular joint dysfunction[15] Thoracic outlet syndrome involving the anterior and mid-scalene region Myofascial pain periscapular muscles and posterior cervical muscles[56] Overuse of posterior cervical and upper shoulder girdle muscles to maintain head in forward posture[56] Forward shoulder posture

ADL = activity of daily living; GH = glenohumeral.

Table 6-15 Interrelationship Between Joints

Structure or Interconnecting Joints	Position of One Joint or Structure	Effect of Position of Other Joint or Structure
STJ and Tibia	STJ pronated	Tibia internally rotated
	STJ supinated	Tibia externally rotated
Tibia and Femur	Internal tibial rotation	Femur internally rotated
	External tibial rotation	Femur externally rotated
Tibiofemoral Joint and the Talocrural Joint	Knee joint flexed, decreasing the angle between tibia and foot	Talocrural joint dorsiflexed
	Knee joint hyperextended, increasing the angle between tibia and foot	Talocrural joint plantarflexed
Femur and Tibia	Femoral anteversion	Tibia internally rotated*
	Femoral retroversion	Tibia externally rotated*
Femur and Patella	Internal femoral rotation	Squinting patellae
	External femoral rotation	Frog-eye patellae
Pelvic Position and the Hip Joint	Pelvis in an anterior pelvic tilt, decreasing the angle between the pelvis and femur	Hip flexed
	Pelvis in a posterior pelvic tilt, increasing the angle between the pelvis and femur	Hip extended
Position of the Pelvis and the Lumbar Spine	Pelvis in an anterior pelvic tilt, flexing the sacrum (nutation) and extending the lumbar spine	Increased lumbar lordosis
	Pelvis in a posterior pelvic tilt, extending the sacrum (counter nutation) and flexing the lumbar spine	Decreased lumbar lordosis

*The patient may attempt to compensate for femoral anteversion by excessively externally rotating the tibia to maintain the feet positioned straight ahead, the opposite is also true for the patient with femoral retroversion.

STJ = subtalar joint.

functional limitations and disability and establishing a plan to work toward correcting or minimizing these faults is an essential role for a clinician. Most soft tissue dysfunctions that have a gradual, insidious onset have, at least, a minimal postural component. This postural component may result in or cause imbalances between agonist and antagonist muscle groups or **inert soft tissue** structures. Clinicians must learn to investigate and observe the entire body and the interrelationships between regions when evaluating a specific body part. Learning to look at the "whole picture" makes someone a more effective clinician and more successful in treating patients.

Documentation of Postural Assessment

Documentation of posture needs to be concise, yet as detailed as possible for the clinician to correlate possible postural impairments to the patient's functional limitations and disability. Table 6-16 presents a sample postural assessment that would be recorded in the impairment section of an initial evaluation. A sample of a standard postural assessment form is provided in Figure 6-16.

The following are guidelines for documenting posture:

- Document the view that is being observed (i.e., anterior, posterior, right lateral, left lateral).
- Quantify each postural deficit using minimum, moderate, or severe and, whenever possible, objectively measure the deficits. When measuring the deficit, note the specific landmarks used, specific positions measured, or any specific techniques used to measure them. This will assist in reproducibility of the measurement.
- Document the side of the body where the deficit occurs. If it involves unequal heights, choose whether to document the higher or lower side and then be consistent with your documentation.
- Use arrow symbols (↑ ↓) to represent increases or decreases regarding asymmetries in height.
- Use greater than (>) and less than (<) symbols to represent regions of muscle mass that are larger or smaller than the contralateral side.
- Document in an outline form (rather than paragraph form) to make the assessment easier to read and identify specific regions quickly.

Table 6-16 Documentation of Impairments Identified in a Full Postural Assessment

View	Characteristics
Anterior	Min pes planus bilateral feet
	Mod bilateral squinting patellae
	Mod bilateral genu valgum
	Min ↑ R ASIS
	Min bilateral IR shoulder, R > L
Posterior	Min bilateral calcaneal valgum
	Mod bilateral genu valgum
	Min ↓ R PSIS
	Min bilateral protraction scapulae, R > L
Right Lateral	Min genu recurvatum
	Mod ant pelvis tilt, 20°
	Min ↑ lumbar lordosis
	Min FHP
Left Lateral	Mod genu recurvatum
	Mod ant pelvis tilt, 20°
	Min ↑ lumbar lordosis
	Min FHP

ASIS = anterior superior iliac spine; FHP = forward head posture; PSIS = superior posterior iliac spine; IR = internal rotation

- Document only postural deficits in the assessment. Identify normal regions as within normal limits.
- Use standard, approved medical abbreviations. .
- Use an asterisk (*) to emphasize a significant finding by placing the * beside the deficit.
- When evaluating an upper quarter condition, include the pelvis, lumbar spine, and all joints proximal to the injury in the postural assessment.
- When evaluating a lower quarter condition, include the lumbar spine, pelvis, and all joints distal to the painful site in the postural assessment.
- Include the entire body in the postural assessment of a patient with a spinal injury.

Inert soft tissue Noncontractile soft tissue, including the joint capsule and ligaments supporting the joint capsule.

Standard Postural Assessment Form

Name: ____________ Painful area: ____________ Duration of symptoms (months): ______

Clinician: ____________ Date: ______

ANTERIOR VIEW

Alignment of plumb line with trunk: ____________

Alignment of plumb line with head: ____________

Calluses, bunions, blisters on feet: ____________

Lower Extremity

Arch Position:	□ pes planus	□ pes cavus	□ neutral
Subtalar Joint:	□ pronated	□ supinated	□ neutral
Tibia Position:	□ medial rotation	□ lateral rotation	□ neutral
Patella Position	□ squinting	□ frog-eyed	□ neutral
Leg Position:	□ genu valgum	□ genu varum	□ neutral

Q-angle: □ left: □ right:

Muscle mass/girth comments: ____________

Other comments: ____________

____

Pelvis/Trunk

Iliac crest symmetry: ____________

ASIS symmetry: ____________

Abdominal muscle mass: ____________

Chest Shape: □ pectus excavatum □ pectus recurvatum □ normal

Shoulder Girdle, Cervical Spine, and Head

Shoulder Position:	□ internally rotated	□ externally rotated	□ neutral
Shoulder Heights:	□ right elevated right	□ depressed	□ neutral
Head Position:	□ side bent	□ rotated	□ neutral

Pectoral muscle mass: ____________

Upper trapezius muscle mass: ____________

POSTERIOR VIEW

Alignment of plumb line with trunk: ____________

Alignment of plumb line with head: ____________

Note calluses, blisters on heels: ____________

Lower Extremity

Calcaneal Position:	□ genu valgum	□ genu varum	□ neutral
Leg Position:	□ genu valgum	□ genu varum	□ neutral

Muscle mass calves: ____________

Muscle mass posterior thighs: ____________

Pelvis/Trunk

Spinal Alignment: □ scoliosis □ neutral

Iliac crest symmetry: ____________

PSIS symmetry: ____________

Gluteal muscle mass: ____________

Shoulder Girdle, Cervical Spine, and Head

Scapula Positions: ____________

Elevation/depression: ____________

Protraction/retraction: ____________

Upward/downward Rotation: ____________

Winging: ____________

Periscapula muscle mass: ____________

Upper trapezius muscle mass: ____________

Shoulder height: ____________

Head Position: □ side bent □ rotated □ neutral

LATERAL VIEW: RIGHT or LEFT (circle which):

Note alignment of following structures relative to plumb line:

Lat. Malleolus:	□ anterior	□ posterior	□ bisecting
Talocrural Joint:	□ plantarflexed	□ dorsiflexed	□ neutral
Lat. Femoral Epicondyle:	□ anterior	□ posterior	□ bisecting
Knee Position:	□ flexed	□ extended	□ neutral
Greater Trochanter:	□ anterior	□ posterior	□ bisecting
Mid-Thorax:	□ anterior	□ posterior	□ bisecting
Acromion Process:	□ anterior	□ posterior	□ bisecting
Cervical Vertebral Bodies:	□ anterior	□ posterior	□ bisecting
External Auditory Meatus:	□ anterior	□ posterior	□ bisecting
Pelvic Position:	□ ant. rotation	□ post. rotation	□ neutral
Shoulder Position:	□ forward	□ neutral	
Head Position:	□ forward	□ neutral	

Lumbar Spine Position: ____________

Thoracic Spine Position: ____________

Cervical Spine Position: ____________

Shoulder/Head: ____________

LATERAL VIEW: RIGHT or LEFT (circle which):

Note alignment of following structures relative to plumb line:

Lat. Malleolus:	□ anterior	□ posterior	□ bisecting
Talocrural Joint:	□ plantarflexed	□ dorsiflexed	□ neutral
Lat. Femoral Epicondyle:	□ anterior	□ posterior	□ bisecting
Knee Position:	□ flexed	□ extended	□ neutral
Greater Trochanter:	□ anterior	□ posterior	□ bisecting
Mid-Thorax:	□ anterior	□ posterior	□ bisecting
Acromion Process:	□ anterior	□ posterior	□ bisecting
Cervical Vertebral Bodies:	□ anterior	□ posterior	□ bisecting
External Auditory Meatus:	□ anterior	□ posterior	□ bisecting
Pelvic Position:	□ ant. rotation	□ post. rotation	□ neutral
Shoulder Position:	□ forward	□ neutral	
Head Position:	□ forward	□ neutral	

Lumbar Spine Position: ____________

Thoracic Spine Position: ____________

Cervical Spine Position: ____________

Shoulder/Head: ____________

FIGURE 6-16 ■ Sample postural assessment form.

REFERENCES

1. Kendall, FP, et al: *Muscles: Testing and Function with Posture and Pain*, ed 5. Baltimore, Lippincott Williams & Wilkins, 2005.
2. Kisner, C, and Colby, LA: *Therapeutic Exercise: Foundations and Techniques*, ed 4. Philadelphia, FA Davis, 2002.
3. Kendall, HO, Kendall, FP, and Boynton, DA: *Posture and Pain.* Huntington, NY, Robert E. Krieger, 1970, pp 15, 153.
4. Norkin, CC: Posture. In Levangie, PK, and Norkin, CC (eds): *Joint Structure and Function: A Comprehensive Analysis*, ed 4. Philadelphia, FA Davis, 2005, pp 479–512,
5. Riegger-Krugh, C, and Keysor, JJ: Skeletal malalignments of the lower quarter: Correlated and compensatory motions and postures. *J Orthop Sports Phys Ther*, 23:164, 1996.
6. Borstad, JD: Resting position variables at the shoulder: Evidence to support a posture-impairment association. *Phys Ther*, 86:549, 2006.
7. Borstad, JD, and Ludewig, PM: The effect of long versus short pectoralis minor resting length on scapular kinematics in healthy individuals. *J Orthop Sports Phys Ther*, 35: 227, 2005.
8. Massie, DL, and Haddox, A: Influence of lower extremity biomechanics and muscle imbalances on the lumbar spine. *Athl Ther Today*, 4:46, 1999.
9. Tibierio, D: Pathomechanics of structural foot deformities. *Phys Ther*, 68:1840, 1988.
10. Whilt, SG, and Sahrmann, SA: A Movement system approach to management of musculoskeletal pain. In Grant, R: *Clinics in Physical Therapy: Physical Therapy of the Cervical and Thoracic Spine.* New York, Churchill Livingstone, 1994.
11. Jull, GA, and Janda, V: Muscles and motor control in low back pain: Assessment and management. In Twomey, LT, and Taylor, JR (eds): *Physical Therapy of the Low Back*, ed 2. New York, Churchill Livingstone, 1994, pp 253–277.
12. Mannheimer, JS, and Rosenthal, RM: Acute and chronic postural abnormalities as related to craniofascial pain and temporomandibular disorders. *Dent Clin North Am*, 35:185, 1991.
13. Krivickas, LS: Anatomical factors associated with overuse sports injuries. *Sports Med*, 24:132, 1997.
14. Novack, C, and Mackinnon, S: Repetitive use and static postures: A source of nerve compression and pain. *J Hand Ther*, 10:151, 1997.
15. Harrison, AL, Barry-Greb, T, and Wojtowicz, G: Clinical measurement of head and shoulder posture variables. *J Orthop Sports Phys Ther*, 23:353, 1996.
16. Garrett, TR, Youdas, JW, and Madson, TJ: Reliability of measuring forward head posture in a clinical setting. *J Orthop Sports Phys Ther*, 17:155, 1993.
17. Raine, S, and Twomey, LT: Head and shoulder posture variations in 160 asymptomatic women and men. *Arch Phys Med Rehabil*, 78:1215, 1997.
18. Peterson, DE, et al: Investigation of the validity and reliability of four objective techniques for measuring forward shoulder posture. *J Orthop Sports Phys Ther*, 25:34, 1997.
19. Greenfield, BH, et al: The influence of cephalostatic ear rods on the positions of the head and neck during positional recordings. *Am J Dentofacial Orthop*, 95:312, 1989.
20. Molhave, A: *A Biostatic Investigation of the Human Erect Posture.* Munkgard, Copenhagen, 1958.
21. Sheir-Neiss, GI, et al: The association of backpack use and back pain in adolescents. *Spine*, 28:922, 2003.
22. Brackley, HM, and Stevenson, JM: Are children's backpack weight limits enough? A critical review of relevant literature. *Spine*, 29:2184, 2004.
23. Kovacs, FM, et al: Effect of firmness of mattress on chronic non-specific low-back pain: randomized, double-blind, controlled multicentre trial. *Lancet*, 362:1599, 2003.
24. Flegal, KM, et al: Overweight and obesity in the United States: Prevalence and trends, 1960–1994. *Int J Obes Relat Metab Disord*, 22:39, 1998.
25. Prentice, AM, and Jebb, SA: Beyond body mass index. *Obesity Rev*, 2:141, 2001.
26. Ferguson, BRL: Limb length discrepancies. *J Am Podiatr Med Assoc*, 82:33, 1992.
27. Gurney, B: Leg length discrepancy. *Gait and Posture*, 15:195, 2002.
28. Beal, MC: A review of the short leg problem. *J Am Osteopath Assoc*, 50:109, 1950.
29. Botte, RR: An interpretation of the pronator syndrome and foot types of patients with LBP. *J Am Podiatr Med Assoc*, 71:243, 1981.
30. Friberg, O, et al: Accuracy and precision of clinical estimation of leg length inequality and lumbar scoliosis: Comparison of clinical and radiographical measurements. *Int Disabil Stud*, 10:45, 1988.
31. Hoyle, DA, Latour, M, and Bohannon, RW: Intraexaminer, interexaminer, and interdevice comparability of leg length measurements obtained with measuring tape and Metrecom. *J Orthop Sports Phys Ther*, 14:263, 1991.
32. Hanada, E, et al: Measuring leg-length discrepancy by the "iliac crest palpation and book correction" method: reliability and validity. *Arch Phys Med Rehabil*, 82:938, 2001.
33. Defrin, R, et al: Conservative correction of leg-length discrepancies of 10 mm or less for the relief of chronic low back pain. *Arch Phys Med Rehabil*, 86:2075, 2005.
34. Hoppenfeld, S: Physical examination of the hip and pelvis. In Hoppenfeld, S (ed): *Physical Examination of the Spine and Extremities.* New York, Appleton-Century-Crofts, 1976, p 165.
35. Krawiec, CJ, et al: Static innominate asymmetry and leg length discrepancy in asymptomatic collegiate athletics. *Man Ther*, 8:207, 2003.
36. Levangie, PK: The association between static pelvic asymmetry and low back pain. *Spine*, 24:1234, 1999.
37. Nijs, J, et al: Clinical assessment of scapular positioning in patients with shoulder pain: State of the art. *J Manip Phys Ther*, 30:68, 2007.
38. Keenan, A, et al: The Foot Posture Index: Rasch analysis of a novel, foot-specific outcome measure. *Arch Phys Med Rehabil*, 88:88, 2007.
39. Redmond, AC, Crossbie, J, and Ouvrier, RA: Development and validation of a novel rating system for scoring standing foot posture: The Foot Posture Index. *Clin Biomech*, 21:89, 2006.
40. Yates, B, and White, S: The incidence and risk factors in the development of medial tibial stress syndrome among naval recruits. *AJSM*, 32:772, 2004.
41. Heath, CM, and Stahili, LT: Normal limits of knee angle in white children—genu varum and genu valgum. *J Pediatr Orthop*, 13:259,1993.

42. Naudie, DDR, Amendola, A, and Fowler, PJ: Opening wedge high tibial osteotomy for symptomatic hyperextension-varus thrust. *Am J Sports Med*, 32:60, 2004.
43. Byl, NN, et al: Postural imbalance and vibratory sensitivity in patients with idiopathic scoliosis: Implications for treatment. *J Orthop Sports Phys Ther*, 26:60, 1997.
44. Weinstin, SL, et al: Health and function of patients with untreated idiopathic scoliosis. A 50-year natural history study. *JAMA*, 289:559, 2003.
45. U.S. Preventive Services Task Force: Screening for idiopathic scoliosis in adolescents: Recommendation statement. *Am Fam Phys*, 71:1975, 2005.
46. DiVeta, J, Walker, ML, and Skibinski, B: Relationship between performance of selected scapula muscles and scapula abduction in standing subjects. *Phys Ther*, 70:470, 1990.
47. Culham, E, and Peat, M: Spinal and shoulder complex posture: Measurement using the 3S pace isotrak. *Clin Rehabil*, 7:309, 1993.
48. Ayub, E: Posture and the upper quarter. In Donatelli, RA (ed): *Physical Therapy of the Shoulder*, ed 2. New York, Churchill Livingstone, 1991.
49. Greenfield, B, et al: Posture in patients with shoulder overuse injuries and healthy individuals. *J Orthop Sports Phys Ther*, 21:287, 1995.
50. Knudsen, HO: *Posture: Sitting, Standing, Chair Design and Exercise.* Springfield, IL, Charles C Thomas, 1988, pp 125, 314–315.
51. Langford, ML: Poor posture subjects a worker's body to muscle imbalance, nerve compression. *Occup Health Saf*, 63:38, 1994.
52. Travell, JG, and Simons, DG: *Myofascial Pain and Dysfunction. The Trigger Point Manual.* Baltimore, Williams & Wilkins, 1984.
53. Kopel, HP, and Thompson, WAL: *Peripheral Entrapment Neuropathies*, ed 2. New York, Robert E. Krieger, 1976.
54. Howell, JW: Evaluation and management of thoracic outlet syndrome. In Donatelli, RA (ed): *Physical Therapy of the Shoulder*, ed 2. New York, Churchill Livingstone, 1991.
55. Willford, CH, et al: The interaction of wearing multifocal lenses with head posture and pain. *J Orthop Sports Phys Ther*, 23:194, 1996.
56. Garrett, TR, Youdas, JW, and Madison, TJ: Reliability of measuring forward head posture in a clinical setting. *J Orthop Sports Phys Ther*, 17:155, 1993.
57. Lee, DG: "Tennis elbow": A manual therapist's perspective. *J Orthop Sports Phys Ther*, 8:134, 1986.

CHAPTER 7

Evaluation of Gait

Monique Mokha, PhD, ATC

Walking has been described as a series of narrowly averted catastrophes where the body falls forward, and then the legs move under the body to establish a new base of support.[1] Watching a toddler walk across the room, struggling to control balance against the force of gravity, demonstrates the intricacy of this learned chain of events. As motor function and coordination develop, walking becomes a subconscious effort. The cyclic actions of gait can, however, develop deviations, or become temporarily or permanently impaired as the result of acute injury, chronic pain, or anatomical and biomechanical abnormalities.

Gait evaluation may be needed to identify underlying causes of functional limitations or of chronic pain related to physical activity. Results can be used to compare a patient's performance to normative data, classify the severity of disability, determine the efficacy of an intervention, enhance performance, assist in shoe selection, and/or identify mechanisms that might be causing gait dysfunction.

Gait analysis is the functional evaluation of a person's walking or running style and is the classic test of function for lower extremity pathology.[2] Gait changes can be subtle or dramatic and can arise from acute or chronic injury or improper biomechanics. Consider, for example, an athlete who limps off the basketball court after suffering an ankle sprain. The trauma to the stabilizing ligaments and pain prohibits the ankle from normal weight bearing, yielding such abnormalities as a shorter stance time and a decreased or absent push-off from the forefoot on the involved leg. This, in turn, alters the mechanics of the knee, the hip, and possibly the lumbar spine. Theoretically, when acute trauma heals normally, normal gait should return. Chronic injuries (e.g., peroneal tendinopathy) or congenital abnormalities (e.g., tarsal coalition) can permanently alter gait. Consequently, altered stresses are created that may lead to injury or pain along the kinetic chain. Finally, an analysis of *running* gait is critical in the athletic patient as pain and/or improper biomechanics may amplify from walking to running. This analysis also yields more sport-specific information.

The results of the gait analysis are most useful if combined and compared with the results from the remainder of the examination (Fig. 7-1). A meaningful assessment requires a keen eye, guided practice, a planned system of observation, and a detailed understanding of the components of walking and running gait.

Gait Terminology

To begin gait analysis, standardized definitions of terminology are needed. Temporal–spatial, or time–distance variables include measures of stride duration, stride length, step length, step width, cadence, and velocity. A **step** is the sequence of events from a specific point in the gait of one

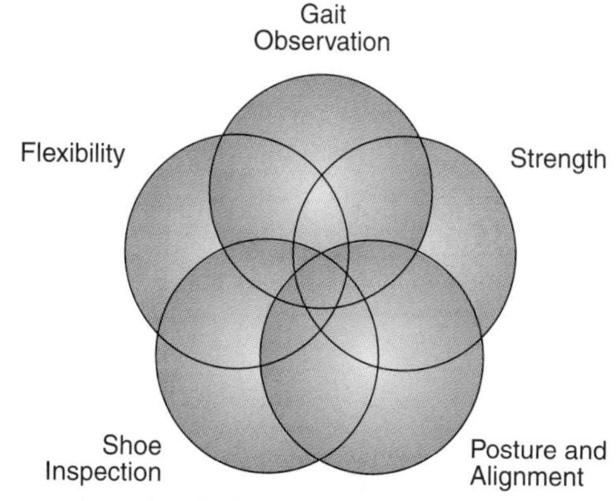

Figure 7-1 ■ Interplay of influences on gait diagnosis. The determination of gait involves the quantification of running mechanics, strength, and flexibility of the lower extremity and lumbar spine, body posture and segmental alignment, and an inspection of footwear.

extremity, initial contact for example, to the same point in the opposite extremity. **Step length** is the linear distance covered by a step. **Step width** is the distance between the points of contact of both feet. Two sequential steps comprise a **stride** (Fig. 7-2).

The temporal (time-based) aspects of gait can be quantified by using a stopwatch and counting the number of steps taken to walk a measured distance. **Cadence** is the number of steps taken per unit time, and is usually expressed in steps per minute. The normal cadence for walking in adults is 107 ± 2.7 steps per minute, with women having a greater cadence than men.[3] Velocity, a valid overall predictor of functional disability during walking, is defined as the distance covered per unit time and is usually expressed in meters per second (m/sec). This yields basic measurements of **gait velocity** (meters per second) and **gait cadence** (steps per minute). Gait velocity correlates highly with walking performance and is commonly measured. The spatial aspects of gait can be quantified by measuring the distance between one foot strike to the next. This yields a basic measurement of a patient's step length.

Stride time is time required to complete a single stride, and **stride length** is the linear distance covered in one stride. The normal step length for the right and left stride is 75 ± 1.6 cm.[3]

Kinetic measures such as **ground reaction force** (GRF) and **center of pressure** (CoP) are derived with the use of force plates, pressure plates, or insoles. Every contact of the foot with the ground generates force yielding vertical, anteroposterior (A/P), and mediolateral (M/L) components (Fig. 7-3).

Vertical GRF provides a good indication of the impacts the body is sustaining, while A/P GRFs give information in the horizontal direction regarding breaking force at initial foot contact, and propulsive force when the foot leaves the surface. Mediolateral GRFs also provide information in the horizontal direction, but rather with regard to force generation and absorption in the frontal plane. GRF magnitudes are typically expressed in body weights, and the largest magnitudes are in the vertical GRF which has a characteristic "m" shape denoting initial contact and toe-off where vertical forces are greatest during stance (Fig. 7-4).

CoP measures are derived from GRFs and can be used to show the path of the pressure point underneath the

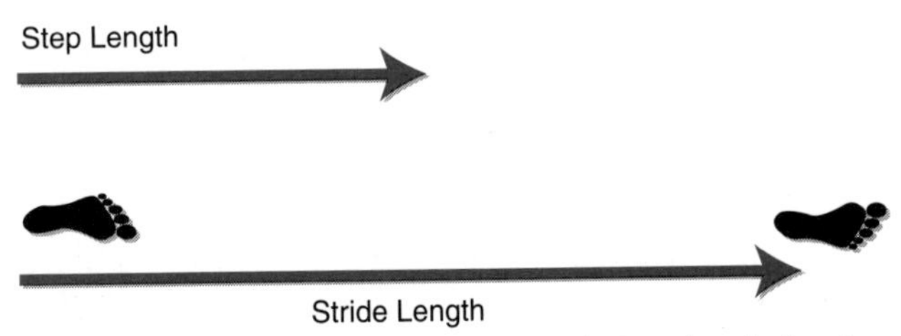

Figure 7-2 ■ Step length versus stride length. Step length describes the distance covered by one limb; stride length describes the distance covered by both limbs during gait.

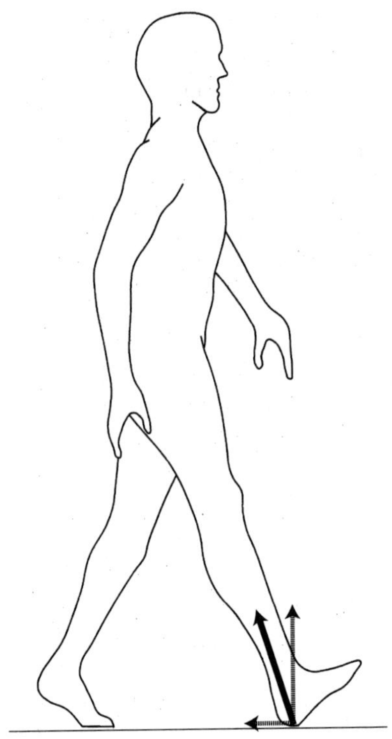

Figure 7-3 ■ Ground reaction forces with horizontal, vertical, and resultant components during walking.

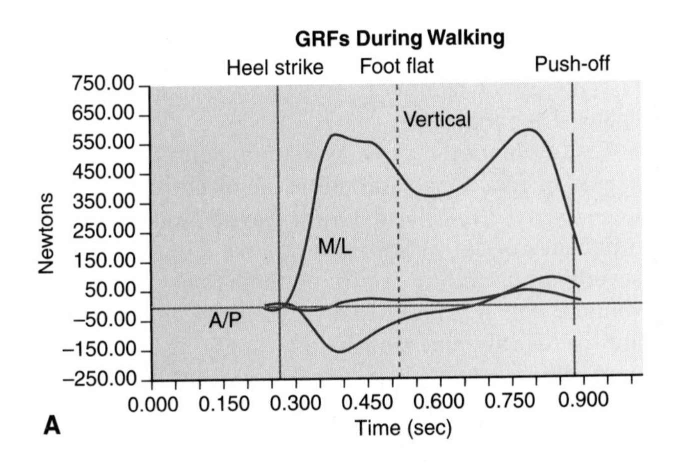

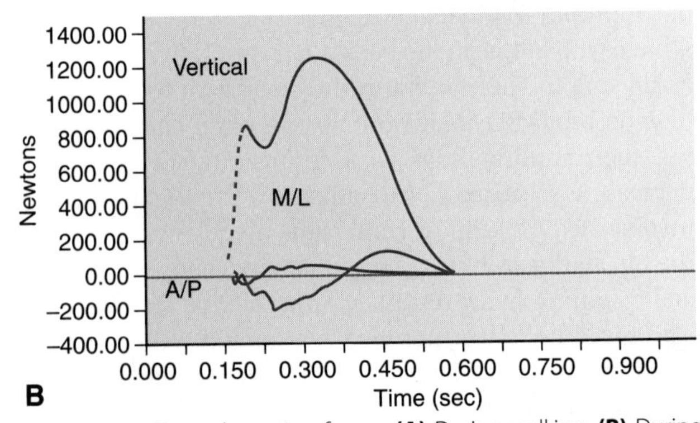

Figure 7-4 ■ Ground reaction forces. **(A)** During walking. **(B)** During running.

foot during gait. CoP paths are altered in the presence of pain, orthotics, different shoe types, barefoot versus shod conditions, different walking or running speeds, and where on the shoe a runner strikes (rear-, mid-, forefoot) (Fig. 7-5).[4]

Walking Gait Phases

During the walking gait cycle each leg alternates between a supportive (stance) and a nonsupportive (swing) phase (Fig. 7-6). While one leg is in the stance phase, the other leg is in the swing phase. At two points in the gait cycle, midstance and terminal stance, the body is supported by a single limb.

Efficient gait incorporates minimal upward and side-to-side motion and maximal forward motion. The path of the **center of gravity** is that of a smooth, sinusoidal curve without sharp breaks. The more efficient the walking gait, the less horizontal motion. The body vertically rises and falls approximately 5 cm and there is a slight lateral motion in

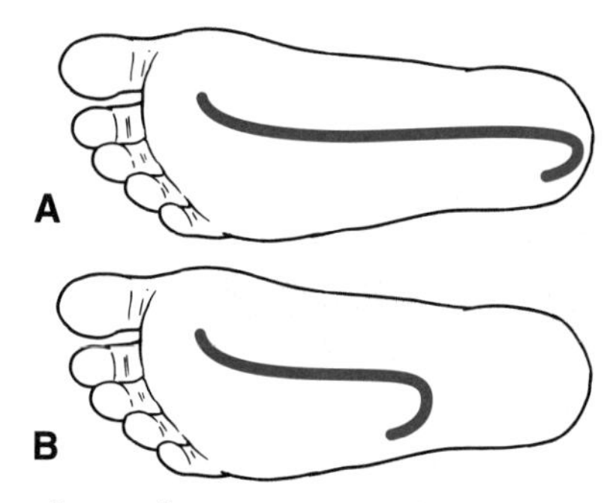

Figure 7-5 ■ Center of pressure patterns for the left foot. **(A)** Rearfoot striker. **(B)** Midfoot striker.

the horizontal plane (Fig. 7-7). As the speed of walking increases, the rotation of the spine is aided by shoulder action, with the opposite arm moving forward as the foot advances. To lengthen the stride, the pelvis rotates on the supporting femur internally rotating the hip joint. At the same time, the swinging limb is rotated externally at the hip to keep the foot aligned with the direction of movement.

The stance and swing phases are further divided into discrete periods. The following sections describe the adult norms for **kinematic**, **kinetic**, and muscle activity measures within each phase.

Stance Phase

A closed kinetic chain is created in the lower extremity during weight bearing, allowing forces from the lower extremity to be transferred to the ground, thereby producing movement.[5] The stance phase, typically lasting 600 ms (0.6 s) consists of two periods of double limb support (initial stance and terminal stance), beginning with initial contact of the foot on the surface and ending as the foot breaks the contact with the ground. Advancement of the body over the supporting limb occurs in the stance phase, constituting approximately 60 percent of the gait cycle. The **stance phase** is the high-energy portion of gait because the descending leg decelerates just before and at the time of the initial contact, thus preventing injury to the heel.

The stance phase involves the transfer of kinetic energy. During the early portion of stance, kinetic energy is absorbed from the ground and transferred up the kinetic chain. During the push-off phase the limb transfers energy to the ground, moving the body forward.[6] Nearly 60 percent

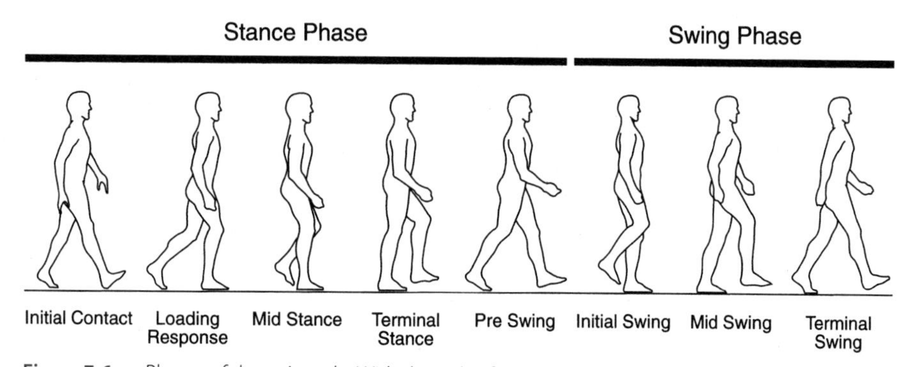

Figure 7-6 ■ Phases of the gait cycle. With the right (facing) limb as an example, two distinct phases occur—the weight-bearing stance phase and the non–weight-bearing swing phase. With the exception of the dual phases of double limb support, one limb is in the stance phase and the other is in the swing phase and vice versa. (Courtesy of Norkin, CC, and Levangie, PK: Joint *Structure and Function: A Comprehensive Analysis*, ed 2. Philadelphia, FA Davis, 1992.)

Step length The distance traveled between the initial contacts of the right and left foot.

Center of gravity The point inside or outside the body where the body is equally balanced or where gravitational pull is concentrated.

Kinematic The characteristics of movement related to time and space (e.g., range of motion, velocity, and acceleration); the effects of joint action.

Kinetic The forces being analyzed; the causes of joint action.

Stance phase The weight-bearing phase of gait, beginning on initial contact with the surface and ending when contact is broken.

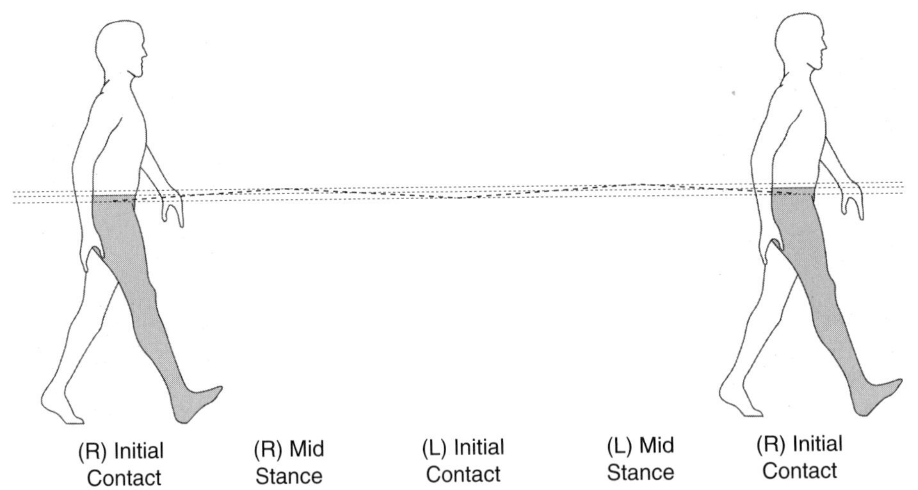

Figure 7-7 ■ Path of the center of gravity during gait. The body's center of gravity, typically located near the L5/S1 joint, moves approximately 2 cm in the frontal plane and 4 cm in the transverse plane during normal gait.

of the body's weight is loaded abruptly (less than 20 ms) onto the limb during early stance phase highlighting the importance of muscle strength and coordination in attenuating shock, preserving gait velocity, and maintaining stability. Five distinct periods occur during the stance phase: initial contact, loading response, midstance, terminal stance, and preswing (Box 7-1).

Initial contact

Initial contact begins with the instant that the foot touches the supporting surface. This contact should occur on the lateral aspect of the heel, then move forward toward the lateral edge of the foot through the loading response and midstance phases and finally diagonally toward the undersurface of the great toe at terminal stance. Although this pattern is similar among individuals, each person's exact pressure pattern is unique.[6]

During initial contact, both limbs are in contact with the ground at the same time. This double-support period represents approximately 20 percent of the total gait cycle.

Loading response

The loading response occurs immediately after initial contact. During this period, the limb reacts to accepting the impact of the body weight. The body weight is then advanced onto the foot by midtarsal and subtalar joint pronation, coupled with internal tibial rotation. The dorsiflexors eccentrically contract to control the ankle plantarflexion that helps to place of the foot on the surface. This period lasts until the opposite extremity has left the surface and double limb support has ended.

Midstance

Midstance begins as the body weight moves directly over the support limb and stationary foot, and concludes when the center of gravity is directly over the foot. At this point, the foot is flat on the surface. The ankle plantarflexors begin activation eccentrically as single limb support begins to control advancement of the tibia over the foot and to stabilize the knee.

Terminal stance

The terminal stance begins as the center of gravity passes over the foot and ends just before the contralateral limb makes initial contact with the ground. The body moves ahead of the supporting foot with the weight shift over the metatarsal heads until the contralateral limb provides a new base of support. As the heel begins to rise, the gastrocnemius continues to contract to begin active plantarflexion.

Preswing

Preswing is the final period of the stance phase, the transitional period of double support during which the limb is rapidly unloaded from the ground and prepared to swing forward. This is the second of the two periods with double limb support in a normal walking gait cycle. Preswing begins with the initial contact of the contralateral limb and ends with the toe-off of the stance limb. With the weight is over the first metatarsophalangeal joint, the ankle plantarflexors act concentrically to generate force for pushing off.

Swing Phase

The low-energy phase of the gait cycle occurs during the acceleration portion, or swing phase, and represents approximately 38 percent of the gait cycle.[5] The **swing phase** begins as soon as the toes leave the surface and terminates when the limb next makes contact with the surface. The swing phase achieves foot clearance and advancing of the trailing limb and limb repositioning for subsequent initial contact. Gravity is working in favor of

Swing phase The non–weight bearing phase of gait; beginning at the instant the foot leaves the surface and ending just before initial contact.

the pendulum swing of the limb by pulling the leg mass down toward the surface. The momentum gained at toe-off helps carry the leg through the swing phase, requiring considerably less energy than that expended in the stance phase.[6] Three distinct periods occur during the swing phase: initial swing, midswing, and terminal swing (Box 7-2).

Initial swing

Initial swing begins at the point when the toes leave the ground creating a propulsive force, and continues until the knee reaches its maximum range of flexion, approximately 60 degrees. The thigh is advanced and the ankle dorsiflexes through concentric contraction to begin toe clearance. The ankle dorsiflexors remain active throughout the swing phases.

Midswing

During midswing, the knee extends from the point of maximum flexion to the point at which the tibia reaches a vertical position perpendicular to the ground. The thigh continues to advance, toe clearance is ensured, and the propulsion force continues to be developed.

Terminal swing

The final period of the swing phase is the terminal swing, which occurs from the end of the midswing to the initial contact period of the stance phase. The momentum gained from toe-off assists in carrying the leg through in a pendulum-like motion. The trunk is erect, the thigh decelerates for heel contact, and the knee extends to create a step length for heel contact.

Muscle Activity During Gait

Understanding muscle activity and necessary available range of motion (ROM) helps in identifying impairments and compensations associated with pathologies. For example, an inability to achieve approximately 60 degrees of weight-bearing knee flexion needed during midstance will result in compensatory strategies to shorten the limb.

Hip

At initial contact, the hip is flexed to approximately 30 degrees and begins its movement to a maximum of 20 degrees of extension as stance continues. In the swing phase, the hip flexes back to 30 degrees, then just before initial contact it begins to extend to place the foot on the ground.

At initial contact, the hip is in a neutral adduction–abduction position and is externally rotated approximately 5 degrees. By early midstance, the maximum adducted position of approximately 5 degrees is achieved to limit side-to-side excursion. Throughout the remainder of stance, the hip abducts to approximately 10 degrees at toe-off. Hip rotation ROM during gait is highly variable across individuals, but the joint typically begins internally rotating by terminal stance. It then reverses its action and externally rotates as the heel begins to rise to a maximal position of 15 degrees during initial swing. During the swing phase, the hip internally rotates to within 3 degrees of neutral and stays relatively constant (± 2 degrees).

During early stance phase, the hip extensors act concentrically while the hip abductors stabilize the joint. Electromyography (EMG) recordings show increasing activity of the lower fibers of the gluteus maximus from initial contact to the middle of loading response that gradually decreases by the end of loading response. The upper fibers of the gluteus maximus and medius increase activity through loading response and gradually decrease by the end of midstance. Moderate activation of the posterior fibers of the tensor fascia lata occurs at the initiation of the loading response while the posterior fibers become active through terminal stance. During preswing, initial swing, and midswing, the hip flexors (adductor longus, rectus femoris, sartorius, iliacus, psoas major) are activated to advance the limb. The adductor longus is activated earliest in terminal stance and continues the longest into early midswing. The hip flexors also function during push-off to aid in toe clearance and positioning the limb in swing phase. The rectus femoris is activated during preswing and persists into early initial swing. The iliacus, sartorius, and gracilis have short periods of activation, primarily during initial swing.

Knee

At initial contact, the knee is near or at full extension. As contact continues, the knee flexes to a maximum of approximately 20 degrees at midstance to assist in force absorption. Toward the end of midstance the knee moves back to near full extension. The knee then flexes to approximately 40 degrees during preswing. It continues to flex following push-off to a maximum of 60 to 70 degrees, then moves toward extension as the leg prepares for initial contact again.

When the knee is extended, stability is derived from its bony alignment and ligamentous support, with the primary restraints occurring against valgus (abduction) and varus (adduction). Knee valgus and varus alignment should remain within 2 to 3 degrees of neutral during stance.

Rotation at the knee during the stance phase ranges between 10 and 20 degrees, primarily occurring during flexion (internal rotation) and extension (external rotation). This coupling of motions is caused by the bony shape of the femoral condyles and tibial plateaus (screw-home mechanism).

Most of the hamstring muscles are active during late midswing or terminal swing to control the acceleration of knee extension and hip flexion as the limb prepares for

Box 7-1
Stance Phase of Gait

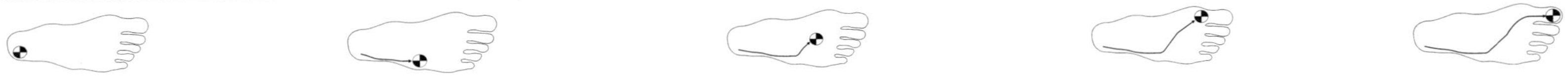

	Initial Contact	Loading Response	Midstance	Terminal Stance	Preswing
Weight-Bearing Surface					
Subtalar Joint	5° Supination	10° Pronation	5° Pronation, supinating toward neutral	5° Supination	10° Supination
Talocrural Joint	Neutral or slightly plantarflexed moving in plantar flexion direction	Reaches maximum of 7° plantarflexion	Reaches maximum of 15° dorsiflexion as lower leg moves anteriorly over foot	5°–10° Dorsiflexion moving toward plantarflexion	0°–20° Plantarflexion
Knee	0° Flexion: Tibia externally rotated	20° Flexion: Tibia internally rotates, tibia begins to externally rotate as the knee extends	20° Flexion to 0°: Tibia externally rotating	5° Flexion to 0°: Tibia externally rotates	0°–40° Flexion: Tibia externally rotates
Hip	30° Flexion: Femur externally rotated	30° Flexion: Femur internally rotating to neutral	25° Flexion to 0°: Femur internally rotated Femur is abducted 5°	0°–10° Extension: Femur externally rotates and adducts	20° Extension to 0° extension: Femur externally rotates with slight abduction

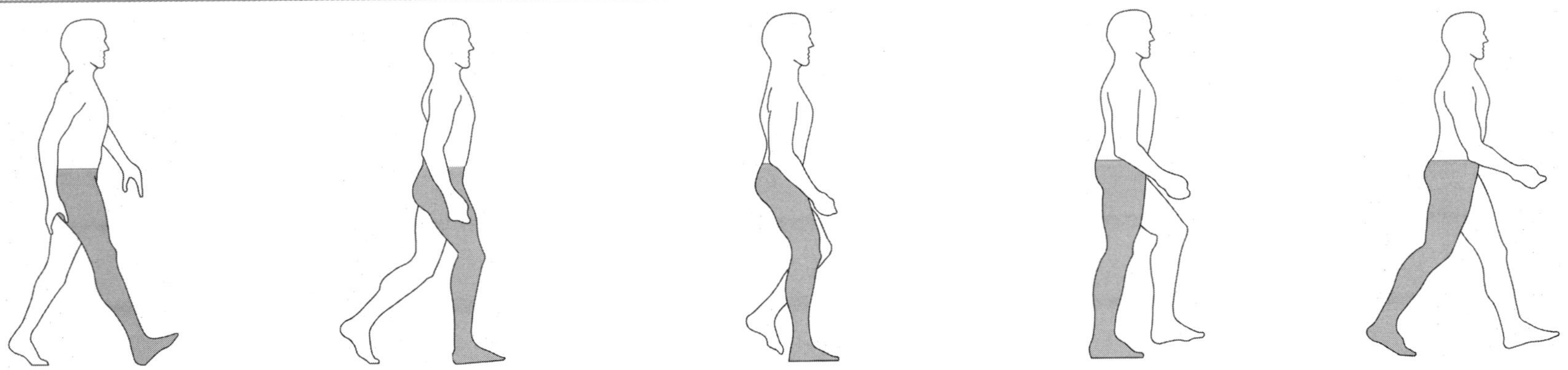

Muscle Activity				
Foot Intrinsics				
Isometric stabilization	Eccentric	Concentric	Concentric	Concentric
Plantarflexors				
Silent	Eccentric	Eccentric	Eccentric to concentric	Concentric
Dorsiflexors				
Eccentric	Eccentric	Concentric, but momentum can carry the talocrural joint through its range of motion.	Isometric	Concentric to silent
Quadriceps				
Concentric	Eccentric	Silent	Silent	Eccentric to silent
Hamstrings				
Eccentric	Isometric stabilization	Isometric	Concentric	Concentric
Hip Adductors				
Eccentric	Eccentric	Isometric	Isometric	Eccentric to control the pelvis
Gluteus Maximus				
Isometric to eccentric	Concentric	Silent	Isometric	Isometric
Gluteus Medius and Minimus				
Eccentric	Isometric or concentric	Concentric	Concentric	Isometric
Iliopsoas				
Eccentric	Isometric stabilization	Eccentric	Eccentric	Concentric

Figures modified from Levangie, PK, and Norkin, CC: *Joint Structure and Function: A Comprehensive Analysis*, ed 4. Philadelphia, FA Davis, 2005.

Box 7-2
Swing Phase of Gait

	Initial Swing	Midswing	Terminal Swing
Limb Position			
Weight-Bearing Surface	⊘	⊘	⊘
Subtalar Joint	Pronating	Neutral	5° Supination
Talocrural Joint	Reaches maximum of 20° rapid dorsiflexion for toe clearance	Neutral	Neutral
Knee	30°–70° Flexion: Tibia internally rotates	30°–0° Flexion: Tibia externally rotates	0°: Tibia externally rotates
Hip	0°–20° Flexion: Femur externally rotates to neutral	20°–30° Flexion: Femur externally rotates	30° Flexion: Femur externally rotates
Muscle Activity			
Foot Intrinsics	Isometric stabilization	Isometric	Isometric stabilization
Plantarflexors	Concentric, reducing muscular activity	Concentric	Isometric

Dorsiflexors		
Concentric until the foot is clear of the ground, then isometric	Isometric	Isometric
Quadriceps		
Concentric	Silent—Momentum carries the limb through the ROM	Concentric to stabilize the knee
Hamstrings		
Concentric to eccentric	Eccentric	Eccentric
Hip Adductors		
Concentric	Isometric	Eccentric
Gluteus Maximus		
Isometric	Eccentric	Eccentric
Gluteus Medius and Minimus		
Isometric	Isometric	Isometric
Iliopsoas		
Concentric	Concentric or silent	Isometric

Figures modified from Levangie, PK, and Norkin, CC: *Joint Structure and Function: A Comprehensive Analysis*, ed 4. Philadelphia, FA Davis, 2005.

initial contact. During early midswing, the short head of the biceps femoris is active to flex the knee enough to assist in toe clearance. As the limb approaches contact from the swing phase, the quadriceps group is acting concentrically to extend the knee. On initial contact the quadriceps eccentrically contract to control flexion. Thereafter, the quadriceps act concentrically to extend the knee as the body's center of mass is raised over the contact limb.

Foot and Ankle

At initial contact, the ankle is in neutral or slightly plantarflexed; as the limb moves into loading response, the ankle plantarflexes to a maximum of 7 degrees. During midstance, terminal stance, and preswing the ankle dorsiflexes to a maximum of 15 degrees as the lower leg traverses anteriorly over the contact foot and as the body weight is transferred to the opposite limb. A rapid dorsiflexion to a neutral position follows push-off to ensure toe clearance. The ankle may then plantarflex slightly during terminal swing in preparation for the next contact.

At initial contact, the dorsiflexors are active eccentrically to control the rate of plantarflexion and foot placement onto the surface. The plantarflexors then fire eccentrically to decelerate the rate of dorsiflexion and progression of the tibia over the stationary foot. Just before weight transfer onto the opposite limb, the plantarflexors act to push-off, aiding in maintaining gait velocity and step length. Finally, to allow for foot clearance after push-off, the dorsiflexors fire concentrically.

At initial contact between the foot and the surface, the subtalar joint pronates as a shock-absorbing mechanism. The inverters, including the posterior tibialis, anterior tibialis, flexor hallucis longus, and flexor digitorum longus, act to slow this motion. The anterior tibialis is quiet (inactive) by midstance. The tibialis posterior becomes active during loading response and remains active throughout the stance phase until early preswing. The peroneus longus and brevis initiate activity when the load goes to the forefoot with their maximum activity occurring during terminal stance.

Running Gait Cycle

Running is a modification of walking, but with two distinct differences: (1) presence of a flight phase during which neither foot is in contact with the supporting surface and (2) absence of a period of double-limb support. As the speed of the run increases, various aspects of the technique, such as arm swing ROM, stride length, cadence, and knee flexion ROM, change in proportion to the speed. Muscular force and speed of contraction requirements change, particularly with the eccentric contractions required to control pronation during the loading response and initiate supination prior to preswing.[7] Less upward and downward motion of the total body also accompanies faster speeds.

During running the stance phase accounts for approximately one third of the cycle (depending on the speed of running) (Fig. 7-8).[8] Greater vertical GRFs are produced during running. Decreased stance phase time (250 ms versus 600 ms) and increased vertical GRFs (2.0 to 6.0 times the body weight versus 0.7 to 0.8 times the body weight) contribute to the greater number of injuries that occur during running versus walking (see Fig. 7-4). In addition, runners classified as low arch runners tend to incur soft tissue injuries such as posterior tibial tendinopathy while high arch runners are more likely to sustain bony injuries such as stress fractures.[9]

Because the critical features occur at a quicker rate, detecting subtle abnormalities with the naked eye can be difficult. Use of a video camera for stop action playback along with a carefully developed observational gait analysis tool can assist in the viewing of events and subsequent diagnosis of technique. Further, evaluation of running on a treadmill is recommended so the observational distance remains constant.

Stance Phase

The running gait cycle begins with the initial contact of the limb in the stance phase. The loading response and the midstance period occur more rapidly during running gait. The end of the stance phase is a significant biomechanical sequence necessary to generate quick, forceful forward propulsion.

At initial contact, the hip is flexed to approximately 50 degrees. From this point, the hip moves toward extension during the remainder of the stance phase. The knee, flexed approximately 30 degrees at initial contact, reaches a maximum range of 50 degrees of flexion during the loading response and then moves into extension through the rest of the stance phase.[10] Full extension is not reached at push-off, and greater extension values are generally associated with faster running speeds.

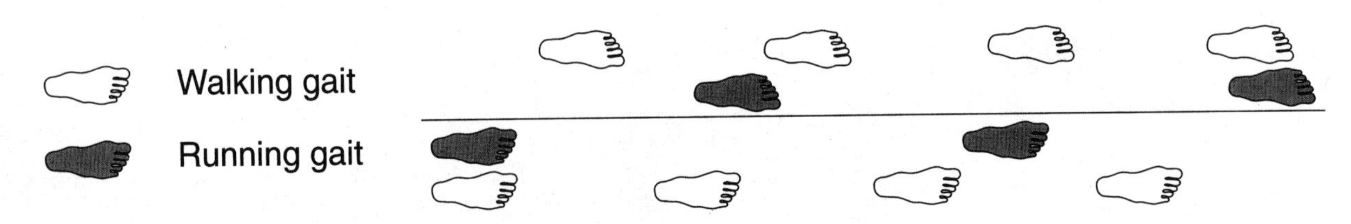

Figure 7-8 ■ Comparison of strides between walking and running gaits. Running requires greater range of motion, balance, and strength compared with walking. Notice the increased stride length and decreased stride width associated with running.

The talocrural joint is dorsiflexed to a maximum range of 25 degrees at the point of initial contact. The subtalar joint is supinated at initial contact, then pronates to allow for adaptation to uneven surfaces and absorption of forces. As the limb continues from midstance to preswing, the talocrural joint plantarflexes and the subtalar joint supinates to form a rigid lever for the athlete to push-off.

Swing Phase

The swing phase clears the non–weight-bearing limb over the ground and positions the foot to accept weight bearing. Because weight-bearing forces are not involved, the probability of injury during the swing phase is less than the weight-bearing stance phase. Most injuries occurring during the swing phase of the running cycle involve the lower extremity muscles that decelerate and control the limb when running. The hamstring muscle group is often strained during the swing phase as it eccentrically contract to slow knee extension.[11]

During the initial swing phase, the hip is in 10 degrees of extension. The hip then flexes during the remainder of the swing period, reaching approximately 50 to 55 degrees of flexion during the terminal swing period.

The knee moves through its greatest ROM during the swing phase and varies on the intensity of running (e.g., jog or sprint). While fully extended at initial swing, the knee can reach 125 degrees of flexion during midswing. Extreme knee flexion is characteristic of sprinters. By increasing the knee flexion angle, the radius of rotation is decreased, reducing the **moment of inertia**, thus making it easier to rotate the limb about the hip joint. In walking or distance running, in which less angular acceleration of the legs is required, knee flexion during the swing phase remains relatively small and the leg's moment of inertia relative to the hip is increased. In terminal swing, the knee extends in preparation for initial contact.

Initially during the swing period, the talocrural joint is at 25 degrees of plantarflexion but proceeds rapidly to 20 degrees of dorsiflexion, where it remains until initial contact during the stance phase. Runners are classified as rearfoot, midfoot, or forefoot strikers, according to the portion of the foot first making contact with the ground.

Factors influencing GRF patterns include running speed, running style, ground surface, and grade of incline.[12] The running shoes worn and the use of orthotics may also affect GRF patterns.[13] Overstriding can be counterproductive to producing speed. GRFs with larger retarding horizontal components are generated. Also, with longer strides, muscles crossing the knee absorb more of the shock that is transmitted upward through the musculoskeletal system, which may translate to additional stress being placed on the knees.[14]

Moment of inertia The amount of force needed to overcome a body's or body part's present state of rotatory motion.

Observational Gait Analysis

The two basic methods for evaluating gait are qualitative assessment and quantitative assessment. In some settings where clinicians are either extensively trained or work in conjunction with a gait or biomechanics laboratory, these techniques can be combined yielding comprehensive results to use for treatment. This chapter focuses on qualitative evaluation using observational gait analysis (OGA). Refer to Box 7-3 for information regarding quantitative analysis.

In most clinical settings gait evaluation is performed qualitatively using minimal equipment. The patient is asked to walk and/or run with and without shoes on a treadmill or designated area where an OGA may be conducted. Qualitative analysis in gait has poor to moderate reliability. This may be improved with experience, by using video so that the motion can be replayed and slowed down, and by using a very specific observational tool. OGA tools have been designed to record information about the critical features of gait (Fig. 7-9). OGA tools for persons with gross gait abnormalities or disabilities are readily available. However, they are often not sensitive enough to allow documentation of milder deviations in other patients. Thus, a small amount of toeing out might qualify as unremarkable on a standard OGA tool, yet in an athletic patient performing repetitive, high-force movements, this could be a vital finding. In addition, an OGA for walking gait will need to be adapted to use with running.

Preparing for observational gait analysis involves developing a plan for gathering gait information. Preplan when and where the patient will be observed, and what materials will be used (e.g., video camera, treadmill, observation tool). Using an OGA tool, such as those found in this chapter, provides a systematic method for observing and documenting gait (Box 7-4). Be cognizant of visual imitations during testing. For example, brightly colored shorts can draw the eyes away and make it difficult to focus on arm swing or knee action. Also, viewing too close or too far away can cause misjudgments in gross or subtle features. Good observation is not limited to the visual inspection of gait. Auditory information about the rhythm or cadence of a patient's gait also offers cues. For example, a hard foot slap or an uneven step length can have auditory components. Symmetry of the fine aspects of gait such as pronation cannot be assumed.[15] Thus, the analysis should always include the left and right sides separately. Lastly, allow the patient should walk or run at a self-selected pace during the evaluation.[16]

The clinical examination findings are compiled to identify underlying impairments. The intervention step involves providing feedback, correcting and changing correctable impairments, and improving function. Specifics will vary

Box 7-3
Quantitative Gait Analysis

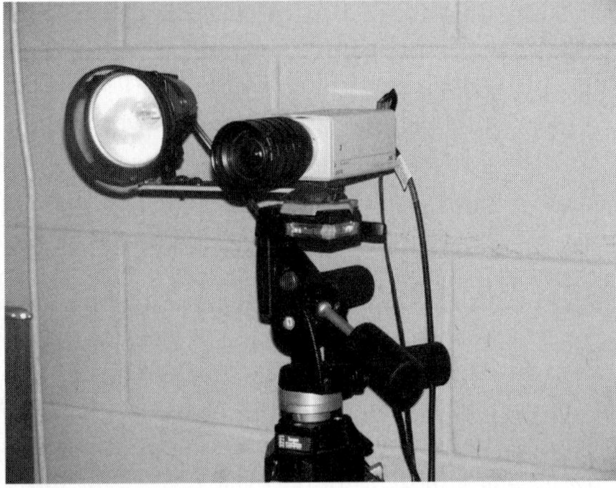

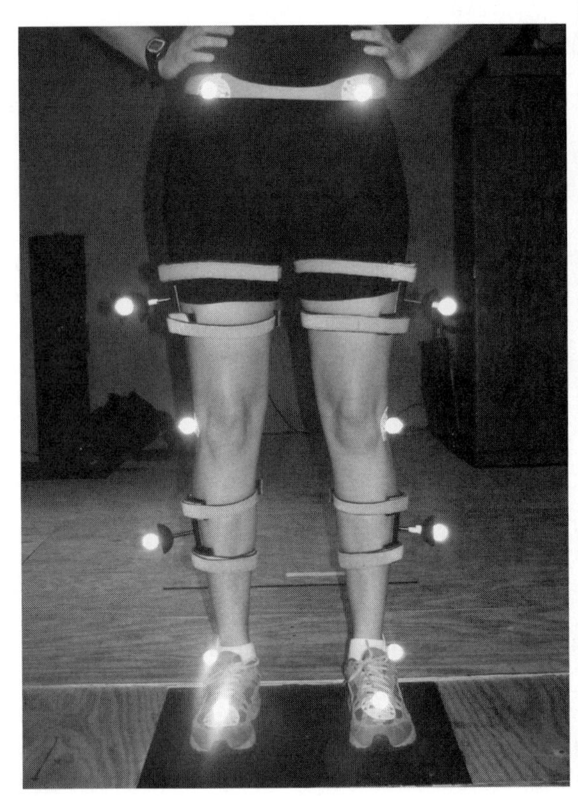

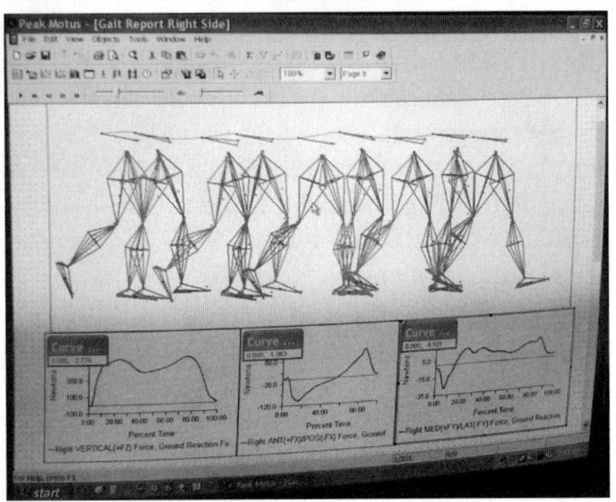

A quantitative gait analysis yields numerical results for the motion, force, and muscle activity characteristics during gait and may be conducted with simple tools such as a stopwatch and camcorder, or with a motion measurement system that may also include instrumented walkways, force plates, pressure mats, and/or electromyography (EMG) capabilities. Other more sophisticated methods include the use of (1) electromechanical instruments such as imbedding pressure-sensitive switches into the patient's shoe or inserts or applying them to the bottom of the foot and (2) optoelectronic techniques such as video capture.

Video capture requires the use of reference markers that are attached to the patient, careful calibration of the video space, a computerized digitizing process of the reference markers, and mathematical equations to yield the results. Motion measurement systems are usually housed in gait analysis laboratories. Angular kinematics, such as knee extension range of motion (ROM) or hip flexion velocity, are measured using electrogoniometry, accelerometry, or optoelectronic techniques. An electrogoniometer is a device that is attached to the body segments for a direct measure of angular displacement (ROM) of a joint. They are available in uniaxial and multiaxial designs. Accelerometers are similar. They are attached to the body segments of interest but directly measure segmental acceleration. Segmental velocities and displacements are then determined.

EMG techniques are used to measure the timing and amplitude of muscle activity, and help to describe the motor performance underlying the kinematic and kinetic characteristics of gait. Surface EMG where electrodes are attached directly to the skin over the muscles of interest is more common in clinical gait analyses. Intramuscular EMG, in which needles are inserted through the skin and into the muscles of interest, is primarily used in gait research.

EMG, force, and pressure plates are typically integrated with a motion measurement system to enable simultaneous acquisition of kinematic, kinetic, and muscle activity information. These systems are also helpful in producing gait reports.

depending on the diagnosis, but may include any or all of the following:

- Cue words or phrases during gait or exercises to improve gait
- Footprints on the floor for visual feedback on technique, or a hand on a body segment for kinesthetic feedback
- Orthotics
- Different shoes
- Strength training exercises
- Flexibility or ROM exercises

Evaluation of gait after an injury or surgical procedure is often complicated because the patient might display a

Observational Gait Analysis Model

Barry University Biomechanics Laboratory, Miami Shores, FL 33161

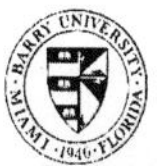

STRENGTH (MMT and Functional)

	Quads	Hams	Hip IR	Hip ER	TA	TP	Peroneals	Gastroc	Core Squat
R	/5	/5	/5	/5	/5	/5	/5	/5	
L	/5	/5	/5	/5	/5	/5	/5	/5	

FLEXIBILITY

	RF (Kendall)	Iliopsoas (Thomas)	Hams (deg)	Gastroc (deg)	IT Band (Ober's)
R					
L					

NONWEIGHT BEARING ALIGNMENT

	Rearfoot	Forefoot	Hallux	Toes	Med Long Arch	LLD	Callus location
R	□ valgus □ varus	□ valgus □ varus	□ valgus □ bunion	□ claw □ hammer	□ planus □ cavus		
L	□ valgus □ varus	□ valgus □ varus	□ valgus □ bunion	□ claw □ hammer	□ planus □ cavus		

FUNCTIONAL STANDING ALIGNMENT

Navicular Drop (mm)	Toe Raise*	SL Squat*	DBL Squat*
R L	R L	R L	

*assess and document stability and/or alignment changes during test

STANDING POSTURE & ALIGNMENT (FRONTAL PLANE)

Achilles	Toe In/Out	Knee (valgus/varus)	Popliteal Creases	Iliac Crests (level, rotation)	Shoulders (level)
□ valgus □ R □ L □ varus □ R □ L	□ in □ R □ L □ out □ R □ L □ WNL	□ valgus □ varum □ recurvatum □ WNL	□ level □ uneven	□ level □ R > L □ L > R	□ level □ R > L □ L > R

STANDING POSTURE & ALIGNMENT (SAGITTAL PLANE)

Knee (recurvatum)	Lumbar	Thoracic	Shoulders	Cervical
□ yes □ no	□ lordosis □ flat	□ kyphosis	□ rounded	□ excessive lordosis

Figure 7-9 ■ Barry University Runner's Clinic OGA.

STANDING POSTURE & ALIGNMENT (TRANSVERSE PLANE)

	Hips	Patellae	Tibia (rotation)
R	□ anteversion □ retroversion	□ alta □ baja □ squint □ frog eye	□ ER □ IR
L	□ anteversion □ retroversion	□ alta □ baja □ squint □ frog eye	□ ER □ IR

DYNAMIC GAIT ASSESSMENT – Initial Contact through Mid-stance

	Location of Initial Contact	Landing Position	Pronation ROM	Pronation Velocity	Stride Length	Trendelenberg
R	□ heel □ lat □ med □ neutral □ midfoot	□ pro □ sup □ neutral	□ >15 □ WNL	□ excessive □ WNL	□ excessive □ inadequate □ WNL	□ yes □ no
L	□ heel □ lat □ med □ neutral □ midfoot	□ pro □ sup □ neutral	□ >15 □ WNL	□ excessive □ WNL	□ excessive □ inadequate □ WNL	□ yes □ no

DYNAMIC GAIT ASSESSMENT – Push-off through Swing

	Hip Flexion Angle	Hip Flexion Velocity	Knee Flexion Angle	Knee Flexion Velocity	Ankle PF Angle	Toe In/Out
R	□ excessive □ inadequate □ WNL	□ excessive □ inadequate □ WNL	□ excessive □ inadequate □ WNL	□ excessive □ inadequate □ WNL	□ excessive □ inadequate □ WNL	□ in □ out
L	□ excessive □ inadequate □ WNL	□ excessive □ inadequate □ WNL	□ excessive □ inadequate □ WNL	□ excessive □ inadequate □ WNL	□ excessive □ inadequate □ WNL	□ in □ out

SHOE WEAR

Brand/Model	Age or Mileage of Shoes	Last Type		Heel Counter Wear/Flexibility	Mid Sole Wear/Flexibility	Location Excessive Wear
			R			
			L			

Evaluator's signature______________________________

Figure 7-9 ■ cont'd

temporary compensation. Because the body is a kinetic chain system, other parts of the body appear to be dysfunctional as they assume compensatory roles (Box 7-5). These deviations result without conscious effort by the patient. Rather, they represent the body's protecting itself after injury or from further injury and subconsciously making gait as efficient as possible.

Observational Gait Analysis Findings

Correlating the findings of the gait analysis with the functional limitations described by the patient and the impairments identified during the clinical examination completes the examination picture. This section describes typical deviations and their associated pathologies.

Box 7-4
Observational Gait Analysis

Using an OGA written tool, the presence or absence of the critical events in the gait cycle can be determined. When preparing for your analysis, refer to the following OGA guidelines:

1. Prepare the area and materials ahead of time.
2. Avoid clutter in the viewing background.
3. Have the patient wear clothing that does not restrict viewing of joints.
4. Ensure that the patient is at a self-selected walking pace; otherwise, gait will be altered.
5. Position yourself in a position to view the individual segments (i.e., if you are observing for forefoot pronation and supination, then squat down so your eyes are in line with the patient's feet).
6. Observe the subject from multiple views (anterior, posterior, and both lateral views) but not from an oblique angle.
7. Look at the individual body parts first, then the whole body, then the individual parts again.
8. Conduct multiple observations or trials.
9. Conduct the analysis with the patient barefoot and wearing shoes.
10. Label all DVDs or videotapes (if used) with pertinent data.

Table 7-1 describes common impairments during the stance phase; Table 7-2 presents impairments to the swing phase.

Excessive pronation

The term *pronation* is often perceived as a pathological motion. However, foot pronation is necessary for shock absorption during the contact phase of gait. Further, a pronated foot in a static position does not necessarily dictate faulty mechanics.[17]

*** Practical Evidence**

Pronating more than approximately 15.5 degrees during running has been linked with increased risk of lower extremity injury (Fig. 7-10).[18]

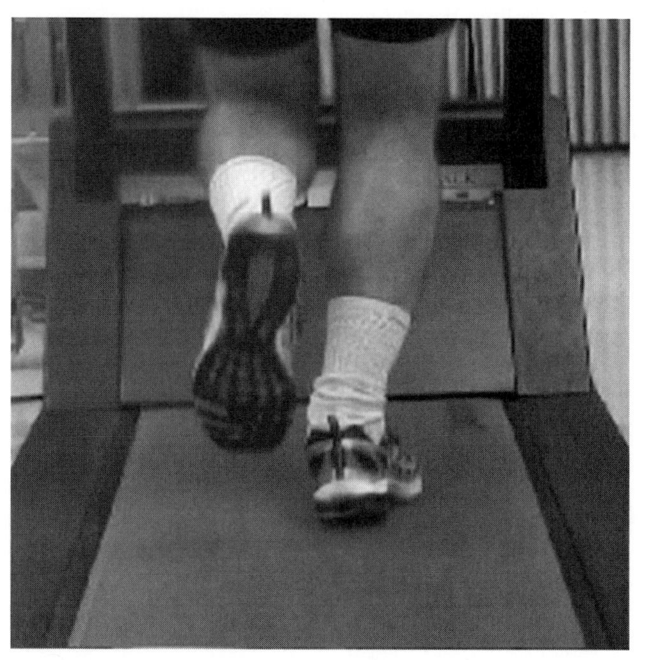

Figure 7-10 ■ Excessive pronation right foot during running.

The tibia is rotated internally during pronation and externally during supination. Disturbance in the coordination of these joint actions imposes abnormal stresses on the tissues possibly altering muscle activity and leading to injury. Increased and prolonged pronation coupled with increased pressure on the medial aspect of the foot during running is associated with the developed of lower leg pain.[19]

Excessive pronation during gait may be related to genu valgum, leg length discrepancy (the foot of the long leg pronates more), pes planus, an imbalance in hip musculature causing a "collapsing" of the limb medially (tight hip adductors and weak hip abductors), and shoes made with softer midsoles (cushioning shoes). A patient who overpronates will also exhibit calcaneal eversion, lowering and elongation of the medial longitudinal arch, increased pressure on the first metatarsophalangeal joint (creating an excessive wear pattern on the corresponding area in the patient's shoe insert), and medial knee pain.

In addition, runners who make initial contact on the central heel versus lateral heel must move through their pronation at a quicker rate. This quickened pronation velocity does not allow the foot adequate shock absorption and may increase the risk for lower extremity injury.[20]

Toe in or toe out

The lower limb should move through the sagittal plane with minimal deviation. Toe-in or toe-out can be witnessed at either midstance or just after push-off. Most often, it is the result of malignment further along the kinetic chain (tibial rotation, hip rotation). Toe-in during midstance can place stress on the lower leg's lateral soft tissues (e.g., peroneus longus) contributing to pain and injury at that site. Toe-out during midstance places the foot in an overpronated position causing stress on the foot's medial and plantar structures. Sometimes toe-out,

Box 7-5
Compensatory Gait Deviations

Gluteus Maximus Gait

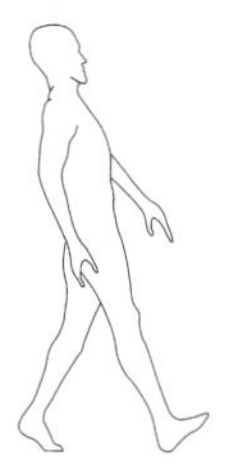

At initial contact, the thorax is thrust posteriorly to maintain hip extension during the stance phase, often causing a lurching of the trunk.

Cause: Weakness or paralysis of the gluteus maximus muscle.

Stiff Knee or Hip Gait

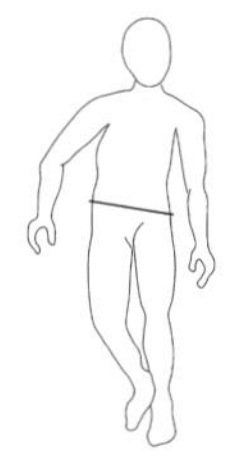

In the swing phase, the affected extremity is lifted higher than normal to compensate for knee or hip stiffness. To accomplish this, the uninvolved extremity demonstrates increased plantarflexion.

Cause: Knee pathologies such as meniscal or ligamentous tears, or hip pathologies such as bursitis or muscle strains that result in a decrease in the ROM.

Trendelenburg's Gait (gluteus medius gait)

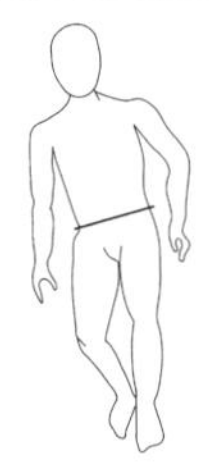

During the stance phase of the affected limb, the thorax lists toward the involved limb. This serves to maintain the center of gravity and prevent a drop in the pelvis on the affected side.

Cause: Weakness of the gluteus medius muscle.

Calcaneal Gait

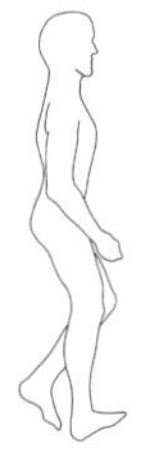

During the stance phase, increased dorsiflexion and knee flexion occur on the affected side, resulting in a decreased step length.

Cause: Paralysis or weakness of the plantarflexors or painful when weight bearing on the forefoot or toes caused by such conditions as blisters, hallucis rigidus, sesamoiditis, or ankle sprains.

Psoatic Limp

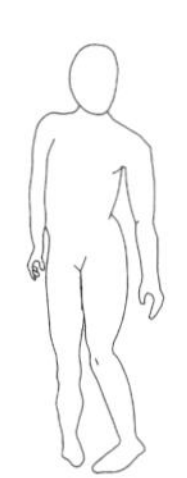

To compensate during the swing phase, lateral rotation and flexion of the trunk occurs with hip adduction. The trunk and pelvic movements are exaggerated.

Cause: Weakness or reflex inhibition of the psoas major muscle (Legg–Perthes disease).

Short Leg Gait

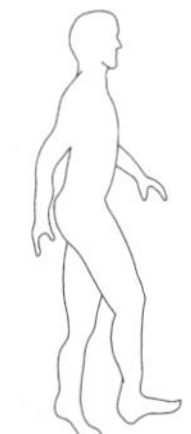

Increased pronation occurs in the subtalar joint of the long leg, accompanied by a shift of the trunk toward the longer extremity.

Cause: True (anatomical) leg length discrepancy; the right (facing) leg is longer.

Steppage Gait (dropfoot)

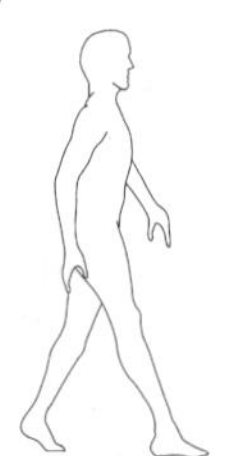

The foot slaps at initial contact, owing to foot drop. During the swing phase, the affected limb demonstrates increased hip and knee flexion to avoid toe dragging, producing a "high-step" pattern.

Cause: Weakness or paralysis of the dorsiflexors.

ROM = range of motion.
Figures modified from Levangie, PK, and Norkin, CC: *Joint Structure and Function: A Comprehensive Analysis*, ed 4. Philadelphia, FA Davis, 2005.

Table 7-1 Effects of Impairments During the Stance Phase of the Gait Cycle

	Compensation			
Impairment	**Initial Contact**	**Loading Response**	**Midstance**	**Terminal Stance**
Decreased Dorsiflexion	Increased subtalar pronation Forefoot abduction	Increased and prolonged midtarsal joint pronation		Decreased ability to toe-off Premature heel rise
Decreased First MTP Joint Motion				Decreased ability to toe-off Premature heel rise
Extrinsic Leg or Thigh Muscle Weakness	Altered position	Increased subtalar joint pronation Increased tibial rotation	Impaired supination	Impaired supination Decreased ability to toe-off
Hip	Toe-out gait			
Rotator Muscle Weakness		Increased rotation of femur and tibia		
Rearfoot Varus	Increased subtalar pronation Increased medial leg or foot stresses	Excessive pronation	Impaired supination	Incomplete resupination with decreased force at toe-off
Rearfoot Valgus	Decreased shock absorption	Decreased subtalar pronation: Heel approaching the vertical position	Decreased ability to accommodate to uneven surfaces	Decreased ability to supinate
Hypomobile First Ray	Altered midfoot and forefoot position	Instability in midtarsal joints and forefoot	Altered distribution of ground reaction forces	Pain or decreased force at toe-off
Plantarflexed First Ray	First ray contacts the ground	Decreased subtalar pronation	Decreased ability to absorb shock	Increased force on first ray
Forefoot Varus	Increased pronation Toe-out gait			
Forefoot Valgus		Decreased ability to absorb shock	Decreased force at toe-off	
Tarsal Coalition	Decreased or absent subtalar joint motion			
Tibial Torsion	Increased compensatory subtalar joint pronation			
Femoral Torsion	Toe-in gait Increased subtalar joint pronation secondary to internal tibial rotation			
Leg Length Discrepancy	Compensatory pronation of the longer leg with compensatory supination of the shorter leg			

MTP = metatarsophalangeal.

Table 7-2 Effects of Impairments during the Swing Phase of the Gait Cycle

	Compensation		
Impairment	**Initial Swing**	**Midswing**	**Terminal Swing**
Hamstring Weakness		Decreased knee flexion leading to shortened step length	
Hip Flexor Weakness	Decreased hip flexion propulsion causing inability to achieve toe clearance; compensatory hip elevation occurs along with a shortened step length		
Hamstring Strain or Sciatic Nerve Pathology			Decreased knee extension and impaired ability to decelerate leg for contact
Leg Length Discrepancy	Hip drop when short side in swing phase		
Hip External Rotator Tightness	Toeing out		

when observed just after push-off, is the result of an excessively pronated foot during stance that has placed the limb more medial (Fig. 7-11). The lower leg compensates by rotating externally, giving the toe-out appearance.

Shortened step length

When pain or weakness is present in the hip, knee, or ankle, a shortened step length can occur. Specifically, an inadequate push-off by the plantar flexors or pull-off by the hip flexors at the end of the stance phase will shorten the time during swing, bringing the leg back to the surface quicker.[21] Thus, a shortened step length is created. Larger forces are present with longer strides. Patients with pain in the lower extremities may shorten the stride so as not to exacerbate their symptoms when absorbing the larger impacts.

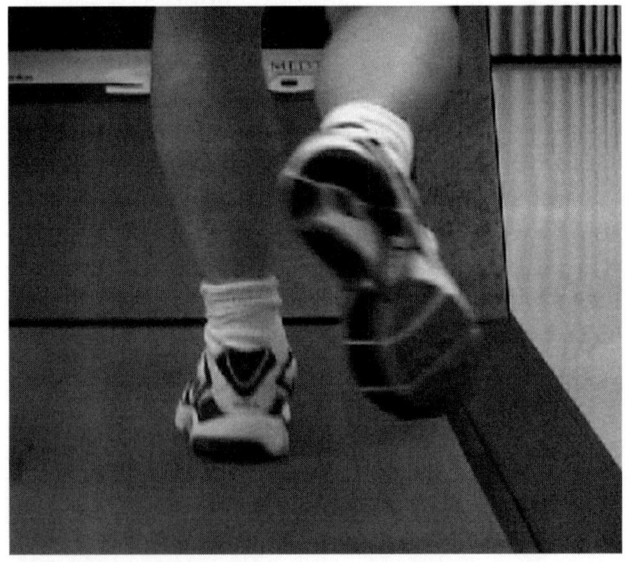

Figure 7-11 ■ Toe-out on right lower leg during running.

Reflex inhibition A reflex arc prohibiting the contraction of a specific muscle or muscle group.

Shortened stance time

When a patient spends less time on one side contacting the ground, this is typically due to pain. Pain can result from an acute or chronic cause giving the antalgic gait pattern, or limp. The shortened stance time is the patient's attempt at avoiding load absorption for any length of time. It may be necessary to fit the patient for crutches and/or fit an athlete with a protective brace if the injury is causing a significant shortened stance time because gait asymmetry can lead to injury or pain elsewhere due to the unequal distribution of load.

Unequal hip height

Unequal hip height, observed from the frontal plane view, could be the result of a leg length discrepancy (the shorter side shows a dropped hip), or perhaps a weak gluteus medius muscle causing a short-leg or Trendelenburg gait, respectively (Fig. 7-12). Since a postural analysis and manual muscle testing will both have been completed by the time the gait analysis occurs, the clinician will know the root of the deviation.

Asymmetrical arm swing

The arm swing occurs primarily to counterbalance the activity of the hips and pelvis during walking and running. Thus, during running, a larger arm swing in the sagittal plane is observed because greater ROM occurs at the pelvis and hips than during walking. When the swing of the left arm is different from the right arm, consider what is being

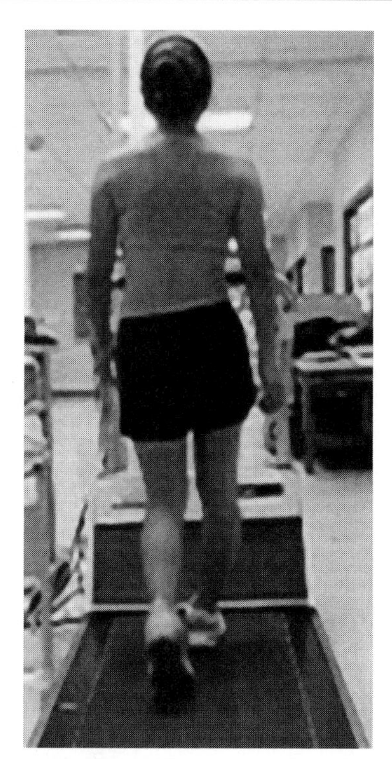

Figure 7-12 ■ Unequal hip height as a result of a leg length discrepancy.

observed in the lower extremity, unless the patient has an upper extremity injury, of course. Leg length discrepancies and spine deformity such as scoliosis can cause an asymmetrical arm swing. If motion is limited or exaggerated on one side of the pelvis or hip, then most likely, arm swing motion will follow suit. This is best observed from the sagittal plane.

Plantarflexed ankle at initial contact

The ankle should be in neutral or very slightly plantarflexed at initial contact. An ankle that remains plantarflexed can be the result of spasticity of the gastrocnemius/soleus complex or denervation of the tibialis anterior preventing active dorsiflexion ("drop foot"). Prolonged or exaggerated plantarflexion is a compensation for pain associated with hamstring or knee pathology.[21] Associated pain and swelling that occur with knee joint pathology cause the patient to maintain the knee in the resting position of slight flexion. This creates space to accommodate swelling and decreases the contact between the femur and tibia which decreases pain. In turn, the patient walks on the toes, or plantarflexes the ankle.

Flat foot stance

A flat-footed gait most likely indicates an ankle sprain or gastrocnemius or soleus sprain. Usually, an absence of initial contact with the heel is observed. Patients often move the center of gravity quickly over the foot, making contact with a flat foot instead. Plantarflexion at the ankle, the open-packed position, is avoided in the terminal stance and preswing phases as the limb is quickly brought into swing phase. Applying load to a smaller surface area (forefoot versus entire foot) is also accomplished helping avoid pain. Shortening the stance phase helps keep weight bearing to a minimum, which helps the patient avoid an exacerbation of symptoms.

Inadequate ankle plantarflexion angle at push off

Plantarflexion at push-off is observed because of the contracting triceps surae. Insufficient plantarflexion at push-off is noted as a weak push-off and may be caused from inadequate strength from the triceps surae (tibial nerve pathology, atrophy), an acute ankle sprain with pain and swelling as limiting factors, or forefoot pathology where the patient is avoiding contact over the area.[21]

Excessive knee flexion angle at contact

The knee is near full extension at contact during normal walking gait. During running, the knee is flexed in the range of 21 to 30 degrees. Patients with a hamstring strain, tight hamstring, or spasm will avoid full extension to prevent lengthening of the affected muscle, thus causing pain. Similarly, sciatic nerve pathology either from a herniated disk or piriformis syndrome will also prevent the knee from being extended at contact to avoid tension on the nerve and a consequent exacerbation of symptoms. Hip adductor strains may also result in a gait that shows a more flexed knee at contact in addition to an internally rotated hip. This is an attempt to keep the muscle in a shortened state so as to avoid pain.

Inadequate knee flexion angle during stance

To absorb shock the knee flexes to about 20 degrees during stance. This flexion is controlled by the eccentric contraction of the quadriceps muscle. Thus, any pathology to this muscle may hinder its ability to control the knee flexion angle leaving it in a more extended position. Joint pain can also limit the flexion angle.

Inadequate knee flexion during swing

The knee is flexed 30 to 60 degrees in the swing phase during walking and more than 90 degrees during fast running speeds. Hamstring related-pathology such as strains, spasms, or sciatica could limit the flexion used during swing.

Inadequate hip extension at terminal stance

The hip extends as the body has body has been propelled forward onto the swing leg in walking and into the air in running. Inadequate hip extension could be the result of a contracture of the hip flexor muscles.[21] The limited extensibility would prevent the hip from achieving the desired extension.

Forward trunk angle

The trunk is relatively upright during walking and running. A forward trunk could indicate low back pathology such as a herniated disk, weak and painful hip flexors, or weak ankle plantarflexors.

REFERENCES

1. Steindler, A: *Kinesiology of the Human Body Under Normal and Pathological Conditions,* ed. 3. Springfield, IL, Charles C Thomas, 1970.
2. Nuber, GW: Biomechanics of the foot and ankle during gait. *Clin Sports Med,* 7:1, 1988.
3. Murray, MP: Walking patterns of men with Parkinsonism. *Am J Phys Med,* 57:278, 1978.
4. Coulter, HC, et al: Effects of custom-molded orthotics on pain and temporal parameters of physically active, symptomatic patients. *Annual Symposium of the Southeast American College of Sports Medicine,* January, 2004.
5. Root, ML, Orient, WP, and Weed, JH: Normal and abnormal function of the foot. *Clinical Biomechanics,* Vol. II. Los Angeles, Clinical Biomechanics Corp, 1977.
6. Adrian, MJ, and Cooper, JM: *Biomechanics of Human Movement,* ed 2. Dubuque, IA, WCB Brown & Benchmark, 1995.
7. Donatelli, R: *The Biomechanics of the Foot and Ankle,* ed 2. Philadelphia, FA Davis, 1996.
8. Slocum, D, and James, S: Biomechanics of running. *JAMA,* 205:97, 1968.
9. Williams, DS, McClay IS, and Hamill, J: Arch structure and injury patterns in runners. *Clin Biomech,* 16:341, 2001.
10. Hamill, J, and Knutzen, KM: *Biomechanical Basis of Human Movement,* ed 3. Philadelphia, Lippincott Williams & Wilkins, 2003.
11. Crossier, J: Factors associated with recurrent hamstring injuries. *Sports Med,* 34:, 2004.
12. Cavanagh, PR, and Lafortune, MA: Ground reaction forces in distance running. *J Biomech,* 13:397, 1980.
13. Putnam, CA, and Kozey, JW: Substantive issues in running. In Vaughan, CL (ed): *Biomechanics of Sport.* Boca Raton, FL, CRC Press, 1989.
14. Derrick, TR, Hamill, J, and Caldwell, GE: Energy absorption of impacts during running at various stride lengths. *Med Sci Sports Exerc,* 30:128, 1998.
15. De Cock, A, et al: Temporal characteristics of foot roll-over during barefoot jogging: Reference data for young adults. *Gait Posture,* 21:432, 2005.
16. Monaghan, K, Delehunt, E, and Caulfield, B: Ankle function during gait in patients with chronic ankle instability compared to controls. *Clin Biomech,* 21:168, 2006.
17. Butler, RJ, Davis, IS, and Hamill, J: Interaction of arch type and footwear on running mechanics. *Am J Sport Med,* 34; 1998, 2006.
18. Willems, TM, et al: Gait-related risk factors for exercise-related lower-leg pain during shod running. *Med Sci Sports Exer,* 39:330, 2007.
19. Williams, DS, et al: Lower extremity kinematic and kinetic differences in runners with high and low arches. *J Appl Biomech,* 17:153, 2001.
20. Willems, TM, et al: A prospective study of gait related risk factors for exercise-related lower leg pain. *Gait Posture,* 23:91, 2006.
21. Kirtley, C: *Clinical Gait Analysis: Theory and Practice.* London, Churchill Livingstone, 2005

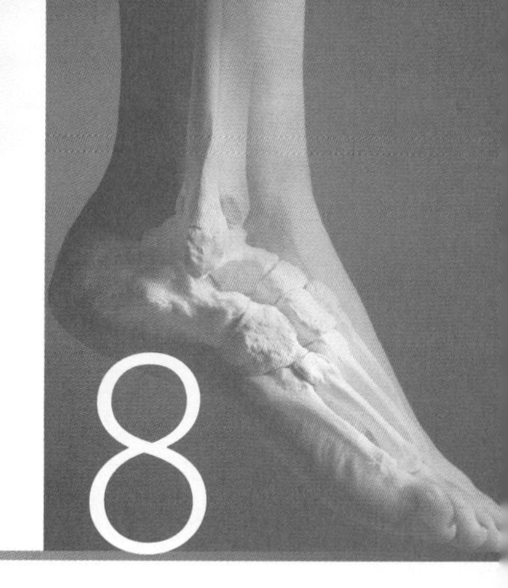

SECTION 2

Regional Examination

CHAPTER 8

Foot and Toe Pathologies

The demands placed on the foot and toes require a delicate balance between the need to provide a rigid platform and an ability to remold itself to adapt to uneven terrain. The foot acts as a rigid lever during the pre-swing phase of gait and as a shock absorber during the initial contact and loading response phases (Fig. 8-1). When running, the foot is required to absorb and dissipate three to eight times the person's body weight.[1]

Biomechanically, the functions of the foot, toes, and ankle are highly interrelated, as is the examination of these areas. The diagnostic techniques for the foot and toes are described in this chapter. The examination of the ankle and leg is discussed in Chapter 9. An examination of the foot and toes should also include the ankle evaluation and vice versa. In addition, many conditions may necessitate examining the entire lower extremity and lumbar region. The functional assessment frequently includes a gait analysis, described in Chapter 7.

Clinical Anatomy

The foot relies on intimate and precise relationships with the various surrounding structures. True one-on-one articulation between its bones is rare, tending to be limited to the joints of the toes. The majority of the remaining bones have multiple articulations with their contiguous structures. Motion and support are provided by the muscles originating off the bones of the foot (intrinsic muscles) and extrinsic muscles originating from the lower leg.

Formed by 26 structural and sesamoid bones, the foot is divided into three regions: the **rearfoot**, the **midfoot**, and the **forefoot** (Fig. 8-2). The **tarsals** consist of the calcaneus, talus, navicular, cuboid, and three cuneiforms. Articulating with the distal tarsals, each of the five **metatarsals** (MTs) leads to the proximal phalanges. Each toe consists of three **phalanges** (proximal, middle, and distal), with the exception of the great toe, which has only two bones (proximal and distal).

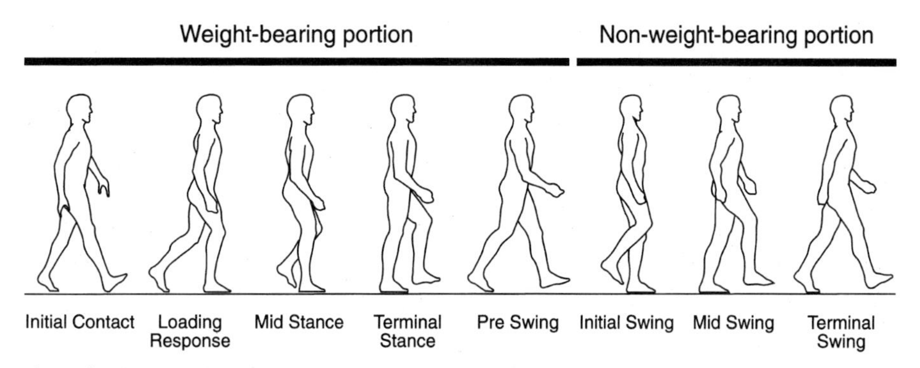

FIGURE 8-1 ■ Phases of gait for the right foot as defined by the Los Ranchos Medical Center system of gait analysis. This system, described in Chapter 7, divides the gait into weight-bearing and non–weight-bearing portions. (Courtesy of Norkin, CC, and Levangie, PK: *Joint Structure and Function: A Comprehensive Analysis*, ed 2. Philadelphia, FA Davis, 1992.)

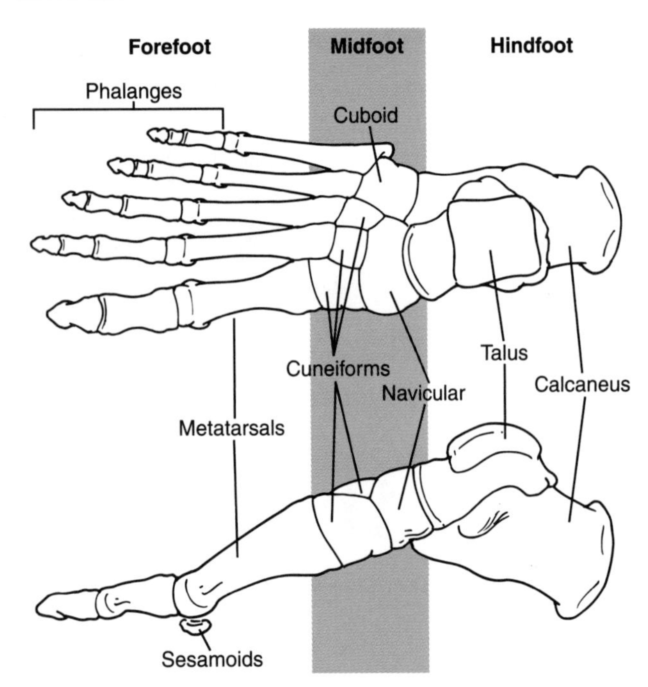

FIGURE 8-2 ■ Anatomical zones of the foot. The talus and calcaneus form the rearfoot; the 3 cuneiforms, the navicular, and the cuboid form the midfoot; and the 5 metatarsals, 14 phalanges, and 2 sesamoid bones form the forefoot.

Rearfoot

The rearfoot, formed by the calcaneus and talus, provides stability and shock absorption during the early stance phase of gait and serves as a lever arm for the Achilles tendon during plantarflexion. The calcaneus is the largest of the tarsal bones. Its most prominent feature is the posteriorly projecting **calcaneal tubercle**. The large size of this tubercle provides a mechanically powerful lever for increasing the muscular force produced by the **triceps surae muscle group** (gastrocnemius and soleus). The large calcaneal body is the origin or insertion for many of the ligaments and muscles acting on the foot and ankle.

Arising off the anterior superior medial surface of the calcaneal body, the **sustentaculum tali** (*tali* is Latin for "shelf") helps support the talus (Fig. 8-3). On the inferior surface of the sustentaculum tali is a groove through which the tendon of the flexor hallucis longus passes. The lateral portion of the anterior calcaneus articulates with the cuboid. Projecting off the lateral side of the calcaneus, the **peroneal tubercle** assists in maintaining the stability and alignment of the peroneal tendons. Here, the peroneal tendons diverge, with the peroneus brevis running superior to the tubercle and the peroneus longus coursing inferior to it.

The distal tibia and fibula form an articular mortise in which the talus sits (Fig. 8-4). The inferior surface of the **talus** is marked by anterior, middle, and posterior ***facets***. These facets provide a surface for weight bearing and serve as the site for ligaments to attach. The superior surface is marked with facets that articulate with the tibia.

The saddle-shaped talus is the interface between the foot and ankle. Its unique shape is necessitated by its five functional articulations: (1) superiorly with the distal end of the tibia, (2) medially with the medial malleolus, (3) laterally with the lateral malleolus, (4) inferiorly with the calcaneus, and (5) anteriorly with the navicular. There is no muscle attachment on the talus, the only axial skeletal bone to have this distinction.

Midfoot

Serving as the shock-absorbing segment of the foot, the midfoot is composed of the **navicular**, three cuneiforms, and the cuboid bones. The **keystone** of the medial longitudinal arch, the navicular, articulates anteriorly with the three cuneiforms, the cuboid laterally, and the talus posteriorly. The medial aspect of the navicular gives rise to the **navicular tuberosity**, the primary insertion for the tibialis posterior muscle.

The **cuboid** articulates with the third cuneiform and navicular medially, the fourth and fifth MTs anteriorly, and the calcaneus posteriorly. A palpable **sulcus** is formed anterior to the cuboid tuberosity and posterior to the base of the fifth MT, where the peroneus longus begins its course along the foot's plantar surface.

Adding to the flexibility of the midfoot and forefoot, the three **cuneiforms** are identified by their relative position on the foot: medial (first), intermediate (second), and lateral (third). Each cuneiform articulates with the navicular posteriorly, the corresponding MT anteriorly, and its contiguous cuneiform medially and laterally. The lateral border of the third cuneiform also articulates with the medial aspect of the cuboid.

Forefoot and Toes

The forefoot and toes, formed by the 5 MTs and 14 phalanges, act as a lever during the preswing phase of gait. The MTs and phalanges are long bones, each having a proximal base, body, and distal head. The MTs are referenced numerically from medial (first) to lateral (fifth). Proximally, the bases of the first three MTs articulate with the corresponding cuneiform, except the second MT, which also articulates with the first cuneiform. The fourth and fifth MTs articulate with the cuboid. Each of the MT heads articulates with the proximal phalanx of the corresponding toe and loosely with the neighboring MT heads (see Fig. 8-3). Like the MT heads, the bases articulate with the contiguous MTs, but with a tighter fit. The toes are numerically referenced as one through five from medial to lateral.

At least three sesamoids are located on the plantar aspect of the great toe. Two are located in the flexor hallucis

Keystone The crown of an arch that supports the structures on either side of it.

Sulcus A groove or depression within a bone.

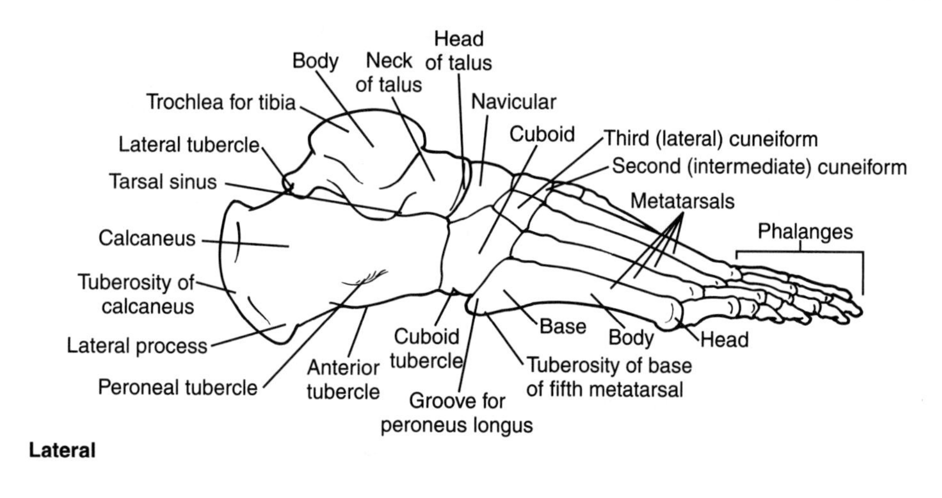

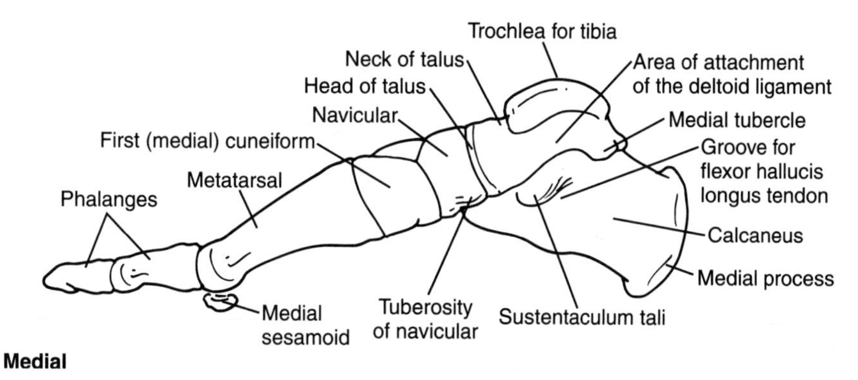

FIGURE 8-3 ■ Anatomy of the foot showing prominent bony landmarks and sites of ligamentous and muscular attachments.

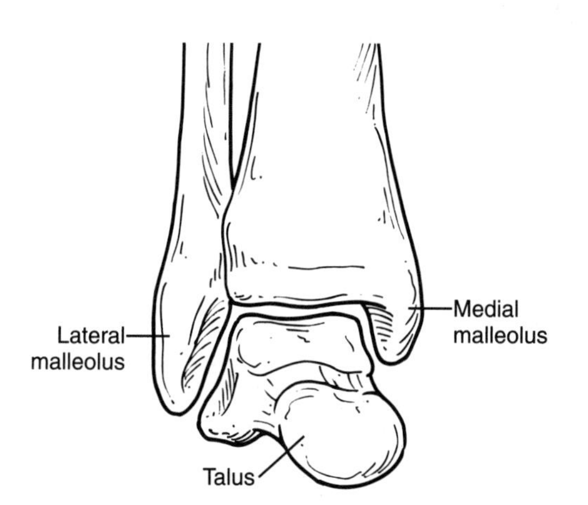

FIGURE 8-4 ■ The ankle mortise. The articulation formed by the talus, tibia, and fibula. The subtalar joint is formed by the articulation between the inferior talus and the superior portion of the calcaneus.

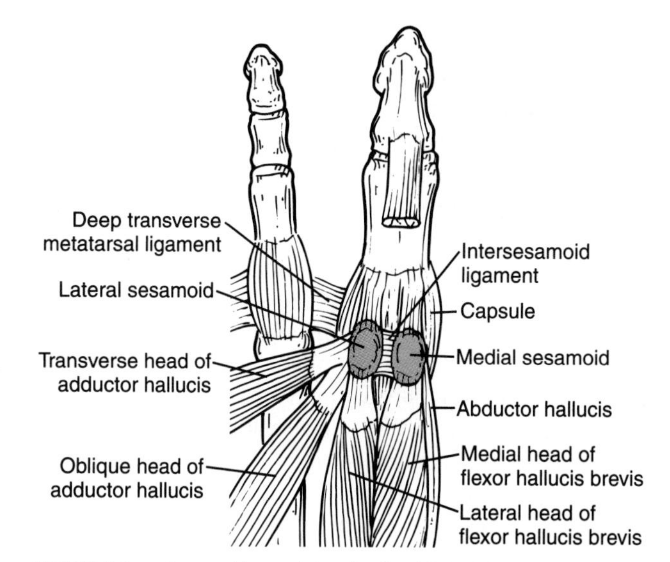

FIGURE 8-5 ■ Sesamoids overlying the first MTP joint.

brevis (FHB) tendon beneath the MTP joint, one medially and one laterally. A third sesamoid is often located on the plantar aspect of the interphalangeal joint. These sesamoids assist in absorbing and redirecting weight-bearing forces, reduce friction, and protect the tendon.[2] Within the FHB tendon, the two sesamoids lie in separate grooves and are bound by the intersesamoid ligament (Fig. 8-5). The medial (tibial) sesamoid is usually larger than the lateral fibular) sesamoid and is therefore more affected by weight bearing.[3]

Articulations and Ligamentous Support

The ligaments joining the tarsal bones of the foot are collectively grouped into three sets: (1) the thin **dorsal tarsal ligaments,** (2) the relatively thick **plantar tarsal ligaments**, and

Table 8-1 Summary of Non–Weight-Bearing and Weight-Bearing Pronation and Supination

	Component Movements of Subtalar Supination/Pronation	
Motion	**Non–Weight Bearing**	**Weight Bearing**
Supination	Calcaneal inversion (or varus)	Calcaneal inversion (or varus)
	Calcaneal adduction	Talar abduction (or lateral rotation)
	Calcaneal plantarflexion	Talar dorsiflexion
		Tibiofibular lateral rotation
Pronation	Calcaneal eversion (or valgus)	Calcaneal eversion (or valgus)
	Calcaneal abduction	Talar adduction (or medial rotation)
	Calcaneal dorsiflexion	Talar plantarflexion
		Tibiofibular medial rotation

(3) the **interosseous** tarsal ligaments that stretch between contiguous bones and interrupt the synovial cavities. The specific names given to these ligaments typically reflect the bones they connect.

Subtalar joint

Located at the junction between the inferior surface of the talus and the superior surface of the calcaneus, the subtalar (talocalcaneal) joint has three articular facets. The posterior articulation is a concave facet on the talus. The anterior and middle articulations are convex talar facets. A sulcus that allows for the attachment of an intra-articular ligament, the tarsal canal, obliquely crosses the talus and calcaneus.

Although often misused, the single plane motion terminology of "inversion" and "eversion" do not accurately describe the joint biomechanics. The subtalar joint is a uniaxial joint with 1 degree of **freedom of movement**, pronation and supination, which occurs around an oblique axis and cuts through all three cardinal planes. Supination and pronation do not occur only at the subtalar joint. Rather, they are the composite motion of the talocrural joint, subtalar joint, midtarsal joints, and distal tibiofibular syndesmosis (see Chapter 9).[4]

Pronation of the foot and ankle influence proximal joint mechanics, causing internal tibial rotation, knee flexion, and hip internal rotation. Supination also changes proximal joint mechanics, resulting in external tibial rotation, knee extension, and hip external rotation.

Talar motions are identified by the direction in which the talar head moves. The bony motion that occurs during subtalar joint motion differs when the extremity is weight bearing and when it is nonweight bearing (Table 8-1). When nonweight-bearing, the calcaneus moves on the talus. When weight bearing the talus moves on the calcaneus.

Because no muscles attach to the talus, the stability of the subtalar joint is derived from ligamentous and bony restraints. The **interosseous talocalcaneal ligament** lies in the tarsal canal. In addition to assisting in maintaining the alignment between the talus and calcaneus, this ligament serves as an axis for talar tilt and divides the subtalar joint into two articular cavities. A second intra-articular ligament, the **ligamentum cervicis**, lies laterally in the tarsal canal. Collateral support is gained from the lateral and medial (deltoid) ankle ligaments. A segment of the deltoid ligament, the **medial talocalcaneal ligament**, provides medial intrinsic support to the subtalar joint, and the **lateral talocalcaneal ligament** provides lateral support. Anterior glide of the talus on the calcaneus is partially restrained by the **posterior talocalcaneal ligament.**

Freedom of movement The number of cardinal planes in which a joint allows motion.

Midfoot

The **talocalcaneonavicular (TCN) joint** and the **calcaneocuboid (CC) joint** represent the junction between the rearfoot and midfoot. The TCN joint is formed by the articulation between the talar head, the posterior aspect of the navicular, and the anterior border of the calcaneus and its sustenaculum tali. The **plantar calcaneonavicular ("spring") ligament** provides soft tissue support to the inferior portion of the joint capsule. Spanning the distance from the sustentaculum tali to the inferior surface of the posterior navicular and blending in with the deltoid ligament of the ankle, this ligament forms a "socket" for the talar head and supports the medial longitudinal arch.

Formed by the anterior border of the calcaneus and the posterior aspect of the cuboid, the CC joint is reinforced by the plantar and dorsal **calcaneocuboid ligaments.** Support is also gained from the **long plantar ligament** and **plantar fascia** that attaches to the three primary weight-bearing points on the foot: medial tubercle of the calcaneus, head of the first metatarsal, and head of the fifth metatarsal.[5]

The **midtarsal joints** are formed by the articulations of the tarsal bones located perpendicular to the long axis of the foot, the talonavicular and calcaneocuboid joints. The midtarsal joints increase the range of motion (ROM) during pronation and supination and allow the forefoot to compensate for uneven terrain. With pronation, the axes of the midtarsal joints become parallel, allowing more mobility.

Supination results in a less parallel orientation of the axes at the midtarsal joints, resulting in increased stability.

Forefoot

The junction between the midfoot and forefoot is demarcated by the **tarsometatarsal joints** (Lisfranc joint). Here the five MTs form gliding articulations with the bones of the midfoot. Proximal and distal **intermetatarsal joints** are formed between the bases and heads of adjacent MTs. Permitting a slight amount of dorsal/plantar glide, the proximal joints are bound together by the plantar, dorsal, and interosseous ligaments. The deep transverse ligament and the interosseous ligament support the distal joints.

A condyloid articulation between the MTs and the toes, the **metatarsophalangeal (MTP) joints** allow flexion and extension, and limited degrees of abduction, adduction, and rotation of the toes. Synovial and fibrous joint capsules surround each MTP joint. The plantar portion of the capsule is reinforced by the plantar fascia and thickened portions of the capsule, the plantar ligament. The medial and lateral joint capsule are reinforced by **collateral ligaments.**

With the exception of the first toe (hallux), each toe has two **interphalangeal (IP) joints**: a proximal interphalangeal (PIP) joint and a distal interphalangeal (DIP) joint. The hallux has only one IP joint. These hinge joints allow only flexion and extension to occur. Similar to the MTP joints, each joint is reinforced by the plantar and dorsal joint capsule and collateral ligaments.

Muscles Acting on the Foot and Toes

The intrinsic foot muscles are those originating on the foot and directly influence the motion of the foot and toes. The extrinsic foot muscles originate on the lower leg or the distal femur. In addition to producing motion at the foot and toes, the extrinsic foot muscles cause motion at the ankle. The gastrocnemius and plantaris also flex the knee.

Intrinsic muscles of the foot

The foot's intrinsic muscles originate and insert from the foot and are grouped into four layers (Table 8-2). The origins, insertions, action, and innervation of the intrinsic muscles are presented in Table 8-3.

Table 8-2 Layers of the Foot's Intrinsic Muscles

Layer	Muscles
1st: Superficial Layer	Abductor hallucis Flexor digitorum brevis Abductor digiti minimi
2nd: Middle Layer	Tendon of flexor hallucis longus Tendons of flexor digitorum longus Quadratus plantae Lumbricals
3rd: Deep Layer	Flexor hallucis brevis Adductor hallucis Flexor digiti minimi brevis
4th: Interosseous Layer	Plantar interossei Dorsal interossei

The **superficial layer** contains the primary abductor of the first toe, the abductor hallucis; the primary abductor of the fifth toe, the abductor digiti minimi; and the secondary flexor of the second through fifth toes, the flexor digitorum brevis (Fig. 8-6). The **middle layer** is formed by the quadratus plantae, a muscle that, when contracted, changes the angle of pull for the flexor digitorum longus and the lumbricals that flex the MTP joints and extend the IP joints. The tendons of the flexor hallucis longus and flexor digitorum longus also pass through this layer. The **deep layer** consists of the secondary flexors of the first and fifth toes, the flexor hallucis brevis and the adductor hallucis and the flexor digiti minimi brevis. The **interosseous layer**, found beneath the deep layer, contains the plantar and dorsal interossei. The three plantar interossei adduct the lateral three toes and the four dorsal interossei abduct the middle three toes (in relation to the second MT).

Extrinsic muscles acting on the foot

Arising from the leg compartments described in Chapter 9 (p. 225), the muscles that cross the talocrural and subtalar joints affect the position of the foot. The flexor hallucis longus assists in plantarflexion and adduction and supination of the foot and ankle. The flexor digitorum longus also plantarflexes the ankle while supinating the foot (Table 8-4).

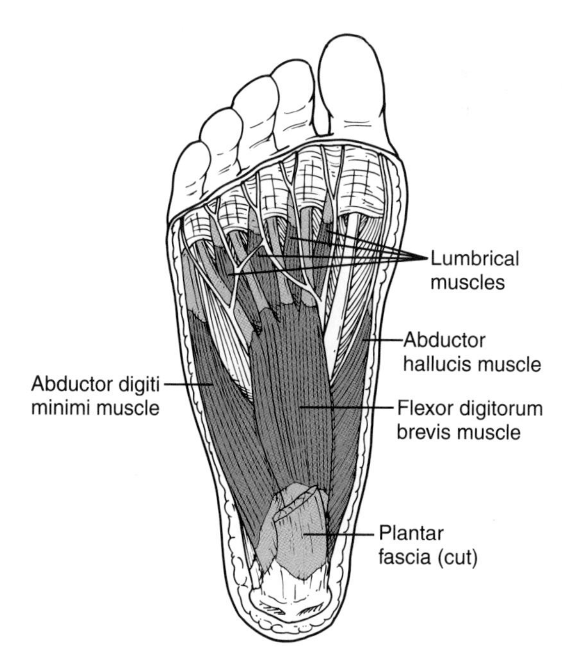

FIGURE 8-6 ■ The superficial layer of the foot's intrinsic muscles is formed by the abductor digiti minimi, the abductor hallucis, and the flexor digitorum brevis muscles. The lumbrical muscles are a component of the middle muscle layer.

Table 8-3 Intrinsic Foot and Toe Muscles

Muscle	Action	Origin	Insertion	Innervation	Root
Abductor Digiti Minimi	Flexion of the 5th MTP joint Abduction of the 5th MTP joint	Lateral portion of the calcaneal tuberosity Proximal lateral portion of calcaneus	Lateral portion of the 5th proximal phalanx	Lateral plantar	S1, S2
Abductor Hallucis	Abduction of the 1st MTP joint Assists in flexion of the 1st MTP joint Assists in forefoot adduction	Medial calcaneal tuberosity Flexor retinaculum Plantar aponeurosis	Plantar surface of the medial base of the 1st toe's proximal phalanx	Medial plantar	L4, L5, S1
Adductor Hallucis	Adduction of the 1st MTP joint Assists in flexion of the 1st MTP joint	Oblique head • Bases of 2nd through 4th metatarsals • Tendon sheath of peroneus longus Transverse head • Plantar surface of 3rd, 4th, and 5th metatarsal heads	Lateral surface of the base of the 1st toe's proximal phalanx	Lateral plantar	S1, S2
Flexor Digiti Minimi Brevis	Flexion of the 5th MTP joint	Plantar surface of the cuboid Base of the 5th metatarsal	Plantar aspect of the base of the 5th proximal phalanx	Lateral plantar	S1, S2
Flexor Digitorum Brevis	Flexion of the 2nd through 5th PIP joints Assists in flexion of the 2nd through 5th MTP joints	Medial calcaneal tuberosity Plantar fascia	Via four tendons, each having two slips, into the medial and lateral sides of the proximal 2nd through 5th phalanges	Medial plantar	L4, L5, S1
Flexor Hallucis Brevis	Flexion of 1st MTP joint	Medial side of the cuboid's plantar surface Slip from the tibialis posterior tendon	Via two tendons into the medial and lateral sides of the proximal phalanx of the first toe	Medial plantar	L4, L5, S1
Interossei, Dorsal	Abduction of the 3rd and 4th digits Assists in flexion of the MTP joints Assists in extension of the 3rd, 4th, and 5th IP joints	Via two heads to the contiguous sides of the metatarsals	Bases of proximal phalanges and associated dorsal extensor mechanism of medial second toe and the lateral 2nd 3rd, and 4th toes.	Lateral plantar	S1, S2
Interossei, Plantar	Adduction of the 3rd, 4th, and 5th digits Assists in MTP joint flexion Assists in extension of the 3rd, 4th, and 5th IP joints	Base and medial aspect of the 3rd, 4th, and 5th metatarsals	Medial portion of the bases of the 3rd, 4th, and 5th proximal phalanges	Lateral plantar	S1, S2
Lumbricals	Flexion of the 2nd through 5th MTP joints Assists in extension of the 2nd through 5th IP joints	Tendons of flexor digitorum longus	Posterior surfaces of the 2nd through 5th toes via the flexor digitorum longus tendons	1st: Medial plantar 2nd to 5th Lateral plantar	1st: L4, L5, S1 2nd to 5th: S1, S2
Quadratus Plantae	Modifies the flexor digitorum longus' angle of pull Assists in flexion of the 2nd through 5th MTP joints	Medial head Medial calcaneus Lateral head Lateral calcaneus	Dorsal and plantar surfaces of the flexor digitorum longus	Lateral plantar	S1, S2

DIP = distal interphalangeal; IP = interphalangeal; MTP = metatarsophalangeal; PIP = proximal interphalangeal.

Table 8-4 Posterior Leg Muscles Acting on the Ankle, Foot, and Toes

Muscle	Action	Origin	Insertion	Innervation	Root
Flexor Digitorum Longus	Flexion of 2nd through 5th PIP and DIP joints Flexion of 2nd through 5th MTP joints Assists in ankle plantarflexion Assists in foot supination	Posterior medial portion of the distal two thirds of the tibia From fascia arising from the tibialis posterior	Plantar base of distal phalanges of the 2nd through 5th toes	Tibial	L5, S1
Flexor Hallucis Longus	Flexion of 1st IP joint Assists in flexion of 1st MTP joint Assists in foot supination Assists in ankle plantarflexion	Posterior distal two thirds of the fibula Associated interosseous membrane and muscle fascia	Plantar surface of the proximal phalanx of the 1st toe	Tibial	L4, L5, S1
Gastrocnemius	Ankle plantarflexion Assists in knee flexion	Medial head • Posterior surface of the medial femoral condyle • Adjacent portion of the femur and knee capsule Lateral head • Posterior surface of the lateral femoral condyle • Adjacent portion of the femur and knee capsule	To the calcaneus via the Achilles tendon	Tibial	S1, S2
Peroneus Brevis	Pronation of foot Assists in ankle plantarflexion	Distal two thirds of the lateral fibula	Styloid process at the base of the 5th metatarsal	Superficial peroneal	L4, L5, S1
Peroneus Longus	Pronation of foot Assists in ankle plantarflexion	Lateral tibial condyle Fibular head Upper two thirds of the lateral fibula	Lateral aspect of the base of the 1st metatarsal Lateral and dorsal aspect of the 1st cuneiform	Superficial peroneal	L4, L5, S1
Plantaris	Ankle plantarflexion Assists in knee flexion	Distal portion of the supracondylar line of the lateral femoral condyle Adjacent portion of the femoral popliteal surface Oblique popliteal ligament	To the calcaneus via the Achilles tendon	Tibial	L4, L5, S1
Soleus	Ankle plantarflexion	Posterior fibular head Upper one third of the fibula's posterior surface Soleal line located on the posterior tibial shaft Middle one third of the medial tibial border	To the calcaneus via the Achilles tendon	Tibial	S1, S2
Tibialis Posterior	Supination of the foot Assists in ankle plantarflexion	Length of the interosseous membrane Posterior, lateral tibia Upper two thirds of the medial fibula	Navicular tuberosity Via fibrous slips to the sustentaculum tali; cuneiforms; cuboid; and bases of the 2nd, 3rd, and 4th metatarsals	Tibial	L4, S1

DIP = distal interphalangeal; IP = interphalangeal; MTP = metatarsophalangeal; PIP = proximal interphalangeal.

The long toe extensors, extensor hallucis longus (EHL), and extensor digitorum longus (EDL) assist in ankle dorsiflexion. The EHL also supinates the foot. The EDL slightly contributes to pronation (Table 8-5).

Arches of the Foot

Serving primarily as shock absorbers to buffer and dissipate the **ground reaction forces,** the three arches of the foot increase its flexibility. Normal arches are more prominent in the non–weight-bearing position than in the weight-bearing position. When non–weight bearing, the medial longitudinal arch is the most noticeable; the lateral longitudinal arch and the transverse arch are less distinct. With weight bearing, the arches flatten as the foot contacts the ground at multiple points: the head of the first MT, the head of the fifth MT, and the calcaneus.

Medial longitudinal arch

Five bones form the prominent medial longitudinal arch: the calcaneus, talus, navicular, first cuneiform, and first MT (Fig. 8-7). The bony, ligamentous, and muscular arrangement of the medial arch allow a greater amount of motion than the other arches of the foot. Serving as the keystone, the navicular is the stabilizing element between the proximal and distal sides of the arch. Because the navicular plays an important role in supporting the medial longitudinal arch, dysfunction of this bone or the structures that support and reinforce the navicular leads to dysfunction of the entire arch.

Ligamentous support of the medial arch is obtained from the plantar calcaneonavicular ("spring") ligament, the long and short plantar ligaments, the deltoid ligament, and the plantar fascia. A **slip** from the spring ligament to the ankle's deltoid ligament also assists in supporting the navicular. A second slip supports the talus.

Primary support of the medial longitudinal arch is obtained from the three slips of the plantar fascia.[1] The central slip, originating off the medial calcaneal tubercle and inserting into the distal plantar aspects of each of the five digits, is the longest and thickest (Fig. 8-8). As the central slip progresses down the length of the foot, it gives rise to medial and lateral slips. The function of the plantar fascia is complemented by most of the foot's intrinsic muscles and ligaments. The plantar fascia is attached to the overlying plantar skin.[6]

The plantar fascia supports the medial and lateral longitudinal arches similar to the way a bow string functions to give the bow a curve. By longitudinally supporting the calcaneus to the MT heads, the plantar fascia bows the foot's long arches. Because of the fascia's attachment on the phalanges, extending the toes draws the calcaneus toward the MT heads. As a result, the arches become further accentuated because of the **windlass effect** (Fig. 8-9).

During static weight bearing, muscles provide little support to the medial arch. However, during walking, a **force couple** is formed between the tibialis anterior and the tibialis posterior, drawing the arch proximally and superiorly to supinate the foot. Dysfunction of this force couple can place additional stress on the foot's bony and soft tissue structures, possibly leading to lower leg pathologies such as medial tibial stress syndrome or tibialis posterior tendinopathy.

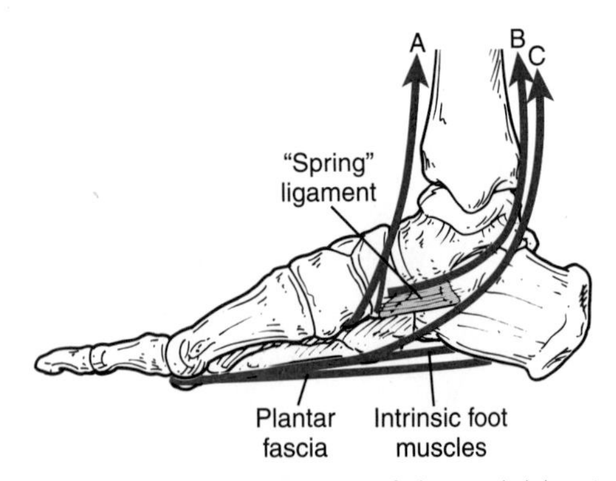

FIGURE 8-7 ■ Soft tissue support of the medial longitudinal arch. Dynamic support is obtained through the **(A)** tibialis anterior, **(B)** tibialis posterior, and **(C)** flexor hallucis longus muscles. The spring ligament is assisted by the plantar fascia and intrinsic foot muscle in bowing the arch.

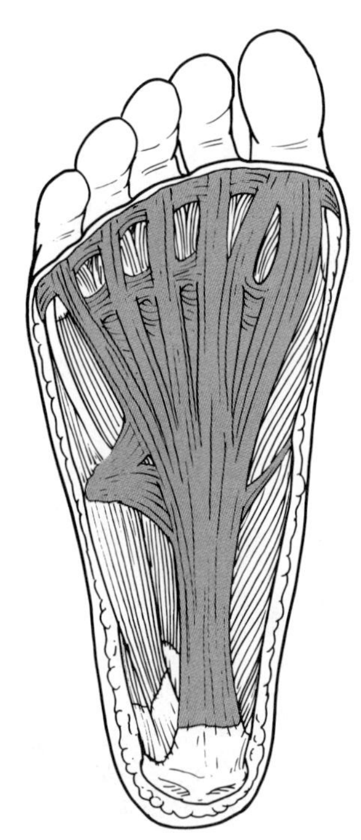

FIGURE 8-8 ■ Plantar fascia. The central slip attaches to each of the five toes. Extending the toes tightens the fascia, increasing the curvature of the medial longitudinal arch.

Slip A distinct band of tissue arising from the main portion of a structure.

Table 8-5 Anterior Leg Muscles Acting on the Ankle, Foot, and Toes

Muscle	Action	Origin	Insertion	Innervation	Root
Extensor Digitorum Brevis	Extension of the 1st though 4th MTP joints Assists in extension of the 2nd, 3rd, and 4th PIP and DIP joints	Distal portion of the superior and lateral portion of the calcaneus Lateral talocalcaneal ligament Lateral portion of the inferior extensor retinaculum	To the dorsal surface of the base of the first phalanx **(termed the extensor hallucis brevis)** Proximal phalanges of the 2nd, 3rd, and 4th toes and to the distal phalanges via an attachment to the extensor digitorum longus tendon	Deep peroneal	L5, S1
Extensor Digitorum Longus	Extension of the 2nd through 5th MTP joints Assists in extending 2nd through 5th PIP and DIP joints Assists in foot pronation Assists in ankle dorsiflexion	Lateral tibial condyle Proximal three fourths of anterior fibula Proximal portion of the interosseous membrane	Via four tendons to the distal phalanges of the 2nd through 5th toes	Deep peroneal	L4, L5, S1
Extensor Hallucis Longus	Extension of the 1st MTP joint Extension of the 1st IP joint Assists in ankle dorsflexion	Middle two thirds of the anterior surface of the fibula Adjacent portion of the interosseous membrane	Base of the distal phalanx of the 1st toe	Deep peroneal	L4, L5, S1
Peroneus Tertius	Pronation of the foot Dorsiflexion of the ankle	Distal one third of the anterior surface of the fibula • Adjacent portion of the interosseous membrane	• Dorsal surface of the base of the 5th metatarsal	Deep peroneal	L4, L5, S1
Tibialis Anterior	Dorsiflexion of the ankle Supination of the foot	Lateral tibial condyle Upper one half of the tibia's lateral surface Adjacent portion of the interosseous membrane	Medial and plantar surface of the 1st cuneiform • Medial and plantar surfaces of the 1st metatarsal	Deep peroneal	L4, L5, S1

DIP = distal interphalangeal; IP = interphalangeal; MTP = metatarsophalangeal; PIP = proximal interphalangeal.

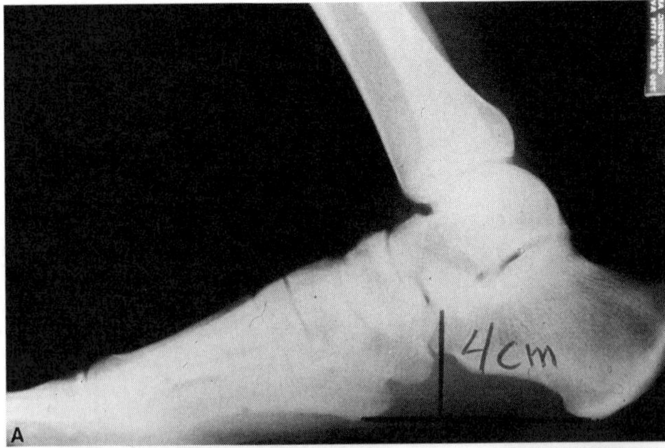

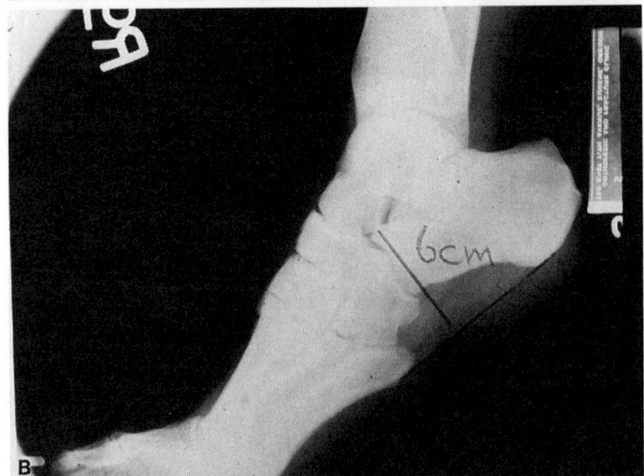

FIGURE 8-9 ■ Windlass effect of the plantar fascia on the medial longitudinal arch of the right foot. (A) The height of the medial arch when the foot is fully weight bearing. (B) Extending the toes causes the plantar fascia to tighten, resulting in an increase in the height of the arch.

Lateral longitudinal arch

Lower and more rigid than the medial longitudinal arch, the lateral arch is composed of the calcaneus, the cuboid, and the fifth MT and is a continuation of the medial longitudinal arch. The arch itself is rarely the site of injury.

Transverse metatarsal arch

The transverse MT arch is formed by the lengths of the MTs and tarsals and is shaped by the concave features along the inferior surface of the MTs. The arch originates at the MT heads and remains present until the point where it fades on the calcaneus (Fig. 8-10). The first and fifth MT heads are the distal weight-bearing structures. The second MT forms the apex of the arch.

Architecturally, the transverse MT arch is supported through a buttress formed by the medial and lateral longitudinal arches, with dynamic support provided by the peroneus longus muscle.[7] Normally, the transverse MT arch is only slightly visible during non–weight bearing, being obscured by the fat pad covering the plantar aspect of the MT heads. During static weight bearing, the arch flattens, with the first MT head and sesamoids bearing 33% of the body weight while the remaining four toes equally assume the rest of the load.

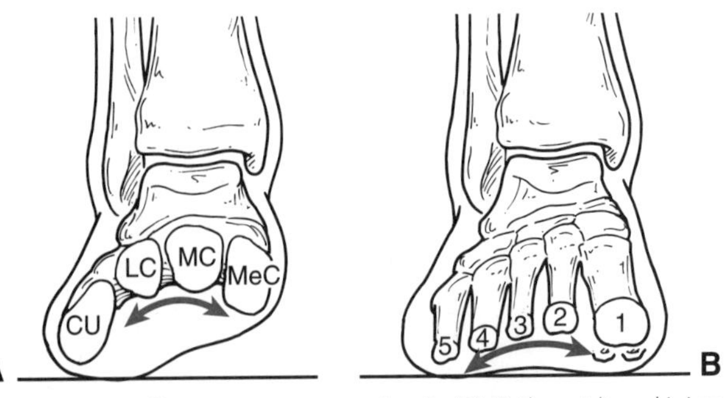

FIGURE 8-10 ■ Transverse metatarsal arch. (A) At the midtarsal joints. (B) At the distal metatarsals. CU = cuboid, LC = lateral cuneiform, MC = middle cuneiform, MeC = medial cuneiform.

The presence of a functional transverse metatarsal arch as a uniquely identified structure of the foot is controversial. The tripod theory (weight distributed between the first MT head, fifth MT head, and the calcaneus) has been questioned as a result of ultrasonic analysis and studies of the forces on the plantar surface of the foot when weight bearing.[8]

Neurologic Anatomy

The sensory and motor nerve supply to the foot is a continuation of the compartmental innervation of the leg described in Chapter 9. The lateral foot is supplied by the **sural nerve**, the dorsal surface of the foot by branches of the **deep and superficial peroneal nerve**, the medial aspect by the **saphenous nerve**, the plantar surface by the **lateral and medial plantar nerve**, and the posterior aspect by the calcaneal branches of the sural nerve and the **tibial nerve**. Each of these peripheral nerves represents more than one nerve root; therefore, neurological sensory testing must be specific to both nerve root dermantomes and peripheral nerve dermatomes.

Vascular Anatomy

The foot's dorsal structures receive their blood supply from the **dorsalis pedis artery**. After crossing the anterior talocrural joint line, the dorsalis pedis artery branches to form the **lateral tarsal artery**. The **arcuate artery**, formed between the distal end of the lateral tarsal and dorsalis pedis artery, supplies the lateral four **rays**. A continuation of the dorsalis pedis artery, the **first dorsal metatarsal artery**, supplies the first ray.

The blood supply to the plantar structures is received from the **posterior tibial artery** that gives rise to several branches. The **medial tibial artery** branches from the posterior tibial artery to supply the medial structures and first ray. The posterior tibial artery terminates in a collateral loop formed with the **deep plantar artery**, the **plantar arch**.

Venous drainage occurs via a dorsal and plantar network that exits the foot via the **medial marginal vein** that drains into the **great saphenous vein** and the **lateral marginal vein,** which drains into the **small saphenous vein**.

Ray The series of bones formed by the metatarsal and phalanges.

Clinical Examination of Foot and Toe Injuries

Examination Map

HISTORY

Past Medical History

History of Present Condition

INSPECTION

Functional observation

General Inspection of the Foot

General Foot Type Classifications
Feiss Line
Assessment of foot position in STNJ

Inspection of the Toes

Pathological toe postures
Posture of the first ray

Inspection of the Medial Structures

Medial longitudinal arch

Inspection of the Lateral Structures

Fifth metatarsal

Inspection of the Dorsal Structures

Long toe tendons

Inspection of the Plantar Surface

Plantar fascia
Medial calcaneal tubercle
Callus/blister formation

Inspection of the Posterior Structures

Achilles tendon
Calcaneus
Retrocalcaneal exostosis

Inspection of Foot and Calcaneal Alignment

Assessment of subtalar joint neutral
Common foot postures assessed in subtalar joint neutral
Position of first tarsometatarsal joint

PALPATION

Palpation of the Medial Structures

First MTP joint
First metatarsal
First cuneiform
Navicular
Talar head
Sustentaculum tali
Calcaneonavicular ligament
Medial talar tubercle
Calcaneus
Tibialis posterior
Flexor hallucis longus
Flexor digitorum longus
Posterior tibial pulse

Palpation of the Lateral Structures

Fifth MTP joint
Fifth metatarsal
Styloid process
Cuboid
Lateral calcaneal border
Peroneal tubercle
Peroneal tendons

Palpation of the Dorsal Structures

Rays
Cuneiforms
Navicular
Dome of the talus
Sinus tarsi
Extensor digitorum brevis
Inferior extensor retinaculum
Tibialis anterior
Extensor hallucis longus
Extensor digitorum longus
Dorsalis pedis pulse

Palpation of the Plantar Structures

Medial calcaneal tubercle
Plantar fascia
Intermetatarsal neuromas
Lateral four metatarsal heads
Sesamoids

JOINT AND MUSCLE FUNCTION ASSESSMENT

Goniometry

Rearfoot inversion and eversion
First metatarsophalangeal abduction
Metatarsophalangeal flexion and extension

Active Range of Motion

Toe flexion
Toe extension

Manual Muscle Tests

Toe flexion
Toe extension

Passive Range of Motion

Toe flexion
Toe extension
Mobility of first ray

JOINT STABILITY TESTS

Stress Testing

Metatarsophalangeal and interphalangeal joints

- Valgus and varus stress testing of the MTP and IP joints

Joint Play Assessment

Intermetatarsal joints
Tarsometatarsal joints
Midtarsal joints

NEUROLOGIC EXAMINATION

L4–S2 Nerve Roots

Tarsal Tunnel Syndrome

Interdigital Neuroma

VASCULAR EXAMINATION

Dorsalis Pedis Pulse

Posterior Tibial Pulse

Capillary Refill

PATHOLOGIES AND SPECIAL TESTS

Foot Type

Navicular drop test

Pes Cavus

Plantar Fasciitis

Test for supple pes planus

Plantar Fascia Rupture

Heel Spur

Tarsal Coalition

Tarsal Tunnel Syndrome

Dorsiflexion-eversion test

Metatarsal Fractures

Acute fractures
Stress fractures

Lisfranc Injury

Phalangeal Fractures

Intermetatarsal Neuroma

Mulder sign

Hallux Rigidus

Hallux Valgus

First MTP Joint Sprains

Sesamoiditis

When examining foot injuries, an evaluation of the ankle complex is often included. In addition, examination of the lower extremity, lumbar region, and gait also may be necessary. Having the patient dressed in shorts during the examination expedites the evaluation of these structures.

History

A detailed and accurate history of recent and prior incidence of foot pain is required to evaluate this body area accurately. An acute onset of symptoms should lead the examiner to suspect bony or soft tissue trauma. Insidious pain may arise from soft tissue degeneration, inflammation of ligamentous or muscular structures, or from a stress fracture.

Past medical history

Multiple influences exist on the development and resolution of foot pain. A thorough exam warrants consideration of these potential causative factors.

- **Seronegative spondyloarthropathies**: Conditions such as rheumatoid arthritis, reactive arthritis, psoriatic arthritis, or inflammatory bowel disease can produce swelling in the foot and ankle. Rheumatoid arthritis can lead to osteophytic growth.[5]
- **Gout:** Associated with elevated levels of uric acid, **gout** attacks tend to localize in the extremities, particularly the great toe. Acute symptoms include redness, swelling, and exquisite pain.
- **Diabetes**: **Peripheral neuropathy** and/or **peripheral arterial disease** affect approximately 30% of people with diabetes who are older than the age of 40.[9] Decreased sensory function can cause the patient to under-recognize the magnitude of the condition. Vascular dysfunction can inhibit the healing process. People with diabetes should be educated regarding frequent foot inspection for tissue breakdown and infections.
- **Chronic heel pain:** Heel pain that does not have a discernible origin could be indicative of **Ewing's sarcoma** or other metastatic tumors.[5]
- **Open wounds**: Has the patient suffered any recent cuts, punctures, or open sores (including soft corns) of the foot, possibly indicating infection?

History of the present condition

- **Location of the pain**: Pain in the foot may arise from trauma or occur secondary to compensation for improper lower leg biomechanics. Pain may be referred from the lumbar or sacral nerve roots, the sciatic nerve, or the femoral nerve or one of their branches (Table 8-6). Other neurologic symptoms such as numbness, burning, or tingling may be the result of peripheral nerve entrapment.[5]
  - **Retrocalcaneal pain**: Pain along the posterior aspect of the calcaneus may result from inflammation of the retrocalcaneal bursa, inflammation, degeneration of the Achilles tendon, or os trigonum pathology (see Chapter 9). Retrocalcaneal bursa pain tends to be isolated to the area between the Achilles and the calcaneus; the pain associated with tendon pathology is more diffuse.
  - **Heel pain**: Pain in the heel may be the result of plantar fasciitis or a heel spur, especially if the pain is located on the medial plantar aspect. In the absence of a mechanism of injury to this area, consider pain referred from the lumbar nerve roots or their peripheral nerves.
  - **Medial arch pain**: The medial arch can be the site of pain for tarsal tunnel syndrome, a midfoot sprain, plantar fasciitis, navicular fracture, or tibialis posterior tendinopathy. Compression of the posterior tibial nerve, **tarsal tunnel syndrome**, radiates a sharp, burning pain and paresthesia to the medial and/or lateral arch (see Chapter 9).
  - **Metatarsal pain**: Pain specifically isolated to a MT that worsens over time can indicate a stress fracture. This pain should be differentiated from pain arising from between the MTs, possibly the result of impingement of the intermetatarsal nerves. The pain caused by both conditions carries the common trait of worsening with activity. **Metatarsalgia** is nondescript pain arising from the MTs.
  - **Great toe pain**: Pain and dysfunction in the great toe can be disabling, causing the patient to walk on the lateral foot to avoid pushing off on the great toe Pathology within the MTP joint, such as **hallux rigidus** or **hallux valgus**, is characterized by diffuse pain throughout the joint during hyperextension and flexion. Pain localized to the plantar surface of the joint may be caused by a sesamoid fracture or inflammation of the sesamoids (**sesamoiditis**). The first MTP joint is often the first part of the body to demonstrate the signs and symptoms of gout, characterized by swelling, redness, and severe pain. Dorsal pain can originate from an ingrown toenail.
  - **Lateral arch pain**: Compression of the posterior tibial nerve as it passes through the tarsal tunnel can cause pain radiating along the lateral arch. Acutely, pain may be isolated to the lateral arch after fractures of the fifth MT or cuboid. Pain arising from peroneal tendon pathology may radiate into the lateral foot (see Chapter 9).

Gout A form of arthritis marked by inflammation and pain in the distal joints.

Ewing's sarcoma A cancerous tumor that forms in the shaft of long bones or, less frequently, in soft tissue and is most prevalent in children and teenagers.

Table 8-6 Possible Pathology Based on the Location of Pain

	Location of Pain					
	Proximal (Calcaneus)	**Distal (Toes)**	**Plantar**	**Dorsal**	**Medial**	**Lateral**
Soft Tissue Pathology	Calcaneal bursitis	Corns	Callus	MTP sprain	Spring ligament sprain	Peroneal tendinopathy*
	Retrocalcaneal bursitis	Hallux rigidus	Plantar fasciitis	Forefoot sprain	Plantar fasciitis	
					Plantar fascia rupture or sprain	
	Achilles tendinopathy*	IP sprain	Plantar fascia rupture		Posterior tibial nerve entrapment (Tarsal tunnel syndrome)	
		MTP sprain	Plantar warts		Tibialis posterior tendinopathy*	
		Ingrown toenail	Intermetatarsal neuroma		1st MTP sprain	
			Tarsal tunnel syndrome			
Bony Pathology	Calcaneal fracture	Phalanx fracture	Sesamoiditis	Metatarsal stress fracture	Navicular stress fracture	Cuboid fracture
	Calcaneal spur	Arthritis or inflammation	Sesamoid fracture	Lisfranc fracture/ dislocation	Bunion	Fifth metatarsal fracture (especially at the base)
	Calcaneal cyst		Heel spur	Talus fracture	Hallux rigidus	Bunionette
				Tarsal coalition	Hallux valgus	

IP = interphalangeal; MTP = metatarsophalangeal.

*Discussed in Chapter 9.

- **Onset and mechanism of injury**: The duration of the symptoms and the presence of pain that worsens or diminishes with specific activities provide insight about the nature of the injury and the tissues involved.
  - **Acute onset:** The acute onset of foot injuries can occur from a rotational force as the foot lands on an uneven surface. These irregular positions place an increased force across the bones and ligamentous structures as they are stressed beyond their end ROM. A direct blow to the phalanges or MTs may result in their fracture. Ligaments can be avulsed from their attachment site if the joint is forced beyond its normal ROM. Although rare, avulsion of muscle attachments may result from forceful contractions as the patient attempts to control motion during activity.
  - **Insidious onset**
    - **Playing surface**: In athletic activities, changing from a playing surface of one density to a surface with a different density may precipitate injury. For example, a change from running on an indoor rubberized track to running outdoors on pavement alters the ground reaction forces and stabilizing requirements that are distributed through the foot, ankle, and lower leg. Moving to a harder surface places an increased load on these structures. Moving to a softer or rubberized surface increases eccentric demand of the muscles because of the surface's rebounding effect.
    - **Distance and duration**: Altering the components of the training regimen may increase or otherwise change the forces placed on the body and hinder the foot's ability to accommodate, resulting in overuse injuries. Ask the patient if he or she has significantly increased the distance, duration, or intensity of training. With increased stresses, the muscles providing dynamic support to the foot become fatigued, resulting in altered biomechanics.
    - **Shoes**: Training shoes that no longer provide adequate support may produce injury-causing forces at the foot. Changing either competitive or casual footwear (such as high heels) may alter the biomechanics of the lower extremity and redistribute forces in the foot. Ask the patient if he or she has been wearing shoes that are excessively worn or of an inappropriate type. Determine if the patient has a new pair of shoes for competition or daily wear. Question the patient regarding the use of orthotics, the reason for their use, the activities during which they are worn, and the last time they were fitted.

✱ Practical Evidence

Wearing high-heeled shoes significantly redistributes the weight-bearing forces on the foot and alters muscular activity up the kinetic chain. The gastrocnemius, especially the lateral portion fatigues, shifting the center of pressure laterally on the foot.[10] Plantarflexion strength and range of motion is reduced, increasing hip flexor muscle activity and increasing forces on the MTP joints and forefoot.[11]

Inspection

During the history-taking process, note any bilateral gross or subtle deformity, swelling, or redness in the foot, toes, and ankle (Fig. 8-11).

Inspect the feet while they are non–weight-bearing and then compare these findings with those obtained while weight bearing and during gait (see Chapter 7). When non–weight-bearing, the foot normally assumes its natural alignment. When weight bearing, the foot reveals the way it compensates for structural abnormalities of the foot, the lower extremity, and the body as a whole. Also inspect the patient's daily casual and participation footwear for irregular wear patterns and for the appropriateness relative to the activity.

Functional observation

The tests of function for the patient involve observing activities that bring on or exacerbate the primary symptoms and observing for deviations. Usually, this begins by watching the patient approach. Note whether the patient

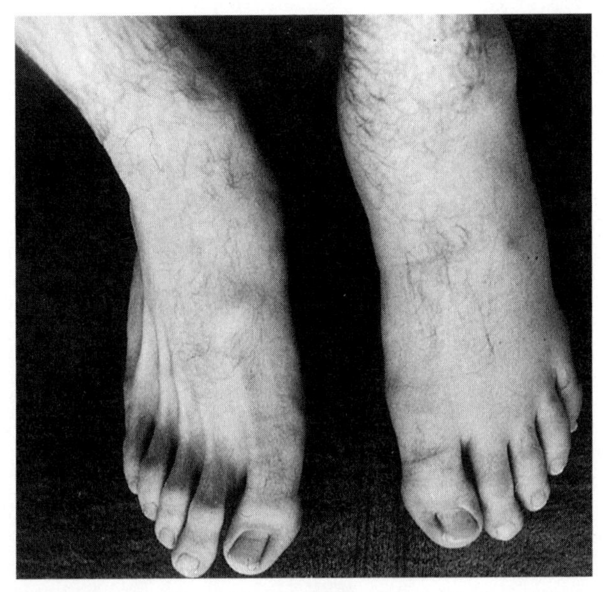

FIGURE 8-11 ■ Swelling of the foot. Without first gathering a history of the injury, it cannot be determined whether this swelling is caused by trauma to the foot or ankle or from a lower leg or knee injury. If the leg is kept in a gravity-dependent position, edema will migrate distally.

was assisted into the facility, is using crutches or a cane, or has any gross gait dysfunction. Subtle gait deviations, described in Chapter 7, may also be problematic. Observe for prolonged pronation as evidenced by a navicular that is still plantarflexing when the heel rises.[12] Walking on the heel to avoid push-off may indicate a metatarsal or phalanx fracture, plantar fasciitis, or great toe pathology. Walking on the lateral foot may indicate pathology to the medial foot structures and walking only on the toes may reflect pathology in the calcaneal or ankle region. Any observed functional limitations serve as the basis for further examination to identify the underlying impairments.

General inspection of the foot

- **Foot type**: Foot structure is classified as **cavus, planus,** or **neutral** through observing the weight-bearing foot from the anterior and posterior views (Inspection Findings 8-1). A gross assessment foot type can be determined using the **Feiss Line** (Special Test 8-1).

A cavus foot is characterized by a high medial longitudinal arch, an adducted forefoot, and an inverted rearfoot. A planus foot has a low and bulging medial longitudinal arch, an abducted forefoot, and an everted rearfoot. Planus foot structure is further classified as either supple or rigid. A rigid planus foot maintains its weight-bearing shape when non–weight bearing. The medial longitudinal arch of a supple planus foot becomes more prominent when non–weight bearing or during a heel raise (see Plantar Fasciitis, p. 198). A normal foot is neither cavus nor planus.

Although a useful classification strategy, this system must be considered relative to the resulting kinematics and pathology. Deviation of a foot from normal represents either a structural foot abnormality or the foot's adaptation to a structural deficit in the leg, pelvis, or spine. Abnormal foot posture may also be the result of neurologic or disease states.

- **Calluses and blisters:** Inspect the foot and toes for blisters and calluses, possibly indicating improperly fitting shoes, poor biomechanics, or underlying bony or soft tissue dysfunction. Blisters may be the result of dermatologic conditions such as **tinea pedis** or indicate areas of increased friction or irritation from the foot rubbing against the shoe. Calluses develop as the result of long-term pressures. The presence of callus under the MT heads may indicate a biomechanical abnormality. Those under the calcaneus are usually the result of an atypical gait pattern.[13]
- **Skin conditions**: Skin conditions can provide evidence to the nature of pain or alteration in gait. Some open skin lesions are contagious and will require the use of Standard Precautions (see Box 1-6).
  - **Tinea pedis: "Athlete's foot"** is a common tinea infection affecting athletes, primarily men and boys (Fig. 8-12). This condition also may be caused by *Candida* or filamentous fungi. Proper bathing, regularly changing socks, and keeping the area dry help prevent the buildup of fungi.[14] Topical corticosteroid agents can be used to provide symptomatic treatment for the lesions. When multiple sites of outbreak occur, systemic oral medication may be prescribed.[14]
  - **Corns**: Also referred to as clavus, a corn is a thickening of the stratum corneum and tends to occur in non–weight-bearing areas. Corns may be sensitive to the touch. Corns should be differentiated from a **callus** in that a callus does not have a central core.
    - **Hard corns** (heloma dura), located in areas that receive excessive pressure, appear as hard, granular nodules on the skin with a hard central core and a defined margin. Hard corns tend to form on the toes and PIP joints.
    - **Soft corns** (heloma molle) form between the toes, most frequently the web space between the fourth and fifth toes.[15] Dampness in the web space moistens the corn, thus keeping it soft and giving it a **macerated** appearance. The moisture together with the dark, warm environment predispose the lesion to infection and **ulceration**.
  - **Plantar warts:** Plantar warts (verruca plantaris), a common dermatologic abnormality affecting the foot's plantar aspect, have a different appearance

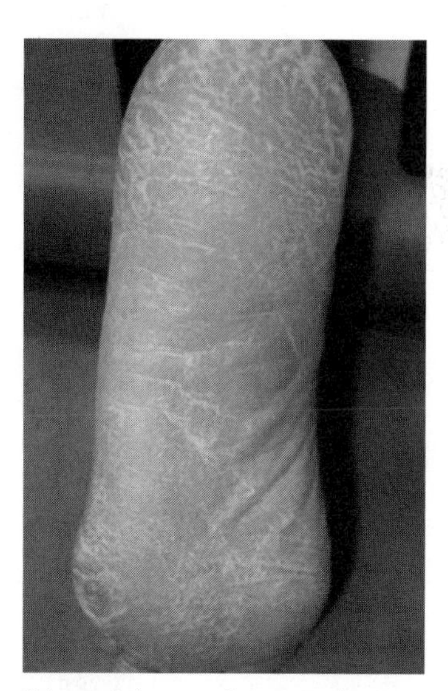

FIGURE 8-12 ■ "Moccasin" type of tinea pedis. Dryness, scaling, and erythema of the plantar and/or lateral foot. (From Barankin B and Freiman A. *Derm Notes: Clinical Dermatology Pocket Guide.* Philadelphia, FA Davis, 2006.)

Tinea pedis A fungal infection of the foot and toes.

Macerated Soft and fluid-soaked.

Ulceration An open sore or lesion of the skin or mucous membrane that is accompanied by inflamed and necrotic tissue.

Inspection Findings 8-1
General Foot Type Classifications (Weight Bearing)

	Pes Planus	Neutral	Pes Cavus
	A	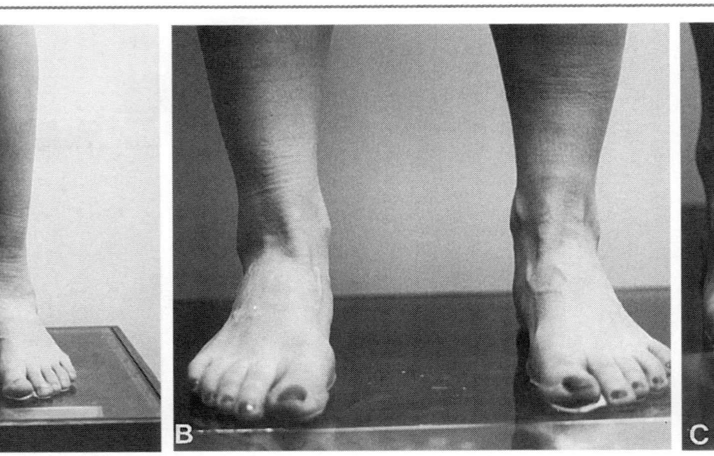	C
Description	Medial bulge; abducted forefoot, everted calcaneus A medial bulge must be present at the talonavicular joint, indicating excessive talar adduction. The medial arch must be low. This is determined by the Feiss line, formed by connecting the points formed by the head of the first MT, the navicular tubercle, and the medial malleolus (see Box 4–1).	The calcaneus is slightly everted. A medial bulge is not present. Feiss line indicates that the most prominent aspect of the navicular is in line with the apex of the medial malleolus and the plantar surface of the first MTP joint.	The calcaneus must be inverted greater than 3° from perpendicular relative to the position of the ground. A medial bulge is not present. Using Feiss' line, the arch must be high.

Special Test 8-1
Feiss Line

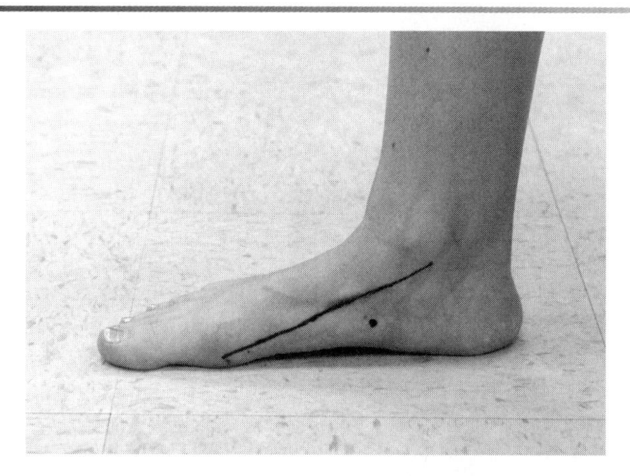

The Feiss line is used to assess static foot structure and provides a general assessment of foot type. With the patient in a weight-bearing position, a line is drawn from the plantar surface of the 1st MT head to the apex of the medial malleolus and the relative position of the navicular tubercle is noted.

Patient Position	Relaxed stance with the weight evenly distributed
Position of Examiner	Positioned at the patient's feet
Evaluative Procedure	Instruct the patient to stand with the feet shoulder-width apart and the weight evenly distributed. With the patient weight bearing, identify and mark the apex of the medial malleolus and the plantar aspect of the head of the 1st MT. Mark the position of the navicular tubercle and note its position relative to the line.
Positive Test	Tubercle above the line: Pes cavus Tubercle intersects the line: Normal Tubercle below the line: Pes planus
Implications	Cavus foot type has reduced shock-absorbing capacity. Planus foot type is often hypermobile.
Comments	The Feiss line can be assessed with the foot non–weight bearing.
Evidence	Evidence is absent in the literature.

MT = metatarsal.

than common warts (verruca vulgaris) (Fig. 8-13). Weight-bearing and the thick callous cause plantar warts to appear to grow inward, creating a dark core within a depression on the bottom of the foot. The central **petechiae** mask the normal **whorls** and skin markings, thus differentiating them from callus. Caused by exposure to the human papilloma virus, usually found in a moist environment (e.g., public showers), plantar warts are usually localized to areas of excessive weight-bearing stresses. However, they may develop anywhere on the plantar aspect of the foot.

Plantar warts are more focal than an ordinary callus, are point tender, and can cause pain during weight-bearing activities and disrupt gait. The patient often complains of the sensation of "stepping on a pebble." Warts may spontaneously appear and disappear. Persistent warts can be successfully treated using over-the-counter wart medication containing salicylic or lactic acid. Severe, widespread, or unrelenting warts may be removed by a physician or podiatrist using cryotherapy, electrocautery, or laser therapy.

Inspection of the toes

- **General toe alignment**: The common toe malalignments are presented in Inspection Findings 8-2.
- **Morton's alignment**: This condition, also referred to as **Morton's toe**, results in a greater amount of force

Petechiae Small, purplish, hemorrhagic spots on the skin.

Whorls Swirl markings in the skin. Fingerprints are images formed by the whorls on the fingertips.

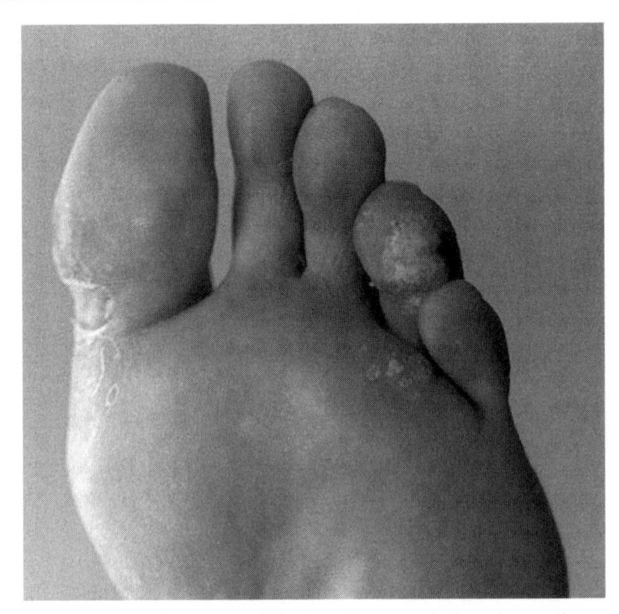

FIGURE 8-13 ■ Plantar warts. This condition results in point tenderness and masks the normal skin markings, thus distinguishing it from callus.

transmitted along the second ray during push-off. A callus may be present under the second MT head. Morton's toe has been associated with increased callus formation, pain, stress fracture, and hallux rigidus.[17,18] Hypertrophy of the second MT was once believed to be a consequence of Morton's toe, but this relationship has not been substantiated.[19]

- **Claw toes:** Claw toes are commonly associated with pes cavus. A callus may be found over the dorsal portion of the PIP joint and on the plantar surface of the MTP joint and, in some cases, on the tips of the toes.
- **Hammer toe:** Hammer toes may develop as either the long toe extensors or long toe flexors substitute for weakness of the primary dorsiflexors or plantarflexors. They often occur after injury, such as a rupture of the plantar fascia, or with neuromuscular disease states. A callus may be located on the dorsal surface of the PIP joint, resulting from friction against the shoe. In most cases, this deformity affects only one ray and may be caused by improperly fitting shoes (especially during the growth years), hereditary factors, elongation of the plantar fascia, or hallux valgus.[20]
- **Hallux valgus:** Hallux valgus is characterized by an abducted first ray at the MTP joint and is associated with a pes planus foot type.[21] Pain and dysfunction may also result from a bunion over the first MTP joint that forms secondary to the valgus deformity or secondary to the dislocation of the first MTP joint's sesamoid bones. The subsequent toe deformity can cause footwear to fit improperly and alter biomechanics (see Hallux Valgus, p. 214).[16]
  - **Bunion**: Formed by the development and subsequent inflammation of a bursa, bunions are characterized by inflammation on the medial aspect of the first MTP joint. Causes of bunions include hallux valgus and poorly fitting shoes. A smaller bunionette, or tailor's bunion, may form on the lateral aspect of the fifth MTP joint.
- **Ingrown toenail (onychocryptosis)**: Most often involving the great toe, the medial and/or lateral aspect of the nail grows into the bed (Fig. 8-14). The areas of ingrowth cause disruption and subsequent infection of the skin surrounding and beneath the nailbed, causing it to appear red and swollen, warranting physician referral.
- **Subungual hematoma:** Localized trauma to the toe can result in the formation of a hematoma beneath the nail, a subungual hematoma (Fig. 8-15). Commonly found in the great toe, the resulting collection of blood turns the nail a dark purple and causes pain from pressure being placed on the involved nerve endings. A subungual hematoma may form secondary to a fracture of the distal phalanx and may be caused by a falling object or other compressive forces. If the lumina is no longer visible, the nail will eventually fall off.

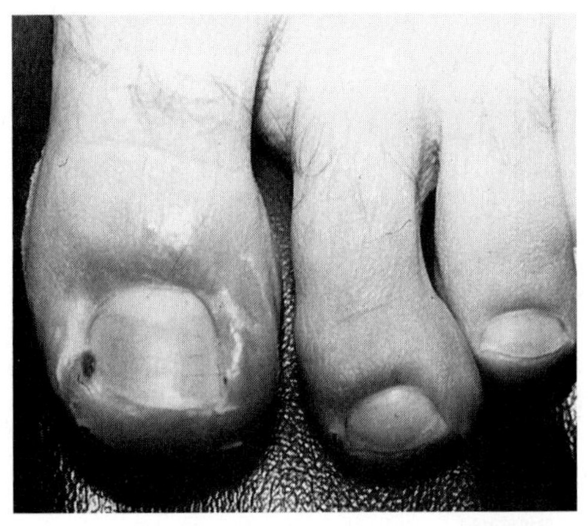

FIGURE 8-14 ■ Ingrown toenail. This painful condition results from abnormal growth patterns of the nail, causing it to imbed within the skin.

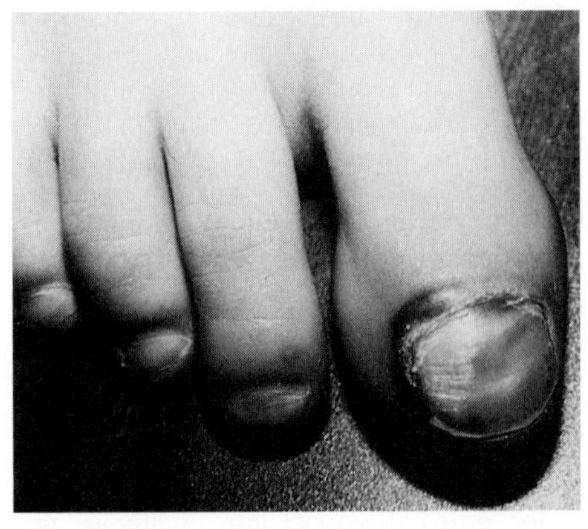

FIGURE 8-15 ■ Trauma to the toe can result in bleeding under the nail, a subungual hematoma. Often, the blood must be drained from beneath the nail.

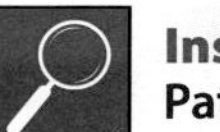

Inspection Findings 8-2
Pathological Toe Postures

	Claw Toes	Hammer Toes	Morton's Toes	Hallux Valgus
Observation				
Illustration			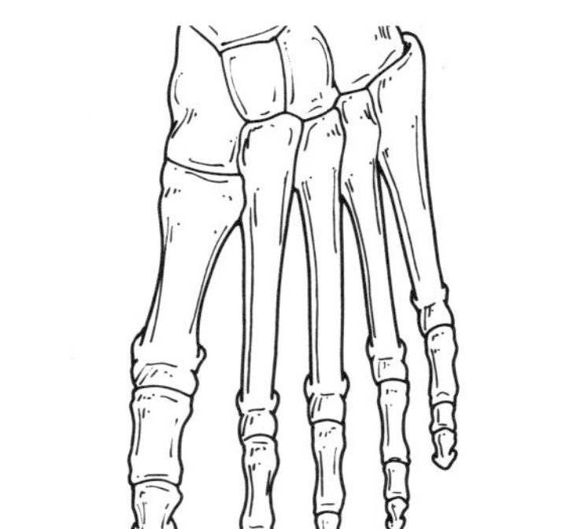 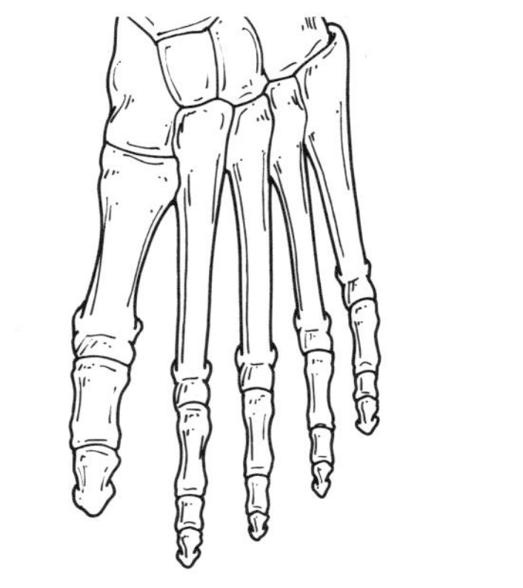	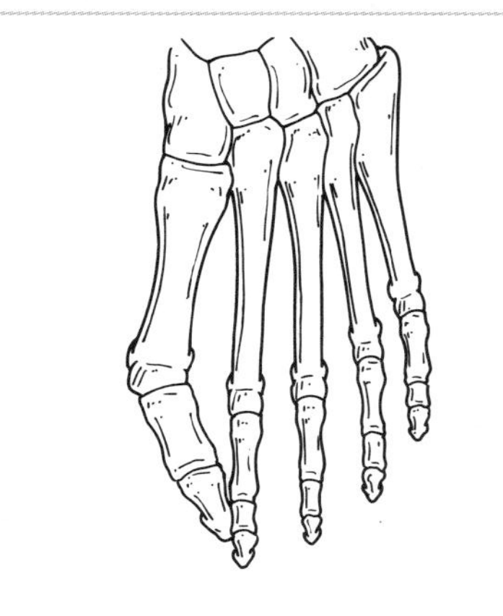
Deviation	Progressive contracture of the interosseous or lumbrical muscles (or both)	Contractures of the associated toe extensors and flexors; inability of the interosseous muscles to hold the proximal phalanx in the neutral position	Although it appears that the 2nd toe is longer than the 1st, Morton's toe is formed by the 1st metatarsal being shorter than the 2nd.	Over time, there is a gradual and subluxation of the 1st MTP joint. A bunion will develop on the medial border of the 1st MTP joint. Lateral displacement of the great toe may interfere with the function of the 2nd toe[16]
Description	Hyperextension of the MTP joint and flexion of the PIP and DIP joints. Claw toes affect the lateral four toes.	Hyperextension of the MTP and DIP joints and flexion of the PIP joints of the lateral four toes	The posture of the foot is normal, but the 2nd toe extends beyond the great toe.	The 1st MTP joint exceeds an angle of 20° in the frontal plane. The 1st and 2nd toes may overlap.

DIP = distal interphalangeal; PIP = proximal interphalangeal; MTP = metatarsophalangeal.

Inspection of the medial structures

- **Medial longitudinal arch**: Spanning from the calcaneus to the first MTP joint, the medial longitudinal arch is more prominent when the foot is non–weight bearing. The relationship between weight-bearing and non–weight-bearing appearance gives a subjective measure of the amount of the foot's flexibility. In the non–weight-bearing position, observe if the arch assumes a planus or cavus posture. A detailed evaluation of the arch is presented in the Pathologies and Related Special Tests Section of this chapter.

Inspection of the lateral structures

- **Fifth metatarsal**: Normally, the foot's lateral border is relatively straight, especially along the shaft of the fifth MT. Note for deviation of the bone's contour, indicative of a fracture.

Inspection of the dorsal structures

The tendons of the long toe extensors and the small mass of the extensor digitorum brevis thinly cover the dorsal surface of the foot laterally. Observe the dorsal aspect of the foot for swelling, discoloration, or abnormal bony alignment.

Inspection of the plantar surface

When inspecting the length of the plantar surface of the foot, pay particular attention to the condition of the skin and the presence of callus formation or blisters, as previously noted. Swelling may be present at the medial calcaneal tubercle in the presence of plantar fasciitis or at the head of the first metatarsal if the sesamoids are pathologically involved. Observe for callus formation. Calluses under the head of the second metatarsal are typical in the presence of a rearfoot varus due to instability at push-off. A "pinch" callus at the medial great toe is associated with a forefoot varus.[22]

Inspection of the posterior structures

- **Achilles tendon**: With the patient weight-bearing, observe the relationship of the Achilles tendon to the tibia. Normally these two structures are aligned. Bowing of the tendon may be an indication of pes planus (Fig. 8-16). Chapter 9 describes Achilles tendon pathology.
- **Calcaneus:** Retrocalcaneal exostosis (also referred to as **Haglund's deformity** or "pump bumps") can be associated with rearfoot varus (Fig. 8-17).

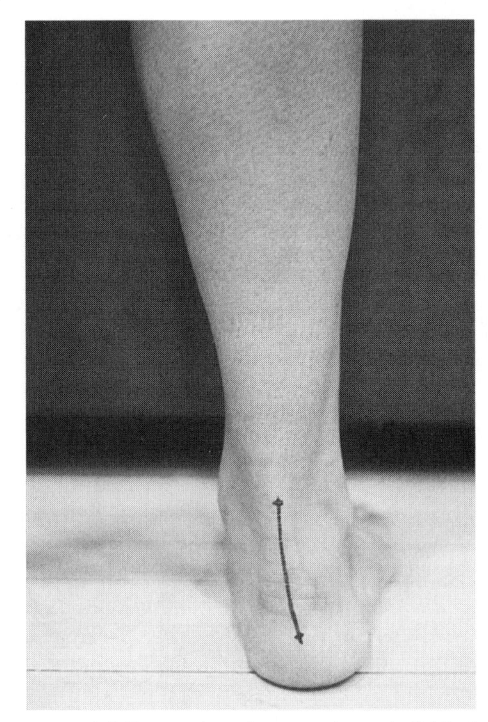

FIGURE 8-16 ■ Achilles tendon alignment in an individual with pes planus. Note the valgus alignment of the calcaneus as noted by the inward bowing of the Achilles tendon.

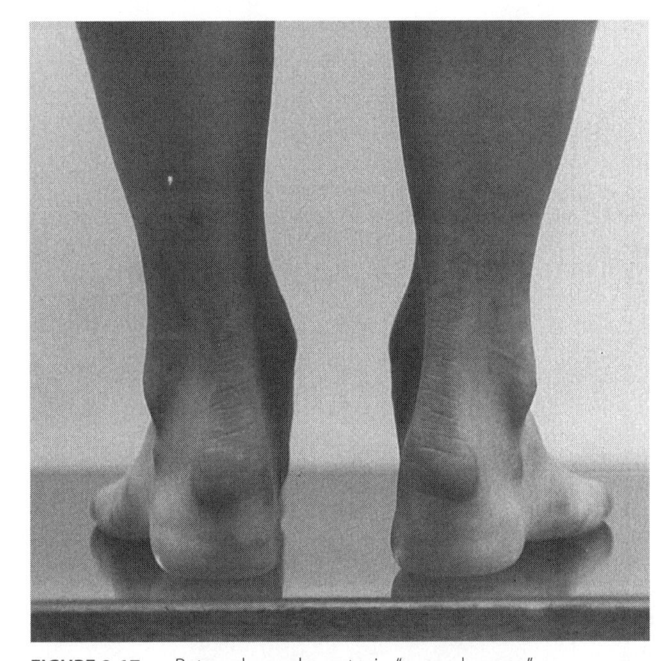

FIGURE 8-17 ■ Retrocalcaneal exostosis, "pump bumps."

Inspection of foot and calcaneal alignment

The controversial concept of a neutral foot position—in which the subtalar joint is neither pronated or supinated—provides a method to examine the static foot. Establishing a **subtalar joint neutral** (STJN) position allows the observation of frontal plane deviations in the rearfoot and forefoot (Special Test 8-2). These deviations alter the gait cycle and place abnormal stress on the foot and proximally along the extremity and into the spine.

Although widely used, the validity of assessing foot alignment has been questioned because it accounts for only frontal plane movement of the more complex subtalar joint and the inter-rater reliability is consistently low, making the usefulness of the quantitative results questionable.[23–25] Calcaneal position in STJN is more reliably measured in weight bearing than in non–weight bearing, but may improve with extensive training.[24,26]

Compare the alignment of the foot when it is weight bearing to when it is non–weightbearing to determine functional adaptations or compensation. Non–weight-bearing

Special Test 8-2
Assessment of Subtalar Joint Neutral

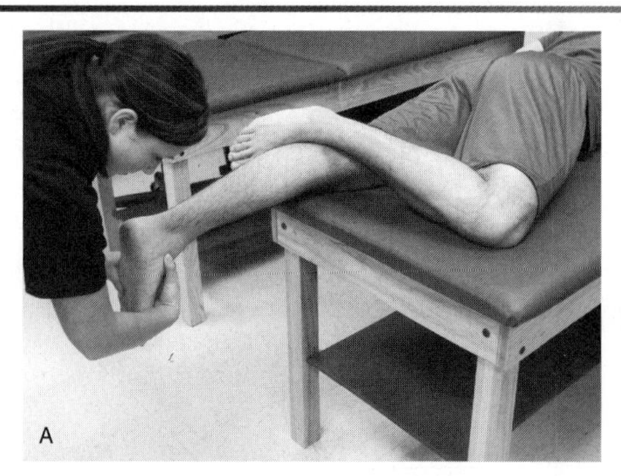
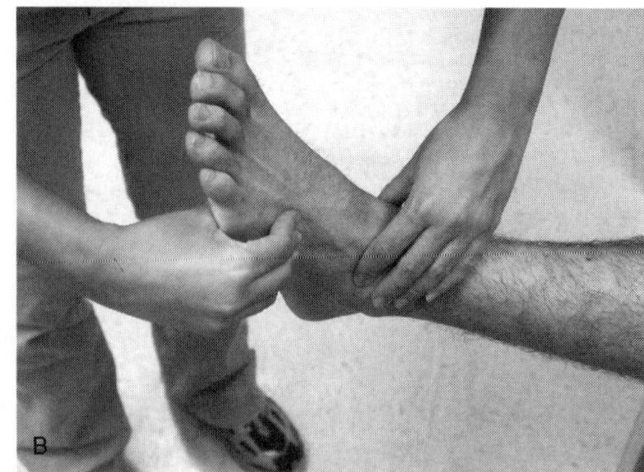

This technique positions the subtalar joint in neutral to allow standardized assessment of rearfoot and forefoot position. **(A)** Patient in the testing position. **(B)** Hand position for palpating the talus and manipulating the forefoot (patient shown supine for clarity).

Patient Position

Prone with foot off the end of the table.

The nontest leg is positioned with the hip flexed, abducted, externally rotated, and the knee flexed (figure 4 position).

Position of Examiner

At the patient's feet

The thumb and index finger at the anterior talocrural joint, palpating the medial and lateral aspects of talar head.

The thumb and index finger of the distal hand grasp the heads of the 4th and 5th metatarsals, gently applying a dorsiflexion pressure until soft-tissue resistance is noted.[27]

Evaluative Procedure

The examiner passively supinates and pronates the foot using the distal hand while palpating talar position with the proximal hand.

Neutral position is found when the talus is symmetrically aligned between the proximal thumb and forefinger. From this position, the postures of the forefoot and rearfoot are noted (see Inspection Findings 8-3).

A goniometric measurement provides an objective assessment of calcaneal position. with the STJ in neutral:

- Align the fulcrum over the proximal calcaneus.
- Position the proximal stationary arm bisecting the lower leg.
- Position the distal movement arm bisecting the calcaneus.

Modification

STJN can be assessed with the patient standing or sitting and the examiner kneeling in front of the patient. The assessment can also be performed with the patient in the supine position.

Comments

Findings from a static foot posture assessment must be interpreted in conjunction with functional assessment.

Evidence

Non–weight bearing

Inter-rater reliability

Not Reliable — Very Reliable
Poor | Moderate | Good
0 0.1 0.2 0.3 0.4 0.5 0.6 0.7 0.8 0.9 1.0

Intra-rater reliability

Not Reliable — Very Reliable
Poor | Moderate | Good
0 0.1 0.2 0.3 0.4 0.5 0.6 0.7 0.8 0.9 1.0

Weight bearing

Inter-rater reliability

Not Reliable — Very Reliable
Poor | Moderate | Good
0 0.1 0.2 0.3 0.4 0.5 0.6 0.7 0.8 0.9 1.0

Intra-rater reliabiltiy

Not Reliable — Very Reliable
Poor | Moderate | Good
0 0.1 0.2 0.3 0.4 0.5 0.6 0.7 0.8 0.9 1.0

assessment is performed with the patient prone and the subtalar joint in neutral to provide a standardized position from which the relative alignment of the rearfoot and forefoot can be observed. Each can be classified as varus, valgus, or neutral (Inspection Findings 8-3).

With the subtalar joint still in the neutral position, assess the tarsometatarsal joint and the first metatarsal for position and mobility (Special Test 8-3). A first ray that is plantarflexed at the tarsometatarsal joint results in the first ray being located inferior to the remaining four rays. Plantarflexed first rays are associated with a cavus foot or can be acquired in the presence of genu varum and may be confused with forefoot valgus. Pes planus is often marked by hypermobility of the first ray at the tarsometatarsal articulation; pes cavus may result in a rigid ray.

- Following assessment of foot position in STJN, observe for compensations with the patient in relaxed stance. For example, an individual with a rearfoot varus assessed in STJN may compensate into a valgus calcaneal position in weight bearing as the medial calcaneal tubercle makes contact with the ground. The findings from this static assessment should be used in concert with the findings from the gait assessment.

PALPATION

To make palpation easier, position the patient so the foot and ankle extend off the end of the table. Include the related ankle structures during the palpation phase of a foot evaluation.

Palpation of the Medial Structures

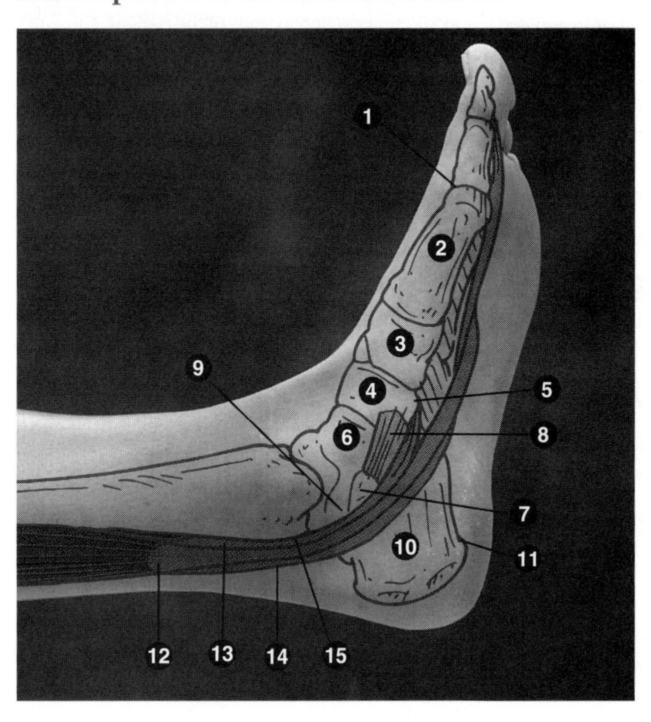

1 First MTP joint: Begin palpating the medial foot by locating the articulation between the proximal phalanx of the first toe and the first MT. Palpate the area for tenderness or increased skin temperature that may indicate acute injury to the ligamentous structures, chronic inflammatory conditions of the tendons or articular structures, or disease states such as **gout**. In the presence of hallux valgus or hallux rigidus, thickening of the synovial capsule, sesamoid pain (see Palpation of the Plantar Structures, p. 181), callus, and crepitus may be noted. These symptoms may also involve the second toe.[16]

2 First metatarsal: From the first MTP joint, palpate the length of the first MT, noting for crepitus, bony deformity, or pain elicited along the shaft. Because the dorsal and medial surfaces and part of the plantar surface of this bone are easily palpated, gross fractures can be identified with relative ease.

3 First cuneiform: Identify the base of the first MT as it articulates with the first cuneiform by the attachment of the tibialis anterior. To make this bone more palpable, ask the patient to actively plantarflex the ankle. The motion causes the base of the first MT to be depressed on the cuneiform, making this junction more palpable.

4 Navicular and 5 navicular tuberosity: Palpate proximally from the first cuneiform to locate its articulation with the medial border of the navicular. The navicular serves as the keystone of the medial longitudinal arch. As such, any dysfunction of this bone results in dysfunction of the arch as a whole. The **navicular tuberosity:** Move posteriorly from the articulation to find the prominent medial navicular tuberosity. The tuberosity may become detached from the bone, resulting in an **accessory navicular**.

6 Talar head: Palpate the talar head, immediately proximal and superior to the navicular. This structure is more easily located by pronating and supinating the midfoot. When the midfoot is pronated, the talar head is more prominent medially.

7 Sustentaculum tali: Palpate the sustentaculum tali, a protrusion off the calcaneus, inferior to the medial malleolus. Serving as an attachment site for the calcaneonavicular ligament and providing inferior support to the talus, the sustentaculum tali is not always easily identifiable.

8 Calcaneonavicular ligament: Palpate the plantar calcaneonavicular ligament from its origin on the sustentaculum

tali to its insertion on the navicular. This ligament, with its very limited extensibility, is the base of the joint capsule of the calcaneotalonavicular joint. In cases of pes planus or midfoot sprains, this ligament may become very tender to the touch or feel thickened.

9 **Medial talar tubercle:** Palpate proximally and superiorly from the calcaneonavicular ligament to locate the small projection off the proximal–medial border of the talus, immediately adjacent to the anterior margin of the medial malleolus. The medial talar tubercle serves as a site of attachment for a segment of the deltoid ligament.

10 **Calcaneus:** From the medial talar tubercle, palpate inferiorly to locate the posterior flare of the calcaneus; continue to palpate to the site of the Achilles tendon attachment.

Medial tendons:

11 **Tibialis posterior:** Palpate the tibialis posterior from its insertion on the medial aspect of the navicular. The tendon will become more prominent if the patient actively supinates the foot.

12 **Flexor hallucis longus:** The bulk of this muscle, hidden beneath the gastrocnemius and soleus muscles, is not palpable until its tendon begins its path posterior to, and around, the medial malleolus. It is difficult to distinguish this tendon from the other structures in the area. As the tendon begins its course along the plantar aspect of the foot, it again is no longer palpable until it inserts on the distal phalanx of the great toe. Resisting flexion of the great toe makes this tendon more prominent as it passes across the plantar aspect of the first MTP joint and courses to its attachment site.

13 **Flexor digitorum longus:** Similar to the flexor hallucis longus, the mass of the flexor digitorum longus is not identifiable as it lies beneath the bulk of the gastrocnemius and soleus muscles. Its tendon is palpable, although not uniquely identifiable, as it passes posterior to, and around, the medial malleolus. As it passes along the plantar aspect of the foot, the tendon is no longer palpable until it inserts on the plantar aspect of the second through fifth toes.

14 **Posterior tibial pulse:** Locate the posterior tibial artery just behind the lateral malleolus.

Palpation of the Lateral Structures

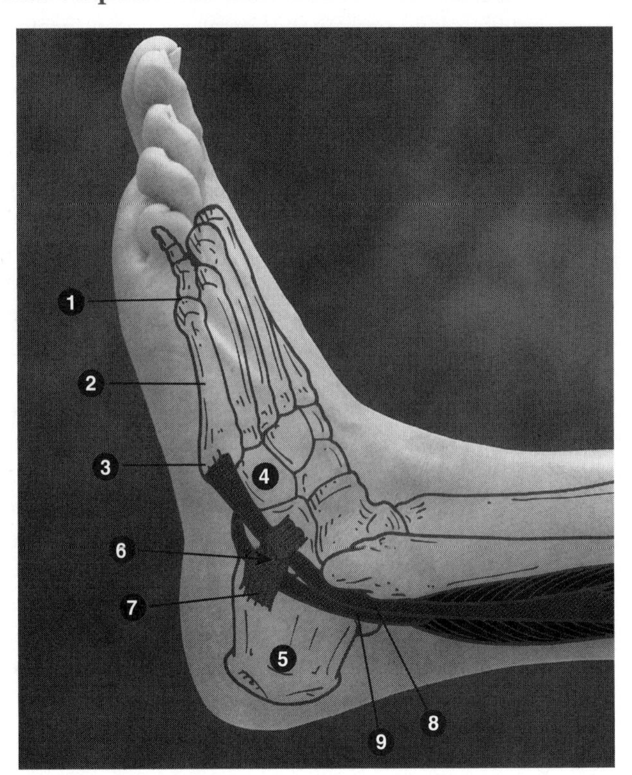

1 **Fifth MTP joint:** Locate the articulation between the fifth toe and fifth MT. Palpate the joint for tenderness arising from ligament or articular damage.

2 **Fifth metatarsal:** From the fifth MTP joint, palpate the length of the fifth MT, noting for pain or discontinuity in the bone's shaft. This structure, especially at its proximal end, is a frequent site of acute injuries and stress fractures.

3 **Styloid process:** The base of the fifth MT is marked by a laterally projecting styloid process (tuberosity), the site where the peroneus brevis tendon attaches. Covered by a bursa, this structure is commonly avulsed as the peroneus brevis tendon is pulled from its attachment.

4 **Cuboid:** Locate the cuboid by palpating immediately proximal to the styloid process. The groove through which the peroneus longus begins to pass on the plantar aspect of the foot is located at the middle portion of the lateral aspect of the cuboid.

5 **Lateral calcaneal border:** From the cuboid, continue to palpate toward the rearfoot. The junction between the cuboid and the calcaneus is often indistinct.

6 **Peroneal tubercle:** The peroneal tubercle is the most prominent bony landmark on the lateral calcaneus, located inferior and anterior to the most distal portion of the lateral malleolus. The peroneal tubercle marks the point where the peroneus longus and brevis tendons diverge after passing posterior and inferior to the lateral malleolus.

7 **Peroneal tendons:** Locate the bony lateral portion of the distal one third of the fibula. The tendons of the peroneus longus and brevis are palpated as a single structure as they course posterior to the distal third of the fibula and pass on the inferior aspect of the lateral malleolus. The tendons' paths split at the peroneal tubercle, with the brevis superiorly and the longus inferiorly. From this point, the peroneus brevis tendon can be palpated to its insertion on the styloid process of the fifth MT. The peroneus longus tendon can be palpated to the point where it passes through the peroneal groove between the fifth MT's styloid process and the anterior margin of the cuboid. Here it disappears on the plantar aspect of the foot. The peroneus longus' insertion can be palpated on the medial and inferior surface of the first cuneiform and lateral head of the first MT. Injury to these structures may result in pain at the base of the fifth MT and cuboid.

Palpation of the Dorsal Structures

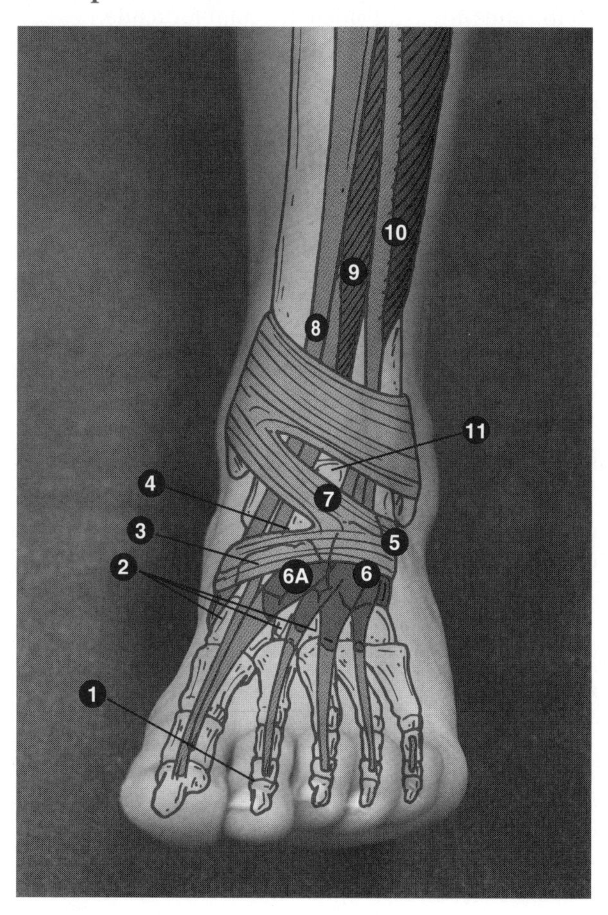

1 **Rays:** Starting with the distal phalanx, palpate the toes and the length of their associated MTs, noting any deformity, crepitus, or pain elicited during the process.

2 **Cuneiforms:** Although the cuneiforms are indistinguishable from each other to the touch, their locations can be approximated relative to the first three MTs. The three cuneiforms each articulate with the first three MTs. The individual cuneiforms can be identified by palpating the length of the medial three MTs to their bases (see Fig. 8-3).

3 **Navicular:** Palpate posteriorly from the cuneiforms to locate the navicular and its prominent medial tuberosity.

4 **Dome of the talus:** Palpate posteriorly and somewhat laterally from the navicular to find the dome of the talus. This structure is more easily located if the foot and ankle are placed in supination and plantarflexion, allowing the dome's lateral border to become palpable from under the ankle mortise.

5 **Sinus tarsi:** Locate the sinus tarsi located anterior to the lateral malleolus. Normally, this landmark appears as a depression just anterior to the lateral malleolus, marking the site of the extensor digitorum brevis muscle. With chronic conditions such as arthritis or after acute trauma, including ankle sprains, tarsal fractures, or dislocations, the sinus may become obscured by swelling (see Fig. 9-19).

6 **Extensor digitorum brevis:** Palpate the origin and proximal muscle belly of the extensor digitorum brevis in the sinus tarsi while the patient is actively extending the toes. The tendinous slips to each of the toes become indistinguishable as they pass under the long toe tendons. The most medial portion of the extensor digitorum brevis muscle and its tendon attaching on the first toe are often referred to as a separate muscle, the **extensor hallucis brevis**.

7 **Inferior extensor retinaculum:** Palpate the inferior extensor retinaculum along its entire length as it traverses the entire upper portion of the foot. As the tendons of tibialis anterior, extensor hallucis longus, and extensor digitorum longus pass over the talus and tarsals, their proximity to the bones during dorsiflexion is maintained by the retinaculum.

8 **Tibialis anterior:** Ask the patient to supinate the subtalar joint and dorsiflex the ankle to make the tibialis anterior tendon more palpable at the point where it inserts on the first cuneiform. As the tendon crosses the talocrural joint, it is easily palpable but quickly loses its identity as it flares into its musculotendinous junction.

9 **Extensor hallucis longus:** Locate the extensor hallucis longus tendon by palpating laterally from the tibialis

anterior tendon. With the great toe actively extended, palpate the tendon's length from the tibialis anterior to its flare into the distal phalanx. Continue to palpate the length of the EHL to its origin on the middle half of the anterior fibula and adjacent interosseous membrane.

10 Extensor digitorum longus: Palpate lateral to the extensor hallucis longus for the tendon of the extensor digitorum longus. Although the central portion of the tendon is difficult to palpate, palpate its individual slips to the lateral four toes, prominent on the dorsal aspect of the foot when the toes are extended.

11 Dorsalis pedis pulse: Locate the dorsalis pedis artery lying between the tendons of extensor hallucis longus and extensor digitorum longus. With the ankle in the neutral position, palpate the dorsalis pedis pulse and compare it with the opposite extremity. A unilateral absence or decreased pulse may indicate a vascular obstruction such as anterior compartment syndrome (see Chapter 9).

Palpation of the Plantar Structures

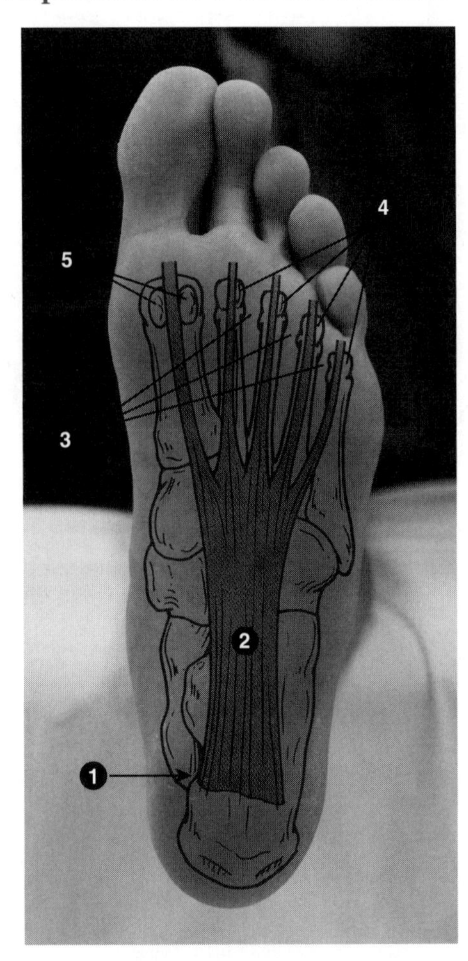

The plantar surfaces of the calcaneus and the MT heads are padded by fatty deposits and overlying thick skin, making it difficult to identify specific bony structures and muscles. The examiner must rely on approximations and functional tests in identifying and determining the source of pain.

1 Medial calcaneal tubercle: Locate the medial calcaneal tubercle by identifying the point where the heel pad begins to thin and merge into the medial longitudinal arch. From this point, move to the medial ridge and apply pressure upward and toward the calcaneus. The medial calcaneal tubercle can also be located by dorsiflexing the ankle and extending the toes to make the plantar fascia more prominent. Then trace the fascia back to its origin on the medial calcaneal tubercle. The anterior ridge of the medial calcaneal tubercle is the attachment site of the plantar fascia and the flexor digitorum brevis muscle. The medial border of this structure is the origin of the abductor hallucis. Pain elicited during palpation of this area may indicate a **plantar fasciitis** or a **heel spur**.

2 Plantar fascia: Palpate the plantar fascia from its origin on the calcaneus through its length and breadth to its attachment on each of the MT heads, noting any painful areas within this structure. Individuals suffering from plantar fasciitis will be tender. An increase in tissue density along the length of the fascia may be noted.

3 Intermetatarsal neuroma: Apply gentle pressure to the area between the MTs. Nerves located in this area can become compressed and painful, resulting in dysfunction of the foot and lower extremity.

4 Lateral four metatarsal heads: Beginning with the first MTP joint, palpate each of the MT heads, noting for the presence and integrity of the transverse arch. The pads under the first and fifth MT heads should be the thickest because they are the primary weight-bearing areas of the forefoot.

5 Sesamoid bones of the great toe: Palpate along the plantar surface of the first MT to reach the first MTP joint. At this point, two small sesamoid bones can be felt in the flexor hallucis brevis tendon. Inflammatory conditions of these bones, **sesamoiditis**, or fractures elicit pain to the touch or while weight bearing, especially during the toe-off phase of gait, when pressure is applied to the ball of the foot and the MTP joint is extended. The onset of sesamoiditis has been linked to rigidity of the first ray (often associated with a cavus foot structure).

Joint and Muscle Function Assessment

The relatively limited amount of motion available to the small IP joints makes it difficult to measure their ROM in a clinically meaningful way. This section describes ROM assessment for the MTP and subtalar joints only. The results should be compared bilaterally and considered in light of

Inspection Findings 8-3
Common Foot Postures Assessed in Subtalar Joint Neutral

	Normal Foot Posture	Forefoot Varus	Forefoot Valgus	Rearfoot Varus	Rearfoot Valgus
Observation	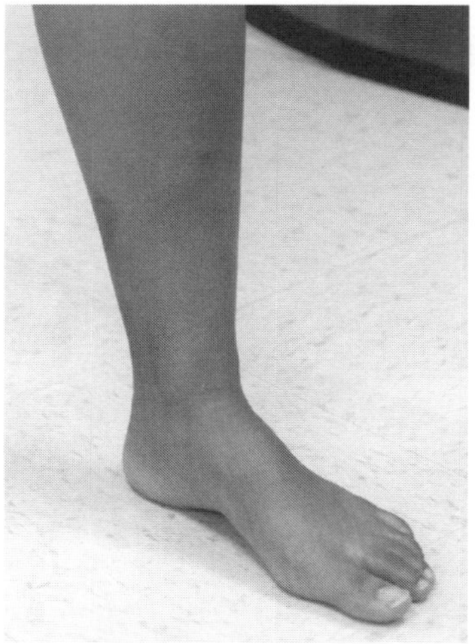	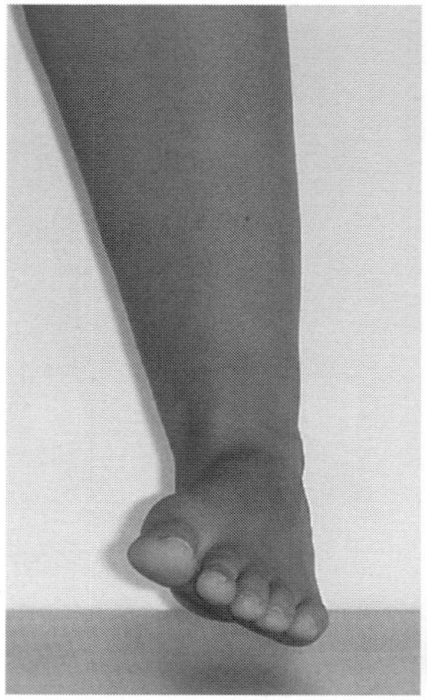	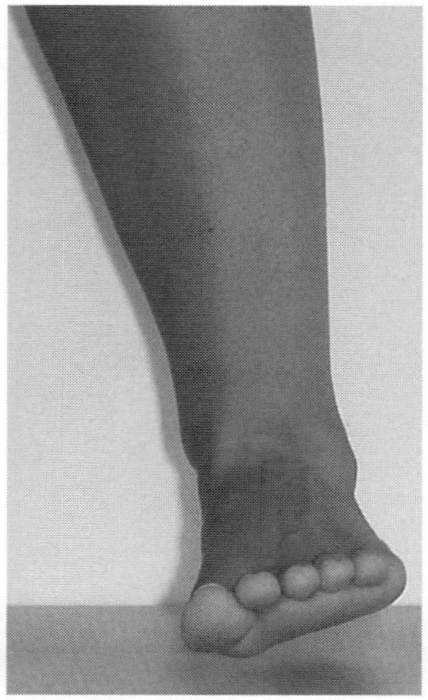	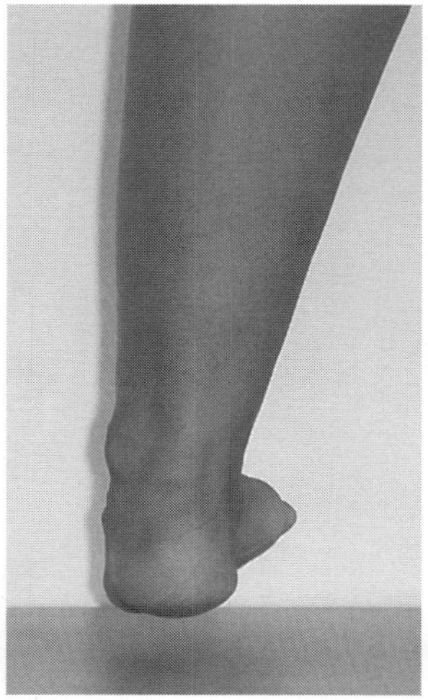	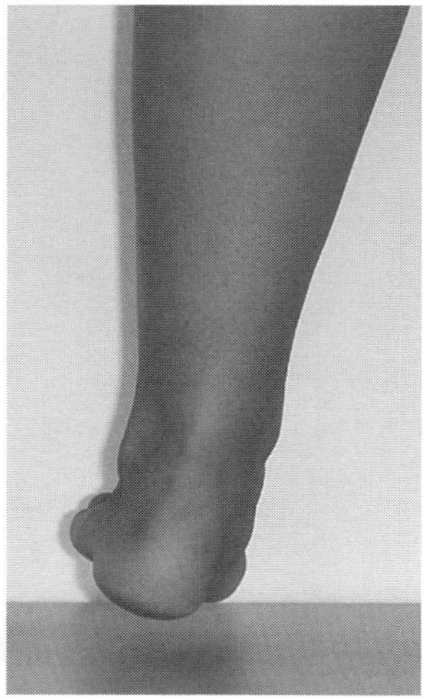
Illustration		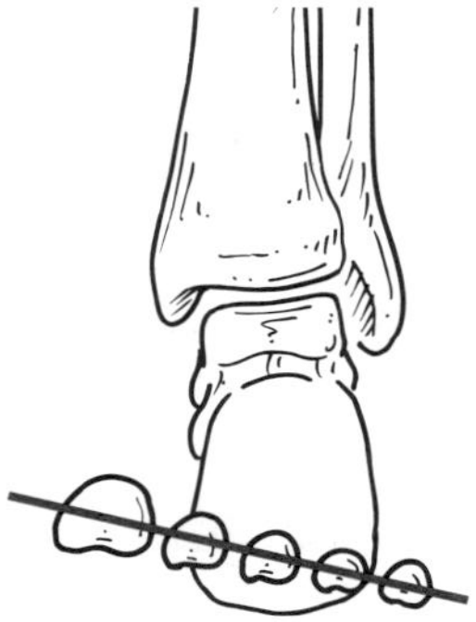	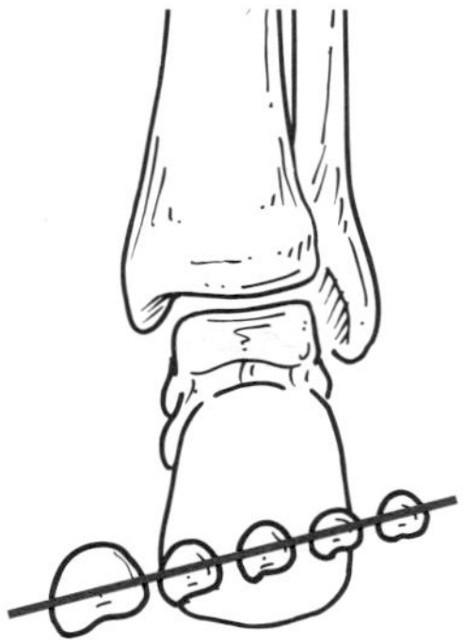	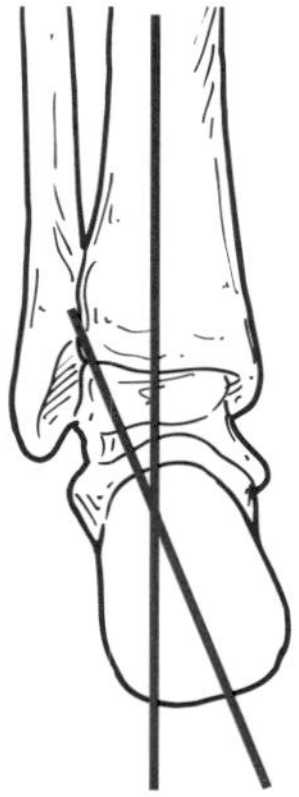	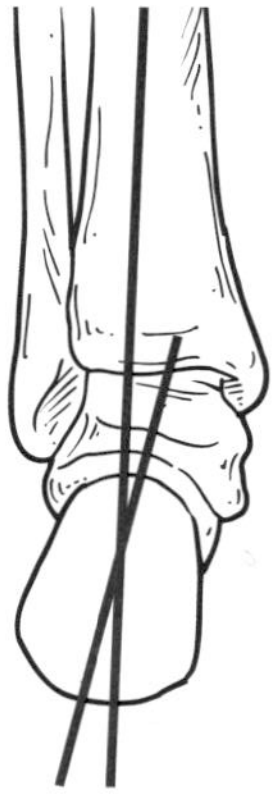

Posture				
Calcaneus is vertical or slightly (<3°) inverted (varus) relative to the long axis of the bisected lower leg. Metatarsal heads are perpendicular to calcaneus.	Metatarsal heads are inverted relative to the rearfoot. Varus of 1–8 degrees of is considered normal.[26]	Metatarsal heads are everted relative to the rearfoot. A plantarflexed first ray will also give the appearance of a forefoot valgus	Calcaneus is inverted relative to the long axis of the bisected lower leg and may be related to a varus alignment of the tibia or a calcaneus that does not completely derotate during development.	Calcaneus is everted relative to the long axis of the tibia and can be associated with a valgus tibial alignment. Rearfoot valgus is rarely observed.
Compensation				
	During static weight bearing, the forefoot compensates by abducting and everting, resulting in a more planus foot. During gait, pronation is excessive and prolonged, as the 1st MT has farther to travel before contacting the ground.	During static weight bearing, the midfoot supinates as the first metatarsal contacts the ground and may give the foot a cavus appearance. During gait, the 1st MT strikes the ground prematurely, resulting in early supination, reducing the shock-absorbing capacity of the limb.	With sufficient subtalar joint mobility, the rearfoot will rapidly and excessively pronate during the early stages of gait.	The rearfoot becomes hypermobile, resulting in increased pronation.

MT = metatarsal.
Observation figures from Donatelli, RA: *Biomechanics of the Foot and Ankle.* Philadelphia, FA Davis, 1990.

Special Test 8-3
Position and Mobility of First Tarsometatarsal Joint

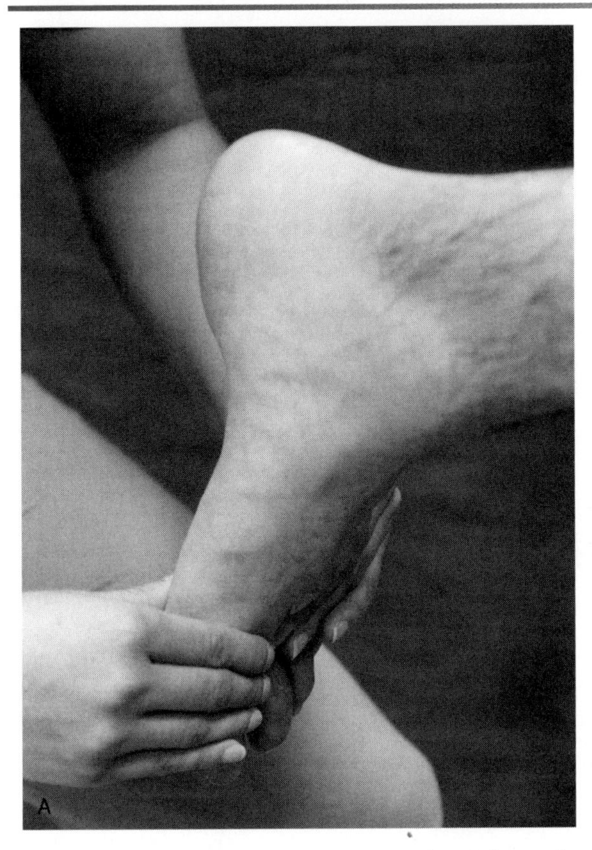

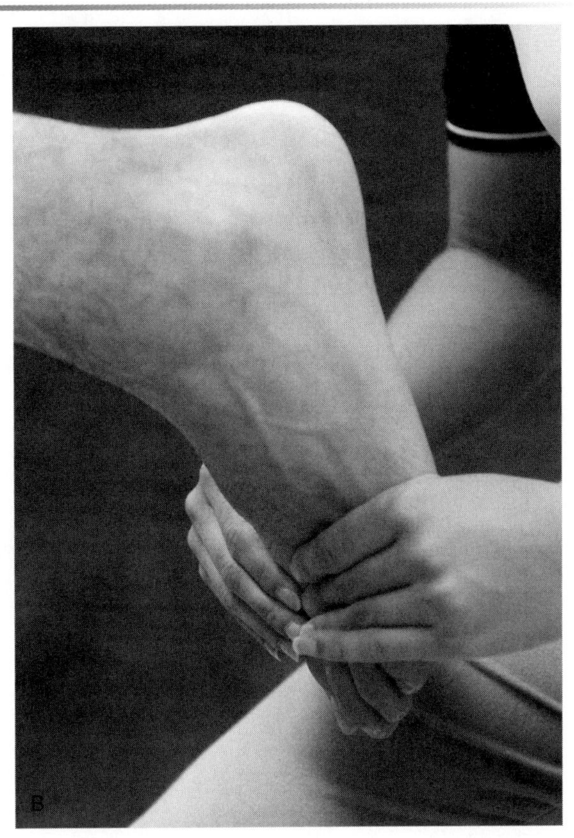

The static position and mobility of the first metatarsal can influence foot mechanics and should be assessed from a non–weight-bearing position with the subtalar joint in neutral. **(A)** Medial view **(B)** Lateral view.

Patient Position	Prone with foot off the end of the table in subtalar joint neutral (see Special Test 8-2). The non–test leg is positioned with the hip flexed, abducted, and externally rotated and the knee flexed (figure 4 position).
Position of Examiner	Using a lumbrical grip on the lateral 4 metatarsal heads while grasping the first metatarsal head allows examination of the metatarsal position.
Evaluative Procedure	Note the resting position of the first metatarsal. Plantarflex and dorsiflex the first ray, noting the amount of mobility in each direction.
Positive Test	A rigid or stiff plantarflexed first ray cannot be brought into a neutral alignment, while a supple plantarflexed first ray has sufficient mobility to realign. A plantar flexed first ray is inferior as compared to the lateral four metatarsal heads.
Implications	A rigid plantarflexed first ray creates early supination, resulting in less shock absorption during gait. Stress fractures or sesamoid pathology may result. A hypermobile first ray may contribute to general metatarsal pain (metatarsalgia) and hallux valgus deformity.[29]
Modification	Use of a ruler for a quantitative assessment is also associated with poor inter-rater reliability (ICC = 0.05; SEM = 1.2 mm).[30]
Comments	A forefoot valgus alignment is easily confused with a plantarflexed first ray.
Evidence	Assessment of first ray mobility has poor inter-rater reliability ((κ) $\le$ .16). The low relationship between results of the manual technique and a more reliable mechanical device indicates that the technique's validity is also suspect.[29] Mechanical measurement of dorsal first ray mobility has poor reliability (ICC = 0.05).[30]

the functional examination to determine pathology at these joints.

The frontal plane measurement of calcaneal inversion and eversion is frequently used to approximate the amount of pronation and supination, even though it captures only a single plane of these complex motion. This reliability of this measurement is generally poor, improving somewhat when performed in weight-bearing.[28,31] Goniometric measurement of rear foot inversion and eversion is presented in Goniometry Box 8-1. Flexion/extension and abduction/adduction of the great toe are presented in Goniometry Boxes 8-2 and 8-3. Assessment of talocrural plantarflexion, dorsiflexion and calcaneal inversion and eversion are described in Chapter 9.

Active range of motion

The greatest ROM occurs at the first MTP joint, allowing 75 to 85 degrees of extension and 35 to 45 degrees of flexion (Fig. 8-18). To prevent compensatory motion of excessive pronation, the first MTP joint must permit at least 60 to 65 degrees of extension. The ROM available to the MTP joints decreases at each subsequent lateral joint. Active motion at the fifth MTP joint is negligible. Few people have volitional control of the abductor hallucis, making visible active great toe abduction minimal. In the presence of a valgus deformity of the great toe, the muscle's ability to abduct the great toe is decreased. It is not clear if this is a cause or a result of the deformity.[32]

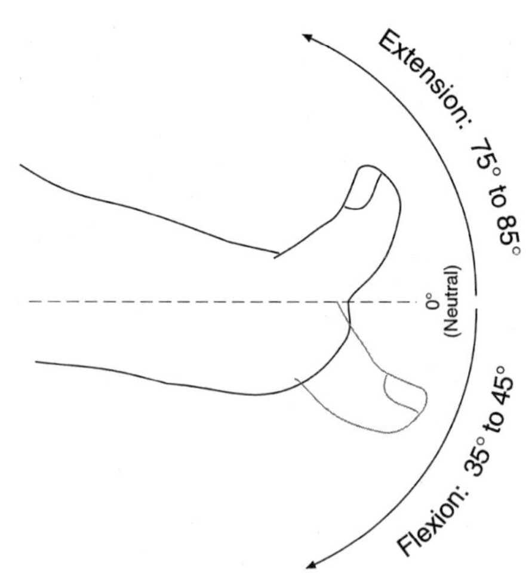

FIGURE 8-18 ■ Active range of motion for flexion and extension of the great toe's metatarsophalangeal joint. The range of motion decreases with each subsequent joint from the first MTP joint to the fifth.

Manual muscle tests

Strength testing of the great toe musculature is conducted separately from that of the muscles of the lateral four toes (Manual Muscle Tests 8-1 and 8-2). When manual muscle testing, the strength of the long toe flexors and extensors

Goniometry Box 8-1
Rearfoot Inversion and Eversion

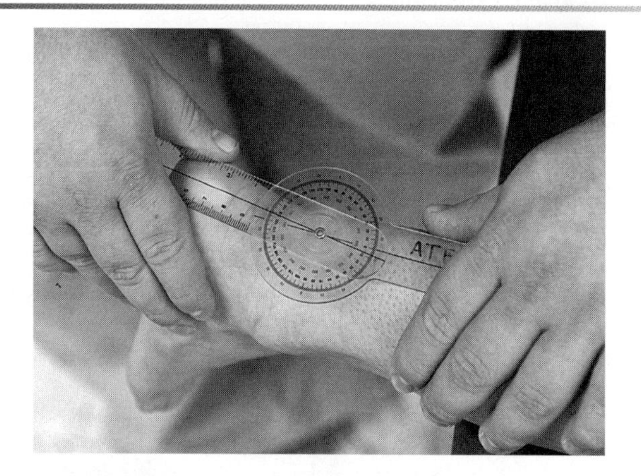

	Inversion 0°–30°	Eversion 0°–5°
Patient Position	Prone with ankle in neutral and STJ in neutral	
Goniometer Alignment		
Fulcrum	The axis is centered over the Achilles tendon with the axis bisecting the malleoli.	
Proximal Arm	The stationary arm is centered over the midline of the lower leg.	
Distal Arm	The movement arm is centered over the midline of the calcaneus.	

STJ = subtalar joint.

Goniometry Box 8-2
First Metatarsophalangeal Abduction

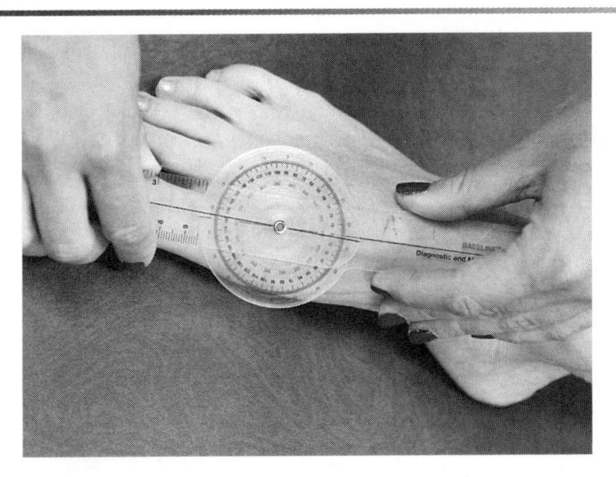

	Passive Abduction
Patient Position	Supine or sitting with the STJ and ankle in neutral
Goniometer Alignment	
Fulcrum	The axis of the goniometer is placed over the dorsal aspect of the MTP joint.
Proximal Arm	The stationary arm is centered over the metatarsal being tested.
Distal Arm	The movement arm is centered over the proximal phalanx.

MTP = metatarsophalangeal; STJ = subtalar joint.

Goniometry Box 8-3
Metatarsophalangeal Flexion and Extension

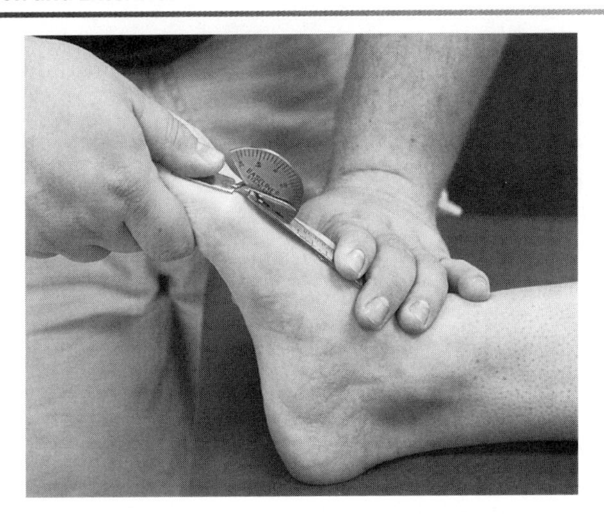

	Flexion 0°–70°	**Extension 0°–30°**
Patient Position	Supine with ankle in neutral	
Goniometer Alignment		
Fulcrum	Position the axis of the goniometer over the dorsal aspect of the MTP joint being tested.	
Proximal Arm	The stationary arm is centered on the midline of the metatarsal.	
Distal Arm	The movement arm is centered on the midline of the proximal phalanx.	

MTP = metatarsophalangeal.

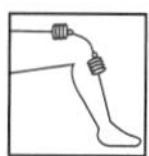

Manual Muscle Test 8-1
Toe Flexion

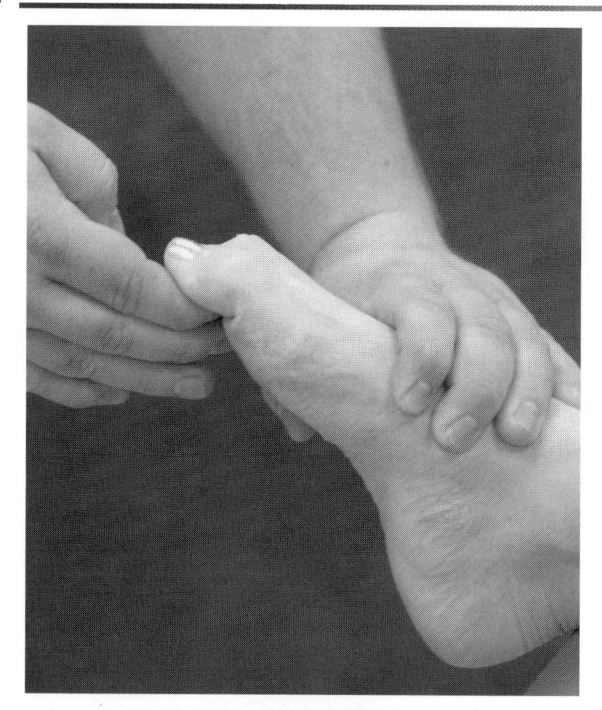

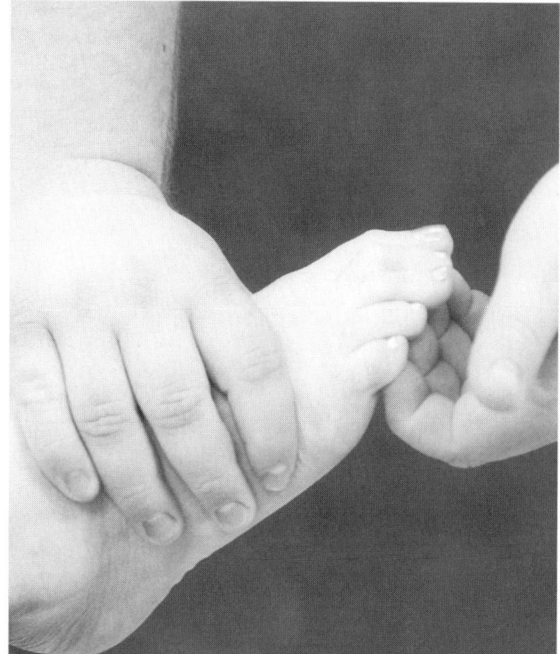

	Great Toe MTP Flexion	Lateral 4 Toes Flexion
Patient Position	Long sitting with the ankle in the neutral position	
Starting Position	The toes are in the neutral position.	
Stabilization	The forefoot is stabilized by grasping the metatarsals proximal to their heads.	
Palpation	Head of the first metatarsal, palpating the flexor hallucis longus	Not applicable (tendons are too deep to palpate).
Resistance	Along the entire length of the toe's plantar aspect	On the plantar aspect of the lateral four toes
Primary Mover(s) (Innervation)	Flexor hallucis longus: IP joint (L4, L5, S1) Flexor hallucis brevis: MTP joint (L4, L5, S1)	Flexor digitorum longus: DIP joint (L5, S1) Flexor digitorum brevis: PIP joint (L4, L5, S1) Flexor digiti minimi brevis: MTP joint of the 5th toe (S1, S2)
Secondary Mover(s) (Innervation)		Dorsal interossei: MTP joint flexion (S1, S2) Plantar interossei: MTP joint flexion (S1, S2) Lumbricals: MTP flexion (1st MTP: L4, L5, S1; 2nd to 5th: S1, S2)
Compensation/ Substitution	IP joint flexion, talocrural plantarflexion	Talocrural plantarflexion
Comments		The toe flexors collectively flex the MTP joints.

IP = interphalangeal; MTP = metatarsophalangeal.

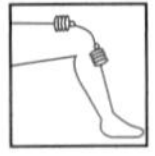

Manual Muscle Test 8-2
Toe Extension

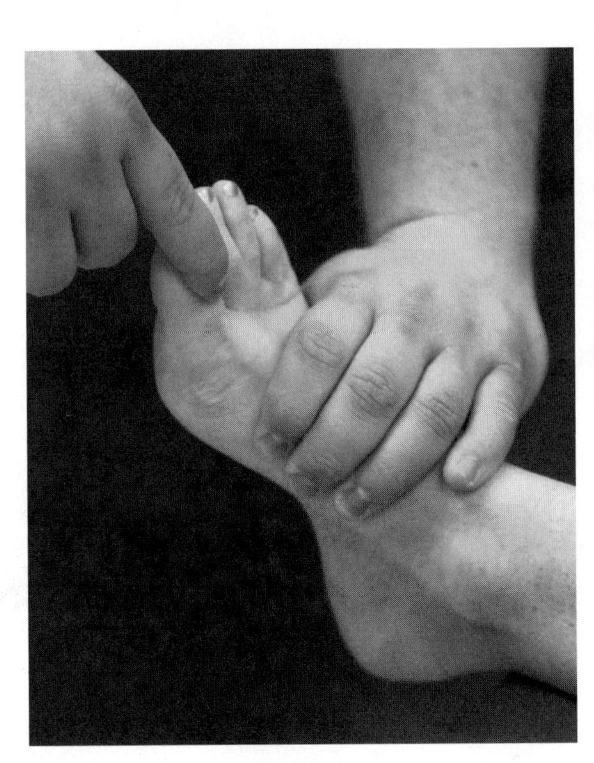

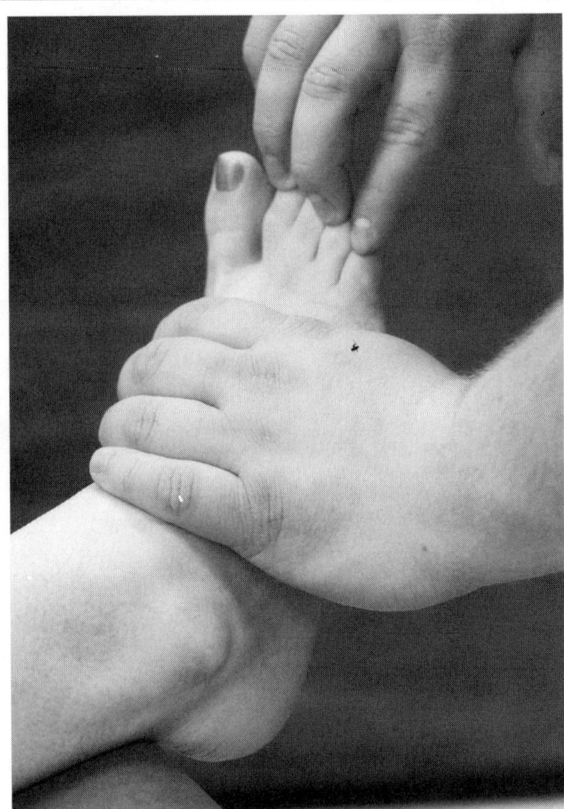

	MTP Extension	Toe Extension
Patient Position	Long sitting with the ankle in the neutral position	
Starting Position	The toes are in the neutral position.	
Stabilization	The forefoot is stabilized by grasping the metatarsals proximal to their heads.	
Palpation	Dorsal surface of the distal first metatarsal	Common extensor tendon on the proximal portion of the dorsum of the foot
Resistance	Dorsal aspect of the proximal phalanx of hallux	Dorsal aspect of the proximal phalanges of toes 2–5
Primary Mover(s) (Innervation)	Extensor hallucis longus (L4, L5, S1) Extensor hallucis brevis (L5, S1)	Extensor digitorum longus (L4, L5, S1) Extensor digitorum brevis (L5, S1) Dorsal interossei: IP joint extension (S1, S2) Plantar interossei: IP joint extension (S1, S2) Lumbricals (IP joint extension)
Compensation/ Substitution	Tibialis anterior	Tibialis anterior

(flexor hallucis longus, flexor digitorum longus, extensor hallucis longus and extensor digitorum longus) should be assessed repetitively to determine the impact of fatigue on the onset of symptoms and/or weakness. Manual muscle testing for the ankle is discussed in Chapter 9.

Passive range of motion

An assessment of passive ROM for each MTP joint can identify tendinous or capsular restrictions to movement. Capsular patterns are identified in Table 8-7. The position of the subtalar joint affects the amount of motion and the firmness of the MTP's end-feel, especially moving into extension. The position of the ankle influences the length of the tendons of the long toe extensors and flexors. The anatomical position, where the talocrural joint is flexed to 90 degrees, is not the biomechanical joint neutral position. Although the neutral position differs from person to person, it tends to be 15 to 20 degrees short of 90 degrees and represents the point where the ATF is most taut. If passive MTP extension is performed with the ankle at 90 degrees, a firm end-feel will develop early, owing to stretching of the long toe flexors. To determine only the end feel for passive toe extension, perform the maneuver with the ankle flexed to 90 degrees. To determine the full joint ROM and capsular end-feel, perform the test with the ankle relaxed.

- **Flexion:** Stabilize the forefoot proximal to the MT heads. To prevent contribution from the IP joints, apply pressure on the dorsal portion of the proximal phalanx (Fig. 8-19). The normal end-feel for flexion is firm owing to tension of the dorsal fibers of the joint capsule and the collateral ligaments. A limitation in great toe MTP extension can increase stresses on the medial structures of the foot and lower leg, including the plantar fascia, flexor hallucis longus, and flexor digitorum longus.

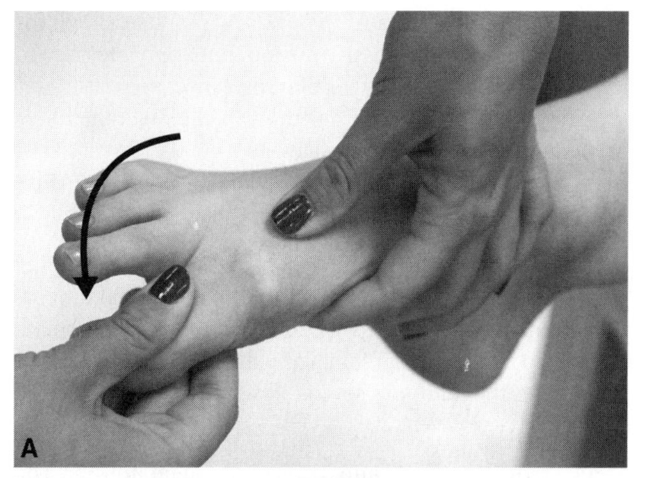

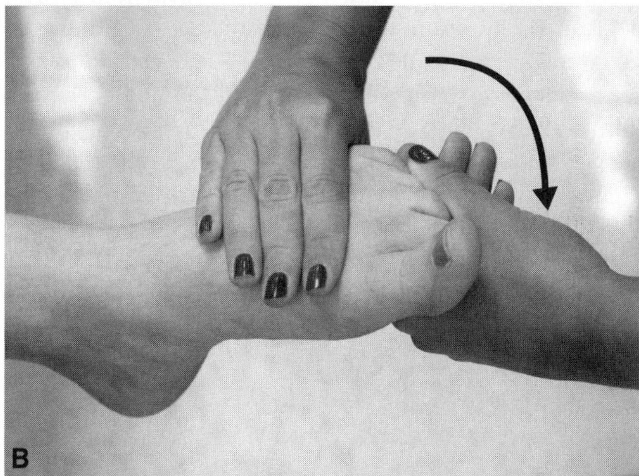

FIGURE 8-19 ■ Passive flexion of the **(A)** great toe and **(B)** lateral four toes.

Table 8-7 Foot and Toe Capsular Patterns and End-Feels

Capsular Patterns	
Midtarsal joint	Dorsiflexion, plantarflexion, adduction, internal rotation
Metatarsophalangeal joint: Great toe	Extension, flexion
Metatarsophalangeal joints: 2nd–5th toes	Flexion, extension
End-feels	
Abduction at the midtarsal joints	Firm: Soft tissue stretch (intrinsic muscles, capsule, and ligaments)
Adduction at the midtarsal joints	Firm: Soft tissue stretch (intrinsic muscles, capsule, and ligaments)
Flexion of the toes	Firm: Tightness of the toe extensors
Extension of the toes	Firm: Tightness of the toe flexors
Abduction of the toes (MTP)	Firm: Soft tissue stretch (intrinsic muscles, capsule, and ligaments)
Adduction of the toes (MTP)	Firm: Soft tissue stretch (intrinsic muscles, capsule, and ligaments)

- Extension: Maintain stabilization as described for measurement of passive flexion, but apply pressure to the proximal phalanx's plantar aspect (Fig. 8-20). A firm end-feel arises from the capsule's plantar fibers and the short flexor muscles.

Joint Stability Tests

With the exception of the MTP and IP joints, identifying subtle hyper- and hypomobilities of the individual foot articulations is difficult. This section describes how to isolate stresses to the ligaments stabilizing the toes and the general integrity of the midfoot's soft tissues.

Stress testing

Metatarsophalangeal and interphalangeal joints. The MTP and IP joints are supported by the medial and lateral collateral ligaments (MCL and LCL). The dorsal and plantar surfaces of these articulations are reinforced by the joint capsule. Passive **overpressure** in flexion, as described in the Passive Range of Motion section of this chapter, is used to determine the integrity of the dorsal joint capsule; passive overpressure in extension evaluates the integrity of the plantar capsule.

The application of a valgus force stresses the MCL of the joint. A varus force stresses the LCLs (Stress Test 8-1). Compare the results of this examination with those obtained when the test is repeated on the same joint on the opposite extremity.

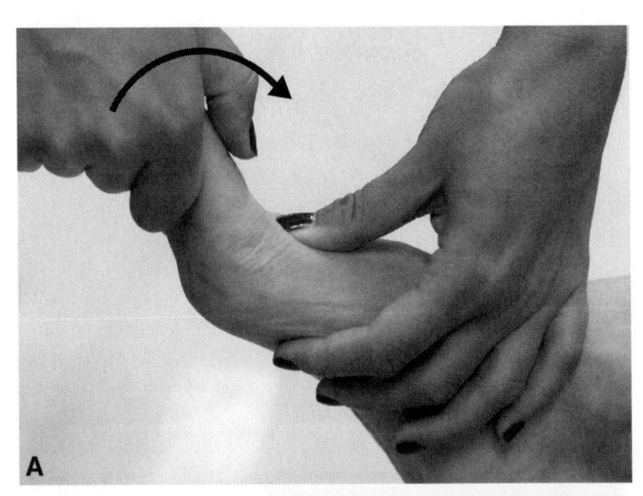

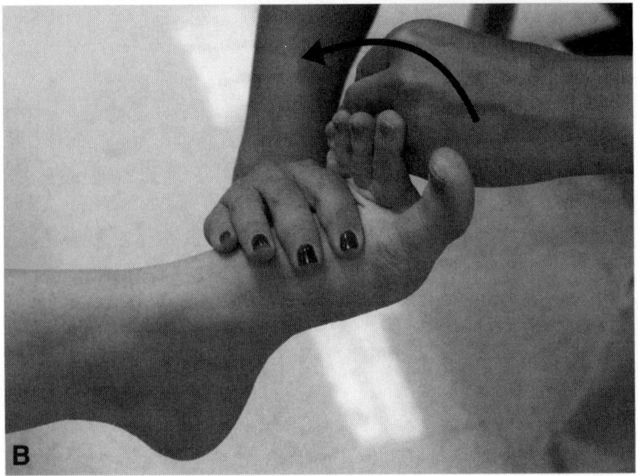

FIGURE 8-20 ■ Passive extension of the (A) great toe and (B) lateral four toes.

Joint play assessment

Intermetatarsal joints. The deep transverse MT ligaments and the interosseous ligaments secure the MT heads in a relatively stable alignment. Forces causing an abnormal amount of glide between any two MT heads can result in trauma to these ligaments. Likewise, immobilization or degenerative changes can result in hypomobility. Testing intermetatarsal glide, thus duplicating the mechanism of injury, can be used to evaluate the integrity of these ligaments (Joint Play 8-1). Compare the amount of glide bilaterally.

Tarsometatarsal joints. The tarsometatarsal joints are evaluated by assessing the amount of motion during dorsal and plantar glide (Joint Play 8-2). The fourth and fifth MTs have more mobility with the cuboid than the remaining proximal MT–cuneiform articulations.

Midtarsal joints. The stability of the midtarsal joints is evaluated via dorsal and plantar glide of the cuneiforms (Joint Play 8-3).

Neurologic Examination

The foot and toes are supplied by the L4 to S2 nerve roots. Neurologic dysfunction of the nerve roots or individual nerves can radiate symptoms to the foot. When neurologic symptoms (e.g., numbness, muscle weakness, hyperflexia, or hyporeflexia) are present, the source of the dysfunction, such as if the lesion involves a spinal nerve root, peripheral nerve, or a branch of the peripheral nerve, must be determined.

To identify nerve root pathology, refer to the Lower Quarter Neurologic Screen in Chapter 1 (Neurologic Screening Box 1-1). Pathologies that can result in local neurologic dysfunction include entrapment of the posterior tibial nerve (tarsal tunnel syndrome) and interdigital neuroma. Peroneal nerve trauma, disc herniations, and anterior compartment syndrome (discussed in Chapter 9) can also radiate symptoms into the foot (Fig. 8-21).

Vascular Examination

The posterior tibial pulse can be palpated just posterior to the medial malleolus. Identifying the pulse is easier when the patient's foot is supinated. Palpate the dorsalis pedis pulse just lateral to the extensor hallicus longus tendon as the artery crosses the talocrural joint line. These pulses,

---

Overpressure A force that attempts to move a joint beyond its normal range of motion.

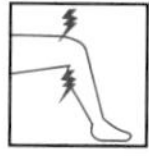

Stress Test 8-1
Valgus and Varus Stress Testing of the MTP and IP Joints

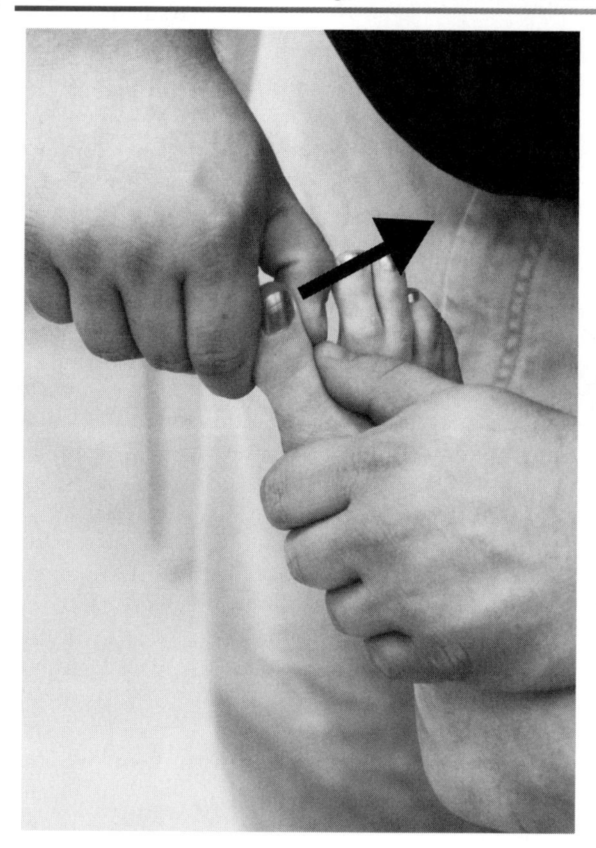

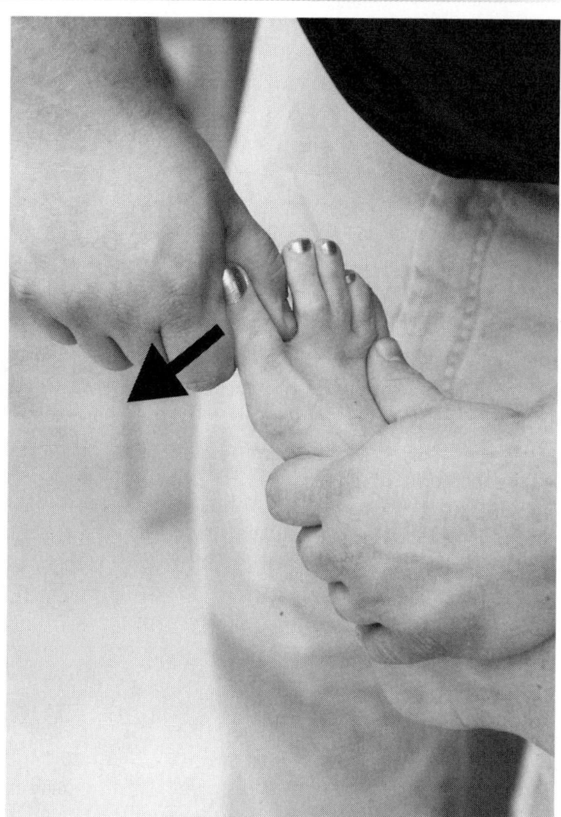

Stress testing of the toe's capsular ligaments: **(A)** Valgus stress applied to the interphalangeal joint; **(B)** varus stress applied to the metatarsophalangeal joint.

Patient Position	Supine or sitting
Position of Examiner	Standing The proximal bone stabilized close to the joint to be tested The bone distal to the joint being tested grasped near the middle of its shaft Care is necessary to isolate the joint being tested while not overlapping the test ligament.
Evaluative Procedure	***Valgus testing (A):*** The distal bone is moved laterally, attempting to open up the joint on the medial side. ***Varus testing (B):*** The distal bone is moved medially, attempting to open up the joint on the lateral side.
Positive Test	Pain or increased laxity or decreased laxity when compared with the same joint on the opposite extremity
Implications	***Valgus test (A):*** MCL sprain, avulsion fracture, or adhesions of the involved joint ***Varus test (B):*** LCL sprain, avulsion fracture, or adhesions of the involved joint
Comments	Increased joint laxity, especially with an empty end-feel, may reflect an associated fracture.
Evidence	Absent or inconclusive in the literature

IP = interphalangeal; LCL = lateral collateral ligament; MCL = medial collateral ligament; MTP = metatarsophalangeal.

Joint Play 8-1
Intermetatarsal Glide Assessment

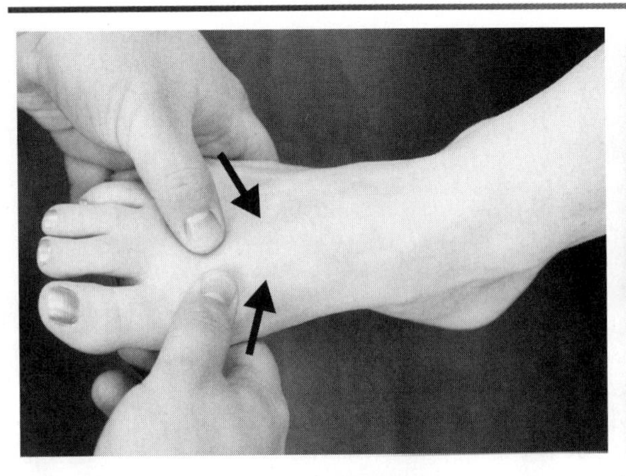

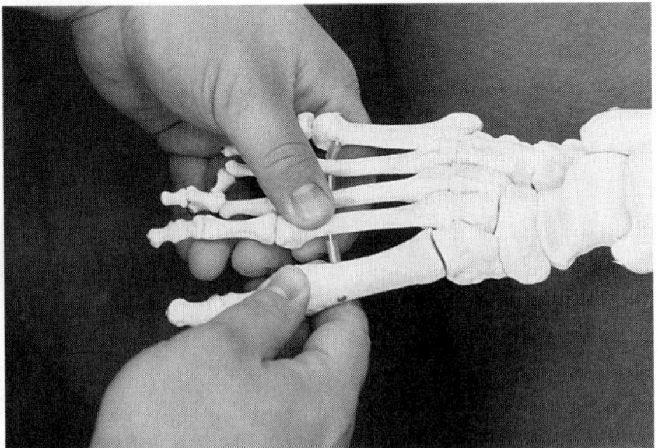

Assessment of the amount of intermetatarsal glide between the 1st and 2nd metatarsal heads. Perform this test for each of the four articulations formed between the five metatarsals.

Patient Position	Supine or sitting on the table with the knees extended
Position of Examiner	Standing in front of the patient's feet One hand grasping the first MT head; the other grasping the second MT head
Evaluative Procedure	Stabilize one of the MT heads while moving the other in a plantar and dorsal direction. This procedure is repeated by moving to the lateral MT heads until all four intermetarsal joints have been evaluated.
Positive Test	Pain or increased glide or decreased glide compared with the opposite extremity
Implications	Trauma to the deep transverse metatarsal ligament, interosseous ligament, or both Pain without the presence of laxity may indicate the presence of a neuroma
Evidence	Absent or inconclusive in the literature

MT = metatarsal.

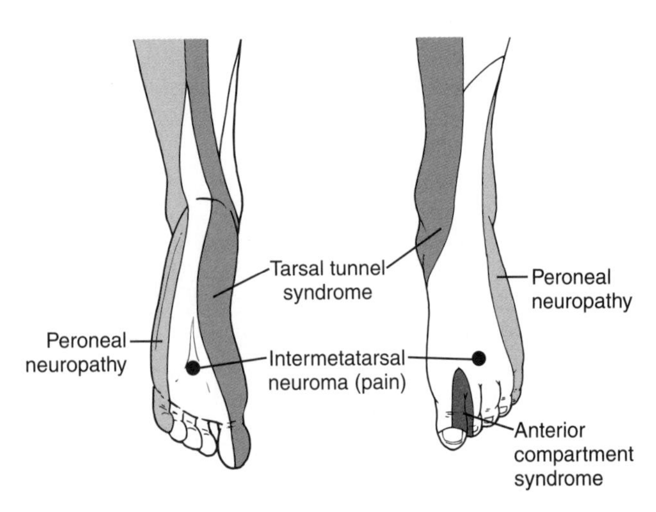

FIGURE 8-21 ■ Peripheral neurologic symptoms in the foot.

especially the posterior tibial pulse, are frequently undetectable in a young, healthy population. In this case, confirm arterial supply by checking capillary refill in the nail bed or on the skin on the dorsum of the foot. Refer to page 178 for more information on palpation of the foot and ankle pulses.

In the absence of trauma, absent or diminished pulses are indicative of peripheral arterial disease. Unexplained edema can be the result of peripheral vascular disease, diabetes, or other disease states.

Pathologies of the Foot and Toes and Related Special Tests

Many of the conditions affecting the normal function of the foot may be traced to improper biomechanics of the foot itself or the result of compensation by the foot for biomechanical deficits elsewhere in the lower extremity.

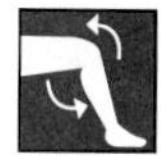

Joint Play 8-2
Tarsometatarsal Joint Play

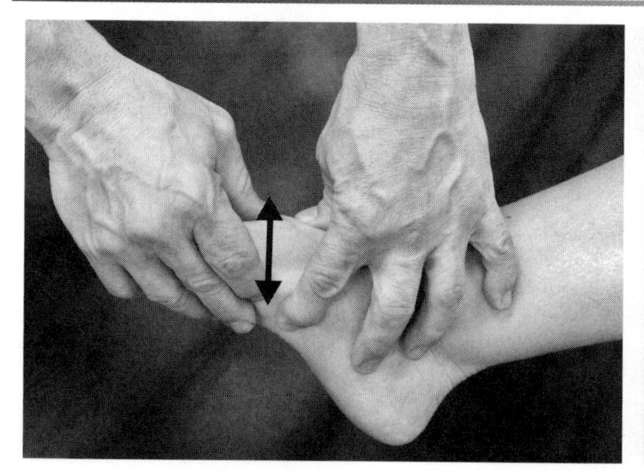

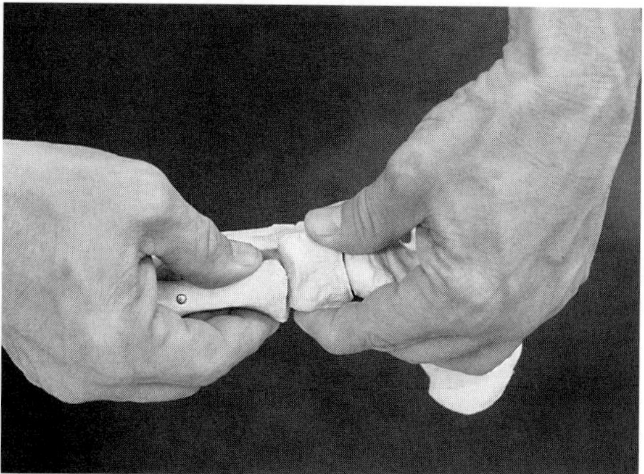

Assessment of the amount of glide between the tarsals and the base of the metatarsals. Perform this test on each of the five tarsometatarsal joints.

Patient Position	Supine or seated The foot is pronated. Knee flexed and the heel stabilized by the edge of the table
Position of Examiner	Standing or sitting in front of the patient's foot One hand gasping the proximal tarsal (e.g., cuneiform, cuboid) The opposite hand gasping the metatarsal being glided
Evaluative Procedure	The metatarsal is glided dorsally on the tarsal and then glided plantarly on the tarsal. Repeat for each joint.
Positive Test	Pain associated with movement Increased or decreased glide relative to the opposite foot
Implications	***Increased glide:*** Ligamentous laxity ***Decreased glide:*** Joint adhesions, articular change causing coalition of the joint
Modification	Wedges or balls may be needed to achieve sufficient proximal stabilization.
Evidence	***Intra-rater reliability***[30] Not Reliable — Very Reliable Poor — Moderate — Good 0 0.1 0.2 0.3 0.4 0.5 0.6 0.7 0.8 0.9 1.0

Influence of Foot Structure on Pathology

Although abnormalities of the foot may be caused by acute trauma or disease states, they more commonly occur congenitally. Many people function normally with pes planus or pes cavus. Increasing or decreasing the height of the arch alters the biomechanical function of the subtalar and midtarsal joints. These conditions are a concern when they become painful or result in pathologic biomechanical dysfunction elsewhere in the lower extremity. Possible ramifications of pes planus include plantar fasciitis, heel spurs, and patellofemoral pain. Pes cavus can predispose an individual to claw toes, MT stress fractures, or a plantar fascia rupture. Abnormal foot posture also increases the patient's risk of developing overuse injuries, especially when the stress is compounded by the rapid increase in activity.[13]

Arch height can be computed via several different methods. The most accurate (and most expensive) is a lateral weight-bearing radiograph of the foot from which the: (1) the height of the medial longitudinal arch,

Joint Play 8-3
Midtarsal Joint Play

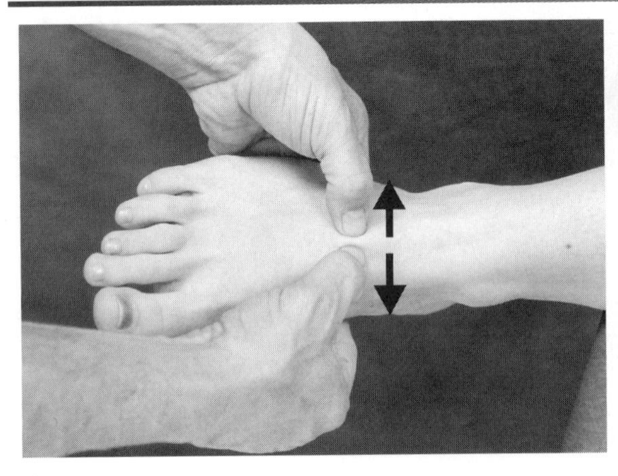

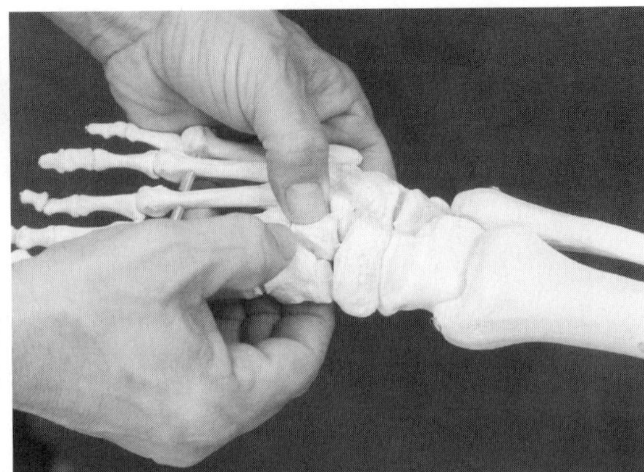

Assessment of the amount of joint glide between the tarsals

Patient Position	Supine or seated Knee flexed and the heel stabilized by the edge of the table
Position of Examiner	Standing or sitting in front of the patient's foot Grasp the plantar and dorsal aspect of one tarsal with the stabilizing hand. The opposite hand grasps the adjacent tarsal in a similar manner.
Evaluative Procedure	One tarsal is glided dorsally and then plantarly on the stabilized adjacent tarsal. Repeat for each tarsal joint.
Positive Test	Pain associated with movement Increased or decreased glide relative to the opposite foot
Implications	***Increased glide:*** Ligamentous laxity ***Decreased glide:*** Joint adhesions, articular changes causing coalition of the joint
Modification	Wedges or balls may be needed to achieve sufficient proximal stabilization.
Evidence	Absent or inconclusive in the literature

(2) the height-to-length ratio, and (3) the calcaneal-first MT angle are determined (Fig. 8-22).[23,33] The height of the arch itself is a less significant finding than the actual change in height that occurs when the foot goes from non–weight bearing to weight bearing as measured by navicular drop (refer to Special Test 8-4).

*** Practical Evidence**

Navicular drop causes increased internal rotation of the tibia on the foot. Excessive navicular drop may cause the anterior cruciate ligament (ACL) to "wind" around the posterior cruciate ligament, potentially predisposing the risk of ACL sprains.[34]

Pes planus

Pes planus is characterized by the lowering of the medial longitudinal arch, giving this condition its colloquial name, "flat feet" (Fig. 8-23). The onset of pes planus can be traced to a congenital origin, biomechanical changes, or acute trauma. Pes planus results in biomechanical changes in all three planes of the foot and ankle, especially affecting the function of the subtalar and calcaneocuboid joints.[35] The lowered arch causes the talus to tilt medially and the navicular to displace inferiorly, making the talus more prominent (talar beaking).

Acute pes planus can occur after trauma to the structures supporting the medial longitudinal ligament, including rupture of the plantar fascia, tears of the plantar ligaments, calcaneonavicular (spring) ligament sprains, or the rupture of the tibialis posterior or tibialis anterior tendon.[1,36–38] Traumatic, symptomatic pes planus can also be related to a fracture of an **accessory navicular** (Fig. 8-24). The accessory navicular is an abnormal osseous outgrowth on the navicular that, when present, serves as a partial attachment site for the tibialis posterior. Loss of the union between the accessory navicular and the navicular

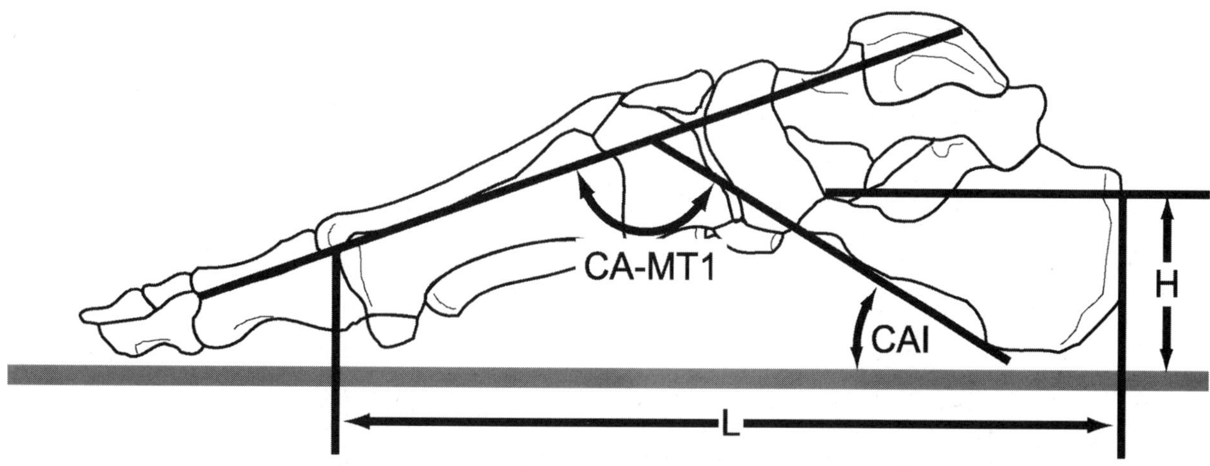

FIGURE 8-22 ■ Calculation of arch height and length taken from a weight-bearing radiograph. H = height; L = length; CA-MT1 = calcaneal 1st metatarsal angle; CAI = calcaneal inclination.

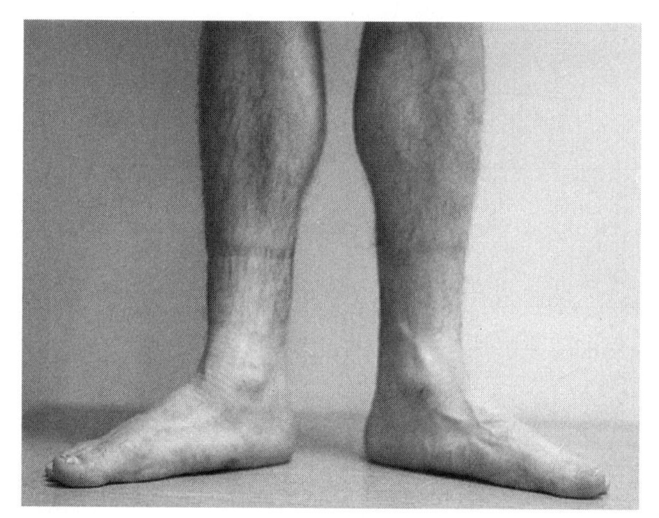

FIGURE 8-23 ■ Pes planus. Note the absence of the medial longitudinal arch.

itself results in a decrease in the effectiveness of the tibialis posterior in supporting the medial arch.

✱ Practical Evidence

There are three types of accessory naviculars: a sesamoid bone in the distal tibialis posterior tendon (type I), an accessory center of ossification (type II), and the cornuate navicular, an enlarged navicular tuberosity (type III). When the accessory navicular is symptomatic the patient will be able to precisely locate the source of pain.[39]

Mechanical factors leading to pes planus include weakness of the tibialis posterior, tibialis anterior, and the toe flexors. Stretching or weakness of the supporting ligaments, especially the calcaneonavicular ligament, results from the plantar–medial displacement of the talus, further increasing the amount of weight-bearing pronation. This weakness may be triggered or exacerbated by compensatory postures to structural abnormalities of the spine and lower extremity.

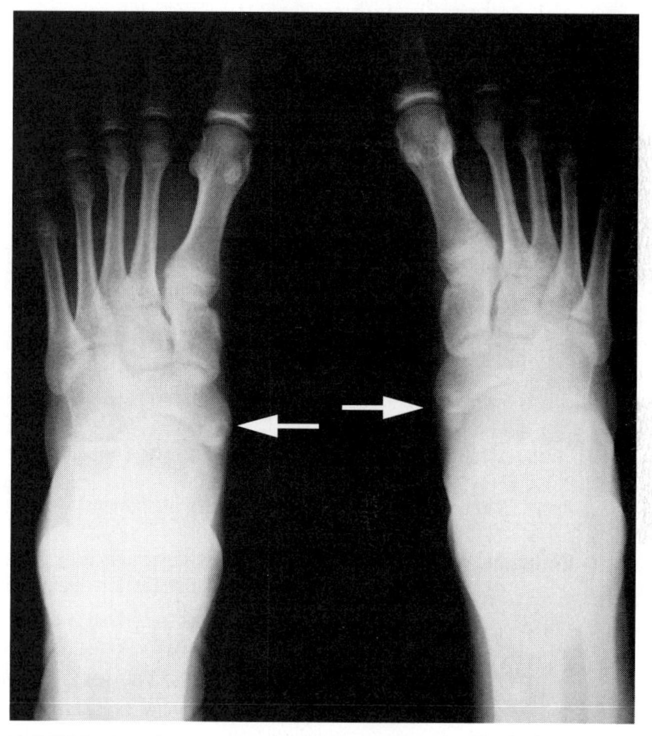

FIGURE 8-24 ■ Accessory navicular. The arrows identify the bony outgrowths associated with an accessory navicular.

Also, compensation may increase over time after a strain or rupture of the posterior tibialis tendon.

Pes planus is classified as being either rigid (structural) or flexible (supple). Rigid pes planus, sometimes associated with tarsal coalition, is marked by the absence of the medial longitudinal arch when the foot is both weight bearing and non–weight bearing. A rigid pes planus foot has less shock-absorbing capacity and, when detected early in life, may respond to surgical intervention. In supple pes planus, the arch appears normal during non–weight bearing but disappears when the foot is weight bearing (refer to Special Test 8-5). A pes planus foot type rarely requires surgical correction.

Special Test 8-4
Navicular Drop Test

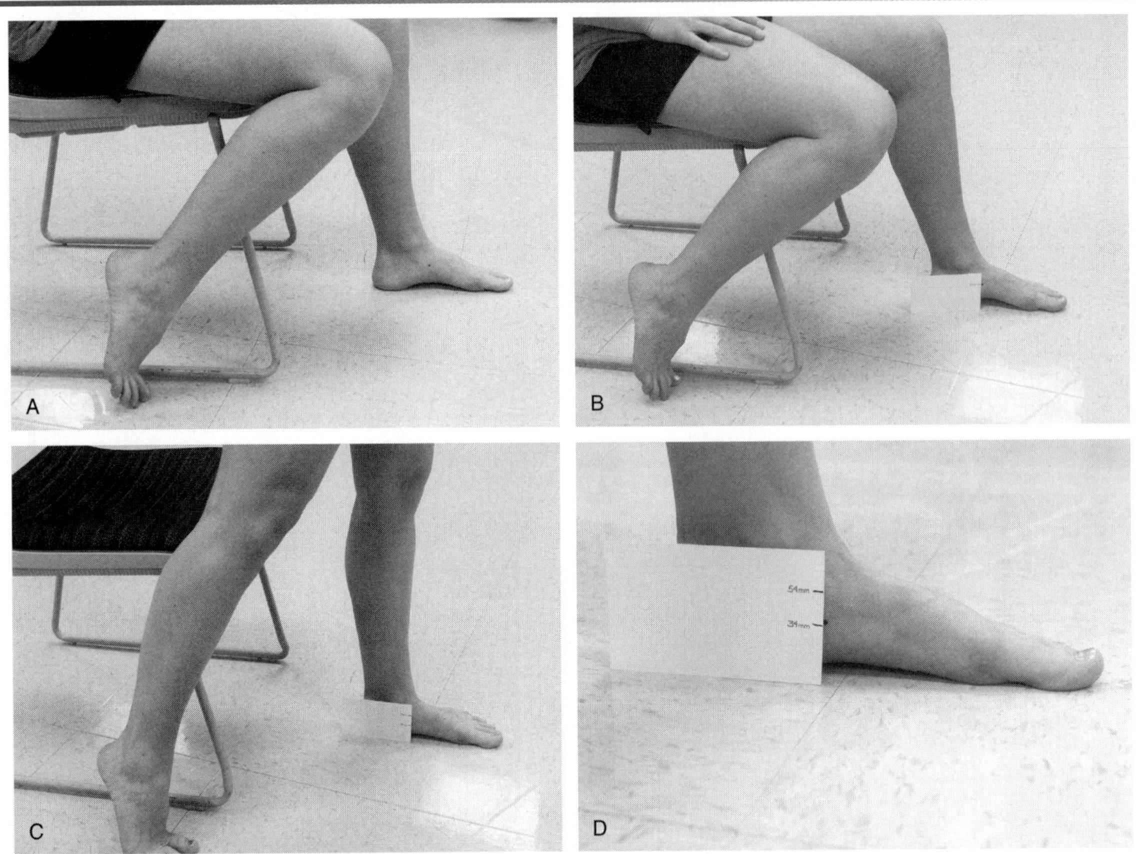

The navicular drop test is used to assess amount of pronation of the foot by measuring the height of the navicular tuberosity while the foot is non–weight bearing to weight bearing and measuring the distance of the inferior displacement. Note that the body weight should be evenly distributed between the two feet (non test leg above was moved for clarity).

Patient Position	Sitting with both feet on a noncarpeted floor
Position of Examiner	Kneeling in front of the patient
Evaluative Procedure	The subtalar joint is placed in the neutral position with the patient's foot flat against the ground, but non–weight bearing. With the patient non–weight-bearing, a dot is placed over the navicular tuberosity **(A)**. While the foot is still in contact with the ground, but non–weight bearing, an index card is positioned next to the medial longitudinal arch. A mark is made on the card corresponding to the level of the navicular tuberosity **(B)**. The patient stands with the body weight evenly distributed between the two feet, and the foot is allowed to relax into pronation. The new level of the navicular tuberosity is identified and marked on the index card **(C)**. The relative displacement (drop) of the navicular is determined by measuring the distance between the two marks in millimeters **(D)**.
Positive Test	The navicular drops greater than 10 mm.[43] Normal values for restricted navicular drop have not been established.
Implications	Limited or excessive pronation
Comments	The relatively static measurement of navicular drop is associated with amount of pronation during gait.
Evidence	Highly variable intra-rater reliabilities (ICC = 0.61–0.96) have been reported and vary with the experience of the clinician.[25,26,28] Reported intra-rater reliabilities range from an ICC of 0.61[25] to 0.96[26] The inter-rater reliability is poor (ICC = 0.57–0.73).[25, 28] A strong relationship exists between excessive forefoot varus (>8°) and an increased navicular drop.[26] The low inter-rater reliability associated with the navicular drop test is related to the low reliability of assessing subtalar joint neutral. The height of the navicular in weight bearing (the second measurement of the navicular drop test) is highly correlated with radiographic measurements of navicular height in weight bearing.[40]

STJ = subtalar joint.

Special Test 8-5
Test for Supple Pes Planus Windlass Test

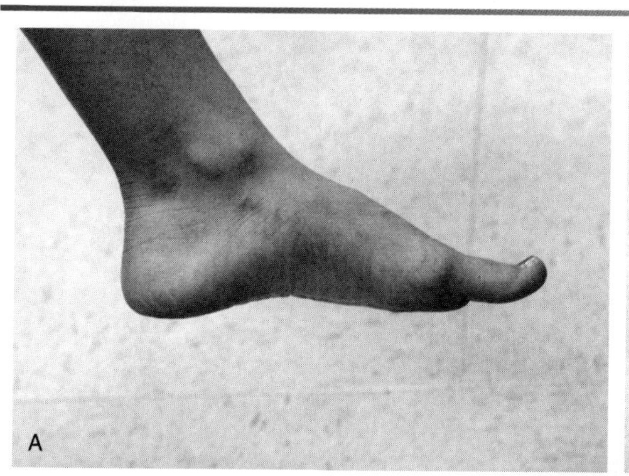

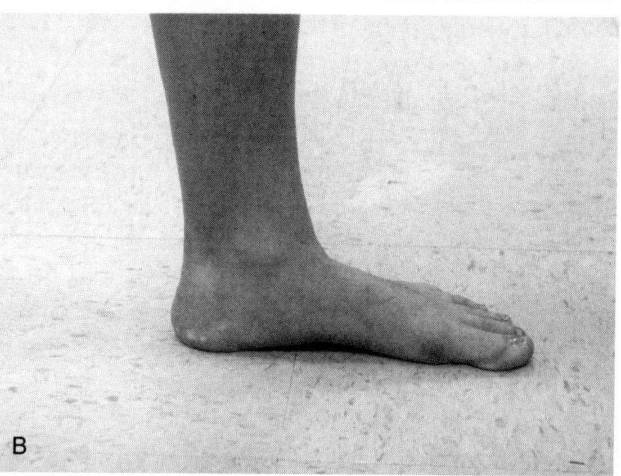

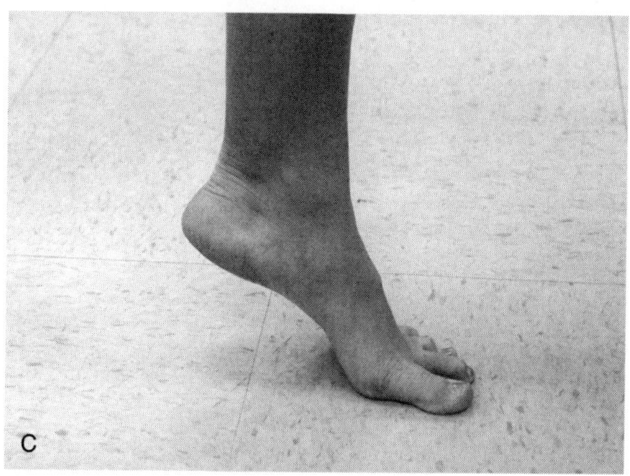

Supple pes planus. The patient displays a normal arch in the non–weight-bearing position **(A)**. In weight bearing, the arch disappears **(B)**. When the patient performs a toe raise, the arch returns by means of the windlass effect **(C)**. In the presence of plantar fasciitis **(C),** the Windlass test, will produce pain.

Patient Position	Sitting on the edge of the examination table
Position of Examiner	Positioned at the patient's foot
Evaluative Procedure	With the patient in a non–weight-bearing position the examiner notes the presence of a medial longitudinal arch **(A).** The examiner instructs the patient to stand so that the body weight is evenly distributed **(B).** The patient is then asked to perform a single-leg heel raise on the limb being tested **(C).** In the presence of supple pes planus note if the arch reappears as the patient performs a toe raise. For the **Windlass test** (used to identify plantar fasciitis), pain may be produced.
Positive Test	The presence of a medial longitudinal arch when non–weight bearing disappears when weight bearing The Windlass test is positive if pain is reproduced during part C.
Implications	If the medial longitudinal arch disappears when weight bearing, a supple pes planus is present. If no arch is present while in a non–weight-bearing position, a rigid pes planus is present. **Windlass test:** Pain during the single-leg heel raise
Comments	This test for supple pes planus is meaningful only when the medial longitudinal arch is present with the patient in a non–weight-bearing position.
Evidence	Negative likelihood ratio

Not Useful — Useful

Very Small | Small | Moderate | Large

1.0 0.9 0.8 0.7 0.6 0.5 0.4 0.3 0.2 0.1 0

The **windlass test** has a high specificity (1.00) but low sensitivity (0.24) indicate that a positive finding is highly related to presence of plantar fasciitis, yet a negative finding is less helpful in ruling out the condition.[53]

Associated pathology frequently responds to proximal muscle strengthening and/or stretching, orthotics, or changes in footwear.

Various assessment techniques can be used to determine the position of the navicular and the extent of its displacement when the foot transitions from non–weight-bearing to weight-bearing status. Measurement of the navicular height in a relaxed stance provides a valid estimate of arch height when compared with a radiograph, especially when normalized to the length of the foot.[40] The **Feiss line** provides an estimation of the position of the navicular relative to a line spanning the distance of the plantar aspect of the first MTP joint and the apex of the medial malleolus (see Special Test 8-1). A quantitative measure of pronation can be calculated via the **navicular drop test** (Special Test 8-4).[41] Navicular drop is the distance between the original height of the navicular (in subtalar joint neutral position) to the final weight-bearing position of the navicular in a relaxed stance.[42] A forefoot varus of greater than 8 degrees is associated with an increased navicular drop, indicating the relationship of forefoot varus to increased pronation.[26]

Supple pes planus may be corrected with the use of firm or soft orthotic material (depending on the specific foot characteristics) to reduce the amount and velocity of navicular drop.[43] Semirigid orthotics or motion-control shoes may be used for pes planus to limit certain biomechanical deficiencies such as excessive pronation.

Pes planus can lead to MT stress fractures, low back pain, and other musculoskeletal problems in the lower extremity and spine.[33] Evidence has also established a relationship between pes planus and a predisposition to anterior cruciate ligament (ACL) sprains. The tibia internally rotates as the navicular drops during pronation, causing the ACL to tighten as it wraps around the posterior cruciate ligament (see Chapter 10).[34]

Pes cavus

Appearing as a high medial longitudinal arch, pes cavus is often a congenital foot deformity. Certain neurologic or disease states such as upper motor neuron lesions or **cerebral palsy** may also result in the acquisition of a cavus foot type.[44] Hypertrophy of the peroneus longus muscle relative to the tibialis anterior has also been associated with cavus deformities.[45] This foot type is associated with a generalized stiffness and impaired ability to absorb ground contact forces. During running, pes cavus results in increased pressure loads on the forefoot and rearfoot.[13] A hypomobile plantar flexed first ray may also contribute to the limited shock-absorbing capability of the cavus foot.

A spreading and apparent drop of the forefoot relative to the rearfoot caused by the depression of the MT heads is noted during inspection of the area (Fig. 8-25). The dorsal pads under the calcaneus and the MT heads appear smaller than in a "normal" foot. The lateral four toes may be clawed. Over time, calluses form over the PIP joints.

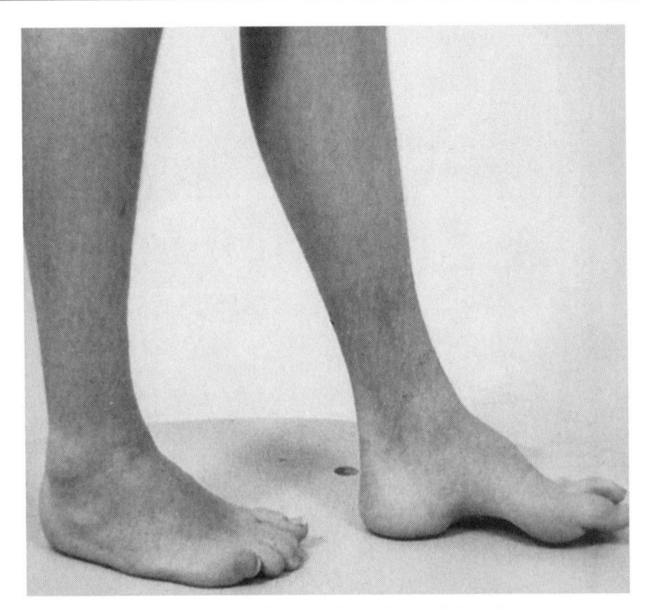

FIGURE 8-25 ■ Pes cavus, abnormally high medial arches.

A cavus foot tends to have decreased ground contact area and be more rigid and have less shock absorbing characteristics than normal or planus foot types.

✱ Practical Evidence

Individuals with cavus feet also tend to experience foot pain more frequently than those with an normal foot type, with the most frequent diagnoses being metatarsalgia and plantar fasciitis.[46]

In the case of problematic pes cavus, treatment approaches are often symptomatic, and soft orthotics or shoes with soft midsoles may be used to maximize available motion and to dissipate forces. Advanced conditions may be corrected through a plantar facial release, a surgical technique in which the plantar fascia is sectioned, allowing for increased foot mobility.[6]

Increased height of the medial longitudinal arch may be a predisposing condition to MT, tibial, and femoral stress fractures.[33] Pes cavus may also be associated with spinal scoliosis, although the cause-and-effect relationship has not been established.[45]

Plantar Fasciitis

Aggravation of the plantar fascia or the junction between the fascia and the first layer of intrinsic muscles can be traced to a single traumatic episode, repeated stress, biomechanical deficits, the presence of a heel spur, nerve entrapment, or Achilles tendon tightness.[2,50] Many cases of

Cerebral palsy A birth-related neurologic defect that results in motor dysfunction.

plantar fascia pathology are not inflammatory, but rather a degenerative process that is better described as plantar **fasciosis.**[5]

Pes planus or pes cavus may predispose an individual to plantar fasciitis.[48] The incidence of plantar fasciitis increases with age and may be associated with the gradual collapse of the medial longitudinal arch.[48] The onset of plantar fasciitis can occur after significant changes in activity intensity and duration, prolonged standing, training errors, weight gain, or in the presence of limited ankle dorsiflexion ROM.[20,49] Bilateral fasciitis may be caused by nerve, vascular, muscular, or connective tissue disease.[51] Biomechanical dysfunction can also be the result of medial heel pain caused by the entrapment of the medial calcaneal nerve or the nerve innervating the abductor digiti quinti muscle.[50]

Plantar fasciitis and heel spurs were once thought to be closely related. It was believed that shortening of the plantar fascia caused an outgrowth (i.e., a heel spur) to appear on the medial calcaneal tubercle. Although heel spurs and plantar fasciitis may occur concurrently, their presence may be coincidental (see the Heel Spurs section of this chapter). Regardless of the relationship between these two conditions, a heel spur has the potential for negatively impacting the foot's biomechanics, leading to plantar fasciitis.

Trauma to the plantar fascia may lead to inflammation, a pulling away of its origin from the calcaneus, a strain of its tissues, or its complete rupture. Inflammation of the fascia may also result in tearing-type injuries secondary to the functional shortening of its tissues. Over time, tightness of the triceps surae muscle group occurs, resulting in a valgus heel position at heel strike and early heel-rise during the latter stages of gait. During push-off, dorsiflexion and supination are restricted, further increasing the tension placed on the plantar fascia. As a result, the triceps surae's ability to produce power is decreased.[52]

The clinical diagnosis of plantar fasciitis is based on the patient's history and physical examination findings.[49] Typically, pain is centralized around the plantar fascia's origin on the medial calcaneal tubercle although the fascia may be tender along its entire length. A common symptom of plantar fasciitis is pain when stepping out of bed in the morning or stepping on the foot after a period of non–weight bearing. Initially, the patient's chief complaint is pain in the heel when resting after activity. Weakness and increased pain may be demonstrated during resisted plantarflexion, especially in single-leg stance (Special Test 8-5). Dorsiflexion also is decreased and painful and pain is increased when the ankle is dorsiflexed and the toes extended.[52] Increased symptoms may also be described when walking barefoot, on the toes, or when climbing stairs.[49] As the condition progresses, pain is experienced with the onset of activity, subsiding during activity because of stretching of the tissues and increased blood flow to the area. In the chronic stage, the pain is almost always constant (Examination Findings 8-1).

Fasciosis The noninflammatory degeneration of fascia.

Radiographs are not useful in determining the presence of plantar fasciitis and the presence or absence of heel spurs is not diagnostic.[49] Magnetic resonance imaging (MRI) or ultrasonic imaging is more useful in the early diagnosis of plantar fasciitis. Each of these methods can identify thickening of the proximal portion of the fascia, localized soft-tissue edema, and edema within the calcaneus.[47,48]

When accompanied by pes planus or pes cavus, plantar fasciitis may be considered a result of the foot's biomechanics. In this event, the biomechanics must be corrected to alleviate the plantar fasciitis.

Chronic plantar fasciitis can lead to tightness of the triceps surae muscle group and vice versa. As the calf muscles tighten during the latter stages of gait, they prematurely plantarflex the foot, increasing and prolonging the tension on the plantar fascia as it attaches at the calcaneal tubercle.[2]

Conservative treatment of plantar fasciitis is effective in 80% of patients and may include dorsiflexion night splints, anti-inflammatory medications, orthotics, heel cups, and stretching of the plantar fascia and the muscles of the lower extremity. Most patients respond well to conservative care, but those suffering from bilateral inflammation respond less favorably.[20,51]

Prefabricated insoles, such as heel cups, combined with a stretching program are five times more effective in controlling symptoms than custom orthotics and stretching.[49] Dorsiflexion splints may be used when the patient is at rest. These devices place the ankle in dorsiflexion to passively maintain the length of the triceps surae and the plantar fascia. Focused stretching of the plantar fascia yields better results than general stretching of the Achilles' tendon.[54]

Physicians may elect to use corticosteroid injections for problem cases, but this technique has been associated with ruptures of the plantar fascia, making corticosteroid iontophoresis a more favorable treatment option.[49] Four weeks of low-Dye taping and acetic acid iontophoresis provide better clinical results than taping and dexamethasone iontophoresis.[55] Extracoporeal shockwave therapy (EWST) has been successfully used in the treatment of plantar fasciitis patients who received conservative treatment for 6 months.[49,56]

Plantar fascia rupture

Forced ankle dorsiflexion and toe extension exerts a tensile force on the plantar fascia.[57] If the force of this stretch is sufficient, the fascia can avulse from its bony attachment on the calcaneus or rupture its central or medial slip.

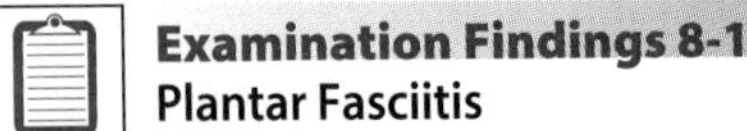

Examination Findings 8-1
Plantar Fasciitis

Examination Segment	Clinical Findings
History	***Onset:*** Acute or insidious ***Pain characteristics:*** Pain centralized near the medial calcaneal tubercle that can spread throughout the fascia. Pain may be described when weight bearing and is worsened after being in a non–weight-bearing position. Symptoms may increase when barefoot, walking on the toes, or when climbing stairs. Initial steps in the morning may be particularly symptomatic. ***Other symptoms:*** Complaints of stiffness after periods of non–weight bearing ***Mechanism:*** **Acute:** Forced dorsiflexion of the ankle combined with toe extension **Insidious:** Increased activity, additional distance when running, changing surface, or using a new or different shoe type or brand. ***Predisposing conditions:*** Pes cavus, pes planus, heel spur, hallux rigidus, forefoot valgus, excessive and prolonged foot pronation, decreased subtalar joint mobility, Achilles tendon or triceps surae tightness, leg length discrepancy, weight gain (including pregnancy), advancing age
Inspection	In some cases, swelling may be noted on the plantar aspect near the calcaneus. Pes planus or pes cavus may be noted.
Palpation	Pain is at or near the origin of the plantar fascia that, on occasion, runs the length of the plantar fascia. Tissue thickening may be palpable in chronic cases.
Joint and Muscle Function Assessment	Pain may be experienced during both active and passive ankle dorsiflexion and toe extension because of the stretch placed on the plantar fascia. ***AROM:*** Decreased ankle dorsiflexion ***MMT:*** Increased pain with test of flexor digitorum brevis ***PROM:*** Decreased ankle dorsiflexion with pain at end range. Pain experienced during passive extension of the MTP joints.
Joint Stability Tests	***Stress tests:*** Not applicable ***Joint play:*** STJ and/or midtarsal hypomobility (see Chapter 9)
Special Tests	Navicular drop, test for supple pes planus
Neurologic Screening	Tinel's sign to rule out posterior tibial nerve entrapment (tarsal tunnel syndrome)
Vascular Screening	No remarkable findings
Functional Assessment	Increased symptoms with push-off phase of gait; may present with heel-only (calcaneal) gait. May observe limited or excessive pronation or early heel-rise. Decreased strength during plantar flexion, especially when weight bearing (e.g., doing single-leg toe raises)
Imaging Techniques	MRI may reveal soft tissue edema and/or heel spur[47] MRI and ultrasonic imaging may be used for early identification of plantar fasciitis by the associated thickening of the proximal structure[48] Radiographic imaging is used to rule out other conditions. Heel spurs may be noted on 50% of symptomatic patients and 20% of patients without plantar fasciitis.[48,49]
Differential Diagnosis	Heel spur, calcaneal fracture/stress fracture, tarsal tunnel syndrome

AROM = active range of motion; MMT = manual muscle test; MRI = magnetic resonance imaging; PROM = passive range of motion.

A low (shallow) calcaneal pitch angle can increase the risk of plantar fascia rupture (see Fig. 8-22)[58,59] and may be associated with a history of plantar fasciitis.[57] The risk of rupture is increased further after corticosteroid injections.[6,20,57]

The patient has immediate difficulty bearing weight secondary to pain and may describe a "tearing" sensation on the plantar aspect of the foot.[57] The terminal stance, midstance, and preswing phases of gait are painful. The area around the medical calcaneal tubercle may be swollen and discolored secondary to soft tissue swelling and bleeding. A palpable defect may be noted on the medial calcaneal tubercle.[5] Soon after the rupture, the patient may demonstrate an acute hammer toe deformity on the involved foot (see Examination Findings 8–1).[20]

Heel Spur

A heel spur is a hook-shaped bony outgrowth (exostosis) located on the medial calcaneal tubercle (Fig. 8-26). This condition was once thought to be the result of increased tension from a shortened plantar fascia, leading to exostosis of its attachment on the calcaneus. However, surgical and radiographic investigations have determined that heel spurs are commonly located at the origin of the short toe flexor muscles rather than on the fascia's attachment site.[51]

✱ Practical Evidence

Radiographic evidence of heel spurs is noted in 15–20% of asymptomatic adults; radiographic evidence of a spur is found in 50% of symptomatic cases of plantar fasciitis.[49,60]

Although plantar fasciitis and a heel spur can occur simultaneously, the cause-and-effect relationship between the two conditions is unclear.[51] Calcaneal pitch angle may be a predictor of heel spurs and plantar fasciitis,[58,59] and, similarly to plantar fasciitis, the prevalence of heel spurs increases with age.[61]

The impairments associated with a heel spur are similar to those of plantar fasciitis (refer to Examination Findings 8–1). However, heel spurs tend to have a gradual onset and the chief complaint is pain during the heel-strike phase of gait. Evaluate the triceps surae muscle group for tightness associated with plantar fasciitis and heel spurs.

Conservative treatment including stretching and changes in footwear is similar to that used for those with plantar fasciitis. Surgical intervention may be required for spurs that do not respond to conservative treatment, are unusually large, or impair neurovascular function.

Tarsal Coalition

A hereditary condition, tarsal coalition is a bony, fibrous, or cartilaginous union between two or more tarsal bones. Tarsal coalition most often affects the calcaneonavicular, talonavicular, or talocalcaneal joints, with 50% of the cases occurring bilaterally.[15,35,62] The resulting impairments and functional limitations depend on the joints involved. Tarsal coalition clinically resembles rigid pes planus when diagnosed in the adolescent and may be related to **peroneal spastic flatfoot**. Joint play assessment reveals restricted subtalar joint motions leading to

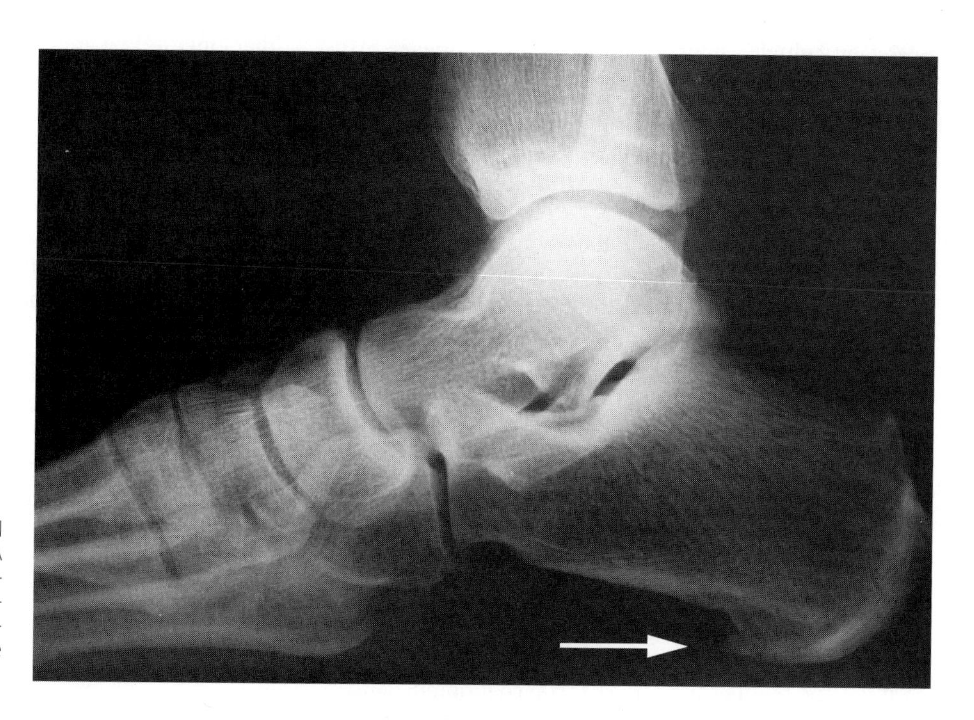

FIGURE 8-26 ■ Radiograph of a heel spur (medial view of the right foot). A form of exostosis, heel spurs are an abnormal bony outgrowth of the calcaneus. Note the hooklike projection arising from the anterior border of the calcaneal tuberosity.

Peroneal spastic flatfoot A lowering of the medial foot caused by spasm of the peroneus longus muscle.

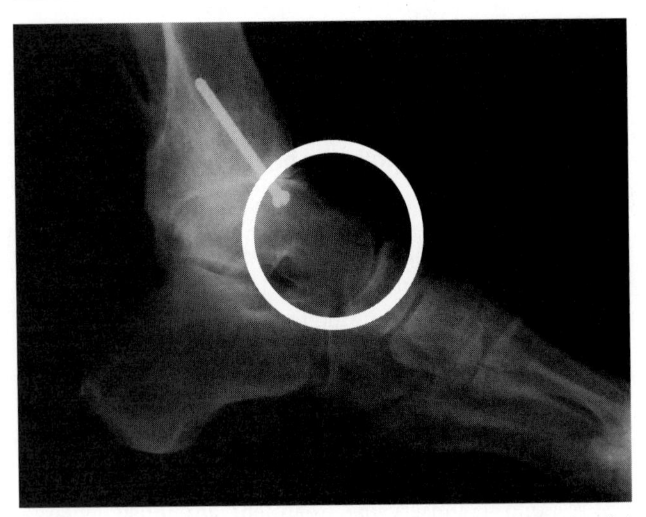

FIGURE 8-27 ■ Talar beaking associated with tarsal coalition (medial view of the left foot). The screw implanted in the tibia is for an unrelated condition.

further stress at the midtarsal area with eventual collapse of the longitudinal arches.

Rigidity of the coalesced bones results in compensatory forces distal and proximal to the subtalar joint. The calcaneus assumes a valgus position relative to the tibia, and the forefoot abducts, the arch flattens, and the navicular overrides the talus to cause **talar beaking** (Fig. 8-27).[35,63] On occasion, spasm and pain result as the peroneals contract, especially the peroneus longus.[35]

Tarsal coalition becomes symptomatic in preteens and teenagers as the bones ossify. The initial finding often follows an inversion ankle sprain, an injury that is predisposed by subtalar joint coalition.[35,64] Age appears to be related to the period during which the joints fuse: the talonavicular joint for children age 3 to 5 years; the calcaneonavicular joint for those age 8 to 12 years; and the talocalcaneal joint for those age 12 to 16 years.[35]

Clinically, tarsal coalition is exhibited as a rigid flatfoot with calcaneal valgus and abduction of the forefoot that is unchanged when the patient is in a weight-bearing position (rigid pes planus) (see Special Test 8-5).[35] In adults, the foot alignment may appear neutral.[65] Palpation over the involved joint may cause pain.

Tarsal coalition is differentiated from other foot pathologies by the limitations in subtalar motion (see Joint Play 9-1 and 9-2). It also can be identified via radiographic examination. A definitive diagnosis of tarsal coalition is made via radiographs for bony fusion, computed tomography (CT), or magnetic resonance imaging (MRI) for cartilaginous or fibrous coalition.[35] Any rigidity in the rearfoot may indicate tarsal coalition, warranting referral to a physician for further evaluation.

If detected in its early stages, tarsal coalition usually responds well to immobilization, the use of orthotics, or both.[35,66] When surgery is performed to release the coalition before any secondary degenerative changes occur, the prognosis is excellent.[67] Fusion is the treatment of choice if degenerative changes are present.

Tarsal Tunnel Syndrome

Tarsal tunnel syndrome (TTS) is caused by the entrapment of the posterior tibial nerve or one of its medial or lateral branches as it passes through the tarsal tunnel. The definition of TTS also includes compressive lesions of the posterior tibial nerve proximal to the retinaculum, under the deep fascia of the leg, and distally under the abductor hallicus muscle.[69]

Anatomically, the tarsal tunnel is bordered anteriorly by the tibia and the talus and laterally by the calcaneus. The flexor retinaculum forms a fibrous roof that is attached to the sheaths of the tibialis posterior, flexor hallicus longus, and flexor digitorum longus tendons (Fig. 8-28).[70] The tunnel itself is compartmentalized by fascial membranes, or septa, which tightly bind the posterior tibial nerve, predisposing it to compressive forces.[69]

Several different factors can cause TTS. Acute TTS may be caused by trauma, including tarsal fracture or dislocation, hyperplantarflexion, or eversion. It can also be the result of overuse injuries. Predisposing conditions include ganglion formation, fibrosis, arthritis, or disease states such as diabetes.[69,71–73] Anatomic factors that may lead to TTS include nonunion fractures of the sustenaculum tali, tarsal coalition, muscle anomalies, or anterior entrapment of the nerve by the extensor hallucis brevis muscle.[74–77] Biomechanically, rearfoot varus coupled with excessive pronation, increased internal rotation of the tibia, and hypermobility of the medial longitudinal arch place an increased stress on the posterior tibial nerve, predisposing it to TTS.[5,78]

The primary patient complaints are diffuse pain, burning, paresthesia, or numbness along the plantar and medial aspect of the foot that increases with activity and decreases with rest. Approximately one third of patients report pain arising from the medial malleolus and radiating into the medial lower leg, midcalf, and, occasionally, the medial heel (Examination Findings 8-2).[70] Cold intolerance and

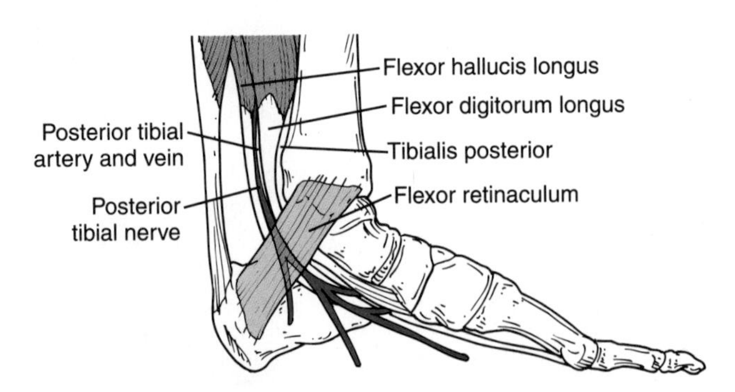

FIGURE 8-28 ■ The tarsal tunnel. The bony surface of the tarsal tunnel is formed by the tibia, talus, and calcaneus, with the roof being formed by the flexor retinaculum.

Examination Findings 8-2
Tarsal Tunnel Syndrome

Examination Segment	Clinical Findings
History	***Onset:*** Acute or insidious ***Pain characteristics:*** Pain, numbness, and paresthesia occur along the plantar or medial aspects of the foot. Symptoms increase with increased activity. ***Other symptoms:*** Cold intolerance of the involved foot may be described. ***Mechanism:*** Compression of the posterior tibial nerve (or its branches) within the tarsal tunnel. This pressure may also involve the vascular structures within the tunnel. A history of a plantarflexion–eversion mechanism injury to the ankle may be described. TTS is also possibly associated with fracture, dislocation, or inflammation of the tarsals or local ganglion formation. ***Predisposing conditions:*** Prior tarsal fracture or dislocation; rearfoot varus; history of eversion ankle injury; excessive pronation during gait; arthritis; nonunion fracture of the sustentaculum tali; inflammation of the extensor retinaculum; tarsal coalition; diabetes
Inspection	Inspection of the non-weight-bearing foot is normally unremarkable. However, in chronic cases, trophic changes of the foot and nails may be noted. Inspection of the medial longitudinal arch reveals pes planus, a condition often associated with TTS.
Palpation	Palpation over the tibial nerve and its branches results in tenderness, especially in the area of the tarsal tunnel behind the lateral malleolus and beneath the flexor retinaculum.
Joint and Muscle Function Assessment	***AROM:*** Motor function of the intrinsic and extrinsic muscles is often normal. ***MMT:*** Normal ***PROM:*** Forced dorsiflexion and eversion may increase symptoms secondary to pressure from the flexor retinaculum and tension on the nerve.
Joint Stability Tests	***Stress tests:*** No remarkable findings ***Joint play:*** Possible hypermobility medial subtalar glide
Special Tests	Dorsiflexion–eversion test for tarsal tunnel syndrome Tinel sign
Neurologic Screening	Hypoesthesia of the posterior tibial nerve distribution. Medial plantar nerve: Medial plantar surface Lateral plantar nerve: Lateral plantar surface Medial calcaneal branch (tibial nerve): Medial calcaneus The Tinel sign may be positive inferior and distal to the medial malleolus. Sharp or dull and two-point discrimination may be decreased along the medial and plantar aspects of the foot.
Vascular Screening	No remarkable findings
Functional Assessment	Increased pain or symptoms during period of maximum pronation such as the midstance phase of gait.
Imaging Techniques	CT, MRI, and ultrasonic imaging can identify space-occupying lesions within the tarsal tunnel.[68]
Differential Diagnosis	Plantar fasciitis, posterior tibialis tendinopathy, talocalcaneal coalition, calcaneal stress fracture
Comments	Symptoms of TTS closely resemble those of other foot maladies, especially plantar fasciitis. Proximal nerve compression may mimic the signs and symptoms of TTS.

AROM = active range of motion; CT = computed tomography; MMT = manual muscle test; MRI = magnetic resonance images; PROM = passive range of motion; TTS = tarsal tunnel syndrome.

increased pain when wearing low-cut or high heel shoes may also be described.[58] Muscle function is often normal. A positive **Tinel's sign** may be elicited along the path of the nerve inferior and distal to the medial malleolus (Fig. 8-29). The **dorsiflexion–eversion test** may also reproduce the symptoms of tarsal tunnel syndrome (Special Test 8-6).[68]

Tarsal tunnel syndrome may be confused with the symptoms produced by plantar fasciitis, but close examination of the symptoms can differentiate between the two.[71] Pain produced by TTS is located along the medial portion of the heel and arch; with plantar fasciitis, pain is localized near the fascia's insertion on the calcaneus. The straight leg raise test can assist in the differential diagnosis between plantar fasciitis and tarsal tunnel syndrome (see Special Test 13-7). Stretching and exercise often decrease plantar fasciitis symptoms, activity increases the pain caused by TTS. A definitive diagnosis of TTS is made via electrodiagnostic studies, MRI, or ultrasonic imaging.[58,69,79]

A complete evaluation of the lower extremity is required to identify the cause of TTS. A common finding is pes planus in which excessive pronation increases the traction stress placed on the nerve. The use of an orthotic or motion control shoe to limit the amount and speed of pronation is recommended.[80] Surgical intervention may be needed to release the compressive forces placed on the posterior tibial nerve. Results are most successful when the compression occurs within the tarsal tunnel itself.[58]

Metatarsal Fractures

Fracture of the MTs can result from direct trauma or overuse; the location of pain and crepitus are indicative of the type of fracture (Fig. 8-30). Acute fractures occur secondary to compressive, tensile, rotational, or crushing forces. Stress fractures have a more insidious and complex onset. The toe flexors assist the foot in dissipating the forces placed on the MTs. Fatigue or general weakness of the toe flexors increases

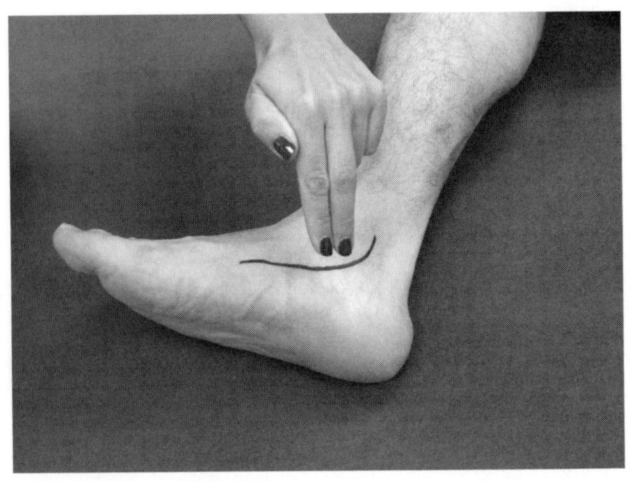

FIGURE 8-29 ■ Location of Tinel's sign for tarsal tunnel syndrome. Tapping over the path of the posterior tibial nerve refers pain into the foot and toes.

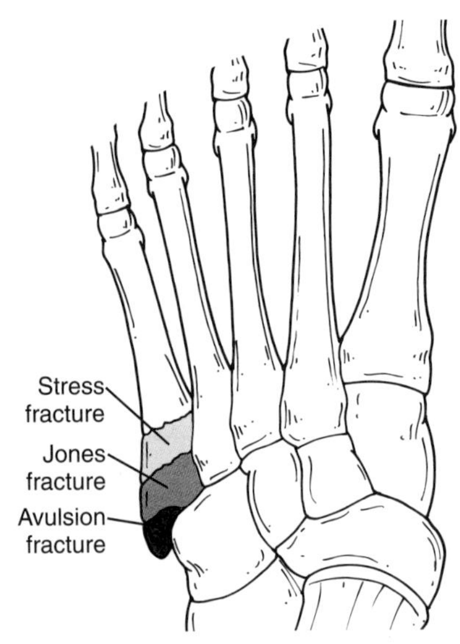

FIGURE 8-30 ■ Fractures of the proximal fifth metatarsal. Avulsion fractures involve the styloid process, "Jones fractures" occur 1 cm distal to the proximal diaphysis, and stress fractures tend to occur distal to that demarcation.

the amount of strain placed on the MTs, increasing the risk of fracture.[81] The presence of diabetes mellitus also increases the risk of MT fracture (Examination Findings 8-3).[82]

Acute fractures

The base of the fifth MT is particularly prone to avulsion fractures (Fig. 8-31). The body counters against inadvertent inversion of the foot and ankle by contracting the peroneals, everting the foot and bringing it back to its proper

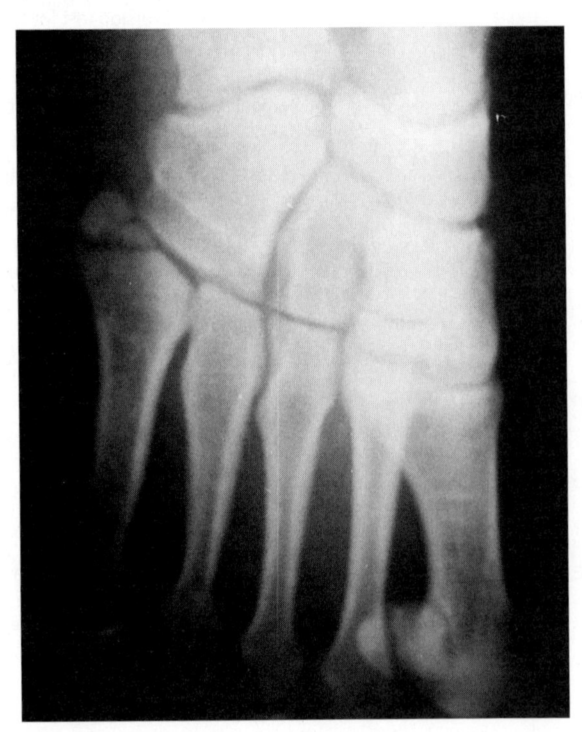

FIGURE 8-31 ■ Fracture of styloid process of the fifth metatarsal (dorsal view of the right foot).

Special Test 8-6
Dorsiflexion-Eversion Test for Tarsal Tunnel Syndrome

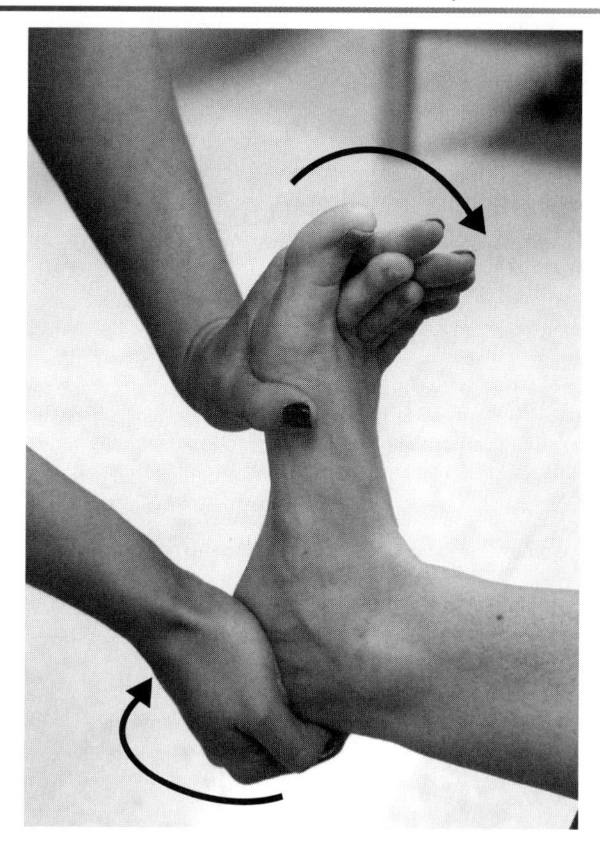

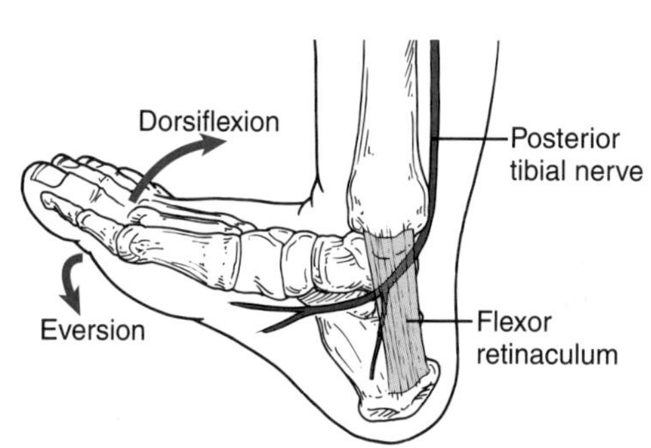

This test places tension on the posterior tibial nerve by replicating the mechanics of pes planus during gait.[68]

Patient Position	Sitting with the legs off the table
Position of Examiner	At the patient's feet
Evaluative Procedure	The examiner passively everts the heel (calcaneus and talus) while passively dorsiflexing the foot and toes. This position is held for 5 to 10 sec.
Positive Test	Provocation of pain and/or paresthesia radiating into the foot
Implications	Posterior tibial nerve dysfunction
Modification	The Tinel sign can be performed over the course of the nerve during this procedure.
Evidence	LR+ = unable to calculate; high probability that the condition is present with a positive test result LR–[77]

Not Useful **Useful**

Very Small | Small | Moderate | Large

1.0 0.9 0.8 0.7 0.6 0.5 0.4 0.3 0.2 0.1 0

Examination Findings 8-3
Metatarsal Fractures

Examination Segment	Clinical Findings
History	***Onset:*** Acute, or in the case of stress fractures, insidious ***Pain characteristics:*** Localized pain occurring along the shaft of the metatarsal, radiating into the intermetatarsal space ***Other symptoms:*** Not applicable ***Mechanism:*** **Acute:** Direct trauma to the metatarsal (e.g., being stepped on), dynamic overload (e.g., avulsion of the peroneus brevis tendon), or rotational (e.g., inversion of the foot). **Insidious:** Repetitive stresses placed along the shaft of the metatarsal or compression arising from the contiguous metatarsals (e.g., "march fracture"). The symptoms typically increase with activity and decrease with rest. ***Predisposing conditions:*** A history of long-term diabetes mellitus. Forefoot valgus, rearfoot varus, rearfoot valgus, pes planus, pes cavus, or Morton's toe may predispose the individual to metatarsal stress fractures. Stress fractures may also be induced by change in footwear, increased intensity or duration of training, and changing running surfaces. Postmenopausal or amenopausal women are at an increased risk of stress fractures.
Inspection	In acute injuries, gross deformity and/or swelling may be visible along the shaft of the bone.
Palpation	Stress fractures may reveal no significant signs, but localized swelling around the painful area may be present. Tenderness and crepitus may be present over the site of acute fractures of maturing stress fractures. A false joint may be present with acutely fractured metatarsals.
Joint and Muscle Function Assessment	***AROM:*** Movements that compress the bone, mainly dorsiflexion of the ankle or rotation of the foot, typically result in pain. ***MMT:*** Contraindicated if acute fracture is suspected. In the presence of a stress fracture, MMT of the muscles of the foot may or may not produce pain. ***PROM:*** Movements that compress the bone, mainly dorsiflexion of the ankle or rotation of the foot, typically result in pain.
Joint Stability Tests	***Stress tests:*** Not applicable ***Joint play:*** Contraindicated if acute fracture is suspected. Hypomobility at adjacent joint may predispose to stress fracture.
Special Tests	Long bone compression test
Neurologic Screening	No remarkable findings
Vascular Screening	No remarkable findings
Functional Assessment	Inability to bear weight or walk Pain during toe-landing or push-off phase of gait.
Imaging Techniques	Bone scans or MRIs are required to definitively diagnose stress fractures in their early stages. The presence of acute fractures must be confirmed via radiographic examination.
Differential Diagnosis	Stress fractures: Interdigital neuromas, tarsal tunnel syndrome Acute fracture: Sprain, dislocation

AROM = active range of motion; MMT = manual muscle test; MRI = magnetic resonance images; PROM = passive range of motion.

orientation. If the force of the contraction is too great, the peroneal brevis tendon can be avulsed from its attachment on the styloid process of the fifth MT. This mechanism, when associated with pain, crepitus, and swelling over the insertion site, strongly suggests a fracture. The location of pain is also indicative of the type of fracture. The signs and symptoms of an avulsion fracture of the fifth MT's styloid process are clinically similar to those of a **Jones' fracture**, a fracture of the fifth MT 1 cm distal to the proximal diaphysis (Fig. 8-32).[83]

The signs and symptoms of an acute fracture may include obvious deformity and the presence of a **false joint** over the fracture site. The suspicion of acute fractures may be further substantiated by the **long bone compression test** (Fig. 8-33). ROM of the joints above and below the fracture site may be limited because of pain.

Management depends on the type and location of the fracture. Any suspected acute fracture to the MTs requires immediate immobilization and non–weight bearing while the patient is referred to a physician. Avulsion fractures may be managed with soft casts and typically require 4 weeks for recovery.[84,85] Fractures of the MT shaft or neck typically require immobilization and weight bearing to tolerance for 4 to 6 weeks.

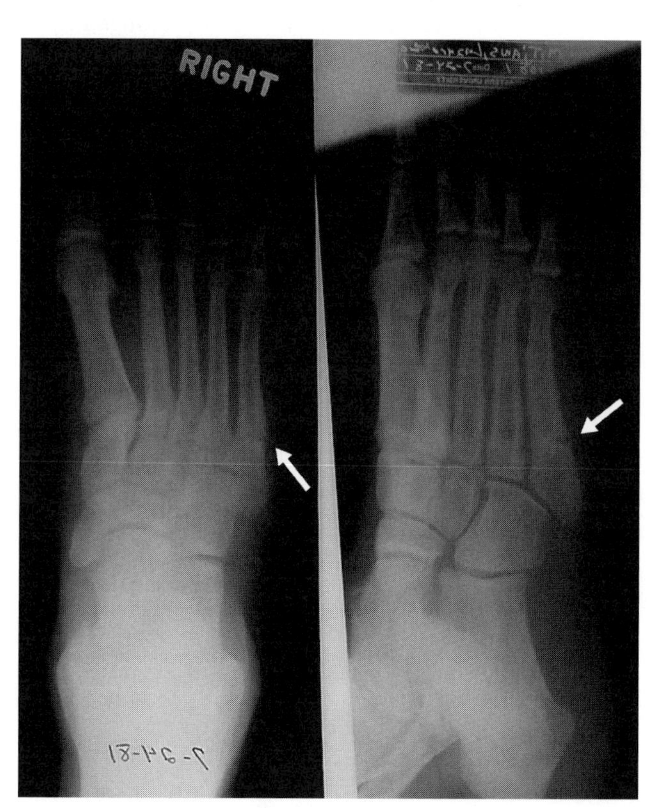

FIGURE 8-32 ■ Radiograph of a Jones' fracture, a fracture of the fifth MT 1 cm distal to the styloid process (dorsal and oblique view of the right foot).

False joint Abnormal movement along the length of a bone caused by a fracture or incomplete fusion.

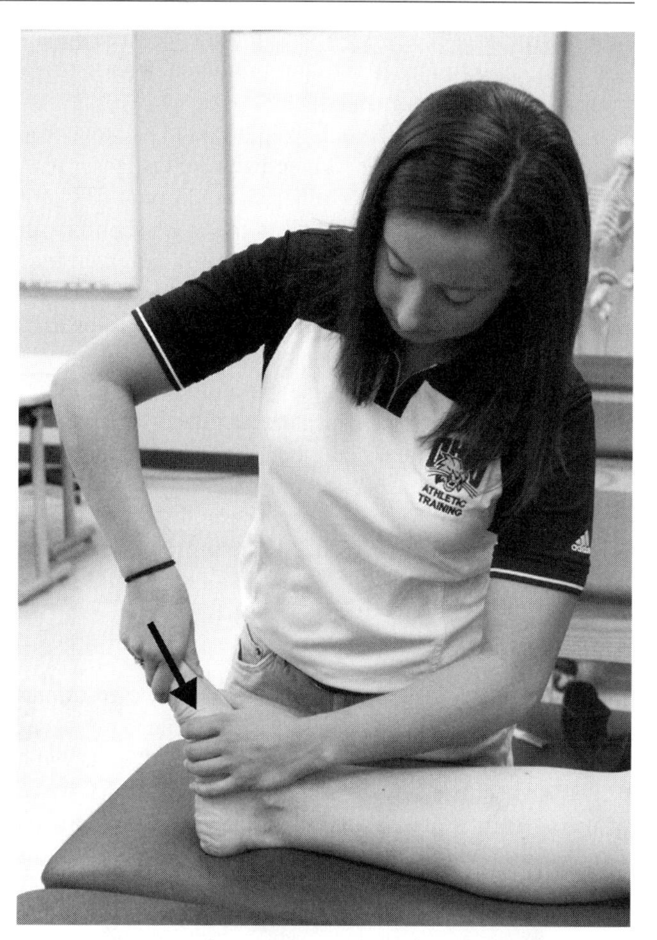

FIGURE 8-33 ■ Long bone compression test for suspected fractures of the metatarsals. A longitudinal force is placed along the shaft of the bone. In the presence of a fracture, compression of the two fragments results in pain and possibly the presence of a "false joint."

In an active population early fixation of Jones' fractures has a superior outcome over immobilization alone.[86] Because of their propensity for a non-union, Jones' fractures require surgical fixation with return to competition expected in 8 weeks. Conservative treatment consists of 8 weeks of immobilization followed by weight bearing in a cast as tolerated.[85]

Stress fractures

Metatarsal, tarsal, and ankle stress fractures are related to biomechanical abnormalities of the foot.[87] Predisposing conditions include dysfunction of the first MTP joint, neuropathy, metabolic disorders (including diabetes and osteoporosis), and rearfoot malalignment.[88] Because of the prevalence of osteoporosis, postmenopausal women are at increased risk of stress fractures.[89] Stress fractures of the foot and ankle occur in relatively predictable patterns.[90]

During weight bearing, hypomobility increases the stress placed on the midfoot and hypermobility increases the amount of stress placed on the forefoot. Over time, the individual begins to experience local pain associated with activity. Stress fractures of the MTs have been termed

"march fractures" because of their prevalence in new military recruits. If unrecognized and untreated, a stress fracture can progress to a gross fracture.

Stress fractures are characterized by a dull pain over the fracture site that increases with activity and decreases with rest. This condition must be differentiated from other foot conditions. Pain may be referred to the MTs secondary to TTS or an intermetatarsal neuroma. In addition, pain may arise from irritation of the interosseous muscles, be caused by an inflammatory condition such as periosteitis, or have a vascular origin.

Stress fractures are managed symptomatically. The patient is withheld from activities that aggravate the fracture site and fitted with a walking boot or instructed to wear stiff-soled shoes. In the case of multiple stress fractures or a stress fracture that fails to heal, the possibility of underlying or contributory pathology such as **osteopenia** must be ruled out.

Lisfranc Injuries

Injury to the Lisfranc joint can include sprains, dislocations, fractures, or fracture dislocations through the tarsometatarsal joints (Fig. 8-34). Lisfranc fractures represent only about 0.2% of all fractures, but up to 20% of these are misdiagnosed or ignored.[92] It is debatable if the tarsometatarsal joint can be dislocated without concurrent fracture.[93] Clinically the signs and symptoms of these conditions may range from subtle to obvious, and frequently the injury is dismissed as a "sprain."[91,92] Because long-term outcomes are poor, a high index of suspicion is necessary for any acute midfoot injury.[91]

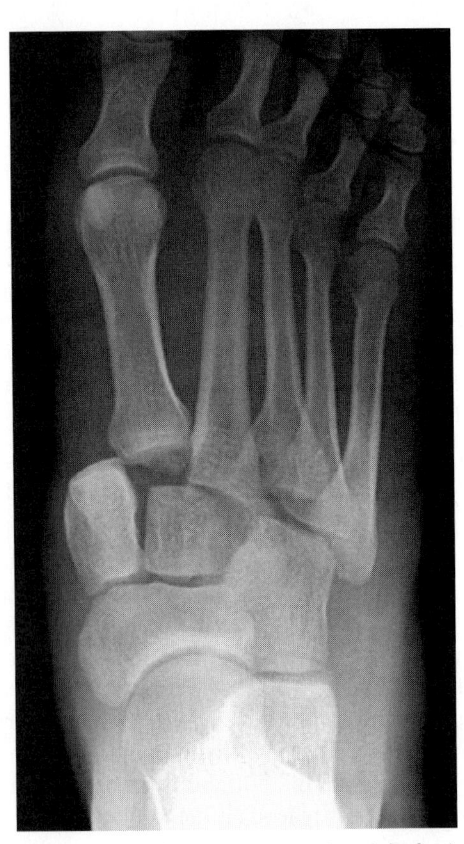

FIGURE 8-34 ■ Lisfranc's fracture (superior view, right foot). Note the lateral displacement of the metatarsals relative to the tarsals.

Fracture-dislocations are often the result of a high-energy mechanism; sprains result from lower-energy forces.[94] Lisfranc fracture-dislocations are commonly the result of an axial load being placed on the foot while the toes are extended (Fig. 8-35). Attempting to rotate (pronate or supinate) the foot while the distal segment is fixed—as in being stepped on—is also a common mechanism. A fracture-dislocation is characterized by severe pain and palpable and potentially visible deformity immediately following the injury. The deformity is quickly obscured by the rapid onset of swelling (Examination Findings 8-4). Radiographs are used to identify the type of fracture and the displacement of the bony surfaces. The injury is classified by the direction and magnitude of displacement of the tarsals using the **Modified Hardcastle** system.[95,96]

*** Practical Evidence**

Following a loading or crushing mechanism to the foot, plantar ecchymosis is indicative of a possible Lisfranc joint injury.[92]

Conservative treatment consisting of prolonged non–weight bearing is warranted when weight-bearing radiographs reveal no displacement.[91] Operative reduction and internal fixation is the typical course of treatment for Lisfranc injuries with bony displacement. Postoperative treatment consists of 8 weeks of non–weight-bearing in a

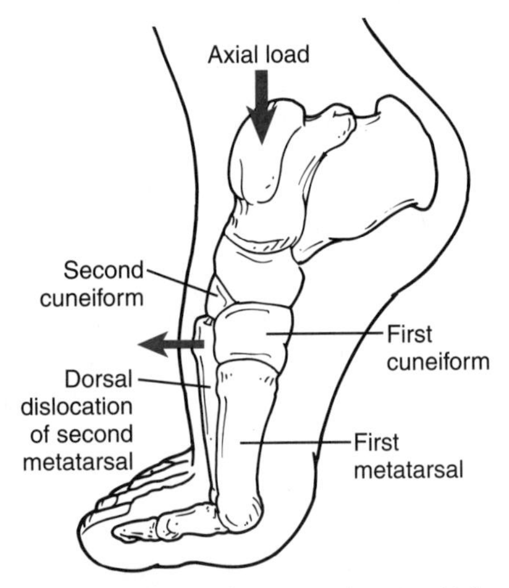

FIGURE 8-35 ■ A mechanism of injury resulting in a Lisfranc fracture-dislocation, an axial load being placed on the rearfoot while weight bearing on extended toes.

Osteopenia Decreased bone density, but less severe than osteoporosis.

Examination Findings 8-4
Lisfranc Injury

Examination Segment	Clinical Findings
History	***Onset:*** Acute ***Pain characteristics:*** Generally severe pain at the time of injury.[91] ***Other symptoms:*** A snapping, popping, or tearing sensation at the time of injury may be reported. ***Mechanism:*** Sudden rotational loading of the TMT joints or axial loading that forces the toes into extension and the foot and ankle into dorsiflexion (e.g., landing from a jump). Rotational loading on a fixed forefoot Crushing force
Inspection	Swelling over the dorsum of the foot In some instances, displacement of the MTs may be noted. Fracture-dislocations are marked by an apparent shortening and widening of the involved foot.
Palpation	Point tenderness over the TMT joints and fractured MTs
Joint and Muscle Function Assessment	***AROM:*** Decreased pronation and supination ***MMT:*** Decreased strength secondary to pain is found during pronation, supination, dorsiflexion, and plantarflexion ***PROM:*** Pain at end range of all motions
Joint Stability Tests	***Stress tests:*** Not applicable ***Joint play:*** Do not perform if fracture is suspected. Increased glide may represent manual displacement of the fracture line.
Special Tests	Not applicable
Neurologic Screening	Local branches of peripheral nerve may be damaged secondary to tensile or compression forces.
Vascular Screening	A crushing mechanism of injury may result in vascular compromise including a compartment syndrome.[92]
Functional Assessment	Inability to bear weight or antalgic gait to minimize weight bearing on involved side
Imaging Techniques	AP, lateral, and oblique radiographs in standing[91]
Differential Diagnosis	Tarsal fracture, MT fracture
Comments	If a compartment syndrome develops, immediate surgical decompression and repair is needed. Because of the poor long-term outcomes and complications of unrecognized, untreated Lisfranc injuries, any suspected Lisfranc joint involvement should be immediately referred to a physician.[91]

AP = anteroposterior; AROM = active range of motion; MMT = manual muscle test; MT = metatarsal; PROM = passive range of motion; TMT = tarsometatarsal.

cast or splint.[93] Ligamentous injury to the Lisfranc joints respond better to **arthrodesis** than open reduction and internal fixation.[97] Unrecognized or untreated Lisfranc joint injury has a morbidly high rate of posttraumatic arthritis and nonunion, malunion, and/or malalignment in bone healing.

Phalangeal Fractures

Phalangeal fractures are the result of a longitudinal force applied to the bone, such as kicking an immovable object, or occur secondary to a crushing force, such as a weight falling on the toes (Fig. 8-36). Impairments associated with a fractured phalanx include deformity, pain, and crepitus. Pain is experienced during toe-off when running or walking. Although phalangeal fractures result in pain and an **antalgic gait**, few treatment options exist. After a fracture has been confirmed via radiographic examination, the treatment consists of rest, the use of a hard-soled shoe to prevent extension of the toes, taping the affected toe to the one next to it ("buddy taping"), and possibly the use of crutches. Surgical intervention may be required if the fracture disrupts the articular surface.

Intermetatarsal Neuromas

Intermetatarsal neuromas, also referred to as plantar neuromas or interdigital neuromas, are caused by the entrapment of a nerve between two MT heads.[98] **Morton's neuroma** is entrapment between the third and fourth MTs. The third common digital (plantar) nerve is most commonly affected.[99,100] The communicating branch of the lateral plantar nerve has also been implicated with Morton's neuroma.[99]

Prolonged pressure on the involved nerve results in a degenerative neuropathy and formation of fibrotic nodules and edema around the nerve. The exact relationship of this buildup and the diagnosis of a neuroma is unclear.[100,101] Over time, **demyelination** of the nerve occurs.[101]

Excessive motion, a thickened and shortened transverse intermetatarsal ligament, and excessive pronation predispose individuals to intermetatarsal neuromas. Activities that increase weight-bearing pressure or compressive pressure in the forefoot, such as wearing pointed-toed and high-heeled shoes, can trigger the signs and symptoms.[100] Women are more likely to be affected with this condition than men. Also, a high likelihood exists for reoccurrence in the same foot.[100,102]

The chief impairments, closely resembling those of a MT stress fracture, include pain in the anterior transverse arch radiating to the toes, the plantar aspect of the foot, and, occasionally, projecting up the ankle and lower leg. Numbness and paresthesia in the digits may also be described. An increase in intermetatarsal pressure during weight bearing on the forefoot increases pain.[103] The symptoms increase when the patient is wearing shoes, especially if the shoes are tight fitting. Patients report relief of the symptoms when

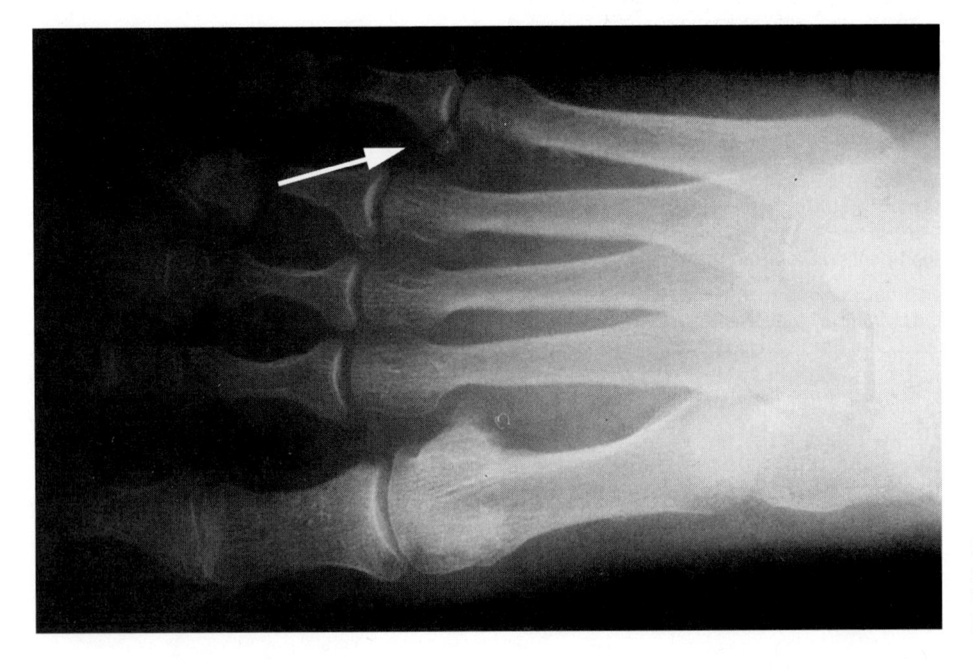

FIGURE 8-36 ■ Fracture of the proximal phalanx of the fifth toe of the right foot. Note the fracture line crossing the proximal medial process.

Arthrodesis Surgical joint fusion.

Antalgic gait A limp or unnatural walking pattern.

Demyelination Loss of a nerve's fatty lining.

Examination Findings 8-5
Intermetatarsal Neuroma

Examination Segment	Clinical Findings
History	***Onset:*** Pain increases with time. ***Pain characteristics:*** Pain originating in the forefoot. As symptoms progress, the pain may radiate proximally. ***Other symptoms:*** Numbness and paresthesia in the forefoot and toes may be reported. ***Mechanism:*** Inflammation of—or around—a plantar nerve ***Predisposing conditions:*** Hypermobility, adhesions in the transverse intermetatarsal ligament, pronated foot type
Inspection	Often unremarkable. Swelling may be noted in the forefoot.
Palpation	Point tenderness between the affected MT heads Pain is increased when squeezing the transverse arch, compressing the MT heads (Mulder sign). A palpable nodule may be noted.
Joint and Muscle Function Assessment	***AROM:*** Unremarkable findings ***MMT:*** Possible increased pain with toe flexion ***PROM:*** Unremarkable findings
Joint Stability Tests	***Stress tests:*** Not applicable ***Joint play:*** Hypermobility of the intermetatarsal joints
Special Tests	Mulder sign
Neurologic Screening	Lower quarter screen to rule out proximal nerve compression
Vascular Screening	No remarkable findings
Functional Assessment	Antalgic gait may be noted.
Imaging Techniques	MRI using a contrast medium Ultrasonic imaging
Differential Diagnosis	Stress fracture, arthritis, metatarsalgia, proximal nerve compression
Comments	Symptoms increase when the patient is wearing footwear, especially pointed-toed shoes, and decrease when non–weight-bearing or walking barefoot.

AROM = active range of motion; MMT = manual muscle test; MT = metatarsal; PROM = passive range of motion.

the footwear is removed. A nodule may be palpated between the involved MT heads. Tenderness may be increased by extending the digits and dorsiflexing the foot during palpation (Examination Findings 8-5). Squeezing the transverse arch, thus compressing the MT heads, replicates the symptoms. The **Mulder Sign** (Special Test 8-7) or the eraser end of a pencil may be used to apply pressure directly to the neuroma, resulting in an increase in the symptoms (Fig. 8-37).[104]

The definitive diagnosis is based on the clinical symptoms and imaging. Ultrasonography is highly reliable in identifying the location and size of intermetatarsal neuromas.[102,105] The temporary alleviation of symptoms following an injection of lidocaine adds in the diagnostic accuracy.

Initial treatment includes modification of footwear (i.e., the patient should avoid wearing shoes that increase symptoms), the use of orthotics to decrease intermetatarsal pressure, and the use of oral antiinflammatory medication.[106,107] Corticosteroid or local anesthetic injections may be used for symptomatic relief. However, this form of treatment seldom resolves a neuroma.[106,108] Surgical excision of the neuroma provides dramatic relief of the symptoms for most patients.[100,106,109]

Hallux Rigidus

Literally meaning "stiff great toe," hallux rigidus is the progressive degeneration of the first MTP joint's articular surfaces with consequences ranging from limited motion

Special Test 8-7
Mulder Sign for Intermetatarsal Neuroma

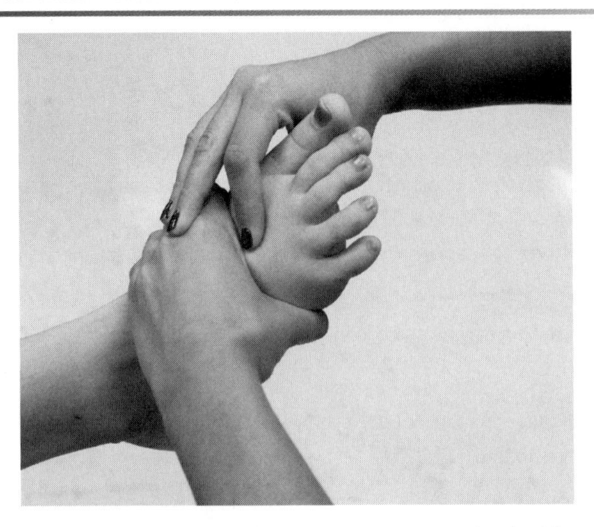

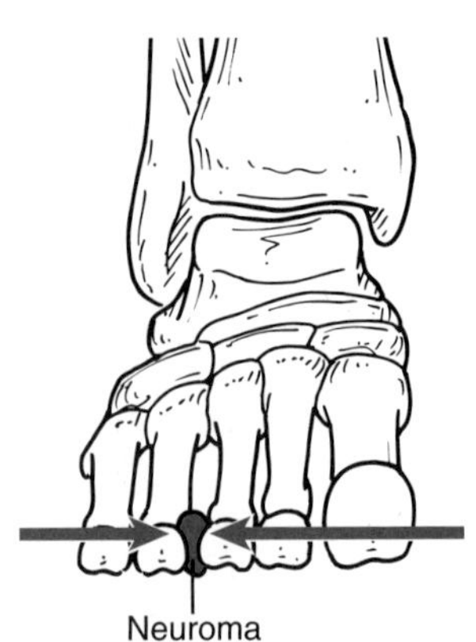

The Mulder sign involves manual compression of the transverse metatarsal arch with pressure applied over the interdigital nerve to reproduce the symptoms associated with an intermetatarsal neuroma.

Patient Position	Long or short sitting
Position of Examiner	Standing at the patient's feet
Evaluative Procedure	Position one hand along the distal fifth metatarsal and the opposite hand along the distal first metatarsal. Apply pressure to compress the transverse arch. Using the thumb and forefinger to apply pressure over the symptomatic interspace between the metatarsals.
Positive Test	A click, pain, and/or reproduction of symptoms
Implications	Intermetatarsal neuroma
Evidence	Absent or inconclusive in the literature

(hallux limitus) or complete **ankylosis** (hallux rigidus) that causes the loss of dorsiflexion.[16,110] The joint degeneration is caused by osteoarthritis; rheumatoid arthritis; gout; and advanced hallux valgus, synovial effusion, or other chondral erosions affecting the articular surfaces.[111–114] The etiology of hallux limitus and rigidus may be related to an irregularly flattened MT head, hypermobility of the first tarsometatarsal joint, or a long first MT leading to degeneration-causing forces on the joint.[110] Hallux rigidus is frequently bilateral and has a strong genetic component.[115] Morton's toe has been associated with hallux rigidus, especially in female dancers.[18]

As the condition progresses, the MT head erodes (chondritis dessicans) or a fracture occurs through the articular surface (osteochondritis dessicans).[112] The axis of joint motion shifts from the center of the MTP to its plantar aspect. If untreated, spastic contractures and fusion of the joint (ankylosis) occur.[112,114] In some cases, the sesamoids located under the first MTP joint may hypertrophy, further decreasing ROM.[112] Irregularity of the joint surfaces results in pain at the first MTP, and vague complaints of lateral

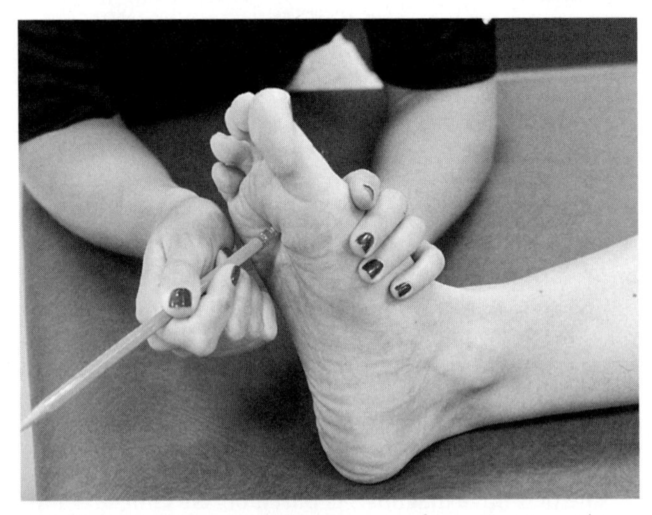

FIGURE 8-37 ■ Determining the presence of an intermetatarsal neuroma. A pencil eraser is used to apply pressure to the intermetatarsal space, compressing the nerve ending.

Ankylosis Immobility of a joint.

Examination Findings 8-6
Hallux Rigidus

Examination Segment	Clinical Findings
History	***Onset:*** Insidious ***Pain characteristics:*** Pain arising from the first MTP joint ***Mechanism:*** Degeneration of the articulating surfaces secondary to repetitive stress. ***Predisposing conditions:*** Flattened MT head, long first MT, hypermobility of the first MTP joint, Morton's alignment
Inspection	Swelling of the first MTP joint, especially after activity. Atrophy of the triceps surae may be noted.
Palpation	Exostosis may be palpable on the dorsal and/or medial aspects of the joint. Hypertrophy of the sesamoids may be noted.
Joint and Muscle Function Assessment	***AROM:*** MTP extension is restricted and painful. ***MMT:*** Extensor hallucis longus: Strength reduced secondary to pain In chronic conditions weakness of the triceps surae group (see Chapter 9) may be noted. ***PROM:*** MTP extension is restricted and painful.
Joint Stability Tests	***Stress tests:*** Hypomobile with valgus and varus stress ***Joint play:*** MTP hypomobility will be noted.
Special Tests	Not applicable
Neurologic Screening	No remarkable findings
Vascular Screening	No remarkable findings
Functional Assessment	Restriction of first MTP extension alters terminal stance and the preswing phases of gait.
Imaging Techniques	Radiographs may reveal osteophytes.
Differential Diagnosis	Arthritis, sesamoiditis, sprain, hallux valgus, gout
Comments	Hallux rigidus often occurs bilaterally.

AROM = active range of motion; MMT = manual muscle test; MT = metatarsal; MTP = metatarsophalangeal; PROM = passive range of motion.

foot pain may be present secondary to compensatory forces. The subsequent loss in ROM affects the terminal stance and preswing phases of gait, which is visible during the functional assessment (see Fig. 8-1). With time, atrophy and associated weakness of the triceps surae will develop (Examination Findings 8-6).

A palpable and painful exostosis may develop on the dorsal aspect of the joint. Extension of the first MTP joint is limited by the phalanx striking the exostosis. Similar to what happens with arthritis, the joint is prone to pain and swelling, especially after activity. Radiographic examination is used to definitively diagnose this condition (Fig. 8-38).

Conservative treatment includes the use of passive ROM exercises to maintain extension in the joint and the use of orthotics to decrease hyperextension forces on the first MTP joint. Fit the patient with shoes having adequate depth and width to accommodate the increased bulk of the forefoot. A rocker sole boot may be prescribed to decrease joint motion.[16]

Corticosteroid injections assist in decreasing inflammation. If the condition progresses to the point where extension is limited and gait is affected, surgical intervention may be required. The most common surgical procedure, a cheilectomy, involves the removal of the distal dorsal aspect of the first MT and the superior half of the joint surface and other areas of exostosis.[116,117] Removal of the bone decreases pain and restores extension to the joint, allowing a more normal gait pattern.

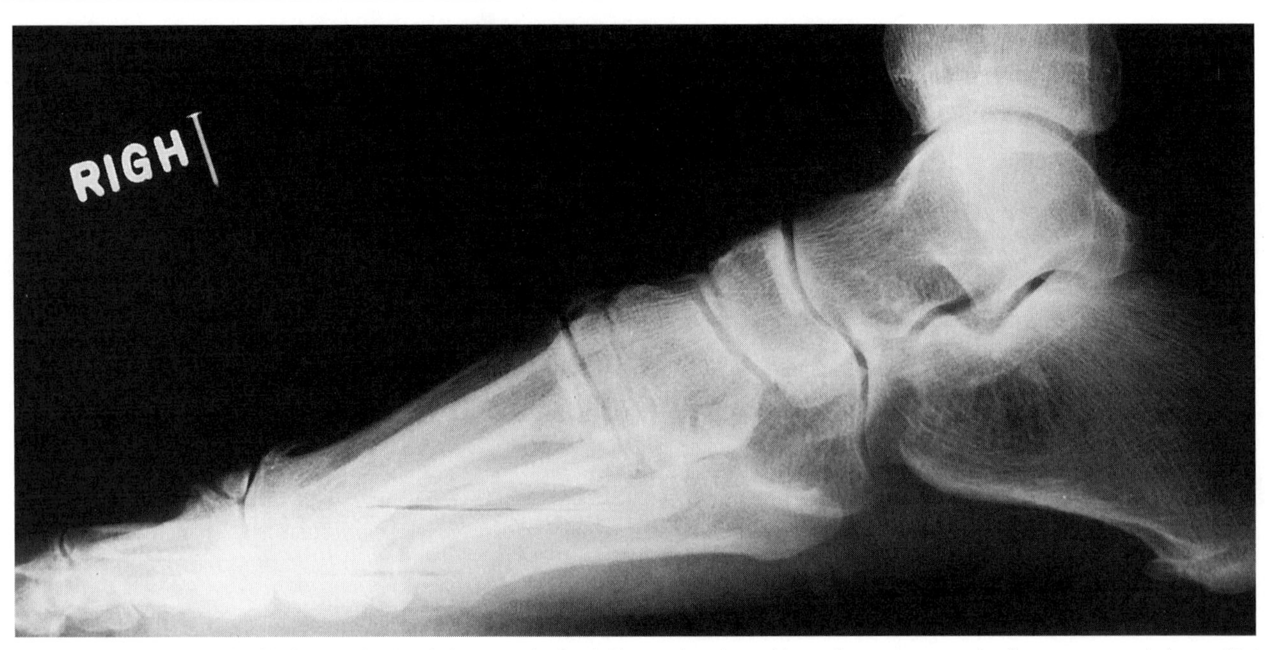

FIGURE 8-38 ■ Radiograph of hallux rigidus (medial view, right foot). The wedge-shaped bony formation over the first metatarsophalangeal joint serves as a mechanical block in limiting extension.

Hallux Valgus

A progressive degeneration and subluxation of the first MTP joint, hallux valgus is characterized by the joint angle being greater than 20 degrees in the frontal plane. As a result, the distal end of the first toe angles laterally, placing a valgus load on the MTP joint (see Inspection Findings 8-2). The valgus deformity may interfere with the function of the second toe. With time a bunion, the enlargement and subsequent ossification of the underlying bursa, will develop over the medial aspect of the joint, causing further pain and dysfunction (Examination Findings 8-7).

In the presence of hallux valgus, the amount of passive first MTP flexion and extension available is indicative of the potential success of surgical repair. Restriction into passive extension while manually maintaining the normal alignment of the great toe suggests that normal range of motion could not be restored by surgical realignment.[16]

Initial management of hallux valgus involves instructing the patient to wear shoes that can accommodate the deformity without increasing pressure on the medial toe.[119] A felt or foam pad can be inserted between the first and second toe to maintain normal alignment. Anti-inflammatory medications may be helpful in further reducing the symptoms.

First Metatarsophalangeal Joint Sprains

Sprains of the first MTP joint usually occur when the foot is planted and the ankle is subsequently dorsiflexed. As the shoe grasps the playing surface, body weight and forward momentum force the first MTP joint into hyperextension. Sprains of the plantar MTP joint capsule and/or the subsequent inflammatory response caused by repetitive hyperextension has been termed "**turf toe**" because of the reportedly high instance of this injury during competition on artificial turf.[120]

Pain in the joint during the push-off phase of gait, active joint motion, or manual resistance, or when attempting quick stops are common complaints of patients with first MTP joint sprains. The joint is painful to the touch and ROM is limited. A radiograph is needed to rule out fracture to the MT or phalanx.

Athletes, especially those who compete barefooted, are also susceptible to varus and valgus sprains of the MTP joints. A varus force is applied to the joint capsule and collateral ligaments when the toes are bent toward the body's midline. An outward bending results in a valgus force being placed on the capsule. On rare occasions, the MTP joint may dislocate.

Management of sprains of the first MTP involves removing aggravating stresses through the use of crutches, a firm shoe insole, or other immobilization device. The physician may prescribe the use of oral or injectable antiinflammatory medications.

Sesamoiditis

Two sesamoids lie within the tendon of the flexor hallucis brevis. These bones provide a mechanical advantage to great toe flexion and absorb and redirect weight-bearing forces. Each of the two FHB sesamoids lies in its own groove on the head of the first MT. As great toe extension increases,

Examination Findings 8-7
Hallux Valgus

Examination Segment	Clinical Findings
History	***Onset:*** Insidious ***Pain characteristics:*** Arising from the first MTP joint ***Mechanism:*** A prolonged valgus stress being placed on the first MTP joint ***Predisposing conditions:*** Improperly fitting shoes; wearing high heels Pes planus Congenital development Diseases such as cerebral palsy, rheumatoid arthritis, or osteoarthritis[118]
Inspection	Valgus angulation of the first toe The first and second toe may overlap. Bunion formation over the medial border of the first MTP joint
Palpation	The medial joint and sesamoids may be tender to the touch. Thickening of the synovial capsule may be noted.
Joint and Muscle Function Assessment	***AROM:*** Pain may be produced during flexion and extension. ***PROM:*** Pain may be produced during flexion and extension. ***MMT:*** Extensor hallucis longus is weak secondary to pain.
Joint Stability Tests	***Stress tests:*** Valgus and varus stress test ***Joint play:*** Hypermobility of the first ray
Special Tests	Not applicable
Neurologic Screening	No remarkable findings
Vascular Screening	No remarkable findings
Functional Assessment	Gait, especially toe-off, may be affected.
Imaging Techniques	Weight-bearing radiographs
Differential Diagnosis	Osteoarthritis, septic arthritis,[119] sesamoiditis, sprain, hallux rigidus, gout
Comments	The sesamoid bones on the plantar surface of the MTP joint may also dislocate. The toe deformity can cause footwear to fit improperly and alter biomechanics.[16]

AROM = active range of motion; MMT = manual muscle test; MTP = metatarsophalangeal; PROM = passive range of motion.

the sesamoids become less stable in their grooves, subjecting them to greater stresses.

Sesamoiditis, an irritation of the bones and soft tissue in the area, and sesamoid fractures are associated with both cavus and planus foot types. In the cavus foot, the sesamoids are subjected to increased forces from the more acute angle of the MT. In the planus foot, the sesamoids are compressed for prolonged periods while the foot attempts to push off on the relatively unstable surface. Bipartate sesamoids are present in up to 25% of the population, and should not be confused with sesamoid fractures on radiographs.[3]

Patients with sesamoid pathology complain of increased symptoms when on their toes, such as during dance or wearing high-heeled shoes, and during the push-off phase of gait (Examination Findings 8-8). Passive MTP extension is painful at end range. Walking on the lateral aspect of the foot to avoid push-off is a typical gait strategy used by those with sesamoid pain. Use of orthotics and appropriate footwear to dissipate forces is the initial intervention for individuals with sesamoid pain. If conservative treatment fails, surgical excision of the sesamoids is the next intervention.

Examination Findings 8-8
Sesamoiditis

Examination Segment	Clinical Findings
History	*Onset:* Acute or insidious *Pain characteristics:* Pain may be described as local to the sesamoids, or more general complaints of pain arising from the great toe may be reported. *Other symptoms:* Pain or snapping may be reported as the hallux extends during gait. The sensation of snapping or cracking may be reported in the event of a sesamoid fracture. *Mechanism:* Repetitive MTP extension, especially when weight bearing *Predisposing conditions:* Cavus or planus foot type
Inspection	Swelling may be noted, especially on the plantar and medial aspects of the joint. A plantarflexed first ray
Palpation	Point tenderness over the involved sesamoid(s)
Joint and Muscle Function Assessment	*AROM:* Pain moving into MTP extension *MMT:* Test for flexor hallucis longus produce pain and weakness secondary to irritation of the sesamoids *PROM:* Pain moving into MTP extension
Joint Stability Tests	*Stress tests:* Not applicable *Joint play:* Decreased MTP joint glide may be present secondary to joint effusion.
Special Tests	Not applicable
Neurologic Screening	Possible positive Tinel sign along the medial branch of the plantar digital nerve
Vascular Screening	No remarkable findings
Functional Assessment	Alteration of gait to avoid weight bearing on the sesamoids; gait may be altered to avoid extending the great toe during toe-off.
Imaging Techniques	AP, medial, and lateral oblique radiographs to rule out fracture CT scans can identify posttraumatic degeneration MRI helps differentiate between a bony stress reaction, fracture, or soft tissue inflammation.[121]
Differential Diagnosis	Sesamoid fracture, hallux valgus, capsular sprain, arthritis, gout, avascular necrosis, chondromalacia[122]
Comments	Edema, inflammation, or displacement of a bipartite sesamoid may place pressure on a digital nerve, producing radicular symptoms.

AP = anteroposterior; AROM = active range of motion; MMT = manual muscle test; PROM = passive range of motion.

Sesamoid fracture

Acute sesamoid fractures are usually the result of eccentric loading during extension and are often accompanied by a popping sensation followed by immediate inability to push-off on the involved great toe.[2] Localized swelling is evident on the plantar surface of the first MTP joint. Exquisite point tenderness is present, and the patient's gait is altered to keep the weight-bearing forces on the lateral portion of the foot.

The medial sesamoid fracture may fragment into as many as four parts. Clinically it is difficult to differentiate between a symptomatic bipartite sesamoid and a sesamoid fracture.[3] The definitive diagnosis of a fractured sesamoid is usually determined via radiographs. The shape and magnitude of comminuted fractures can be determined using 3D CT scans.[2]

Conservative treatment consists of protected weight bearing and the use of a metatarsal pad.[2] Removal, or sesamoidectomy, of the symptomatic sesamoid results in good outcomes if conservative treatment fails or aggressive management is indicated in the early stage of treatment.[123]

On-Field Evaluation of Foot Injuries

Although it is possible for an athlete to walk off the playing area with a fracture, especially if it involves the toes, significant trauma to the foot and toes usually results in the athlete's inability to bear weight without pain. The location of the pain and mechanism of injury act as a guide for on-field injury evaluation. Not all of the steps described in this section apply to all injuries.

With any sign or symptom indicating a bony fracture or joint dislocation, terminate the evaluation, splint the foot and ankle, and refer the athlete to a physician. The inability to bear weight without pain as well as the inability to push off or hop on the involved foot also indicates the need to keep the athlete from further competition. After the athlete is moved to the sideline or the sports medicine facility, the remaining evaluation proceeds, as described earlier in this chapter.

Equipment Considerations

Only the most severe cases, based on the degree of pain, reports of a "crack" or "pop," or obvious trauma such as bleeding through the shoe, warrant removal of the shoe or sock while the patient is on the playing surface. (Chapter 9 provides a description of removing footwear and ankle braces.)

On-Field History

Question the athlete about his or her history relating to the mechanism of injury, the location of the pain, any sounds associated with its onset, and the athlete's willingness and ability to bear weight on the injured limb. Pain may also radiate to the foot from the lumbar or sacral plexus or after trauma to the peroneal nerve or anterior compartment syndrome.

On-Field Inspection

Observe the posture of the athlete. Is the individual remaining down on the field or court or is the athlete hopping off or being assisted off the playing surface? The shoe itself will prohibit a direct inspection of the foot. If the footwear is removed while the athlete is still on the field, note the integrity of the joints, any gross deformity of the long bones, or the presence of gross swelling or discoloration.

If a significant injury such as a fracture or dislocation is evident during the initial inspection, perform a secondary survey to rule out the presence of unrecognized trauma. Then immobilize the body part and refer the athlete for medical evaluation.

On-Field Palpation

With the exceptions of the plantar and superior aspects of the calcaneus and the talus, the bones of the foot are relatively subcutaneous, assisting in the identification of crepitus or other deformities through palpation.

- **Bony palpation:** The presence of a fracture or dislocation must be ruled out:
  - Palpate the lengths of the five rays to rule out discontinuity in the bony shafts or joints.
  - Palpate the tarsals, calcaneus, talus, and the medial and lateral malleoli for point tenderness or crepitus that may indicate a gross or avulsion fracture or dislocation.
- **Soft tissue palpation:** The forces placed on the foot can be sufficient to significantly strain or rupture its tendons, fascia, or ligaments.
  - **Plantar fascia:** Palpate the length of the plantar fascia to identify areas of point tenderness. Pain arising from the medial calcaneal tubercle may signify a rupture of the plantar fascia.
  - **Anterior musculature:** Palpate the anterior musculature. Hyperplantarflexion of the ankle or an eccentric contraction of the tibialis anterior can result in a strain, rupture, or avulsion of its tendon, leading to tenderness of these structures. This mechanism may also result in a fracture of an accessory navicular.
  - **Medial musculature**: Palpate the tibialis posterior, flexor hallicus longus, and flexor digitorum longus, which pass posterior to the medial malleolus. These tendons may be impinged by eversion of the subtalar joint. The tibialis posterior may be strained secondary to an eccentric contraction following to an inversion mechanism.
  - **Posterior musculature**: Palpate the posterior musculature. Achilles tendon ruptures are common in activities that require explosive starts or eccentrically load the triceps surae muscles. (Refer to Chapter 9 for more information on this condition.)
  - **Lateral musculature**: Palpate the peroneal tendons as they pass posterior to the lateral malleolus. An inversion and plantarflexion mechanism followed by contraction of the peroneals can result in an avulsion of the peroneus brevis attachment from the styloid process of the fifth MT.

On-Field Range-of-Motion Tests

ROM testing during this phase of the evaluation is most likely limited to active flexion and extension of the toes, pronation and supination of the foot, and plantarflexion and dorsiflexion of the ankle. If these can be performed without pain or signs of a fracture or dislocation, the athlete can attempt to bear weight, as described in Chapter 3.

On-Field Management of Foot Injuries

Except in rare circumstances, most foot injuries do not require the athlete to be transported directly from the playing field to the hospital. Acute trauma such as Achilles tendon ruptures, ankle fractures, and ankle dislocations are discussed in Chapter 9.

Plantar Fascia Ruptures

Splint suspected plantar fascia ruptures with the foot and ankle in a slightly plantarflexed position or instruct the athlete not to bear weight. Fit the athlete with crutches and refer the individual to a physician or doctor of podiatric medicine.

Fractures and Dislocations

Remove athletes from the field in a non–weight-bearing manner if a fracture or dislocation is suspected. After further evaluating the athlete on the sideline, immobilize his or her foot, fit the athlete for crutches, render appropriate immediate treatment, and refer the patient to a physician.

REFERENCES

1. Huang, CK, et al: Biomechanical evaluation of longitudinal arch stability. *Foot Ankle*, 14:353, 1993.
2. Mouhsin, E, et al: Acute fractures of medial and lateral great toe sesamoids in an athlete. *Knee Surg Sports Traumatol Arthrosc*, 12:463, 2004.
3. Richardson, EG: Hallucal sesamoid pain: Causes and surgical treatment. *J Am Acad Orthop Surg*, 7:270, 1999.
4. Mueller, MJ: The ankle and foot complex. In Levangie, PK and Norkin, CC (eds): *Joint Structure and Function: A Comprehensive Analysis*, ed 4. Philadelphia, FA Davis, 2005, pp. 437–434.
5. Aldridge, T: Diagnosing heel pain in adults. *Am Fam Physician*, 70:332, 2004.
6. Kitaoka, HB, Luo, ZP, and An, K: Effect of plantar fasciotomy on stability of arch of foot. *Clin Orthop*, November:344, 1997.
7. Thordarson, DB, et al: Dynamic support of the human longitudinal arch. A biomechanical evaluation. *Clin Orthop*, July:165, 1995.
8. Kanatli, U, Yetkin, H, and Bolukbasi, S: Evaluation of the transverse metatarsal arch of the foot with gait analysis. *Arch Orthop Trauma Surg*, 123:148, 2003.
9. Gregg, EW, et al: Prevelence of lower-extremity disease in the US adult population ≥40 years of age with and without diabetes: 1999-2000 National Health and Nutrition Examination Survey. *Diabetes Care*, 26:1591, 2003.
10. Gefen, A, et al: Analysis of muscular fatigue and foot stability during high-heeled gait. *Gait Posture*, 15:56, 2002.
11. Esenyel, M, et al: Kinetics of high-heeled gait. *J Am Podiatr Med Assoc*, 93:27, 2003.
12. Payne, C: Sensitivity and specificity of the functional hallux limitus test to predict foot function. *J Am Podiatr Med Assoc*, 92:269-271,2002.
13. Sneyers, CJL, et al: Influence of malalignment of feet on the plantar pressure patterns in running. *Foot Ankle Int*, 16:624:1995.
14. Weinstein, A, and Berman, B: Topical treatment of common superficial tinea infections. *Am Fam Physician*, 65:2095, 2002.
15. Freeman, DB: Corns and calluses resulting from mechanical hyperkeratosis. *Am Fam Physician*, 65:2277, 2002.
16. Mann, RA: Disorders of the first metatarsophalangeal joint. *J Am Acad Orthop Surg*, 3:34-43, 1995.
17. Krivickas, LS: Anatomical factors associated with overuse sports injuries. *Sports Med*, 24:132, 1997.
18. Ogilvie-Harris, DJ, Carr, MM, and Fleming, PJ: The foot in ballet dancers: The importance of second toe length. *Foot Ankle Int*, 16:144, 1995.
19. Grebing, BR, and Coughlin, MJ: Evaluation of Morton's theory of second metatarsal hypertrophy. *J Bone Joint Surg*, 86(A): 1375, 2004.
20. Acevedo, JI, and Beskin, JL: Complications of plantar fascia rupture associated with corticosteroid injection. *Foot Ankle Int*, 19:91, 1998.
21. Klaue, K, Hansen, ST, and Masquelet, AC: Clinical, quantitative assessment of first tarsometatarsal mobility in the sagittal plane and its relation to hallux valgus deformity. *Foot Ankle*, 15:9, 1994.
22. Tiberio, D: Pathomechanics of structural foot deformities. *Phys Ther*, 68:1840, 1988.
23. Razeghi, M, and Batt, ME: Foot type classification: A critical review of current methods. *Gait Posture*, 15:282, 2002.
24. Smith-Oricchio, K, and Harris, BA: Interrater reliability of subtalar neutral, calcaneal inversion and eversion. *J Orthop Sports Phys Ther*, 21:10, 1990.
25. Picciano, AM, Rowlands, MS, and Worrell, T: Reliability of open and closed kinetic chain subtalar joint neutral positions and navicular drop test. *J Orthop Sport Phys Ther*, 18:553; 1993.
26. Buchanan, KR, and Davis, I: The relationship between forefoot, midfoot, and rearfoot static alignment in pain-free individuals. *J Orthop Sports Phys Ther*, 35:559, 2005.
27. Elveru, RA, et al: Methods for taking subtalar joint measurements. *Phys Ther*, 68:678, 1988.
28. Scll, KE, et al: Two measurement techniques for assessing subtalar joint position: A reliability study. *J Orthop Sports Phys Ther*, 19:162, 1994.
29. Glasoe, WM, et al: Comparison of two methods used to assess first-ray mobility. *Foot Ankle Int*, 23:248, 2002.
30. Glascoe, WM, et al: Criterion-related validity of a clinical measure of dorsal first ray mobility. *J Orthop Sports Phys Ther*, 35:589, 2005.
31. Incel, NA, et al: Muscle imbalance in hallux valgus: An electromyographic study. *Am J Phys Med Rehabil*. 82:345, 2003.
32. Buckley, RE, and Hunt, DV: Reliability of clinical measurement of subtalar joint movement. *Foot Ankle Int*, 18:229, 1997.
33. Saltzman, CL, Nawoczenski, DA, and Talbot, KD: Measurement of the medial longitudinal arch. *Arch Phys Med Rehabil*, 76:45, 1995.
34. Allen, MK, and Glasoe, WM: Metrecom measurement of navicular drop in subjects with anterior cruciate ligament injury. *J Athl Train*, 35:403, 2000.
35. Kulik, SA, and Clanton, TO: Tarsal coalition. *Foot Ankle Int*, 18:286, 1996.
36. Borton, DC, and Saxby, TS: Tear of the plantar calcaneonavicular (spring) ligament causing flatfoot. A case report. *J Bone Joint Surg Br*, 79:641, 1997.
37. Rule, J, Yao, L, and Seeger, LL: Spring ligament of the ankle: Normal MR anatomy. *Am J Roentgenol*, 161:1241, 1993.
38. Kitaoka, HB, Luo, Z, and An, K: Three-dimensional analysis of flatfoot deformity: Cadaver study. *Foot Ankle Int*, 19:447, 1998.
39. Miller, TT: Painful accessory bones of the foot. *Semin Musculoskel Imaging*, 6:153, 2002.

40. Menz, HB, and Munteanu, SE: Validity of 3 clinical techniques for the measurement of static foot posture in older people. *J Orthop Sport Phys Ther*, 35:279, 2005.
41. Hewett, TE, Myer, GD, and Ford, KV: Anterior cruciate ligament injuries in female athletes. Part 1, mechanisms and risk factors. *Am J Sport Med*, 34:299, 2006.
42. Brody, D: Techniques in the evaluation and treatment of the injured runner. *Orthop Clin North Am*, 13:542, 1982.
43. Mueller, MJ, Host, JV, and Norton, BJ: Navicular drop as a composite measure of excessive pronation. *J Am Podiatr Med Assoc*, 83:198, 1993.
44. Ramcharitar, SI, Koslow, P, and Simpson, DM: Lower extremity manifestations of neuromuscular diseases. *Clin Podiatr Med Surg*, 15:705, 1998.
45. Carpintero, P, et al: The relationship between pes cavus and idiopathic scoliosis. *Spine*, 19:1260, 1994.
46. Burns, J, et al: The effect of pes cavus on foot pain and plantar pressure. *Clin Biomech*, 20:877, 2005.
47. Zhu, F, et al: Chronic plantar fasciitis: Acute changes in the heel after extracorporeal high-energy shock wave therapy—Observations at MR imaging. *Radiology*, 234:206, 2005.
48. Akfirat, M, Sen, C, and Gunes, T: Ultrasonic appearance of the plantar fasciitis. *J Clin Imaging*, 27:353, 2003.
49. Cole, C, Seto, C, and Gazewood, J: Plantar fasciitis: Evidence-based review of diagnosis and therapy. *Am Fam Physician*, 72:2237, 2005.
50. Sammarco, GJ, and Helfrey, RB: Surgical treatment of recalcitrant plantar fasciitis. *Foot Ankle Int*, 17:520, 1996.
51. Powell, M, et al: Effective treatment of plantar fasciitis with dorsiflexion night splints: A crossover prospective randomized outcomes study. *Foot Ankle Int*, 19:10, 1998.
52. Kibler, WB, Goldberg, C, and Chandler, TJ: Functional biomechanical deficits in running athletes with plantar fasciitis. *Am J Sports Med*, 19:66, 1991.
53. De Garceau, D, et al: The association between diagnosis of plantar fasciitis and windlass test. *Foot Ankle Int*, 24:251, 2003.
54. DiGiovanni, BF, et al: Plantar fascia-specific stretching exercise improves outcomes in patients with chronic plantar fasciitis. *J Bone Joint Surg*, 88(A):1775, 2006.
55. Osborne, HR, and Allison, GT: Treatment of plantar fasciitis by low-Dye taping and iontophoresis – short-term results of a double blinded, randomized placebo controlled clinical trial of dexamethasone and acetic acid. *Br J Sports Med*, 40:545, 2006.
56. Kudo, P, et al: Randomized, placebo-controlled, double-blind clinical trial evaluating the treatment of plantar fasciitis with an extracorporeal shockwave therapy (ESWT) device: A North American confirmatory study. *J Orthop Res*, 24:115, 2006.
57. Saxena, A, and Fullem, B: Plantar fascia rupture in athletes. *Am J Sports Med*, 32:662, 2004.
58. Bailie, DS, and Kelikian, AS: Tarsal tunnel syndrome: Diagnosis, surgical technique, and functional outcome. *Foot Ankle Int*, 19:65, 1998.
59. Prichasuk, S, and Subhadrabandhu, T: The relationship of pes planus and calcaneal spur to plantar heel pain. *Clin Orthop*, Sept:192, 1994.
60. Leach, RE, Seavey, MS, and Salter, DK: Results of surgery in athletes with plantar fasciitis. *Foot Ankle Int*, 7:156, 1986.
61. Riepert, T, et al: Estimation of sex on the basis of radiographs of the calcaneus. *Forensic Sci Int*, 77:133, 1996.
62. Stormont, DM, and Peterson, HA: The relative incidence of tarsal coalition. *Clin Orthop*, 181:24, 1983.
63. Clarke, DM: Multiple tarsal coalitions in the same foot. *J Pediatr Orthop*, 17:777, 1997.
64. Kelo, MJ, and Riddle, DL: Examination and management of a patient with tarsal coalition. *Phys Ther*, 78:518, 1998.
65. Varner, KE, and Michelson, JD: Tarsal coalition in adults. *Foot Ankle Int*, 21:669, 2000.
66. Vincent, KA: Tarsal coalition and painful flatfoot. *J Am Acad Orthop Surg*, 6:274, 1998.
67. O'Neill, DB, and Micheli, LJ: Tarsal coalition: A followup of adolescent athletes. *Am J Sports Med*, 17:544, 1989.
68. Kinoshita, M, et al: The dorsiflexion-eversion test for diagnosis of tarsal tunnel syndrome. *J Bone Joint Surg*, 83(A):1835, 2001.
69. Frey, C: Magnetic resonance imaging and the evaluation of tarsal tunnel syndrome. *Foot Ankle Int*, 14:159, 1993.
70. Mann, RA: Tarsal tunnel syndrome. In Mann, RA, and Coughlin, MJ (eds): *Surgery of the Foot and Ankle*. St. Louis, Mosby-Year Book, 1993, p. 554.
71. Jackson, DL, and Haglund, B: Tarsal tunnel syndrome in athletes. Case reports and literature review. *Am J Sports Med*, 19:61, 1991.
72. Stefko, RM, Lauerman, WC, and Heckman, JD: Tarsal tunnel syndrome caused by an unrecognized fracture of the posterior process of the talus (Cedell fracture). *J Bone Joint Surg Am*, 76:116, 1994.
73. Sammarco, GJ, Chalk, DE, and Feibel, JH: Tarsal tunnel syndrome and additional nerve lesions in the same limb. *Foot and Ankle*, 14:71, 1993.
74. Myerson, MS, and Berger, BI: Nonunion of a fracture of the sustentaculum tali causing a tarsal tunnel syndrome: A case report. *Foot Ankle Int*, 16:740, 1995.
75. Sammarco, GJ, and Conti, SF: Tarsal tunnel syndrome caused by an anomalous muscle. *J Bone Joint Surg Am*, 76:1308, 1994.
76. Kanbe, K, et al: Entrapment neuropathy of the deep peroneal nerve associated with the extensor hallicus brevis. *J Foot Ankle Surg*, 34:560, 1995.
77. Kinoshita, M, et al: The dorsiflexion-eversion test for diagnosis of tarsal tunnel syndrome. *J Bone Joint Surg*, 83(A):1835, 2001.
78. Daniels, TR, Lau, JT, and Hearn, TC: The effects of foot position and load on tibial nerve tension. *Foot Ankle Int*, 19:73, 1998.
79. Masciocchi, C, Catalucci, A, and Barile, A: Ankle impingement syndromes. *Eur J Radiol*, 27(S1):S70, 1998.
80. Mann, RA, and Baxter, DE: Diseases of the nerves. In Mann, RA, and Coughlin, MJ (eds): *Surgery of the Foot and Ankle*, ed 6. St Louis, CV Mosby, 1992, p. 543.
81. Sharkey, NA, et al: Strain and loading of the second metatarsal during heel-lift. *J Bone Joint Surg Am*, 77:1050, 1995.
82. Wolf, SK: Diabetes mellitus and predisposition to athletic pedal fracture. *J Foot Ankle Surg*, 37:16, 1998.
83. Kavanaugh, JH, et al: The Jones' fracture revisited. *J Bone Joint Surg*, 60A:776, 1978.
84. Weiner, BD, Linder, JF, and Giattini, JF: Treatment of fractures of the fifth metatarsal: A prospective study. *Foot Ankle Int*, 18:267, 1997.
85. Clapper, MF, O'Brien, TJ, and Lyons, PM: Fractures of the fifth metatarsal: Analysis of a fracture registry. *Clin Orthop*, June: 238, 1995.
86. Mologne, TS, et al: Early screw fixation versus casting in the treatment of acute Jones fractures. *Am J Sports Med*, 33:970, 2005.

87. Brukner, P, et al: Stress fractures: A review of 180 cases. *Clin J Sport Med*, 6:85, 1996.
88. Weinfeld, SB, Haddad, SL, and Myerson, MS: Metatarsal stress fractures. *Clin Sports Med*, 16:319, 1997.
89. Kaye, RA: Insufficiency stress fractures of the foot and ankle in postmenopausal women. *Foot Ankle Int*, 19:221, 1998.
90. Muthukumar, T, Butt, SH, and Cassar-Pullicino, VN: Stress fractures and related disorders in foot and ankle: Plain films scintigraphy, CT, and MR imaging. *Semin Musculoskel Radiol*, 9:210, 2005.
91. Sands, AK, and Grose, A: Lisfranc injuries. *Injury, Int J Care Injured*, 35:S-B71, 2004.
92. Perron, AD, Brady, W, and Keats, TE: Orthopedic pitfalls in the ED: Lisfranc fracture-dislocation. *Am J Emerg Med*, 19:71, 2001.
93. Rajapakse, B, Edwards, A, and Hont, T: A single surgeon's experience of treatment of Lisfranc joint injury. *Injury, Int J Care Injured*, 37:914, 2006.
94. Hatem, SF, Davis, A, and Sundaram, M: Midfoot sprain: Lisfranc ligament disruption. *Orthopedics*, 28:75, 2005.
95. Talarico, RH, et al: Fracture dislocations of the tarsometatarsal joints: Analysis of interrater reliability in using the modified Hardcastle Classification System. *J Foot Ank Surg*, 45:300, 2006.
96. Kavanagh, EC, and Zoga, AC: MRI of trauma to the foot and ankle. *Semin Musculoskel Imag*, 10:308, 2006.
97. Ly, TV, and Coetzee, JC: Treatment of primarily ligamentous Lisfranc joint injuries: Primary arthrodesis compared with open reduction and internal fixation. *J Bone Joint Surg*, 88(A):514, 2006.
98. Thompson, FM, and Deland, JT: Occurrence of two interdigital neuromas in one foot. *Foot Ankle*, 14:15, 1993.
99. Frank, PW, Bakkum, BW, and Darby, SA: The communicating branch of the lateral plantar nerve: a descriptive anatomic study. *Clin Anat*, 9:237, 1996.
100. Wu, KK: Morton's interdigital neuroma: A clinical review of its etiology, treatment, and results. *J Foot Ankle Surg*, 35:112, 1996.
101. Bourke, G, Owen, J, and Machet, D: Histological comparison of the third interdigital nerve in patients with Morton's metatarsalgia and control patients. *Aust N Z J Surg*, 64:421, 1994.
102. Levine, SE, et al: Ultrasonographic diagnosis of recurrence after excision of an interdigital neuroma. *Foot Ankle Int*, 19:79, 1998.
103. Holmes, GB: Quantitative determination of intermetatarsal pressure. *Foot Ankle*, 13:532, 1992.
104. Mulder, JD: The causative mechanism in Morton's metatarsalgia. *J Bone Joint Surg*, 33(B):94-5,1951.
105. Sobiesk, GA, et al: Sonographic evaluation of interdigital neuromas. *J Foot Ankle Surg*, 36:364, 1997.
106. Bennett, GL, Graham, CE, and Mauldin, DM: Morton's interdigital neuroma: A comprehensive treatment protocol. *Foot Ankle Int*, 16:760, 1995.
107. Nunan, PJ, and Giesy, BD: Management of Morton's neuroma in athletes. *Clin Podiatr Med Surg*, 14:489, 1997.
108. Rasmussen, MR, Kitaoka, HB, and Patzer, GL: Nonoperative treatment of plantar interdigital neuroma with a single corticosteroid injection. *Clin Orthop*, May:188, 1996.
109. Coughlin, MJ, and Pinsonneault, T: Operative treatment of interdigital neuroma: A long-term follow-up study. *J Bone Joint Surg*, 83(A):1321, 2001.
110. Vanore, JV, and Corey, SV: Hallux limitus, rigidus, and metatarso-phalangeal joint arthrosis. In Marchinko, DE (ed): *Comprehensive Textbook of Hallus Abducto Valgus Reconstruction*. Chicago, Mosby, 1993, pp. 209–221.
111. Ahn, TK, et al: Kinematics and contact characteristics of the first metatarsophalangeal joint. *Foot Ankle Int*, 18:170, 1997.
112. Camasta, CA: Hallux limitus and hallux rigidus: Clinical examination, radiographic findings, and natural history. *Clin Podiatr Med Surg*, 13:432, 1996.
113. Weinfeld, SB, and Schon, LC: Hallux metatarsophalangeal arthritis. *Clin Orthop*, Apr:9, 1998.
114. Lichniak, JE: Hallux limitus in the athlete. *Clin Podiatr Med Surg*, 14:407, 1997.
115. Coughlin, M, and Shurnas, P: Presentation at the Advanced Foot and Ankle Course, San Francisco, May 23–25, 2002.
116. Mackay, DC, Blyth, M, and Rymaszewski, LA: The role of cheilectomy in the treatment of hallux rigidus. *J Foot Ankle Surg*, 36:337, 1997.
117. Iqbal, MJ, and Chana, GS: Arthroscopic cheilectomy for hallux rigidus. *Arthroscopy*, 14:307, 1998.
118. Marchinko, DE: The complex deformity known as hallux abducto valgus. In Marchinko, DE (ed): *Comprehensive Textbook of Hallus Abducto Valgus Reconstruction*. Chicago, CV Mosby, 1993, pp. 1–5.
119. Paige, NM, and Nouvong, A: The top 10 things foot and ankle specialists wish every primary care physician knew. *Mayo Clin Proc*, 81:818, 2006.
120. Tewes, DP, et al: MRI findings of acute turf toe. A case report and review of anatomy. *Clin Orthop*, July:200, 1994.
121. Ashman, CJ, Klecker, RJ, and Yu, JS: Forefoot pain involving the metatarsal region: Differential diagnosis with MR imaging. *RadioGraphics*, 21:1425, 2001.
122. Kanatli, U, et al: Absence of the medial sesamoid bone associated with metatarsophalangeal pain. *Clin Anat*, 19:634, 2006.
123. Lee, S, et al: Evaluation of hallux alignment and functional outcome after isolated tibial sesamoidectomy. *Foot Ankle Int*, 26:803, 2005.

CHAPTER 9

Ankle and Leg Pathologies

The ankle's muscular, capsular, and bony structures must absorb and dissipate normal and abnormal forces. Ankle sprains are frequently cited as the most common sports-related injuries and have a high reinjury rate secondary to chronic laxity of the ligaments and/or the subsequent loss of the joint's sense of position caused by injury to proprioceptors.[1,2] Seemingly minor injuries, such as contusions, can have severe consequences resulting from compression of the neurovascular structures of the ankle, foot, and toes. Trauma or dysfunction of the ankle and leg muscles can lead to biomechanical changes, causing gait deviations that lead to further injury. Different foot types are associated with gait pattern deviations that may redistribute stresses on bones and demands on the muscles of the lower extremity Discussion and examination of the ankle must also include the rearfoot, midfoot, and fifth metatarsal (MT) because of the ligamentous and muscular attachments to these structures (Chapter 8).

Clinical Anatomy

The leg is formed by the tibia and fibula (Fig. 9-1). A normal anatomic relationship between the tibia and fibula is required for proper biomechanics of the knee proximally and the ankle and foot distally. These bones function to distribute the weight-bearing forces along the limb, allowing the junction of the distal tibia, fibula and talus, the **ankle mortise**, to produce the range of motion (ROM) needed for walking and running (Fig. 9-2).

Confusion exists when the terms inversion and eversion are used to describe the motion of the foot and ankle. Motions of the subtalar and talocrural joints are described either by their individual single cardinal plane nature (inversion/eversion, dorsiflexion/plantarflexion, or abduction/adduction) or by the composite motions of pronation and supination that occur around an oblique axis. Pronation comprises dorsiflexion, abduction, and eversion, with supination resulting from plantarflexion, adduction and inversion (see Table 8-1). Closed-chain pronation causes internal tibial rotation, knee flexion, and internal rotation of the femur at the hip. Closed-chain supination results in external tibial rotation, knee extension, and external rotation at the hip.

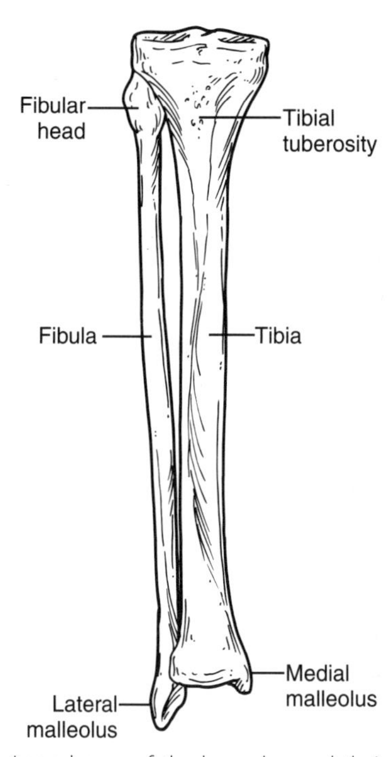

FIGURE 9-1 ■ Long bones of the lower leg and their primary bony landmarks.

The **tibia** is the primary weight-bearing bone of the leg. Its slightly concave distal articular surface forms the roof of the ankle mortise; the medial malleolus forms the shallow medial border of the mortise and provides a broad site for the attachment of the **deltoid ligaments**.

Many of the muscles acting on the ankle, foot, and toes originate off the anterolateral and posterior borders of the tibial shaft. The relatively flat anteromedial border is covered only by skin, predisposing the periosteum to contusions in

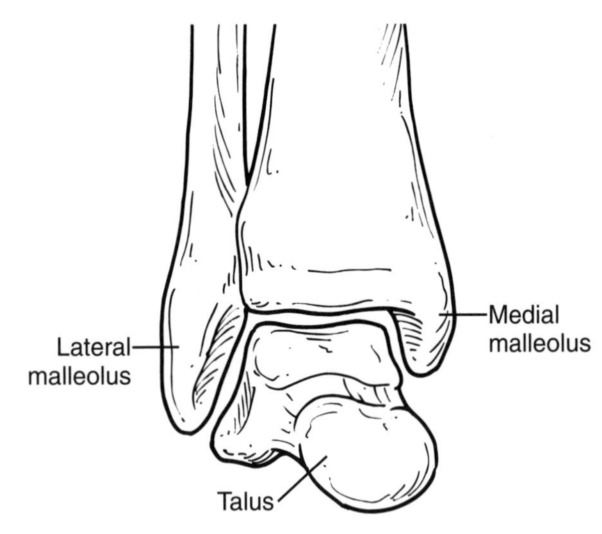

FIGURE 9-2 ■ Ankle mortise—the articulation formed by the distal articular surface of the tibia and its medial malleolus, the fibula's lateral malleolus, and the talus.

this area. The periosteum of the tibial shaft may become inflamed at the sites of muscular attachment secondary to overuse syndromes. The **interosseous membrane** arises off the length of the lateral tibial border and attaches to the length of the medial fibula, binding the bones together.

Lateral to the tibia is the **fibula**. A long, thin bone, the fibula (1) serves as a site of muscular origin and attachment, (2) serves as a site of ligamentous attachment, (3) provides lateral stability to the ankle mortise, and (4) serves as a pulley to increase the efficiency of the muscles that run posteriorly to it.

The amount of force transmitted through the fibula has been reported to range from 0 to 12% of the total body weight.[3,4] Clinically, the percentage of body weight carried along this bone is inconsequential because the end result is that trauma to the fibula decreases its ability to serve in its previously described roles.

With the exception of the fibular head, the upper two thirds of the fibular shaft is protected by overlying muscle. The peroneal nerve, which innervates the leg's anterior and lateral compartments, is closely associated with the fibular head (Fig. 9-3). Protected only by skin, the common peroneal nerve passes posterior to the fibular head, making it vulnerable to injury at this site. The distal one third of the fibula, a common fracture site, becomes more superficial and begins to thin immediately proximal to the lateral malleolus.

The lateral malleolus provides a site of attachment for the lateral ankle ligaments. The lateral malleolus extends farther distally than the medial malleolus does, forming the lateral wall of the ankle mortise. The lateral malleolus is mechanically superior at limiting eversion than the medial malleolus is at limiting inversion due to its greater length and anterior position. The lateral ankle is a common site for sprains, possibly resulting in avulsion of the ligaments from the lateral malleolus, especially when the ankle is inverted.

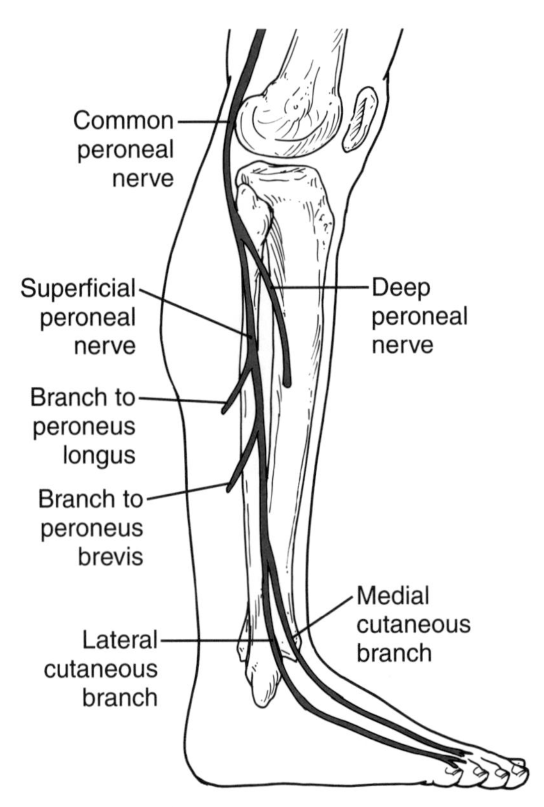

FIGURE 9-3 ■ Path of the peroneal nerve. The common peroneal nerve courses behind the fibular head, exposing it to potential injury. Trauma at this site causes a weakness in eversion and dorsiflexion.

The superior articulating portion of the **talus**, the **trochlea**, is quadrilateral in shape and almost entirely covered with articular cartilage. Its anterior surface is broader than its posterior surface (Fig. 9-4). The medial and lateral borders of the talus articulate with the corresponding malleoli. The superior talar surface is concave, creating a snug articulation with the slightly convex shape of the distal tibia.[5] Its inferior surface articulates with the calcaneus, forming the subtalar joint.

Related Bony Structures

The insertion of the Achilles tendon on the **calcaneal tubercle** provides the foot with a mechanical advantage. Forming a long lever arm, the calcaneus provides increased power during gait (see Fig. 8–1). The large body of the calcaneus also provides a site of attachment for some of the ankle's ligaments.

The **navicular** bone is located anterior to the talus along the foot's medial arch. This bone serves as one of the insertion sites for the tibialis posterior muscle. It also supports the medial longitudinal arch via the plantar calcaneonavicular ("spring") ligament. Positioned along the lateral longitudinal arch, the **cuboid** is anterior to the calcaneus. The base of the **fifth metatarsal** articulates with the anterolateral portion of

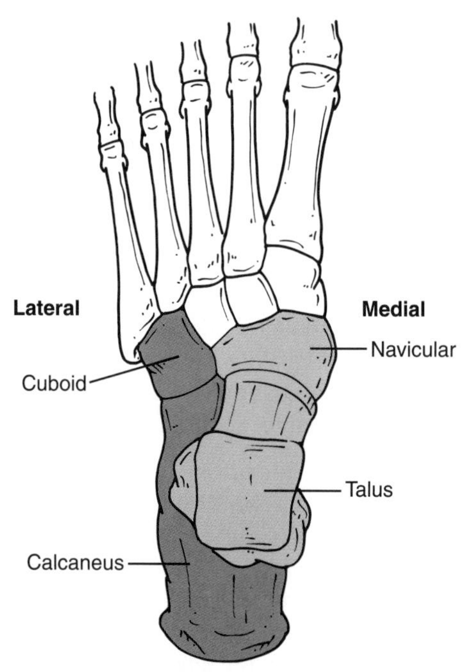

FIGURE 9-4 ■ View of the superior articular surface of the talus (left foot). Its wide anterior edge fits tightly in the mortise when the ankle is dorsiflexed.

the cuboid. The fifth MT serves as the site of attachment for the peroneus brevis and, along with the cuboid, provides a passageway for the route of the peroneus longus along the foot's plantar aspect.

Articulations and Ligamentous Support

Isolated movements of a single joint in a single plane do not occur during functional movements of the ankle complex. Pure uniplanar injuries are almost nonexistent because of the ankle's intimate anatomic relationship with the structures of the foot. The majority of injuries to the ankle involve the lateral structures, resulting from an inversion stress accompanied by plantarflexion of the foot.

Talocrural joint

Formed by the articulation between the talus, tibia, and fibula, the talocrural joint is a close-fitting articulation, especially as it nears its **closed-packed position** of full dorsiflexion. A modified **synovial hinge joint**, the talocrural articulation has one degree of freedom of movement: dorsiflexion and plantarflexion. The axis of rotation runs obliquely, connecting the points just distal to the inferior tips of the lateral and medial malleolus (Fig. 9-5).

The talocrural joint is surrounded by a joint capsule that is thicker posteriorly than anteriorly. Most of the ligaments described in this section are actually areas of increased density in the capsule. Tearing of the ankle ligaments usually results in damage to the joint capsule and irritation of the synovial lining,[5] with the exception of the calcaneofibular ligament, which is extracapsular.

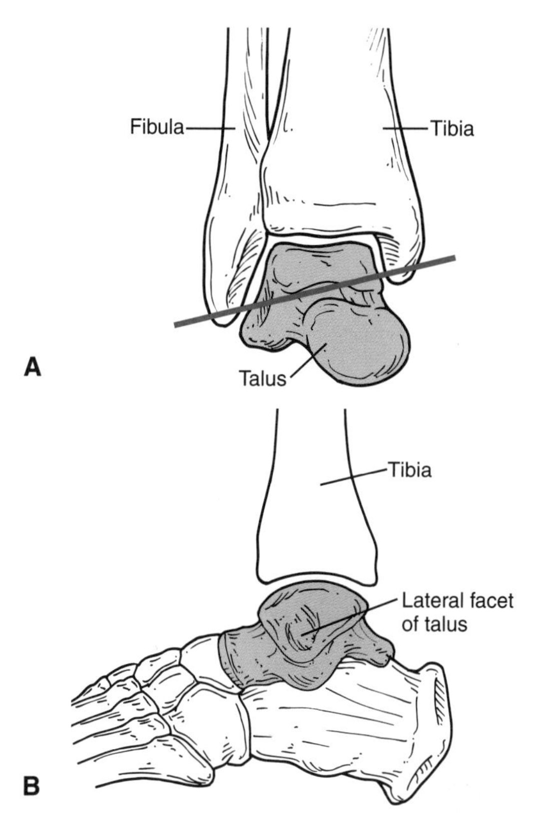

FIGURE 9-5 ■ The right talocrural joint in the (A) transverse and (B) frontal planes. The axis of motion in the transverse plane is indicated.

When non–weight-bearing the joint's ligamentous and tendinous structures are the primary restraints limiting rotation and translation of the talus within the ankle mortise. When weight-bearing the architecture of the joint's articular surfaces limit these motions.[6]

Lateral ankle ligaments. Three ligaments provide lateral support to the talocrural joint so that at least one is taut regardless of the relative position of the talocalcaneal unit (Fig. 9-6). The **anterior talofibular (ATF) ligament** originates off the anterolateral surface of the lateral malleolus, following a path to the talus near the sinus tarsi. The ATF is oriented parallel to the long axis of the leg when the foot is plantarflexed.[7] This ligament is tight during plantarflexion, limiting anterior translation of the talus on the tibia, and resists inversion and internal rotation of the talus within the mortise.

The **calcaneofibular (CF) ligament** is an extracapsular structure with an attachment on the outermost portion of the lateral malleolus. It courses inferiorly and posteriorly to its insertion on the calcaneus.[8] The CF ligament is the primary restraint of talar inversion within the midrange of talocrural motion.

Arising from the posterior portion of the lateral malleolus, the **posterior talofibular (PTF) ligament** takes an

Closed-packed position The point in a joint's range of motion at which its bones are maximally congruent; the most stable position of a joint.

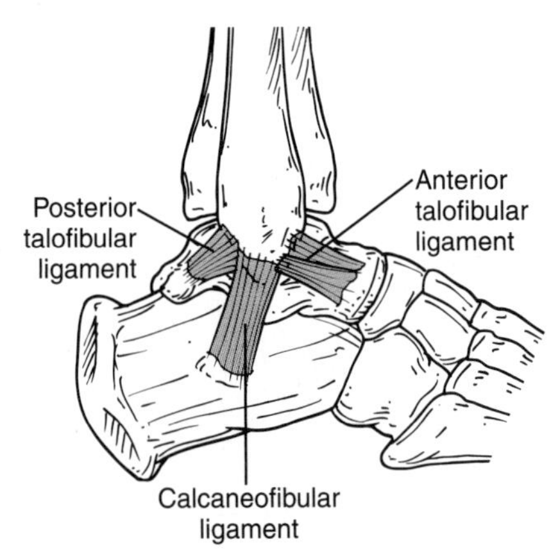

FIGURE 9-6 ■ Lateral ankle ligaments. The calcaneofibular ligament is an extracapsular structure; the anterior and posterior talofibular ligaments are thickenings in the joint capsule.

inferior and posterior course to attach on the talus and calcaneus. This is the deepest and strongest of the three lateral ligaments and is responsible for limiting posterior displacement of the talus on the tibia.

Medial ankle ligaments. Four individual ligaments collectively form the **deltoid ligament** that supports the medial aspect of the ankle (Fig. 9-7). The **anterior tibiotalar (ATT) ligament** originates off the anteromedial portion of the tibia's malleolus and inserts on the superior portion of the medial talus. The **tibiocalcaneal (TC) ligament** arises from the apex of the medial malleolus to attach on the calcaneus directly below the medial malleolus. The **posterior tibiotalar (PTT) ligament** spans the posterior aspect of the medial malleolus, attaching on the posterior portion of the talus. As a group, these three ligaments prevent eversion of the talus. The **tibionavicular (TN) ligament** runs beneath and slightly posterior to the ATT ligament, inserting on the medial surface of the navicular to limit lateral translation and lateral rotation of the tibia on the foot. The ATT and TN ligaments are taut when the subtalar joint is plantarflexed. The TC and PTT ligaments tighten during dorsiflexion.

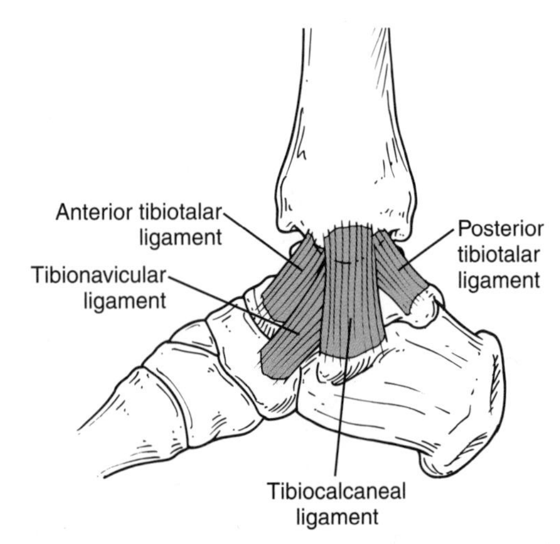

FIGURE 9-7 ■ Medial deltoid ankle ligament group showing the four individual ligaments.

The subtalar joint

The subtalar, or talocalcaneal, joint provides 1 degree of freedom of movement around a single oblique axis. The motions of the subtalar joint, the talocrural joint, and the midtarsal joints combine to produce the functional motions of pronation and supination. The incongruent nature of the subtalar joint makes isolated cardinal plane movement impossible, although calcaneal motion is frequently described as either inversion or eversion, the most observable component of pronation and supination. (Chapter 8 provides more information about the subtalar joint.)

Distal tibiofibular syndesmosis

The integrity of the ankle mortise relies on the functional relationship between the tibia and fibula. This union is a **syndesmosis joint** in which a convex facet on the fibula is buffered from a concave tibial facet by dense, fatty tissue. The syndesmosis is maintained by the inferior **anterior and posterior tibiofibular (tib-fib) ligaments**, and an extension of the interosseous membrane the **crural interosseous (CI) ligament** (Fig. 9-8).[5,9]

This structural arrangement allows for rotation and slight spreading of the mortise while still maintaining joint stability and allowing the fibula to glide inferiorly during weight bearing, deepening the ankle mortise and tightening the interosseous membrane.[5] The CI ligament functions as a fulcrum to motion at the lateral malleolus, so a small amount of malleolar movement results in a large amount of movement at the tibiofibular joint.[10] During dorsiflexion, the distal fibula moves laterally away from the tibia and glides superiorly, bringing the interosseous membrane and tibiofibular ligaments into a more horizontal alignment. When the ankle is plantarflexed, the fibula is

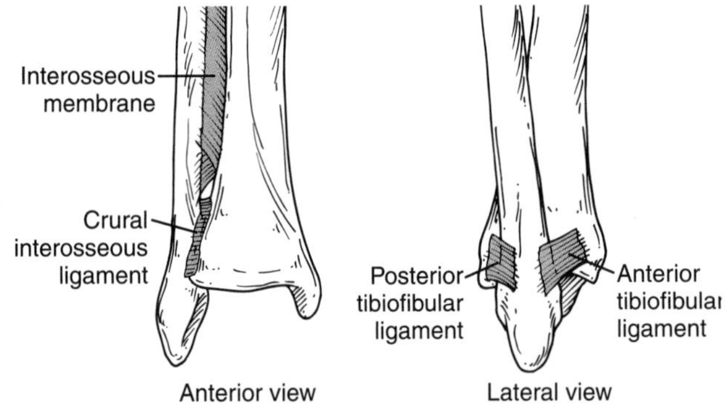

FIGURE 9-8 ■ Distal tibiofibular syndesmosis of the right ankle with the talus removed for clarity. The anterior view shows the role of the interosseous membrane and the crural interosseous ligament in maintaining lateral restraint of the fibula. The lateral view shows the role of the tibiofibular ligaments in preventing anterior and posterior displacement of the fibula on the tibia.

Syndesmosis joint A relatively immobile joint in which two bones are bound together by ligaments.

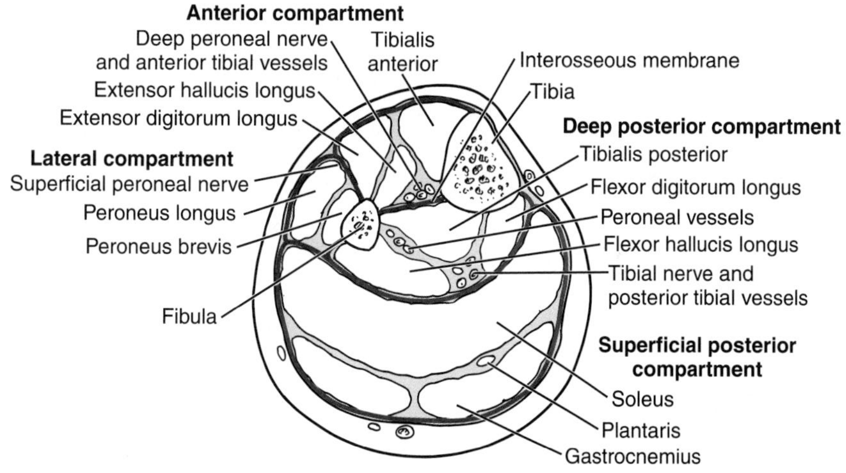

FIGURE 9-9 ■ Cross section of the left leg, indicating the muscles and neurovascular structures located in each of the four compartments. "Vessels" refer to the associated artery, vein, and lymphatic vessel.

pulled inferiorly and medially toward the tibia and the ligamentous structures take a vertical alignment, with the CI ligament acting as a spring to reunite the bones.[5,11] Forced eversion or dorsiflexion can result in a widening of the ankle mortise, with possible injury to the ligaments supporting the syndesmosis.

Interosseous membrane

The interosseous membrane, a strong fibrous tissue acting to fixate the fibula to the tibia, also serves as part of the origin for many of the muscles acting on the foot and ankle. A small proximal opening allows passage of the deep peroneal nerve and anterior tibial artery to pass through. Distally, the membrane blends into the anterior and posterior tibiofibular ligaments to support the distal tibiofibular syndesmosis joint.

Muscles of the Leg and Ankle

The leg is divided into four compartments: the anterior, lateral, superficial posterior, and deep posterior (Fig. 9-9). Each compartment contains muscles, nerves, and blood vessels that are tightly encased by fascial linings. Because of this fixed volume, intracompartmental injury can result in the accumulation of fluids that increase the pressure within the compartment, obstructing the flow of blood to and from the area and placing pressure on the nerves. The action, origin, insertion, and innervation of each muscle are described in Table 9-1.

Anterior compartment structures

The muscles of the anterior compartment, the tibialis anterior, the extensor hallucis longus (EHL), the extensor digitorum longus (EDL), and the peroneus tertius all act as dorsiflexors at the ankle (Fig. 9-10). The most superficial of these muscles, the **tibialis anterior**, is the prime mover for ankle dorsiflexion and supination, providing approximately 80% of the ankle's dorsiflexion power.[12] In addition to their functions at the toes, the **extensor hallucis longus** assists during supination, and the **extensor digitorum longus** contributes to pronation. The **peroneus tertius** runs parallel with the fifth tendon of the EDL, but its attachment on the dorsal surface of the fifth MT causes this muscle to make a stronger contribution to pronation than dorsiflexion.

Crossing the anterior portion of the ankle mortise is the extensor retinaculum, whose superior and inferior bands give it a Z shape (Fig. 9-11). The retinaculum serves to secure the distal tendons of the muscles of the anterior compartment as they cross the talocrural joint, preventing a

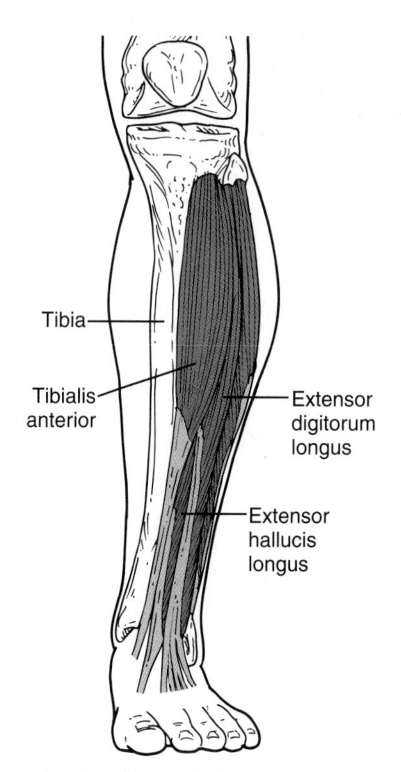

FIGURE 9-10 ■ Muscles of the anterior compartment of the left leg: the tibialis anterior, extensor hallucis longus, and extensor digitorum longus. The peroneus tertius is not shown.

Table 9-1 Muscles Acting on the Foot and Ankle

Muscle	Action	Origin	Insertion	Nerve	Root
Extensor Digitorum Longus	Extension of the 2nd through 5th MTP joints Assists in extending the 2nd through 5th PIP and DIP joints Assists in STJ and midtarsal pronation* Assists in ankle dorsiflexion	Lateral tibial condyle Proximal three-fourths of anterior fibula Proximal portion of the interosseous membrane	Via four tendons to the distal phalanges of the 2nd through 5th toes	Deep peroneal	L4, L5, S1
Extensor Hallucis Longus	Extension of the 1st MTP joint Extension of the 1st IP joint Assists with dorsiflexion Assists with supination**	Middle two-thirds of the anterior surface of the fibula Adjacent portion of the interosseous membrane	Base of the distal phalanx of the 1st toe	Deep peroneal	L4, L5, S1
Flexor Digitorum Longus	Flexion of the 2nd through 5th PIP and DIP joints Flexion of the 2nd through 5th MTP joints Assists in ankle plantarflexion Assists in STJ and midtarsal supination**	Posterior medial portion of the distal two-thirds of the tibia From fascia arising from the tibialis posterior	Plantar base of distal phalanges of the 2nd through 5th toes	Tibial	L5, S1
Flexor Hallucis Longus	Flexion of the 1st IP joint Assists in 1st MTP joint flexion Assists in STJ and midtarsal supination** Assists in ankle plantarflexion	Posterior distal two thirds of the fibula Associated interosseous membrane and muscular fascia	Plantar surface of the proximal phalanx of the 1st toe	Tibial	L4, L5, S1
Gastrocnemius	Ankle plantarflexion Assists in knee flexion	Medial head • Posterior surface of the medial femoral condyle • Adjacent portion of the femur and knee capsule Lateral head • Posterior surface of the lateral femoral condyle • Adjacent portion of the femur and knee capsule	To the calcaneus via the Achilles tendon	Tibial	S1, S2

Peroneus Brevis	STJ and midtarsal pronation* Assists in ankle plantarflexion	Distal two-thirds of the lateral fibula	Styloid process at the base of the 5th metatarsal	Superficial peroneal	L4, L5, S1
Peroneus Longus	STJ and midtarsal pronation* Assists in ankle plantarflexion	Lateral tibial condyle Fibular head Upper two thirds of the lateral fibula	Lateral aspect of the head of the 1st metatarsal Lateral and dorsal aspect of the 1st cuneiform	Superficial peroneal	L4, L5, S1
Peroneus Tertius	STJ and midtarsal pronation* Assists in ankle dorsiflexion	Distal one third of the anterior surface of the fibula Adjacent portion of the interosseous membrane	Dorsal surface of the base of the 5th metatarsal	Deep peroneal	L4, L5, S1
Plantaris	Ankle plantarflexion Assists in knee flexion	Distal portion of the supracondylar line of the lateral femoral condyle Adjacent portion of the femoral popliteal surface Oblique popliteal ligament	To the calcaneus via the Achilles tendon	Tibial	L4, L5, S1
Soleus	Ankle plantarflexion	Posterior fibular head Upper one-third of the fibula's posterior surface Soleal line located on the posterior tibial shaft Middle one-third of the medial tibial border	To the calcaneus via the Achilles tendon	Tibial	S1, S2
Tibialis Anterior	Ankle dorsiflexion STJ and midtarsal supination**	Lateral tibial condyle Upper one-half of the tibia's lateral surface Adjacent portion of the interosseous membrane	Medial and plantar surfaces of the 1st cuneiform Medial and plantar surfaces of the 1st metatarsal	Deep peroneal	L4, L5, S1
Tibialis Posterior	Assists in ankle plantarflexion STJ and midtarsal supination**	Length of the interosseous membrane Posterior, lateral tibia Upper two-thirds of the medial fibula	Navicular tuberosity Via fibrous slips to the sustentaculum tali, cuneiforms, cuboid, and bases of the 2nd, 3rd, and 4th metatarsals	Tibial	L4, L5, S1

DIP = distal interphalangeal; IP = interphalangeal; MTP = metatarsophalangeal; PIP = proximal interphalangeal; STJ = subtalar joint.
*Calcaneal eversion.
**Calcaneal inversion.

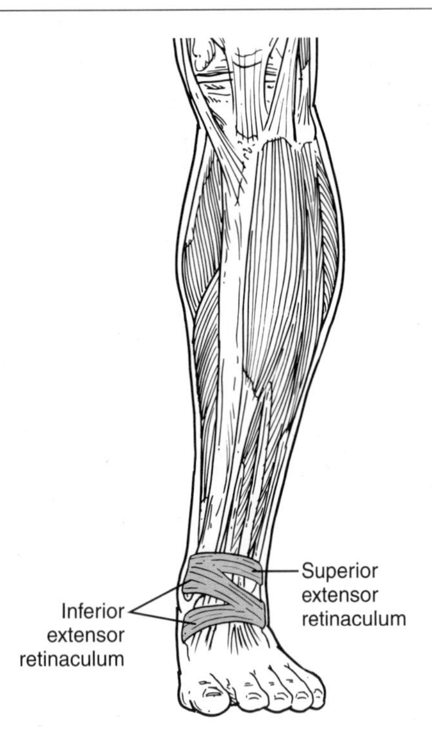

FIGURE 9-11 ■ Extensor retinaculum formed by the inferior and superior bands. These structures prevent the tendons of the anterior compartment from bowing during dorsiflexion and toe extension.

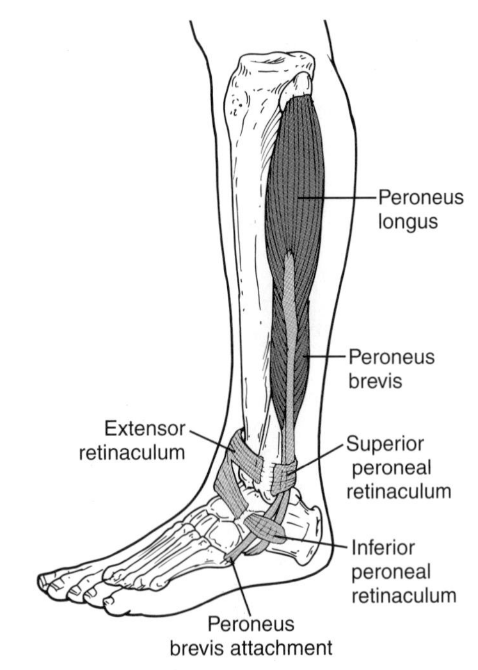

FIGURE 9-12 ■ Muscles of the lateral compartment: the peroneus longus and brevis. The superior and inferior peroneal retinacula maintain the alignment of the peroneal tendons so that their angle of pull plantarflexes and everts the ankle.

bowstring effect during dorsiflexion or toe extension. The medial portion of the inferior band holds the tibialis anterior and extensor hallucis longus close to the dorsum of the foot. A loop on the lateral border of the retinaculum wraps around the four tendinous slips of the extensor digitorum longus, holding them laterally and against the dorsum of the foot.

Branching off the **common peroneal nerve** near the fibular head and into the anterior compartment, the **deep peroneal nerve** runs from the upper portion of the fibula along the interosseous membrane behind the tibialis anterior. This nerve and its subsequent branches innervate most of the muscles located within the anterior compartment and on the dorsum of the foot. Supplying the anterior compartment with blood, the **anterior tibial artery** passes through the superior portion of the interosseous membrane to follow the path taken by the deep peroneal nerve. A branch of the anterior tibial artery, the **dorsalis pedis artery**, supplies blood to the dorsum of the foot.

Lateral compartment structures

The peroneus longus and peroneus brevis form the bulk of the lateral compartment. As a group, these muscles are strong evertors of the ankle and contribute to plantarflexion (Fig. 9-12). The **peroneus longus** is the most superficial of these muscles, with its belly covering all but the most inferior portion of the peroneus brevis and its tendon. The **peroneus brevis** lies beneath the peroneus longus as the tendons pass behind the lateral malleolus where they share a common synovial sheath. The peroneal tendons are held in position posterior to the malleolus primarily by the **superior peroneal retinaculum** and, to a lesser extent, the **inferior peroneal retinaculum.**[2,12] Their paths diverge as they clear the retinaculum and approach the peroneal tubercle. At this point, each tendon has its own synovial sheath.[2] The peroneus brevis tendon courses to the styloid process on the base of the fifth MT, while the peroneus longus tendon runs a more inferior path along the plantar aspect of the foot to attach to the head of the first MT and first cuneiform. A small sesamoid bone, the **os peroneum**, may be located in the peroneus longus tendon just proximal to and at the level of the cuboid.[2] The **peroneus quartus**, a small muscle that arises from the peroneus brevis and inserting on the retrotrochlear eminence on the calcaneus, is present in less than 7% of the population.[13] Adding little to the function of the foot and ankle, the peroneus quartus is often injured concurrently with other structures.[2,13]

The lateral compartment contains the **superficial peroneal nerve**, which innervates the peroneus longus, peroneus brevis, and in some cases the peroneus tertius. Arising off the **posterior tibial artery**, the peroneal artery runs lateral to the interosseous membrane, supplying blood to the lateral compartment and lateral ankle.

Superficial posterior compartment structures

The gastrocnemius and soleus form the **triceps surae muscle group** because of the three heads of the two muscles (the gastrocnemius has two heads) (Fig. 9-13). The **gastrocnemius** and **plantaris** are two-joint muscles originating on the posterior aspect of the femoral condyles. The **soleus**, arising off the posterior tibia, is the only member of

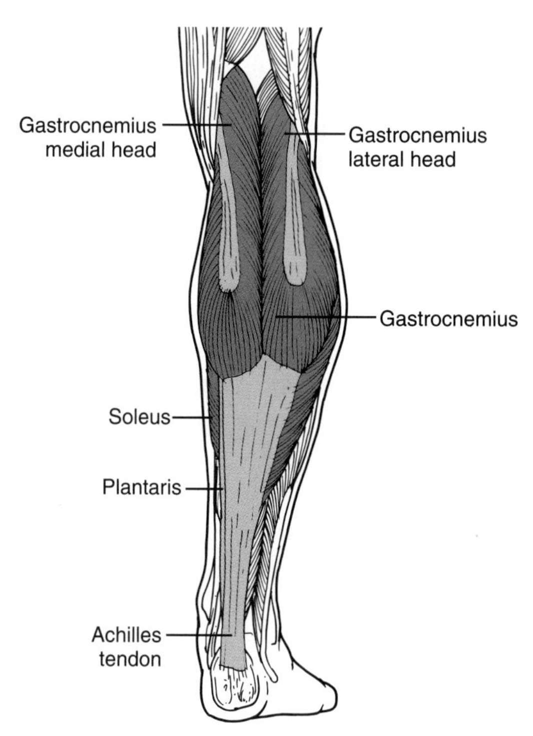

FIGURE 9-13 ■ Muscles of the superficial posterior compartment: the gastrocnemius, soleus, and plantaris. The gastrocnemius and soleus muscles are collectively referred to as the "triceps surae" because of the three heads they form.

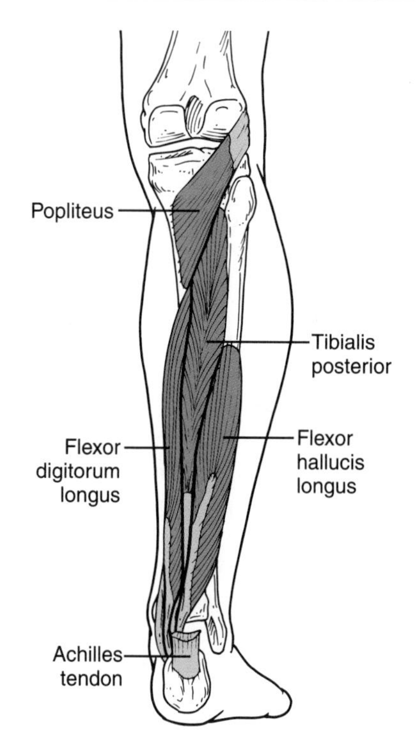

FIGURE 9-14 ■ Muscles of the deep posterior compartment: the tibialis posterior, flexor hallucis longus, and flexor digitorum longus. The superficial muscles have been removed to show the deep compartment. A common mnemonic, "Tom, Dick, And Nervous Harry," is used to describe the structures that pass behind the medial malleolus: tibialis posterior, flexor digitorum longus, tibial artery, tibial nerve, and the flexor hallucis longus.

the triceps surae group to cross only one joint. The gastrocnemius, soleus, and plantaris have a common insertion on the calcaneus via the Achilles tendon. The gastrocnemius and soleus are prime movers during plantarflexion. The gastrocnemius is most active in plantarflexing the ankle when the knee is extended.

Coursing between the medial and lateral heads of the gastrocnemius and running deep to lie between the soleus and the tibialis posterior (located in the deep posterior compartment) is the longest branch of the sciatic nerve, the **tibial nerve**. Supplying the innervation for all of the muscles in the superficial and deep posterior compartment, branches of the tibial nerve continue to the plantar aspect of the foot after coursing around the medial malleolus. The **posterior tibial artery**, arising from the tibial artery follows the same course as the tibial nerve.

Deep posterior compartment structures

The **tibialis posterior** is the only muscle of the deep posterior compartment that does not act on the toes (Fig. 9-14). Because of its angle of pull, this muscle is a primary adductor of the forefoot while also assisting in plantarflexion and inversion and generates significant tension during running as it controls pronation.[12] The remaining two muscles of the deep posterior compartment, the **flexor digitorum longus** and the **flexor hallucis longus**, act primarily to flex the toes and secondarily act to plantar flex and invert the ankle. These muscles pass through the tarsal tunnel formed behind the medial malleolus, predisposing them to repetitive mechanical irritation and inflammation (see Tarsal Tunnel Syndrome, p. 202).

Bursae

Two major bursae are associated with the leg and ankle. The **subtendinous calcaneal** (retrocalcaneal) **bursa** is found between the Achilles tendon and the calcaneus, decreasing friction between these two structures. Lying between the posterior aspect of the Achilles tendon and the skin is the **subcutaneous calcaneal bursa**, which protects the Achilles tendon from direct trauma and decreases friction from the skin and footwear.

Neurologic Anatomy

The neurologic innervation described for each of the four compartments arises from the lumbar and sacral plexes (see Chapter 13). The motor nerves for the leg muscles are presented in Table 9-1. The common peroneal nerve diverges at the fibular head, with the deep peroneal nerve innervating the muscles of the anterior compartment and the superficial peroneal nerve innervating the muscles of the lateral compartment (see Fig. 9-3). The tibial nerve, deep and well-protected until it becomes superficial at the medial ankle, passes through the deep posterior compartment and divides into the medial and lateral plantar nerves at the flexor retinaculum at the medial ankle. The sural nerve, arising from both the common peroneal and tibial nerves, provides sensory input from the posterior and lateral leg and the lateral foot. The saphenous nerve, originating off of the femoral nerve, innervates the skin on the medial ankle and foot. The motor nerves and the sural and saphenous nerves (sensory nerves) contribute to the ankle's proprioception (Fig. 9-15).

Vascular Anatomy

Arterial and venous systems of the leg are described for each of the four compartments. The leg's venous system is divided into superficial and deep components. The deep veins are associated with the major arteries and are described in each of the compartmental anatomy portions of this section.

The superficial venous return network is formed by two large veins, the **great** and **small saphenous veins.** Originating in the area of the foot's medial longitudinal arch, the great saphenous vein accepts tributaries that primarily sprout from the foot and posterior leg. Once passing the knee joint and traversing the length of the thigh, the great saphenous vein empties into the femoral vein. Originating near the fifth toe, the small saphenous vein courses up the posterior aspect of the leg and primarily receives blood from the superficial posterior compartment.

Assisted by **perforating veins**, most of the veins in the legs are positioned in a manner that allows muscle contractions to squeeze venous blood through a series of one-way valves from the distal extremity toward the heart. Rehabilitation programs using active muscle contractions and electrical stimulation "muscle milking" techniques exploit this anatomic trait.

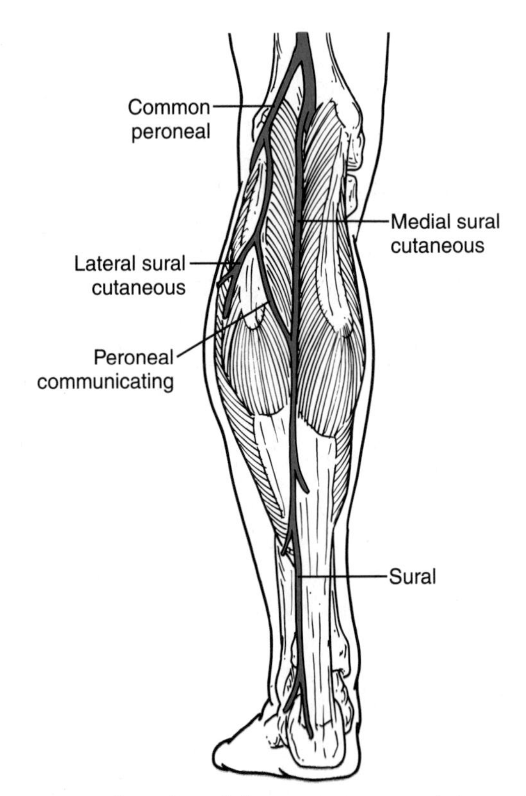

FIGURE 9-15 ■ Illustration of the motor nerves and the sural and saphenous nerves (sensory nerves) of the foot and ankle.

Clinical Examination of the Ankle and Leg

The ankle and leg are influenced by joints distal and proximal, necessitating possible inclusion of the foot, knee, hip, and spine in the examination process. The lower extremities must be exposed to facilitate this examination.

History

During the history-taking process for a patient with an ankle or leg injury, location of pain, the onset and mechanism of injury, the duration of the symptoms, and any previous history of injury to the involved or uninvolved limb must be established. For patients reporting a history of chronic ankle instability, the use of a self-reporting instrument such as the **Foot and Ankle Disability Index** provides a reliable descriptor of how the impairment affects daily life.[14] The patient's responses to this questioning guide the remainder of the history-taking process and form the framework on which the rest of the examination is based.

Past Medical History

Question the patient and, if available, review the patient's medical file regarding the history of injury to both the involved and uninvolved extremities and the lumbar spine. Patients with a history of previous ankle sprains may demonstrate excess laxity and decreased proprioception. Osteoarthritis may develop secondary to repetitive stresses, and rheumatoid arthritis can result in pain and dysfunction. **Peripheral vascular disease** can cause swelling in the foot and ankle. Individuals with diabetes may have associated neuropathy and prolonged tissue healing times.

History of the Present Condition

Other injuries to the lower extremity or lumbar spine may present with biomechanical changes in gait, predisposing different tissues to abnormal stresses. For example, patients with lateral ankle sprains often ambulate with a toe-only gait on the involved side to position the talocrural joint in its resting position. This, in turn, causes adaptive shortening of the Achilles' tendon, predisposing it to injury when a more normal gait is assumed.

- **Location of the pain** (Table 9-2): Ask the patient to specifically identify the location of pain so that the subsequent portions of the evaluation emphasize the suspected structures involved (Fig. 9-16). In the leg, a well-localized, specific pain may be indicative of bone

Examination Map

HISTORY

Past Medical History

History of the Present Condition

Mechanism of Injury

INSPECTION

Functional Observation

Inspection of the Lateral Structures

Peroneal muscle group

Distal one-third of fibula

Lateral malleolus

Inspection of the Anterior Structures

Sinus tarsi

Malleoli

Talus

Inspection of the Medial Structures

Medial malleolus

Medial longitudinal arch

Inspection of the Posterior Structures

Gasctrocnemius/soleus

Achilles tendon

Bursae

Calcaneus

PALPATION

Palpation of the Fibular Structures

Common peroneal nerve

Peroneal muscle group

Fibular shaft

Anterior tibiofibular ligament

Posterior tibiofibular ligament

Interosseous membrane

Superior peroneal retinaculum

Palpation of the Lateral Ankle

Lateral malleolus

Calcaneofibular ligament

Anterior talofibular ligament

Posterior talofibular ligament

Inferior peroneal retinaculum

Peroneal tubercle

Cuboid

Base of fifth metatarsal

Peroneus tertius

Palpation of the Anterior Structures

Anterior tibial shaft

Tibialis anterior

Extensor hallucis longus

Dome of the talus

Extensor retinacula

Sinus tarsi

Palpation of the Medial Structures

Medial malleolus

Deltoid ligament

Sustentaculum tali

Spring ligament

Navicular

Navicular tuberosity

Tibialis anterior

Tibialis posterior

Flexor hallucis longus

Flexor digitorum longus

Palpation of the Posterior Structures

Gastrocnemius and soleus

Achilles tendon

Subcutaneous calcaneal bursa

Calcaneus

Subtendinous calcaneal bursa

JOINT AND MUSCLE FUNCTION ASSESSMENT

Goniometry

Plantarflexion/dorsiflexion

Rearfoot inversion/eversion

Active Range of Motion

Plantarflexion

Dorsiflexion

Inversion

Eversion

Manual Muscle Tests

Tibialis anterior

Peroneus longus and brevis

Gastrocnemius and soleus

Tibialis posterior

Passive Range of Motion

Plantarflexion

Dorsiflexion

Inversion

Eversion

JOINT STABILITY TESTS

Stress Testing

Inversion stress test

Eversion stress test

Joint Play Assessment

Medial talar glide

Lateral talar glide (Cotton test)

Distal tibiofibular glide

NEUROLOGIC EXAMINATION

Lower Quarter Screen

Common peroneal nerve

Tibial nerve

VASCULAR EXAMINATION

Dorsalis Pedis Pulse

Posterior Tibial Pulse

Capillary Refill

PATHOLOGIES AND SPECIAL TESTS

Ankle Sprains

Lateral ankle sprain

Distal tibiofibular syndesmosis

- Squeeze test

Medial ankle sprains

Ankle and Leg Fractures

Os Trigonum Injury

Achilles Tendon Pathology

Achilles tendon tendinopathy

Achilles tendon rupture

- Thompson test

Peroneal Tendon Pathology

Medial Tibial Stress Syndrome

Stress Fractures

- Bump test

Compartment Syndromes

Deep Vein Thrombosis

Table 9-2 Possible Trauma Based on the Location of Pain

	Location of Pain			
	Lateral	**Anterior**	**Medial**	**Posterior**
Soft Tissue	Lateral ankle ligament sprain	Extensor retinaculum sprain	Deltoid ligament	Triceps surae strain
	Syndesmosis sprain	Syndesmosis sprain	Capsular impingement	Achilles tendinopathy
	Capsular impingement	Tibialis anterior or long toe extensor strain	Tibialis posterior strain	Achilles tendon rupture
	Subluxating peroneal tendons	Tibialis anterior or long toe extensor tendinopathy	Tibialis posterior tendinopathy	Subtendinous calcaneal bursitis
	Peroneal muscle strain	Anterior compartment syndrome	Posterior tibial nerve compression (tarsal tunnel syndrome)	Subcutaneous calcaneal bursitis
	Peroneal tendinopathy	Interosseous membrane trauma		Deep vein **thrombophlebitis**
	Interosseous membrane trauma	Anterior tibiofibular ligament sprain		Posterior tibiofibular ligament sprain
	Peroneal nerve trauma			
Bony	Lateral ligament avulsion from malleolus, talus, and/or calcaneus.	Tibial stress fracture	Medial ligament avulsion	Calcaneal fracture
		Frank tibial fracture		
	Lateral malleolus fracture	Talar fracture	Medial malleolus avulsion	Arthritis
	Fibular stress fracture	Talar osteochondritis	Medial malleolus fracture	Os trigonum trauma
	Frank fibular fracture			
	Fifth MT fracture	Arthritis	Arthritis	
	Peroneal tendon avulsion	Periostitis		
	Arthritis			

MT = metatarsal.

pathology while more diffuse pain points to soft tissue. The leg and ankle may also be areas of referred pain arising from anterior compartment syndrome, tarsal tunnel syndrome, the peroneal nerve, and sciatic nerve or lumbar nerve root impingement.

- **Onset:** Identify the onset of symptoms to determine if there has been acute trauma such as a sprain, strain, fracture, or if there has been a gradual onset of symptoms as with overuse syndromes.
- **Injury mechanism:** In the case of macrotrauma, determine the mechanism of injury to identify the general area of the structures affected and the type of injury involved (Table 9-3). Chronic or insidious disorders require more in-depth questioning to determine the factors surrounding the cause of pain.
- **Type and severity of pain:** Determine the patient's rating of pain at its extremes using a visual analog or numeric rating scale. Question the patient regarding the type of pain. Burning pain may indicate nerve involvement. Sharp, localized pain may be associated with bone pathology.
- **Pain pattern:** Pose specific questions to determine how the symptoms are aggravated by certain activities. How are these symptoms affecting athletic participation or normal daily activities? Does the pain pattern change throughout the day? Is the onset of pain associated with fatigue? Leg pain that begins during activity and increases to the point that activity must be discontinued is consistent with exertional compartment syndrome.
- **Changes in activity and conditioning regimen:** Gain an understanding of the patient's recent activity, or changes in activity, to understand better the cause of chronic or insidious conditions. For overuse injuries, establish whether the patient has:
  - Significantly increased the duration, intensity, frequency, or type (i.e., added hills) of exercise. When available, the athlete's personal training log is useful in determining excessive increases in exercise intensity.

Thrombophlebitis Inflammation of a vein and the subsequent formation of blood clots.

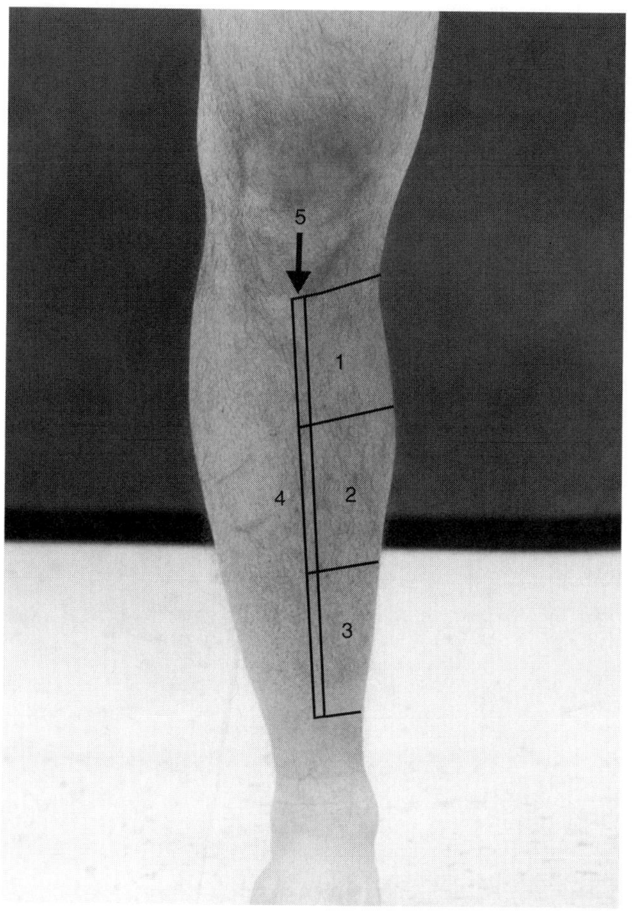

FIGURE 9-16 ■ Pain zones and anatomic correlations.

- Changed shoe brands or styles or is wearing old, worn-out shoes.
- Switched from participating on a surface of one texture and density to one of a different type.
- Recently begun wearing orthotics, changed the type of orthotic worn, or recently discontinued the use of orthotics.

Inspection

Much of the observation phase occurs while the patient is not weight bearing. These results are then compared with the weight-bearing findings. Begin by observing both lower extremities, noting redness, pallor, tendon discontinuity or other obvious deformity. The amount of swelling should be objectively measured via girth or volumetric measurements (see p. 302).[15,16]

Functional assessment

Observe the patient performing the task or activity that produces symptoms to begin to identify the underlying impairments. Gait abnormalities frequently contribute to or result from ankle and leg pathology. The functional assessment that determines willingness to bear weight may begin as the patient enters the facility or walks off the field. Observe for gait deviations such as an antalgic gait or external rotation of the limb on the involved side, suggesting a lack of ankle dorsiflexion caused by pain or restriction. Different foot postures also impact gait and the relative demands on the tissues of the leg and foot (see Chapter 8).

Inspection of the lateral structures

- **Peroneal muscle group:** Inspect the length of the peroneal muscle group. The tendons may be seen as they course posteriorly and inferiorly around the lateral malleolus, being held in position by the superior and inferior peroneal retinacula (see Fig. 9-12). The tendons will become more visible if the patient is able to actively pronate the foot and ankle.
- **Distal one third of the fibula:** Note the contour and symmetry of the distal one third of the fibula as it becomes superficial proximal to the lateral malleolus. Any discontinuity in the bone's shaft or the formation of edema over this portion of the shaft may indicate a possible fracture.
- **Lateral malleolus:** The lateral malleolus is covered only by skin, making its shape easily identifiable.

Table 9-3 Mechanism of Ankle Injury and the Resulting Tissue Damage

Uniplanar Motion	Tensile Forces	Compressive Forces
Inversion	Lateral structures: Anterior talofibular ligament, calcaneofibular ligament, posterior talofibular ligament, lateral capsule, and peroneal tendons; lateral malleolus fracture	Medial structures: Medial malleolus, deltoid ligament, and posterior tibial nerve, tibial artery, tibial vein.
Eversion	Medial structures: Deltoid ligament, tibialis posterior, and long toe flexors, posterior tibial nerve, tibial artery	Lateral structures: Lateral malleolus and lateral capsule
Plantarflexion	Anterior structures: Anterior capsule, long toe extensors, tibialis anterior, and extensor retinaculum Lateral structures: Anterior talofibular ligament	Posterior structures: Posterior capsule, subtendinous calcaneal bursa, subcutaneous calcaneal bursa, os trigonum, and talus fracture
Dorsiflexion	Posterior structures: Triceps surae, Achilles tendon, tibialis posterior, flexor hallucis longus, flexor digitorum longus Lateral structures: Posterior talofibular ligament, peroneal tendons	Anterior structures: Anterior capsule, syndesmosis, and extensor retinaculum, anterior talus

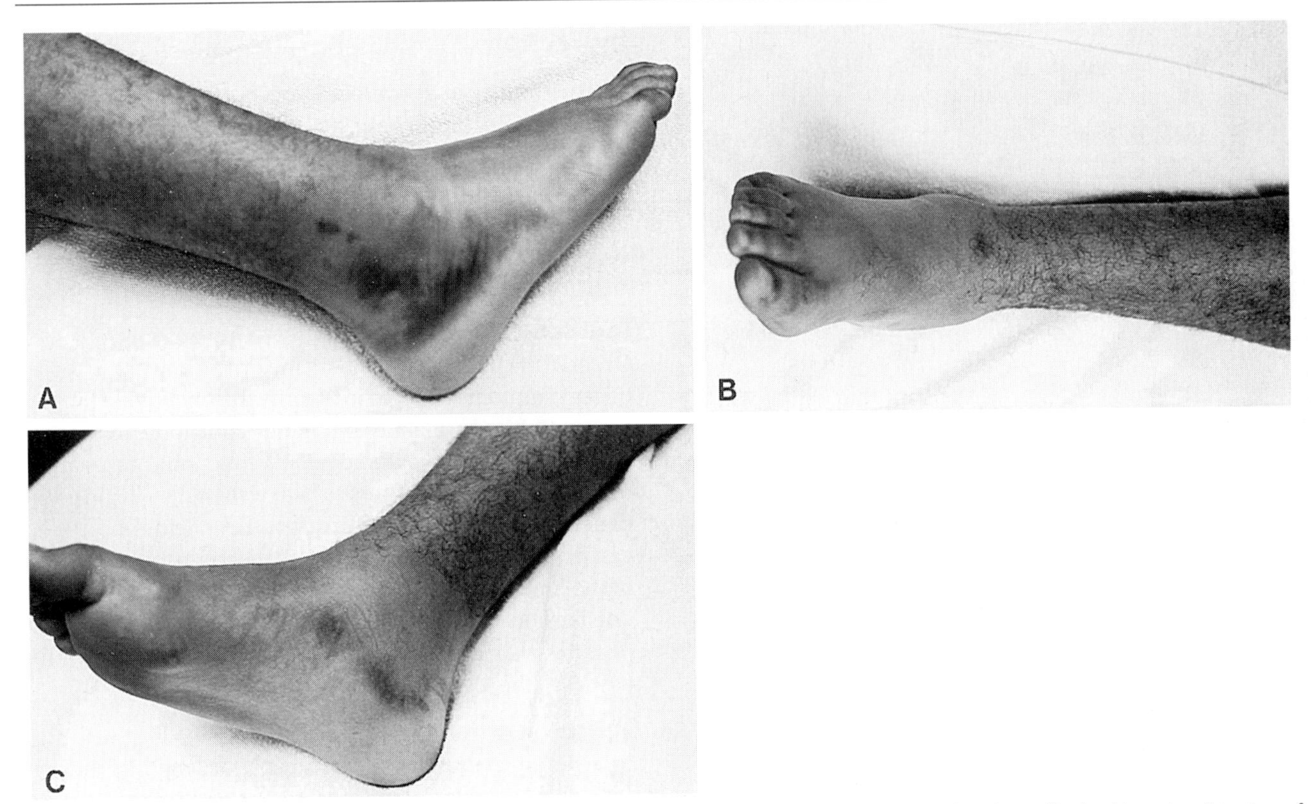

FIGURE 9-17 ■ Damage to the lateral ankle capsule can result in the collection of edema around and distal to the malleolus. Note the distortion of the normal ankle contours and medial formation of ecchymosis.

Even mild ankle sprains can result in swelling that obscures the malleolus and peroneal tendons (Fig. 9-17). Any formation of ecchymosis around and distal to the lateral malleolus may signify acute trauma such as a sprain or fracture, although it will not occur immediately.

Inspection of the Anterior Structures

- **Appearance of the anterior leg:** Inspect the anterior leg for skin color and edema. Anterior compartment syndrome may present with reddened or shiny skin or pitting edema. If these signs coincide with paresthesia in the web space between the first and second toes, decreased dorsiflexion strength, and/or absence of the dorsalis pedis pulse, immediately refer the patient to a physician or emergency room.
- **Sinus tarsi:** Observe the sinus tarsi, an indentation formed over the anterolateral aspect of the talus, noting for its normally concave shape. After injury to the anterior talofibular ligament or fractures about the ankle, the area fills with fluid, resulting in loss of its normal indentation in the proximal foot (Fig. 9-18).[17] The amount of fluid collection can be quantified using girth or volumetric measurements (see Special Test 2-1).
- **Contour of the malleoli:** Observe the malleoli, which should be prominent as they project from the distal tibia and fibula. Swelling can obscure these structures.

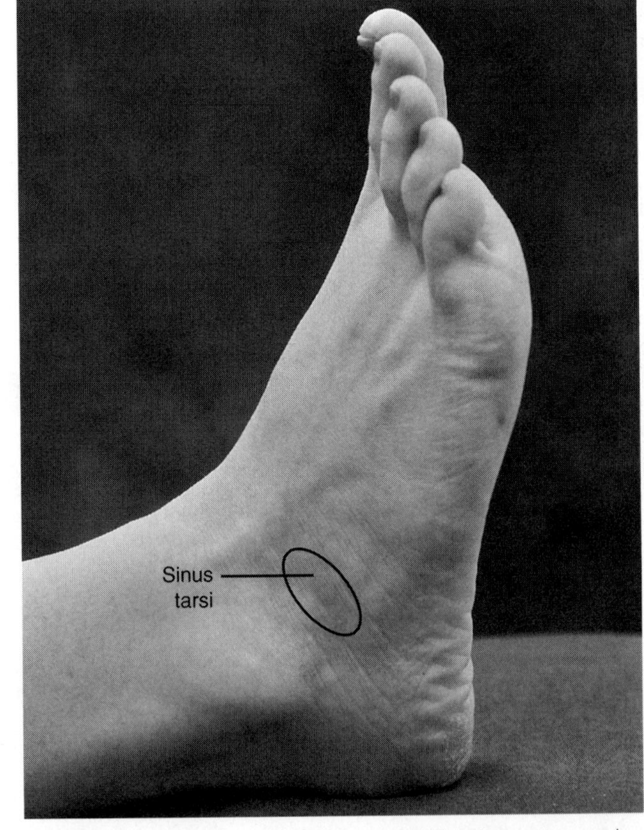

FIGURE 9-18 ■ Location of the left sinus tarsi. This depression may become swollen and painful secondary to trauma to the foot or ankle.

Edema between the tibia and fibula in the distal one third of the interosseous membrane may indicate a syndesmotic sprain.

- **Talus:** If possible, observe the bilateral symmetry of the tali while the patient is weight bearing. In the case of leg length discrepancies, one foot has a prominent medial talus caused by pronation of the longer leg; the shorter leg maintains a somewhat neutral or supinated position (see Fig. 6–9).

Inspection of the medial structures

- **Medial malleolus:** Similar to the lateral malleolus, the medial malleolus is superficial, with little soft tissue covering it. Its appearance should be distinct without obvious deformity or the presence of edema.
- **Medial longitudinal arch:** If the patient is capable of bearing weight, observe the appearance of the medial longitudinal arch, which should be maintained with the patient both bearing weight and non–weight bearing. If this arch is not adequately supported, the medial aspect of the talus rotates inward and the navicular drops inferiorly (pes planus). Excessive protrusion of the talus can be seen from the anterior and posterior views. Leg pain, such as periostitis or tendinopathy of the tibialis anterior or tibialis posterior muscles, is often associated with this alignment. The supporting muscles may be predisposed to fatigue or pain developing at their tibial origins as they attempt to control excessive medial motion of the talus and the associated drop in the medial longitudinal arch.

  Pes cavus, a high medial arch, results in a supinated foot, and a potential predisposition to lateral ankle sprains or stress fractures caused by limited shock-absorbing capacity.

Inspection of the Posterior Structures

- **Gastrocnemius–soleus complex:** Bilateral comparison should indicate calf musculature of approximately equal size, shape, and mass. Atrophy may be present if the leg has been immobilized or the S1 or S2 nerve root or if the sciatic nerve or tibial nerve portion of the sciatic nerve is impaired. Tearing of the muscle may result in depressions in the skin, especially at the musculotendinous junction with the Achilles tendon. Unexplained redness and swelling of the posterior calf could indicate **deep vein thrombosis**.
- **Achilles tendon:** The prominent Achilles tendon is visble as it tapers from the musculotendinous junction to its insertion on the calcaneus. Achilles tendon ruptures may present with a visible defect if the tear occurs in its middle or distal portion.
- **Bursae:** Inspect the calcaneal bursae for swelling, redness, or other signs of inflammation or infection.
- **Calcaneus:** The calcaneus is normally very distinct, with little soft tissue covering its medial and lateral borders. The presence of a thickened area at the insertion of the Achilles tendon is sometimes associated with retrocalcaneal pain. This thickening, an exostosis, may be caused by footwear rubbing on this area, possibly associated with subcutaneous calcaneal bursitis (see Chapter 8).

PALPATION

Palpation of the Fibular Structures

1 Common peroneal nerve: Palpate over the common peroneal nerve as it passes behind the lateral portion of the fibular head and then branches into its deep and superficial branches.

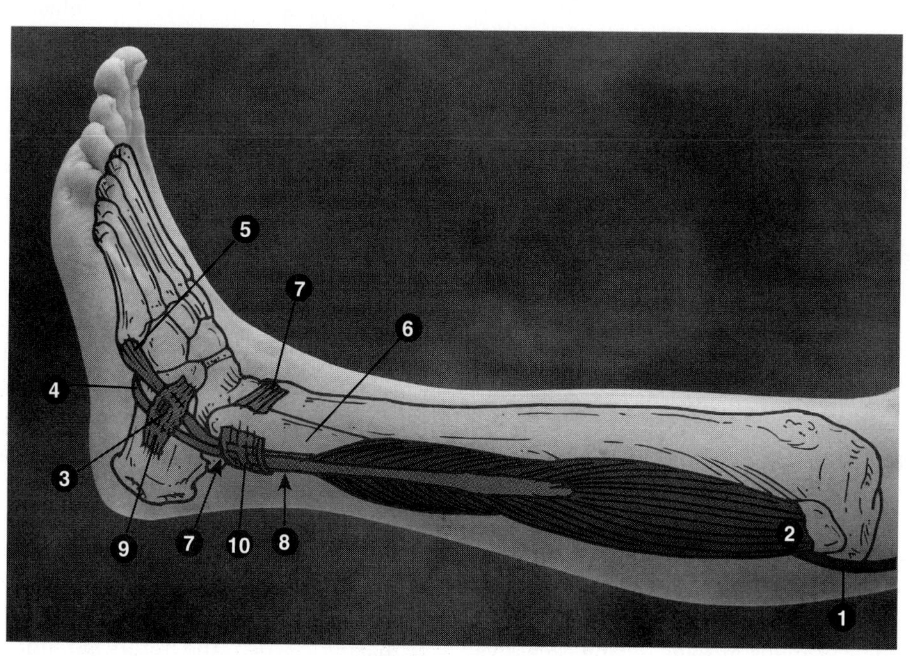

2 Peroneal muscle group: Locate the peroneus longus muscle from its origin on the fibular head and palpate the muscle belly along the upper two thirds of the lateral fibula. The tendons of both the peroneus longus and brevis are palpable along the distal one third of the fibula and as they course posterior to the lateral malleolus.

3–5 Peroneal tubercle: As the peroneal tendons approach the **(3)** peroneal tubercle, they diverge so that the **(4) peroneus longus tendon** passes through the groove in the cuboid and is no longer palpable as it continues to the head of the first metatarsal. The acute angle of the peroneus longus tendon as it changes course at the cuboid is a common site of rupture.[18] The **(5) peroneus brevis tendon** travels a shorter distance to its attachment on the base of the fifth MT.

6 Fibular shaft: Begin by locating the fibular head and palpate along the length of the shaft over the bulk of the peroneals until the bone reemerges along its distal third. Apply gentle pressure over the distal one third of the fibular shaft, noting any pain and discontinuity in the bone, indicative of a fracture.

7 Anterior and posterior tibiofibular ligaments: Locate the attachment of the anterior and posterior tibiofibular ligaments on the fibula just superior to the lateral malleolus. Palpate anteriorly along the length of the anterior tib-fib ligament to its attachment on the anterolateral portion of the tibia. Direct palpation of the posterior tib-fib ligament is difficult because of the peroneal tendons. Tenderness along these structures or the interosseous membrane may indicate a syndesmotic ankle sprain.

8 Interosseous membrane: An area of the interosseous membrane may be palpated in the ankle syndesmosis between the distal fibula and tibia. Begin palpating the posterior tibiofibular joint line, just superior to the lateral malleolus and progress superiorly until the fibula becomes covered by the mass of the peroneal muscles.

9 Superior peroneal retinaculum: Palpate the superior peroneal retinaculum as it projects off of the superior portion of the lateral malleolus. This structure may be painful after an acute tear or stretching.

Palpation of the Lateral Ankle

1 Lateral malleolus: The lateral ligamentous structures may be avulsed from their origin on the malleolus or their insertion on the talus or calcaneus through the tensile forces associated with inversion. Avulsion fractures result in point tenderness, swelling, and crepitus. The distal portion of the lateral malleolus may be "knocked off" by the calcaneus or talus during excessive eversion of the calcaneus.

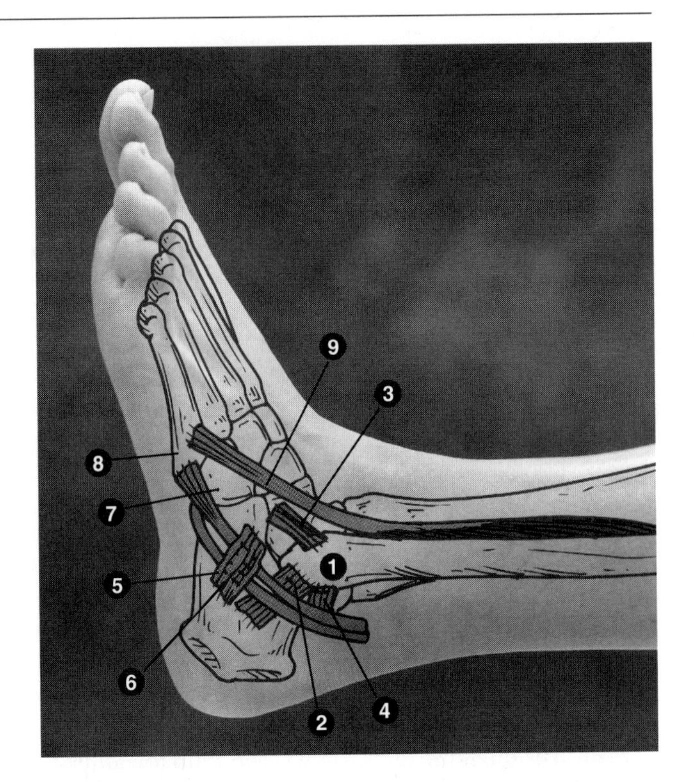

2 Calcaneofibular ligament: Locate the origin of the CF ligament on the distal tip of the malleolus. The ligament becomes palpable as it leaves the malleolus and crosses the joint space, taking an oblique posterior course to the peroneal tubercle. Tenderness of the CF ligament during palpation of an acute an lateral ankle sprain is highly indicative of a CF sprain.

3 Anterior talofibular ligament: Locate the origin of the CF ligament and move anteriorly on the malleolus to find the origin of the ATF ligament on the inferior portion of the anterolateral malleolus. Running a course somewhat parallel to the plantar surface of the foot when the foot is in neutral position, the ATF ligament attaches on the anterolateral aspect of the talus near the sinus tarsi. The ATF ligament is not normally distinctly palpable. Tenderness tends to be more widespread during the initial examination and becomes more focal to the ATF in the days following the injury.

4 Posterior talofibular ligament: From the origin of the calcaneofibular ligament, move upward and posteriorly around the malleolus to locate the PTF ligament. This ligament is not directly palpable, but pressure should be applied over the point of its insertion on the posterior portion of the talus. In most cases, the PTF ligament is damaged only in severe ankle sprains or dislocations.

5 Inferior peroneal retinaculum: Palpate the space between the posterior portion of the lateral malleolus and the calcaneus for pain elicited over the superior peroneal retinaculum where the peroneal tendons pass beneath it. Follow the length of the tendons to locate the inferior peroneal retinaculum immediately below the lateral malleolus, along the lateral aspect of the calcaneus. Tears in these structures, especially the superior retinaculum, result in dislocating or subluxating peroneal tendons.

6 Peroneal tubercle: Feel for a small nodule located anterior to the attachment of the CF ligament and inferior to the distal tip of the lateral malleolus. The peroneal tubercle marks the point on the calcaneus where the peroneus longus and brevis tendons diverge. In cases of peroneal tendinopathy or rupture of the distal peroneal retinaculum, this area is tender to the touch.

7 Cuboid: Palpate anteriorly from the peroneal tubercle to locate the cuboid as it lies proximal to the base of the fifth MT. The cuboid is rarely injured but may become tender secondary to ligamentous injury such as a sprain of the cuboid–metatarsal joint or inflammation of the peroneal tendons.

8 Base of the fifth metatarsal: Palpate anteriorly from the cuboid to find the base of the fifth MT and its laterally projecting flare, the styloid process. This structure may be avulsed from the shaft after the forceful contraction of the peroneus brevis muscle as the muscle attempts to counteract inversion of the ankle.

9 Peroneus tertius: Locate the peroneus tertius where it rises from the distal half of the anterior surface of the fibula. Palpate distally along the length of the muscle belly and tendon to the insertion point on the dorsal aspect of the base of the fifth MT. The tendon is most palpable as it crosses the joint anterior to the lateral malleolus. It is identifiable by being the most lateral of the muscles on the anterior aspect of the lower leg. The peroneus tertius is absent in 5% to 17% of the population, but those individuals who are lacking a peroneus tertius are not at an increased risk of experiencing a lateral ankle sprain.[19]

Palpation of the Anterior Structures

1 Anterior tibial shaft: Locate the patellar tendon's attachment on the tibial tuberosity. The anteromedial portion of the tibia is subcutaneous and therefore palpable along its length to its medial malleolus. Note tenderness arising from the anteromedial ridge of the tibia where the tibialis anterior and long toe extensors originate, as well as to the periosteum and posterior border of the shaft along the origins of the tibialis posterior, flexor hallucis longus, and flexor digitorum longus. These areas may become inflamed secondary to overuse and improperly described as "shin splints" (Box 9-1).

2 Tibialis anterior: Locate the origin of the tibialis anterior on the anterolateral portion of the proximal tibia and palpate distally along the length of the muscle belly. Near the distal one third of the medial tibia, the belly begins to merge into a thick, round tendon. Palpate the tendon to its insertion on the medial cuneiform and first MT.

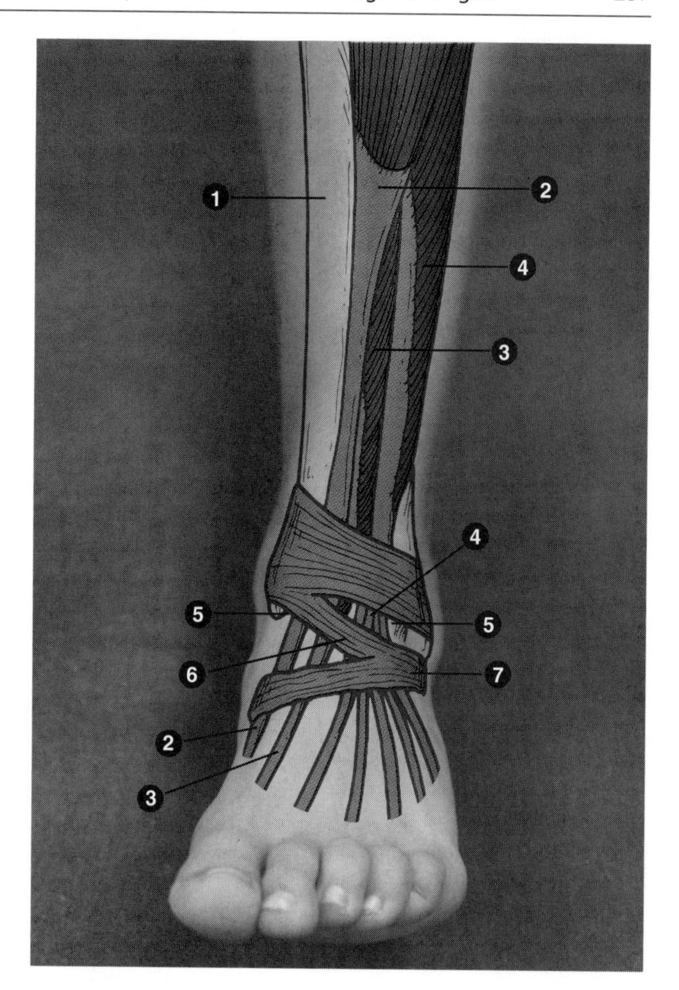

3 Extensor hallucis longus: Have the patient actively extend the great toe to make the EHL tendon palpable at its insertion. Continue to palpate the length of the EHL as it passes lateral to the tibialis anterior to its origin on the middle half of the anterior fibula and adjacent interosseous membrane. The tendon eventually becomes obscured by the tibialis anterior muscle.

Box 9-1
Shin Splints

The term "shin splints" has been used to describe nondescript leg pain. Pathologies leading to leg pain include (1) tibialis anterior and/or long toe extensor tendinopathy, (2) tibialis posterior and/or long toe flexor tendinopathy, (3) periostitis, (4) tibial stress fractures, (5) fibular stress fractures, (6) exertional compartment syndrome, (7) inflammation of the interosseous membrane, (8) popliteal artery entrapment, (9) strain of the tibialis anterior or tibialis posterior, and (10) deep vein thrombosis.

The diagnosis of "shin splints" lacks the accuracy and specificity required to develop a management plan for the patient's condition.[20] Avoid using the term shin splints. Rather, identify the underlying pathology that produces the pain and the resulting impairments.

4 Extensor digitorum longus: Locate the tendon of the extensor digitorum longus lateral to the extensor hallucis longus. Active extension of the toes causes the EDL tendons to stand out on the dorsal aspect of the toes and foot. Palpate the individual slips on the lateral four toes up though its common tendon.

5 Dome of the talus: Have the patient plantarflex the ankle to allow the anterior dome of the talus to be exposed from under the ankle mortise. Pain along this area is common with ankle synovitis and impact injuries to the ankle joint.

6 Extensor retinacula: Palpate the extensor retinacula for signs of tenderness as the tendons pass under them (see Fig. 9-13). The superior extensor retinaculum is palpated along the anterior aspect of the distal leg, just proximal to the tibiofibular joint. The inferior extensor retinaculum is palpated laterally beginning at the area of the inferior peroneal retinaculum and proceeds across the dorsum of the foot to the medial aspect of the midfoot. The retinacula may become traumatically injured during forceful, sudden dorsiflexion, or the tendons passing under it may become inflamed secondary to friction.

7 Sinus tarsi: Locate the sinus tarsi between the lateral malleolus and the neck of the talus. This area may become swollen and painful to the touch following ATF ligament injury, arthritic changes in the ankle, or fracture of the talus (see Fig. 9-19).

Palpation of the Medial Structures

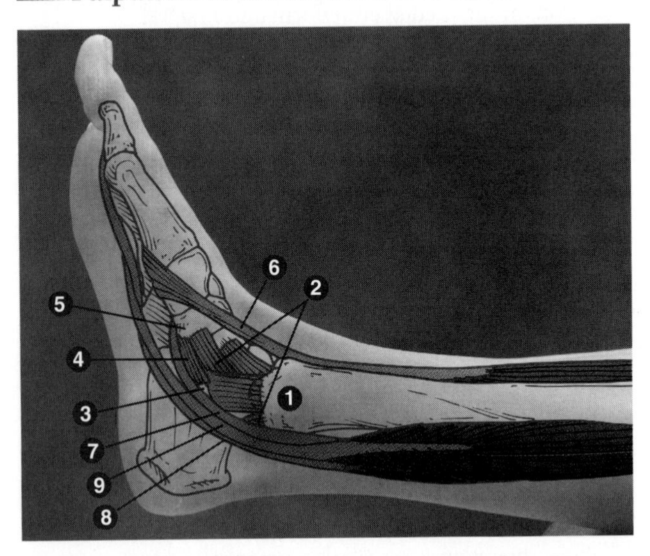

1 Medial malleolus: Palpate the entire border of the medial malleolus, noting any pain that may be elicited at the attachment sites of the medial ligaments or crepitus possibly indicating a fracture. Continue to palpate up the posteromedial tibial border, noting any pain that arises along the periosteal lining.

2 Deltoid ligament: Palpate the mass of the deltoid ligament as it encircles the distal medial malleolus. Clinically, the individual ligaments forming this complex cannot be distinguished from each other except by their relative location on the joint.

3 Sustentaculum tali: Palpate approximately one finger's width inferior from the medial malleolus to locate the calcaneal sustentaculum tali. This structure supports the talus and is an attachment site for the spring ligament.

4 Spring ligament: Locate the spring ligament's origin on the sustentaculum tali and palpate along its route distally to its insertion on the navicular. The spring ligament becomes stretched in cases of chronic pes planus or torn following acute pronation or rotation of the forefoot.

5 Navicular and navicular tuberosity: Identify the navicular tuberosity (tubercle) by the attachment of the tibialis posterior. Palpate the navicular bone for signs of tenderness that possibly indicate tibialis posterior tendinopathy, a sprain of the spring ligament, or a stress fracture. Pain elicited during palpation of this structure can also indicate an inflamed accessory navicular.

6 Tibialis anterior: From the insertion of the tibialis anterior on the medial and plantar surfaces of the first cuneiform and first metatarsal, identify the tendon and palpate proximally along its length.

7 Tibialis posterior: The belly of the tibialis posterior is not distinctly palpable as it lies under the gastrocnemius and soleus muscles. Its tendon passes behind and around the medial malleolus and becomes most palpable at its insertion on the navicular tuberosity.

8 Flexor hallucis longus: Palpate the FHL tendon as it begins its path behind and around the medial malleolus. Note that it is difficult to distinguish this tendon from the other structures in the area. As the tendon begins its course along the plantar aspect of the foot, it is no longer palpable until it inserts on the distal phalanx of the great toe. The FHL often becomes inflamed in individuals who engage in repetitive push-off activities, such as ballet dancers.[12]

9 Flexor digitorum longus: Similar to the flexor hallucis longus, palpate the FDL tendon, although not uniquely identifiable, as it passes behind and around the medial malleolus. After it passes along the plantar aspect of the foot, the tendon is again palpable as it inserts on the plantar aspect of the second through fifth toes.

Palpation of the Posterior Structures

1 Gastrocnemius-soleus complex: Palpate the gastrocnemius from its dual origin on the lateral and medial femoral condyles. Giving rise to a large muscle mass, the belly of the gastrocnemius is palpated in its entirety as it forms the bulk of the posterior calf musculature. The soleus, which is covered by the gastrocnemius muscle, is not always directly palpable.

2 Achilles tendon: From its attachment on the calcaneus, palpate the length of the Achilles tendon proximally to where it blends with the triceps surae muscle group. This tendon should feel firm and ropelike, with a gradual, symmetrical increase in its width as you progress proximally. Palpate the Achilles tendon and its musculotendinous junction for signs of tendinopathy or an Achilles tendon rupture, in which a gap in the tendon may be felt.

3 Subcutaneous calcaneal bursa: Isolate the subcutaneous calcaneal bursa, located between the posterior aspect of the Achilles tendon and the skin, by pinching the skin that overlies the tendon. In chronic inflammatory conditions, this bursa may be enlarged and thickened, forming "pump bumps" (see Fig. 8-18).

4 Calcaneus: Locate the posterior flare of the calcaneus and continue to palpate to the site of the Achilles tendon attachment. The calcaneal dome is located just anterior to the subtendinous calcaneal bursa. Pain elicited from adolescent patients during palpation of this area may indicate calcaneal apophysitis near the Achilles tendon's insertion on the calcaneus (see Chapter 8).

5 Subtendinous calcaneal bursa: Isolate this structure between the posterior aspect of the calcaneus and the anterior portion of the Achilles tendon by squeezing the soft tissue on either side of the Achilles tendon.

Joint and Muscle Function Assessment

The ROM available to the talocrural joint can be affected by muscular tightness, bony abnormalities, or soft tissue constraints. To allow for proper gait, the talocrural joint must provide 10 degrees of dorsiflexion during walking and 15 degrees during running as the opposite limb goes from the stance to the swing phase. When dorsiflexion is limited, one manner that the foot compensates is by increasing pronation during the weight-bearing phases of gait. This compensation results in biomechanical changes in the lower extremity that predisposes the individual to overuse injuries.

For the purposes here, plantarflexion and dorsiflexion are defined as the movement taking place at the talocrural joint, and inversion and eversion describe the single frontal plane calcaneal motion occurring at the subtalar joint (Table 9-4; see Table 9-1 for nerve innervations). The shape of the subtalar joint precludes true single plane motion. Pronation and supination better describe the collective movements of the subtalar and midtarsal articulations. However, the most apparent components of supination and pronation are, respectively, calcaneal inversion and eversion. These terms and measurements are often used to quantify the amount of supination and pronation. The use of goniometric measurements for plantarflexion and dorsiflexion and inversion and eversion is described in Goniometry Box 9-1. Rearfoot inversion and eversion are presented in Goniometry Box 8-1 (p. 185).

Active range of motion

- **Plantarflexion and dorsiflexion:** Spanning a range of 70 degrees, normal active ROM occurs as 20 degrees of dorsiflexion and 50 degrees of plantarflexion from the neutral position (see Goniometry Box 9-1).
- **Inversion and eversion:** A component of pronation and supination, rear foot inversion and eversion accounts for a total of 25 degrees with the predominant movement being 20 degrees of inversion from the neutral position and 5 degrees of eversion from neutral (see Goniometry Box 8-2).

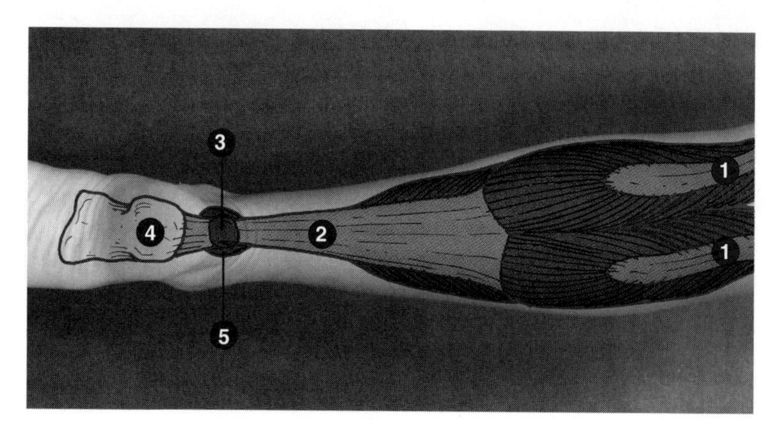

Table 9-4 Muscles Contributing to Uniplanar Foot and Ankle Movements

Dorsiflexion	Inversion
Extensor digitorum longus	Extensor hallucis longus
Extensor hallucis longus	Flexor digitorum longus
Peroneus tertius	Flexor hallucis longus
Tibialis anterior	Tibialis anterior
	Tibialis posterior
Plantarflexion	**Eversion**
Flexor digitorum longus	Extensor digitorum longus
Flexor hallucis longus	Peroneus brevis
Gastrocnemius	Peroneus longus
Peroneus brevis	Peroneus tertius
Peroneus longus	
Plantaris	
Soleus	
Tibialis posterior	

Manual muscle tests

When the patient presents with a complaint having a gradual onset of symptoms, performing repetitive tests or examining the patient postexercise when the muscles are fatigued may provide more applicable results. Because the ankle plantarflexor group is so powerful, it is often necessary to test these muscles using a unilateral heel-raise. The patient is asked to perform a set of 10 toe raises holding onto a sturdy object for balance (Fig. 9-19). Weakness in the plantarflexor group is evidenced by the inability to complete the test, leaning forward, or bending the knee when the gastrocnemius is being isolated.

As with the functional examination, strength of individual muscles should be assessed using repeated measurements to determine the impact of fatigue on strength or an increase in symptoms. Manual Muscle Tests 9-1, 9-2, 9-3, and 9-4 include testing of the muscles originating in the anterior, posterior, and deep posterior compartments. Manual muscle tests of the long toe flexors and extensors are presented in Boxes 8-1 and 8-2 (pp. 187 and 188).

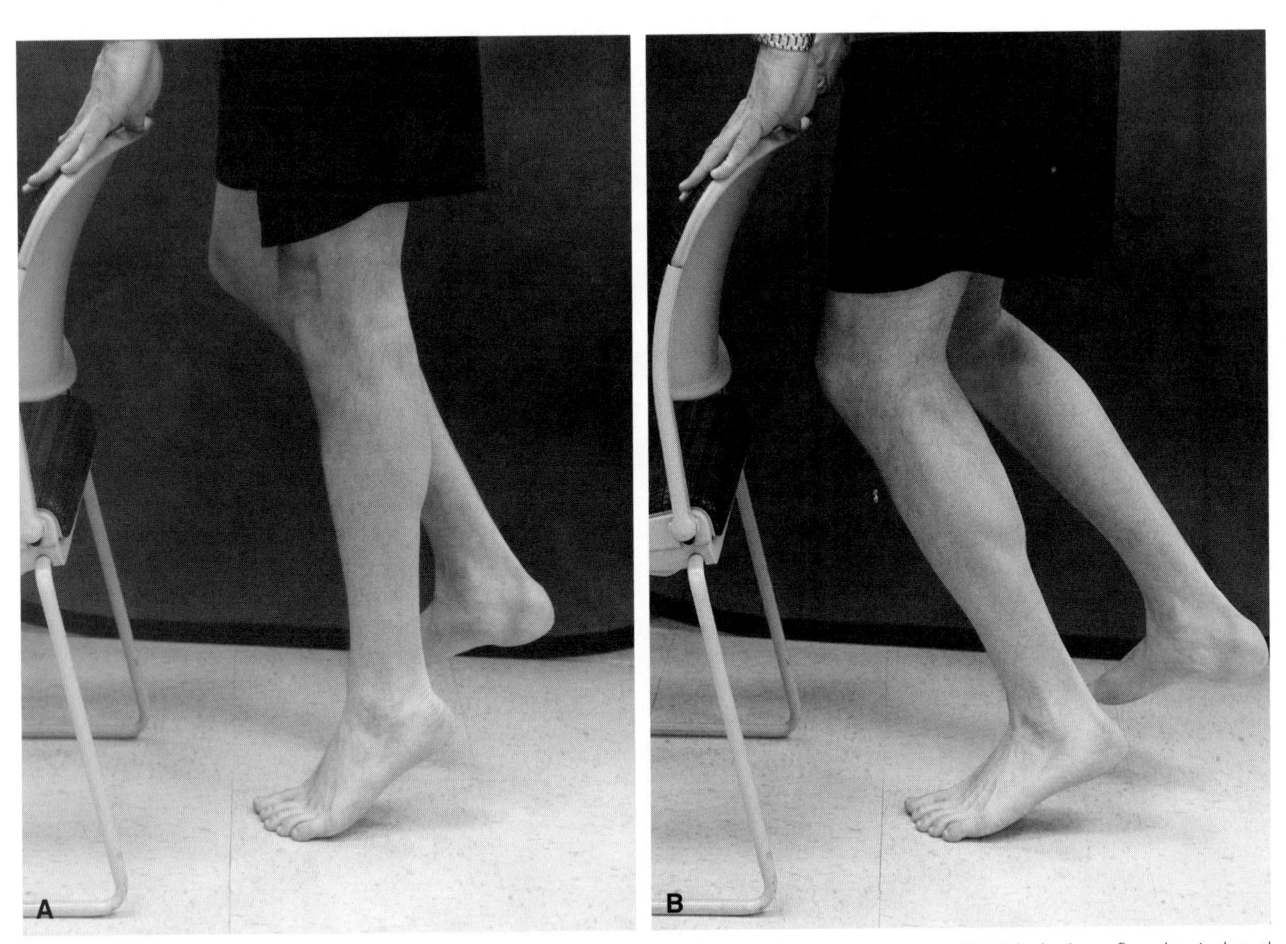

FIGURE 9-19 ■ Heel-raise test for plantarflexion. (A) With the knee extended to include the gastrocnemius. (B) With the knee flexed to isolate the soleus muscle.

Goniometry Box 9-1
Ankle Plantarflexion/Dorsiflexion

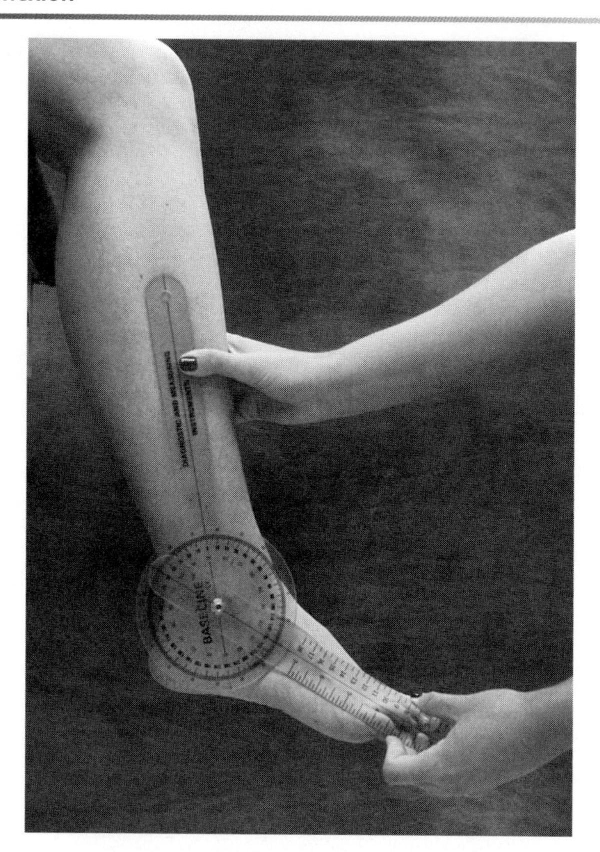

Dorsiflexion 0–20 **Plantarflexion 0–50**

Patient Position	Sitting with the knee flexed to 90°, the ankle in anatomical position, and the foot in 0° of inversion and eversion
Goniometer Alignment	
Fulcrum	The axis is centered over the lateral malleolus.
Proximal Arm	The stationary arm is aligned with the long axis of the fibula.
Distal Arm	The movement arm is aligned parallel with the bottom of the foot.
Modification	Dorsiflexion may be measured with the patient prone and the knee flexed to 90°.
Comment	Avoid extending the toes or twisting the foot. Measuring dorsiflexion with the knee extended assesses for limitation in dorsiflexion secondary to gastrocnemius tightness, which may be clinically useful. Measurements are relative to the ankle at 90° (anatomical position).

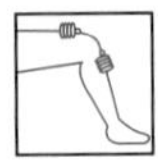

Manual Muscle Test 9-1
Dorsiflexion and Supination

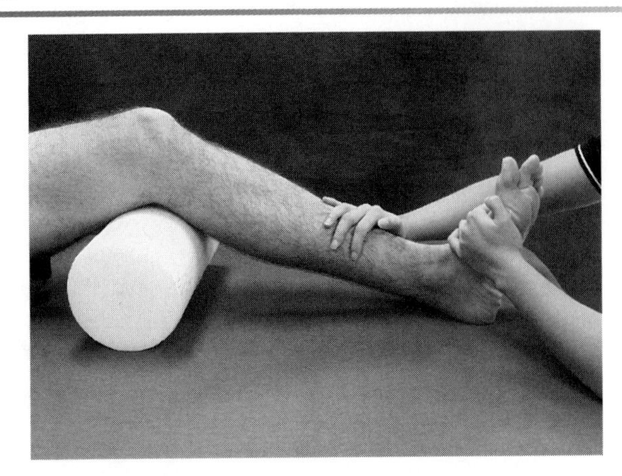

Patient Position	Seated
Starting Position	The knee is flexed. The foot is positioned in plantarflexion and eversion.
Stabilization	Distal tibia, preventing knee extension and femoral external rotation
Palpation	Muscle belly of anterior tibialis or its tendon (the most medial tendon on the anterior aspect of the talocrural joint)
Resistance	Medial aspect of the dorsum of the foot
Primary Mover(s) (Innervation)	Tibialis anterior (L4, L5, S1)
Secondary Mover(s) (Innervation)	Extensor hallucis longus (L4, L5, S1) Extensor digitorum longus (L4, L5, S1) Peroneus tertius (negligible contribution) (L4, L5, S1)
Substitution	Knee extension Toe extension
Comment	Ensure that the toes are relaxed to reduce the contribution of extensor hallucis longus and extensor digitorum longus.

ROM = range of motion.

Passive range of motion

The extensive soft tissue arrangement of the talocrural and subtalar joint results in a firm end-feel owing to tissue stretch (Table 9-5). Damage to the ligamentous or capsular structures may result in a hard end-feel as bone contacts bone.

- **Plantarflexion and dorsiflexion:** Dorsiflexion is measured once with the knee extended to determine the overall influence of the triceps surae group and then again with the knee flexed to determine the influence of the soleus. The normal end-feel for both plantarflexion and dorsiflexion is firm, owing to soft tissue stretch of the anterior joint capsule, deltoid ligament, and ATF ligament during plantarflexion and of the

Table 9-5 Talocrural Joint Capsular Patterns and End-Feels

Capsular Pattern Talocrural Joint: Plantarflexion, Dorsiflexion	
Plantarflexion of the talocrural joint	Firm – soft tissue stretch
Dorsiflexion of the talocrural joint	Firm – soft tissue stretch
Capsular Pattern Subtalar Joint: Supination, Pronation	
Inversion of the subtalar joint	Firm – soft tissue stretch
Eversion of the subtalar joint	Firm – soft tissue stretch

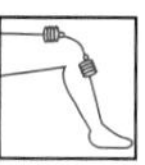

Manual Muscle Test 9-2
Eversion and Pronation

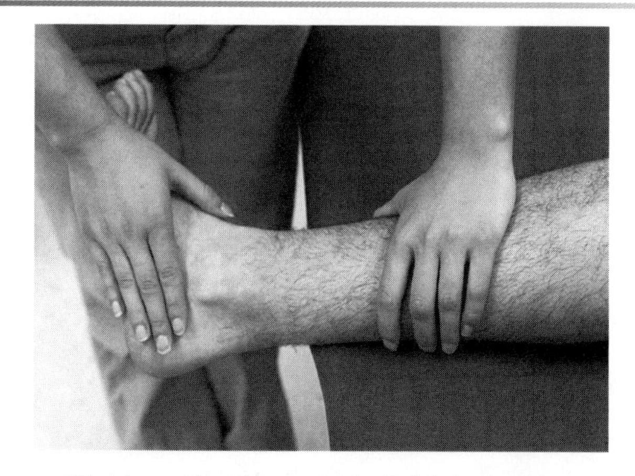

Patient Position	Side-lying on the side opposite the limb being tested The opposite hip is flexed
Starting Position	The test foot is off the end of the table in slight plantarflexion.
Stabilization	Lower leg
Palpation	Posterior aspect of the lateral malleolus; proximal portion of the fibula
Resistance	Lateral border of the foot
Primary Mover(s) (Innervation)	Peroneus longus (L4, L5, S1) Peroneus brevis (L4, L5, S1)
Secondary Mover(s) (Innervation)	Extensor digitorum longus (L4, L5, S1)
Substitution	Plantarflexors Toe extension
Comment	Avoid toe extension to decrease the contribution of the extensor digitorum longus.

Achilles tendon during dorsiflexion. After injury, the amount of ROM lost is greater during plantarflexion than in dorsiflexion. However, loss of dorsiflexion is more debilitating in the long term because of the resultant changes in gait mechanics.

- **Inversion and eversion:** The calcaneal inversion and eversion components of subtalar pronation and supination are assessed and measured with the patient prone. The tibia and fibula are stabilized to prevent hip or leg rotation. The normal end-feel during neutral inversion is firm secondary to soft tissue stretch from the lateral ankle ligaments (especially the CF ligament) and the peroneus longus and brevis muscles. A hard end-feel may be present during eversion if the calcaneus contacts the fibula. The end-feel may be firm because of stretching of the medial joint capsule and musculature. After injury, the capsular pattern loss is greater for inversion than for eversion.

Joint Stability Tests

ROM tests place stress on the ligaments of the ankle complex, especially during passive ROM testing (see Table 9-3). Although several manual stress tests are used to identify laxity in the lateral ankle ligaments, their ability to differentiate between the individual ligaments and the relative severity of the trauma is unclear.[21] While these tests may identify ankle laxity, they may lack the specificity to identify which ligaments are involved, owing to individual tissue properties and variations in torque applied during the testing procedure.[21] Joint stability tests (stress testing and special tests) are most accurate when they are performed 4 to 7 days following the injury. Prior to this time pain, swelling, and patient apprehension contaminate the results.[7] Ankle arthrometers, instruments designed to quantify the amount of laxity, provide an intrarater reliability between 0.71 and 0.94, but their validity remains unclear.[22]

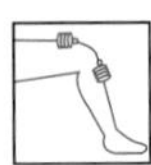

Manual Muscle Test 9-3
Plantarflexors

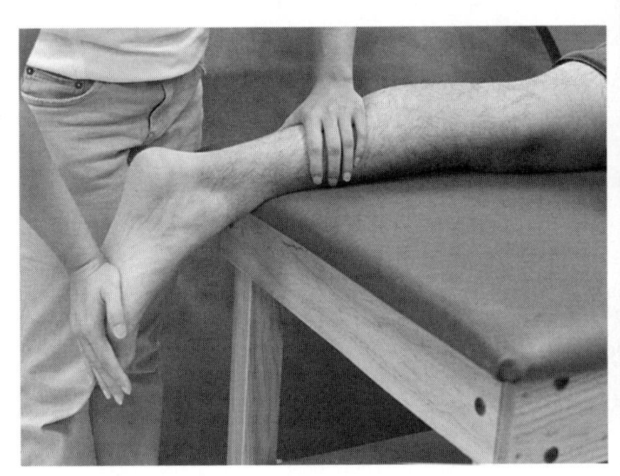

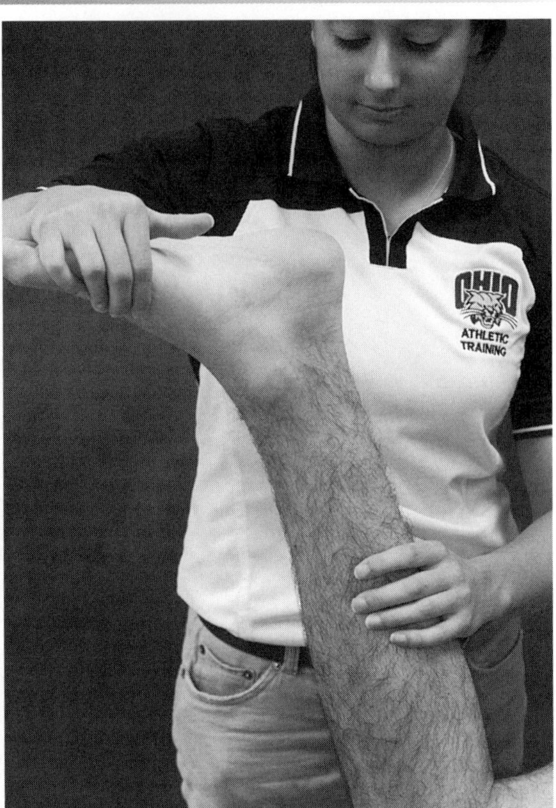

Patient Position	Prone
Starting Position	***Gastrocnemius:*** **(A)** The knee is extended with the foot off the table ***Soleus:*** **(B)** The knee is flexed past 30°
Stabilization	Proximal to the ankle
Palpation	***Gastrocnemius:*** Posterior leg just distal to the knee joint line. ***Soleus:*** Midleg anterior to the gastrocnemius
Resistance	Plantar aspect of the rear- and midfoot
Primary Mover(s) (Innervation)	Gastrocnemius (S1, S2) Soleus (S1, S2)
Secondary Mover(s) (Innervation)	Flexor digitorum longus (L5, S1) Flexor hallucis longus (L4, L5, S1) Tibialis posterior (L4, L5, S1)
Substitution	Hamstrings: Avoid knee flexion
Comment	Avoid toe flexion to reduce the contribution of flexor hallucis longus and flexor digitorum longus. Avoid inversion to reduce the contribution of tibialis posterior. Because the plantarflexors are a strong muscle group, single-leg heel raises may provided a better indicator of strength.

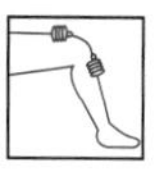

Manual Muscle Test 9-4
Rearfoot Inversion

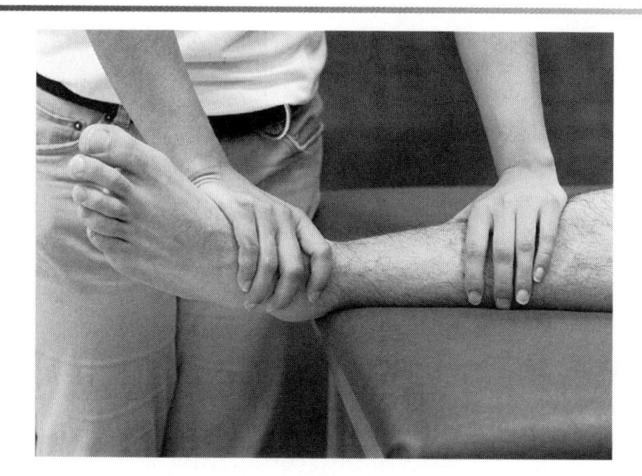

Patient Position	Side-lying on the side opposite being tested The opposite hip is flexed.
Starting Position	The test foot is off the end of the table with the ankle in the resting position.
Stabilization	Medial aspect of the distal leg
Palpation	Posterior margin of the medial malleolus
Resistance	Medial border of the foot (navicular, medial cuneiform)
Primary Mover(s) (Innervation)	Tibialis posterior (L4, L5, S1)
Secondary Mover(s) (Innervation)	Flexor digitorum longus (L5, S1) Flexor hallucis longus (L4, L5, S1)
Substitution	Plantarflexors Toe flexors
Comment	Avoid toe flexion to reduce the contribution of flexor hallucis longus and flexor digitorum longus.

Stress testing

Test for anterior talofibular ligament instability. The combined motions of ankle plantarflexion and subtalar supination place a strain on the ATF ligament as it prevents anterior translation of the talus relative to the ankle mortise. The **anterior drawer test** is used to determine the integrity of the ATF (Stress Test 9-1).[26,27]

Test for calcaneofibular ligament instability. The **inversion stress test** (talar tilt test) is used to determine if the calcaneofibular ligament has been injured (Stress Test 9-2). This test also stresses the anterior and posterior talofibular ligaments and may reveal instability in the subtalar joint.[28]

Tests for deltoid ligament instability. The distal projection of the lateral malleolus limits the amount of ankle eversion, but rotation of the talocrural and/or subtalar joint may injure the deltoid ligament.[29] The **eversion stress test** (Stress Test 9-3) is used to evaluate injury to the deltoid ligament group. The **external rotation test** (Kleiger's test) is used to determine injury to the deltoid ligament caused by a rotational stress or injury to the syndesmosis, with the results differentiated by the location of pain (Special Test 9-1).

Joint play testing

Joint play assessment is indicated at the proximal (see Chapter 8) and distal tibiofibular joints, the talocrural joint or the subtalar joint. Hypermobility at any of these joints confirms the presence of a sprain.

Subtalar joint play. The talocrural joint may become restricted following a period of immobilization (Joint Play 9-1). A restriction in posterior talar glide, common following a period of immobilization, is functionally demonstrated by a limitation in dorsiflexion. Restricted subtalar medial glide may be a causative factor in limited pronation during ambulation.

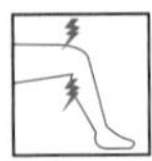

Stress Test 9-1
Anterior Drawer Test

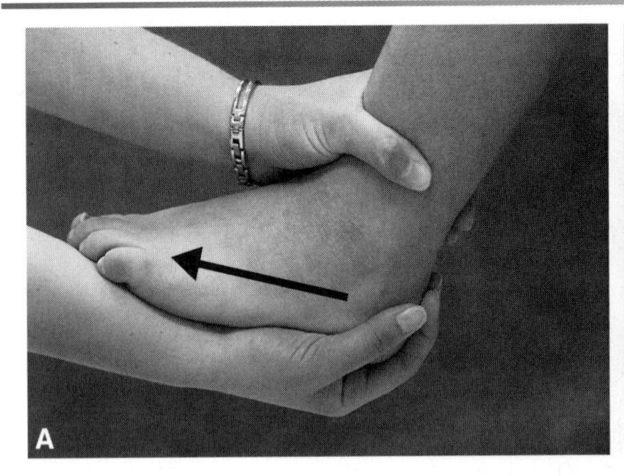

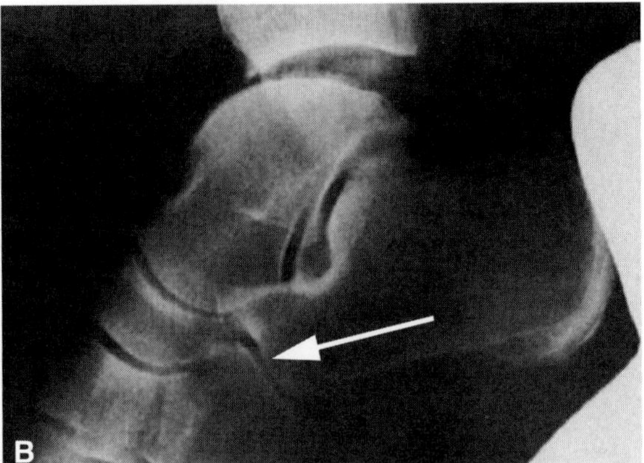

(A) Anterior drawer test to check the integrity of the anterior talofibular ligament. **(B)** Radiographic view of a positive anterior drawer test. Note the anterior displacement of the talus relative to the tibia. (**B** Courtesy of Donatelli, RA: *Biomechanics of the Foot and Ankle*. Philadelphia, FA Davis, 1990.)

Patient Position	Sitting over the edge of the table with the knee flexed to prevent gastrocnemius tightness from influencing the outcome of the test
Position of Examiner	Sitting in front of the patient One hand stabilizes the leg, taking care not to occlude the mortise. The other hand cups the calcaneus while the forearm supports the foot in a position of slight plantarflexion (10°–20° from the anatomical position).[7,23]
Evaluative Procedure	The calcaneus and talus are drawn forward while providing a stabilizing force to the tibia.
Positive Test	The talus slides anteriorly from under the ankle mortise compared with the opposite side (assuming it is normal). There may be an appreciable "clunk" as the talus subluxates and relocates, or the patient may describe pain.
Implications	Sprain of the anterior talofibular ligament and the associated capsule
Modification	The test may be performed with the patient supine, but the knee must be kept in a minimum of 30° flexion to eliminate the influence of the gastrocnemius muscle. The tibia can be pushed posteriorly as the calcaneus is drawn anteriorly.
Comments	Pain or apprehension can result in the patient contracting the triceps surae, thereby produce false-negative results. Do not apply over-pressure in an attempt to overcome this response.[24] The anterior drawer test is useful in differentiating an intact ATFL from an isolated ATFL sprain, but is less sensitive in differentiating an ATFL sprain from a more diffuse lateral ankle sprain involving the CFL.[25]
Evidence	***Inter-rater reliability***

Not Reliable — Very Reliable
Poor | Moderate | Good
0 0.1 0.2 0.3 0.4 0.5 0.6 0.7 0.8 0.9 1.0

Positive likelihood ratio

Not Useful — Useful
Very Small | Small | Moderate | Large
0 1 2 3 4 5 6 7 8 9 10

Negative likelihood ratio

Not Useful — Useful
Very Small | Small | Moderate | Large
1.0 0.9 0.8 0.7 0.6 0.5 0.4 0.3 0.2 0.1 0

ATFL = anterior talofibular ligament; CFL = calcaneofibular ligament.

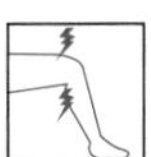

Stress Test 9-2
Inversion (Talar Tilt) Stress Test

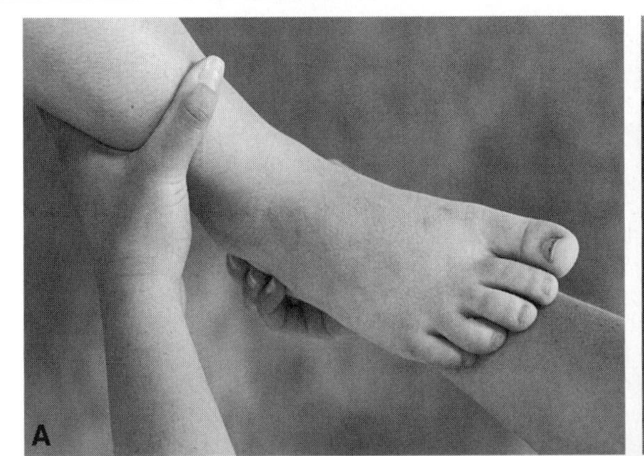

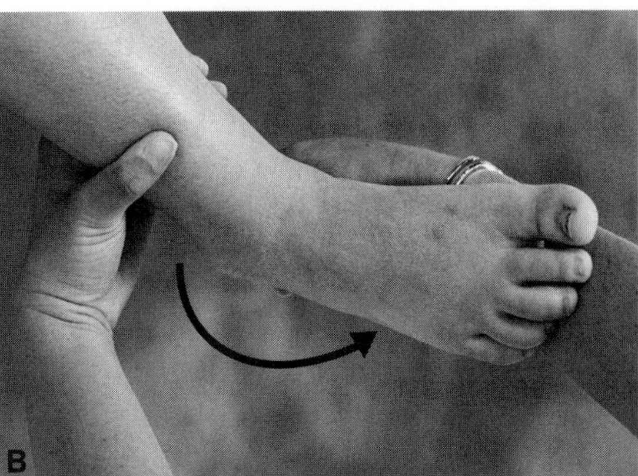

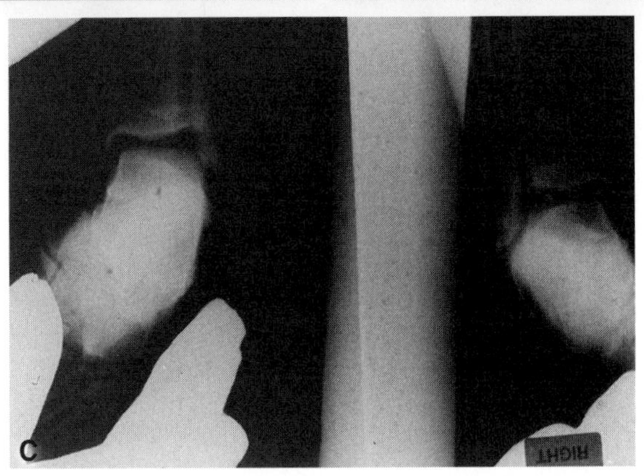

(A and B) Inversion stress test (talar tilt test) to check the integrity of the calcaneofibular ligament. **(C)** Radiograph of an inversion stress.

Patient Position	Supine or sitting with legs over the edge of a table
Position of Examiner	In front of the patient One hand grasps the calcaneus and talus as a single unit and maintains the foot and ankle in 10° of dorsiflexion to isolate the calcaneofibular ligament.[25] The opposite hand stabilizes the leg; the thumb or forefinger is placed along the calcaneofibular ligament so that any gapping of the talus away from the mortise can be felt.
Evaluative Procedure	The hand holding the calcaneus provides an inversion stress by rolling the calcaneus medially, causing the talus to tilt.
Positive Test	The talus tilts or gaps excessively (i.e., greater than 10°) compared with the uninjured side; or pain is produced.
Implications	Involvement of the calcaneofibular ligament, possibly along with the anterior talofibular and posterior talofibular ligaments
Modification	Inversion can be assessed with the ankle in different positions in the ROM to stress specific ligaments.
Comments	When the severity of injury is being based on the relative laxity, a history of injury and residual laxity to the uninvolved ankle mask the magnitude of the current trauma.[7,25]
Evidence	The specificity of 0.68 for combined ATFL and CFL sprains.[25]

ATFL = anterior talofibular ligament; CFL = calcaneofibular ligament.

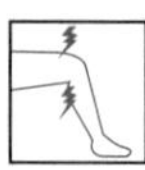

Stress Test 9-3
Eversion (Talar Tilt) Stress Test

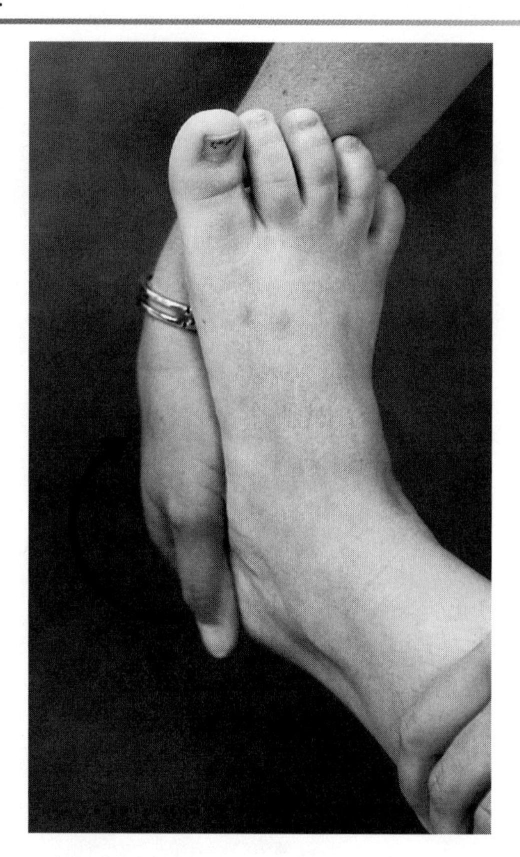

Eversion stress test to determine the integrity of the deltoid ligament, especially the tibiocalcaneal ligament.

Patient Position	Supine or sitting with legs over the edge of a table
Position of Examiner	In front of the patient One hand grasps the calcaneus and talus as a single unit and maintains the ankle in a neutral position.
Evaluative Procedure	The opposite hand stabilizes the leg. The thumb or forefinger may be placed along the deltoid ligament so that any gapping of the talus away from the mortise can be felt. The hand holding the calcaneus rolls it laterally, tilting the talus and causing a gap on the medial side of the ankle mortise.
Positive Test	The talus tilts or gaps excessively as compared with the uninjured side, or pain is described during this motion.
Implications	Deltoid ligament sprain
Comments	Pain at the distal syndesmosis may indicate a distal tibiofibular sprain.
Evidence	Absent or inconclusive in the literature

Special Test 9-1
External Rotation Test (Kleiger's Test)

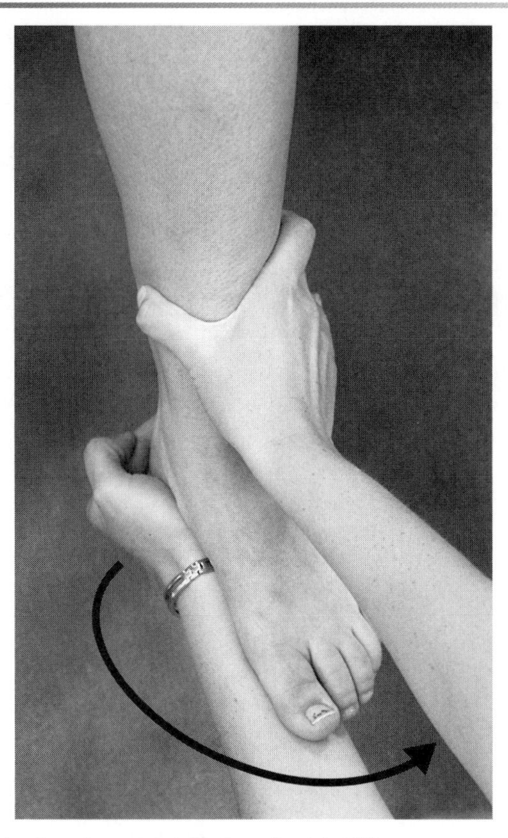

External rotation (Kleiger's) test for determination of rotatory damage to the deltoid ligament or the distal tibiofibular syndesmosis. The implication is based on the area of pain that is elicited. Externally rotating the talus (1) places a lateral force on the fibula (2), spreading the syndesmosis and stretching the deltoid ligament (3).

Patient Position	Sitting with legs over the edge of the table
Position of Examiner	In front of the patient One hand stabilizes the leg in a manner that does not compress the distal tibiofibular syndesmosis. The other hand grasps the medial aspect of the foot while supporting the ankle in a neutral position.
Evaluative Procedure	The foot and talus are externally rotated, while maintaining a stable leg. To stress the syndesmosis, place the ankle in dorsiflexion. To stress the deltoid ligament, place the ankle in neutral position or slightly plantarflexed.
Positive Test	***Deltoid ligament involvement:*** Medial joint pain. The examiner may feel displacement of the talus away from the medial malleolus. ***Syndesmosis involvement:*** Pain is described in the anterolateral ankle at the site of the distal tibiofibular syndesmosis.
Implications	Medial pain is indicative of trauma to the deltoid ligament. Pain in the area of the anterior or posterior tibiofibular ligament should be considered syndesmosis pathology unless determined otherwise (e.g., malleolar fracture). Fracture of the distal fibula
Comments	Pain arising from the distal tibiofibular syndesmosis during this test is associated with a prolonged recovery time.[28]
Evidence	***Inter-rater reliability***

Not Reliable — **Very Reliable**

Poor | Moderate | Good

0 0.1 0.2 0.3 0.4 0.5 0.6 0.7 0.8 0.9 1.0

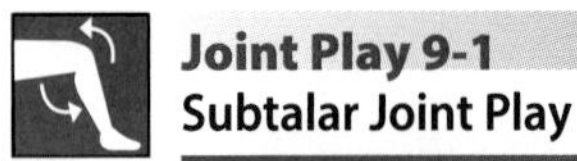

Joint Play 9-1
Subtalar Joint Play

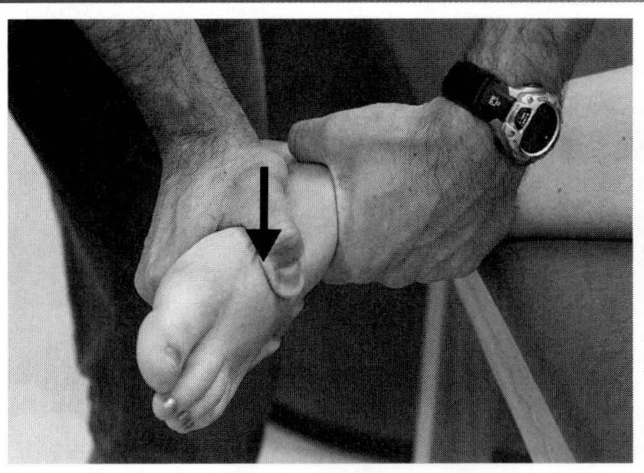

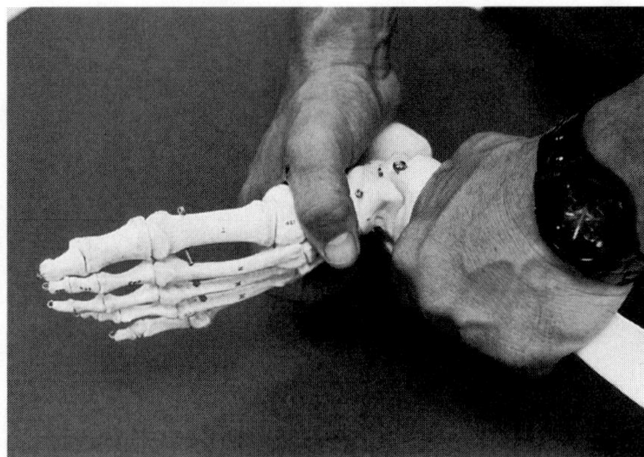

After stabilizing the talus in the mortise, the amount of medial and lateral movement at the subtalar joint is assessed (lateral glide shown).

Patient Position	***Medial glide:*** Side-lying on test limb. STJ in neutral (see p. 177 for finding STJ neutral position). ***Lateral glide:*** Side-lying on non-test limb. STJ in neutral. A towel may be placed under the distal tibia.
Position of Examiner	Stabilizing talus in the mortise The opposite hand cups the calcaneus.
Evaluative Procedure	Force is applied to move the talus medially and laterally.
Positive Test	Increased or decreased medial or lateral translation of the talus relative to the opposite side.
Implications	Results are compared relative to the opposite (uninjured) ankle: Hypomobile medial glide is associated with decreased pronation/calcaneal eversion. Hypomobile lateral glide is associated with decreased supination/calcaneal inversion.
Comments	Hypermobile medial glide is commonly associated with lateral ankle sprains.[28]
Evidence	Absent or inconclusive in the literature

STJ = subtalar joint.

Lateral translation of the talus in the ankle mortise is evaluated using the **Cotton Test** (Joint Play 9-2). The external rotation test identifies syndesmosis pathology by forcing the talus and calcaneus against the lateral malleolus, causing it to be displaced laterally and posteriorly stressing the syndesmosis (see Special Test 9-2, p. 259).

Test for distal tibiofibular syndesmosis instability. Injury to the distal tibiofibular syndesmosis, the anterior tibiofibular ligament, the interosseous membrane, and the posterior tibiofibular ligament may be identified through overpressure at the end of dorsiflexion ROM or by placing an external rotation force on the talus. During forced dorsiflexion, the wider anterior border of the talus is wedged into the talocrural joint, causing the fibula to move slightly away from the tibia. If the syndesmosis has been traumatized, pain will be elicited. **Distal tibiofibular joint play** is used to identify the anterior–posterior stability of the distal syndesmosis (Joint Play 9-3).

Neurologic Testing

Neurologic dysfunction can occur secondary to compression proximal to the leg, compartment syndromes, or direct trauma. The common peroneal nerve or its superficial or deep branches is most prone to trauma (Table 9-6). Figure 9-20 presents the distribution of neurologic symptoms around the ankle and foot. A lower quarter screen may also be required to rule out neurologic symptoms

Table 9-6 Mechanisms of Injury of the Common Peroneal Nerve

Mechanism	Causal Factor
Lesion	Fracture of the fibular head
Concussive	Contusion to the superior lateral portion of the leg
Compression	Knee braces or elastic wraps, especially when combined with cryotherapy
Internal Pressure	Prolonged squatting (e.g., baseball or softball catcher)
Entrapment	Exertional compartment syndromes (branches of the common peroneal nerve)
Traction	Varus stress to the knee, hyperextension of the knee, plantarflexion and inversion of the ankle

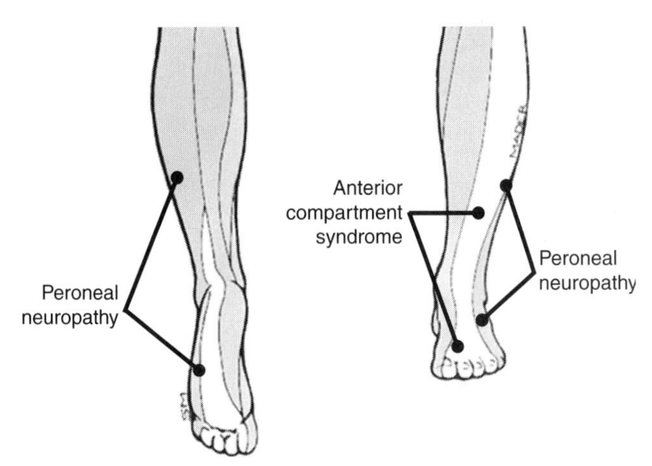

FIGURE 9-20 ■ Local neuropathies of the ankle and leg. These findings should also be matched with those of a lower quarter neurologic screen.

arising from the lumbar or sacral plexus (see Neurologic Screening Box 1-2).

Vascular Assessment

Vascular compromise can result from an acute or chronic increase in compartmental pressure or may be the result of bony fracture or joint dislocation of a leg structure anywhere proximal to the ankle. Prolonged impaired circulation can result in tissue necrosis.

- **Posterior tibial artery:** Palpate the posterior tibial artery, located between the flexor digitorum longus and flexor hallucis longus tendons as they pass behind the medial malleolus. Supplying blood to the foot, the presence of this pulse must be established after any significant lower extremity bone fracture or joint dislocation. Note that swelling along the medial joint line may mask the presence of this pulse and make its detection difficult.

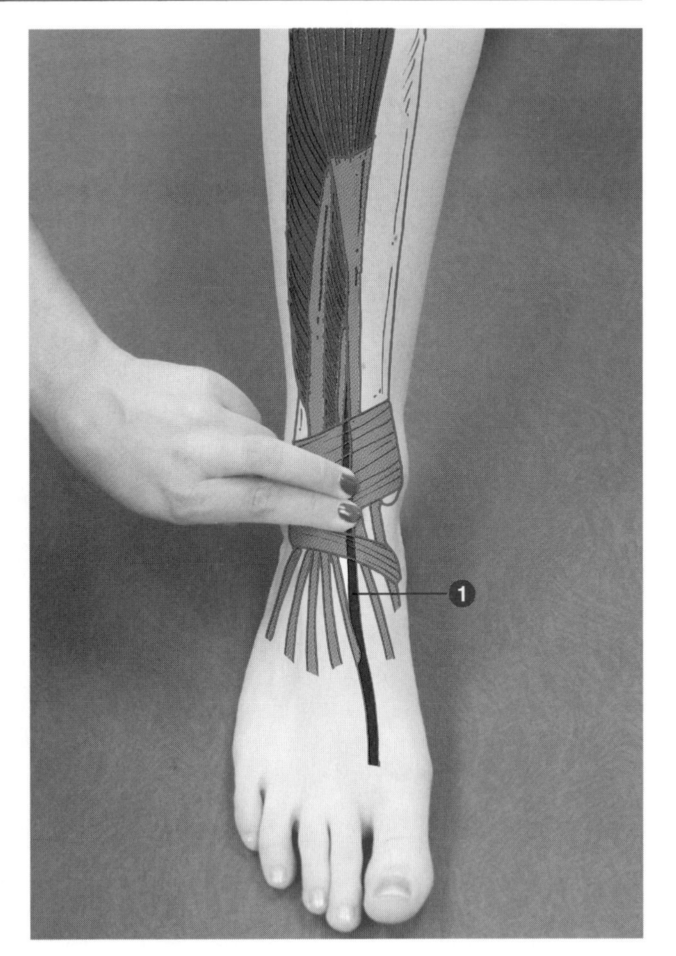

1 **Dorsalis pedis artery:** A branch of the anterior tibial artery, the dorsalis pedis pulse may be palpated between the extensor digitorum longus and extensor hallucis longus tendons as they pass over the cuneiforms. The presence of this pulse after lower extremity fracture or dislocation and in those individuals suspected of having an anterior compartment syndrome must be established. This pulse is not readily detectable in all people. In the absence of a pulse on the involved side, make sure that the pulse is identifiable on the uninvolved extremity.

Pathologies and Related Special Tests

Although sprains are the predominant type of injury suffered by the leg and ankle, the evaluation process must not discount other potential injuries. Other acute injuries to this body area include fractures, dislocations, and tendon ruptures. In addition, many overuse conditions affect the leg. Historically, all emergency room visitations for acute ankle trauma routinely underwent radiographic examination. In many cases, the results were negative for a fracture. The Ottawa Ankle Rules were developed to help discriminate among those signs and symptoms that are more highly suggestive of fracture and thus reduce the number

Joint Play 9-2
Cotton Test (Lateral Talar Glide)

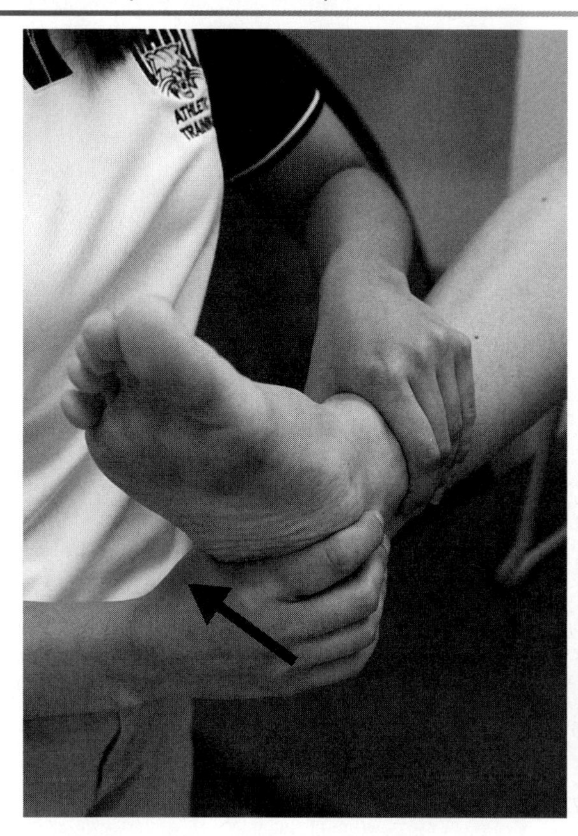

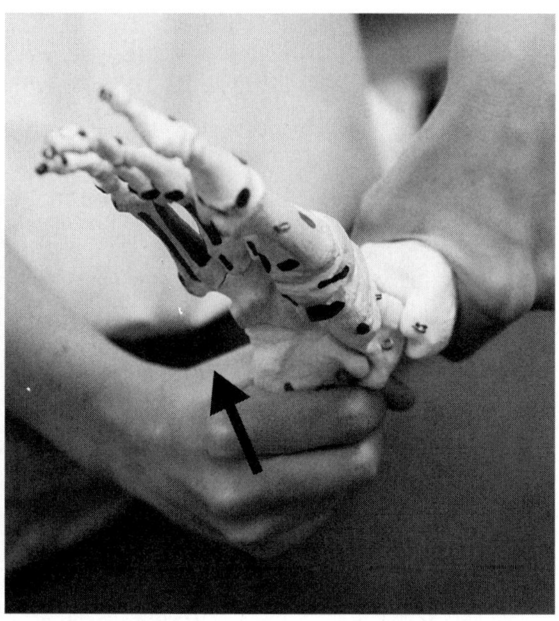

The Cotton test assesses the amount of lateral translation of the talus within the ankle mortise.

Patient Position	Supine or short sitting with the ankle in the neutral position
Position of Examiner	One hand grasps the ankle mortise just proximal to the tibotalar joint line, stabilizing the distal leg, but not compress the distal tibiofibular syndesmosis. The opposite hand cups the calcaneus and talus.
Evaluative Procedure	Force is applied to move the talus laterally.
Positive Test	Increased lateral translation of the talus relative to the opposite side Pain[29]
Implications	Distal tibiofibular syndesmosis sprain
Comments	There is a relationship between an arthroscopically confirmed diagnosis tibiofibular syndesmosis sprain and a positive Cotton test.[29]
Evidence	Absent or inconclusive in the literature

of unneeded and costly routine radiographs (see Ankle and Leg Fractures, p. 260).

Ankle Sprains

Most ankle sprains occur secondary to excessive supination, causing trauma to the lateral ligament complex as the calcaneus inverts and the talus abducts in a closed chain. A lesser yet significant percentage of ankle sprains involves the medial ankle ligaments and the distal tibiofibular syndesmosis. Because of the close association of many of the ankle ligaments with the joint capsule, ligament injury often results in trauma to the capsule. Ankle sprains are complicated by fractures of the ankle mortise, avulsion of the ligaments from their attachment site, dislocation of the talus, or nerve involvement.[31]

Joint Play 9-3
Distal Tibiofibular Joint Play

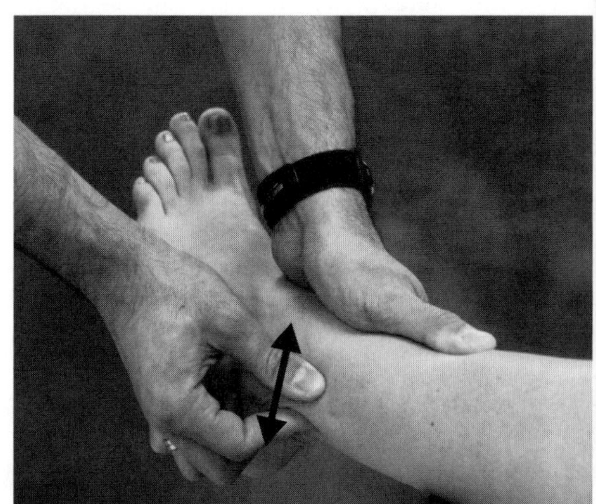

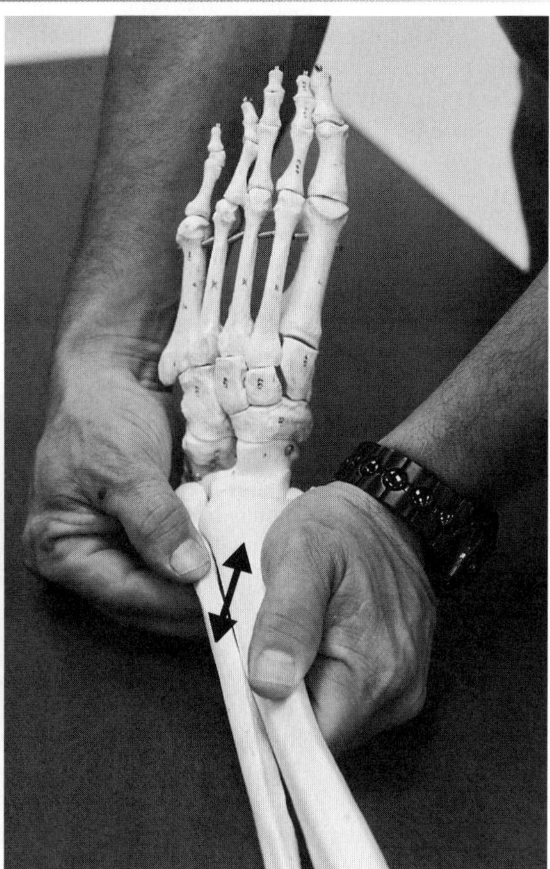

This joint play test identifies the amount of anterior–posterior play in the distal tibiofibular syndesmosis.

Patient Position	Supine or short sitting with the ankle relaxed into plantar flexion
Position of Examiner	Grasping the fibula at the lateral malleolus and stabilizing the tibia
Evaluative Procedure	Pressure is applied to obliquely move the fibula anteriorly and then posteriorly relative to the tibia.
Positive Test	Pain arising from the syndesmosis or increased motion relative to the uninvolved side[30]
Implications	Sprain of the distal tibiofibular syndesmosis
Modification	The distal fibula can be compressed ("squeezed") to identify lateral play based on the amount of movement.
Comments	Pain is a more reliable indicator of syndesmotic trauma than increased motion.[30]
Evidence	Absent or inconclusive in the literature

Lateral ankle sprains

The ankle complex is least stable when it is in the **open-packed position** of plantarflexion and inversion (supination) while the foot is non–weight bearing, resulting in a sprain of the lateral ankle ligaments. The inversion component of supination is most commonly used to describe mechanism of injury to the lateral ankle ligament complex. Many athletic skills require extreme amounts of supination, thereby predisposing the ankle to injury.

A sudden, forceful supinatory force to the foot and ankle can tear the lateral ligaments, with the specific structures involved depending on the position of the talocrural joint and the amount of force applied to the structures. Because it becomes taut when the foot and ankle are supinated, the anterior talofibular ligament is the most commonly sprained ankle ligament. If the amount of supination is sufficient or if the ankle is near its neutral position, the calcaneofibular ligament also may be traumatized. Significantly more force is required to invert the ankle in its dorsiflexed, closed-packed position, primarily stressing the lateral malleolus and posterior talofibular ligament (Examination Findings 9-1).

Anatomic and physiologic factors predisposing individuals to lateral ankle sprains include decreased proprioceptive ability, decreased muscular strength, and a lack of muscular coordination, all factors associated with a history of multiple ankle sprains.[33,39] Tightness of the Achilles tendon or the triceps surae muscle group creates an increased risk of sprains to the lateral ligament complex by placing the ankle complex in a plantarflexed, open-packed resting position.

The primary clinical finding of an lateral ankle sprain is a history of inversion, plantarflexion, and/or rotation (see Table 9-3). A sensation of tearing or "popping" may also be described. Pain is localized along the lateral ligament complex and sinus tarsi. Because the anterior talofibular and posterior talofibular ligaments are capsular structures, tears of these ligaments can produce rapid, diffuse swelling. Being extracapsular, the calcaneofibular ligament produces relatively little edema when it is damaged. Sprains of the posterior talofibular rarely occur in isolation. Trauma to the PTF ligament is usually associated with significant ligament disruption of the calcaneofibular and anterior talofibular ligaments.[7]

*** Practical Evidence**

The accuracy and usefulness of the clinical findings for a lateral ankle sprain improve with time.[25] Five days following the injury, pain elicited during palpation of the ATF ligament, lateral ecchymosis, and a positive anterior drawer is 96% specific in detecting ligament ruptures.[37]

Palpation elicits tenderness along the involved ligament. The associated joint capsule and the sinus tarsi may become tender.[17] Special attention must be paid to pain and crepitus elicited over the origin and insertion of the ligament, indicating a possible avulsion fracture. Pain is demonstrated during the movements of inversion or plantarflexion, as described in the Joint and Muscle Function Assessment and the Joint Stability Testing sections of this chapter.

The severity and relative damage associated with moderate ankle sprains are often underestimated, and other trauma that is caused by the injury mechanism may be overlooked.[40] Excessive inversion can place compressive forces on the medial structures; exert a tensile force on the peroneal tendons and peroneal nerve; and involve the Achilles tendon, tibialis posterior, extensor digitorum brevis, and calcaneocuboid ligament.[31] The subtalar joint is often sprained at the same time as the lateral ankle ligaments.[25]

Inverting the talus can impinge the medial ligaments, medial joint capsule, and the structures passing beneath the medial malleolus, especially the tibialis posterior tendon. Excessive inversion of the talus and calcaneus can result in the fracture of the distal medial malleolus, base or styloid process of the fifth MT, or avulse the lateral ligaments from their site of origin or insertion (Fig. 9-21).

Chronic lateral ankle instability is classified as either mechanical, functional, or both.[1,6] Mechanical instability is

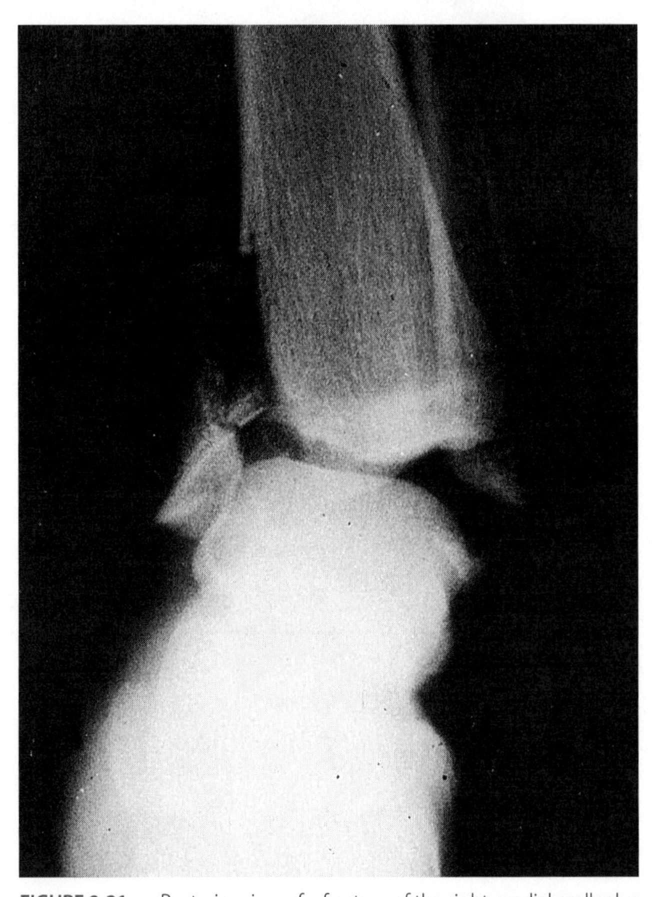

FIGURE 9-21 ■ Posterior view of a fracture of the right medial malleolus caused by excessive inversion of the ankle.

characterized by gross laxity to one or more of the ankle's joints or insufficiency of the supporting structures. Functional instability involves repeated ankle sprains in individuals who have normal findings during ligamentous stress tests and is associated with proprioceptive and neuromuscular deficits, decreased strength, and/or postural control.[6]

Moderate to severe ankle sprains result in recurrence rates greater than 70%, with approximately 60% of those affected experiencing residual deficits on athletic performance.[41] Basketball players with a history of ankle sprains are five times more likely to suffer an ankle sprain than a player who has no history of sprain.[33] Two theories have been suggested to account for this[42]: (1) the loss of the ligament's ability to passively support and protect the joint in conjunction with a reflex arc that is too slow to evoke a contraction in the peroneal muscles, limiting the force and speed of inversion[43]; and (2) decreased proprioceptive ability of the capsule, ligaments, and peroneal muscles.[44,45]

Chronic or severe lateral ankle sprains often result in a number of secondary conditions. After a sprain of the anterior talofibular and calcaneofibular ligaments, the anterolateral capsule may develop a dense area of thickened connective tissue that becomes impinged between the lateral malleolus and calcaneus when the foot and ankle are dorsiflexed and everted.[46] Bone bruises, accumulations of blood within the talus, navicular, and calcaneus,[47] and longitudinal tears of the peroneus brevis tendon[48] are also associated with lateral ankle sprains. Recurrent pain behind the lateral malleolus following a significant lateral ankle sprain or in the presence of chronic lateral ankle instability is highly suggestive of a peroneal tendon lesion and/or subluxation.

Lateral ankle sprains may produce an associated talar or tibial **chondral lesion** (osteochondral defect) caused by the combination of inversion, plantarflexion, and talar rotation that compress the superior medial articulating cartilage of the talus against the tibia.[36] These small fractures, not easily identified on standard radiographic examination, share a common trait of pain of unidentified origin, reports of pain "deep in the ankle" and tenderness along the superior anteromedial (tibial) portion of the ankle mortise (Fig. 9-22). The use of magnetic resonance imaging (MRI) and CT scans has improved the accuracy in diagnosing chondral lesions.[49,50] If this condition goes unrecognized, osteochondritis dissecans of the talocrural joint is likely to develop.[51,52]

Traction injuries to the peroneal nerve can affect the sensory and motor function of the leg and ankle. Decreased sensory function may be present in the involved ankle immediately after forceful plantarflexion and inversion. After a severe sprain, inhibition of sensory and motor function can extend as far as the hip.[53]

Added care is necessary when evaluating apparent ankle sprains in adolescents. Patients displaying excessive laxity require referral to a physician to rule out epiphyseal fractures.

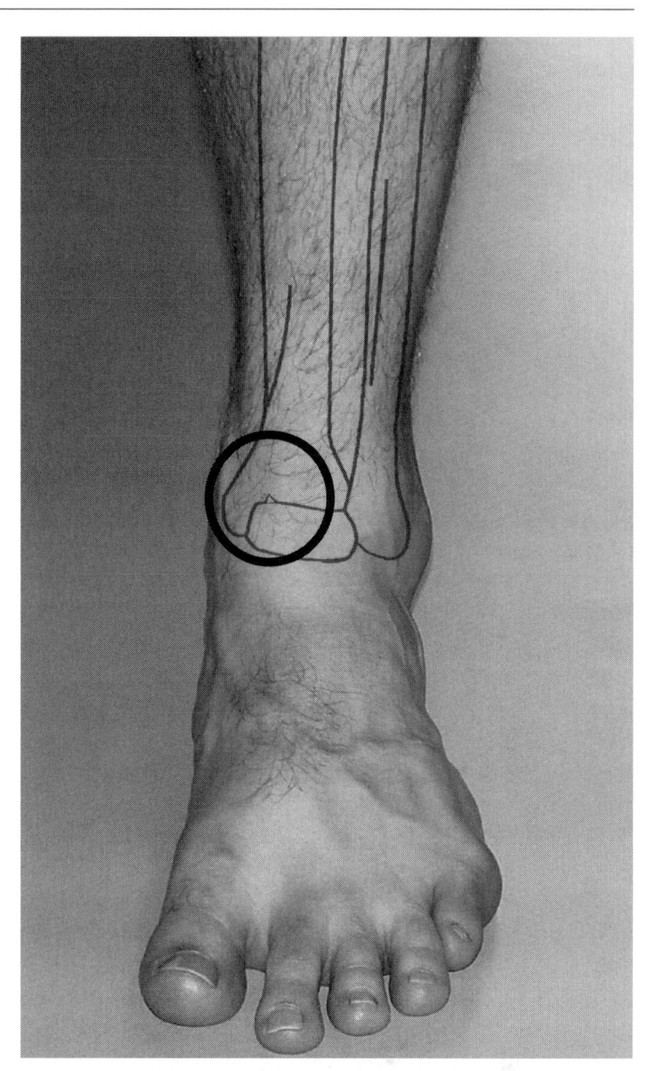

FIGURE 9-22 ■ Location of a tibial osteochondral lesion following an lateral ankle sprain. As the talus inverts, its superomedial border may contact the tibia with sufficient force to cause a bony defect in either the tibia or talus.

Tape and braces have been used to prevent recurrence of ankle sprains. However, a complete rehabilitation program is required for all ankle sprains. Implementing early ROM exercises and other forms of mobilization have been shown to decrease pain and swelling while increasing overall ROM.[54,55] Early mobilization does result in more residual subjective complaints but has little long-term detrimental effect on athletic performance.[56] Chronic ankle instability can be repaired using a variety of surgical reconstruction techniques with varying amounts of success.[57] For complete ruptures of the lateral ligaments, operative treatment yields improved results relative to conservative treatments.[58]

Syndesmosis sprains

Injury to the tibiofibular syndesmosis has been estimated to account for 10% of all ankle sprains and as high as 18% of ankle sprains in professional football players.[60] Although

Examination Findings 9-1
Lateral Ankle Sprains

Examination Segment	Clinical Findings
History	***Onset:*** Acute ***Pain characteristics:*** Lateral aspect of the ankle around the area of the malleolus and sinus tarsi ***Other symptoms:*** An associated "pop" may be reported. ***Mechanism:*** Supination (calcaneal inversion), plantarflexion, or talar rotation in any combination ***Predisposing conditions:*** A history of ankle sprain leading to decreased proprioceptive ability, decreased strength, and/or a lack of muscular coordination[32,33,34] Achilles tendon and/or triceps surae tightness; tarsal coalition Pes cavus/supinated foot type Overweight as indicated by high Body Mass Index[34,35]
Inspection	Findings include swelling around the lateral joint capsule, which may spread to the dorsum of the foot and into the sinus tarsi. Ecchymosis may be present around the lateral malleolus.
Palpation	Pain is elicited along the involved ligaments, but may be diffuse during the initial examination.[25] The sinus tarsi may be sensitive to the touch Crepitus at the site of ligamentous origin or insertion may indicate an avulsion fracture
Joint and Muscle Function Assessment	***AROM:*** Pain on the lateral side of the ankle during plantarflexion and inversion indicates stretching of the lateral ligaments. Pain medially indicates a pinching of the medial structures. ***MMT:*** Peroneals are weak and painful. Extensor digitorum longus is weak and painful. ***PROM:*** Motion produces pain along the ligaments, primarily: – Inversion and plantarflexion: Anterior talofibular ligament, calcaneofibular ligament – Inversion, neutral position: calcaneofibular ligament – Inversion and dorsiflexion: posterior talofibular ligament
Joint Stability Tests	***Stress tests:*** Positive inversion stress test and/or anterior drawer test results in laxity and/or pain ***Joint play:*** Increased medial glide at the subtalar joint.
Special Tests	Squeeze test to rule out a fracture of the distal fibula

Neurologic Screening	Repeated lateral ankle sprains may result in neuropathy of the peroneal and/or sural nerves.[1] Sensory testing of the peroneal nerve distribution if neurologic symptoms are present.
Vascular Screening	Within normal limits
Functional Assessment	Gait observation reveals antalgic gait with shortened stance phase on involved side and ankle maintained in resting position of slight plantarflexion Single-leg balance testing may be diminished.[1]
Imaging Techniques	MR images may detect an osteochondral lesion on the superomedial talus or the inferior tibial articulating surface.[36] Patients with negative radiographs who still experience pain after 2–4 weeks of conservative rehabilitation should be referred for bone scan, MR, or CT imaging.[36] Ultrasonic images have a LR+ of 2.55 and a LR– of 0.13 in determining lateral ligament ruptures.[37] Stress radiographs have a LR+ of 2.34 and LR–1 of 0.45 in determining lateral ligament ruptures.[37]
Differential Diagnosis	Syndesmotic ankle sprain, subluxating peroneal tendon, tear of the peroneus brevis tendon, peroneal strain, subtalar joint sprain, lateral malleolus fracture, medial malleolus fracture, osteochondral fracture of the talus, Jones' fracture
Comments	An avulsion fracture of the lateral ligaments from the malleolus, impingement of the medial joint capsule, impingement of the structures beneath the medial malleolus, and possible fracture of the medial malleolus or base of the 5th MT can occur concurrently with a lateral ankle sprain. Subtalar joint hypermobility is associated with talocrural instability in approximately 66% of cases, although it is unclear if this is causative or a result of pathology.[28] A chondral defect may be present in the articulating surfaces of the superior portion of the anteromedial talus and/or the inferior portion of the anteromedial tibia. Adolescents displaying ankle instability should be referred for radiographic examination to rule out the possibility of an epiphyseal injury. Persistent anterolateral ankle pain following lateral ankle sprains may indicative abnormal synovial thickening.[38]

AROM = active range of motion; CT = computed tomography; LR+ = positive likelihood ratio; LR- = negative likelihood ratio; MMT = manual muscle test; MR = magnetic resonance; PROM = passive range of motion; MT = metatarsal.

representing only a small percentage of all ankle sprains, syndesmotic ankle sprains are associated with significantly longer time lost from activity compared with other types of ankle sprains.

During excessive external rotation of the talus or forced dorsiflexion, the talus places pressure on the fibula, causing the distal syndesmosis to spread. The lateral displacement of the distal fibula can result in a sprain of the anterior and posterior tibiofibular ligaments, the interosseous membrane, and the crural interosseous ligament (Fig. 9-23).

Syndesmosis sprains, also referred to as "high" ankle sprains, are attributed to playing on artificial surfaces, but research does not substantiate this claim.[11] Other factors contributing to the occurrence of syndesmotic ankle sprains include **collision sports** where the mechanism of injury involves planting the foot and "cutting" so that the talus is externally rotated and the foot is dorsiflexed. Another common mechanism is being fallen on while lying on the ground, causing forced dorsiflexion and external rotation of the foot. Syndesmotic and deltoid ligament sprains often occur concurrently.[11]

Pain is located primarily on the anterior aspect of the ankle and proximally along the interosseous membrane and is intensified during forced dorsiflexion, the **external rotation test** (Special Test 9-1), or the **squeeze test** (Special Test 9-2).[29,61] Pain is often reported during palpation of the anterior and posterior tibiofibular ligaments (Examination Findings 9-2). The widening of the ankle mortise results in instability of the ankle as the talus is allowed a greater amount of glide within the joint. Other clinical findings include provocation of symptoms when the patient is weight bearing and moving the ankle into dorsiflexion and relieved when a compressive force is applied during the same movement (the **dorsiflexion–compression test**). When a syndesmotic sprain is suspected, palpate the entire length of the fibula for pain and crepitus. The forces required to produce a syndesmotic sprain may also be sufficient to fracture the fibula (Fig. 9-24). The fracture can occur in the proximal one third of the fibula, a **Maisonneuve fracture**, a spiral fracture of the proximal one-third of the fibula with concurrent disruption of the distal tibiofibular syndesmosis.

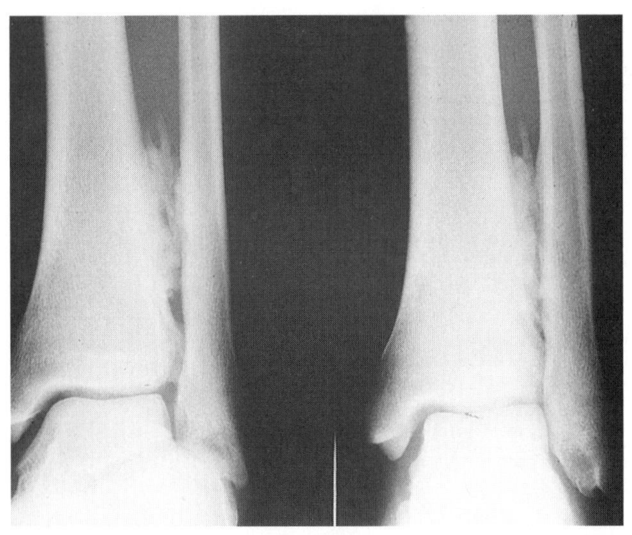

FIGURE 9-23 ■ Radiograph of a syndesmosis sprain. Note the wide gap between the tibia and fibula on the left image versus the image on the right. This injury results from the wide anterior border of the talus being forced into the mortise during hyperdorsiflexion, from external rotation of the foot, or both.

Syndesmotic sprains require a longer recovery period than lateral ankle sprains do. Patients also may benefit from a period of non–weight-bearing activity or immobilization.[11,60] Over time, **heterotopic ossification** or **synostosis** of the interosseous membrane may develop, prolonging pain during the push-off phase of gait.[11] If heterotopic ossification develops, surgery may be required.[62]

Medial ankle sprains

The strength of the deltoid ligament and the mechanical advantage of the longer lateral malleolus limit eversion. Because of the small amount of eversion (i.e., 5°) normally associated with the subtalar joint, the primary mechanism for damage to this ligament group is external rotation of the talus in the ankle mortise. These anatomic and biomechanical properties result in a low rate of deltoid ligament sprains, with reports from 3% to 15% of all ankle sprains. Deltoid sprains are frequently associated with other ankle pathology including syndesmotic sprains and malleolar fractures.[7,63] Because of its close association with the spring ligament, the stability of the medial longitudinal arch requires evaluation when a sprain of the deltoid ligament is suspected.

Physical examination findings can identify trauma to the medial ligaments.[64] Pain is present along the medial joint line, especially the anterior portion, and swelling tends to be more localized than that associated with lateral ankle sprains (Examination Findings 9-3). If an eversion mechanism is described, the lateral malleolus should be carefully evaluated for the presence of a "knock-off" fracture (Fig. 9-25). Stress radiographs are indicated if the anteroposterior radiographs are negative for mortise disruption (less than 4 mm distance between medial malleolus and talus).[64]

Eversion may also cause an avulsion of the medial malleolus. A bimalleolar fracture (**Pott's fracture**) may be caused by a similar mechanism and carries with it the increased potential complication of a nonunion of the medial malleolus if surgical intervention is not performed. Intraarticular trauma to the talus and tibia may also be present.

Collision sports Individual or team sports relying on the physical dominance of one athlete over another. By their nature, these sports involve violent physical contact.

Synostosis The union of two bones though the formation of connective tissue.

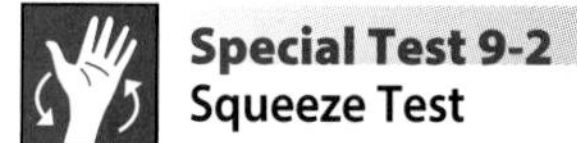

Special Test 9-2
Squeeze Test

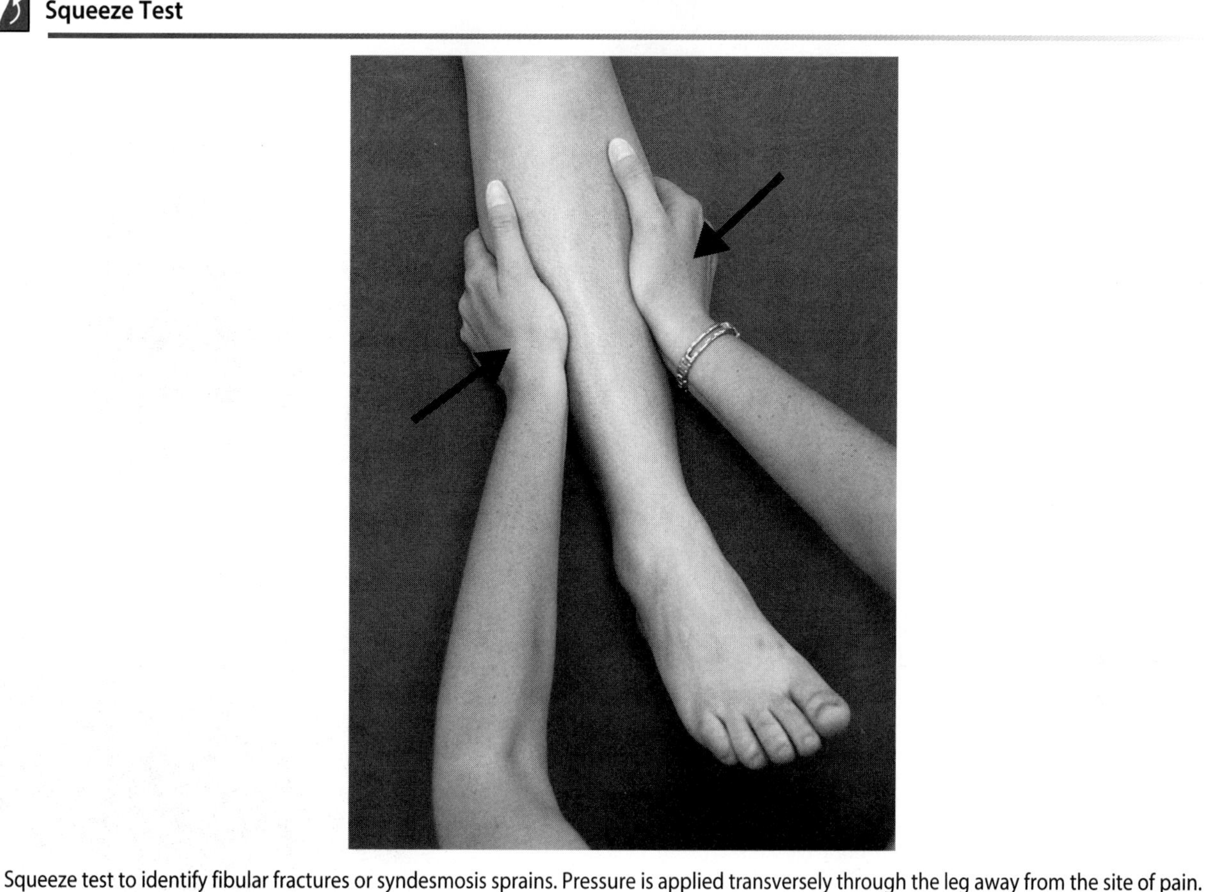

Squeeze test to identify fibular fractures or syndesmosis sprains. Pressure is applied transversely through the leg away from the site of pain.

Patient Position	Lying with the knee extended
Position of Examiner	Standing next to, or in front of, the injured leg; the evaluator's hands cupped behind the tibia and fibula away from the site of pain
Evaluative Procedure	Gently squeeze (compress) the fibula and tibia, gradually adding more pressure if no pain or other symptoms are elicited. Progress toward the injured site until pain is elicited.
Positive Test	Pain is elicited, especially when it is away from the compressed area.
Implications	**(A)** Gross fracture or stress fracture of the fibula when pain is described along the fibular shaft **(B)** Syndesmosis sprain when pain is described at the distal tibiofibular joint
Comments	Avoid applying too much pressure too soon into the test. Pressure should be applied gradually and progressively. The test is infrequently positive, even in the presence of other clinical findings indicative of a syndesmosis sprains. Its usefulness is limited.[29]
Evidence	***Inter-rater reliability*** Not Reliable — Very Reliable Poor | Moderate | Good 0 0.1 0.2 0.3 0.4 0.5 0.6 0.7 0.8 0.9 1.0

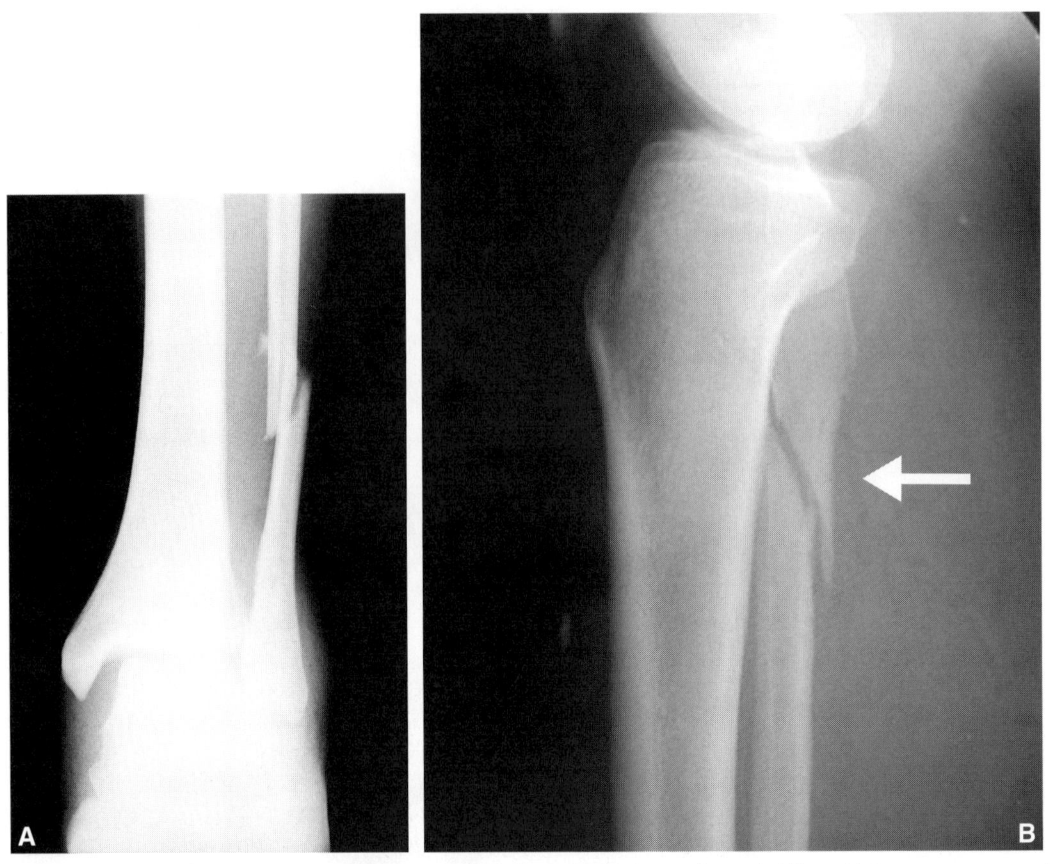

FIGURE 9-24 ■ (A) Fracture of the fibula concurrent with a sprain of the distal tibiofibular syndesmosis. When this fracture occurs proximally on the fibula, it is termed a Maisonneuve fracture (B).

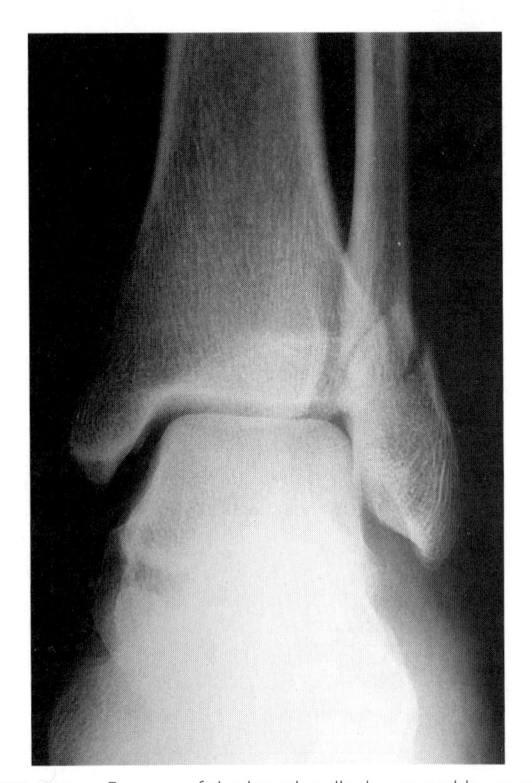

FIGURE 9-25 ■ Fracture of the lateral malleolus caused by excessive eversion of the ankle (anterior view of the left ankle). This type of fracture to the lateral malleolus is more common as it extends farther inferiorly than does the medial malleolus.

Ankle and Leg Fractures

Acute fractures and dislocations of the leg, especially those involving the tibial shaft, often exhibit obvious gross deformity (Fig. 9-26). Significant force is required to fracture the tibial shaft, but inversion, eversion, or rotational forces

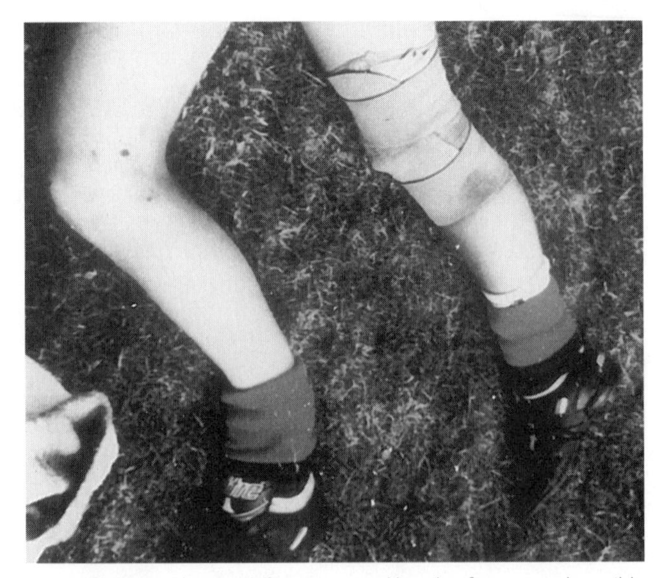

FIGURE 9-26 ■ Obvious deformity caused by a leg fracture and possible ankle dislocation.

Examination Findings 9-2
Syndesmotic ("High") Ankle Sprains

Examination Segment	Clinical Findings
History	***Onset:*** Acute ***Pain characteristics:*** Anterior portion of the distal tibiofibular syndesmosis ***Mechanism:*** External rotation of the talus within the ankle mortise and/or dorsiflexion Forced hyperdorsiflexion or hyperplantarflexion Internal rotation of the talus ***Predisposing conditions:*** Activities on surfaces that have a high coefficient of friction between the shoe and playing surface (e.g., artificial turf), especially when sharp cutting or pivoting is required.
Inspection	Swelling present over the distal tibiofibular syndesmosis, but is less prominent and wide spread as compared to lateral ankle sprains.[9]
Palpation	Pain over the distal tibiofibular syndesmosis Pain possibly elicited over the anterior and posterior tibiofibular ligaments Palpation of the length of the fibula to rule out the presence of fibular fracture
Joint and Muscle Function Assessment	***AROM:*** Motion is restricted and pain is elicited, especially with dorsiflexion and eversion, but pain is also present at the end ranges of plantarflexion and inversion. Any attempt at rotating the foot increases the pain anteriorly. ***MMT:*** Anterior tibialis, posterior tibialis may be weak and painful. Resisted testing in all directions can be inhibited by pain in more severe syndesmotic sprains ***PROM:*** All motions are limited by pain with the greatest decreases noted in dorsiflexion and eversion. Passive dorsiflexion may increase pain
Joint Stability Tests	***Stress tests:*** No significant findings ***Joint play:*** Anterior/posterior tibiofibular joint play. Distal fibular translation test[30]
Special Tests	External rotation test Dorsiflexion-compression test Squeeze test
Neurologic Screening	Within normal limits
Vascular Screening	Within normal limits
Functional Assessment	Gait assessment may reveal shortened swing on the contralateral side to avoid full dorsiflexion. Toe gait on involved side.
Imaging Techniques	Standard mortise view to evaluate the talocrural angle and amount of talar tilt Stress test with external rotation of the ankle is better than standard mortise view to detect separation of tibiofibular syndesmosis.[59]
Differential Diagnosis	Lateral ankle sprain, fibular fracture, deltoid sprain
Comments	Heterotopic ossification or synostosis of the interosseous membrane may develop over time. Syndesmosis sprains often occur concurrently with deltoid ligament sprains. The presence of a Maisonneuve fracture should be ruled out Syndesmotic sprains have an increased recovery time relative to other types of ankle sprains.

AROM = active range of motion; MMT = manual muscle test; PROM = passive range of motion.

Examination Findings 9-3
Medial Ankle Sprains

Examination Segment	Clinical Findings
History	***Onset:*** Acute ***Pain characteristics:*** Medial border of the ankle and foot, radiating from the medial malleolus ***Mechanism:*** Eversion and/or rotation ***Predisposing conditions:*** Activities such as soccer that load the medial aspect of the foot.
Inspection	Swelling around the medial joint capsule
Palpation	Pain around the deltoid ligaments Crepitus at the site of ligamentous origin or insertion may indicate an avulsion fracture
Joint and Muscle Function Assessment	***AROM:*** Pain on the medial side of the ankle during plantarflexion indicates stretching of the anterior tibiotalar and/or or the tibionavicular ligaments. Pain during dorsiflexion indicates trauma to the posterior tibiotalar ligament. Lateral pain may indicate a pinching of the lateral ligaments and/or trauma to the lateral malleolus. ***MMT:*** Posterior tibialis pain and weakness ***PROM:*** Motion produces pain along the ligaments, as described in the Ligamentous and Capsular Testing section of this chapter (also see Table 9-2).
Joint Stability Tests	***Stress tests:*** Eversion stress test ***Joint play:*** Cotton test Talonavicular glide (see Chapter 8)
Special Tests	External rotation test Squeeze test to rule out a fracture of the distal fibula
Neurologic Screening	Posterior tibial nerve
Vascular Screening	Within normal limits
Functional Assessment	Decreased strength or medial pain during most motions secondary to stretching of the medial ligaments Gait evaluation reveals shortened midstance phase and/or supinated gait as the patient avoids pronation. Increased pain during midstance phase of gait.
Imaging Techniques	Radiographs are used to rule out bony trauma and evaluate the width of the ankle mortise; stress images may be obtained. MRI may be ordered to ascertain soft tissue trauma.
Differential Diagnosis	Posterior tibialis strain, fibular fracture, distal syndesmosis sprain, medial malleolus fracture, posterior tibial neuropathy
Comments	The anterior fibers of the deltoid ligament tend to be most frequently involved in medial ankle sprains.[7] Excessive calcaneal eversion can result in a fracture of the lateral malleolus, talar dome, or disruption of the syndesmosis. An external rotation mechanism warrants a careful evaluation of the syndesmosis.

AROM = active range of motion; MMT = manual muscle test; MRI = magnetic resonance imaging; PROM = passive range of motion.

can fracture the fibula and/or malleoli. Fractures involving the talus and calcaneus will produce more subtle findings and may mimic those of a sprain. Trauma involving the fibula may also disrupt the interosseous membrane, causing a Maisonneuve fracture (see Fig. 9-24B).[65] When only the shaft of the fibula is fractured it is referred to as a Hugier or high Dupuytren fracture. Fractures of the ankle mortise can result in a dislocation of the talus and rupture of the associated ligaments. Stress fractures are discussed on page 273.

The patient (or others in the vicinity of the injury) report an audible snap or crack at the time of injury. Pain is

Examination Findings 9-4
Ankle and Leg Fractures

Examination Segment	Clinical Findings
History	***Onset:*** Acute ***Pain characteristics:*** Sharp and localized. ***Other symptoms:*** Not applicable ***Mechanism:*** Direct blow, inversion or eversion stress ***Predisposing conditions:*** Not applicable
Inspection	May or may not present with visible deformity. Swelling and ecchymosis may be present.
Palpation	Point tender, possible crepitus, possible palpable deformity.
Joint and Muscle Function Assessment	***AROM:*** Assess the patient's willingness to move the knee and ankle. ***MMT:*** Do not perform if a fracture is suspected. ***PROM:*** Do not perform if a fracture is suspected.
Joint Stability Tests	***Stress tests:*** Do not perform if a fracture is suspected. ***Joint play:*** Do not perform if a fracture is suspected.
Special Tests	Bump test Squeeze test (do not perform in the presence of an obvious fracture).
Neurologic Screening	Within normal limits
Vascular Screening	Within normal limits
Functional Assessment	None required.
Imaging Techniques	Radiograph CT or MRI to detect talar fractures.
Differential Diagnosis	Lateral ankle sprain, talocrural joint dislocation, subtalar dislocation, deltoid ligament sprain, compartment syndrome.
Comments	Management depends on involved bone and the extent of deformity. Leg and ankle fractures may be emergent. Management for shock may be required. See "On-Field Examination" for footwear removal instructions.

AROM = active range of motion; MMT = manual muscle test; PROM = passive range of motion.

reported at the fracture site, possibly radiating up the leg and extremity. Palpation, which should not be performed over obvious fractures may reveal crepitus or discontinuity along the bone shaft (Examination Findings 9-4).

Although long bone fractures normally result in immediate dysfunction and an inability to bear weight, those suffering from fibular fractures may be capable of walking. In cases in which deformity or other signs of a gross fracture are absent, the squeeze test may be used to confirm a fibular fracture.

Historically, radiographs were routinely performed for all emergency room visits for foot and ankle trauma to rule out the presence of a fracture, thereby increasing the costs associated with the visit. The Ottawa Ankle Rules use palpation findings and the patient's ability to bear weight to determine the need for radiographs (Box 9-2).[25,66] When the Ottawa Ankle Rules are followed it is unlikely that a fracture will be missed.[67,68]

Anteroposterior and lateral radiographs are used to rule out or more precisely identify fractures involving the tibia and/or fibula. Fractures involving the articular surface, especially the talus which is difficult to clinically diagnose, are more readily identified using CT or MR imaging.[69] The presence of radiographic stress findings (external rotation force) are not well correlated with physical examination findings such as point tenderness, ecchymosis, and swelling.[64] See Management of Leg Fractures and Ankle Dislocations, p. 283.

Box 9-2
Modified Ottawa Ankle Rules

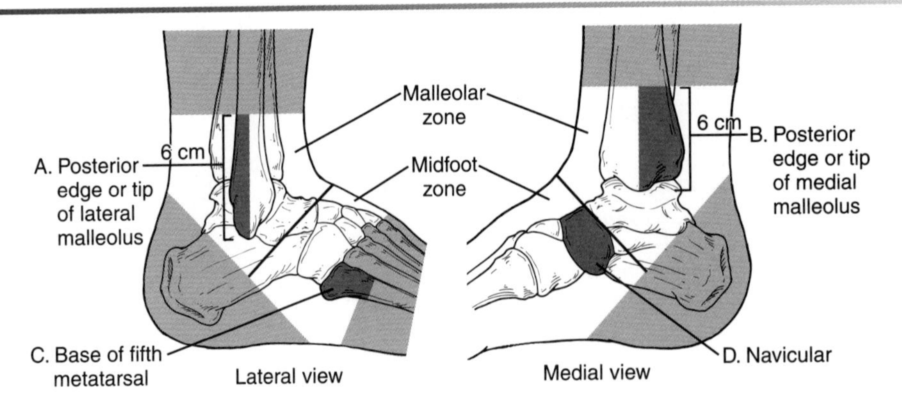

Description

The Ottawa Ankle Rules provide evaluative criteria to identify when the patient should be referred for radiographs.

Criteria for Radiographic Referral

The patient's inability to walk four steps both immediately following the injury and at the time of examination.

Ankle radiographs should be ordered if pain is elicited during palpation of Zone A or B.

Foot radiographs should be ordered if pain is elicited during palpation of Zone C or D.

Modification

Zones A and B are changed to include pain over the midline of the medial and lateral malleoli.[25,70]

Evidence

Designed to have a high sensitivity so that fractures are not missed, the Ottawa Ankle Rules have a high negative predictive value when applied to a skeletally mature population. If the rules are followed, it is highly likely that a fracture will not be missed.[67,68] The conservative nature of the rules results in a relatively low specificity (0.26–0.48), indicating that many patients are still referred for radiographs who do not have a fracture. With the modification relating to the location of the malleolar pain, the specificity is improved to 0.42–0.59.[25,70]

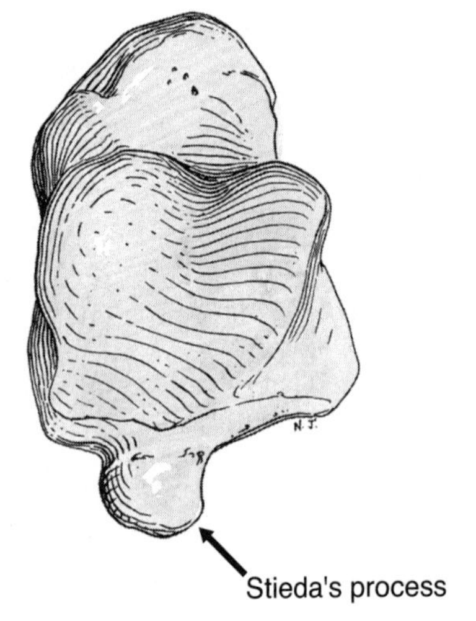

FIGURE 9-27 ■ Stieda's process. A posterior projection off the talus.

Os Trigonum Injury

An os trigonum is formed when **Stieda's process** separates from the talus (Fig. 9-27).[71,72] Stieda's process first appears between the ages of 8 and 13 years, normally fusing within 1 year after its appearance.[73,74] Developmentally, an os trigonum occurs in approximately 7% of the population when the secondary center of ossification fails to fuse the process to the talus (Fig. 9-28). A traumatic os trigonum is formed by a nonunion fracture or stress fracture of Stieda's process.[73,74] Athletes, particularly those whose activity requires sustained plantarflexion, such as dancers, are at an increased risk of sustaining an injury to this structure.[72,75,76]

Symptoms arise when an os trigonum impinges on surrounding tissues. Os trigonum syndrome (also referred to as **talar compression syndrome**) may involve: (1) an inflammation of the posterior joint, (2) inflammation of the ligaments surrounding the os trigonum, (3) a fracture of

Examination Findings 9-5
Os Trigonum Syndrome

Examination Segment	Clinical Findings
History	***Onset:*** Acute or insidious; pain is increased with activity Sudden onset of pain may suggest a fracture ***Pain characteristics:*** Posterior aspect of the talus, anterior to the Achilles tendon. ***Mechanism:*** Acute: forced hyperplantarflexion. Chronic or insidious: repetitive activity usually involving plantarflexion ***Predisposing conditions:*** The presence of an nonunited lateral tubercle on the posterior aspect of the talus (os trigonum)
Inspection	Swelling possibly observed anteromedial and anterolateral to the Achilles tendon
Palpation	Pain elicited when palpating the posterior talus, anterior to the Achilles tendon
Joint and Muscle Function Assessment	***AROM:*** Pain with plantarflexion ***MMT:*** Gastrocnemius and soleus testing may reproduce symptoms. Pain when performing a heel raise. ***PROM:*** Pain with forced plantarflexion, compressing the structures. Pain with forced dorsiflexion, stretching the structures.
Joint Stability Tests	***Stress tests:*** No significant findings ***Joint play:*** No significant findings
Special Tests	Not applicable
Neurologic Screening	Within normal limits
Vascular Screening	Within normal limits
Functional Assessment	Decreased push-off during ambulation. May demonstrate limited capacity to plantarflex for those activities that require it (e.g., ballet, gymnastics).
Imaging Techniques	A definitive diagnosis is made with correlation of findings with the presence of an os trigonum on plain film radiographs or MRI.
Differential Diagnosis	Achilles tendinopathy, tibialis posterior tendinopathy, flexor hallucis longus tendinopathy, peroneal tendon subluxation, lateral ankle instability, arthritis, tarsal tunnel syndrome, tarsal coalition, talus fracture

AROM = active range of motion; MMT = manual muscle test; PROM = passive range of motion.

the os trigonum, or (4) pathology involving the Stieda's process.[71] As the talocalcaneal unit moves into inversion and plantarflexion and the midtarsal joints pronate, the posterior talocalcaneal ligament tightens against Stieda's process. Subtalar and midtarsal joint pronation causes the os trigonum or Stieda's process to become compressed between the tibia and calcaneus.[71]

Inflammatory conditions of the os trigonum become symptomatic after activity, repetitive microtrauma, or other local inflammatory conditions.[77] Os trigonum fractures are characterized by the sudden onset of pain after forced plantarflexion or dorsiflexion. Swelling lateral or medial to the Achilles tendon may be noted. During palpation, tenderness is reported anterior to the Achilles tendon and posterior to the talus. Placing the ankle in plantarflexion may produce pain during ROM testing (Examination Findings 9-5). Plain film radiographs are used to identify the presence of an os trigonum.[78]

The treatment protocol is based on the patient's symptoms. A walker boot or cast with no weight bearing or partial weight bearing is used until the patient can ambulate without pain and a normal gait pattern. Patients can return to their activities after restoring full pain-free ROM and strength to the leg. The use of a viscoelastic heel may be helpful to absorb ground reaction forces. If the condition becomes chronic, the evaluation and use of a permanent

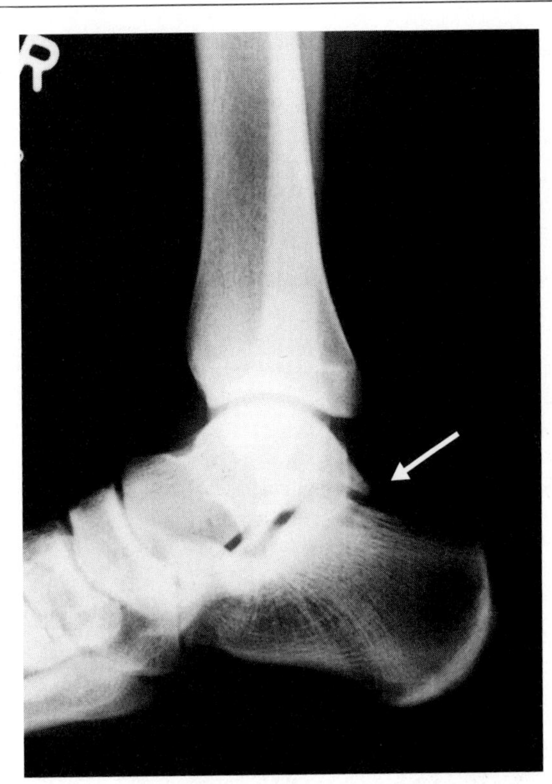

FIGURE 9-28 ■ Radiograph of an os trigonum (medial view of the right ankle). The arrow indicates the location of the os trigonum, a fracture of Stieda's process. A fracture line can be seen at the midpoint on the process.

orthotic to control foot motion may be warranted or surgical removal of the os trigonum may be required.

Achilles Tendon Pathology

Because of its dual association with the two prime plantarflexors, the gastrocnemius and the soleus, any injury to the Achilles tendon results in decreased plantarflexion strength. The decrease in plantarflexion strength may cause significant changes in gait, impairing the patient's ability to walk, run, and jump normally.

Achilles tendinopathy

The Achilles tendon is a poorly vascularized structure, receiving limited blood supply from the posterior tibial artery. The distal avascular zone, 2 to 6 cm proximal to its insertion on the calcaneus, is the most common site of tendon pathology, including inflammation and rupture (Fig. 9-29).[80,81] The tendon's response to aggravating forces is impeded by the poor blood supply in the area, causing delayed healing.

The poor vascular supply of the Achilles tendon itself brings into question if inflammation is even possible within the tendon's substance, as the available blood supply may not be sufficient to provide a widespread inflammatory response. The tendon is, however, surrounded by a highly vascular structure, the **paratenon**. Inflammation of the paratenon, **peritendinitis**, produces pain and forms adhesions with the underlying tendon.[81,82] In chronic cases, peritendinitis can

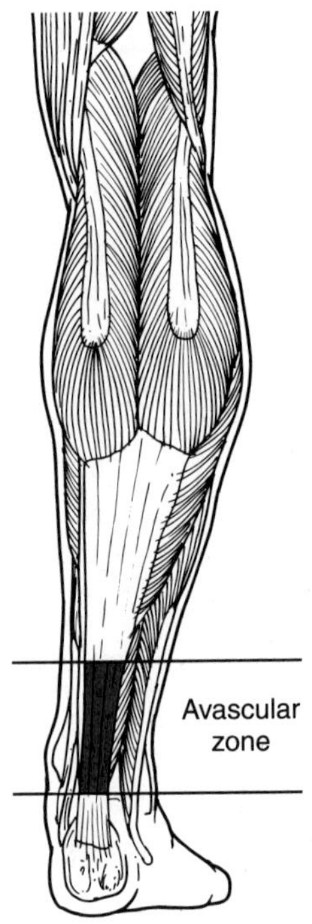

FIGURE 9-29 ■ Achilles tendon avascular zone. The distal 6 cm of the tendon, devoid of a significant blood supply, is a common site of tendinosis.

cause the paratenon to become fibrotic and **stenosed**.[12] **Tendinosis** describes the degeneration of the tendon's substance, starting with microscopic tears and necrotic areas within the tendon as the result of decreased blood flow through the paratenon.[12] Although this breakdown is not always a precursor to a tendon rupture, tendinosis represents a progressive degeneration of the tendon[81]:

Peritendinitis → Tendinosis → Tendon rupture

Tendon ruptures are not always complete. Approximately 20% of peritendinitis cases are associated with a partial rupture of the Achilles tendon, especially along the tendon's lateral border.[12,81] Unlike frank ruptures, partial ruptures can occur in otherwise young, well-conditioned individuals (see Achilles tendon ruptures).[81]

Anatomic factors that lead to the onset of Achilles tendon pathology include tibial varum, calcaneovalgus, hyperpronation, and tightness of the triceps surae and the hamstring muscle groups.[81] Running mechanics, an increase in the duration and intensity of running, the type of shoe, running surface, weak plantarflexion strength, and increased dorsiflexion (greater than 9°) can result in Achilles peritendinitis.[79] Achilles tendinopathy may also have an acute onset as the result of a direct blow to the tendon. Certain antibiotic medications such as fluoroquinolone (e.g., ciprofloxacin) have been associated with Achilles tendon pathology, including tendon ruptures.[83] Age and gender are the strongest predictors of

Stenosed Narrowing of a structure; stenosis.

Achilles tendon injury. As age increases, so does the risk of Achilles tendon pathology, especially in males, who have three times the risk of developing symptoms than that of females.[84,85]

Individuals suffering from Achilles tendinopathy describe pain or "burning" radiating along the length of the tendon, although it is common for the patient to be relatively asymptomatic with the exception of a palpable nodule within the distal tendon. The area may be tender to the touch and crepitus may be elicited, particularly with active ROM. This condition may be the result of or may result in tightness of the triceps surae muscle group (Examination Findings 9-6). MRI is useful in definitively diagnosing the pathology leading to Achilles tendon pain and identifying the predisposition to ruptures.[83]

Most cases of Achilles tendinopathy are traced to overuse syndromes and repeated eccentric loading of the tendon. Individuals with foot rigidity are predisposed to this condition because gait must be modified to compensate for a valgus or varus rearfoot. Improperly fitting footwear may cause friction between the heel counter and the tendon, and shoes with a rigid sole may not permit adequate ROM in the midfoot and forefoot, altering the biomechanics of the foot, ankle, and leg.

Oral antiinflammatory medications are often prescribed for those with acute or moderate inflammatory conditions, and heel lifts may be added to reduce the stresses placed on the Achilles tendon. In advanced cases, immobilization may be required, but the strength of the triceps surae muscle group is slow to return after this technique.[86] Corticosteroid injections may be used to control chronic or severe inflammation, but there is an increased risk of suffering an Achilles tendon rupture for 1 week after the injection.[85,87]

Stretching of the Achilles tendon and triceps surae and hamstrings has long been considered an important component of the therapeutic exercise program. The triceps surae can be strengthened, focusing on eccentric demands, as pain diminishes. A progressive return to activity includes instruction in the proper method of warming up, continued flexibility exercises, monitoring of shoewear and activity surfaces, and the application of ice after exercise.

Achilles tendon rupture

Forceful, sudden contractions, such as when a defensive back or basketball player changes direction or when a gymnast dismounts from a piece of apparatus, results in a large amount of tension developing within the Achilles tendon. If this tension becomes too great, the tendon fails, resulting in an Achilles tendon rupture (Examination Findings 9-7).

Two theories attempt to account for the onset of Achilles tendon ruptures: (1) chronic degeneration of the tendon and (2) failure of the inhibitory mechanism of the musculotendinous unit.[88] As described in the Achilles Tendinopathy section, the Achilles tendon is poorly vascularized and the body is unable to keep pace with the tendon's breakdown (tendinosis). As a result, the tendon weakens. In the final stages of the degenerative process, a rupture occurs.[81,88] When the triceps surae's inhibitory mechanism fails, an excessive force (e.g., stepping in a hole) or a forceful muscle contraction (e.g., an explosive push-off) results in the rupture of the tendon. In both types of mechanisms, the rupture tends to occur in the tendon's avascular zone (the distal 2 to 6 cm).[88]

Although this injury can occur in either gender or in any age group, Achilles tendon ruptures tend to be most prominent in men older than age 30 years.[85] A complete rupture typically occurs in more sedentary individuals who perform episodic strenuous activity. Previous or current tendinosis, age-related changes in the tendon, and **deconditioning** may play roles in the onset of tendon ruptures.[12,89] Healthy and unhealthy tendons can be ruptured through direct trauma or by forceful concentric muscle contraction or eccentric loading of the tendon.[89]

The risk of tendon rupture is also increased for approximately 1 week after corticosteroid injections directly into the tendon.[84,85] Although there are case reports of Achilles tendon rupture after corticosteroid injections in humans, there are no rigorous long-term studies that evaluate the risk of rupture with or without steroid injections.[90] Injections in the paratenon have been demonstrated to be effective without increasing the long-term rate of tendon rupture.[90,91]

Achilles tendon ruptures are characterized by the inability to push off with the injured leg during ambulation or perform a heel raise. The patient usually assumes a stiff-legged gait pattern characterized by external rotation of the extremity and reports the sensation of being "kicked," followed by severe pain.[88] If the lesion occurs in the tendon's midsubstance, the defect may be observable or palpable, although palpation is not a reliable indicator of a tendon defect.[92] As swelling develops, the defect will become difficult to see or palpate (Fig. 9-30). Although the tendon may be completely ruptured, the patient is still able to actively plantarflex the ankle through contraction of the peroneals, long toe flexors, and tibialis posterior muscles, but the strength of the contraction is markedly diminished. Clinically, the presence of a complete Achilles tendon rupture is confirmed through the **Thompson test** (Special Test 9-3).[18,88,93] MRI can be used to identify partial tendon tears.[83]

Complete Achilles tendon ruptures are managed conservatively with casting or dorsiflexion night splints for a minimum of 8 weeks or through open or minimally invasive surgery.[94] The primary advantage of conservative care is the absence of wound problems and decreased medical costs. Disadvantages include an increased rate of re-rupture, decreased muscle function, and patient dissatisfaction compared to surgical repair.[94–96]

The advantages of surgical repair include a reported re-rupture rate of less than 5 percent; a speedier return to pre-injury activity; and a good return of plantarflexion

---

Deconditioning The loss of once existing cardiovascular or muscular endurance and strength.

Examination Findings 9-6
Achilles Tendinopathy

Examination Segment	Clinical Findings
History	***Onset:*** Insidious or the result of trauma to the Achilles tendon ***Pain characteristics:*** Along the length of the Achilles tendon ***Other symptoms:*** May describe "squeaking" sensation. ***Mechanism:*** Tendinitis is typically an acute onset relating to a sudden, large increase in load or a blow to the Achilles tendon. Tendinosis results from repetitive stressors and subsequent local tissue degeneration. Improperly fitting shoe rubbing against the tendon may also activate the inflammatory response. ***Predisposing conditions:*** Tibial varum; calcaneal valgum; hyperpronation or other forms of foot rigidity; tightness of the triceps surae muscle group; risk increases with age, especially in the male population Decreased strength of the plantarflexors and increased dorsiflexion ROM [79] Sudden change in the duration and/or intensity of training Ankle sprains or other foot/ankle pathology resulting in toe-only gait and subsequent shortening of the Achilles' tendon
Inspection	Possible visible edema along the length of the tendon; the tendon on the involved leg may appear thicker than on the opposite leg A discrete nodule may be seen and felt along the distal tendon.[12]
Palpation	Pain elicited during palpation of the tendon, especially 2 to 6 cm proximal to the tendon's insertion on the calcaneus.[12] Crepitus may be evident with active motion
Joint and Muscle Function Assessment	***AROM:*** Pain and crepitus during plantarflexion and dorsiflexion. Dorsiflexion range of motion possibly diminished secondary to Achilles tendon tightness ***MMT:*** Plantarflexion (gastrocnemius and soleus) is painful and/or weak ***PROM:*** Pain at end range of dorsiflexion, resulting from stretching the tendon; dorsiflexion may be decreased
Joint Stability Tests	***Stress tests:*** Not applicable ***Joint play:*** Hypomobile lateral glide of the talus
Special Tests	None
Neurologic Screening	Within normal limits
Vascular Screening	Within normal limits
Functional Assessment	Decreased push-off during gait
Imaging Techniques	MR images can identify partial tears or thickening of the tendon.
Differential Diagnosis	Subcutaneous calcaneal bursitis; subtendinous calcaneal bursitis
Comments	Approximately 20% of Achilles tendinopathy cases also have a partial tear of the tendon.

AROM = active range of motion; MR = magnetic resonance; MMT = manual muscle test; PROM = passive range of motion.

Examination Findings 9-7
Achilles Tendon Rupture

Examination Segment	Clinical Findings
History	***Onset:*** Acute ***Pain characteristics:*** Achilles tendon and/or lower portion of the gastrocnemius ***Other symptoms:*** The patient often reports the sensation of being kicked. Audible "pop" may be described. ***Mechanism:*** Forceful plantarflexion with eccentric loading, usually the result of eccentric loading or plyometric contraction of the calf musculature ***Predisposing conditions:*** A possible relationship between a history of Achilles tendinitis and a rupture of the tendon History of corticosteroid injections to the tendon Advancing age Male gender
Inspection	A defect may be visible in the Achilles tendon or at the musculotendinous junction, but rapid swelling may obscure this; discoloration may be present around the tendon. The patient is unable to bear weight on the involved extremity because of pain.
Palpation	A palpable defect in the Achilles tendon, although it may quickly become obscured by swelling Pain elicited along the tendon and lower gastrocnemius–soleus muscle group
Joint and Muscle Function Assessment	***AROM:*** Plantarflexion may possibly still be present owing to the tibialis posterior, plantaris, peroneals, and long toe flexors, although the patient may complain of pain during this motion and during dorsiflexion (secondary to stretching the Achilles tendon). ***MMT:*** Weak or absent plantarflexion (gastrocnemius and/or soleus) ***PROM:*** Pain during dorsiflexion An empty end-feel may be obtained secondary to patient apprehension.
Joint Stability Tests	***Stress tests:*** Not applicable ***Joint play:*** Not applicable
Special Tests	Thompson test
Neurologic Screening	Within normal limits
Vascular Screening	Within normal limits
Functional Assessment	Unable to perform a heel-rise or push-off during gait
Imaging Techniques	MRI Ultrasonic imaging
Differential Diagnosis	Posterior tibial tendon rupture; plantaris tendon rupture; triceps surae strain; Achilles tendinopathy; deep vein thrombosis
Comments	This injury tends to occur more frequently in males older than age 30 years, but any age group is susceptible. The status of the dorsalis pedis pulse should be monitored.

AROM = active range of motion; MMT = manual muscle test; MRI = magnetic resonance imaging; PROM = passive range of motion.

Special Test 9-3
Thompson Test for Achilles Tendon Rupture

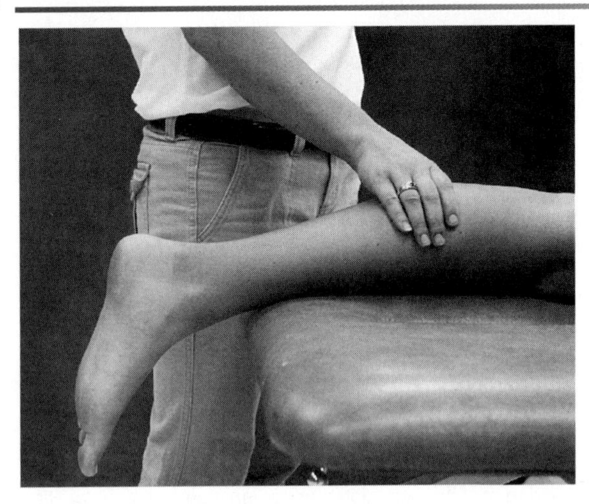

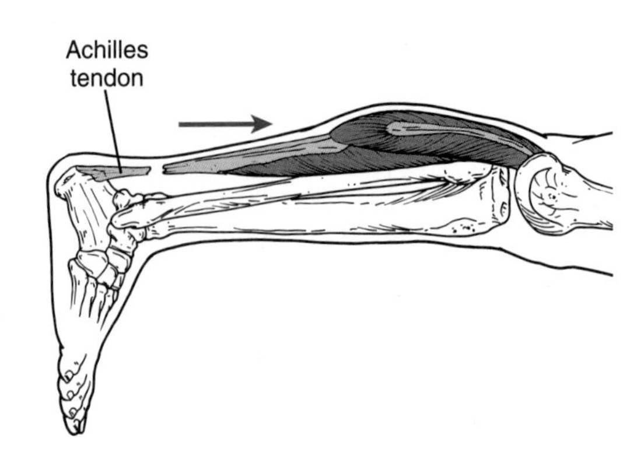

Thompson test for an Achilles tendon rupture. When the Achilles tendon is intact, squeezing the calf muscle results in slight plantarflexion. A positive Thompson test occurs when the calf is squeezed but no motion is produced in the foot, indicating a tear of the Achilles tendon.

Patient Position	Prone, with the foot off the edge of the table
Position of Examiner	At the side of the patient with one hand over the muscle belly of the calf musculature
Evaluative Procedure	The examiner squeezes the calf musculature while observing for plantarflexion of the foot.
Positive Test	When the calf is squeezed, the foot does not plantarflex.
Implications	The Achilles tendon has been ruptured.
Evidence	Positive likelihood ratio[9]

Not Useful — Useful
Very Small | Small | Moderate | Large
13.7
0 1 2 3 4 5 6 7 8 9 10

Negative likelihood ratio

Not Useful — Useful
Very Small | Small | Moderate | Large
1.0 0.9 0.8 0.7 0.6 0.5 0.4 0.3 0.2 0.1 0

strength, power, and endurance.[94–96] Most disadvantages are caused by surgical complications, including wound healing. The skin around the Achilles tendon is very thin with little subcutaneous tissue. Its limited blood supply makes the incision site prone to wound complications.

Peroneal Tendon Pathology

Forceful, sudden dorsiflexion and eversion or plantarflexion and inversion may stretch or rupture the superior peroneal retinaculum which restrains the peroneal tendons behind the lateral malleolus. All cases of peroneal tendon dislocation are associated with a torn or stretched superior peroneal retinaculum.[2,48] Rare cases also involve the inferior peroneal retinaculum (see Fig. 9-12). When these tendons lose their alignment from behind the lateral malleolus and slip anteriorly, the peroneals, which are normally plantarflexors, become dorsiflexors (Fig. 9-31). The dislocation process starts proximally and, with time, progresses distally.[98]

Anatomically, a flattened or convex fibular groove predisposes peroneal subluxations by lessening the bony channel through which the tendons pass.[98,99] Pes planus, rearfoot valgus, recurrent ankle sprains, and laxity of the peroneal retinaculum all contribute to the onset of subluxating peroneal tendons (Examination Findings 9-8).[18]

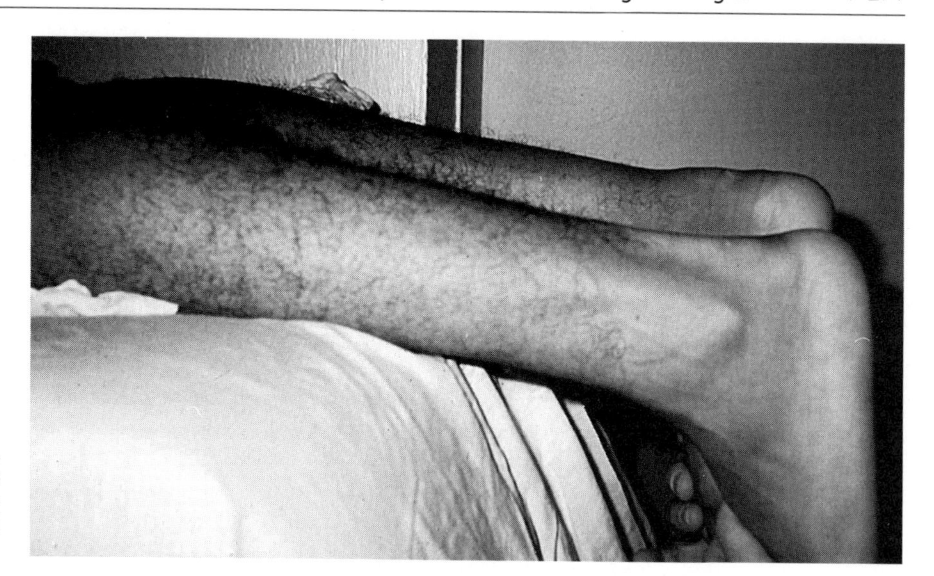

FIGURE 9-30 ■ Ruptured Achilles tendon. The patient's right (far) Achilles tendon has been ruptured. Note the depression proximal to the calcaneus and the involved swelling.

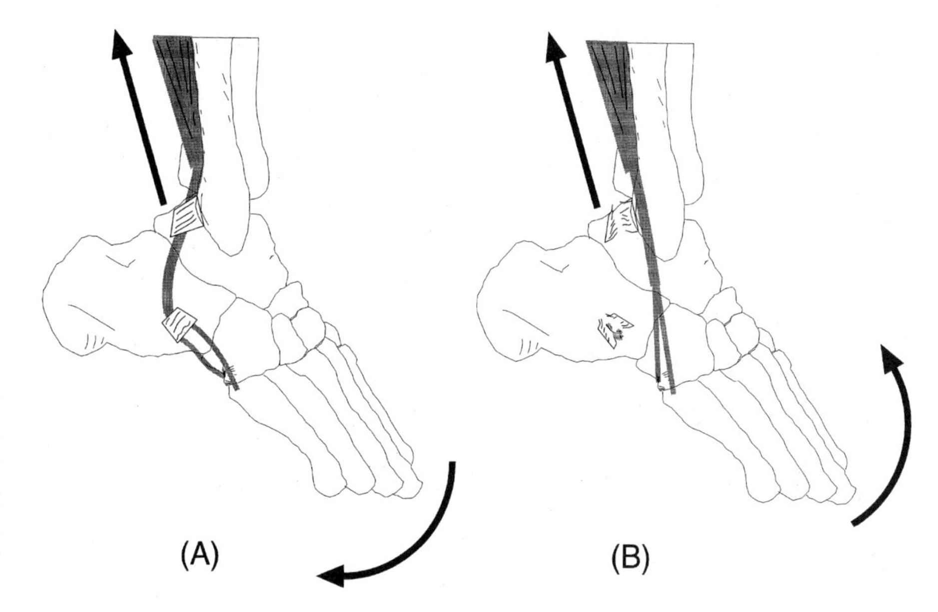

FIGURE 9-31 ■ Illustration showing biomechanical changes with subluxating peroneal tendon. (A) When the peroneal retinacula is intact, the peroneals serve as plantarflexors of the foot. (B) Subluxating peroneal tendons, caused by the rupture or stretching of the retinacula, change the angle of pull to that of a dorsiflexor.

The peroneal tendons may be observed or palpated as they dislocate from the groove behind the lateral malleolus as they snap into and out of position during active plantarflexion and dorsiflexion or active eversion (Fig. 9-32).[18] This biomechanical change alters the biomechanics of the foot and ankle, resulting in pain and dysfunction. Peroneal dislocations are classified into one of four groups[2]:

I Superior peroneal retinaculum is torn from its fibular insertion

II Superior retinaculum and fibrocartilaginous ridge are avulsed from the lateral fibula

III Superior retinaculum is torn from the lateral fibula, the fibrocartilaginous ridge is avulsed, and flake fractures occur on the lateral malleolus

IV Superior retinaculum is torn from its calcaneal insertion

Full or partial thickness longitudinal tears may appear in the tendons.[99–101] Longitudinal tears of the peroneus brevis tendon are frequently associated with chronic lateral ankle instability.[48,102] During an inversion mechanism of an ankle sprain the peroneus longus tendon pulls the anterior portion of the peroneus brevis tendon over the sharp posterior fibular ridge as it subluxates from the groove.[12,48] These ruptures contribute to future subluxations, dislocations, and peroneal tendinopathy.[99–101,103,104] Ultrasonic images can be used to detect chronic subluxation, and kinematic MRIs can be used to identify positional subluxations.[97,105,106] Clinically, peroneus brevis tears and subluxations are differentiated from chronic lateral ankle instability based on the description and location of the symptoms.[48] In the presence of peroneus brevis tendon disorders the patient will describe lateral instability with associated pain on the posterior portion of the malleolus. Patients with chronic ankle instability will complain of

Examination Findings 9-8
Subluxating Peroneal Tendons

Examination Segment	Clinical Findings
History	***Onset:*** Acute or insidious In the case of tendon tears, several months may elapse between the initial injury and the report of symptoms.[2] ***Pain characteristics:*** Behind the lateral malleolus in the area of the superior peroneal retinaculum, across the lateral malleolus, length of the peroneal tendons, and, in rare cases, at the site of the inferior peroneal retinaculum ***Other symptoms:*** Ankle instability accompanied by snapping of the tendon is often reported [2,48] ***Mechanism:*** Forceful dorsiflexion and eversion or plantarflexion and inversion ***Predisposing conditions:*** A flattened or convex fibular groove, pes planus, hindfoot valgus Recurrent lateral ankle sprain Laxity of the peroneal retinaculum
Inspection	Swelling and ecchymosis may be isolated behind the lateral malleolus (see functional tests). After 24 hours post-dislocation the swelling becomes diffuse.[2] The tendons may be seen to sublux during resisted eversion.
Palpation	Tenderness behind the lateral malleolus, over the peroneal tendons, and perhaps over the site of the inferior peroneal retinaculum (see functional tests) Involvement of the peroneus longus may result in pain following the tendon's course through the foot. Palpate the area behind the lateral malleolus during peroneal MMT to identify abnormal movement of the peroneal tendons.
Joint and Muscle Function Assessment	***AROM:*** The peroneal tendon may be seen, felt, or heard as it subluxates while the foot and ankle move from plantarflexion and inversion to dorsiflexion and eversion and back. ***MMT:*** Peroneals: Symptoms may be reproduced. ***PROM:*** No significant clinical findings are noted.
Joint Stability Tests	***Stress tests:*** No significant findings ***Joint play:*** No significant findings
Special Tests	None
Neurologic Screening	Within normal limits
Vascular Screening	Within normal limits
Functional Assessment	Reproduction of symptoms with movements involving rapid change of direction
Imaging Techniques	An avulsion fracture of the lateral ridge of the distal fibula confirms the diagnosis of a peroneal tendon subluxation or dislocation.[12] MRI is used to identify tendon lesions. Tears may be identified by a "boomerang" appearance.[2] Ultrasonic imaging has a specificity of 0.85, accuracy of 0.90, and a positive predictive value of 0.80 in identifying peroneal tendon lesions.[97]
Differential Diagnosis	Longitudinal tear of the tendon, os peroneum syndrome, lateral ankle sprain, fibular fracture, calcaneal process fracture, talar fracture, osteochondritis dessicans
Comments	Longitudinal tears of the tendon tend to occur concurrently with the onset of dislocation/subluxation.

AROM = active range of motion; MMT = manual muscle test; MRI = magnetic resonance imaging; PROM = passive range of motion.

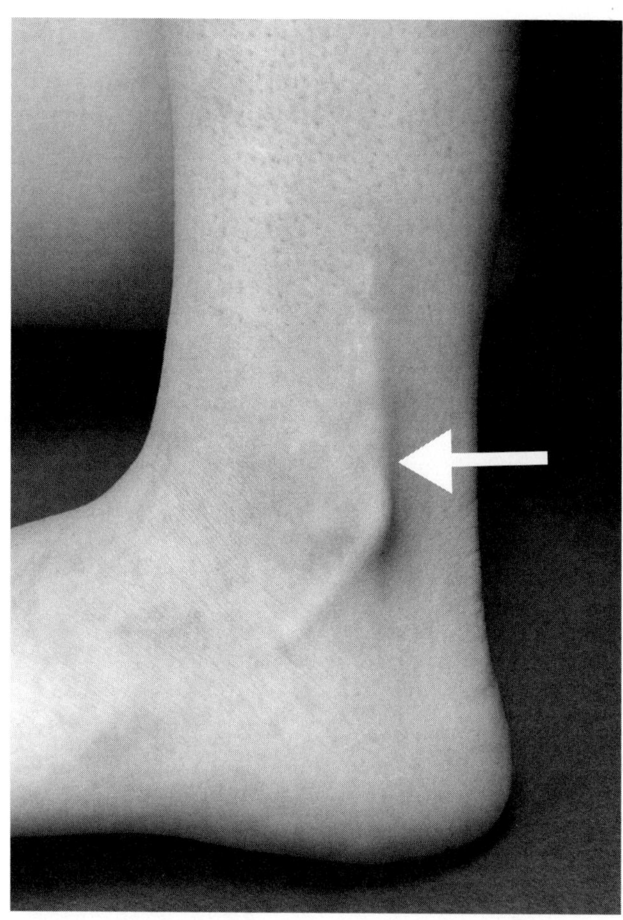

FIGURE 9-32 ■ Observable peroneal dislocation. In some instances the peroneal tendon can be observed as it subluxates from the fibular groove.

the ankle "giving way" and pain in the anterior aspect of the ankle. Peroneus longus tears tend to afflict older individuals and also result in pain through the foot and lateral ankle.[2]

The peroneus longus' sesamoid, the **os peroneum** can be the cause of several painful conditions about the foot and ankle. Generally termed as "painful os peroneum syndrome" (POPS), pain and dysfunction can be associated with an acute or chronic fracture, a multipartite os peroneum (the os peroneum being in two or more pieces), or a tear or rupture of the peroneus longus tendon. In rare instances POPS can be caused by the os peroneum contacting a large peroneal tubercle.[2,107] Clinically, POPS is characterized by increased lateral pain during a single stance heel rise, inversion stress test, and resisted plantarflexion of the first ray.[107]

In cases in which the retinaculum is stretched, the degree of subluxation may be controlled by rehabilitation exercises, taping, and the use of a felt pad over the peroneal groove to assist in holding the tendons in place. However, after the retinaculum has been stretched, it does not return to its original length. When the retinacula have been completely disrupted or pain and dysfunction become great, surgery is required to deepen the fibular groove,[108] repair the involved retinaculum,[18,104] or both.[98] Surgery to repair the soft tissue structures is usually necessary for patients with recurrent peroneal tendon dislocations.[109] If the subluxation is not reduced, chronic ankle instability, pain, and decreased strength impair ankle function.

Medial Tibial Stress Syndrome

Medial tibial stress syndrome (MTSS), a periostitis at the posterior medial border of the tibia, results from repetitive overuse, such as running. Estimated to account for around 15% of all running injuries,[113] the onset of MTSS is attributed to training errors (training on a hard surface, increasing load too quickly), incorrect shoe wear, muscle fatigue, or biomechanical abnormalities. Women are more susceptible than men.[92,113] Prolonged pronation, measured either via static observation, an excessive navicular drop (see p. 196) or more sophisticated gait measures, is a key feature associated with the development of this condition.[92,110–114] A bone stress reaction, MTSS may be a precursor to stress fractures, and bone scans in individuals with MTSS reveal uptake of the radionucleotide in the involved region (see Chapter 5).[112]

Patients with MTSS describe a gradual onset of symptoms, consistent with many overuse injuries (Table 9-7). Early in the progression, patients describe pain at the beginning of an exercise session that subsides as activity continues but returns when the activity is over. As the condition progresses, pain occurs throughout exercise and leads to a change in activity level. The diffuse pain at the posteromedial tibial border covers a broad spans (greater than 5 cm), not the localized tenderness associated with stress fractures. Palpation at the medial and distal posteromedial border is painful. Repetitive testing of the long toe flexors, posterior tibialis or soleus may replicate symptoms that emerge with fatigue of these muscles (Examination Findings 9-9).

Conservative treatment consisting of rest from the offending activities is typically effective. Controlling excessive pronation through adequate footwear or orthotics also provides relief.

Stress Fractures

Leg stress fractures involve the tibia, fibula, and talus and represent the accumulation of microtraumatic forces. Having symptoms of gradual onset, common complaints includes isolated pain along the shaft of the bone. In the case of fibular stress fractures, pain occurs proximal to the lateral malleolus and increases with activity and subsides with rest. During activity, decreased muscular strength and cramping may be reported. Palpation may reveal crepitus in well-developed stress fractures and point tenderness isolated to a single spot along the shaft of the bone. In many cases, the painful area is visually unremarkable (Examination Findings 9-10). A narrow tibial shaft, high degree of hip external rotation, osteopenia, osteoporosis, and pes cavus are common predisposing factors for stress fractures.[116,117] Immature stress fractures are not visible on

Table 9-7 Differential Findings of Stress Fractures, Medial Tibial Stress Syndrome, Acute Compartment Syndrome, and Chronic Exertional Compartment Syndrome

Finding	Stress Fracture	Medial Tibial Stress Syndrome	Acute Compartment Syndrome	Chronic Exertional Compartment Syndrome
Symptom Characteristics	Localized over the involved area of the bone	More diffuse along the posteromedial border of the middle or distal one-third of the tibia.	Severe pain in the involved compartment of the leg Numbness on the dorsum of the foot, especially the web space between the 1st and 2nd toes (anterior) Dorsalis pedis pulse may be diminished (anterior)	Pain in the involved compartment of the leg Numbness on the dorsum of the foot, especially the web space between the 1st and 2nd toes Dorsalis pedis pulse diminished
Onset	Following changes in footwear or playing surfaces or increases in intensity, duration, or frequency of activity	Following changes in footwear or playing surfaces or increases in intensity, duration, or frequency of activity	Acute following trauma to the anterior leg Acute during exercise but symptoms not decreasing with rest	Symptoms increasing in proportion to exercise resulting in inability to continue. Pain possibly limiting activity after symptoms begin
Pain Patterns	Increased with activity decreased with rest Possibly progressing to constant pain	Initially, pain at the start of activity possibly diminishing with continued participation; pain possibly increasing again at the end of activity Pain decreasing with rest	Unremitting pain most likely prohibiting activity	Pain increasing with activity Pain decreasing with rest
Positive Findings	Bump test may be positive	Pain with palpation over the posteromedial tibia Pain during toe raises Pain during resisted plantarflexion, inversion, or dorsiflexion	Pain with active or resisted motion of the compartment's muscles Pain with passive stretching of the compartment's muscles	Pain after or during exercise
Negative Test Results	AROM MMT PROM	AROM PROM		Most test results negative if the individual has not been exercising recently
Definitive Diagnosis	Bone scan Radiograph MRI	Bone scan may show periosteal irritation.	Intracompartmental pressure minus diastolic BP is $\geq$30 mm Hg. Pain that does not subside with rest	Increased intracompartmental pressure after activity Pain that subsides with rest

AROM = active range of motion; PROM = passive range of motion; MMT = manual muscle test.

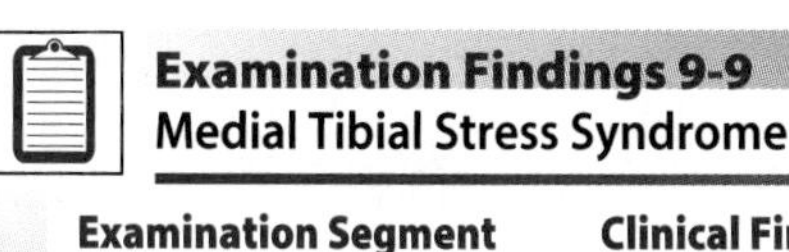

Examination Findings 9-9
Medial Tibial Stress Syndrome

Examination Segment	Clinical Findings
History	***Onset:*** Insidious ***Pain characteristics:*** Diffuse posteromedial tibial pain that increases as activity prolongs. May describe pain at rest. ***Mechanism:*** Overuse/repetitive stress ***Predisposing conditions:*** Increased pronation[110,111]
Inspection	Pes planus Rearfoot and/or forefoot varus when assessed in subtalar joint neutral
Palpation	Diffuse tenderness along posteromedial border of tibia. May have diffuse swelling.
Joint and Muscle Function Assessment	***AROM:*** Unremarkable ***MMT:*** Symptoms reproduced with multiple repetitions of testing involved muscle(s): Posterior tibialis, soleus, flexor digitorum longus, flexor hallucis longus ***PROM:*** Increased pain with ankle dorsiflexion, pronation, or toe extension
Joint Stability Tests	***Stress tests:*** Not applicable ***Joint play:*** Not applicable
Special Tests	Navicular drop test
Neurologic Screening	Within normal limits. Complaints of paresthesia warrant consideration of another diagnosis.
Vascular Screening	Within normal limits
Functional Assessment	Gait observation reveals excessive pronation.
Imaging Techniques	Radiographs and bone scans to differentiate from stress fractures
Differential Diagnosis	Tibial stress fracture, deep posterior exertional compartment syndrome, deep vein thrombosis, popliteal artery entrapment syndrome[112]

standard radiographic examination until bony callus formation has begun, typically around 3 weeks after the onset of symptoms. An early suspicion of a stress fracture requires the use of diagnostic techniques such as bone scans to detect increased bone metabolic activity for definitive diagnosis. In advanced (mature) stress fractures symptoms may be elicited through the squeeze test or the **bump test** (Special Test 9-4), although these tests have limited value. The signs and symptoms of stress fractures may mimic those of medial tibial stress syndromes and compartment syndromes.

✱ Practical Evidence

Medial tibial stress syndrome (MTSS), the low end of the bone stress–failure continuum, is marked by periostitis or symptomatic periosteal remodeling of the middle and distal third of the medial tibia.[20] The site of early MTSS is often correlated with the long-term development of stress fractures and may be more prevalent in individuals who demonstrate a pronatory foot type.

Dancers and athletes who jump, such as basketball players, are disposed to developing stress fractures in the anterior cortex of the tibia, an area prone to nonunion fractures. The fracture area can be visualized on radiographs, but are "cold" or negative on bone scans, producing "the dreaded black line".[20]

Tuning forks have been advocated as an inexpensive alternative to identifying the presence of stress fractures. A vibrating tuning fork is placed on the shaft of the suspected bone. In the presence of a stress fracture the vibration would cause pain. With a positive likelihood ratio of 2.3, a positive findings improves the probability that a stress fracture is present by a small amount. The negative likelihood ratio of 0.75 indicates that a negative test does little to eliminate a stress fracture as a potential diagnoses.[118]

Pain guides the management of patients with stress fractures. Many individuals respond to rest and antiinflammatory medication. Advanced cases may require casting or a walker boot (Fig. 9-33).

Examination Findings 9-10
Leg and Ankle Stress Fractures

Examination Segment	Clinical Findings
History	***Onset:*** Insidious or chronic, secondary to repetitive running and/or jumping ***Pain characteristics:*** Along the shaft of the tibia or fibula; localized during or after exercise; may be described as a localized "ache" while at rest. ***Mechanism:*** No definitive origin of pain. The history possibly indicates a sudden increase in the duration, frequency, or intensity of exercise or a change in playing surface or shoe wear. ***Predisposing conditions:*** Individuals having a narrow tibial shaft, an externally rotated hip and/or pes cavus/supinated foot type have a higher rate of injury, osteopenia, osteoporosis, menstrual irregularity [110]
Inspection	Normally unremarkable; however, localized swelling is possible in advanced stages. Inspect the foot for postural deviations.
Palpation	Pain along the fracture site
Joint and Muscle Function Assessment	***AROM:*** All functional test results may be normal in the acute stages of stress fractures. ***MMT:*** In maturing stress fractures or immediately after exercise, decreased strength may be evident secondary to inflammation of the muscles near the site of the stress fracture. ***PROM:*** Unremarkable findings
Joint Stability Tests	***Stress tests:*** Not applicable ***Joint play:*** Not applicable
Special Tests	The squeeze test is performed for advanced fibular stress fractures. The bump test is performed for advanced fibular, tibial, calcaneal, or talar stress fractures, but has suspect validity. Navicular drop test (see p. 196).
Neurologic Screening	Within normal limits
Vascular Screening	Vascular screening is not normally indicated.
Functional Assessment	Shortened stance phase on the involved side. Restricted or excessive/prolonged pronation may be noted.
Imaging Techniques	Radiographic evaluation is typically normal in immature stress fractures. A "V"-shaped defect, the "dreaded black line" visible on tibial radiographs often determines the need for surgical correction.[115]
Differential Diagnosis	Medial tibial stress syndrome, exertional compartment syndrome
Comments	Early stages of stress fractures may clinically resemble those of periostitis. Early signs of stress fractures appear on bone scans. Stress fractures do not appear on standard radiographic examination for 4 to 6 wk after the onset of symptoms. History of disordered eating and/or malnutrition.

AROM = active range of motion; MMT = manual muscle test; PROM = passive range of motion.

Special Test 9-4
Bump Test for Leg Stress Fractures

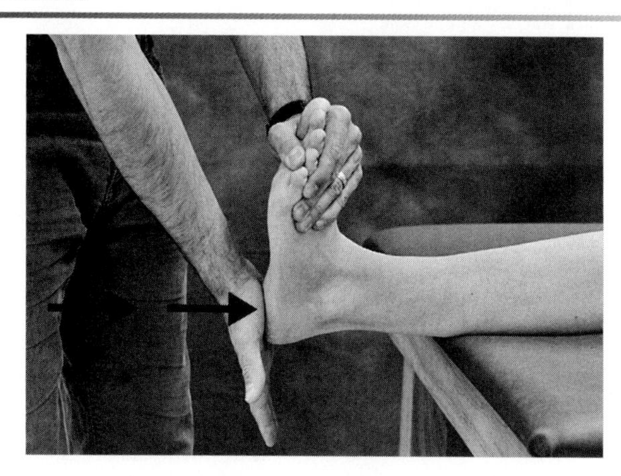

Bump test to identify stress fractures of the leg or talus. The examiner's hand is bumped against the patient's foot. The subsequent shock elicits pain in areas of stress fractures. Note that this test is not definitive, but should not be used in the presence of an obvious fracture.

Patient Position	Sitting with the involved leg off the end of the table and the knee straight, or lying supine The ankle in its neutral position
Position of Examiner	Standing in front of the heel of the involved leg The posterior portion of the leg is stabilized with the nondominant hand.
Evaluative Procedure	Bumps the calcaneus using the palm of the dominant hand
Positive Test	Pain emanating from fracture of the calcaneus, talus, fibula, or tibia
Implications	Possible advanced stress fracture
Evidence	Inconclusive or absent in the literature

Compartment Syndromes

Resulting from increased pressure within the compartment, compartment syndromes threaten the integrity of the leg, foot, and toes by obstructing the neurovascular network (primarily the deep peroneal nerve, capillaries, and anterior tibial artery) contained within this compartment. The combination of bony borders and dense fibrous fascial lining of the compartments result in poor elastic properties to accommodate for expansion of the intracompartmental tissues. When the compartment pressure exceeds **capillary perfusion pressure**, the local tissues do not receive an adequate supply of oxygen. The lack of oxygen leads to ischemia of the tissues and, if not treated, cell death.[119]

Compartment syndromes are classified as traumatic, acute exertional, or chronic exertional. Traumatic anterior compartment syndrome occurs from intracompartmental hemorrhage caused by a blow to the anterolateral or lateral portion of the leg. The subsequent bleeding and edema cause an increased pressure within the compartment, obstructing the neurovascular network to and from the dorsum of the foot, resulting in ischemic destruction of the involved tissues.

Exertional compartment syndromes can have an acute or chronic onset, with symptoms occurring during or after exercise. **Chronic exertional compartment syndrome** (CCS), also referred to as **recurrent compartment syndrome** or **intermittent claudication**, occurs secondary to anatomic abnormalities obstructing blood flow in exercising muscles. Many exertional compartment syndromes are related to an increased thickness of the fascia that inhibits venous outflow but not arterial inflow.[120] Other

Capillary perfusion pressure Pressure within the capillaries that forces blood out into the surrounding tissues.

Claudication Pain caused by inadequate venous drainage or poor arterial innervation.

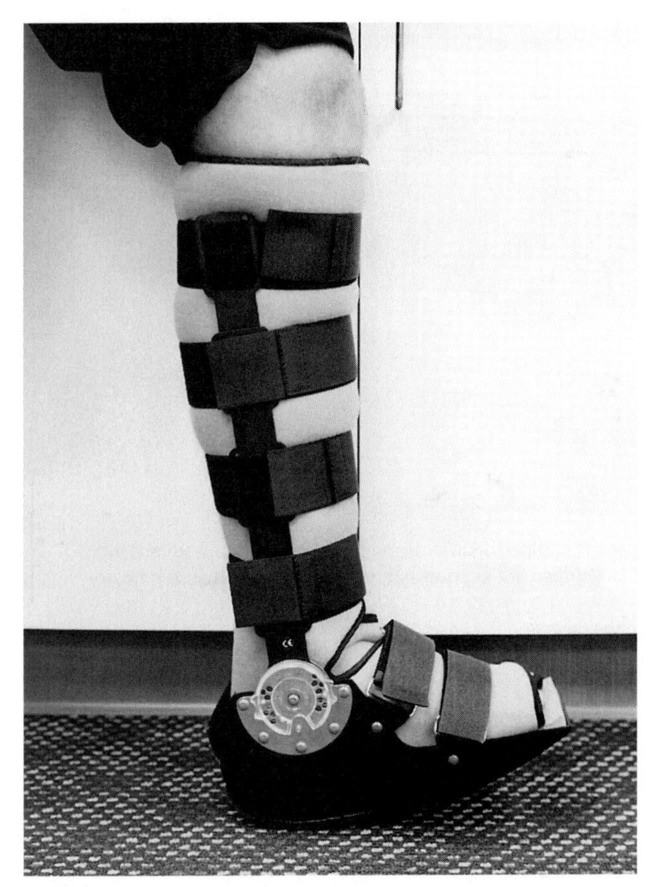

FIGURE 9-33 ■ A walker boot. Walker boots allow for controlled range of motion, earlier stable weight bearing, and the ease of removal for rehabilitation.

anatomic factors that predispose an individual to CCS include[121]:

- Herniation of muscle, occluding the neurovascular network as it transverses the interosseous membrane
- Fascia's failing to accommodate the increase in muscle volume during exercise
- Excessive hypertrophy of the muscles within an otherwise normal fascial network
- Increased capillary permeability
- Postexercise fluid retention
- Decreased venous return

Compartmental syndromes have are been associated with tibial fractures,[122–125] anticoagulant therapy,[126] and diabetes.[127] The use of knee braces[128] and wearing high-heeled shoes or athletic shoes that have an increased heel height[129] have also been implicated in the onset of exertional compartment syndromes.

The signs, symptoms, and pathology of acute and chronic exertional syndromes are similar. However, acute exertional compartment syndromes occur without prior symptoms and do not have a history of traumatic injury to the compartment.[119]

The "five P's" are used to describe the signs and symptoms of compartment syndromes:

- Pain
- Pallor (redness)
- Pulselessness
- Paresthesia
- Paralysis

The identification and management of a compartment syndrome should not be delayed because all of the five P's are not present.[119] Pain is localized within the affected compartment and is often disproportionate with the other findings of the examination. Numbness occurs in the web space between the first and second toes, possibly involving the dorsal and lateral aspects of the foot.[119] Sensory changes and paralysis are usually not noted until ischemia has been present for 1 hour.[125] Pain is increased during active, passive, and resisted foot movement with decreased strength being noted during resisted dorsiflexion. A drop foot gait (see Chapter 8) may also be observed (Examination Findings 9-11 and 9-12).

The presence of the dorsalis pedis pulse must be established in the involved limb (see Vascular Testing, p. 251). Because this pulse is not detectable in all individuals, both limbs must be examined. If the pulse is present in the uninvolved extremity but not in the involved extremity, then it can be deduced that blood flow to the foot has been compromised. The dorsalis pedis pulse will remain palpable in all but the most advanced cases of compartment syndromes. Although the blood pressure within the tibial artery may be sufficient to produce a palpable dorsalis pedis pulse, the pressure increase may be great enough to inhibit flow within the smaller vessels and capillaries.[121] Muscle is relatively resilient to ischemic conditions up to 4 hours duration; after 8 hours of ischemia irreversible muscle damage will occur.[125] Individuals having a higher diastolic blood pressure are able to withstand higher compartmental pressures without permanent tissue damage than those having a lower diastolic pressure.[125]

Compartment syndromes can be fully developed even though a patient still has normal pulses and full capillary refill. The tissue must be ischemic for approximately 1 hour before paresthesia and paralysis develop. The most important clinical finding of compartment syndromes is severe pain with passive stretching of the muscles within the compartment.[119] Compartment syndromes evoking decreased pulses, paresthesia, or paralysis of the involved muscles are medical emergencies requiring immediate referral for medical treatment. Chronic compartment syndromes usually present symptoms during exercise that subsequently subside with rest.

The diagnosis of compartment syndromes is based on the differential pressure between the diastolic blood pressure and intracompartmental pressure. A difference of 30 mm Hg may require a fasciotomy.[123,126] Compartmental

Examination Findings 9-11
Traumatic Compartment Syndrome

Examination Segment	Clinical Findings
History	***Onset:*** Traumatic ***Pain characteristics:*** Severe pain Anterolateral portion of the leg, which is described as "achy," "sharp," or "dull" Other complaints such as muscle tightness, cramping, swelling, weakness, or the inability to exercise owing to pain ***Other symptoms:*** Numbness may develop in the dorsum of the foot, especially in the web space between the first and second toes (anterior). ***Mechanism:*** Direct trauma to the anterolateral or lateral leg Inversion mechanism that avulses peroneals ***Predisposing conditions:*** Anatomic factors that inhibit the expansion of the involved compartment, tibial fracture, anticoagulant therapy, calcaneal fractures
Inspection	The anterior compartment may appear shiny and swollen. In advanced cases, possible discoloration of the dorsum of the foot may be present.
Palpation	The involved compartment is hard and edematous to the touch, the area is painful to the touch.
Joint and Muscle Function Assessment	***AROM:*** Decreased (or absent) ability to dorsiflex the ankle or extend the toes (anterior) Diminished or painful eversion (lateral) ***MMT:*** Not indicated ***PROM:*** Pain during passive motion secondary to stretching of the muscles in the involved compartment, creating pressure within
Joint Stability Tests	***Stress tests:*** Not applicable ***Joint play:*** Not applicable
Special Tests	There are no clinical tests for these conditions. Anterior compartment syndrome is confirmed by measuring the intracompartmental pressure.
Neurologic Screening	Anterior compartment: Paresthesia may be present in the web space between the 1st and 2nd toes and possibly on the dorsum of the foot Lateral compartment: Paresthesia may be present along the lateral distal leg and dorsum of the foot.
Vascular Screening	The presence of a normal dorsalis pedis pulse should be determined.
Functional Assessment	Extreme pain with ambulation. Drop foot gait may be observed (anterior).
Imaging Techniques	Radiographic images may be taken to determine the presence of a bony fracture causing the increased compartmental pressure.
Differential Diagnosis	Tibial fracture, fibular fracture
Comments	Do not apply a compression wrap during the treatment of anterior compartment syndrome because the wrap will increase the intracompartmental pressure and exacerbate the condition. Elevation is also contraindicated as it decreases vascular pressure.

AROM = active range of motion; MMT = manual muscle test; PROM = passive range of motion.

Examination Findings 9-12
Exertional Compartment Syndrome

Examination Segment	Clinical Findings
History	***Onset:*** Acute or chronic; gradual presentation of symptoms ***Pain characteristics:*** Pain in the involved compartment, which is described as "achy," "sharp," or "dull" Pain resolves with cessation of activity. ***Other symptoms:*** Reports of muscle tightness, cramping, swelling, and weakness Numbness is possibly described in the dorsum of the foot, especially in the web space between the first and second toes (anterior compartment) Inability to exercise secondary to severity of symptoms ***Mechanism:*** Symptoms are reported during or after running or other prolonged activity. ***Predisposing conditions:*** Anatomic factors that inhibit the expansion of the compartment, anticoagulant therapy, diabetes, prophylactic and functional knee braces, high-heeled shoes
Inspection	The compartment may appear swollen when symptomatic. A dull sheen may be noted (anterior). Deep posterior compartment involvement will have no visible findings.
Palpation	The involved compartment is hard and edematous to the touch; the area is painful to the touch.
Joint and Muscle Function Assessment	***AROM:*** Decreased (or absent) function in muscles of the involved compartment. Anterior: Inability to dorsiflex the ankle or extend the toes. ***MMT:*** Weakness is noted during testing muscles in the involved compartment. Anterior: Dorsiflexion, supination/inversion Deep posterior: Plantarflexion, toe flexion, supination/inversion Lateral: Pronation/eversion ***PROM:*** Increased pain with stretch of muscles in the involved compartment
Joint Stability Tests	***Stress tests:*** Not applicable ***Joint play:*** Not applicable
Special Tests	There are no clinician tests for these conditions. Exertional anterior compartment syndrome is confirmed by measuring the intracompartmental pressure before, during, and after activity.
Neurologic Screening	Anterior compartment: Numbness may be present in the web space between the 1st and 2nd toes and possibly on the dorsum of the foot. Lateral compartment: Paresthesia may be present along the lateral distal leg and dorsum of the foot. Deep posterior compartment: Paresthesia may be present at the medial calcaneus.
Vascular Screening	The presence of a normal dorsalis pedis pulse should be determined.
Functional Assessment	Antalgic gait. Drop foot gait may be observed if anterior compartment is involved.
Imaging Techniques	Angiography may be used to determine the vascular integrity of the extremity.
Differential Diagnosis	Tibial or fibular stress fracture, medial tibial stress syndrome
Comments	Bilateral involvement in chronic compartment syndromes is common. Findings may be unremarkable if the patient is asymptomatic at the time of the examination. Clinical findings are more apparent if the patient exercises until symptoms appear and then the physical examination conducted.

AROM = active range of motion; MMT = manual muscle test; PROM = passive range of motion.

pressures can also be monitored during exercise, an invasive technique performed in a medical facility. Increases of more than 15 mm Hg when resting, 30 mm Hg 1 minute after exercise, or 20 mm Hg 5 minutes postexercise are diagnostic signs of an exertional compartment syndrome.[119] MRI mages may also be used to detect exertional compartment syndromes.[130]

After surgical fasciotomy of the compartments of the involved leg, the initial treatment and rehabilitation involve adequate healing of the incision site because increased compartmental pressure and decreased blood flow may delay the healing process.[131] After wound healing has been established, therapeutic exercise to restore ROM and strength to the lower extremity is begun. The patient is progressed with functional activities to return to full activity.

Deep Vein Thrombosis

A deep vein thrombosis (DVT), a blood clot, is a potentially life-threatening condition because of the associated risk of pulmonary embolism if the clot should dislodge. Risk factors for developing a DVT include a range of traumatic, congenital, and disease states (Table 9-8).[132] Several conditions can mimic the symptoms of deep vein thrombosis including large or ruptured popliteal cyst, hematoma, tendinitis, osteoarthritis, sciatica, and cellulitis.[132,133]

Palpation reveals warmth, tightness of the calf musculature, and pain. **Homans' sign**, exacerbation of symptoms with the knee flexed and forceful, passive dorsiflexion of the ankle, is widely described as a examination technique to detect DVT; however, its low sensitivity and lack of specificity make it an unreliable indicator.[132,134] A suspicion of a DVT based on physical examination and associated risk factors warrants immediate medical referral. A definitive diagnosis is made using ultrasonic images.[132]

On-Field Examination of Leg and Ankle Injuries

The goals of the on-field evaluation of patients with these injuries include ruling out fractures and dislocations, determining the athlete's weight-bearing status, and identifying the best method for removing the athlete from the field.

Equipment Considerations

The nature of competitive athletics brings with it ever more specialized footwear, braces, and types of tape. Although designed to protect athletes from injury while also improving performance, these devices may hinder the evaluation and management of acute injuries.

Footwear removal

After a gross fracture or dislocation has been ruled out, the athlete's shoe must be removed so a thorough examination of the injury can be conducted after the athlete has reached the sideline. Most shoes may be easily removed by completely unlacing them, spreading the sides, and pulling the tongue down to the toes (Fig. 9-34). The athlete is asked to plantarflex the foot, if possible. The shoe is removed by sliding the heel counter away from the foot and then lifting the shoe up and off the foot. Apprehensive athletes may be allowed to remove the shoe themselves. If a fracture or dislocation is suspected, the examiner should loosen the shoe enough to allow for palpation of the dorsalis pedis and posterior tibial pulses and transport the athlete with the shoe in place and the leg splinted. Metal cleats or spikes may need to be removed prior to immobilization or transportation.

Tape and brace removal

Prophylactic devices such as tape or ankle braces must be removed to allow for the complete examination of the foot

Table 9-8 Risk Factors for Developing Deep Vein Thrombosis

Strong	Moderate	Weak
Knee or hip arthroplasty	Arthroscopic knee surgery	Aging
Major surgery	Cerebrovascular accident	Bed rest over 3 days
Pelvis, femur, or tibia fracture	Chemotherapy	Laparoscopic surgery
Significant trauma	Congestive heart failure	Obesity
Spinal cord injury	Hormone replacement therapy	Pregnancy
	Malignant cancer	Prolonged sitting
	Oral contraceptives	Varicose veins
	Pregnancy (postpartum)	
	Previous history of thromboembolism	
	Respiratory failure	

Adapted from Eskelin, MK, Lotjonen, JM, and Mantysaari, MJ: Chronic exertional compartment syndrome: MR imaging at 0.1 T compared with tissue pressure measurement. *Radiology*, 206:333, 1998.

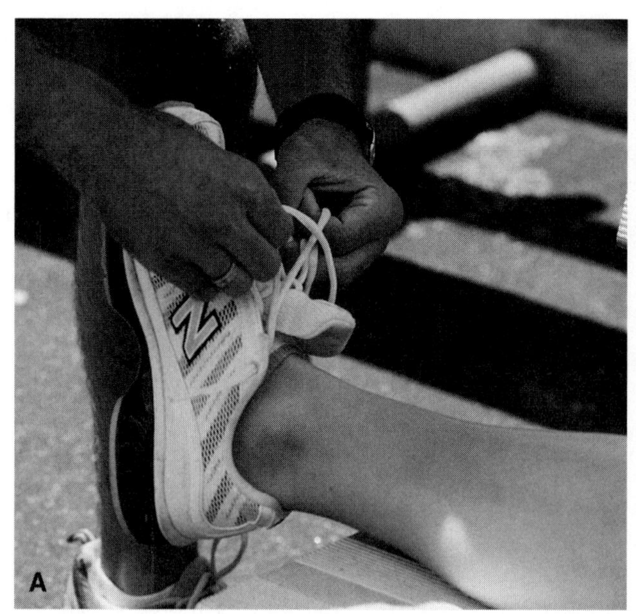
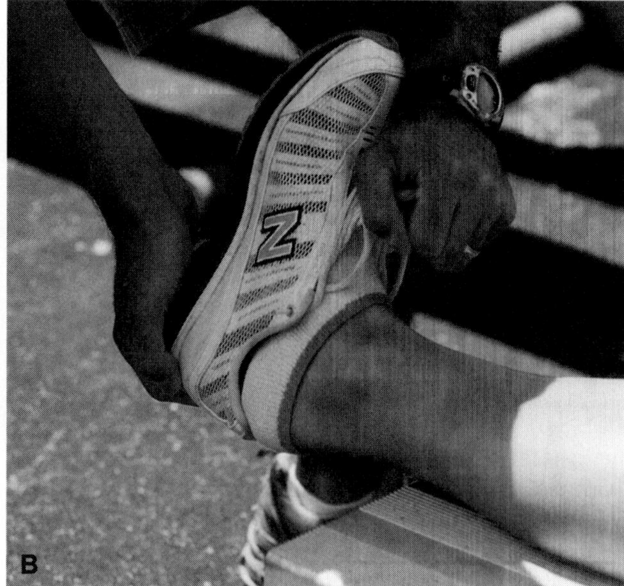

FIGURE 9-34 ■ Removing the shoe following a foot or ankle injury. (A) After completely removing the laces, withdraw the tongue and (B) slide the shoe from the foot.

and ankle. Braces tightened by laces or Velcro straps may be removed in a manner such as described for shoe removal. Ankle tape can be removed by cutting along a line parallel to the posterior portion of the malleolus on the side of the leg opposite the site of pain. The cut is then continued along the plantar aspect of the foot.

On-Field History

In the absence of gross deformity, the mechanism of injury and the associated sounds and sensations can help to identify the underlying pathology or a direct blow to the leg.

- **Mechanism of injury:** Identify the injurious forces placed on the ankle, keeping in mind that the injury may involve multiple forces (e.g., inversion and plantarflexion) or a direct blow to the leg.
  - **Inversion:** Rolling the talus and calcaneus inward exerts tensile forces on the lateral aspect of the ankle and compressive forces on the medial aspect. Lateral ankle sprains, lateral ligament avulsions, and medial malleolar fractures are associated with this mechanism.
  - **Eversion:** Excessive eversion of the talus and calcaneus places tensile forces on the medial aspect of the ankle and compression on the lateral aspect. Syndesmotic ankle sprains and fractures of the lateral malleolus and fibula are also associated with this mechanism.
  - **Rotation:** Rotational forces can lead to syndesmotic sprains or fracture of the tibia, fibula, or both.
  - **Dorsiflexion:** Forced dorsiflexion can strain or rupture the Achilles tendon or cause the distal tibiofibular syndesmosis to separate.
  - **Plantarflexion:** Although this mechanism is rare, forced plantarflexion can traumatize the extensor retinaculum and anterior joint capsule and its associated ligaments.
- **Associated sounds and sensations:** Ascertain for any sounds or sensations. A "snap" or "pop" may be associated with a ligament rupture or bony fracture. An audible snap or pop is also associated with an Achilles tendon rupture and may be described as being "kicked in the calf." Radiating pain or numbness in the anterior ankle and leg can indicate anterior compartment syndrome or trauma to the peroneal nerve.

On-Field Inspection

During on-field inspection of ankle and leg injuries, any gross bony or joint injury must be ruled out before progressing to the other elements of the evaluation. Examine the contour and alignment of the leg, foot, and ankle, noting any discontinuity or malalignment of the structures that may indicate a fracture or dislocation.

On-Field Palpation

Assuming normal alignment of the leg, the evaluation proceeds to palpation of the bony structures and related soft tissue.

- **Bony palpation:** Begin by palpating the length of the tibia and fibula and continuing on to the talus, the remaining tarsals, and the MTs. Note any deformities, crepitus, or areas of point tenderness, especially in areas where pain is described. If a disruption of a long bone or joint is felt, splint the joint and transport the athlete to a hospital.

- **Soft tissue palpation:** Perform a quick yet thorough evaluation of the major soft tissues, emphasizing the ligamentous structures for point tenderness and the tendons for signs of rupture.

On-Field Range of Motion Tests

After the possibility of a gross fracture or dislocation has been ruled out, the athlete's ability to move the limb and subsequently bear weight must be established.

- **Willingness to move the involved limb:** If the athlete displays normal alignment of the limb, observe his or her willingness to move the injured body part through the full ROM. This task should be performed with a minimal amount of discomfort. If the athlete has no ability or is unwilling to move the involved limb, use assistance to remove the athlete from the field.
- **Willingness to bear weight:** If the athlete describes no pain and there are no signs of restriction in the ROM, assist the athlete to the standing position, bearing weight on the uninvolved leg. Assistance is provided by assuming position under the athlete's arm on the involved side, giving some support. The athlete should walk off the field, attempting to place as little weight as possible on the involved limb.

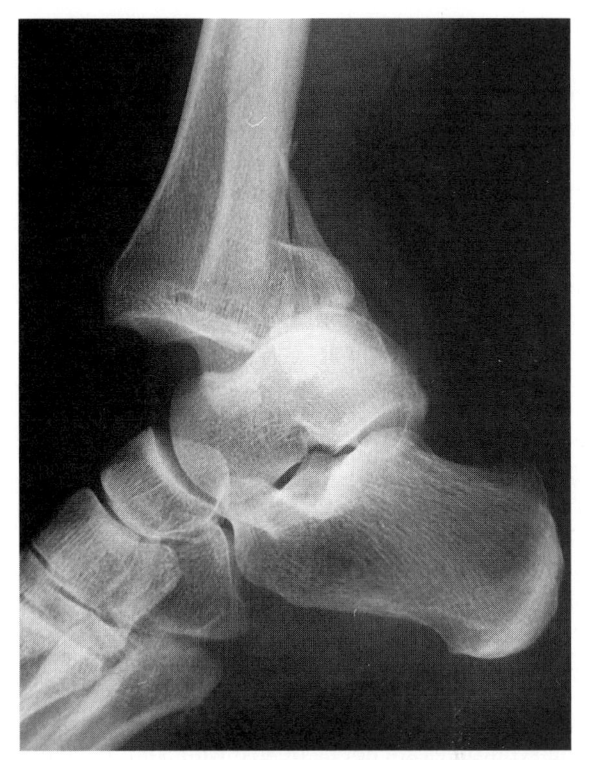

FIGURE 9-35 ■ Posterior ankle dislocation (medial view of the right ankle). Often the talus displaces anteriorly relative to the tibia. This radiograph shows the talus being displaced posteriorly relative to the tibia. Note the fracture of the malleolus caused by the wide anterior talar border's being forced into the mortise.

Initial Management of On-Field Injuries

This section describes the emergency management procedures for major trauma occurring to the ankle and lower extremity. Most ankle injuries (e.g., sprains, Achilles tendon ruptures) are managed on the sidelines or in athletic training rooms. On-field care involves ruling out the presence of a fracture or neurovascular deficit, keeping the injured body from bearing weight, and removing the athlete from the playing field.

Ankle Dislocations

Resulting from excessive rotation combined with inversion or eversion, dislocations of the talocrural joint result in major disruptions of the joint capsule and associated ligaments. Associated fractures of the malleoli, long bones, or talus often occur. Resulting in immediate pain in the ankle and leg and loss of function, the patient may also report an audible snap or crack. The foot and ankle may be grossly malaligned. If the defect is not visible, the superior portion of the talus may be palpated as it protrudes anteriorly and medially from the ankle mortise (Fig. 9-35). The evaluation also must confirm the presence of the distal pulses and include a secondary survey of the ankle mortise and long bones for possible fracture (Fig. 9-36).

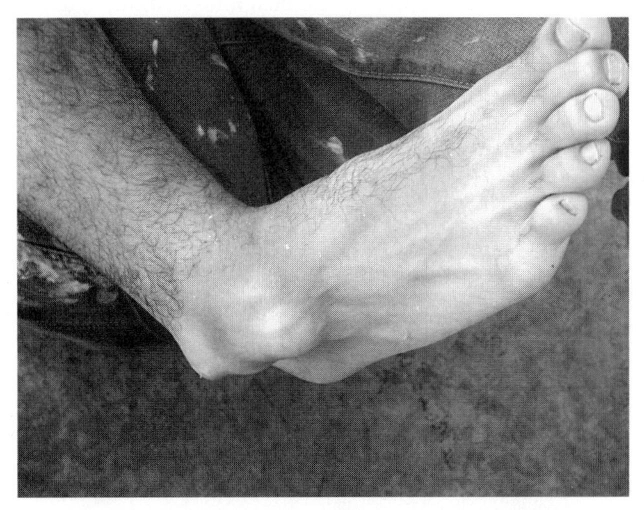

FIGURE 9-36 ■ Ankle fracture–dislocation. Note the irregular contour beneath the lateral malleolus.

Management of leg fractures and ankle dislocations

Any obvious fracture or joint dislocation should immediately be immobilized using a moldable or vacuum splint (see Box 2-2). In most cases, it is recommended that the shoe be left in place while the athlete is being transported to the hospital. It may be more safely removed in the emergency room after further diagnostic tests, such as radiographic examination, to determine the full extent of the injury (Fig. 9-37). The laces and tongue of the shoe are loosened and the sock is cut to permit palpation of the dorsalis pedis and the posterior tibial pulses, which are then compared bilaterally and continually monitored.

Management of an open fracture involves controlling bleeding and immobilizing the fracture. The area around the open fracture should be packed with sterile bandages without causing any further disruption at the fracture site. After bleeding is controlled, the extremity can be immobilized in the position in which it is found, the pulses continually monitored, and the athlete transported to a medical facility.

Nondisplaced fibular or tibial fractures may be treated by simple casting. Comminuted or displaced fractures often require the use of internal or external fixation devices to realign and stabilize the fracture sites. A fracture of the distal fibula involving the syndesmosis may require an internal fixation device or a screw to maintain the alignment of the fibula with the tibia during the healing process and to prevent subsequent rotational instabilities of the talus (Fig. 9-38).[135]

Compartment Syndrome

Unlike other acute soft tissue injuries, suspected compartment syndromes are not be treated with compression. The use of external compression devices, such as wraps or compression boots, increase the pressure within the compartment, exacerbating the condition. If acute gross hemorrhage is present or distal pulses are absent, the athlete must be immediately referred for medical intervention. If, at the time of the injury, the athlete does not display signs of intracompartmental hemorrhage but there is reason to suspect such a response, provide the athlete with a list of the danger signs and symptoms (see Table 9-7) and instruct the athlete about contacting a physician if the symptoms worsen.

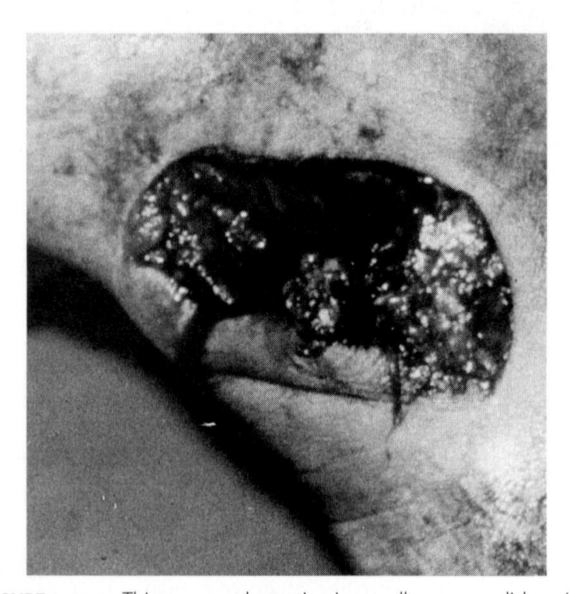

FIGURE 9-37 ■ This apparent laceration is actually an open dislocation of the talus.

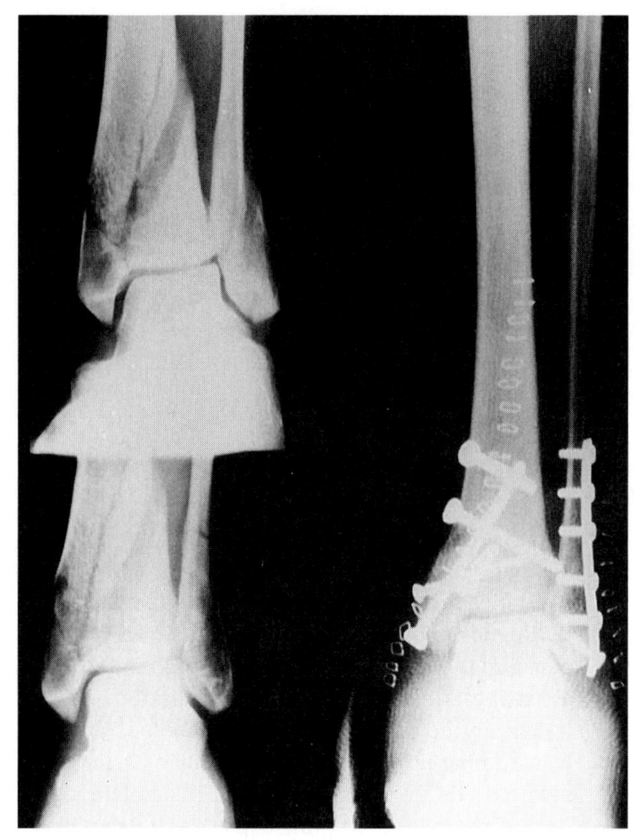

FIGURE 9-38 ■ Radiograph showing screws and plates used to set a fracture of the ankle joint.

REFERENCES

1. Hertel, J: Functional instability following lateral ankle sprain. *Sports Med*, 29:361, 2000.
2. Sammarco, GJ, and Mangone, PG: Diagnosis and treatment of peroneal tendon injuries. *Foot Ank Surg*, 6:197, 2000.
3. Garrick, JM: The frequency of injury, mechanism of injury, and epidemiology of ankle sprains. *Am J Sports Med* 5:241, 1971.
4. Takebe, K, et al: Role of the fibula in weight-bearing. *Clin Orthop* 184:2899, 1984.
5. Norkus, SA, and Floyd, RT: The anatomy and mechanisms of syndesmotic ankle sprains. *J Athl Train*, 36:68, 2001.
6. Hertel, J: Functional anatomy, pathomechanics, and pathophysiology of lateral ankle instability. *J Athl Train*, 37:364, 2002.
7. Lynch, SA: Assessment of the injured ankle in the athlete. *J Athl Train*, 37:406, 2002.
8. Burks, RT, and Morgan, J: Anatomy of the lateral ankle ligaments. *Am J Sports Med* 22:72, 1994.
9. Wuest, TK: Injuries to the distal lower extremity syndesmosis. *J Am Acad Orthop Surg*, 5:172, 1997.
10. Mueller, MJ: The ankle-foot complex. In Levangie, PK and Norkin, CC (eds): *Joint Structure and Function: A Comprehensive Analysis*, ed 4. Philadelphia, FA Davis, 2005, p. 437.
11. Doughtie, M: Syndesmotic ankle sprains in football: A survey of National Football League athletic trainers. *J Athl Train*, 34:15, 1999.
12. Jones, DC: Tendon disorders of the foot and ankle. *J Am Acad Orthop Surg*, 1:87, 1993.

13. Zammit, J, and Singh, D: The peroneus quartus muscle. Anatomy and clinical relevance. *J Bone Joint Surg*, 85:1134, 2003.
14. Hale, SA, and Hertel, J: Reliability and sensitivity of the Foot and Ankle Disability Index in subjects with chronic instability. *J Athl Trng*, 40:35, 2005.
15. Mawdsley, RH, Hoy, DK, and Erwin, PM: Criterion-related validity of the figure-of-eight method of measuring ankle edema. *J Orthop Sports Phys Ther*, 30:149, 2000.
16. Peterson, EJ, et al: Reliability of water volumetry and the figure of eight method on subjects with ankle joint swelling. *JOSPT*, 29:609, 1999.
17. Breitenseher, MJ, et al: MRI of the sinus tarsi in acute ankle injuries. *J Comput Assist Tomogr*, 21:274, 1997.
18. Copeland, SA: Rupture of the Achilles tendon: A new clinical test. *Ann R Coll Surg Engl*. 72:270, 1990.
19. Witvrouw, WE, et al: The significance of peroneus tertius muscle in ankle injuries: A prospective study. *Am J Sports Med*, 34:1159, 2006.
20. Beck, BR: Tibial stress injuries. An aetiological review for the purposes of guiding management. *Sports Med*, 26:265, 1998.
21. Fujii, T, et al: The manual stress test may not be sufficient to differentiate ankle ligament injuries. *Clin Biomech*, 15:619, 2000.
22. Kerkhoffs, GMMJ, et al: Two ankle joint laxity testers: Reliability and validity. *Knee Surg Sports Traumatol Arthrosc*, 13:699, 2005.
23. Corazza, F, et al: Mechanics of the anterior drawer test at the ankle: The effects of ligament viscoelasticity. *J Biomech*, 38:2118, 2005.
24. Tohyama, H, et al: Anterior drawer test for acute anterior talofibular ligament injuries of the ankle: How much load should be applied during the test? *Am J Sports Med*, 31:226. 2003.
25. Vela, L, Tourville, TW, and Hertel, J: Physical examination of acutely injured ankles: An evidence-based approach. *Athletic Therapy Today*, 8:13, 2003.
26. van Dijk, CN, et al: Physical examination is sufficient for the diagnosis of sprained ankles. *J Bone Jt Surg* (Br), 78-B:958, 1996.
27. van Dijk, CN, et al: Diagnosis of ligament rupture of the ankle joint. Physical examination, arthrography, stress radiography and sonography compared in 160 patients after inversion trauma. *Acta Orthop Scand*, 67:566,1996.
28. Hertel, J, et al: Talocrural and subtalar instability after lateral ankle sprain. *Med Sci Sports Exer*, 31:;1501, 1999.
29. Alonso, A, Khoury, L, and Adams R: Clinical tests for ankle syndesmosis injury: reliability and prediction of return to function. *J Orthop Sports Phys Ther*, 27:276, 1998.
30. Beumer, A, Swierstra, BA, and Mulder, PG: Clinical diagnosis of syndesmotic ankle instability. Evaluation of stress tests behind the curtains. *Acta Orthop Scand*, 73:667, 2002.
31. Fallat, L, Grimm, DL, and Saracco, JA: Sprained ankle syndrome: Prevalence and analysis of 639 acute injuries. *J Foot Ankle Surg*, 37:280, 1998.
32. Olmsted-Kramer, LC, and Hertel, J: Preventing recurrent lateral ankle sprains: An evidence-based approach. *Athletic Therapy Today*, 9:19, 2004.
33. McKay, GD, et al: Ankle injuries in basketball: injury rate and risk factors. *Br J Sports Med*, 35:103, 2001.
34. Tyler, TF, et al: Risk factors for noncontact ankle sprains in high school football players. The role of previous ankle sprains and body mass index. *Am J Sports Med*, 34:471, 2006.
35. McHugh, MP, et al: Risk factors for noncontact ankle sprains in high school athletes. The role of hip strength and balance ability. *Am J Sports Med*, 34:464, 2007.
36. Stone, JW: Osteochondral lesions of the talar dome. *J Am Acad Orthop Surg*, 4:63, 1996.
37. van Dijk, CN, et al: Diagnosis of ligament rupture of the ankle joint. Physical examination, arthrography, stress radiography and sonography compared in 160 patients after inversion trauma. *Acta Orthop Scand*, 67:566, 1996.
38. Molloy, S, Solan, MC, and Bendall, SP: Synovial impingement in the ankle. A new physical sign. *J Bone Joint Surg*, 85-B:330, 2003.
39. Hertel, J, and Kaminski, T: Second international ankle symposium summary statement. *J Orthop Sports Phys Ther*, 35:A-2, 2005.
40. Frey, C, et al: A comparison of MRI and clinical examination of acute lateral ankle sprains. *Foot Ankle Int*, 17:533, 1996.
41. Yeung, MS, et al: An epidemiological survey on ankle sprains. *Br J Sports Med*, 28:112, 1994.
42. Johnson, MB, and Johnson, CL: Electromyographic response of peroneal muscles in surgical and nonsurgical injured ankles during sudden inversion. *J Orthop Sports Phys Ther*, 18:497, 1993.
43. Isalov, E: Response of peroneal muscles to sudden inversion of the ankle during standing. *Int J Sport Biomech*, 2:100, 1986.
44. Freeman, MAR: Treatment of ruptures of the lateral ligament of the ankle. *J Bone Joint Surg Br*, 47:661, 1965.
45. Freeman, MAR, et al: The etiology and prevention of functional instability of the foot. *J Bone Joint Surg Br*, 47:678, 1965.
46. Meislin, RJ, et al: Arthroscopic treatment of synovial impingement of the ankle. *Am J Sports Med*, 21:186, 1993.
47. Pinar, H, et al: Bone bruises detected by magnetic resonance imaging following lateral ankle sprains. *Knee Surg Sports Traumatol Arthrosc*, 5:113, 1997.
48. Karlsson, J, and Wiger, P: Longitudinal split of the peroneus brevis tendon and lateral ankle instability: Treatment of concomitant lesions. *J Athl Train*, 37:463, 2002.
49. Taga, I: Articular cartilage lesions in ankles with lateral ligament injury: An arthroscopic study. *Am J Sports Med*, 21:120, 1993.
50. Loomer, R, et al: Osteochondral lesions of the talus. *Am J Sports Med*, 21:13, 1993.
51. Bassett, FH: A simple surgical approach to the posteromedial ankle. *Am J Sports Med*, 21:144, 1993.
52. Verhagen, RAW, et al: Prospective study on diagnostic strategies in osteochondral lesions of the talus. J Bone Joint Surg, 87-B:41, 2005.
53. Bullock-Saxton, JE: Local sensations and altered hip muscle function following severe ankle sprain. *Phys Ther*, 74:17, 1994.
54. Dettori, JR, et al: Early ankle mobilization, part I: The immediate effect on acute, lateral ankle sprains (a randomized clinical trial). *Mil Med*, 159:15, 1994.
55. Eiff, MP, Smith, AT, and Smith, GE: Early mobilization versus immobilization in the treatment of lateral ankle sprains. *Am J Sports Med*, 22:83, 1994.
56. Dettori, JR, and Basmania, CJ: Early ankle mobilization, part II: A one-year follow up of acute, lateral ankle sprains (a randomized clinical trial). *Mil Med*, 159:20, 1994.
57. Schmidt, R, et al: Anatomical repair of lateral ligaments in patients with chronic ankle instability. *Knee Surg Sports Traumatol Arthrosc*, 13:231, 2005.

58. Punenburg, ACM, et al: Treatment of ruptures of the lateral ankle ligaments: A meta-analysis. *J Bone Joint Surg*, 82(A):761, 2000.
59. Candal-Couto, et al: Instability of the tibio-fibular syndesmosis: have we been pulling in the wrong direction? *Injury*, 35:814, 2004.
60. Boytim, MJ, Fischer, DA, and Neumann, L: Syndesmotic ankle sprains. *Am J Sports Med*, 19:294, 1991.
61. Teitz, CC, and Harrington, RM: A biomechanical analysis of the squeeze test for sprains of the syndesmotic ligaments of the ankle. *Foot Ankle Int*, 19:489, 1998.
62. Veltri, DM, et al: Symptomatic ossification of the tibiofibular syndesmosis in professional football players: A sequela of the syndesmotic ankle sprain. *Foot Ankle Int*, 16:285, 1995.
63. Garrick, JG, and Requa, RK: Role of external support in the prevention of ankle sprains. *Med Sci Sports Exerc*, 5:200, 1973.
64. McConnell, T, Creevy, W, and Tornetta, P: Stress examination of supination external rotation-type fibular fractures. *J Bone Joint Surg*, 86A:2171, 2004.
65. Nielson, JH: Correlation of interosseous membrane tears to the level of the fibular fracture. *J Orthop Trauma*, 18:68, 2004.
66. Stiell, IG, et al: The "real"Ottawa Ankle Rules. *Ann Emerg Med*, 27:103, 1996.
67. Bachmann, LM, et al: Accuracy of Ottawa ankle rules to exclude fractures of the ankle and mid-foot: Systematic review. *Br J Med*, 326:417, 2003.
68. Nugent, PJ: Ottawa Ankle Rules accurately assess injuries and reduce reliance on radiographs. *J Fam Pract*, 53:785, 2004.
69. Bhanot, A, et al: Fracture of the posterior process of talus. *Injury*, 35:1341, 2004.
70. Leddy, JJ, et al: Prospective evaluation of the Ottawa ankle rules in a university sports medicine center. With a modification to increase specificity for identifying malleolar fractures. *Am J Sports Med*, 26:158, 1998.
71. Blake, RL, Lallas, PJ, and Ferguson, H: The os trigonum syndrome. A literature review. *J Am Podiatr Med Assoc*, 82:154, 1992.
72. Ihle, CL, and Cochran, KM: Fracture of the fused os trigonum. *Am J Sports Med*, 10:47, 1982.
73. Sarrafin, S: *Anatomy of the Foot and Ankle*. Philadelphia: J.B. Lippincott, 1983, p. 47.
74. Brodsky, AE, and Khalil, M: Talar compression syndrome. *Am J Sports Med*, 14:472, 1986.
75. Paulos, LE, et al: Posterior compartment fracture of the ankles: A commonly missed athletic injury. *Am J Sports Med*, 11:439, 1983.
76. McDougall, A: The os trigonum. *J Bone Joint Surg Br*, 37:257, 1955.
77. Karasick, D, and Schweitzer, ME: The os trigonum syndrome: Imaging features. *Am J Roentgenol*, 166:125, 1996.
78. Masciocchi, C, Catalucci, A, and Barile, A: Ankle impingement syndromes. *Eur J Radiol*, 27(S1):S70, 1998.
79. Mahieu, NN, et al: Intrinsic risk factors for the development of Achilles tendon overuse injury. A prospective study. *Am J Sports Med*, 34:1, 2006.
80. Ahmed, IM, et al: Blood supply of the Achilles tendon. *J Orthop Res*, 16:591, 1998.
81. Scioli, MW: Achilles tendinitis. *Orthop Clin North Am*, 25:177, 1994.
82. Puddu, G, et al: A classification of Achilles tendon disease. *Am J Sports Med*, 4:145, 1976.
83. Gillet, P, et al: Magnetic resonance imaging may be an asset to diagnose and classify fluorouinolone-associated Achilles tendinitis. *Fundam Clin Pharmacol*, 9:52, 1995.
84. Astrom, M, and Rausing, A: Chronic Achilles tendinopathy. A survey of surgical and histopathic findings. *Clin Orthop*, Jul:151, 1995.
85. Astrom, M: Partial rupture in chronic Achilles tendinopathy. A retrospective analysis of 342 cases. *Acta Orthop Scand*, 69:404, 1998.
86. Alfredson, H: Achilles tendinosis and calf muscle strength. The effect of short-term immobilization after surgical treatment. *Am J Sports Med*, 26:166, 1998.
87. Shrier, I, Matheson, GO, and Kohl, HW 3rd: Achilles tendonitis: Are corticosteroid injections useful or harmful? *Clin J Sport Med*, 6:245, 1996.
88. Leppilahti, J, and Orava, S: Total achilles tendon rupture: A review. *Sports Med*, 25:79, 1998.
89. Saltzman, C, and Bonar, S: Tendon problems of the foot and ankle. In Lutter, LD, Mizel, MS, and Pfeffer, GB (eds): *Orthopaedic Knowledge Update: Foot and Ankle*. Rosemont, IL: American Academy of Orthopaedic Surgeons, 1994, p. 271.
90. Shrier, I, Matheson, GO, and Kohl, HW: Achilles tendonitis: Are corticosteroid injections useful or harmful? *Clin J Sports Med*, 6:245, 1996.
91. Read, MT: Safe relief of rest pain that eases with activity in achillodynia by intrabursal or peritendinous steroid injection: The rupture rate was not increased by these steroid injections. *Br J Sports Med*, 33:134, 1996.
92. Bennet, JE, et al: Factors contributing to the development of medial tibial stress syndrome in high school runners. *J Orthop Sports Phys Ther.* 31:504, 2001.
93. Maffulli, N: The clinical diagnosis of subcutaneous tear of the Achilles tendon. A prospective study in 174 patients. *Am J Sports Med*, 26:266, 1998.
94. Fierro, NL, and Sallis, RE: Achilles tendon rupture. Is casting enough? *Postgrad Med*, 98:145, 1995.
95. Troop, RL, et al: Early motion after repair of Achilles tendon ruptures. *Foot Ankle Int*, 16:705, 1995.
96. Nistor, L: Surgical and non-surgical treatment of the Achilles tendon rupture. *J Bone Joint Surg*, 63A:394, 1981.
97. Grant, TH, et al: Ultrasound diagnosis of peroneal tendon tears. *J Bone Joint Surg*, 87(A):1788, 2005.
98. Kumai, T, and Benjamin, M: The histological structure of the malleolar groove of the fibula in man: Its direct bearing on the displacement of peroneal tendons and their surgical repair. *J Anat*, 203:257, 2003.
99. Schweitzer, ME, et al: Using MR imaging to differentiate peroneal splits from other peroneal disorders. *Am J Roentgenol*, 168:129, 1997.
100. Yao, L: MR Findings in peroneal tendonopathy. *J Comput Assist Tomogr*, 19:460, 1995.
101. Krause, JO, and Brodsky, JW: Peroneus brevis tendon tears: Pathophysiology, surgical reconstruction, and clinical results. *Foot Ankle Int*, 19:271, 1998.
102. Steensma, MR, Anderson, JG, and Bohay, DR: Update on diseases and treatment of the peroneal tendon, including peroneal tendon tear, subluxating peroneal tendon, and tendinosis. *Curr Opin Orthop*, 16:60, 2005.
103. Boles, MA, et al: Enlarged peroneal process with peroneus longus tendon entrapment. *Skeletal Radiol*, 26:313, 1997.

104. Mason, RB, and Henderson, JP: Traumatic peroneal tendon instability. *Am J Sports Med*, 24:652, 1996.
105. Magnano, GM, et al: High-resolution US of non-traumatic recurrent dislocation of the peroneal tendons: A case report. *Pediatr Radiol*, 28:476, 1998.
106. Shellock, FG, et al: Peroneal tendons: Use of kinematic MR imaging of the ankle to determine subluxation. *J Magn Reson Imaging*, 7:451, 1997.
107. Sobel, M, et al: Painful os peroneum syndrome: A spectrum of conditions responsible for plantar lateral foot pain. *Foot Ankle Int*, 15:112, 1994.
108. Kollias, SL, and Ferkel, RD: Fibular grooving for recurrent peroneal tendon subluxation. *Am J Sports Med*, 25:329, 1997.
109. Karlsson, J, Eriksson, BI, and Sward, L: Recurrent dislocation of the peroneal tendons. *Scand J Med Sci Sports*, 6:242, 1996.
110. Rauh, M, et al: Epidemiology of stress fracture and lower-extremity overuse injury in female recruits. *Med Sci Sports Exer*, 38:1571, 2006.
111. Willems, TM, et al: A prospective study of gait related risk factors for exercise-related lower leg pain. *Gait & Posture*, 23:91, 2006.
112. Edwards, PH, Wright, ML, and Hartman, JF: A practical approach for the differential diagnosis of chronic leg pain in the athlete. *Am J Sports Med*, 33:1241, 2005.
113. Yates, B, and White, S: The incidence and risk factors in the development of medial tibial stress syndrome among naval recruits. *Amer J Sports Med*, 32:772, 2004.
114. Willems, TM, et al: Gait-related risk factors for exercise-related lower-leg pain during shod running. *Med Sci Sports Exer*, 39:339, 2007.
115. Varner, KE, et al: Chronic anterior midtibial stress fractures with athletes treated with reamed intramedullary nailing. *Am J Sport Med*, 35:1071, 2005.
116. Giladi, M, et al: Stress fractures. Identifiable risk factors. *Am J Sports Med*, 19:647, 1991.
117. Saltzman, CL, Nawoczenski, DA, and Talbot, KD: Measurement of the medial longitudinal arch. *Arch Phys Med Rehabil*, 76:45, 1995.
118. Lesho, EP: Can tuning forks replace bone scans for identification of tibial stress fractures? *Mil Med*, 162:802, 1997.
119. Sollsteimer, GT, and Shelton, WR: Acute atraumatic compartment syndrome in an athlete: A case report. *J Athl Train*, 32:248, 1997.
120. Turnipseed, WD, Hurschler, C, and Vanderby, R, Jr: The effects of elevated compartment pressure on tibial arteriovenous flow and relationship of mechanical and biochemical characteristics of fascia to genesis of chronic anterior compartment syndrome. *J Vasc Surg*, 21:810, 1995.
121. Pedowitz, RA, and Gershuni, DH: Diagnosis and treatment of chronic compartment syndrome. *Crit Rev Phys Rehabil Med*, 5:301, 1993.
122. McQueen, MM, Christie, J, and Court-Brown, CM: Acute compartment syndrome in tibial diaphyseal fractures. *J Bone Joint Surg Br*, 78:95, 1996.
123. McQueen, MM, and Court-Brown, CM: Compartment monitoring in tibial fractures: The pressure threshold for decompression. *J Bone Joint Surg Br*, 78:99, 1996.
124. Heckman, MM, et al: Compartment pressure in association with closed tibial fractures. The relationship between tissue pressure, compartment, and the distance from the site of the fracture. *J Bone Joint Surg Am*, 76:1285, 1994.
125. Whitesides, TE, and Heckman, MM: Acute compartment syndrome: Update on diagnosis and treatment. *J Am Acad Orthop Surg*, 4:209, 1996.
126. McQueen, M: Acute anterior compartment syndrome. *Acta Chir Belg*, 98:166, 1998.
127. Chautems, RC, et al: Spontaneous anterior and lateral tibial compartment syndrome in a type I diabetic patient. *J Trauma*, 43:140, 1997.
128. Jerosch, J, et al: Secondary effects of knee braces on the intracompartmental pressure in the anterior tibial compartment. *Acta Orthop Belg*, 61:37, 1995.
129. Jerosch, J, et al: Influence on the running shoe sole on the pressure in the anterior tibial compartment. *Acta Orthop Belg*, 61:190, 1995.
130. Eskelin, MK, Lotjonen, JM, and Mantysaari, MJ: Chronic exertional compartment syndrome: MR imaging at 0.1 T compared with tissue pressure measurement. *Radiology*, 206:333, 1998.
131. Schepis, A, Gill, SS, and Foster, TA: Fasciotomy for exertional anterior compartment syndrome: Is lateral compartment release necessary? *Am J Sports Med*, 27:430, 1999.
132. Riddle, DL, and Wells, PS: Diagnosis of lower-extremity deep vein thrombosis in outpatients. *Phys Ther*. 84:729, 2004.
133. Curl, WW: Popliteal cysts: Historical background and current knowledge. *J Am Acad Orthop Surg*, 4:129, 1996.
134. Urbano, FL: Homans' sign in the diagnosis of deep vein thrombosis. *Hospital Physician*, March:22, 2001.
135. Michelson, J: Controversies in ankle fractures. *Foot and Ankle*, 14:170, 1993.

CHAPTER 10

Knee Pathologies

The knee complex, formed by the tibiofemoral, tibiofibular, and patellofemoral joints, has little bony support and must rely on soft tissue structures to control the forces transmitted through the joints. The tibiofemoral joint is located between the body's two longest lever arms, the femur and tibia; these long lever arms exert extreme forces on ligaments and tendons. For stability the knee relies on static stabilizers rather than dynamic support and is more stable when the extremity is weight-bearing than when it is not.

This chapter discusses injury to the knee and related muscles. The patella, as it relates to the knee joint proper, is described in this chapter. Conditions that are exclusive to the patellofemoral articulation are described in Chapter 11, and injury to the quadriceps and hamstring muscle groups are addressed in Chapter 12. Foot, ankle, hip, and trunk mechanics (and pathomechanics) alter the biomechanical function of the knee. In the case of chronic knee injuries these areas should also be examined.

Clinical Anatomy

The term "tibiofemoral joint" seems to imply that the knee involves only the articulation between the tibia and femur. In fact, the femur, menisci, and tibia all must function together. The patellofemoral mechanism must also function properly to ensure adequate tibiofemoral mechanics. The superior tibiofibular joint, although not a part of the knee articulation, may also impact the knee but is functionally more influenced by the ankle joint.[1]

The length of the **femur**, the longest and strongest bone in the body, is approximately one quarter of the body's total height.[2] The femur's posterior aspect is demarcated by the **linea aspera,** a bony ridge spanning the length of the shaft (Fig. 10-1). As the femur reaches its distal end, the shaft broadens to form the medial and lateral condyles.

The **medial and lateral condyles** are convex structures covered with articular hyaline cartilage that articulate with the tibia via the menisci. These structures have a discrete anteroposterior curvature that is convex in the frontal plane. The articular surface of the medial condyle is longer than that of the lateral condyle and flares outward posteriorly. The condyles share a common anterior surface, then diverge posteriorly, becoming separated by the deep **intercondylar notch**. An anterior depression forms the **femoral trochlea** through which the patella glides as the knee flexes and extends. The lateral and medial epicondyles arise off the condyles. The **lateral epicondyle** is wider and emanates from the femoral shaft at a

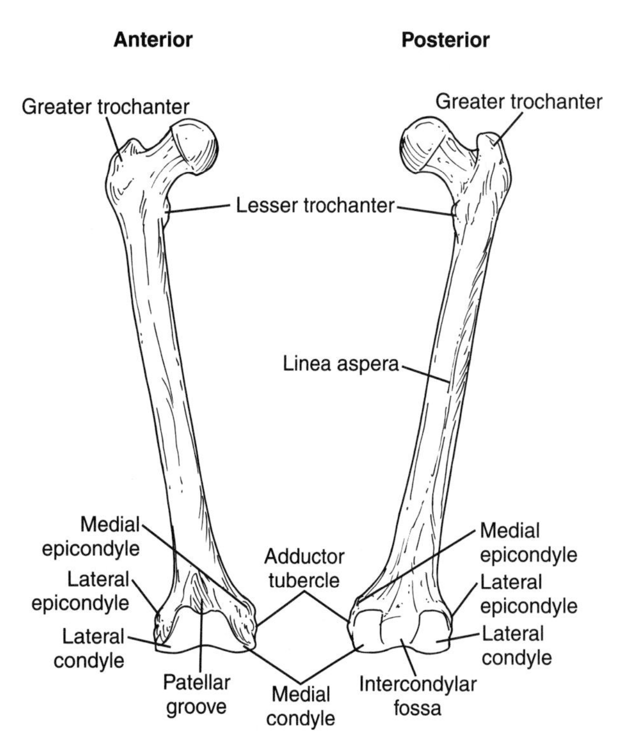

FIGURE 10-1 ■ Anterior and posterior view of the femur. Note that the single anterior articular surface on the condyles of the femur diverges posteriorly to form a lateral and medial compartment of the knee joint.

lesser angle than the **medial epicondyle**. The **adductor tubercle** arises off the superior crest of the medial epicondyle. These prominences serve as attachment sites for tendons to improve the mechanical advantage of the muscle.

The **medial and lateral tibial plateaus** correspond to the femoral condyles. The medial tibial plateau is concave in both the frontal and sagittal planes. The lateral articular plateau is concave in the frontal plane and convex in the sagittal plane. To accommodate for the flare of the femur's medial condyle the medial tibial plateau is 50% larger than the lateral plateau. Intercondylar eminences, raised areas between the tibial plateaus that match the femur's intercondylar notch, separate the two condyles (Fig. 10-2). The **tibial tuberosity**, the site of the patellar tendon's distal attachment, is located on the proximal portion of the anterior tibia.

Two bones outside the tibiofemoral articulation directly affect the knee's function and stability. The **patella**, a sesamoid bone located in the patellar tendon, improves the mechanical function of the quadriceps during knee extension, dissipates the forces received from the **extensor mechanism**, and protects the anterior portion of the knee. Several of the soft tissues on the lateral aspect of the knee attach to the fibular head. Fracture of the proximal fibula or injury to the proximal **tibiofibular syndesmosis** can affect the stability of the knee.

Articulations and Ligamentous Support

The presence of the medial and lateral articular condyles classifies the tibiofemoral joint as a double condyloid articulation, capable of three degrees of freedom: (1) flexion and extension, (2) internal and external rotation, and (3) abduction and adduction.[1] Anterior and posterior translation also occur between the tibia and the femur. The joint may be hypermobile after a sprain or hypomobile secondary to the formation of scar tissue (arthrofibrosis). Hypomobility may occur if a ligament replacement graft is placed too tightly or as the result of scar tissue formation. Hyper- or hypomobility of one or more ligament significantly affects the function of the remaining ligaments.[3]

Joint capsule

A fibrous joint capsule surrounds the circumference of the knee joint. Along the medial, anterior, and lateral aspects of the joint, the capsule arises superior to the femoral condyles and attaches distal to the tibial plateau. Posteriorly, the capsule inserts on the margins of the femoral condyles above the joint line, and inferiorly, to the posterior tibial condyle. Medially, the stability of the joint is reinforced by the medial collateral ligament (MCL), medial patellofemoral ligaments, and medial patellar retinaculum; laterally the joint is augmented by the lateral collateral ligament (LCL), lateral patellar retinaculum, lateral patellofemoral ligament, and iliotibial band; posteriorly by the posterolateral corner (oblique popliteal ligament and arcuate ligaments); and anteriorly by the patellar tendon. Further reinforcement is gained from other tendons that cross the knee joint.

A **synovial capsule** lines the articular portions of the fibrous joint capsule. The synovium surrounds the articular condyles of the femur and tibia medially, anteriorly, and laterally. On the posterior portion of the articulation, the synovial capsule invaginates anteriorly along the femur's intercondylar notch and the tibia's intercondylar eminences, excluding the cruciate ligaments from the synovial membrane (Fig. 10-3). The cruciate ligaments' isolation from the synovial fluid explains their limited healing properties.

Collateral ligaments

The **medial collateral ligament** (MCL) is the primary medial stabilizer of the knee and consists of a deep layer and superficial layer. The **deep layer** is a thickening of the joint capsule and is attached to the medial meniscus. Separated from the deep layer by a bursa, the **superficial layer,**

FIGURE 10-2 ■ Articular structure of the knee. The articulation between the femoral and tibial condyles is enhanced by the menisci. The tubercles of the intercondylar eminence align with the intercondylar notch.

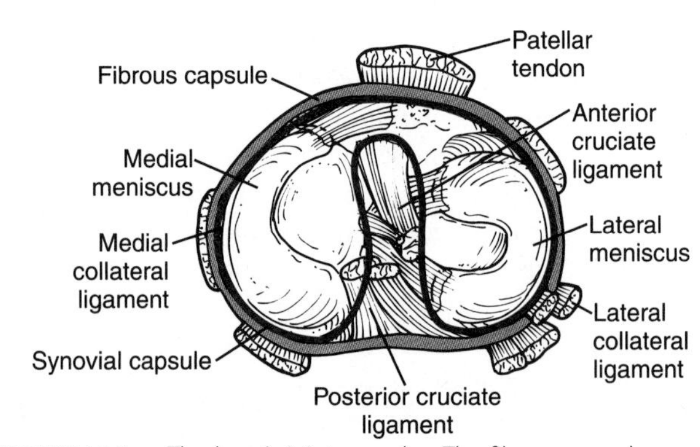

FIGURE 10-3 ■ The knee's joint capsules. The fibrous capsular membrane completely envelops the bony surface of the knee. The synovial capsular membrane surrounds the medial and lateral articular surfaces but excludes the cruciate ligaments.

Extensor mechanism The mechanism formed by the quadriceps and patellofemoral joint responsible for causing extension of the lower leg at the knee joint.

approximately 1.5 cm wide, arises from a broad band just below the adductor tubercle and follows a superoposterior to inferoanterior path across the joint line to deep to the pes anserine tendons (Fig. 10-4).[4] As a unit, the two layers of the MCL are tight in complete extension. As the knee is flexed to the midrange, its anterior fibers are taut; in complete extension, the posterior fibers are tight. The MCL primarily acts to protect the knee against valgus forces while also providing a secondary restraint against external rotation of the tibia and anterior translation of the tibia on the femur, when the anterior cruciate ligament is torn.

Unlike the MCL, the **lateral collateral ligament** (LCL) does not attach to the joint capsule or meniscus.[5] This cordlike structure arises from the lateral femoral epicondyle, sharing a common site of origin with the lateral joint capsule, and inserts on the proximal aspect of the fibular head (Fig. 10-5). The LCL is the primary restraint against varus forces when the knee is in the range between full extension and 30 degrees of flexion. This structure also provides a primary restraint against external tibial rotation and a secondary restraint against internal rotation of the tibia on the femur.[6] The lateral knee system is stronger than the medial structures because it is subjected to increased stress during the initial contact phase of gait when the knee is extended and weight bearing, placing varus forces on the joint.[6]

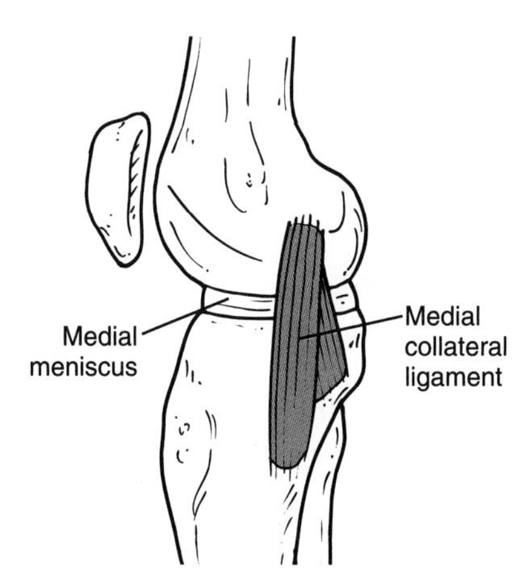

FIGURE 10-4 ■ Medial collateral ligament. Arising from a broad band on the medial femoral epicondyle just below the adductor tubercle, it tapers inward to attach on the medial tibial plateau. Consisting of two layers separated by a bursa, the deep layer is continuous with the medial joint capsule and has an attachment on the medial meniscus.

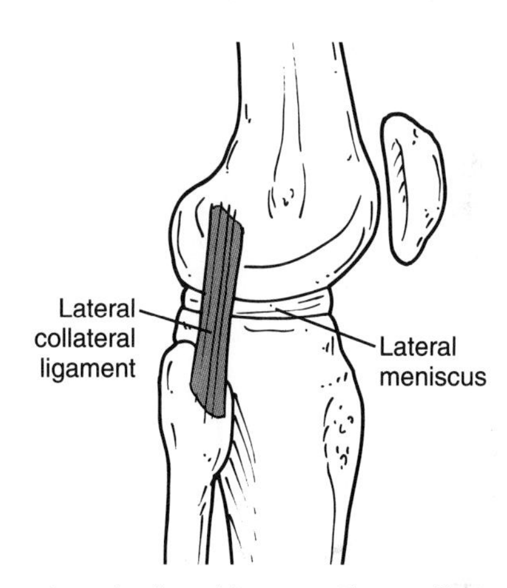

FIGURE 10-5 ■ Lateral collateral ligament. This ropelike structure originates from the lateral femoral epicondyle and attaches to the apex of the fibular head. The lateral collateral ligament is an extracapsular structure.

Cruciate ligaments

The cruciate ligaments, although intraarticular, are located outside of the synovial capsule (see Fig. 10-3). Jointly, the cruciates also help to stabilize the knee against valgus and varus forces.

Anterior cruciate ligament. The **anterior cruciate ligament** (ACL) arises from the anteromedial intercondylar eminence of the tibia, travels posteriorly, and passes lateral to the posterior cruciate ligament (PCL) to insert on the medial wall of the lateral femoral condyle (Fig. 10-6). The ACL serves as a static stabilizer against:

1. Anterior translation of the tibia on the femur
2. Internal rotation of the tibia on the femur
3. External rotation of the tibia on the femur
4. Hyperextension of the tibiofemoral joint

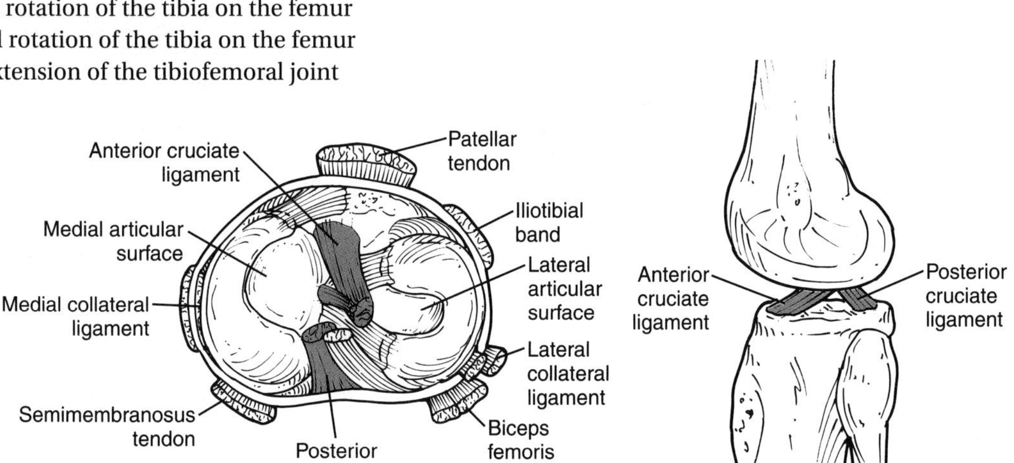

FIGURE 10-6 ■ Cruciate ligaments. The ligaments are named according to their relative attachment on the tibia. **(A)** Superior view referencing the cruciate ligaments to each other and to other supportive structures about the knee. **(B)** Lateral view of the cruciate ligaments.

The ACL has two discrete segments: an **anteromedial bundle** and a **posterolateral bundle** which are named for their attachment site on the tibia.[7] As the knee moves from extension into flexion, a juxtaposition of the ACL's attachment sites occurs. When the knee is fully extended, the femoral attachment of the anteromedial bundle is anterior to the attachment of the posterolateral bundle. When the knee is flexed, the relative positions are reversed, causing the ACL to wind upon itself (Fig. 10-7). This leads to varying portions of the ACL being taut as the knee moves through its range of motion (ROM). When the knee is fully extended, the posterolateral bundle is tight; when the knee is fully flexed, the anteromedial bundle is taut. Because different portions of the ACL are taut at different points in the ROM, the ligament must be stressed in multiple knee positions.

The amount of strain placed on the ACL is influenced by the type of movement and the subsequent translation of the tibia. During passive ROM (PROM), the amount of strain placed on the ACL is minimized when the tibia remains in the neutral position. In the final 15 degrees of extension, internally rotating the tibia greatly increases the strain placed on the ACL; externally rotating the tibia decreases the strain relative to internal rotation, but is still greater than the strain with the tibia in neutral. Both valgus and varus stresses increase the strain on the ACL during PROM (Fig. 10-8).[8] During active open-chain knee extension when the pull of the quadriceps translates the tibia anteriorly the amount of strain placed on the ACL is greatest between 0 and 30 degrees of flexion.[9] Adding resistance, through the arc of knee extension, significantly increases the amount of strain as the knee extends from 45 to 0 degrees of flexion.[9]

Posterior cruciate ligament. The PCL arises from the posterior aspect of the tibia and takes a superior and anterior course, passing medially to the ACL, to attach on the lateral portion of the femur's medial condyle. The PCL, stronger and 120% to 150% wider than the ACL, is a primary stabilizer of the knee.[10–13] The PCL has two distinct components: the **anterolateral** and **posteromedial** bundles, bands named relative to their tibial insertions, although three and four bundles have been described in the PCL.[13,14] As an entire unit, the PCL is the primary restraint against posterior displacement of the tibia on the femur and a secondary restraint against external tibial rotation. The anterolateral bundle is taut when the knee is flexed and loosens when the knee is extended; the posteromedial bundle is relatively lax when the knee is flexed and tightens when the knee extended.[12,13,15] The PCL receives its limited blood supply from the middle geniculate artery.[12]

Although the PCL offers significant support against posterior forces on the knee joint, its function is augmented by the meniscofemoral ligaments (ligaments of Humphrey and Wrisberg) and the posterolateral structures of the knee, specifically the posterolateral corner.[1,16] A combined injury to the PCL and posterolateral structures results in greater posterior laxity than when either structure is affected alone.[17,18] When the knee is near extension, the primary restraint against posterior displacement of the tibia on the femur is obtained from the popliteus, posterior capsule, and other joint structures.[15]

During the **screw home mechanism**, the PCL and ACL wind upon each other in flexion and unwind in extension. Damage to the PCL can result in an inherently unstable

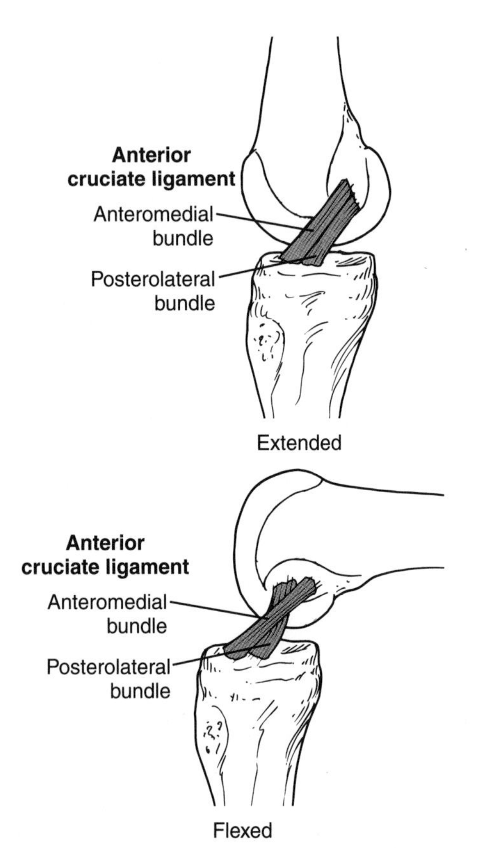

FIGURE 10-7 ■ Biomechanics of the anterior cruciate ligament. When the knee is fully extended, the femoral attachment site of the anteromedial bundle (A) is proximal to the attachment site of the posterolateral bundle (P). When the knee is flexed, these attachment sites juxtapose their positions, causing the anterior cruciate to wind upon itself.

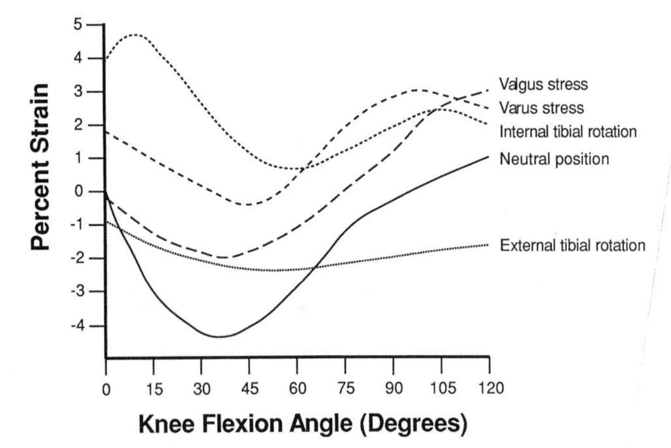

FIGURE 10-8 ■ Strain placed on the anterior cruciate ligament through the passive range of motion. Altering the relative alignment of the tibia to the femur increases the strain on the ligament throughout the range of motion.

knee, not only in the frontal plane but also in the transverse plane because the stable axis of tibial rotation is no longer present.

Posterolateral corner

The posterolateral corner (PLC), also known as the lateral complex and posterolateral complex, has been referred to as "the dark side of the knee" for its varied and relatively poorly understood anatomy (Fig. 10-9).[5,19,20] Consisting of both dynamic and static stabilizers, the PLC is integral in providing stability against varus stress, external tibial rotation, and anterior and posterior forces about the knee. The combined contributions of the anatomical elements of this structure are greater than the sum of the combined parts; the integrity of its individual elements can be disrupted with relatively little joint instability. However, if multiple structures are disrupted profound instability can result (see Posterolateral Rotary Instability, p. 342).[5]

The **popliteofibular ligament** (also referred to as the short external lateral ligament, the popliteofibular fascicles, fibular origin of the popliteus, and the popliteofibular fibers), is a Y-shaped structure with origins from the tibia and fibula, and inserting on the femur, is a key stabilizer against posterior translation, varus forces, and external rotation.[5,6,20–22]

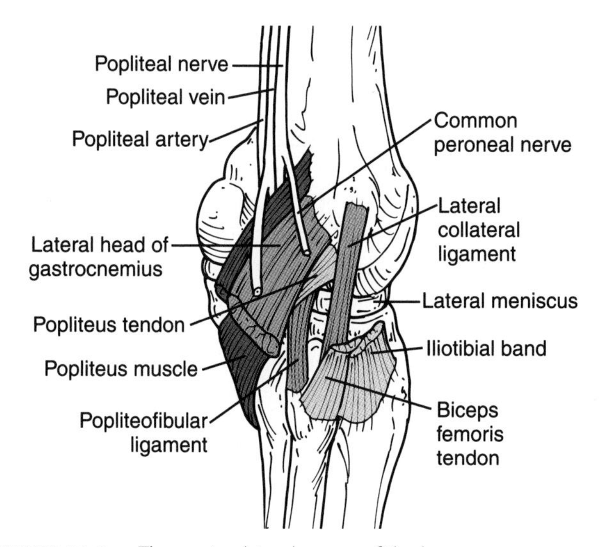

FIGURE 10-9 ■ The posterolateral corner of the knee.

Layers of the Knee's Posterolateral Corner

Layer	Structures
I (Superficial)	Lateral fascia
	Iliotibial band
	Biceps femoris tendon
II (Middle)	Patellar retinaculum
	Patellofemoral ligament
III (Deep)	Joint capsule
	Lateral collateral ligament*
	Arcuate ligament
	Popliteofibular ligament
	Fabellofibular ligament
	Popliteus tendon

*Sometimes grouped into the middle layer.[5]

The **popliteus complex** is formed by the popliteus muscle and its tendon, the popliteofibular ligament, popliteotibial fascicle, and the popliteomeniscal fascicles. The popliteus muscle has attachments to the posterior horn, and middle posterior portions of the lateral meniscus and helps resist external tibial rotation between 20 to 130 degrees of knee flexion.[20] The **arcuate ligament** provides further support to the posterolateral joint capsule.[5] Arising from the fibular head, the arcuate ligament passes over the popliteus muscle, where it diverges into the intercondylar area of the tibia and the posterior aspect of the femur's lateral epicondyle. The arcuate ligament assists the cruciate ligaments in controlling posterolateral rotatory instability. Injury to this area results in increased external rotation of the tibia on the femur.

The **fabella**, when present, lies within the lateral head of the gastrocnemius muscle. Although its actual significance to the structure and function of the knee is unclear, when the fabella is present, a fabellofibular ligament attaches from the fabella to the fibular head, increasing the thickness of the tissues in the posterolateral corner of the knee.[5,20]

Proximal tibiofibular syndesmosis

The proximal tibiofibular syndesmosis, a relatively immobile joint where the proximal tibia and fibula are bound together by ligaments. The proximal syndesmosis is more stable than the distal tibiofibular syndesmosis because of the alignment between the fibular head and the indentation on the proximal tibia. The superior tibiofibular joint is stabilized by the superior anterior and posterior tibiofibular ligaments and, to a lesser degree, by the interosseous membrane. Anterior displacement of the fibula is partially blocked by a bony outcrop from the tibia. Therefore, most fibular instabilities tend to occur posteriorly, possibly affecting the common peroneal nerve because of its proximity to the articulation (Fig. 10-10).

The Menisci

The anatomic differences between the articular surfaces of the tibia and femur is partially resolved by the presence of the fibrocartilaginous medial and lateral menisci. The menisci serve to:

1. Deepen the articulation and fill the gaps that normally occur during the knee's articulation, increasing load transmission over a greater percentage of the joint surfaces
2. Improve lubrication for the articulating surfaces
3. Provide shock absorption
4. Increase passive joint stability
5. Limit the extremes of flexion and extension
6. Serve as proprioceptive organs

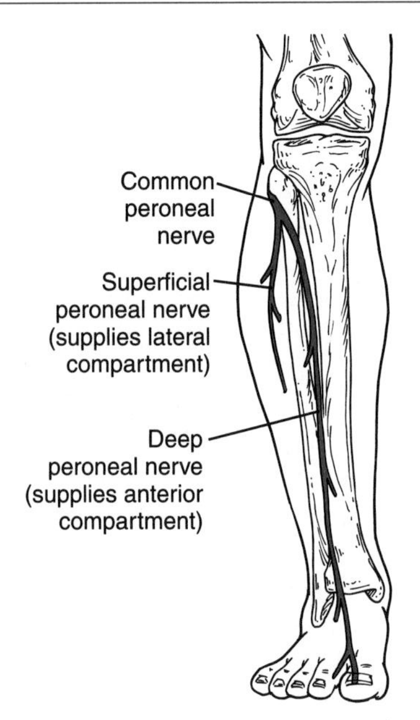

FIGURE 10-10 ■ The common peroneal nerve and its branches.

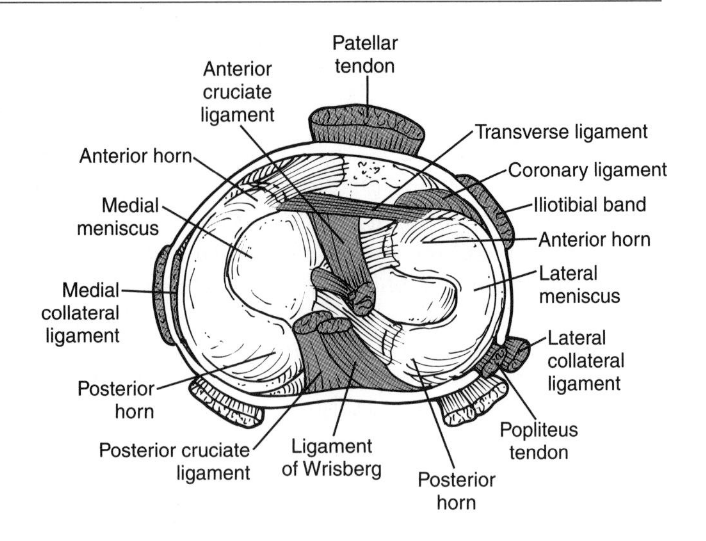

FIGURE 10-11 ■ Superior view of the medial and lateral meniscus and their associated ligamentous structures (right knee shown). The peripheral border of the menisci is fixated to the tibia by the coronary ligament.

When viewed in cross section, the menisci are wedge shaped, with their outer borders thicker than their inner rims. When viewed from above, this wedge creates a concave area on the tibia to accept the femur's articulating surfaces. Because of this geometry, the knee is more stable when it is bearing weight than when it is not.

The entire meniscus is vascularized at birth, but by the age of 9 months the inner third becomes avascular. By the age of 10 years, the menisci reach the vascular profile seen in adulthood.[23] The menisci also become less resistant to stress with aging due to degeneration and dehydration.

Each meniscus is divided into an anterior, middle, and posterior third (Fig. 10-11). The anterior and posterior portions of the menisci are marked by the horns, the area of the menisci most frequently torn. The menisci have a narrow **vascular (red) zone** along their outer rim and the anterior and posterior horns and an **avascular (white) zone** formed by the inner portion of the meniscus. A thin, lightly vascular **pink zone** has been described between the red and white zones. Approximately 10% to 25% of the outer portion of the lateral meniscus and 10% to 30% of the medial meniscus is vascularized.[23] Because of the presence of an active blood supply via the medial, lateral, and middle geniculate arteries, meniscal tears occurring within the vascular zone have an improved chance of healing compared to tears in the avascular zone, which rely on nutrients being delivered through the synovial fluid. These zones cannot be differentiated via standard or contrast imaging techniques and must be visually identified during surgery.[24]

The central portion of the meniscus is relatively denervated, but the anterior and posterior horns do contain sensory nerves that provide proprioceptive feedback during the extremes of flexion (posterior horns) and extension (anterior horns).[23] Meniscal lesions become painful when the adjacent and richly innervated joint capsule becomes irritated or distended by edema.

The **medial meniscus** resembles a half crescent, or C shape, that is wider posteriorly than it is anteriorly. The **lateral meniscus** is more circular in shape, but the size, thickness, shape, and mobility are different than those of the medial meniscus.[25] Both menisci are attached at their peripheries to the tibia via the **coronary ligament**. The **anterior horns** of each meniscus are joined by the **transverse ligament** and connected to the patellar tendon via **patellomeniscal ligaments**.

The lateral meniscus, smaller and more mobile than the medial meniscus, attaches to the lateral aspect of the medial femoral condyle via the **meniscofemoral ligaments** (the **ligament of Wrisberg** and the **ligament of Humphrey**) and to the popliteus muscle via the joint capsule and coronary ligament. Attaching the **posterior horn** of the lateral meniscus to the femur, the orientation of the meniscofemoral ligaments mimics that of the PCL.[1]

During knee extension, patellomeniscal ligaments pull the lateral meniscus anteriorly, distorting its shape in the anteroposterior plane. In the early degrees of flexion, the popliteus pulls the lateral meniscus posteriorly; in the later ROM, the meniscofemoral ligament pulls the posterior horn medially and anteriorly.[26] During passive flexion the menisci are displaced posteriorly and laterally, with the anterior horn moving more than the posterior horn, with maximum displacement occurring at 90 degrees of flexion.[27] Because of its relative lack of mobility and its attachment to the MCL, the medial meniscus tends to be injured from acute trauma while the lateral meniscus tends to suffer degenerative tears.

Muscles Acting on the Knee

The muscles acting on the knee primarily serve to flex or extend it. The flexor musculature has the secondary responsibility of rotating the tibia. The flexors attaching on the tibia's medial side internally rotate it, and those attaching on the lateral side externally rotate it. The muscles acting on the knee, their origins, insertions, and innervation are presented in Table 10-1.

Anterior muscles

The **quadriceps femoris** muscle group consists of four muscles, the **vastus lateralis**, **vastus intermedius**, **vastus medialis**, and **rectus femoris**. Each of the quadriceps femoris muscles has a common insertion on the tibial tuberosity via the patellar tendon (Fig. 10-12). The vastus medialis has two discrete groups of fibers arising from the medial femoral condyle and the fascia of the adductor magnus. Separated by a fascial plane, the muscle is divided into the vastus medialis longus and the vastus medialis oblique (VMO). As a group, the quadriceps femoris extends the knee. The rectus femoris, a two-joint muscle, also serves as a hip flexor, especially when the knee is flexed. During knee extension, the VMO guides the patella medially.

Posterior muscles

The **semitendinosus**, **semimembranosus**, and **biceps femoris** are collectively known as the **hamstring muscle group**. They act as a unit to flex the knee and extend the hip (Fig. 10-13). With attachments to the iliotibial band, Gerdy's tubercle, the LCL, and posterolateral capsule, the biceps femoris serves to rotate the tibia externally and help protect the knee against varus stresses.[6] The semimembranosus and semitendinosus act to internally rotate the tibia. Because its function is redundant with the semimembranosus, the semitendinosis is a good candidate as a graft source for ACL reconstruction. The hamstring muscles also decrease the shear forces that stress the ACL when the knee is flexed beyond 20 degrees.[28,29]

The posterolateral corner of the knee is reinforced by the **popliteus** muscle which provides both dynamic and static stabilization to the knee, resisting posterior tibial translation, static external tibial rotation, dynamic internal tibial rotation, and buffers against varus forces (see Fig. 10-6).[6] In an open kinetic chain, the popliteus causes internal rotation of the tibia on the femur; in a closed kinetic chain, the popliteus externally rotates the femur on the tibia. Responsible for unscrewing the knee from its locked position in extension, its remaining influence on knee flexion is slight. However, when the patient is bearing weight with the knee partially flexed, the popliteus assists the PCL in preventing posterior displacement of the tibia on the femur. Because of the close association between the popliteus muscle and the other structures in the posterolateral corner of the knee, trauma to this muscle will weaken the entire complex.[6]

A diamond-shaped **popliteal fossa** is formed by the leg's posterior musculature (Fig. 10-14). Although its inner boundaries are largely devoid of muscles (with the exception of the popliteus), the popliteal fossa contains the popliteal artery and vein; the tibial, common peroneal, and posterior femoral cutaneous nerve; and the small saphenous vein.

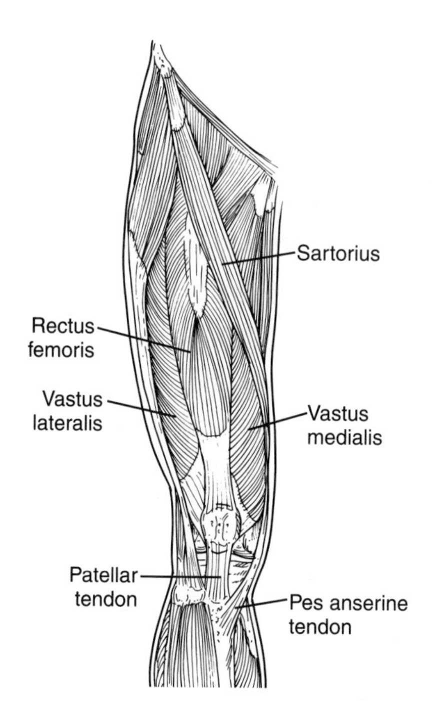

FIGURE 10-12 ■ Anterior muscles acting on the knee. The vastus lateralis, rectus femoris, vastus intermedius (hidden beneath the rectus femoris), and vastus medialis share a common insertion via the patellar tendon.

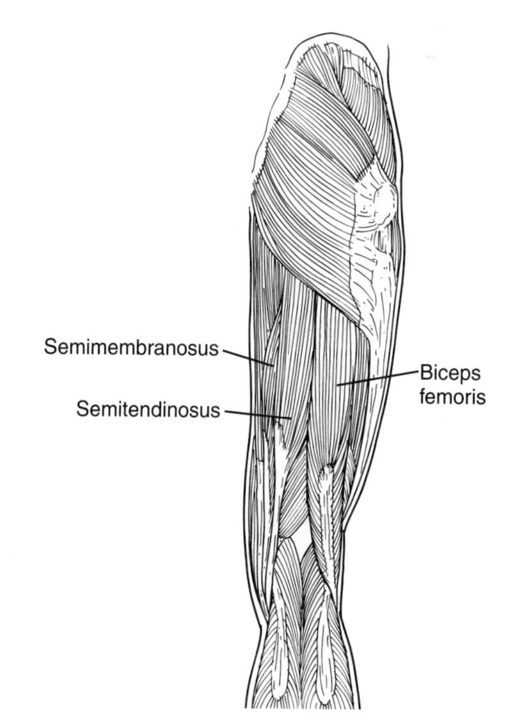

FIGURE 10-13 ■ Posterior muscles acting on the knee. In addition to flexing the joint, the biceps femoris externally rotates the tibia while the semimembranosus and semitendinosus internally rotate it.

Table 10-1 Muscles Acting on the Knee

Muscle	Action	Origin	Insertion	Innervation	Root
Biceps Femoris	Knee flexion External tibial rotation Long head • Hip extension • Hip external rotation	Long head • Ischial tuberosity • Sacrotuberous ligament Short head • Lateral lip of the linea aspera • Upper two-thirds of the supracondylar line	Lateral fibular head Lateral tibial condyle	Long head • Tibial Short head • Common peroneal	Long head S1, S2, S3 Short head L5, S1, S2
Gastrocnemius	Assists knee flexion Ankle plantarflexion	Medial head • Posterior surface of the medial femoral condyle • Adjacent portion of the femur and knee capsule Lateral head • Posterior surface of the lateral femoral condyle • Adjacent portion of the femur and knee capsule	To the calcaneus via the Achilles tendon	Tibial	S1, S2
Gracilis	Knee flexion Internal tibial rotation Hip adduction	Symphysis pubis Inferior ramus of the pubic bone	Proximal portion of the antero-medial tibial flare	Obturator (posterior)	L3, L4
Popliteus	Open chain • Internal tibial rotation • Knee flexion *Closed chain* External femoral rotation Knee flexion	Lateral femoral condyle Oblique popliteal ligament	Posterior tibia superior to the soleal line Fascia covering the soleus	Tibial	L4, L5, S1
Rectus Femoris	Knee extension Hip flexion	Anterior inferior iliac spine Groove located superior to the acetabulum	To the tibial tubercle via the patella and patellar ligament	Femoral	L2, L3, L4
Sartorius	Knee flexion Internal tibial rotation Hip flexion Hip abduction Hip external rotation	Anterior superior iliac spine	Proximal portion of the antero-medial tibial flare	Femoral	L2, L3

Semimembranosus	Knee flexion Internal tibial rotation Hip extension Hip internal rotation	Ischial tuberosity	Posteromedial portion of the tibia's medial condyle	Tibial	L5, S1
Semitendinosus	Knee flexion Internal tibial rotation Hip extension Hip internal rotation	Ischial tuberosity	Medial portion of the tibial flare	Tibial	L5, S1, S2
Vastus Intermedius	Knee extension	Anterolateral portion of the upper two-thirds of the femur Lower one-half of the linea aspera	To the tibial tubercle via the patella and patellar ligament	Femoral	L2, L3, L4
Vastus Lateralis	Knee extension	Proximal interochanteric line Greater trochanter Gluteal tuberosity Upper one-half of the linea aspera	To the tibial tubercle via the patella and patellar ligament	Femoral	L2, L3, L4
Vastus Medialis	Knee extension Oblique portion • Patellar stabilization	Longus portion • Distal one-half of the intertrochanteric line • Medial portion of the linea aspera Oblique portion • Tendons from adductor longus and adductor magnus	To the tibial tubercle via the patella and patellar ligament	Femoral	L2, L3, L4

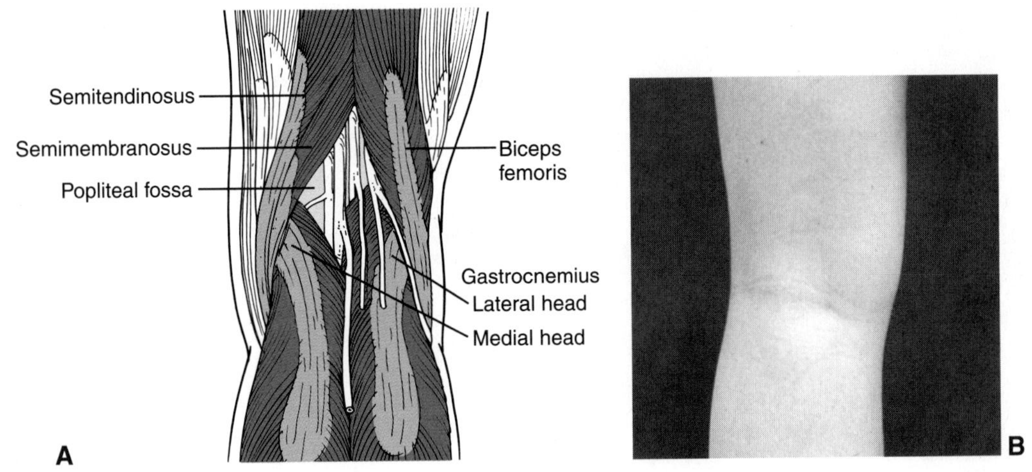

FIGURE 10-14 ■ Popliteal fossa of the right knee. **(A)** Anatomical reference and **(B)** surface anatomy.

Pes anserine muscle group

The **gracilis, sartorius**, and **semitendinosus** muscles form the pes anserine muscle group. In addition to flexing the knee, the pes anserine group internally rotates the tibia when the foot is not planted on the ground. When the foot is planted, the pes anserine externally rotates the femur on a fixed tibia.

The gracilis and semitendinosus muscles are relatively straightforward in their anatomic orientation. However, the sartorius muscle is an unusual one. Although its belly is located on the anterior aspect of the femur, it is a flexor of the knee joint because the sartorius muscle crosses the knee posterior to its axis (see Fig. 10-12). With an origin proximal and anterior to the hip joint, the sartorius muscle also assists in flexion, external rotation, and abduction of the hip.

Iliotibial band

The **iliotibial band** (IT band) is an extension of the **tensor fasciae latae** (a small muscle originating from the **anterior superior iliac** crest) and gluteus maximus muscular fascia. The IT band travels down the lateral aspect of the femur to on **Gerdy's tubercle** on the anterolateral tibia and attaches to the lateral patellar retinaculum and the biceps femoris tendon through divergent slips.[30] Although the tensor fasciae latae and IT band make a relatively insignificant contribution to knee motion, the deep fibers of the IT band attach to the lateral joint capsule and function as an anterolateral knee ligament, playing a significant role in knee stability and patellofemoral pathology.[6,31]

The angle between the IT band and tibia varies according to the relative position of the leg, which, in turn, alters the knee's biomechanics. When the knee is fully extended, the IT band is anterior to or, located over, the lateral femoral epicondyle. When the knee is flexed beyond 30 degrees, the IT band shifts behind the lateral femoral epicondyle, giving it an angle of pull as if it were a knee flexor, exerting an external rotation and posterior force on the tibia (Fig. 10-15). This posterior shift is greatly influenced by the biceps femoris, which has a fibrous expanse attaching to the IT band. During contraction of the biceps femoris, the IT band is drawn posteriorly.

The screw home mechanism

The unequal sizes of the femoral condyles and the tightening of the cruciate ligaments as they wind upon themselves during flexion necessitates a locking mechanism as the knee nears its final degrees of extension.[32] As the knee is extended to its terminal range, the lateral meniscus serves as a pivot point. The medial femoral condyle has a larger surface area than the lateral condyle. As the knee extends, the articular distance on the lateral femoral condyle is expended, and the medial articulation continues to glide, resulting in external rotation of the tibia with the lateral meniscus serving as the pivot point.

During extension of a non–weight-bearing knee, complete motion is achieved by the tibia externally rotating 5 to 7 degrees on the femur. However, when bearing weight, the

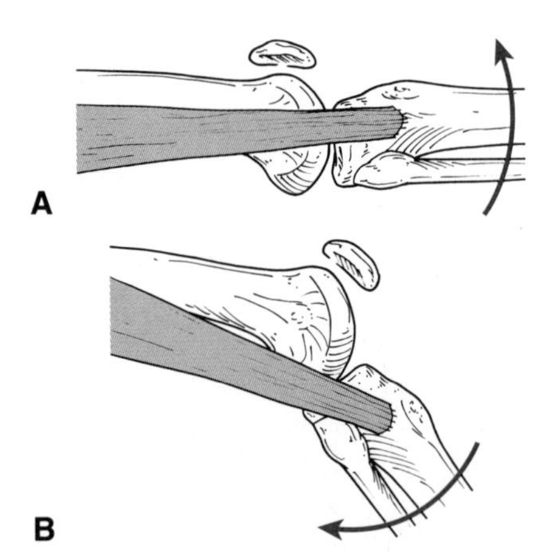

FIGURE 10-15 ■ The iliotibial band's dynamic line of pull in flexion and extension. **(A)** When the knee is fully extended, the iliotibial band's angle of pull is that of a knee extensor. **(B)** When it is flexed past 30°, it assumes an angle of flexor.

tibia is relatively fixed so the terminal ROM is accomplished by a combination of the tibial external rotation and femoral internal rotation. To initiate flexion, the knee must be unlocked by the tibia internally rotating relative to the femur. When not bearing weight, this is accomplished by the popliteus muscle; when bearing weight, unlocking occurs by contraction of the popliteus, semimembranosus, and semitendinosus muscles.

Neurologic Anatomy

The primary neurologic and vascular structures serving the knee and points distal pass through the popliteal fossa. The knee is supplied primarily by the L3, L4, L5, S1, and S2 nerve roots. The knee is innervated by the anterior cutaneous branches of the femoral nerve and the infrapatellar branch of the saphenous nerve anteriorly, the saphenous nerve medially, the posterior cutaneous branches of the cluneal nerve posteriorly, and the sural cutaneous nerve (via the common peroneal nerve) laterally.

Vascular Anatomy

The popliteal artery and vein are separated from the posterior capsule by a layer of adipose tissue. Within the popliteal fossa the popliteal artery sprouts five geniculate arteries (two superior, two inferior, and middle). The geniculate arteries provide collateral circulation to the knee.[33] The anterior tibial artery and lateral femoral circumflex artery provide further blood supply to the anterior and lateral portions of the knee.

Because of the intimacy of the neurovascular structures to the knee joint proper, damage to these structures must be ruled out in the presence of a tibiofemoral dislocation. The popliteal artery is attached to the adductor hiatus proximal and to the soleus muscle distal to the knee joint line, making it particularly prone to trauma.[33]

Clinical Examination of Knee Injuries

The patient is evaluated while wearing shorts to permit inspection and palpation of the muscles originating off the femur and pelvis. The patella is described in this section only as it relates to tibiofemoral function. The examination of patellofemoral conditions is presented in Chapter 12.

History

Blows to the knee place compressive forces on the joint structures at the point of the blow, tensile forces on the side opposite the blow, and shear forces across the joint. Rotatory forces about the knee, such as those experienced when an athlete cuts to change direction, place tensile forces about the joint capsule and cruciate ligaments. The menisci may also be torn by this mechanism secondary to impingement and shearing between the articular condyles. The need for radiographs of the knee to rule out fracture can be determined using the **Ottawa Knee Rules** (see Chapter 11).

Past Medical History

- **Past history of injury:** A past history of injury for both the involved and uninvolved knee must be established. Previous injury can result in chronic inflammation secondary to internal derangement or biomechanical dysfunction. Nonsurgical ligament and capsule sprains may have healed with a great deal of scar tissue, restricting the ROM, or with excess laxity, both of which predispose the knee to reinjury. Surgical conditions involving grafts or **primary repairs** are also subject to reinjury.
- **Injury to related body areas:** Advancing age contributes to the risk of injury, especially to articular cartilage as it becomes less hydrated and has fewer strengthening collagenous cross links. Previous injury to the low back, lower leg, foot and/or ankle may alter mechanics at the knee, inviting pathological changes. Consider the gait adapted by the individual with a sprained ankle. This type of sustained ankle plantarflexion during ambulation places the knee in a prolonged flexed position, altering compressive forces.
- **General medical conditions:** For conditions of chronic or insidious onset, determine if the patient has a history of systemic or local inflammatory diseases such as osteoarthritis, rheumatoid arthritis, or gout.[34] Knee osteoarthritis is a common source of knee pain in post-college aged individuals (see Chapter 4).

*** Practical Evidence**

Aging itself puts certain tissues at the knee at risk. Articular cartilage reaches its maximum tensile strength between the ages of 20 and 30, and its strength dramatically declines with increasing age, making it more susceptible to shearing injury with rotational forces.[35]

History of the Present Condition

- **Location of pain:** Tears of the collateral ligaments or the anteromedial or anterolateral capsule normally result in pain directly corresponding to the area of trauma. Pain arising from the ACL may be described as being "beneath the kneecap" or "inside the knee," and pain from the PCL may mimic that caused by a strain of the medial or lateral origin of the gastrocnemius. Tears to the vascular zone of the menisci can present with joint line pain. Tears in the avascular zone may be described as pain or, more commonly, as popping, clicking, or locking within the knee. Posterior knee

Primary repair The process of surgically repairing a soft tissue injury, usually by suturing the ends together.

Examination Map

HISTORY

Past Medical History

History of the Present Condition

Mechanism of Injury

INSPECTION

Functional Assessment

Girth Measurements

Inspection of the Anterior Structures

Patella

Patellar tendon

Quadriceps muscle group

Tibiofemoral alignment

Tibial tuberosity

Inspection of the Medial Structures

General medial aspect

Vastus medialis

Inspection of the Lateral Structures

General lateral structure

Fibular head

Posterior sag of tibia

Hyperextension

Inspection of the Posterior Structures

Hamstring muscle group

Popliteal fossa
- Baker's cyst

PALPATION

Palpation of the Anterior Structures

Patella

Patellar tendon

Tibial tuberosity

Quadriceps tendon

Quadriceps muscle group
- Vastus medialis
- Rectus femoris
- Vastus lateralis

Sartorius

Palpation of the Medial Structures

Medial meniscus and joint line

Medial collateral ligament

Medial femoral condyle and epicondyle

Medial tibial plateau

Pes anserine tendon and bursa

Semitendinosus

Gracilis

Palpation of the Lateral Structures

Joint line

Fibular head

Lateral collateral ligament

Popliteus

Biceps femoris

Iliotibial band

Palpation of the Posterior Structures

Popliteal fossa

Hamstring muscle group
- Biceps femoris
- Semimembranosus
- Semitendinosus

Determination of Intracapsular versus Extracapsular Swelling

JOINT AND MUSCLE FUNCTION ASSESSMENT

Goniometry

Flexion

Extension

Active Range of Motion

Flexion

Extension

Manual Muscle Tests

Quadriceps

Hamstrings

Sartorius

Passive Range of Motion

Flexion

Extension

JOINT STABILITY TESTS

Stress Testing

Anterior instability
- Anterior drawer test
- Lachman's test
- Prone Lachman's test

Posterior instability
- Posterior drawer test
- Godfrey's test

Medial instability
- Valgus stress test: 0° flexion
- Valgus stress test: 25° flexion

Lateral instability
- Valgus stress test: 0° flexion
- Valgus stress test: 25° flexion

Joint Play Assessment

Proximal tibiofibular syndesmosis

NEUROLOGIC EXAMINATION

Lower Quarter Screen

Common Peroneal Nerve

VASCULAR EXAMINATION

Distal Capillary Refill

Distal Pulse

Posterior tibial artery

Dorsal pedal artery

PATHOLOGIES AND SPECIAL TESTS

Uniplanar Knee Sprains

Medial collateral ligament
- Valgus stress test

Lateral collateral ligament
- Varus stress test

Anterior cruciate ligament
- Anterior drawer test
- Lachman's test
- Prone Lachman's test
- Quadriceps active test

Rotational Knee Instabilities

Anterolateral rotatory instability
- Pivot shift test
- Jerk test
- Slocum drawer test
- Crossover test
- Slocum ALRI test
- Flexion–rotation drawer test

Anteromedial rotatory instability
- Slocum drawer test
- Crossover test
- Lachman's test
- Valgus stress test

Posterolateral rotatory instability
- External rotation (dial) test
- External rotation recurvatum test
- Posterolateral drawer test
- Reverse-pivot shift
- Dynamic posterior shift test

Meniscal Tears

McMurray's test

Apley's compression/distraction test

Thessaly test

Osteochondral Lesions

Wilson's test

Iliotibial Band Friction Syndrome

Nobel compression test

Ober's test

Popliteus Tendinopathy

Tibiofemoral Joint Dislocations

Table 10-2 Possible Pathology Based on the Location of Pain

	Location of Pain			
	Lateral	**Anterior**	**Medial**	**Posterior**
Soft Tissue	LCL sprain Lateral joint capsule sprain Superior tibiofibular syndesmosis sprain Lateral patellar retinaculum irritation* Biceps femoris strain Biceps femoris tendinopathy Popliteal tendinopathy IT band friction syndrome Lateral meniscus tear	ACL sprain (emanating from "inside" the knee) Patellar tendinopathy* Patellar tendon rupture (partial or complete)* Patellar bursitis* Patellofemoral joint dysfunction* Quadriceps contusion Fat pad irritation* Quadriceps tendon rupture*	MCL sprain Medial joint capsule sprain Medial patellar retinaculum irritation* Pes anserine bursitis or tendinopathy Semitendinosus strain Semitendinosus tendinopathy Semimembranosus strain Semimembranosus tendinopathy Medial meniscus tear	PCL sprain Posterior capsule sprain Gastrocnemius strain Hamstring strain Popliteus tendinopathy Popliteal cyst Medial/lateral meniscal tear (posterior horn)
Bony	Fibular head fracture Osteochondral fracture Osteochondritis dissecans Lateral femoral condyle contusion Lateral tibial plateau Contusion Epiphyseal fracture in pediatric patients	Patellar fracture Tibial plateau fracture Sinding-Johansen-Larsen disease* Osgood-Schlatter disease (in adolescents)* Patellar dislocation or subluxation* Chondromalacia	Osteochondral fracture Osteochondritis dissecans Medial femoral condyle contusion Medial tibial plateau Contusion	

*Discussed in Chapter 11.
ACL = anterior cruciate ligament; IT = iliotibial; LCL = lateral collateral ligament; MCL = medial collateral ligament; PCL = posterior cruciate ligament.

pain can represent a PCL tear or popliteal (Baker's) cyst (Table 10-2).[34]

- **Mechanism of injury:** Forces delivered to the knee in the frontal or sagittal plane when the knee is extended have less of a rotational component than blows received at an angle or when the knee is flexed. Forces delivered in a straight planar motion usually result in more isolated injuries to the ligamentous tissues. Rotational stresses may more commonly injure multiple ligamentous and meniscal tissues. A description of an acute, non–contact-related onset most likely reflects a rotational stress that was placed on the knee, as occurs when a person changes directions while running or pivoting (Table 10-3).
- **Weight-bearing status at the time of injury:** Rotational injuries may further be identified by establishing the weight-bearing status of the involved limb. A foot that was planted at the time of injury fixates the tibia, allowing the femur to rotate on it. This effect is magnified by certain types of shoe wear such as cleats.
- **Associated sounds or sensations:** Determine the sensations and any associated sounds (e.g., "pop" or "snap") experienced at the time of the injury. After ruling out a patellar dislocation, subluxation, or fracture, these sounds may indicate a tear of one of the cruciate ligaments.[36] Patients often report the knee "giving way." With true giving way, the knee buckles during weight bearing, likely indicating a meniscal injury or ligamentous instability. The sensation of giving way without actual buckling is usually related to pain, quadriceps weakness or inhibition, or patellofemoral joint disease.

True locking, the inability to fully extend the knee, indicates an unstable meniscal tear, subluxation of the posterior horn of the meniscus,[37] or loose body such as an osteochondral fragment within the joint that wedges between the femur and tibia, locking the joint. Patients may report catching or crepitation as locking. These symptoms often more accurately indicate patellofemoral joint disease.

- **Onset of injury:** Ligamentous injuries most often present with an acute onset related to a specific episode. Injuries having an insidious onset are most likely to involve inflammation of the muscles and tendons acting

Table 10-3 Mechanism of Knee Injuries and the Resultant Soft Tissue Damage

Force Placed on the Knee	Tensile Forces	Compressive Forces
Valgus	Medial structures: MCL, medial joint capsule, pes anserine muscle group, medial meniscus	Lateral meniscus
Varus	Lateral structures: LCL, lateral joint capsule, IT band, biceps femoris	Medial meniscus
Anterior Tibial Displacement	ACL, IT band, LCL, MCL medial and lateral joint capsules	Posterior portion of the medial and lateral meniscus
Posterior Tibial Displacement	PCL, meniscofemoral ligament(s), popliteus, medial and lateral joint capsules	Anterior portion of the medial and lateral meniscus
Internal Tibial Rotation	ACL, anterolateral joint capsule posteromedial joint capsule, posterolateral joint capsule, LCL	Anterior horn of the medial meniscus Posterior horn of the lateral meniscus
External Tibial Rotation	Posterolateral joint capsule, anteromedial joint capsule, MCL, PCL, LCL, ACL	Anterior horn of the lateral meniscus Posterior horn of the lateral meniscus
Hyperextension	ACL, posterior joint capsule, PCL	Anterior portion of the medial and lateral meniscus
Hyperflexion	ACL, PCL	Posterior portion of the medial and lateral meniscus

ACL = anterior cruciate ligament; IT = iliotibial; LCL = lateral collateral ligament; MCL = medial collateral ligament; PCL = posterior cruciate ligament.

on the knee, may be the result of patellar maltracking, or may represent degenerative changes within the knee. As with chronic foot and ankle injuries, chronic knee pain may arise secondary to training errors, foot type, shoe type, postural deviations, hip pathology, and foot biomechanics. Meniscal injuries may be acute or have an insidious onset, as is often the case with the lateral meniscus.

Inspection

As much of the inspection process as possible is performed while the patient is weight bearing. Any observations of an antalgic gait or other gait deviations are also noted. Following a capsular or ligamentous knee injury there is a natural inclination to maintain the knee in the resting position of 30 degrees of flexion, shortening the stance phase of gait, and minimizing stresses on the involved structures. Shortening of the stride length is also indicative of functional shortening of the hamstrings.

Functional assessment

The patient is observed while performing those tasks that are problematic to start the process of identifying the impairments that accompany these functional limitations. With knee sprains and resulting joint instability, the patient may display and describe apprehension and/or decreased speed with tasks requiring abrupt change of direction. Osteoarthritis symptoms may be associated with any weight-bearing activity. Limitations in knee motions may manifest themselves in tasks such as going upstairs. A limitation in knee flexion may manifest itself in difficulty going up stairs. The results of this task analysis are then used during the remainder of the examination process to determine the underlying impairments.

Girth measurements

Chronic conditions or ongoing reevaluations of existing conditions must include a determination of the amount of fluid in and around the knee joint and atrophy of the quadriceps muscle groups. To be objective, these measurements must be made in a consistent and reproducible manner (Special Test 10-1). Following disuse secondary to trauma, including surgery, the volume of the quadriceps muscles significantly reduces relative to the uninvolved limb, but this decrease is not typically seen in the hamstring or adductor muscles. Within the quadriceps group, all muscles tend to atrophy at the same rate, but the vastus medialis and rectus femoris lose slightly more volume.[38] Note that the muscles of the dominant thigh may naturally be hypertrophied relative to the nondominant thigh and measurements are more accurate in lean individuals, especially when performed by the same examiner.[39,40]

Inspection of the anterior structures

- **Patella:** Observe the patella, normally found resting above the femoral trochlea, evenly aligned with the medial and lateral aspects of the knee. Shifting of the patella away from its central position on the trochlea may indicate **patellar malalignment or dislocation**. Patellar dislocations normally occur laterally. A unilaterally high-riding patella, when accompanied by

Special Test 10-1
Girth Measurements

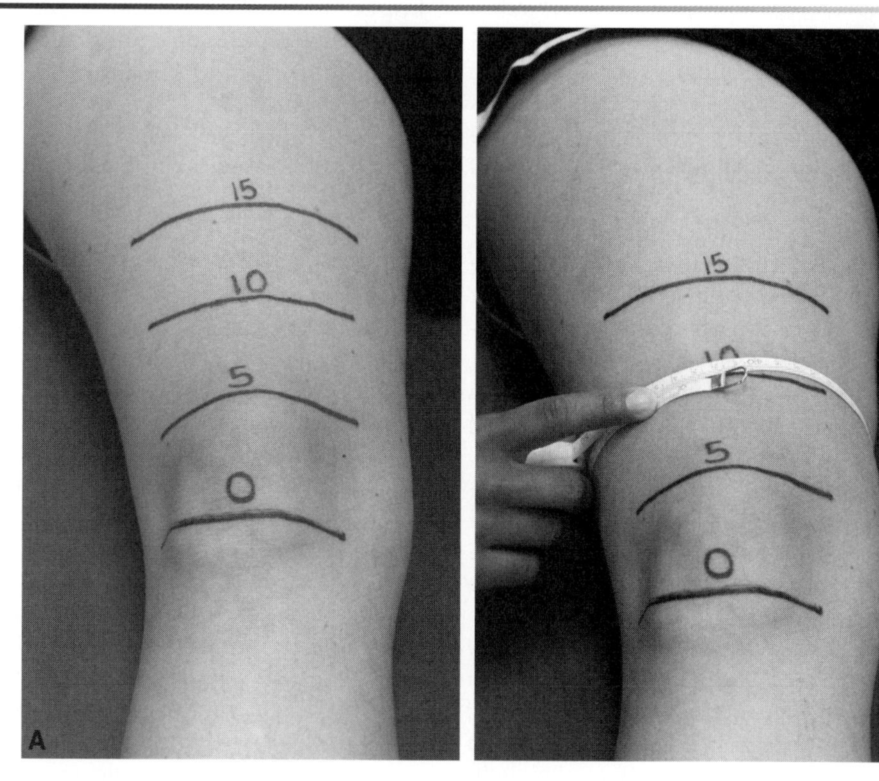

The girth about the knee is determined by identifying the joint line (0 mark) and measuring above and below the joint line. Measurements are made around the joint line and then at consistent intervals up the quadriceps group.

Patient Position	Supine or standing (the patient should be in the same position each time a measurement is taken)
Position of Examiner	Standing next to the patient
Evaluative Procedure	The joint line is identified and measured at the 0-inch mark. Measurements are taken at 5-, 10-, and 15-cm intervals above the joint line. Measurements are taken at 15 cm below the joint line.
Positive Test	A difference of ±1 cm compared bilaterally
Implications	Increased girth on the injured side across the joint line: Edema Decreased muscular girth on the injured side: Atrophy
Modification	The measurement increments can be increased for taller individuals and decreased for shorter people.
Comments	Standardization of the measurements is required for accurate results (e.g., the patient in the same position, same landmarks). The muscular girth of the dominant leg may be naturally hypertrophied relative to the nondominant leg. In the case of migrating edema, ankle and calf girth measurements should also be taken. There is only a slight to moderate relationship between strength and girth in the overall population.
Evidence	Intra-rater correlation: Not Reliable — Very Reliable Poor / Moderate / Good 0 0.1 0.2 0.3 0.4 0.5 0.6 0.7 0.8 0.9 1.0 Inter-rater correlation: Not Reliable — Very Reliable Poor / Moderate / Good 0 0.1 0.2 0.3 0.4 0.5 0.6 0.7 0.8 0.9 1.0

spasm of the quadriceps muscle group, indicates a **ruptured patellar tendon** (see Chapter 11). The actual tendon defect may be obliterated by swelling.

- Normally there are concave depressions on both sides of the patella when the patient is supine and the knee extended. A loss of these depressions is indicative of intra-articular effusion.[34]
- **Patellar tendon:** Note any swelling over or directly around the patellar tendon, possibly indicating tendinopathy or bursitis. Swelling on both sides that masks the definition of the tendon may indicate inflammation of the underlying fat pad.
- **Quadriceps muscle group:** Compare the mass and tone of the quadriceps muscle groups bilaterally and confirm any apparent deficits through girth measurements. Note any discoloration, swelling, or loss of continuity within the quadriceps group.
- **Alignment of the femur on the tibia:** Observe the angle at which the medial tibia and femur articulate (do not confuse this with the Q-angle). The normal angle ranges from 180 to 185 degrees on the line formed by the lateral aspect of the knee. An angle of greater than 185 degrees is termed **genu valgum** ("knock knees"); an angle less than 175 degrees is termed **genu varum** ("bowlegs") (Inspection Findings 10-1). In older individuals, varus deformity may be associated with osteoarthritis of the medial articulating surfaces and a valgus alignment can suggest osteoarthritis of the lateral articulating surfaces.[34]
- **Tibial tuberosity:** Look for possible enlargement of the tibial tuberosity. In adolescent patients, enlargement could indicate Osgood-Schlatter's disease (see Chapter 7). A history of this condition may result in residual enlargement of the tibial tuberosity into adulthood, but it is not typically implicated in future pathology (Fig. 10-16).

Inspection of the medial structures

- **Medial aspect:** Inspect the medial aspect of the knee joint, noting any swelling or discoloration along the tibia, knee joint line, femur, or pes anserine tendon.
- **Vastus medialis**: Observe the vastus medialis with particular attention to the oblique fibers. The VMO should display normal muscle tone and girth compared with that of the opposite limb. This muscle group is the first to atrophy after a knee injury, possibly as the result of disuse or an increase of intracapsular fluid that inhibits its normal function.[41]

Inspection of the lateral structures

- **Lateral aspect:** Inspect the lateral aspect of the tibia, joint line, and femur for swelling or discoloration.
- **Fibular head:** Note the head of the fibula, normally aligned at an equal height compared with the opposite side. With the knee flexed, the biceps femoris tendon and LCL may be visible. Swelling around the fibular head may encroach on the common peroneal nerve.
- **Posterior sag of the tibia:** With the patient lying supine and the knees flexed to 90 degrees, observe the relative positions of the tibia. In PCL-deficient knees, the tibia on the involved side drops or "sags" posteriorly (Fig. 10-17). The influence of gravity is increased by flexing the patient's hips to 90 degrees (Godfrey's test). A straightedge placed along the patella and the anterior aspect of the tibia helps to bilaterally compare the amount of sagging. If the involved tibial tuberosity sits in a more lateral position than on the uninvolved side, damage to the posterolateral corner may be present.
- **Hyperextension:** View the standing patient from the side. Hyperextension, or **genu recurvatum,** is indicated by the posterior bowing of the knee (see Inspection Findings 10-1). Acquired genu recurvatum, especially

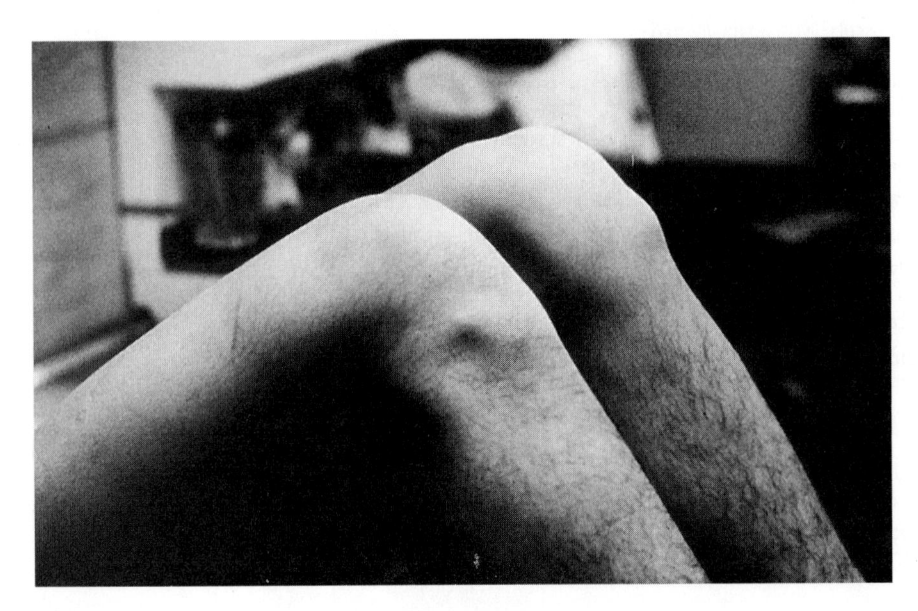

FIGURE 10-16 ■ Residual enlargement of the tibial tuberosity caused by Osgood–Schlatter disease in youth.

Inspection Findings 10-1
Tibiofemoral Alignment

	Normal	Genu Valgum	Genu Varum	Genu Recurvatum
	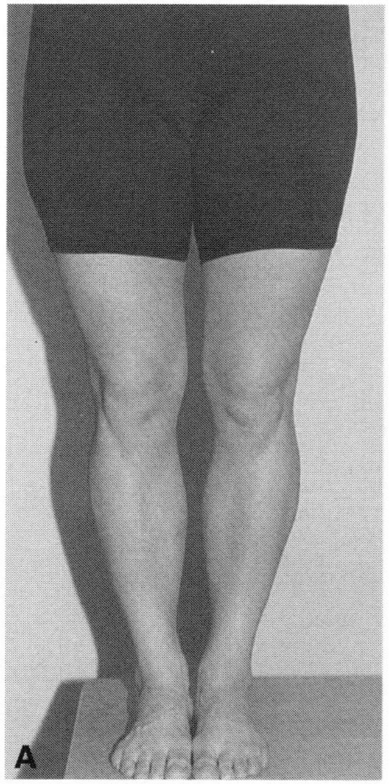 A	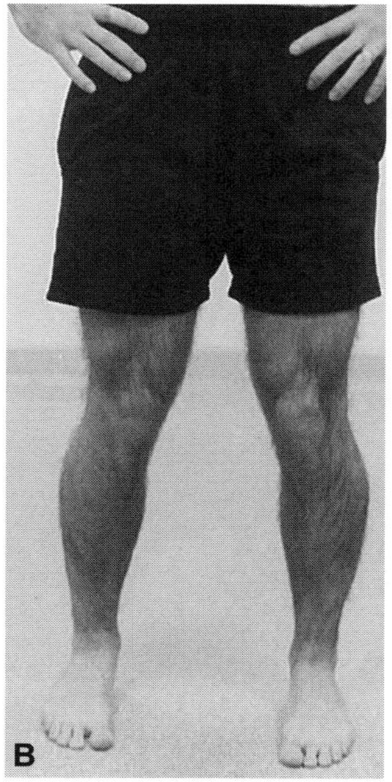 B	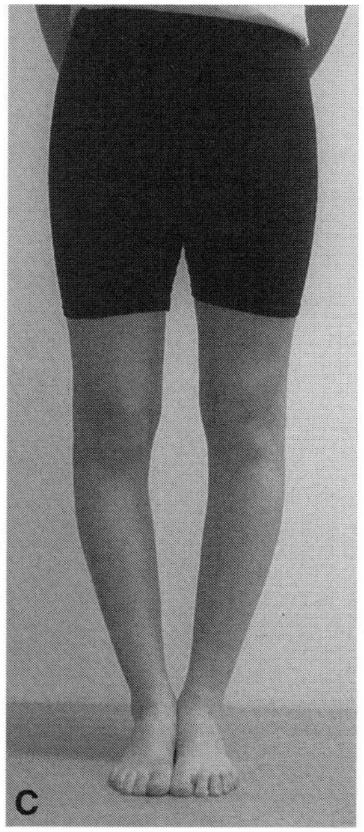 C	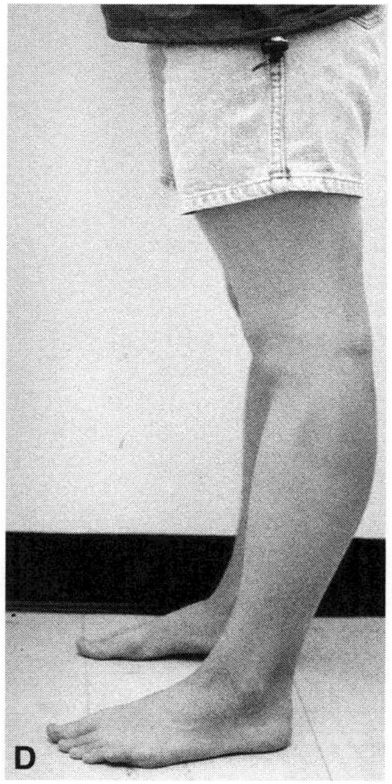 D
Description		Tibia is angled medially more than 5° relative to the femur	Tibia is angled laterally more than 5° relative to the femur	Tibiofemoral extension greater than 0°
Potential Causes		Degeneration of the lateral meniscus Structural or acquired hip abnormalities Excessive foot pronation	Degeneration of the medial meniscus Structural or acquired hip abnormalities Excessive foot supination	Rupture of the ACL or PCL
Consequences		Increased compressive forces on the lateral joint structures Increased tensile forces on the medial joint structures Increased foot pronation Internal tibial rotation Medial patellar position Internal femoral rotation	Increased tensile forces on the lateral joint structures Increased compressive forces on the medial joint structures Increased foot supination External tibial rotation Lateral patellar position External femoral rotation	Increased strain on the ACL and/or PCL Increased contact pressure between the patella and femur

ACL = anterior cruciate ligament; PCL = posterior cruciate ligament.

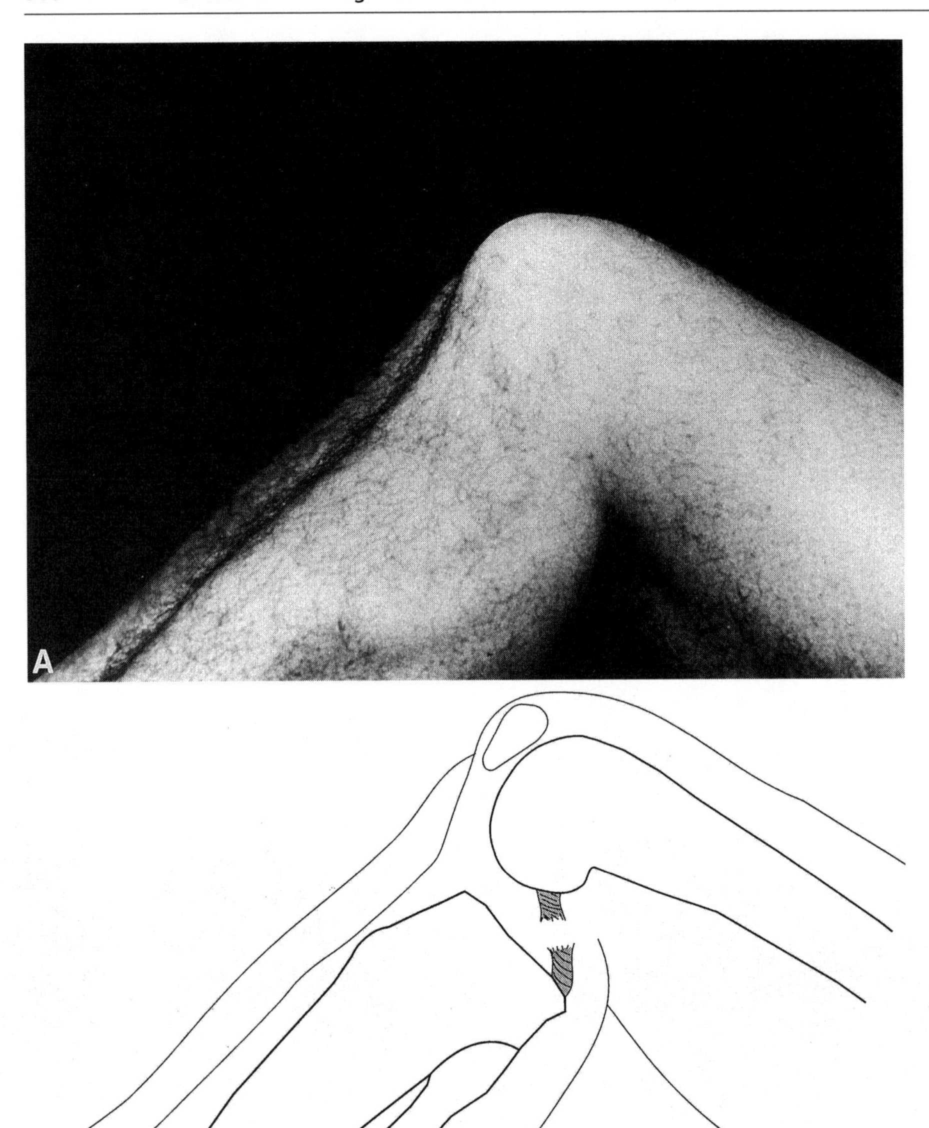

FIGURE 10-17 ■ (A) Posterior tibial sag indicating posterior cruciate ligament deficiency. Note the downward displacement of the tibia. (B) Illustration showing the posterior displacement of the tibia that is caused by tearing of the posterior cruciate ligament (the anterior cruciate ligament has been removed for clarity).

when occurring unilaterally, can indicate an ACL sprain or PCL sprain.

Inspection of the posterior structures

- **Hamstring muscle group:** Observe the length of the hamstring group for signs of a contusion, such as ecchymosis and edema. This signs may also be associated with strains, which are described in Chapter 8.
- **Popliteal fossa:** Inspect the popliteal fossa for signs of swelling or discoloration that can indicate capsular trauma, tears of the distal hamstring tendon or the heads of the gastrocnemius muscle, or a cyst.

Medially the bursae associated with the semimembranosus tendon and the medial head of the gastrocnemius may be interconnected to the synovial lining of the knee. The structure of this junction allows fluids to flow from the joint capsule into the bursa, but not in the reverse direction forming a **Baker's cyst.**[42] By definition, Baker's cysts involve only the bursa of the semimembranosus and medial head of the gastrocnemius. Other cysts may form in the popliteal fossa, often involving the popliteus muscle. Popliteal cysts may not be grossly visible and could require magnetic resonance imaging (MRI) for positive identification.

The cyst itself is often not the cause of a patient's problem but is more indicative of pathology within the knee itself. Popliteal cysts tend to develop in the presence of osteoarthritis, meniscal tears (in particular the posterior horn of the medial meniscus), ligament sprains, or other conditions that produce synovitis in the joint capsule.[42,43] Patients may describe these cysts as "coming and going," a cycle explained by the relative amount of knee effusion, resulting in aching in the fossa and may report "fullness" in the knee during flexion and extension. When the cyst extends into the triceps surae muscles (the gastrocnemius and soleus), the signs and symptoms may mimic that of phlebitis (pseudothrombophlebitis).[42,44]

PALPATION

Palpation is performed to confirm the findings of the inspection portion of the evaluation process and further identify traumatized tissues, although many of the most often injured tissues cannot be palpated. The knee should be palpated in 90 degrees of flexion when possible.[34]

Palpation of the Anterior Structures

1 Patella: Begin palpating the patella at its superior patellar pole where the quadriceps muscle group inserts, noting for areas of point tenderness. Progress centrally down the patella to reach the inferior pole and the origin of the patellar tendon. Return to the starting point on the superior pole by palpating up the medial and lateral patellar borders. In the adolescent, pain at the inferior border may be associated with Sindig–Larson–Johanson disease (see Chapter 11).

With the knee extended and the quadriceps relaxed, palpate the patella to ensure its proper alignment in the femoral trochlea and its freedom of movement. A dislocated patella can occur with or without the patellar tendon rupturing. A rigid, displaced patella accompanied by the inability or unwillingness to extend the knee indicates a patellar dislocation.

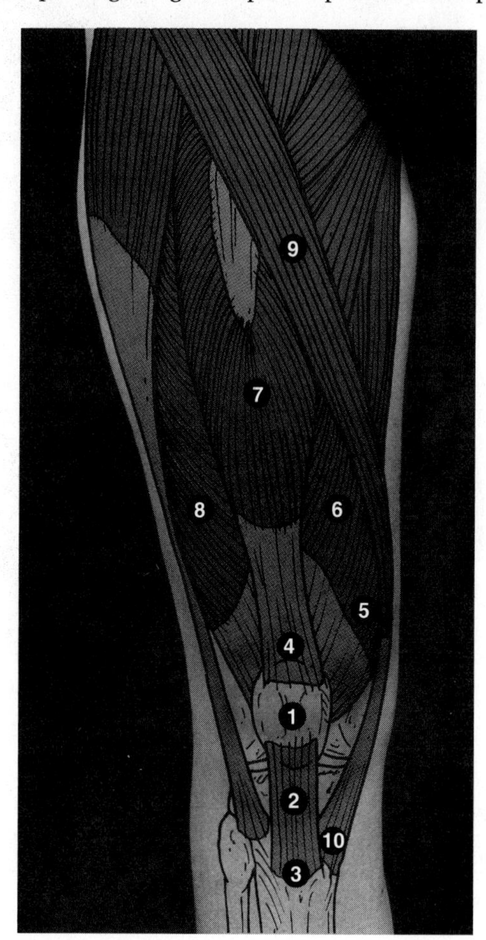

2 Patellar tendon: Palpate the length of the patellar tendon from its insertion at the tibial tuberosity to the inferior aspect of the patella. The patellar tendon normally feels broad and ropelike. A chronic tendinopathy often results in palpable nodules within the mass of the tendon. The tendon can also be palpated while the patient performs active ROM of the knee, noting any crepitus indicating patellar tendinopathy.

3 Tibial tuberosity: Palpate the patellar tendon's attachment site on the tibia. The tibial tuberosity is normally a smooth, rounded protrusion. With adolescent patients, sensitivity and roughness of the tuberosity indicate an inflammation of the tibial tuberosity's growth center, **Osgood–Schlatter** disease. Pain in mature patients may be caused by a contusion or inflammation.

4 Quadriceps tendon: From the superior aspect of the patella, palpate the quadriceps tendon as it attaches across the length of the patella's superior pole. Note that the suprapatellar pouch of the joint capsule and the suprapatellar fat pad lie deep to the quadriceps tendon. Fluids tend to accumulate because of the large capsular redundancy.

5–8 Quadriceps muscle group: Palpate the oblique fibers of the vastus medialis **(5),** the length of the vastus medialis **(6),** the rectus femoris **(7),** and the vastus lateralis muscles **(8)** (the vastus intermedius is not directly palpable), searching for point tenderness, defect, or spasm.

9–10 Sartorius: Palpate the **(9)** sartorius muscle from its origin on the anterior superior iliac spine (ASIS) to its insertion as a part of the pes anserine tendon **(10).**

Palpation of the Medial Structures

1 Medial meniscus and joint line: Place the knee in at least 45 degrees of flexion to locate the joint lines. Palpate on either side of the proximal aspect of the patellar tendon until the indentation formed by the femur and tibia is located. Palpate medially and posteriorly along the joint line, noting any crepitus or pain that may indicate possible meniscal, ligamentous, or capsular trauma. Externally rotating the tibia makes the border of the medial meniscus more palpable.

2 Medial collateral ligament: Many sprains of the MCL occur at the origin or insertion of the ligament. Palpate the length of the MCL from its origin on the medial femoral condyle, just below the adductor tubercle, progressing inferiorly to its insertion on the medial tibial flare that can be located up to 7 cm distal to the joint line. The medial portion of the joint line is covered by the MCL. Note the close relationship between the tendons of the pes anserine group and the MCL.

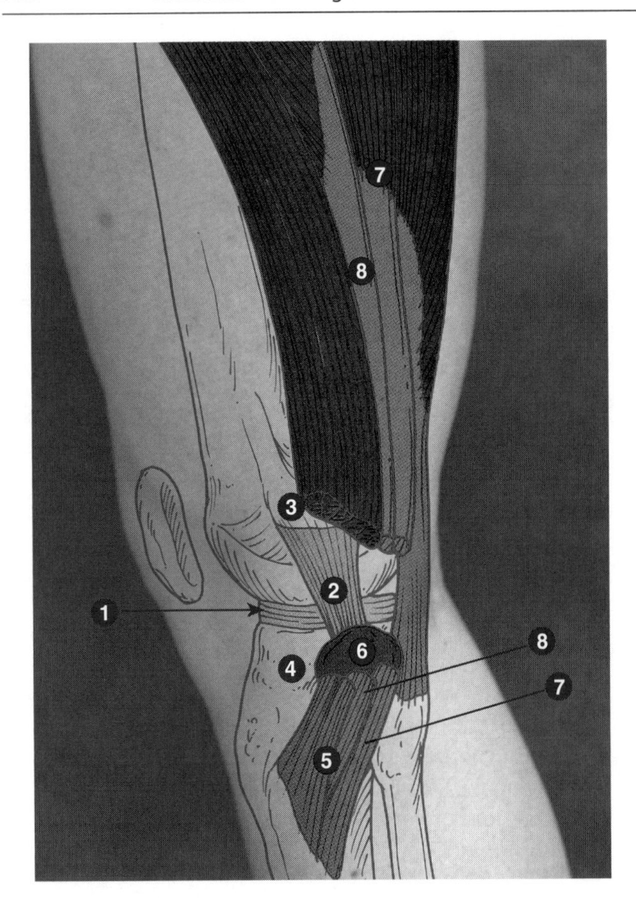

3 **Medial femoral condyle and epicondyle:** Flex the knee beyond 90 degrees to better expose the articulating surface of the condyle immediately above the anteromedial joint line. The adductor tubercle, the attachment site for the adductor longus, projects off of the medial femoral condyle. Injuries with rotational or loading type mechanisms may cause bone bruising or osteochondral fracture, causing pain in the condyles.

4 **Medial tibial plateau:** Locate the medial tibial plateau inferior to the joint line. After palpating along its length, proceed inferiorly to locate the medial tibial flare, a structural necessity to disperse compressive forces at the articulation.

5 **Pes anserine tendon and bursa:** Locate the medial tibial flare, the common site of attachment for the gracilis, sartorius, and semitendinosus muscles. Palpate the common insertion of these tendons located just medial to the tibial tuberosity. These structures and the overlying pes anserine bursa may become inflamed because of direct blows or overuse. The pes anserine bursa may be more easily identified midway between the tibial tuberosity and the anterior aspect of the medial joint line if the tibia is slightly internally rotated.[34]

6 **Semitendinosus tendon:** From the pes anserine attachment, palpate the semitendinosus tendon, the most medial tendon of the hamstring group, to its muscular belly.

7 **Gracilis:** Palpate the thin, ropelike gracilis, located immediately anterior to the semitendinosus tendon, from its insertion to the point that it is lost in the mass of the adductor group.

Palpation of the Lateral Structures

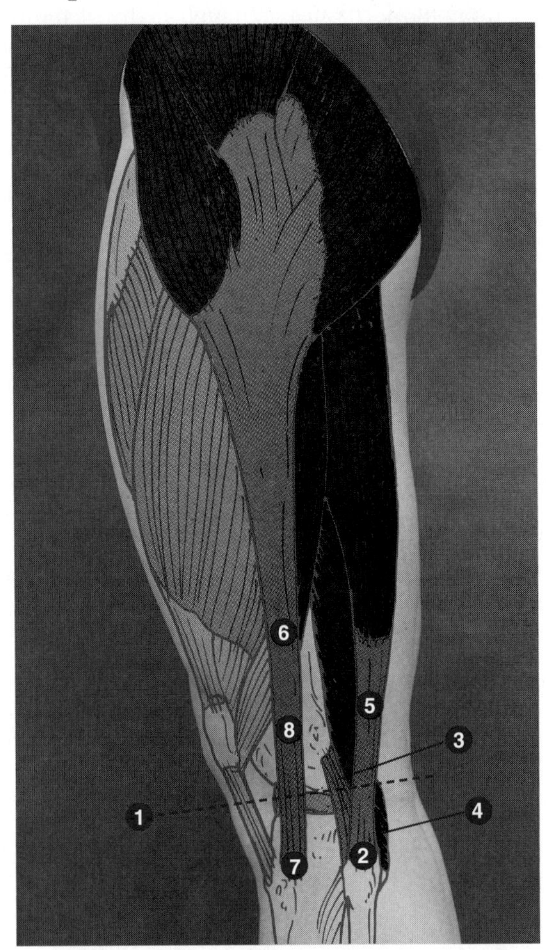

1 **Joint line:** Position the knee in at least 45 degrees of flexion to locate the anterolateral joint line. Begin palpating the joint line lateral to the patellar tendon and progress posteriorly. Pain along the joint line may indicate meniscal pathology. Internally rotating the tibia makes the lateral meniscus more palpable.

2 **Fibular head:** Locate the fibular head below and slightly posterior to the lateral joint line. Two ropelike structures may be felt arising from the fibular head. The LCL projects off its superior portion; slightly posterior to this structure is the insertion of the biceps femoris tendon.

3 **Lateral collateral ligament:** Place the knee in 90 degrees of flexion and externally rotate and abduct the hip (i.e., cross the ankle of the involved leg over the opposite leg) to make the LCL more identifiable. Because it is a separate structure from the joint capsule, the LCL is easily identified as it arises from the fibular head and courses to the lateral femoral condyle.

4 **Popliteus:** Palpate a small portion of the anterior popliteus tendon, posterior to the LCL just above the joint line. Provide slight resistance to knee flexion to make the tendon more prominent.

5 **Biceps femoris:** Flex the knee to 25 degrees and ask the patient to externally rotate the lower leg to make the biceps tendon easily palpable (note that as the tendon crosses the joint line, it may become confused with the IT band). The biceps femoris tendon inserts on the fibular head, posterior to the insertion of the LCL. Continue palpating the biceps femoris tendon to its muscular belly.

6 **Iliotibial band:** Palpate the IT band located anterior to the biceps femoris tendon at its insertion on Gerdy's tubercle **(7)** just lateral to the tibial tuberosity. The IT band becomes more identifiable during resisted flexion past 30 degrees. Palpate the IT band upward to the tensor fasciae latae, noting any increased sensitivity, especially as it passes over the lateral femoral condyle, possibly indicating iliotibial band friction syndrome.

Palpation of the Posterior Structures

1 **Popliteal fossa:** Trauma to this area or edema within this space can occlude neurovascular structures, resulting in referred pain, inhibition of nerve transmission, or disruption of blood flow to or from the lower leg, possibly mimicking the signs and symptoms of thrombophlebitis.[42,43]

With the patient prone, palpate the popliteal fossa for the presence of a cyst, most commonly found on the medial part of the fossa under the medial head of the gastrocnemius and semimembranosus tendon (Baker's cyst). The cyst is usually more prominent during palpation with the knee extended. The cyst may feel firm with the knee extended and soft when the knee is flexed, **Foucher's sign.**[42] Cysts may also be found laterally and are associated with the popliteus tendon (see Inspection of the Posterior Structures, p. 306).

2–5 **Hamstring muscle group:** Palpate the length of the biceps femoris **(2)** on the lateral aspect of the knee and the semimembranosus **(3)** and semitendinosus **(4)** muscles on the medial side of the knee to their common origin on the ischial tuberosity **(5)** noting for point tenderness, spasm, or defect.

6–7 Heads of the gastrocnemius: Palpate the lateral **(6)** and medial heads **(7)** of the gastrocnemius muscle.

8 Popliteal artery: Palpate the pulse associated with this artery. This pulse is most notable in the inferior portion of the popliteal fossa with the knee flexed.

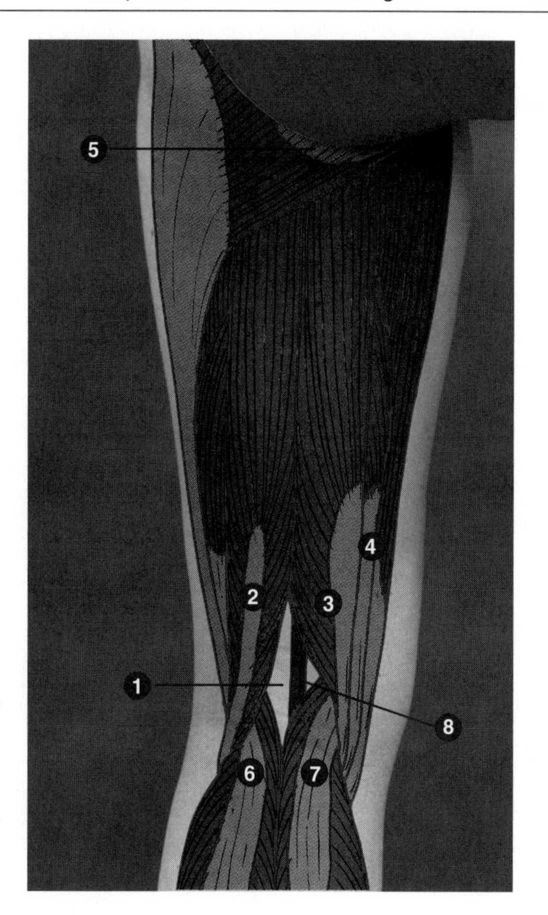

Determination of Intracapsular versus Extracapsular Swelling

Pathology to the knee can result in the formation of swelling within the joint capsule (effusion) or outside of the capsule (extracapsular swelling/edema). The onset of swelling provides important insight to the nature of the underlying condition. The rapid onset of effusion suggests a tear of one of the knee's major ligaments or a fracture of the knee's articular surface. More slowly forming edema is indicative of a meniscal tear, inflammatory conditions, or a less significant ligamentous sprain.[34]

Joint effusion is identified by the ability to manually move ("milk") the fluid from one side of the knee to the other via the **Sweep test** (Special Test 10-2). An effusion can cause the patella to "float" over the femoral trochlea as indicated by the **ballotable patella test** (Special Test 10-3). Localized edema tends to represent extra-articular swelling.[34]

Joint effusion is caused by two different mechanisms. Acute injuries leading to effusion usually indicate a sprained ACL or capsule possibly resulting from the dislocation of the patella, a fractured tibial plateau, or an osteochondral fracture. If aspirated, the fluid would most likely be dark red because of bleeding from these

Special Test 10-2
Sweep Test for Intracapsular Swelling/Effusion

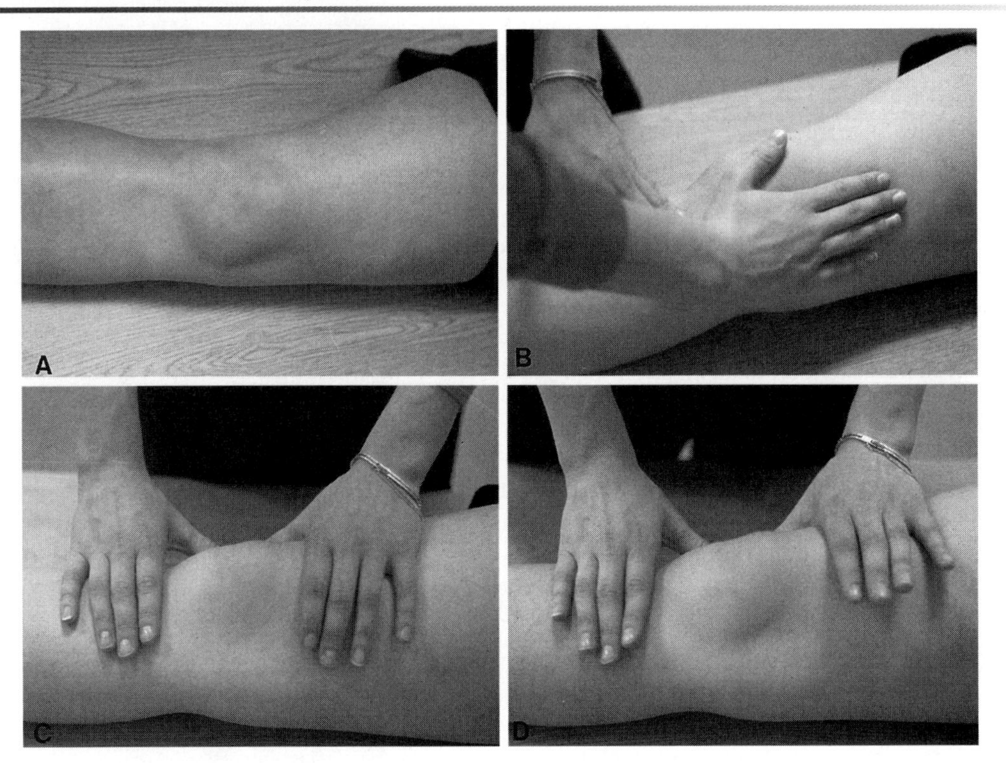

Sweep test to determine the presence of intracapsular swelling.

Patient Position	Lying supine with the knee extended
Position of Examiner	Standing lateral to the patient
Evaluative Procedure	Assuming that the fluid is on the medial side of the knee **(A)**: **(B)** The edema is stroked ("milked") proximally and laterally. **(C)** The normal contour of the knee is restored. **(D)** When pressure is applied on the lateral aspect of the knee, a fluid bulge immediately appears on the medial aspect.
Positive Test	Reformation of edema on the medial side of the knee when pressure is applied to the lateral aspect
Implications	Swelling within the joint capsule, indicating possible anterior cruciate ligament trauma, osteochondral fracture, synovitis, meniscal lesion, or patellar dislocation
Modification	If swelling is more prevalent on the lateral aspect of the knee, the steps are performed on the lateral side of the knee joint.
Evidence	Inconclusive or absent in the literature

structures (**hemarthrosis**). In chronic conditions, knee joint effusion is caused by the inflammatory response producing excess synovial fluid such as in arthritic knees, a mensical tear in the avascular zone, or with chondromalacia patella and yields a clear and straw-colored fluid. If the joint were infected the fluid would be cloudy.

Hemarthrosis Blood within a joint cavity.

*** Practical Evidence**

The rapid onset of effusion, indicating a hemarthrosis, is strongly associated with an ACL sprain, a patellar dislocation, or an osteochondral fracture.[45]

Special Test 10-3
Ballotable Patella

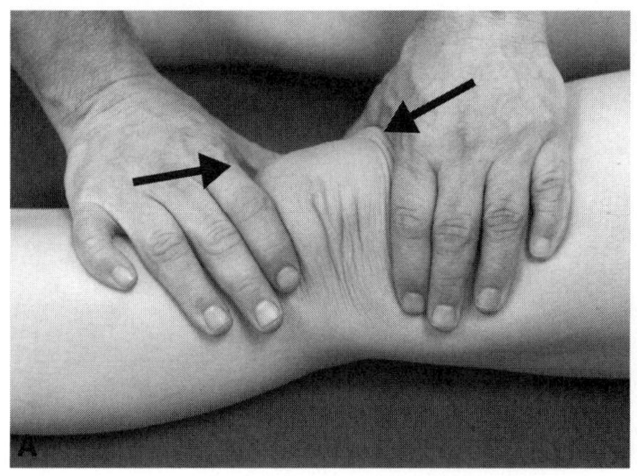

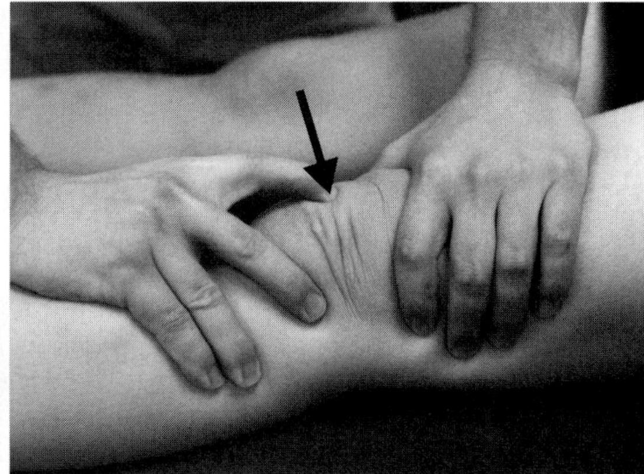

Excess fluid is manually moved inferior to the patella. In the presence of knee effusion, the patella will "float" over the femoral trochlea when the knee is extended.

Patient Position	Supine The knee is extended and the quadriceps are relaxed.
Position of Examiner	Standing to the side being tested
Evaluative Procedure	**(A)** The superior hand pushes any fluid in the superior portion of the knee inferiorly toward the patella. The opposite hand pushes any fluid in the inferior portion of the knee superiorly toward the patella. **(B)** A finger is used to press the patella down towards the patellar groove.
Positive Test	The patella fails to "bounce back" after being depressed.
Implications	Effusion within the joint capsule
Comments	Knee effusions, especially those of rapid onset, are associated with fractures or cruciate ligament sprains.
Evidence	Inconclusive or absent in the literature

Extracapsular edema is often caused by inflammation of the soft tissues surrounding the joint, possibly indicating inflamed bursae or a contusion. Venous insufficiencies may affect the knee in addition to the entire lower extremity, causing the build-up of edema.

Joint and Muscle Function Assessment

The only voluntary movements available at the knee joint are flexion and extension and tibial internal and external rotation. The motions of flexion and extension are easily measured and quantified, but tibial rotation is less accurately measured. The use of a goniometer to measure knee flexion and extension is described in Goniometry Box 10-1. Loss of knee extension can occur following ACL surgery and flexion may be lost following PCL reconstruction.[46] Extension loss may be the result of scar tissue formation in the anterior intercondylar notch ("Cyclops lesion"), fibrous nodules creating a mechanical block, or capsulitis. Focal capsulitis may take the form of a synovial plica (see Chapter 7), contusion, or MCL or LCL sprain. Diffuse capsulitis is a more general reaction to trauma and may lead to arthrofibrosis, extra-articular scarring that restricts both flexion and extension.[46]

Active range of motion

- **Flexion and extension:** The normal arc of motion for knee flexion and extension is 135 to 145 degrees, with the majority of the motion occurring as flexion. A fully extended knee normally is at 0 degrees, but in certain cases may be as great as 10 or more degrees beyond 0 (genu recurvatum). Knee flexion may be limited by tightness of the rectus femoris, in which case a fully extended hip can limit the amount of flexion available at the knee.
- **Internal and external rotation:** To allow for full ROM during knee flexion and extension, the tibia must internally and externally rotate on the femur. Observe and bilaterally compare the rotation of the tibial tuberosity to estimate the amount of internal and external rotation that occurs during active knee flexion and extension.

Goniometry Box 10-1
Knee Flexion/Extension

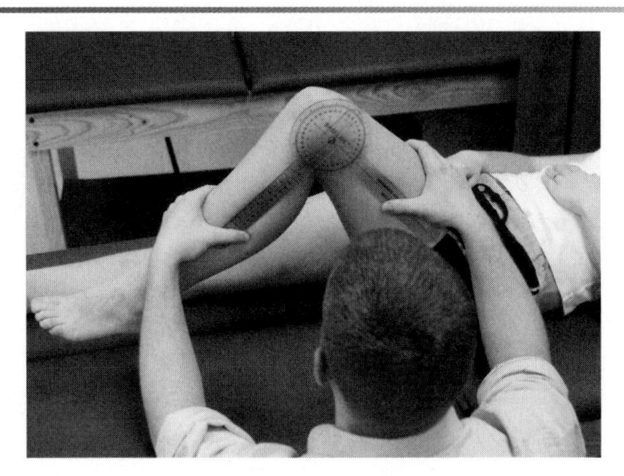

Flexion (0° to 135°–145°)/Extension (0°–10°)

Patient Position	Lying supine. Knee flexion and extension may also be measured with the patient supine and a bolster placed under the distal femur.
Goniometer Alignment	
Fulcrum	Centered over the lateral femoral epicondyle
Proximal Arm	The stationary arm is centered over the midline of the femur, aligned with the greater trochanter.
Distal Arm	The movement arm is centered over the midline of the fibula, aligned with the lateral malleolus.
Comments	Knee flexion can be assessed with the patient prone and using the same landmarks to assess the length of the two-joint rectus femoris muscle.

Manual muscle testing

The leg muscles must be relaxed when manual muscle testing the hamstring group to minimize contributions from the gastrocnemius as a knee flexor. Performing the same test with the tibia internally and externally rotated magnifies contributions from the semimembranosus/semitendinosus and biceps femoris respectively. The quadriceps (Manual Muscle Test 10-1) and hamstrings (Manual Muscle Test 10-2) are tested as a group. The function of the sartorius can be relatively isolated (Manual Muscle Test 10-3).

Passive range of motion

An equal amount of flexion and extension is lost with capsular involvement (Table 10-4).

- **Extension:** Extension is assessed with the tibia slightly elevated by placing a **bolster** under the distal tibia with the patient in the supine position. Extension produces a firm end-feel because the posterior capsule and the cruciate ligaments stretch. Tightness of the hamstring group may limit extension, especially in cases in which the knee has been flexed for extended periods because of stiffness, swelling, or immobilization. A flexion contracture may also limit extension as evidenced by an early firm end-feel.
- **Flexion:** Flexion is assessed with the patient supine and the hip flexed to remove the influence of excessive rectus femoris tightness. Restrictions in the flexion ROM in

Bolster A support used to maintain the position of a body part.

Table 10-4 Knee Capsular Pattern and End-Feels

Capsular Pattern: Flexion, Extension	
End-Feels:	
Extension	Firm: Stretch of the posterior capsule; ACL; PCL
Flexion	Soft: Soft tissue approximation between the triceps surae and the hamstrings. Firm: Stretch of the rectus femoris.
Internal tibial rotation	Firm: Capsular stretch; LCL; IT band
External tibial rotation	Firm: Capsular stretch; MCL; LCL; Pes anserine

ACL = anterior cruciate ligament; IT = iliotibial; LCL = lateral collateral ligament; MCL = medial collateral ligament; PCL = posterior cruciate ligament.

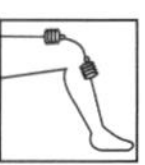

Manual Muscle Test 10-1
Knee Extension

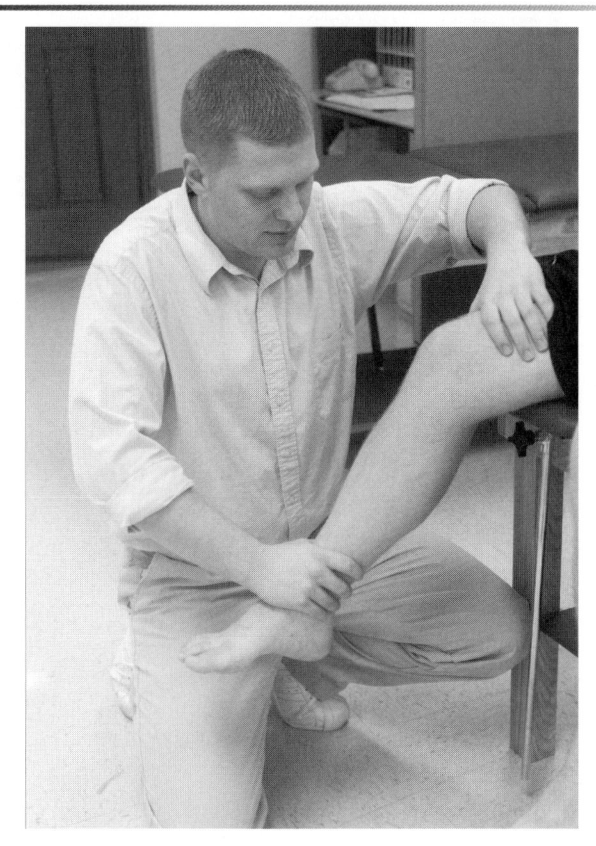

Patient Position	Seated
Starting Position	Knee flexed
Stabilization	Distal femur
Palpation	Proximal to the patella
Resistance	Distal tibia, proximal to the ankle
Primary Mover(s) (Innervation)	Vastus lateralis (L2, L3, L4) Vastus medialis (L2, L3, L4) Vastus intermedius (L2, L3, L4) Rectus femoris (L2, L3, L4)
Secondary Mover(s) (Innervation)	Not applicable
Substitution	Ankle dorsiflexion Hip extension

the supine position suggest joint capsule adhesions or effusion. Flexion measured in the prone position with the rectus femoris stretched over the hip and knee joints more closely reflects the effect of muscular tightness on the joint. The normal end-feel for flexion is soft because of the approximation of the gastrocnemius group with the hamstrings or the heel striking the buttock.

Joint Stability Tests

Ligamentous stability of the knee may occur in one plane, either as anteroposterior instability in the frontal plane or as valgus-varus instability in the sagittal plane. It may also occur as a multidirectional rotatory instability. This section presents tests for uniplanar instabilities. Tests for rotatory

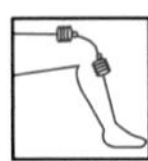

Manual Muscle Test 10-2
Knee Flexion

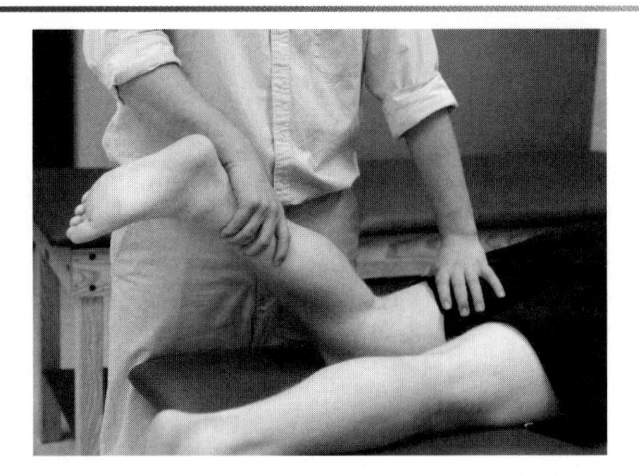

Patient Position	Prone
Starting Position	Knee extended
Stabilization	Femur
Palpation	Mid-belly of medial and lateral hamstrings
Resistance	Distal tibia
Primary Mover(s) (Innervation)	***Biceps femoris:*** Long head—tibial (S1, S2, S3); short head—common peroneal (L5, S1, S2) ***Semimembranosus:*** Tibial (L5, S1) ***Semitendinosus:*** Tibial (L5, S1, S2)
Secondary Mover(s) (Innervation)	Gastrocnemius
Substitution	Hip flexion Ankle plantarflexion
Comments	Internally rotating the leg will emphasize contributions from the semimembranosus and semitendinosus. Externally rotating the leg will emphasize contribution from the biceps femoris.

instabilities are discussed in the Pathologies and Related Special Tests section of this chapter.

Stress testing

Tests for anterior instability. Two basic tests attempt to displace the tibia anteriorly on the femur thus assessing the relative stability of the ACL. The ACL provides 86% of the restraint against anterior translation.[48] In the case of a complete ACL disruption, further displacement is limited by the posterior capsule, the deep layer of the MCL, and the posterolateral complex.

The anterior drawer test involves placing the knee in 90 degrees of flexion and attempting to translate the tibia anteriorly (Stress Test 10-1). The anterior drawer test is particularly sensitive to tears in the anteromedial bundle of the ACL.[49–52] The line of pull from the hamstrings compliments the function of the ACL, possibly masking an otherwise positive test result (Fig. 10-18). The hamstrings, however, do not replicate the function of the ACL as the knee nears extension.[29]

Factors limiting the anterior drawer test include:

1. The need to overcome the effects of gravity while moving the tibia anteriorly
2. Guarding by the hamstring group, masking anterior displacement of the tibia on the femur
3. Effusion within the capsule, providing resistance to movement or the inability to flex the knee to 90 degrees

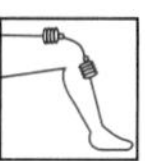

Manual Muscle Test 10-3
Isolating the Sartorius

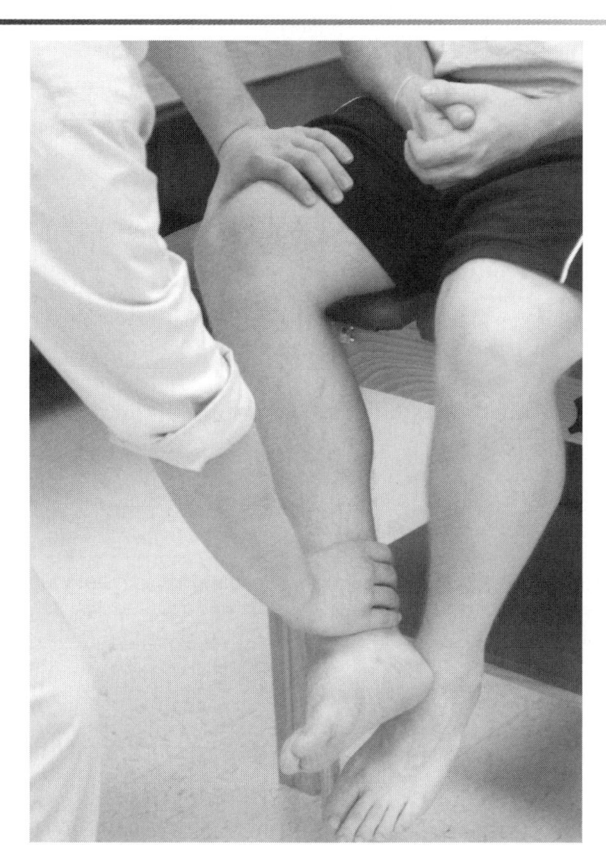

Patient Position	Seated
Starting Position	The heel of the leg being tested is positioned over the anterior talocrural joint with the patient sitting over the edge of the table.
Stabilization	Distal femur
Palpation	Just inferior to the anterior superior iliac spine
Resistance	Medial aspect of the distal tibia and medial ankle The patient attempts to slide the heel up the opposite tibia while the clinician resists hip flexion, hip abduction, hip external rotation, and knee flexion.
Primary Mover(s) (Innervation)	Sartorius (L2, L3)
Secondary Mover(s) (Innervation)	Secondary movers include the hamstring muscle group, hip external rotators, gracilis, and hip flexors.
Substitution	Hip flexion without external rotation or abduction indicates substitution by the rectus femoris and/or iliopsoas.[47]

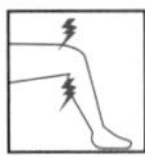

Stress Test 10-1
Anterior Drawer Test for Anterior Cruciate Ligament Instability

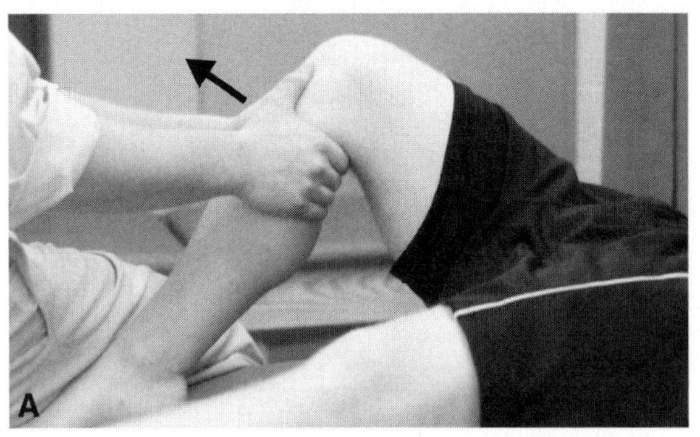

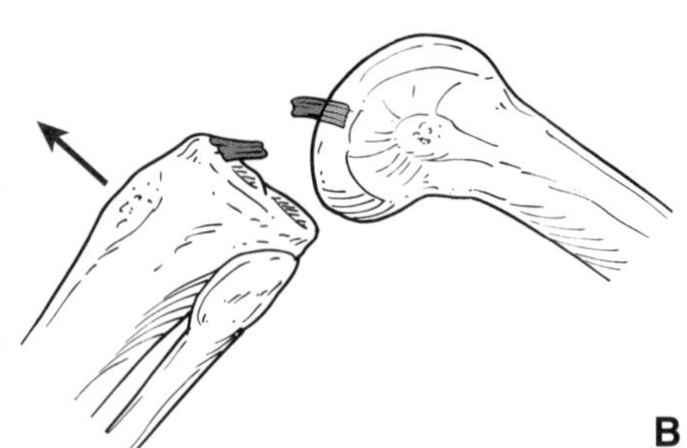

The anterior drawer test for anterior cruciate laxity **(A)**. Schematic representation of tibial displacement in a positive test **(B)**. The anterior drawer test is also used to identify interior joint play.

Patient Position	Lying supine Hip flexed to 45° and the knee to 90°
Position of Examiner	Sitting on the examination table in front of the involved knee, grasping the tibia just below the joint line of the knee. Thumbs are placed along the joint line on either side of the patellar tendon. The index fingers are used to palpate the hamstring tendons to ensure that they are relaxed.
Evaluative Procedure	The tibia is drawn anteriorly.
Positive Test	An increased amount of anterior tibial translation compared with the opposite (uninvolved) limb or the lack of a firm end-point
Implications	A sprain of the anteromedial bundle of the ACL or a complete tear of the ACL
Modification	The patient is seated to remove the posterior sag of the tibia that would be caused by PCL injury. The examiner is kneeling with the patient's lower leg stabilized between the examiner's knees. The tibia is translated anteriorly.
Comments	The hamstring muscle group must be relaxed to ensure proper test results. Too much flexion can result in false-negative result due to tibial plateau and the posterior horns of the menisci contacting the femoral condyle.
Evidence	Positive likelihood ratio Not Useful — Useful Very Small / Small / Moderate / Large 87.9 0 1 2 3 4 5 6 7 8 9 10 Negative likelihood ratio Not Useful — Useful Very Small / Small / Moderate / Large 1.0 0.9 0.8 0.7 0.6 0.5 0.4 0.3 0.2 0.1 0

ACL = anterior cruciate ligament; PCL = posterior cruciate ligament.

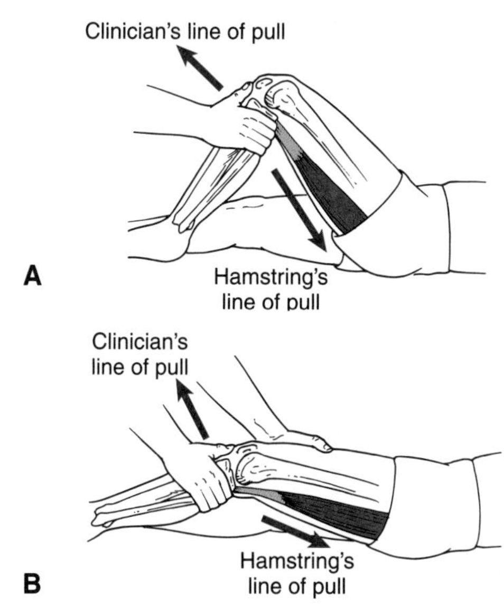

FIGURE 10-18 ■ Biomechanics of the (A) anterior drawer test and (B) Lachman's test for anterior cruciate laxity. (A) During the drawer test contraction of the hamstring group pulls the tibia posteriorly, the direction opposite the line of pull, potentially masking a positive result. (B) The joint position used during the Lachman's test (20° of flexion) alters the hamstring's force vector, thereby reducing the possibility of a false-negative result.

4. The geometry of the articular condyles, causing the triangular shape of the menisci to form a block against anterior movement of the tibia, similar to a doorstop's wedging against the bottom of a door.
5. Flexing the knee to 90 degrees, causing anterior displacement of the tibia, masking the amount of further displacement during the drawer test[53]
6. Reduced sensitivity to lesions located in the posterolateral bundle.[54]

When compared to the Lachman's, the anterior drawer's low specificity makes it less helpful in determining the presence of ACL damage. A negative anterior drawer test, however, is predictive in ruling out an ACL tear.[55]

A modification of the anterior drawer test, the **Lachman's test**, tends to isolate the posterolateral bundle of the ACL because the knee is flexed to 20 degrees (Stress Test 10-2 and see Fig. 10-8). Several modifications of the Lachman's test have been proposed to help accommodate for differences in size, strength, and stature between the clinician and patient (Fig. 10-19). When compared to the gold standard of viewing the ACL through an arthroscope, the Lachman's combined sensitivity and specificity makes it the best examination technique for detecting whether or not an ACL sprain is present.[55,56]

*** Practical Evidence**

When compared with the pivot shift and the anterior drawer, the Lachman's has a high negative predictive value: a negative Lachman's result is highly predictive of an intact ACL.[57,58]

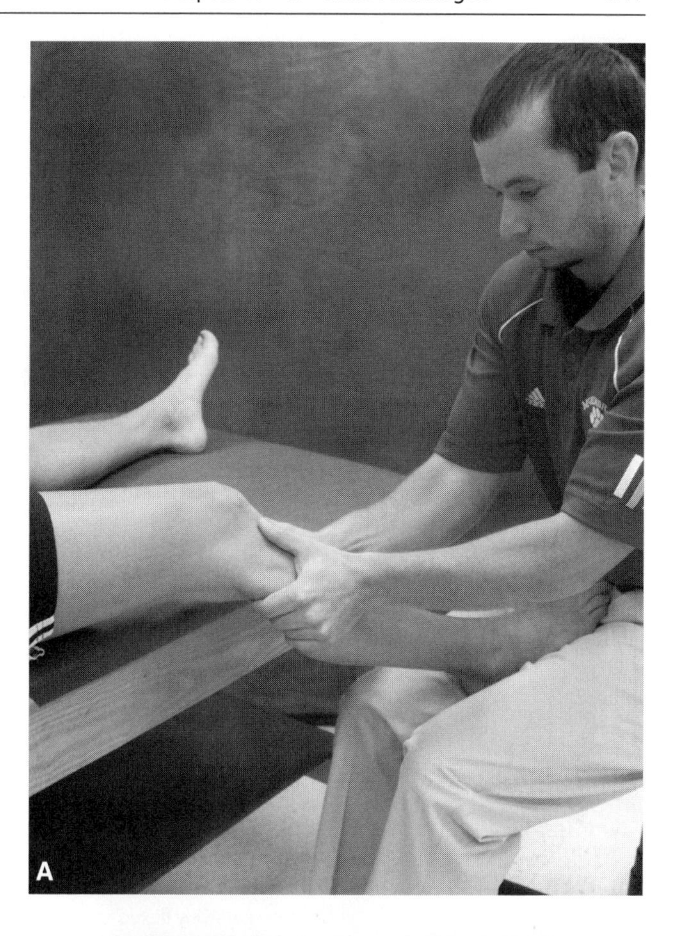

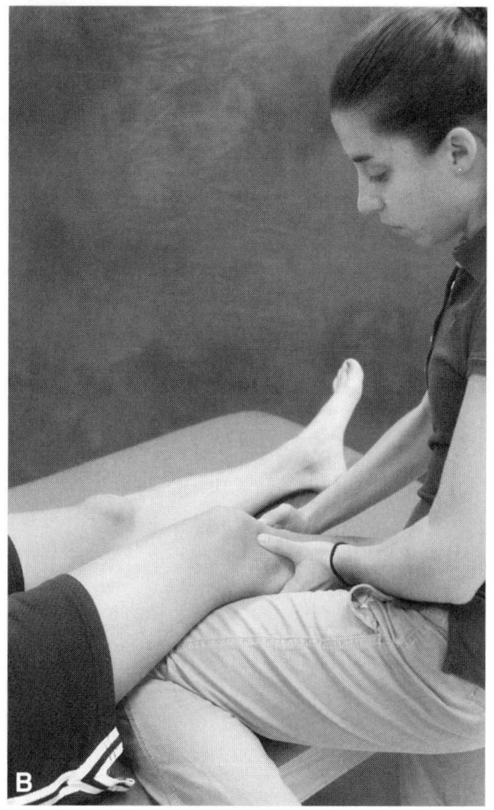

FIGURE 10-19 ■ (A, B) Modifications of the Lachman's test.

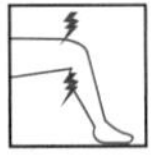

Stress Test 10-2
Lachman's Test for Anterior Cruciate Ligament Laxity

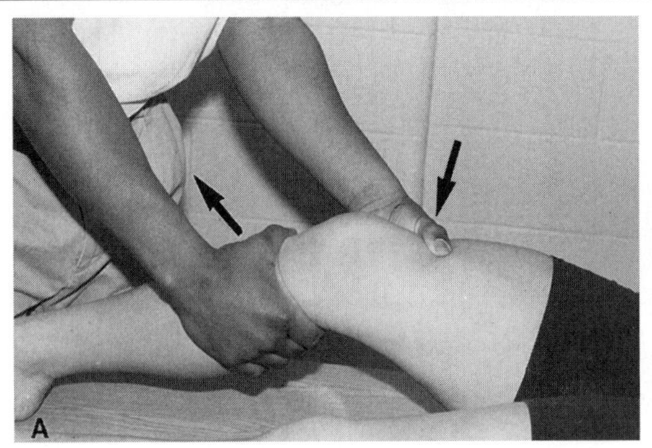

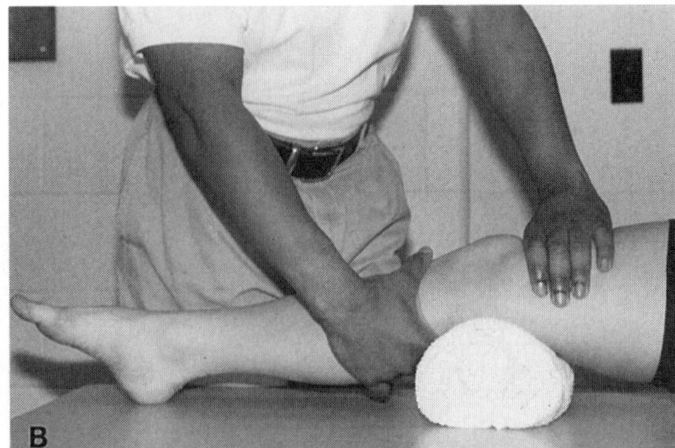

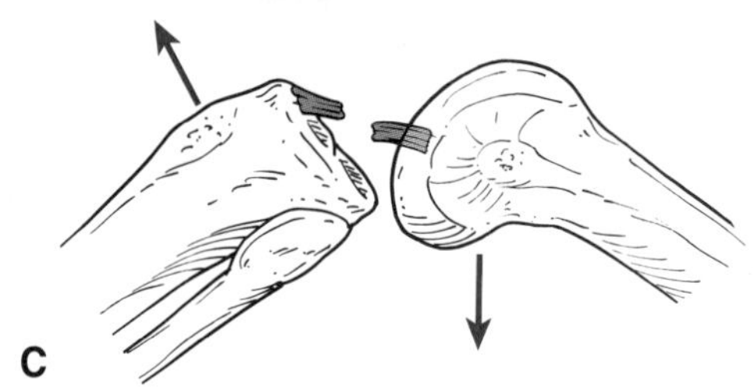

The Lachman's test **(A)** and modification of the Lachman's test **(B)**. Schematic representation of tibiofemoral translation in the presence of ACL deficiency **(C)**.

Patient Position	Lying supine The knee passively flexed to 20°–25°
Position of Examiner	One hand grasps the tibia around the level of the tibial tuberosity and the other hand grasps the femur just above the level of the condyles.
Evaluative Procedure	While the examiner supports the weight of the leg and the knee is flexed to 20°–25°, the tibia is drawn anteriorly while a posterior pressure is applied to stabilize the femur.
Positive Test	An increased amount of anterior tibial translation compared with the opposite (uninvolved) limb or the lack of a firm end-point
Implications	Sprain of the ACL, sprain of the posterolateral bundle of the ACL
Modification	As shown in **B** above, placing a rolled towel beneath the knee may assist in stabilizing the femur.
Comments	See Stress Test Box 10-3, the prone Lachman's test.
Evidence	Positive likelihood ratio

Not Useful — Useful

Very Small | Small | Moderate | Large

12.4 – 93.0

0 1 2 3 4 5 6 7 8 9 10

Negative likelihood ratio

Not Useful — Useful

Very Small | Small | Moderate | Large

1.0 0.9 0.8 0.7 0.6 0.5 0.4 0.3 0.2 0.1 0

ACL = anterior cruciate ligament.

Performing the Lachman's test requires a firm grasp to manipulate the tibia and femur. In many cases, athletes or other large patients have heavy, muscular legs, making it difficult to perform this test. In these cases, the femur may be rested on a tightly rolled towel or stabilized by an assistant.[59] Another method is to abduct the patient's leg off the side of the table and flex the knee to 25 degrees. One hand stabilizes the femur on the table and the foot is supported between the examiner's legs.[60]

In each of these modifications, the tibia is drawn forward in a way similar to the drawer test procedure. The art of manual ACL and PCL testing can be quantified by instrumented **arthrometers** (Fig. 10-20). Arthrometers measure the amount of tibial translation in a more accurate, quantitative, reproducible manner and are less prone to the physical limitation faced by the clinician when performing the anterior drawer or Lachman's test.[61–65] However, as with other clinical testing procedures, the reliability of instrumented arthrometers is correlated with the skill and experience of the individual performing the test.[65–67]

A knee demonstrating an apparently positive anterior drawer or Lachman's test result must also be screened for PCL insufficiency. If the PCL is deficient, tests for ACL insufficiency may appear positive as the tibia is relocated anteriorly from its posteriorly subluxed position on the femur.[68,69]

The **prone Lachman's test** (reverse Lachman, alternate Lachman) can be used to differentiate abnormal tibiofemoral glide caused by tears of the ACL from that caused by PCL deficiencies.[68] This test places the patient in the prone, rather than the supine position, preventing the posterior tibial sag resulting from the supine position (Stress Test 10-3).

Tests for posterior instability. Tests for damage of the PCL attempt to determine the amount of posterior displacement of the tibia on the femur relative to the uninvolved side. This motion places stress primarily on the PCL, followed by the arcuate ligament complex and the anterior joint capsule.

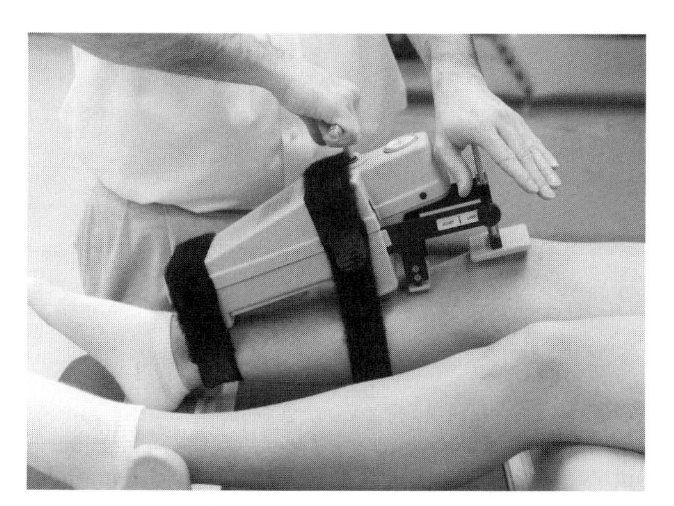

FIGURE 10-20 ■ Instrumented testing of the anterior cruciate ligament using the KT-1000TM arthrometer.

A posterior sag of the tibia may be evidenced when the flexed knee is viewed from the lateral side (see Fig. 10-17). Using the same positioning as the anterior drawer, the **posterior drawer test** attempts to displace the tibia posteriorly (Stress Test 10-4). **Godfrey's test** uses gravity to increase the posterior sag as noted during the inspection process (Stress Test 10-5). The following grading system is used for PCL sprains[70,71]:

Grade	Clinical Signs	Posterior Displacement
I	Palpable but diminished step-off between tibia and femur	0–5 mm
II	Step-off is lost; the tibia cannot be pushed beyond the medial femoral condyle.	5–10 mm
III	Step-off is lost; the tibia can be pushed beyond the medial femoral condyle.	>10 mm

Tests for medial instability. When the knee is fully extended, the MCL is assisted in limiting valgus stress by the posterior oblique ligament, posteromedial capsule, cruciate ligaments, and the muscles crossing the medial joint line. When the knee is flexed to 25 degrees, the MCL is the primary structure for resisting valgus forces.[1]

The **valgus stress test** is performed once with the knee fully extended and again with the knee is flexed to 25 degrees (Stress Test 10-6). Valgus laxity demonstrated on a fully extended knee indicates a major disruption of the medial supportive structures and the presence of an empty end-feel indicates a possible rupture of the cruciate ligaments or fracture of the distal femoral epiphysis in younger patients.[72] Placing the knee in approximately 25 degrees of flexion isolates the stress to the MCL.

Tests for lateral instability. The **varus stress test** is used to determine the integrity of the LCL, lateral joint capsule, IT band, posterior lateral complex, cruciate ligaments, and lateral musculature when it is performed in complete extension (Stress Test 10-7). When the knee is flexed to 25 degrees and the varus stress reapplied, the LCL is better isolated. A positive varus stress test result when the knee is fully extended may also indicate a distal femoral epiphysis fracture in a younger patient.

Joint play assessment

The anterior and posterior drawer tests also are used to identify the amount of anteroposterior glide between the tibia and femur (see Stress Tests 10-1 and 10-4).

Assessment of proximal tibiofibular syndesmosis stability. The proximal tibiofibular syndesmosis is of concern because of the attachment of the LCL and biceps femoris to the fibular head. Instability of the syndesmosis most commonly caused by a glancing blow to the superior fibula results in altered biomechanics and decreased lateral stability secondary to abnormal movement between the fibula and tibia (Joint Play 10-1).

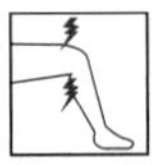

Stress Test 10-3
Prone Lachman's Test

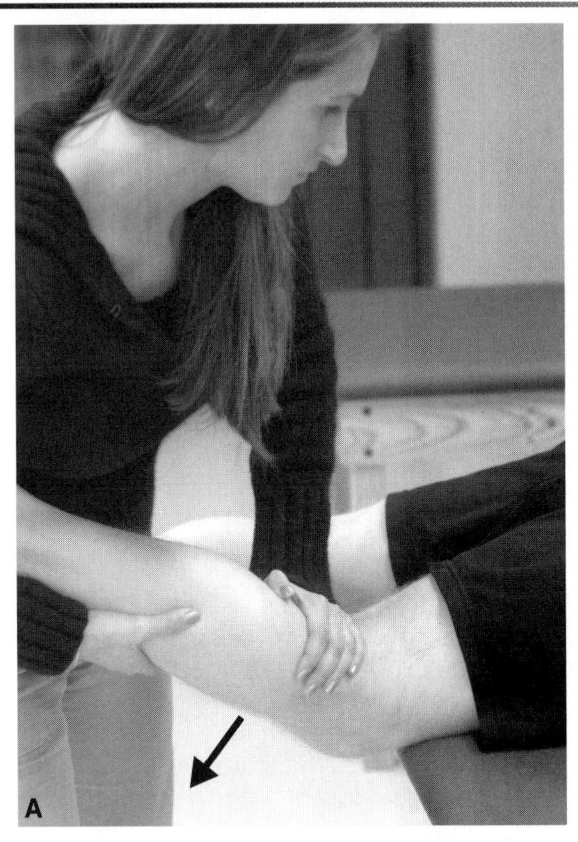

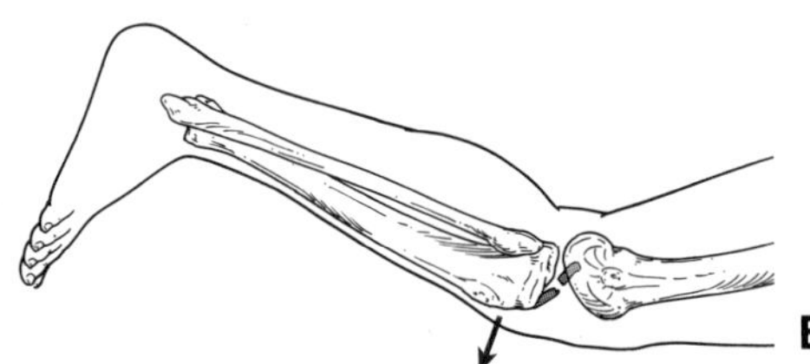

Prone Lachman's test to differentiate between anterior tibial glide caused by ACL versus PCL laxity and may be easier to perform than the Lachman's Test for individuals with small hands or patients with large legs.

Patient Position	Prone, the leg is hanging off the table The knee passively flexed to 30°
Position of Examiner	Positioned at the legs of the patient so that the examiner supports the ankle
Evaluative Procedure	A downward pressure is placed on the proximal portion of the posterior tibia as the examiner notes any anterior tibial displacement.
Positive Test	Excessive anterior translation relative to the uninvolved knee indicates a sprain of the ACL.
Implications	Positive test results found in the anterior drawer and/or Lachman's test and in the alternate Lachman's test indicate a sprain of the ACL. A positive anterior drawer test and/or Lachman test result and a negative alternate Lachman's test result implicate a sprain in the PCL.
Evidence	Inconclusive or absent in the literature

ACL = anterior cruciate ligament; PCL = posterior cruciate ligament.

Neurologic Testing

A neurologic examination is required when referred pain to the knee is suspected, the proximal tibiofibular joint displays laxity, the patient demonstrates posterolateral instability, or after a dislocation of the tibiofemoral joint. In addition, knee pain can be radicular in nature, arising from proximal nerves such as the sciatic nerve or obturator nerve that refers to medial knee. Neurologic involvement may also be associated with swelling within the popliteal fossa or lateral joint line. In addition, local or distal neurologic involvement may occur after

Stress Test 10-4
Posterior Drawer Test for Posterior Cruciate Ligament Laxity

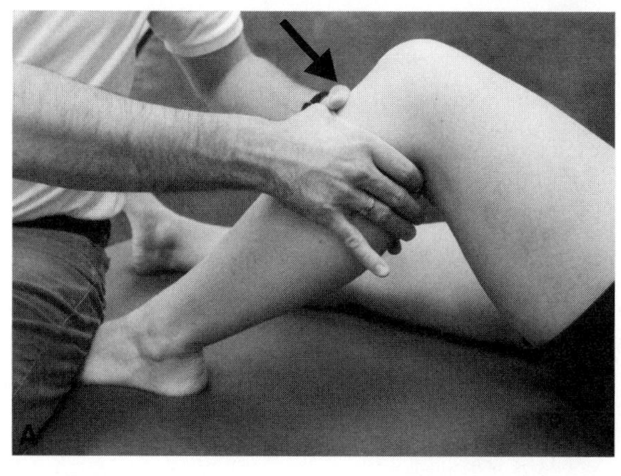

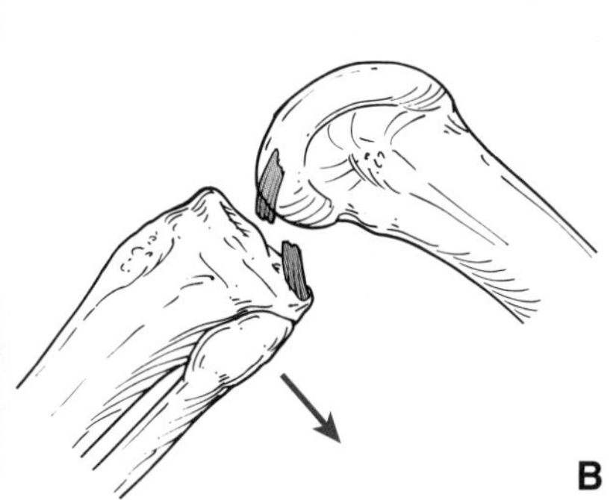

Posterior drawer test for PCL instability. **(A)** The tibia is moved posteriorly relative to the femur. **(B)** Translation of the tibia on the femur in the presence of a PCL tear. The posterior drawer test is also used to assess posterior joint play.

Patient Position	Lying supine The hip flexed to 45° and the knee flexed to 90°
Position of Examiner	Sitting on the examination table in front of the involved knee The patient's tibia stabilized in the neutral position
Evaluative Procedure	The examiner grasps the tibia just below the joint line of the knee with the fingers placed along the joint line on either side of the patellar tendon. The proximal tibia is pushed posteriorly.
Positive Test	An increased amount of posterior tibial translation compared with the opposite (uninvolved) limb or the lack of a firm end-point
Implications	A sprain of the PCL
Modification	To identify injury to the posterolateral corner of the knee, perform the posterior drawer test at 30° of flexion. The drawer test may also be performed with the tibia internally and externally rotated. In isolated PCL tears there will be decreased tibial translation with the tibia internally rotated.[13]
Comments	Increased posterior translation relative to the uninvolved knee at 30° but not at 90° implicates injury to the posterolateral corner. Increased posterior translation relative to the uninvolved knee at 30° and at 90° indicates injury to the PCL.[5]
Evidence	Inconclusive or absent in the literature

PCL = posterior cruciate ligament.

surgery (Fig. 10-21). (Refer to Box 1-1 for a lower quarter screen.)

Tibiofibular trauma can also damage the common peroneal nerve, which is superficial at the fibular head. Distal symptoms include paresthesia along the dorsum of the foot and the lateral leg and foot and an inability or weakness in active dorsiflexion and eversion.

Vascular Testing

An examination of distal pulses (posterior tibial artery, dorsal pedal artery) is indicated if a dislocation of the tibiofemoral joint is suspected.

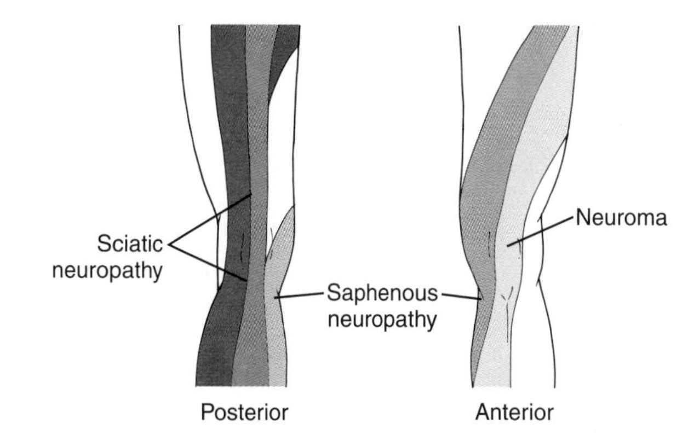

FIGURE 10-21 ■ Local neuropathies of the knee. These findings should also be correlated with a lower quarter neurologic screen.

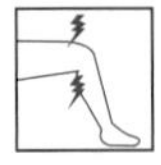

Stress Test 10-5
Godfrey's Test for Posterior Cruciate Ligament Instability

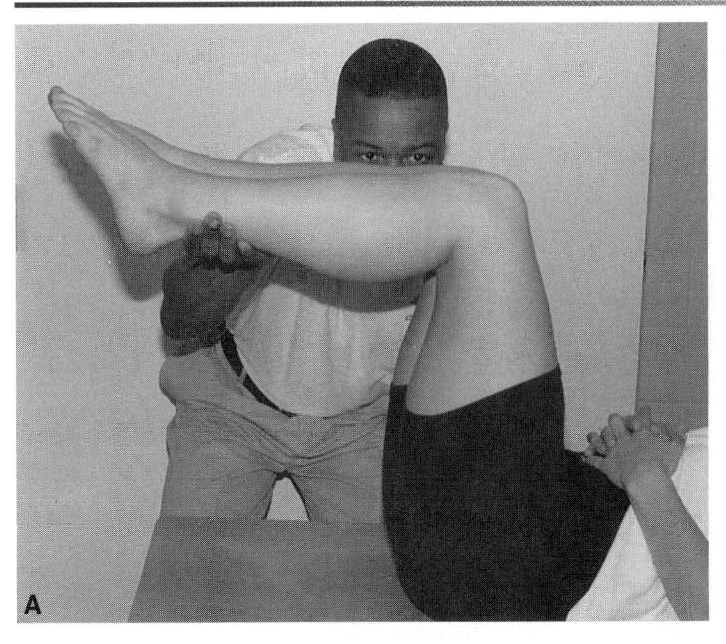

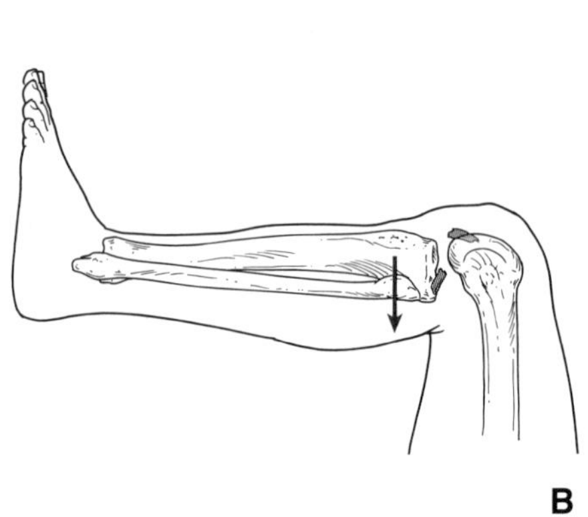

Godfrey's test for posterior cruciate ligament laxity. Note the downward displacement of the left (facing) tibia.

Patient Position	Lying supine with the knees extended and legs together
Position of Examiner	Standing next to the patient
Evaluative Procedure	Lift the patient's lower legs and hold them parallel to the table so that the knees are flexed to 90°. Observe the level of the tibial tuberosities.
Positive Test	A unilateral posterior (downward) displacement of the tibial tuberosity
Implications	A sprain of the PCL
Modification	A straight-edge (such as a ruler) can be placed between the patella and tibia to better visualize the posterior sag.
Comments	The lower leg must be stabilized as distally as possible; supporting the tibia proximally prevents it from sagging posteriorly. An assistant may be used to hold the distal legs.
Evidence	Inconclusive or absent in the literature

ACL = anterior cruciate ligament; IT = iliotibial; LCL = lateral collateral ligament; MCL = medial collateral ligament.

Stress Test 10-6
Valgus Stress Test for Medial Collateral Ligament Instability

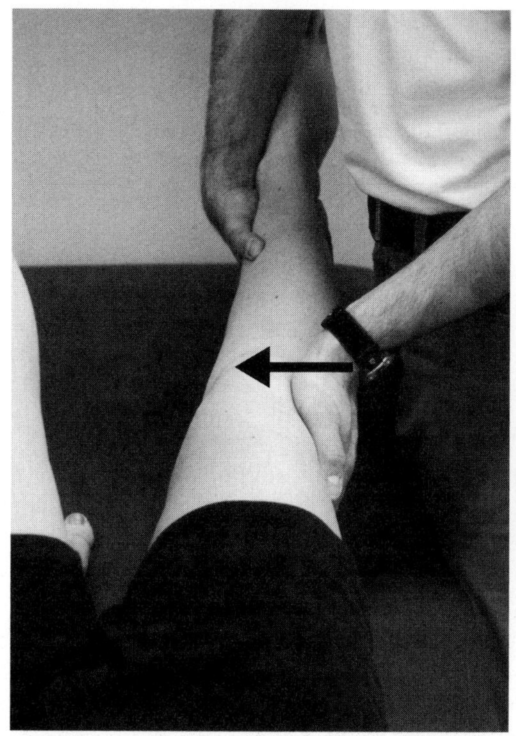

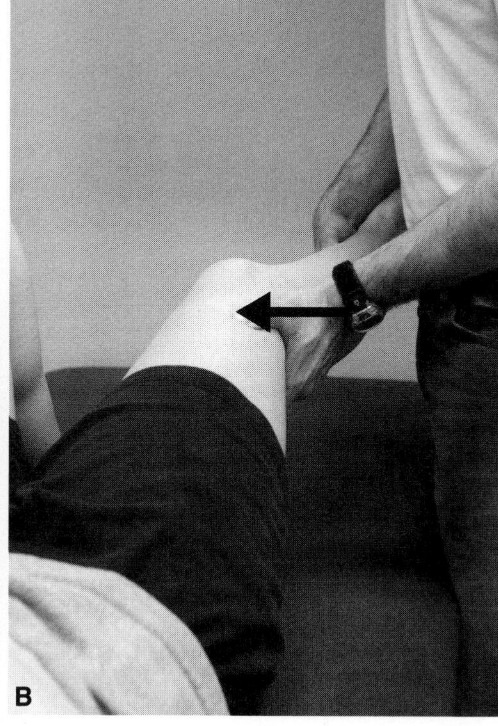

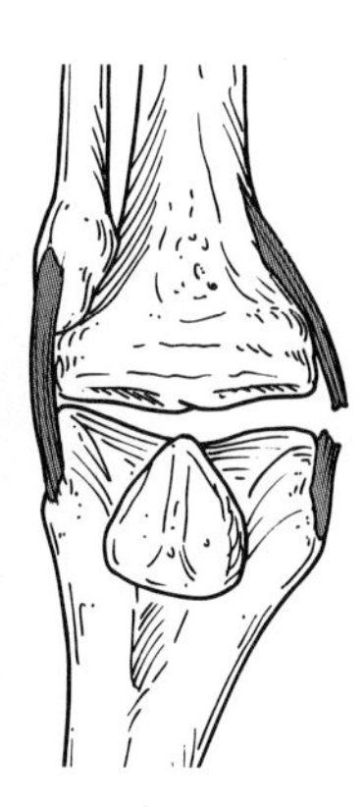

Valgus stress test **(A)** in full extension to determine the integrity of medial capsular restraints and cruciate ligaments, **(B)** with the knee flexed to 25° to isolate the medial collateral ligament, and **(C)** schematic representation of the opening of the medial joint line.

Patient Position	Lying supine with the involved leg close to the edge of the table
Position of Examiner	Standing lateral to the involved limb One hand supports the medial portion of the distal tibia while the other hand grasps the knee along the lateral joint line. To test the entire medial joint capsule and other restraining structures, the knee is kept in complete extension. To isolate the MCL, the knee is flexed to 25°.
Evaluative Procedure	A medial (valgus) force is applied to the knee while the distal tibia is moved laterally.
Positive Test	Increased laxity, decreased quality of the end-point, and/or pain compared with the uninvolved limb
Implications	In complete extension: A sprain of the MCL, medial joint capsule, and possibly the cruciate ligaments, distal femoral epiphyseal fracture In 25° flexion: A sprain of the MCL
Modification	To promote relaxation of the patient's musculature, the thigh may rest on the table with the knee flexed over the side edge of the table.[73] The patient's leg may be held against the clinician's torso to improve the amount of stress applied to the MCL.
Comments	When testing the knee in full extension, it is recommended that the thigh be left on the table, preventing shortening of the hamstring muscle group. The apprehension test (see Chapter 11) should be performed before valgus stress testing in patients who have a history of patellar dislocations or subluxations.
Evidence	Inconclusive or absent in the literature

MCL = medial collateral ligament.

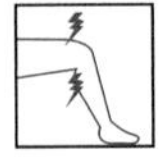

Stress Test 10-7
Varus Stress Test for Lateral Collateral Ligament Instability

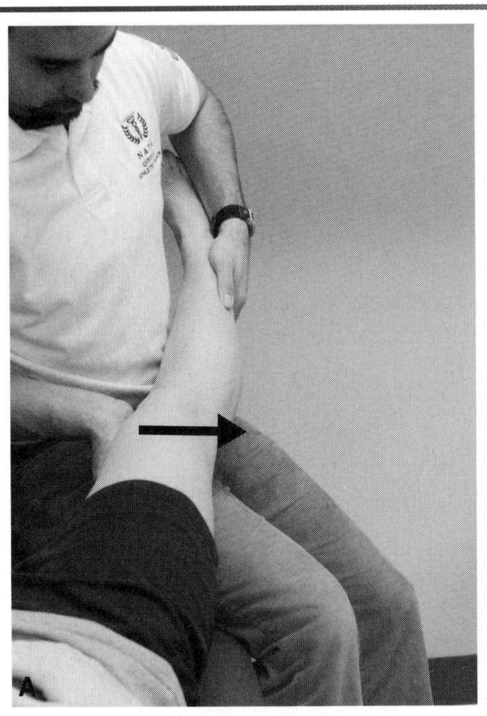

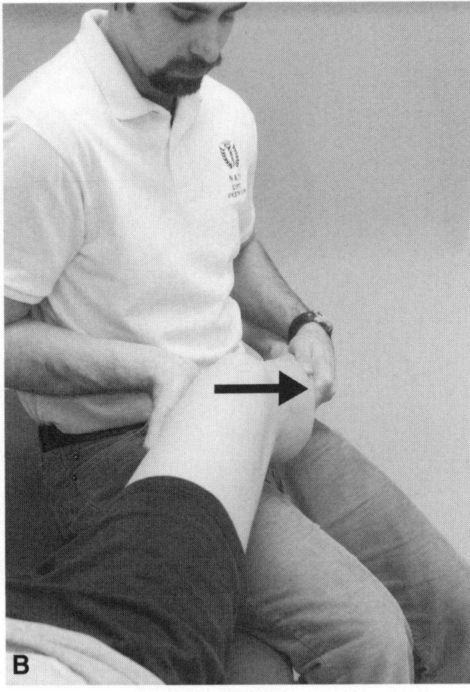

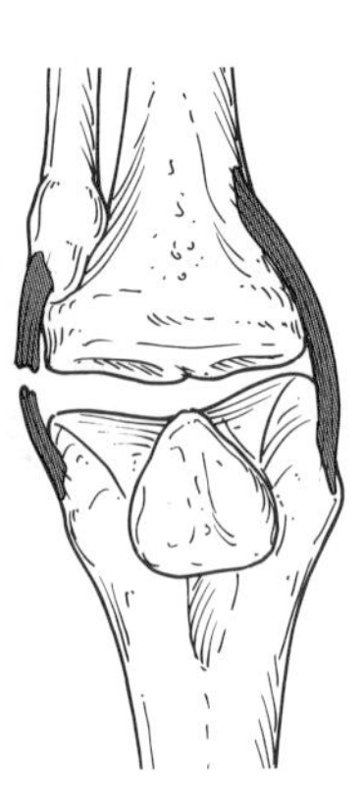

Varus stress test **(A)** in full extension to determine the integrity of lateral capsular restraints, **(B)** with the knee flexed to 25°–30° to isolate the lateral collateral ligament, and **(C)** schematic representation of the opening of the medial joint line.

Patient Position	Lying supine with the involved leg close to the edge of the table
Position of Examiner	Sitting on the table One hand supports the lateral portion of the distal tibia, while the other hand grasps the knee along the medial joint line. To test the entire lateral joint capsule and other restraining structures, the knee is kept in complete extension. To isolate the LCL, the knee is flexed to 25°.
Evaluative Procedure	A lateral (varus) force is applied to the knee while the distal tibia is moved inward.
Positive Test	Increased laxity, decreased quality of the end-point, and/or pain compared with the uninvolved limb
Implications	In complete extension: A sprain of the LCL, lateral joint capsule, cruciate ligaments, and related structures, indicating possible rotatory instability of the joint, distal femoral epiphyseal fracture In 25° of flexion: A sprain of the LCL
Modification	The patient is supine. The examiner is standing to allow the patient's abducted thigh to rest on the table for improved stabilization and relaxation during the varus stress.
Comments	Avoid hip external rotation during the maneuver. The varus force must be applied perpendicular to the ligament in both testing positions.
Evidence	Inconclusive or absent in the literature

LCL = lateral collateral ligament.

Joint Play 10-1
Proximal Tibiofibular Syndesmosis

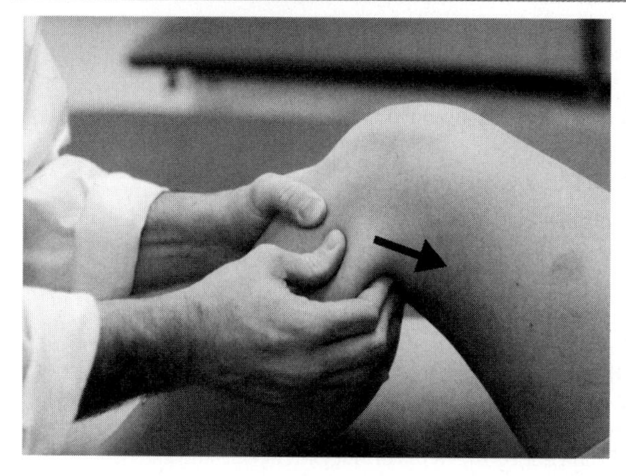

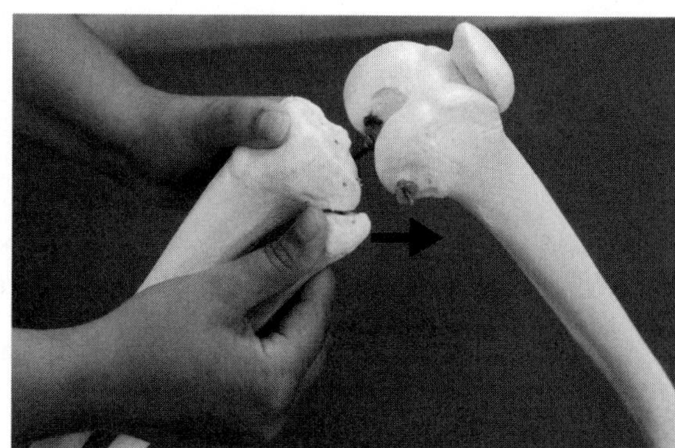

The fibular head is manually manipulated to determine its anterior/posterior stability.

Patient Position	Lying supine with the knee passively flexed to approximately 90°
Position of Examiner	Standing lateral to the involved side
Evaluative Procedure	One hand stabilizes the tibia while the other hand grasps the fibular head. While stabilizing the tibia, the examiner attempts to displace the fibular head anteriorly and then posteriorly.
Positive Test	Any perceived hyper- or hypomobility of the fibula on the tibia compared with the uninvolved side and/or pain elicited during the test
Implications	An anterior fibular shift indicates damage to the proximal posterior tibiofibular ligament; posterior displacement reflects instability of the anterior tibiofibular ligament of the proximal tibiofibular syndesmosis. Hypomobility may alter proximal and distal joint mechanics.
Comments	Damage to the common peroneal nerve is frequently associated with a proximal tibiofibular syndesmosis sprain.
Evidence	Inconclusive or absent in the literature

Pathologies of the Knee and Related Special Tests

Trauma to the knee may result from a contact-related mechanism, through rotational forces placed on the knee while bearing weight, or secondary to overuse. Knee injuries suffered by school-aged athletes (including college students) are most likely to be the result of a single traumatic episode. A small portion of this population and a larger percentage of older athletes are likely to suffer from degenerative changes within the knee.

Uniplanar Knee Sprains

Uniplanar knee sprains present with instability in only one of the body's cardinal planes. Damage to the MCL or LCL leads to valgus or varus instability in the frontal plane. Trauma to the ACL or PCL results in instability in the sagittal plane where the tibia shifts anteriorly or posteriorly relative to the femur. This type of injury involves damage that is isolated to a single structure. When multiple structures are involved (e.g., the ACL and lateral joint capsule), a multiplanar or rotatory instability results.

Medial collateral ligament sprains

The MCL is damaged as the result of tensile forces, most commonly a valgus stress caused by a blow to the lateral aspect of the knee. Noncontact valgus loading or a rotational force being placed on the knee can also injure the MCL (Examination Findings 10-1). The valgus stress test (see Stress Test 10-6) performed in complete extension and 25 degrees of flexion is used to manually determine the integrity of the MCL. When the knee is fully extended, the valgus force is dissipated by the superficial and deep layers of the MCL, the anteromedial and posteromedial joint

Examination Findings 10-1
Medial Collateral Ligament Sprain

Examination Segment	Clinical Findings
History	***Onset:*** Acute ***Pain characteristics:*** Medial aspect of the knee, on, above, or below the joint line, depending on the location of the damage ***Mechanism:*** A valgus force to the knee or, less commonly, external rotation of the tibia ***Predisposing conditions:*** Increased foot fixation on the ground (e.g., cleats)
Inspection	Immediate inspection of an MCL injury may produce unremarkable findings. Over time, edema may be present along the medial aspect of the knee.
Palpation	Tenderness along the length of the MCL from its origin below the adductor tubercle to the insertion on the medial tibial flare
Joint and Muscle Function Assessment	***AROM:*** Pain with possible loss of motion during the terminal ranges of flexion and extension; greater loss of ROM when the MCL is torn proximal to the joint line because of greater capsular involvement[74] ***MMT:*** Decreased flexion and extension strength secondary to pain, with flexion being more painful than extension ***PROM:*** Pain and possible loss of motion during the terminal ranges of flexion and extension
Joint Stability Tests	***Stress tests:*** Valgus laxity in complete extension indicates involvement of the MCL and medial capsular structures. An empty end-feel strongly suggests an associated sprain of the ACL and/or PCL. Valgus laxity in 25° of flexion indicates involvement of the MCL. ***Joint play:*** No remarkable findings
Special Tests	Slocum drawer test for laxity of the anteromedial capsule (see p. 336)
Neurologic Screening	Common peroneal nerve and its branches (L4/L5)
Vascular Screening	Within normal limits
Functional Assessment	Increased pain during midstance phase of gait secondary to femur internally rotating on tibia, increasing valgus forces. Acute: Antalgic gait secondary to pain and instability Chronic instability: Functional limitation in changing direction (cutting) to the opposite side.
Imaging Techniques	T1 and T2-weighted MRI [4] Plain film radiographs may be ordered to rule out epiphyseal fractures in children or avulsion fractures in adults.
Differential Diagnosis	ACL, PCL, medial meniscal tear, semimembranosus strain, pes anserine strain, pes anserine bursitis, common peroneal neuropathy, distal femoral epiphyseal fracture
Comments	Adolescent patients displaying the valgus laxity should be referred to a physician to rule out injury to the epiphyseal plate. If a rotational force is suspected, laxity is displayed in complete extension, or the Slocum drawer test result is positive, pathology to the ACL and PCL should be ruled out. The patella should be checked for lateral stability prior to valgus stress testing (see Special Test 11-3 on Patellar Apprehension) An associated bone bruise, OCD or common peroneal nerve contusion may occur secondary to lateral compressive forces

ACL = anterior cruciate ligament; AROM = active range of motion; MCL = medial collateral ligament; MMT = manual muscle test; PCL = posterior cruciate ligament; PROM = passive range of motion.

capsule, and the tendons of the pes anserine group. When the knee is flexed beyond 20°, the superficial layer of the MCL becomes more responsible for resisting valgus forces. Ruptures of the deep layer of the MCL are almost always associated with a rupture of the superficial layer.[4] Instrumented testing of valgus laxity is highly correlated to findings on MR images and radiographs.[4,72]

Medial collateral ligament sprains may occur in isolation, but because of the deep layer's communication with the medial joint capsule and medial meniscus, concurrent injury to these structures must always be suspected. Fluid escaping from the knee joint to the area around the MCL is an indirect sign of a complete rupture of the deep layer of the MCL.[4]

*** Practical Evidence**

A complete tear of the MCL, marked by the medial joint line opening 8–15 mm and marked by an empty end-feel strongly suggests that the ACL and/or PCL have also been ruptured.[72]

Extreme valgus forces or rotational forces placed on the knee at the time of injury may also lead to the involvement of the ACL.[74] Fractures of the distal femoral physis can mimic a third-degree MCL sprain in growing patients.[75] As described in Chapter 11, patellar dislocations can occur secondary to a valgus force placed on the knee. Therefore, all MCL sprains must include an evaluation of the patella for lateral instability before stress testing.

Most MCL injuries are managed nonoperatively, even when surgical repair of other structures, including the ACL, is warranted.[4,76,77] The ligament lies within the soft tissue matrix of the medial aspect of the knee and enjoys an adequate blood supply for healing. An aggressive functional rehabilitation program provides long-term stability against valgus forces.[76] Successful nonoperative rehabilitation of the MCL includes protecting the joint from valgus stress while healing, providing an optimal healing environment within the MCL through a controlled restoration of ROM, and adequate strengthening and proprioceptive training of the lower extremity. Use of a knee brace with the ability to limit ROM may be indicated in grade II and III injuries to control further injurious stress and provide the restoration of motion without compromising healing within the ligament.[73,78]

Operative treatment for injuries of the MCL has been shown to have a high complication rate, including postoperative stiffness and patellofemoral dysfunction.[79] Clinicians need to be aware of these potential complications whenever treating a patient after surgical repair of the MCL so any symptoms found during the evaluation can be properly treated.

Lateral collateral ligament sprains

Resulting from a blow to the medial knee that places tensile forces on the lateral structures or by internal rotation of the tibia on the femur, LCL sprains result in varus laxity of the knee. The extracapsular nature of the LCL gives it a normally "springy" end-feel. A varus stress test result that feels empty when compared with the contralateral side should be considered a positive result for an LCL sprain (Examination Findings 10-2).

Because a varus force with concurrent tibial rotation can cause damage to other structures, injuries to the posterolateral corner, ACL and/or PCL, and posterolateral rotatory instability must be suspected in patients suffering from LCL injury. Because of the relative proximity of the peroneal nerve, patients suspected of having suffered an injury to the lateral or posterolateral aspect of the knee require careful evaluation of distal function of the common and superficial peroneal nerve, especially if an associated fracture of the fibular head is suspected.[80]

Although the LCL is an extracapsular and extraarticular structure, the ligament still relies on synovial fluid for much of its nutrition.[81] The LCL's relatively poor healing properties and the ligament's importance in providing rotational stability to the knee often necessitate early surgical repair or late reconstruction.[82]

Anterior cruciate ligament sprains

Injury to the ACL results from a force causing an anterior displacement of the tibia relative to the femur (or the femur being driven posteriorly on the tibia), from noncontact-related rotational injuries, or from hyperextension of the knee. Unlike injury to other ligaments, the majority of ACL sprains arise from noncontact-related torsional stress, such as what occurs when an athlete cuts or pivots.[49,50] Hamstring strains may occur secondary to the sudden eccentric contraction of the muscles in an attempt to restrict anterior translation of the tibia (Examination Findings 10-3).

Associated with the injury mechanism, the patient may describe hearing or sensing a "pop" within the knee joint and an immediate loss of knee function. Bystanders may also report hearing the pop as the ACL ruptures. Swelling occurs rapidly secondary to trauma of the medial geniculate artery, the ACL's primary blood supply. Normally this hemarthrosis remains within the fibrous capsule, but trauma to the capsule results in diffuse swelling that may **extravasate** distally over time. Intracapsular swelling combined with the tension placed on the ACL limits the ROM (see Fig. 10-8). Laxity of the ACL may be confirmed through Lachman's test and the anterior drawer test. However, clinical laxity is not a strong predictor of functional ability.[86]

The rotatory forces placed on the knee make "isolated" trauma to the ACL unlikely. Instability of the knee is greatly increased when trauma also damages one or more of the other ligaments or the menisci.[45,87] As is described in the Rotatory Instabilities section of this chapter, the degree of

Extravasate Fluid escaping from vessels into the surrounding tissue.

Examination Findings 10-2
Lateral Collateral Ligament Sprain

Examination Segment	Clinical Findings
History	***Onset:*** Acute ***Pain characteristics:*** Lateral joint line of the knee, fibular head, or femoral condyle, depending on the location of the sprain. ***Mechanism:*** Varus force placed on the knee or excess internal tibial rotation
Inspection	Swelling, if present, is likely to be localized especially when trauma is isolated to the LCL, because it is an extracapsular structure.
Palpation	Palpation eliciting tenderness along the length of the LCL and possibly the lateral joint line
Joint and Muscle Function Assessment	***AROM:*** Pain and loss of motion may be experienced during knee flexion and at terminal extension. ***MMT:*** Pain and weakness when assessing knee flexion and extension ***PROM:*** Pain and loss of motion may be experienced during the terminal ROMs, although lack of such pain does not conclusively rule out LCL trauma.
Joint Stability Tests	***Stress tests:*** Varus laxity in complete extension indicates involvement of the lateral capsular structures and possibly the cruciate ligaments.[20] Varus laxity in 25°–30° of flexion isolates the LCL ***Joint play:*** Tibiofibular joint play
Special Tests	Slocum drawer test for laxity of the anterolateral capsule (see p. 336)
Neurologic Screening	Common peroneal nerve and its branches (L4/L5)
Vascular Screening	Within normal limits
Functional Assessment	Antalgic gait secondary to pain.
Imaging Techniques	A coronal, T2-weighted MRI can demonstrate tearing of the LCL and/or associated meniscal injury.
Differential Diagnosis	Posterolateral corner injury, posterolateral rotatory instability, lateral meniscus tear, lateral head of gastroc strain, biceps femoris strain, iliotibial band inflammation, tibiofibular sprain, fibular head fracture, distal femoral epiphysis fracture
Comments	The LCL has a normal "spring" when a varus force is applied, making bilateral comparison essential. Adolescent patients displaying varus laxity require a referral to a physician to rule out possible epiphyseal plate trauma. For patients who have reported a rotatory mechanism of injury or who display LCL laxity through either a varus stress or a positive Slocum drawer test result, anterolateral rotatory instability must be suspected.

AROM = active range of motion; LCL = lateral collateral ligament; MRI = magnetic resonance image; PROM = passive range of motion.

anterior displacement of the tibia is increased and an anterior subluxation of the tibial condyles results when the anteromedial or anterolateral joint capsules, pes anserine, biceps femoris, or IT band are also traumatized.

Several intrinsic and extrinsic factors predisposing factors to ACL injuries have been suggested (Table 10-5).[88,89] Most predisposing factors share the common trait of causing internal tibial rotation, thus placing an additional stress on the ACL. Females may be particularly predisposed to ACL trauma (Box 10-1).

Because PCL deficiency can replicate positive test results for ACL involvement as the tibia is returned to its normal position, tests for PCL tears need to be performed to rule out such false-positive results.

The term "partially torn ACL" is a misnomer. Because the bands of the ACL wind upon each other, even partial trauma to an individual band results in biomechanical dysfunction, instability, and increased stress on the remaining fibers, predisposing them to future injury. Knees with partial tears of the ACL, typically involving the anteromedial bundle, may initially appear stable during manual stress testing but degrade to demonstrate signs of clinical instability as the remaining ligament fibers adaptively lengthen secondary to increased stress loads.[54]

The long-term consequence of an ACL-deficient knee include instability, meniscal degeneration, chondral surface damage, and osteoarthritis.[96] Patients who perform physical activities that do not involve cutting or pivoting on a planted foot may not experience pain or dysfunction, although proprioceptive function in a single-limb stance is decreased in the presence of an ACL-deficient knee.[99] Patients who have a history of an ACL tear are seven times more likely to develop moderate-to-severe clinical OA and have 105 times greater chance of developing radiographically diagnosed OA than those without a history of an ACL tear.[96]

The rehabilitation program for a patient with an ACL-deficient knee focuses on restoring ROM, lower extremity strength, and proprioception.[99] The use of a functional knee brace may be helpful, although the efficacy of these devices has not been substantiated.

Table 10-5 Potential Factors Predisposing Individuals to Anterior Cruciate Ligament Injury

Extrinsic to the Knee	Intrinsic to the Knee
Sport-specific body motions, such as landing from a jump or side-step cutting maneuvers	Joint laxity[88] Limb alignment[88]
Muscle strength	Narrow intercondylar notch width[90,97,98]
Muscle fatigue[90]	Small size of the ACL[88]
Muscular activation and coordination[90]	Genu recurvatum[93,94]
Athletic skill coordination[88]	
The shoe–surface interface[88,89]	
Hyperpronation of the foot (navicular drop)[91,92,93]	
Anterior pelvic tilt[94]	
Anteverted femur[94]	
Wider pelvis to femoral length ratio[90]	
Menstrual cycle[95]	
History of an immediate family member (sibling, child, or parent) suffering an ACL tear.[96]	
Female[90]	

ACL = anterior cruciate ligament.

Box 10-1
Anterior Cruciate Ligament Injuries in Females

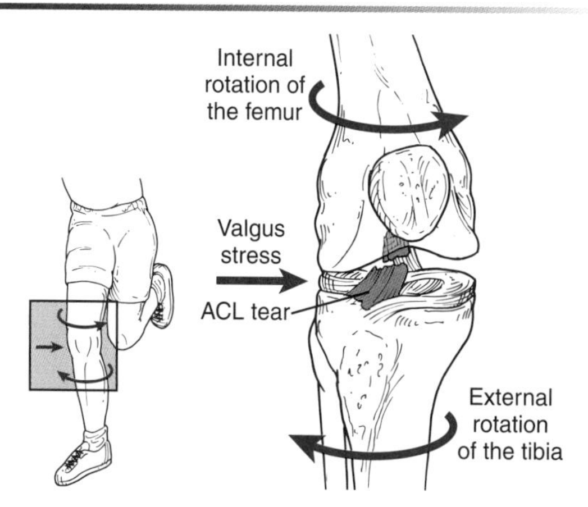

The increased popularity of women's athletics has attracted a large number of female athletes into the world of sports. Although the expected increase in participation of female athletes would normally give rise to an increased number of injuries, female athletes have experienced a disproportionately high rate of noncontact ACL injuries relative to their male counterparts.[90]

Although women normally have an increased amount of anterior tibial translation compared with men, this fails to account for the high incidence rate.[28] The intrinsic and extrinsic factors presented in Table 10-5 that preload the ACL and predispose individuals to ACL injuries also hold true for women. Changes in muscle activation patterns, increased rate of fatigue, and biomechanical differences in landing from a jump and cutting appear to contribute to the increased rate of ACL injuries in females.[90,102] Also, females, on average, have narrower intercondylar notch widths, which may partially account for the higher noncontact ACL injury rate in female athletes.[98]

The influence of the menstrual cycle as a predisposition to ACL injury remains under dispute. Hormone-dependent changes occur throughout the menstrual cycle that may alter physical performance, such as decreasing reaction time and viscoelastic tissue properties. The risk of sustaining an ACL injury appears to be increased during the first days of the menstrual period.[103]

Examination Findings 10-3
Anterior Cruciate Ligament Sprain

Examination Segment	Clinical Findings
History	***Onset:*** Acute ***Pain characteristics:*** Within the knee joint, sometimes described as "pain" or a "pop" under the kneecap Diffuse pain throughout the joint after injury ***Other symptoms:*** Not applicable ***Mechanism:*** Rotation of the knee while the foot is planted (tensile forces), a blow that drives the tibia anterior relative to the femur or the femur posterior relative to the tibia (shear force), or hyperextension ***Predisposing conditions:*** See Table 10-5. Shoe wear and/or playing surfaces that increase foot fixation
Inspection	Rapid effusion, often in the suprapatellar area, that forms within hours after the onset of injury
Palpation	For isolated ACL injuries, pain is not normally reported during palpation (other than that resulting from a contusion caused by the traumatic force). The sweep and ballotable patella test results are positive if intracapsular effusion is present.
Joint and Muscle Function Assessment	***AROM:*** Pain or intracapsular swelling may prohibit any meaningful ROM tests; pain is expected to be greatest at the extremes of the ROM. ***MMT:*** Pain and/or limitation during flexion and extension, possibly precluding this portion of the examination's being conducted in the acute stage of injury Pain and/or weakness during MMT for the hamstrings ***PROM:*** Pain likely throughout the ROM (especially at the extremes) and possibly intensified when the tibia is internally or externally rotated
Joint Stability Tests	***Stress tests:*** Lachman's test Anterior drawer test Prone Lachman's test ***Joint play:*** Anterior glide of the tibia on the femur is assessed using anterior drawer. Posterior glide of the tibia is assessed using the posterior drawer test [83]

Special Tests	Pivot shift test Flexion–rotation drawer[84] Slocum drawer Crossover test Slocum ALRI test
Neurologic Screening	Within normal limits
Vascular Screening	Within normal limits
Functional Assessment	The extent of disability is influenced by the secondary restraints that are also injured. Acute: Antalgic gait (shortened stance time), inability to climb or descend stairs (tending to lead with the uninvolved leg); inability to achieve full extension secondary to quadriceps inhibition resulting from effusion Chronic: Complaints of instability with change of direction
Imaging Techniques	Four-view radiographic series: AP, lateral, skyline, tunnel[85] Coronal and sagittal T1- and T2-weighted MR images
Differential Diagnosis	PCL sprain, meniscus tear, hamstring strain, strain of the gastrocnemius origin, osteochondral fracture, patellar dislocation
Comments	The anterior drawer and Lachman's tests may not produce positive test results in the hours after the onset of the injury because of muscle guarding. Trauma to the PCL may produce false-positive results for ACL insufficiency. Chronic instability can lead to meniscal degeneration.

ACL = anterior cruciate ligament; ALRI = anterior lateral rotatory instability; AP = anteroposterior; AROM = active range of motion; MMT = manual muscle test; MR = magnetic resonance; PCL = posterior cruciate ligament; PROM = passive range of motion; ROM = range of motion.

Anterior cruciate ligament deficient patients who perform activities involving cutting and pivoting will most likely benefit from ACL reconstruction. Several donor tissue options are available, including **autografts** and **allografts**. The use of an accelerated rehabilitation program involving early return of ROM, early weight bearing, and restoration of muscular function has been found to decrease the time lost after surgery.[100] Accelerated programs have also been found to decrease surgical morbidity, including postoperative stiffness and patellofemoral pain.[101]

Posterior cruciate ligament sprains

Uniplanar PCL injury results from the tibia being driven posteriorly on the femur or from hyperflexion or hyperextension of the knee when the joint is distracted (e.g., when the heel steps in a hole). Landing on the anterior tibia while the knee is flexed can drive the tibia posteriorly, stressing the PCL. If the foot is dorsiflexed when falling on the knee, much of the force is directed toward the patellofemoral joint, thereby sparing the PCL (Examination Findings 10-4). However, if the foot is plantarflexed, the resulting force is delivered to the PCL when the tibial tuberosity makes contact with the ground or another stationary object (Fig. 10-22).[12]

Immediately after the onset of injury, the patient may be relatively asymptomatic or may display the signs and symptoms of a strain of the medial head of the gastrocnemius or a sprain of the posterior capsule.[104,107] Over time, symptoms such as pain in the posterior knee, weakness of the hamstring and quadriceps muscle groups, and reduced ROM during flexion become evident. Initially knee ROM may be equal to that of the opposite limb if there is an isolated PCL sprain, but noticeable deficits will be noted if multiple structures are damaged.[104] The posterior drawer and sag tests are highly reliable and sensitive in identifying the presence of chronic PCL sprains.[108] The **quadriceps active test** can identify grade II and III PCL tears (Special Test 10-4).[104] Isolated PCL trauma results in greater posterior instability as the knee is flexed from 0 to 90 degrees.[5] The LCL, posterolateral corner, and MCL are secondary restraints to posterior tibial displacement of the tibia on the femur, especially in the presence of a PCL-deficient knee.[104]

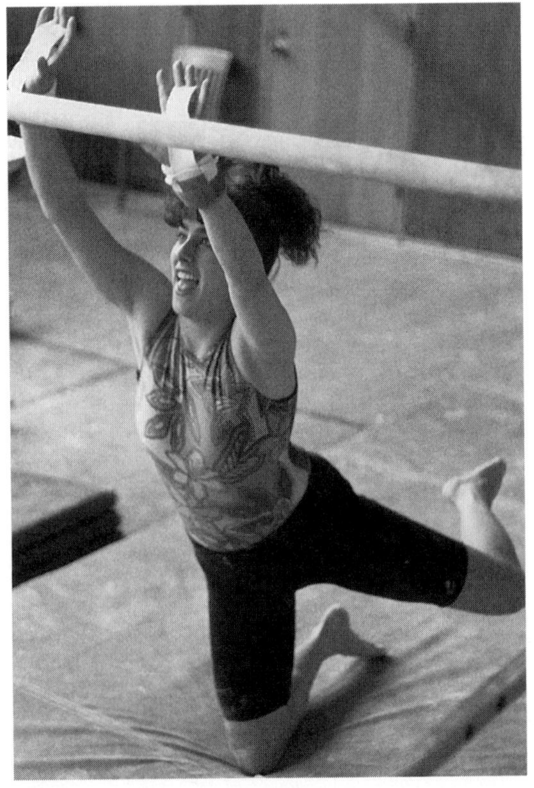

FIGURE 10-22 ■ Mechanism for posterior cruciate ligament (PCL) trauma. Landing on a bent knee and plantarflexed foot forces the tibia posteriorly relative to the femur.

PCL tears are often asymptomatic and go unreported and/or undiagnosed. Isolated PCL sprains increase the amount of posterior tibial translation, but do not increase the varus rotation or external tibial rotation.[20] Instability is greatest when there is concurrent damage to both the PCL and the knee's posterolateral structures.[17,18] The presence of a partial or complete tear of the PCL can be identified via MRI.[108] PCL sprains must also be evaluated for posterolateral corner deficiencies (see p. 339).

Statically, joint loading, joint congruency, and muscular activity can compensate for PCL deficiency. The strength of the quadriceps muscle group soon returns after a PCL sprain to assist the popliteus in providing muscular compensation against posterior tibial displacement.[16,69,109] Actual posterior laxity does not always result in knee dysfunction.[110] Patients treated nonsurgically can regain full function and independence and may often return to athletic competition unhindered by the ligamentous deficit.[106,110] If the PCL deficiency is not identified or not appropriately treated changes in the structure and function of the ACL, meniscus, and weight-bearing surfaces will occur over time, potentially leading to chronic joint instability, alteration in the gait pattern, muscle activation patterns, and reduced muscle strength.[106,109,111] The long-term consequence of these conditions is the early onset of osteoarthritis and increased joint laxity.

Rotational Knee Instabilities

Unlike uniplanar knee instabilities, rotatory (multiplanar) instabilities involve abnormal internal or external rotation at the tibiofemoral joint. The types of instabilities are named based on the relative direction in which the tibia subluxates on the femur. When this type of instability

Allograft The tissues used to replace the ligament obtained from a cadaver.

Autograft The tissues used to replace the ligament harvested from the patient's body (e.g., bone-patellar tendon-bone, hamstring tendon).

Examination Findings 10-4
Posterior Cruciate Ligament Sprain

Examination Segment	Clinical Findings
History	***Onset:*** Acute ***Pain characteristics:*** Within the knee joint radiating posteriorly, although pain may not be immediately experienced. Unlike ACL tears, the patient may not report feeling a "pop" at the time of injury.[13] ***Mechanism:*** Posterior displacement of the tibia on the femur (effect magnified when the foot is plantarflexed) Knee hyperflexion Knee hyperextension ***Predisposing conditions:*** Quadriceps weakness
Inspection	Effusion may not be present initially, but may develop over time. A posterior sag of the tibia may be noted.
Palpation	Tenderness may be elicited in the popliteal fossa if the sprain involves the posterior capsular structures or popliteus muscle; otherwise, no pain or abnormalities are usually noted.
Joint and Muscle Function Assessment	***AROM:*** Acutely, normal ROM present; pain and restrictions possible as the knee nears full flexion ***MMT:*** Pain when performed near terminal flexion Quadriceps strength may be diminished in patients with chronic PCL sprains. ***PROM:*** Pain produced as the knee nears 90° of flexion and with overpressure during flexion, especially in the presence of a partial PCL tear
Joint Stability Tests	***Stress tests:*** Posterior drawer test; Godfrey's sign, external rotation test ***Joint play:*** Posterior glide of the tibia is assessed using the posterior drawer test.[83] Anterior glide of the tibia on the femur is assessed using anterior drawer.
Special Tests	Quadriceps active test See also special tests for posterolateral rotatory instability (pp. 342–343)
Neurologic Screening	Within normal limits
Vascular Screening	Within normal limits
Functional Assessment	Acute: Antalgic gait secondary to avoidance of full extension Chronic sprain: May avoid full extension during ambulation. With damage to the posterolateral complex, the patient may demonstrate impairment during push off on the involved extremity.
Imaging Techniques	Anteroposterior, lateral, sunrise, and tunnel views may be ordered. Avulsion fractures may be noted of the PCL tibial insertion.[104] Posterior drawer stress radiograph[105] MR images are accurate in identify the location of an acute tear and for identifying concomitant trauma about the knee.[104]
Differential Diagnosis	Strain of the medial head of the gastrocnemius, posterior capsule sprain, ACL, posterolateral complex sprain, meniscus tear
Comments	Individuals with moderate PCL sprains as measured by instrumented testing display few functional differences (e.g., during ambulation and landing from a jump) as compared to those with normal knee stability.[106]

AROM = active range of motion; MMT = manual muscle test; PCL = posterior cruciate ligament; PROM = passive range of motion.

Special Test 10-4
Quadriceps Active Test

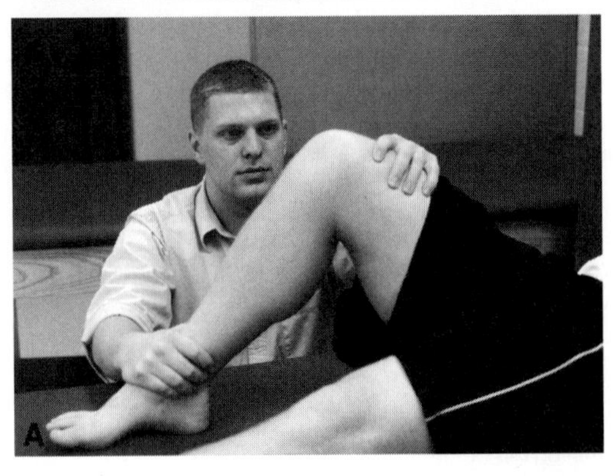

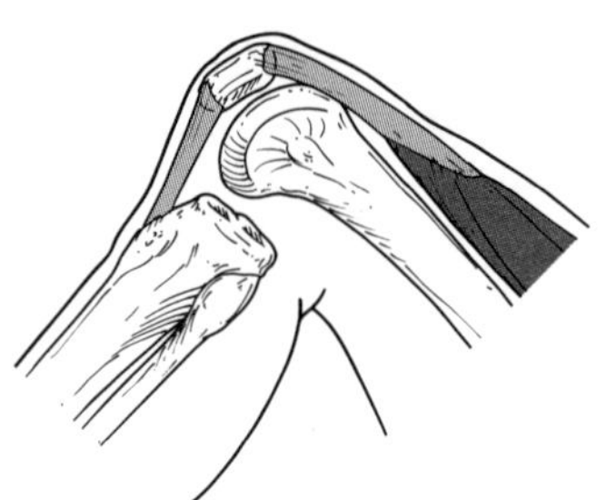

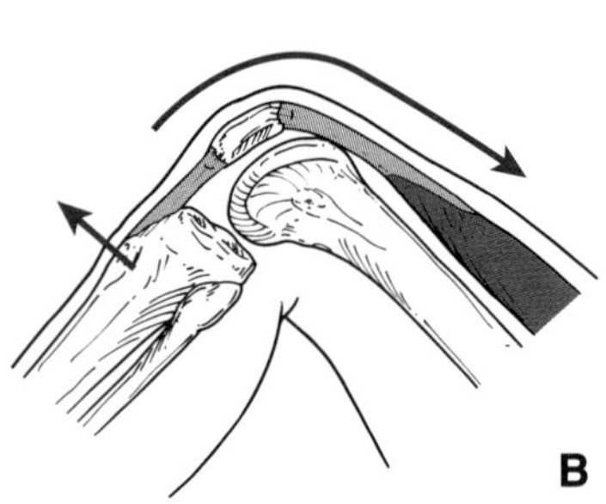

In the presence of a posterior tibial sag, contraction of the quadriceps muscle group will cause the tibia to shift back to its normal resting position.

Patient Position	Lying supine with the knee flexed to 90°
Position of Examiner	At the side of the patient One hand stabilizes the distal tibia and the opposite hand stabilizes the distal femur.
Evaluative Procedure	**(A)** While resisting knee extension the patient is asked to slide the foot forward by contracting the quadriceps. The examiner observes for anterior translation of the tibia.
Positive Test	Anterior translation of the tibia on the femur **(B)**
Implications	Grade II or III PCL sprain[104]
Comments	Interpretation of the results of this test is more accurate in the presence of higher-grade or chronic PCL lesions.[104]
Evidence	Inconclusive or absent in the literature

occurs, the axis of tibial rotation is shifted in the direction opposite that of the subluxation. The four categories of rotatory instability are presented in Box 10-2.

Rotatory instabilities result when multiple structures are traumatized, often as the result of rotational forces placed on the knee. The tests for laxity of the individual structures may produce only mildly positive results. However, when the combined laxity of each structure is summed, the degree of instability is marked.

Any injury to the knee's ligaments is suspect for causing rotatory instability. Therefore, any injury to the cruciate or collateral ligaments, the IT band, the joint capsule, or the biceps femoris must be presumed as potentially resulting in rotational instability.[30] Clinically, patients suffering from rotatory instability report the feeling of the knee "giving way," decreased muscle strength, diminished performance, and a lack of confidence in the stability of the joint. Tests for rotatory instability are not performed as part of an on-field examination. These tests will often only produce positive results when the patient is under anesthesia.

Anterolateral rotatory instability

The most common rotational instability of the knee, an anterolateral rotary instability (ALRI), results in a greater displacement of the tibia because of trauma to both the ACL and the lateral extraarticular restraints.[112] Disruption of the LCL, IT band, biceps femoris, and lateral meniscus accentuates the amount of anterior tibial displacement and internal tibial rotation. Many special tests exist for determining the presence of ALRI, each with its own merits and limitations. The large number of tests probably reflects their relatively low reliability.

Three tests specific to this pathology are discussed here: the **pivot shift**, the Slocum ALRI test, and the flexion–rotation drawer. In addition, two tests, the Slocum drawer test and the crossover test, may be used to determine the presence of either ALRI or anteromedial rotatory instability (AMRI). A positive result for any one of the following techniques is sufficient to warrant further examination by an orthopedic physician.

A derivation of the anterior drawer test, the **Slocum drawer test** attempts to isolate either the anteromedial or

Box 10-2
Classification of Rotational Knee Instabilities

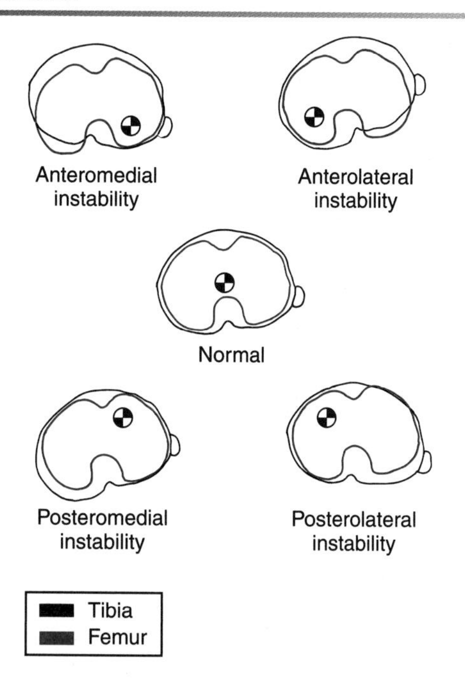

The tibial articulating surface is shown in solid lines, and the femoral articular surfaces in shaded lines. The type of instability is described based on the displacement of the tibia relative to the femur. Note that the axes of rotation are approximated.

Instability	Tibial Displacement	Pathologic Axis	Structural Instability
Anteromedial	Medial tibial plateau subluxates anteriorly.	Posterolateral, resulting in abnormal external tibial rotation	ACL, anteromedial capsule, MCL, pes anserine, medial meniscus, posteromedial capsule
Anterolateral	Lateral tibial plateau subluxates anteriorly.	Posteromedial, resulting in abnormal internal tibial rotation	ACL, anterolateral capsule, LCL, IT band, biceps femoris, lateral meniscus, popliteus, posterolateral capsule
Posteromedial	Medial tibial plateau subluxates posteriorly.	Anterolateral, resulting in abnormal internal tibial rotation	Posterior oblique ligament, MCL, semimembranosus, anteromedial capsule
Posterolateral	Lateral tibial plateau subluxates posteriorly.	Anteromedial, resulting in abnormal external tibial rotation	Posterolateral complex, LCL, biceps femoris

ACL = anterior cruciate ligament; IT = iliotibial; LCL = lateral collateral ligament; MCL = medial collateral ligament.

the anterolateral joint capsule (Special Test 10-5). Internally rotating the tibia checks for the presence of ALRI; externally rotating it checks for AMRI.

The **crossover test** is a semifunctional test used to determine the rotational stability of the knee (Special Test 10-6). This test is not as exacting as other tests for ligamentous instability, but it has the advantage of replicating a sport-specific skill, albeit in slow motion. Although primarily used to determine the presence of ALRI, the crossover test may be modified to test for AMRI by stepping behind with the uninvolved leg.

Used to evaluate ALRI, the **pivot shift test** (also known as the lateral pivot shift) duplicates the anterior subluxation and reduction that occurs during functional activities in ACL-deficient knees (Special Test 10-7). The tibia is internally rotated and a valgus force is applied to the joint while the knee is moved from extension into flexion. In the presence of a torn ACL, the tibia is displaced anteriorly when the knee is near full extension. When the knee reaches the range of 30 to 40 degrees of flexion, the IT band changes its line of pull from an extensor to a flexor and causes the tibia to relocate, resulting in an appreciable "clunk." Although

Special Test 10-5
Slocum Drawer Test for Rotational Knee Instability

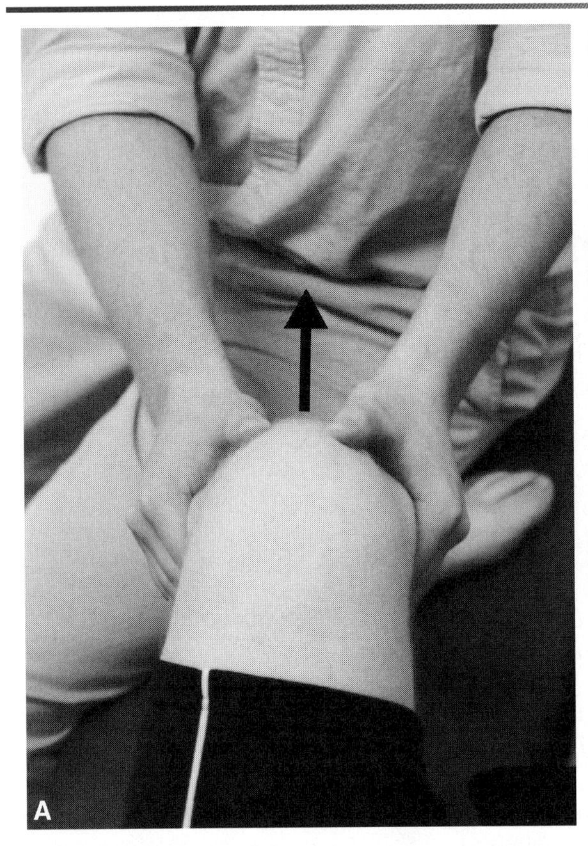

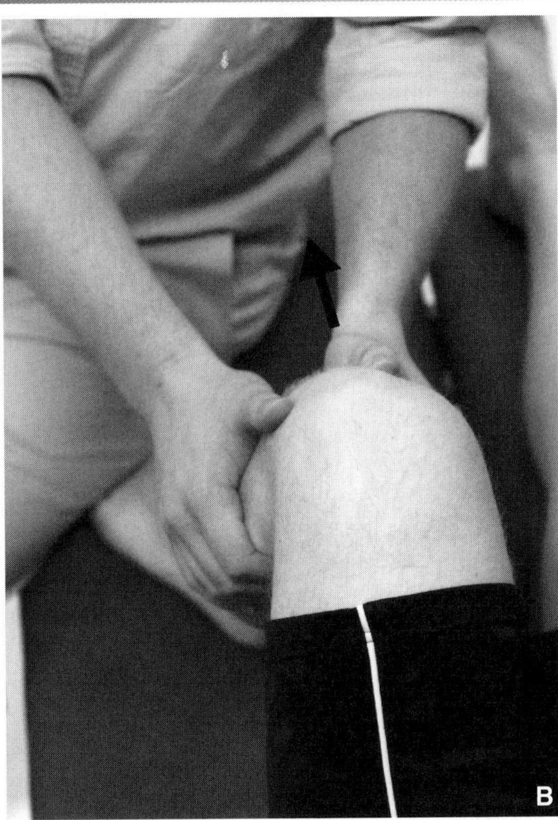

Slocum drawer test with the tibia internally rotated to isolate the lateral capsular structures **(A)** and with the tibia externally rotated to isolate the medial capsule **(B)**.

Patient Position	Lying supine with the knee flexed to 90°
Position of Examiner	Sitting on the patient's foot: **(A)** The tibia is internally rotated to 25° to test for anterolateral capsular instability. **(B)** The tibia is externally rotated to 15° to test for anteromedial capsular instability.
Evaluative Procedure	The tibia is drawn anteriorly.
Positive Test	An increased amount of anterior tibial translation compared with the opposite (uninvolved) limb or the lack of a firm end-point
Implications	**(A)** Test for anterolateral instability: Damage to the ACL, anterolateral capsule, LCL, IT band, popliteus tendon, posterolateral complex, lateral meniscus **(B)** Test for anteromedial instability: Damage to the MCL, anteromedial capsule, ACL, posteromedial capsule, pes anserine, medial meniscus
Comments	Excessive tibial rotation can cause a false-negative test due to wedging of the menisci in the joint space.
Evidence	Inconclusive or absent in the literature

ACL = anterior cruciate ligament; IT = iliotibial; LCL = lateral collateral ligament; MCL = medial collateral ligament.

Special Test 10-6
Crossover Test for Rotational Knee Instability

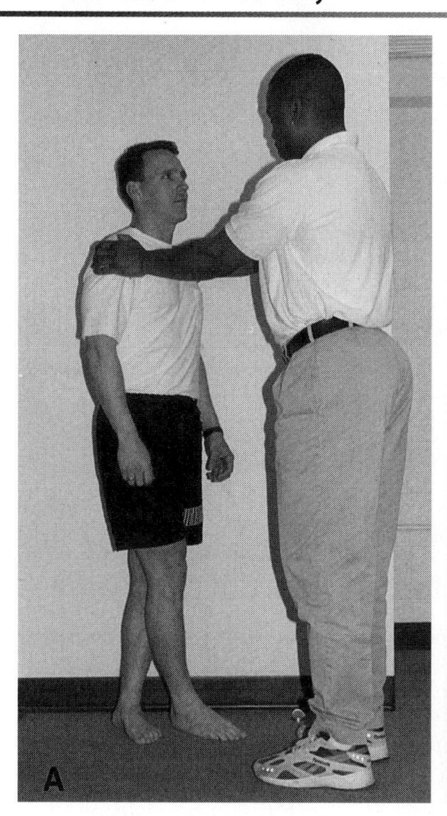

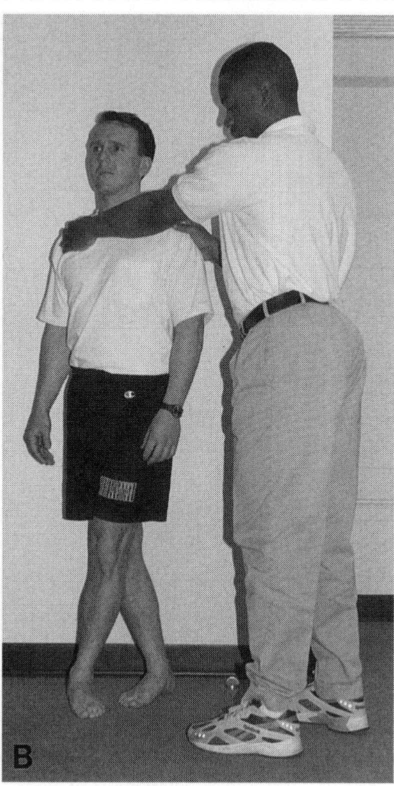

Crossover test: Stepping in front of the injured leg determines the presence of anterolateral rotatory instability **(A)**. Stepping behind the injured leg determines anteromedial rotatory instability **(B)**. Note that patient's left leg is being tested.

Patient Position	Standing with the weight on the involved limb
Position of Examiner	Standing in front of the patient
Evaluative Procedure	**(A) ALRI**: The patient steps across and in front with the uninvolved leg, rotating the torso in the direction of movement. The weight-bearing foot remains fixated. **(B) AMRI**: The patient steps across and behind with the uninvolved leg rotating the torso in the direction of movement. The weight-bearing foot remains fixated.
Positive Test	Patient reports pain, instability, or apprehension.
Implications	**(A) ALRI**: Instability of the lateral capsular restraints **(B) AMRI**: Instability of the medial capsular restraints
Comments	This test can be used as a prelude to assessing the patient's ability to perform a more functional cutting maneuver.
Evidence	Inconclusive or absent in the literature

ALRI = anterolateral rotatory instability; AMRI = anteromedial rotatory instability.

Special Test 10-7
Pivot Shift Test for Anterolateral Knee Instability–Jerk Test

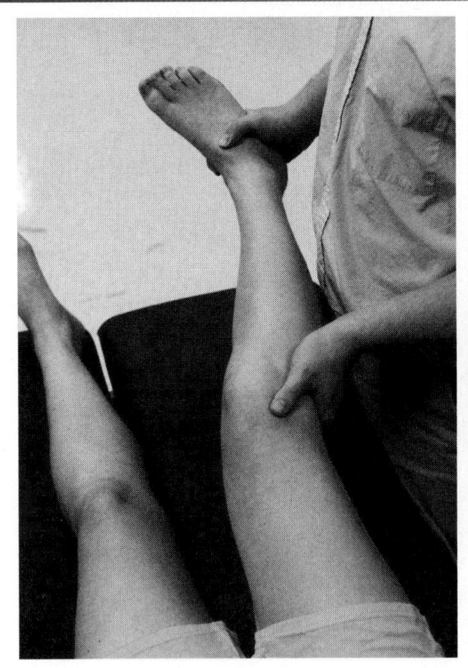

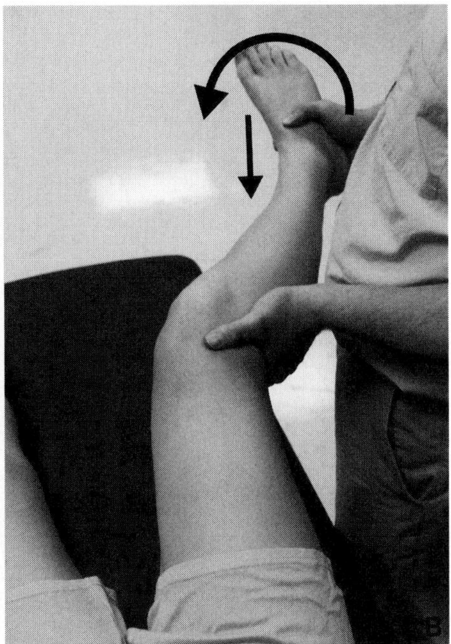

When positive, the pivot shift test (lateral pivot shift) reproduces the subluxation/reduction of the tibia on the femur experienced during gait.

Patient Position	Lying supine with the hip passively flexed to 30°
Position of Examiner	Standing lateral to the patient, the distal lower leg and/or ankle is grasped, maintaining 20° of internal tibial rotation. The knee is allowed to sag into complete extension **(A)**. The opposite hand grasps the lateral portion of the leg at the level of the superior tibiofibular joint, increasing the force of internal rotation.
Evaluative Procedure	While maintaining internal rotation, a valgus force is applied to the knee while it is slowly flexed **(B)**. To avoid masking any positive test results, the patient must remain relaxed throughout this test.
Positive Test	The tibia's position on the femur reduces as the leg is flexed in the range of 30°–40°. Jerk Test: During extension, the anterior subluxation is felt in the same range.
Implications	ACL, anterolateral capsule, LCL, biceps femoris, lateral meniscus, popliteus, posterolateral capsule
Modification	The **jerk test** is a modification of the lateral pivot shift test: The patient's hip is flexed to 45° and the knee flexed to 90°. A valgus and internal rotation force is applied as the knee is extended.
Comments	Meniscal involvement may limit ROM to produce a false-negative test result. Muscle guarding can produce a false-negative result. This test is most reliable when performed by a physician while the patient is under anesthesia.
Evidence	Positive likelihood ratio Not Useful — Useful Very Small · Small · Moderate · Large 93.0 0 1 2 3 4 5 6 7 8 9 10 Negative likelihood ratio Not Useful — Useful Very Small · Small · Moderate · Large 1.0 0.9 0.8 0.7 0.6 0.5 0.4 0.3 0.2 0.1 0

ACL = anterior cruciate ligament; IT = iliotibial; ROM = range of motion.

positive findings with the pivot shift are associated with an ALRI, the test also has a high positive predictive value for diagnosing an ACL sprain. A positive pivot shift almost always indicates damage to the ACL.[66,84,113] The **jerk test** is a variant of the pivot-shift test, but determines subluxation and reduction as the knee goes from flexion into extension (see Special Test 10-7). Drawer-type pivot shift tests are more sensitive than other rotational tests of the knee because they can be administered without significantly increasing pain and muscle spasm.[84]

*** Practical Evidence**

In consolidating the evidence of examination techniques for the anterior cruciate ligament, a positive pivot shift is the most predictive of an ACL tear and a negative Lachman's is most predictive in ruling out a rupture.[57,114]

During the **Slocum ALRI test**, the weight of the patient's limb is used to fixate the femur while the knee is flexed and a simultaneous valgus force is applied (Special Test 10-8). As the knee reaches 30 to 50 degrees of flexion, a subluxation of the tibia is reduced. This test is not as sensitive as the lateral pivot shift but is useful when dealing with large or heavy patients.

The **flexion–rotation drawer test** (FRD) involves the stabilization of the tibia, resulting in the relative subluxation of the femur (Special Test 10-9). In the presence of ALRI, lifting and supporting the distal lower leg causes the femur to displace posteriorly and rotate externally. The test then identifies the subsequent reduction of the femur relative to the tibia.

Anteromedial rotatory instability

O'Donohue described a triad injury involving the ACL, MCL, and medial meniscus, resulting in AMRI. Recently this definition has been revised, with the lateral meniscus being involved in this type of injury more frequently than the medial one.[115] As described in the ALRI section, the variants of the Slocum drawer test and the crossover test may be used to determine the presence of AMRI. In addition, isolated tests for ACL and MCL insufficiency yield positive test results.

Posterolateral corner injuries

While a purely varus force can injure the LCL, a combined mechanism of knee hyperextension and varus stress or hyperextension and external tibial rotation can result in trauma to the structures of the posterolateral corner of the knee. The resulting tissue damage allows the lateral tibial plateau to externally rotate around a medially-shifted axis, causing a posterior subluxation relative to the femur.[6] The greater the number of structures involved, including the ACL or PCL, the more significant the resulting instability (Table 10-6).

Posterolateral corner injuries are particularly difficult to evaluate in the acute setting and frequently require general anesthesia to produce the most accurate results (Examination Findings 10-5).[6,116] Because isolated injuries to the posterolateral corner are rare or nonexistent, injury to the ACL and PCL must also be ruled out.[5]

Table 10-6 Posterolateral Corner Instabilities Relative to Injured Tissues[5]

Loss of Integrity in these Tissues	Resulting Instability
LCL and Posterolateral Complex	Slight increase posterior tibial translation at all angles of flexion Increase in external rotation with posterior force at all angles Increased varus rotation at 30° of flexion
PCL, LCL, Posterolateral Complex	Increased posterior translation at all angles of flexion Increased varus rotation in response to varus force, especially at 60° of flexion Increased external rotation

LCL = lateral collateral ligament; PCL = posterior cruciate ligament.

Posterolateral rotatory instability involves the anterior displacement of the lateral femoral condyle relative to the tibia (the tibia externally rotating relative to the femur). The amount of external tibial rotation varies greatly from person to person and increases with the amount of knee flexion.[117] This motion is produced when the axis of rotation shifts medially toward the medial meniscus.

The patient often reports a history of external tibial rotation or knee hyperextension and describes knee instability. Pain is localized to the posterolateral aspect of the knee, but tension on the medial structures and the change in the rotational axis may produce pain in the medial knee.[118] The patient may describe the sensation of the knee's giving way during activity or static stance. The patient may respond favorably to heel lifts or high-heeled shoes that prevent the knee from fully extending during gait.[6] To prevent subluxation, the tibia may be maintained in internal rotation during gait.

Pain and instability make participation in strenuous activities difficult or impossible. Swelling forms rapidly and the lack of contained edema strongly suggests a complete posterolateral corner injury.[116]

Non–weight-bearing ROM is not affected. In most cases the patient will be unable to bear weight in the presence of acute posterolateral corner injury. With time and as swelling diminishes, the tibia externally rotates on the femur when the knee is extended, resulting in a varus thrust or hyperextended varus thrust of the involved leg during gait.[5]

Several other special tests have been documented to identify trauma to the posterolateral corner of the knee and/or PLRI. These techniques are based on replicating the subluxation and/or reduction of the tibia on the femur. Those tests that reproduce tibial subluxation are the

Special Test 10-8
Slocum Anterolateral Rotatory Instability (ALRI) Test

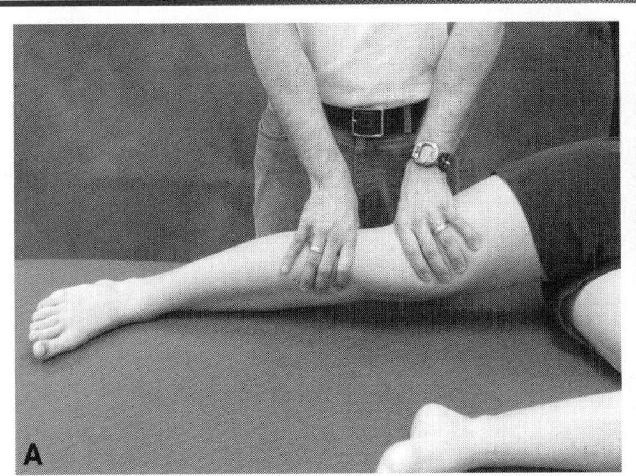

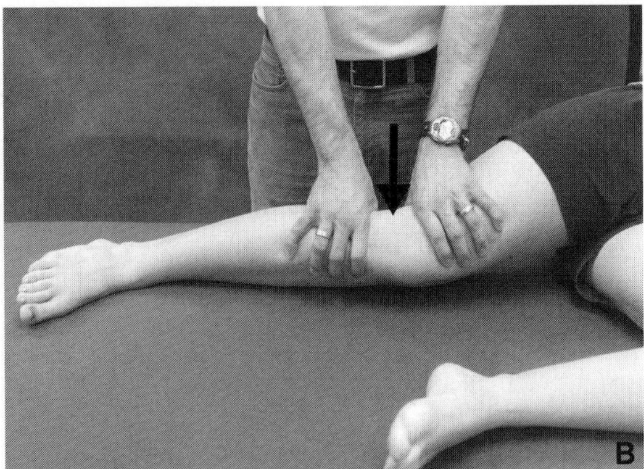

A modification of the valgus stress test, the Slocum ALRI accentuates the amount of internal tibial rotation, causing the tibial plateau to subluxate.

Patient Position	**(A)** Lying on the uninvolved side The uninvolved leg is flexed at the hip and knee, positioning it anterior to the involved extremity. The involved hip is externally rotated. The involved leg is extended with the medial aspect of the foot resting against the table to provide stability.
Position of Examiner	Standing behind the patient, grasping the knee on the distal aspect of the femur and the proximal fibula
Evaluative Procedure	A valgus force is placed on the knee, causing it to move into 30°–50° of flexion **(B)**.
Positive Test	An appreciable "clunk" or instability as the lateral tibial plateau subluxates or pain or instability is reported.
Implications	Tear of the ACL, LCL, anterolateral capsule, arcuate ligament complex, biceps femoris tendon and/or IT band
Comments	Muscle guarding can produce false-negative results. This test should be performed with caution and, if performed, should be done so only at the end of the examination.
Evidence	Inconclusive or absent in the literature

ACL = anterior cruciate ligament; IT = iliotibial; LCL = lateral cruciate ligament.

external rotation (Dial) test (Special Test 10-10),[119,120] **external rotation recurvatum test** (Special Test 10-11), and the **posterolateral drawer test** (Special Test 10-12). The **reverse-pivot shift** (Special Test 10-13) and **dynamic posterior shift test** (Special Test 10-14) cause reduction of a subluxated tibia.

Posterolateral corner injuries are usually managed surgically. Reconstruction using an allograft technique has demonstrated improved outcomes over a primary repair.[12]

Meniscal Tears

Acute meniscal tears result from rotation and flexion of the knee, impinging the menisci between the articular condyles of the tibia and femur. Because of its greater mobility, the lateral meniscus may develop tears secondary to repeated stress, presenting with an insidious onset. Historically, the majority of meniscal tears were believed to involve the medial meniscus. However, contemporary research has reversed this thought.[123,124] Many lateral meniscal tears, often asymptomatic, are associated with ACL sprains. Improved soft tissue imaging, such as the MRI, is now detecting lateral meniscal tears that once may have gone undetected (Examination Findings 10-6).

Classic symptoms of meniscal tears involve "locking" or "clicking" (or both) in the knee, pain along the joint line, and the knee giving way during activity. Locking can occur secondary to a tear or subluxation (hypermobility) of the posterior horn of the medial or lateral meniscus.[37] Patients may describe a rotational mechanism combined with flexion and a valgus or varus stress. Pain may not be described if the tear occurs in the avascular zone of the

Special Test 10-9
Flexion–Rotation Drawer Test for Anterolateral Rotatory Instability

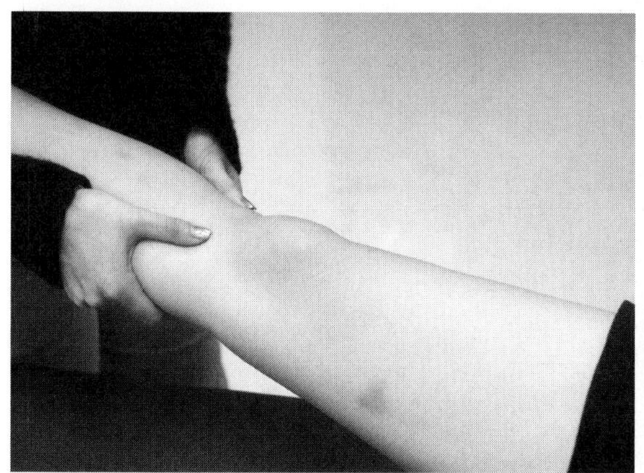

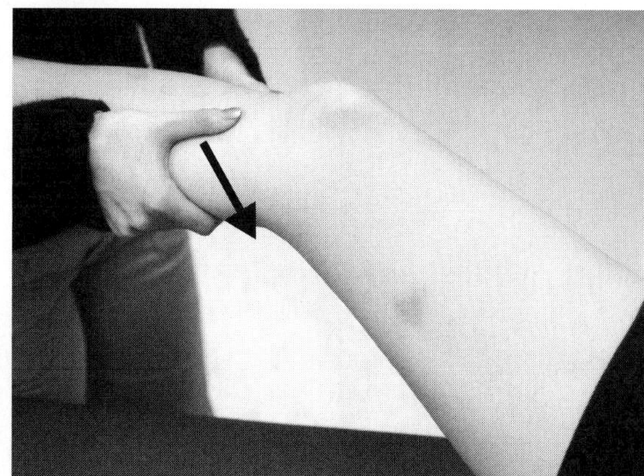

The flexion–rotation drawer replicates the femur relocating itself on the tibia as seen in a closed kinetic chain.

Patient Position	Lying supine The clinician lifts the calf and ankle so that the knee is flexed to approximately 25°. Heavier patients may require that the tibia be supported between the examiner's arm and torso.
Position of Examiner	Standing lateral and distal to the involved knee
Evaluative Procedure	The tibia is depressed posteriorly to the femur.
Positive Test	The femur is relocating itself on the tibia by moving anteriorly and internally, rotating on the tibia.
Implications	Tears of the ACL, LCL, anterolateral capsule, arcuate ligament complex, biceps femoris tendon.
Modification	A valgus stress and axial compression along the tibial shaft can be applied as the knee is slowly flexed.
Evidence	Inconclusive or absent in the literature

ACL = anterior cruciate ligament; IT = iliotibial; LCL = lateral cruciate ligament.

meniscus. Meniscal lesions may mimic the symptoms of patellofemoral dysfunction. Chapter 11 discusses the differential diagnosis between these two conditions.

Two evaluative tests, **McMurray's test** (Special Test 10-15) and **Apley's compression and distraction test** (Special Test 10-16), are frequently used to determine the presence of meniscal tears although their clinical usefulness is debatable because of the degree of inaccuracy when compared to the gold standard of MRI or arthroscopy. The McMurray's test was originally intended to identify tears in the posterior horn of the meniscus. Most clinical research has assessed its ability to identify lesions to any part of the meniscus, possibly explaining its limited clinical value.[125]

The **Thessaly test**, a dynamic, weight-bearing procedure has reported high predictive values for identifying meniscal tears (Special Test 10-17).[122] The absence of physical examination findings essentially rules out meniscal pathology, more so for the medial meniscus than the lateral meniscus.[126]

Although joint line pain is a more accurate predictor of a meniscal tear than either the McMurray's test or Apley's compression test, no single finding, or combination of signs, symptoms, and findings, reliably detects meniscal injury.[127] The patient's functional status, combined with the associated signs and symptoms, may be the best criteria for determining trauma to these structures and disability caused by the injury. The summation of physical examination findings for diagnosing meniscal injuries have a positive likelihood ratio of 2.5 to 9.5, adding a moderate amount of confidence that positive findings rule in the clinical diagnosis. Negative findings decrease the likelihood that a meniscal lesion is present by a small to moderate amount (negative likelihood ratio of 0.15 to 0.32).[34]

The types of meniscal tears are based on the orientation and etiology of the defect (Fig. 10-23). Tearing can occur as the result of excessive forces being placed on healthy tissues or otherwise normal forces being exerted on a degenerating meniscus. Degenerative tears are most prevalent in

Examination Findings 10-5
Posterolateral Rotatory Instability

Examination Segment	Clinical Findings
History	***Onset:*** Most have an acute onset, although chronic cases are possible. ***Pain characteristics:*** Along the posterolateral knee and popliteal area Chronic conditions may produce medial joint line pain. ***Other symptoms:*** Sensation of the knee "giving way" ***Mechanism:*** Posterolaterally directed blow to the medial tibia while the knee is in extension, producing hyperextension, rotation, and varus force Noncontact knee hyperextension and varus force Noncontact knee hyperextension and external tibial rotation ***Predisposing conditions:*** PCL, LCL sprain Genu varum [13] Tibiofemoral dislocation
Inspection	Swelling of the posterolateral knee Swelling possibly more diffuse because of tearing in the capsule Possible hyperextension and/or varus alignment of the involved knee when weight bearing The tibia may be held in internal rotation during gait.[6]
Palpation	Tenderness and swelling possible along the posterolateral capsule, lateral knee, and popliteal fossa A palpable defect may be felt in the biceps femoris tendon.[116]
Joint and Muscle Function Assessment	***AROM:*** Acutely, normal ROM; pain and restrictions possible as the knee nears full flexion Motions may be inhibited by pain especially as the knee moves back into a flexed position ***MMT:*** Knee flexion with the tibia internally rotated, making the popliteus more active Biceps femoris (rule out a secondary tear to the tendon) ***PROM:*** Pain produced as the knee nears 90° of flexion and with hyperextension

Joint Stability Tests	***Stress tests:*** Varus stress test at 0°: PLC, ACL, PCL Varus stress test at 30°: Isolated LCL injury Lachman's test Anterior drawer Alternate Lachman test Posterior drawer at 30° and 90° ***Joint play:*** Anterior glide of the tibia on the femur is assessed using the anterior drawer test. Posterior glide of the tibia is assessed using the posterior drawer test.[83]
Special Tests	Godfrey's sign Pivot shift External rotation test (Dial test) Posterolateral drawer test External rotation recurvatum test
Neurologic Screening	The peroneal nerve may become secondarily involved, resulting in paresthesia along the lateral leg and foot.[20] Manual muscle tests of the tibialis anterior and extensor hallicus longus may be indicated to rule out peroneal nerve trauma.
Vascular Screening	Required after suspected posterolateral dislocation (see p. 332)
Functional Assessment	Possible varus thrust or hyperextension varus thrust during gait[5,6] Complaints of lateral posterior knee instability Hyperextension results in disability and instability when ascending or descending stairs or walking on inclines[5]
Imaging Techniques	T1-weighted coronal oblique MR images can help identify trauma to the posterolateral structures including the fibular head. MRI is also used to rule out bone contusions and trauma to the LCL. Radiographs may be ordered to rule out an avulsion fracture of the capsule from the lateral tibial plateau (segond fracture), avulsion fracture of the fibular head, or an avulsion fracture of Gerdy's tubercle.[5] Stress radiographs will indicate a widening of the lateral joint line.
Differential Diagnosis	Avulsion fracture of the fibular head; lateral meniscus tear; ACL sprain; LCL sprain; PCL sprain; tibiofemoral dislocation; physeal fracture
Comments	Posterolateral instability is typically found concurrently with a tear of the anterior or posterior cruciate ligament.

ACL = anterior cruciate ligament; AROM = active range of motion; LCL = lateral collateral ligament; MR = magnetic resonance; MMT = manual muscle test; PCL = posterior cruciate ligament; PLC = posterolateral corner; PROM = passive range of motion; ROM = range of motion.

the posterior horn. **Meniscal cysts** are frequently associated with longitudinal meniscal tears and become symptomatic because of localized swelling (Fig. 10-24).[23] After a longitudinal tear along the periphery of the meniscus, breaches are formed in the joint capsule that fills with synovial fluid. Meniscal cysts, typically painless and immobile, are often found coincidentally during MRI scanning or arthroscopic examination.[43]

Most commonly involving the lateral meniscus, a **discoid meniscus** has increased thickness and covers a larger area of the tibia.[25] The size, shape, and stability of a discoid meniscus can cause instability leading to catching or locking during movement ("snapping knee syndrome"). A Wrisberg type discoid meniscus has only the ligament of Wrisberg as a posterior stabilizer, potentially leading to an unstable fixation of the meniscus on the tibia and creating locking or catching of the knee during flexion and extension as the meniscus dislocates.[37]

Patients who clinically present with locking or catching of the knee and demonstrate decreased range of motion with associated pain and swelling may require surgical correction of the torn meniscus.[23] Standard surgical options include a partial meniscectomy where only the torn fragment is removed or meniscal repair where tears in the vascular portion of the meniscus are fixated using sutures, staples, or anchors, although experimental procedures involving grafts and adhesives are being performed. Total meniscectomies where the entire meniscus is removed are rarely performed.[128]

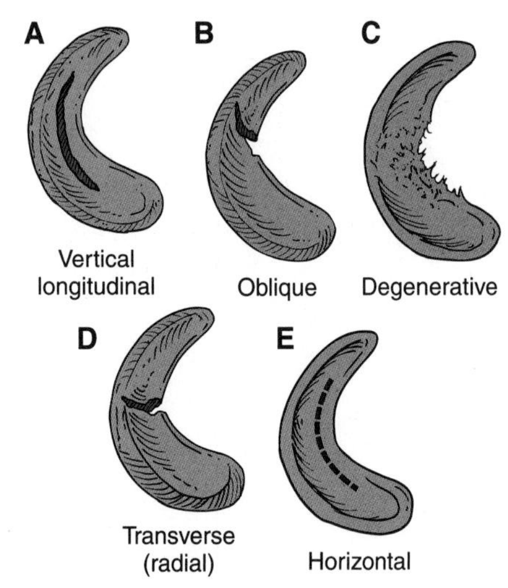

FIGURE 10-23 ■ Classifications of meniscal tears.

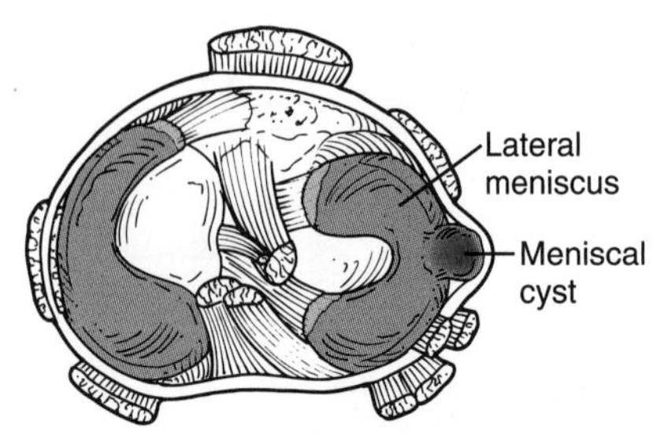

FIGURE 10-24 ■ Meniscal cysts.

Osteochondral Lesions

Osteochondral lesions are used to describe a series of disorders including osteochondral defects and osteochondritis desiccans that involve a joint's articular cartilage and underlying subchondral bone.[129] Osteochondral defects (OCDs) are fractures of the articular cartilage and underlying bone that are typically caused by compressive and shear forces (Fig. 10-25). Eighty percent of knee OCDs involve the medial femoral condyle.[130] The lateral femoral condyle, tibial articulating surface, and patella are also susceptible to OCDs.[131] Males are affected three times more frequently than females.[131]

The signs and symptoms of OCDs are often masked by those of a concurrent injury, although the OCD itself is often asymptomatic (Examination Findings 10-7). Symptomatic OCDs are characterized by complaints of diffuse pain within the knee, a "locking" sensation, and the knee's giving way. A "clunking" sensation may also be described. Pain is increased during weight-bearing activities. In addition, an increase in pain and a decrease in strength are noted in closed kinetic chain activities relative to open chain motions. **Wilson's test** can be used as a clinical evaluation tool for the presence of OCDs on the knee's articular surface (Special Test 10-18). A definitive diagnosis must be made with radiographic examination or MRI.

Osteochondral defects can be managed conservatively, with the outcome largely dependent on the location of the defect with respect to the weight-bearing surface. Activity is modified to reduce painful stresses placed on the knee. When conservative treatment fails, surgical repair of the defect may be required. Surgical intervention can include simple débridement or procedures such as abrasion arthroplasty, subchondral drilling, or microfracture techniques to stimulate fibrocartilage formation in the defect. Newer surgical interventions include autogenous

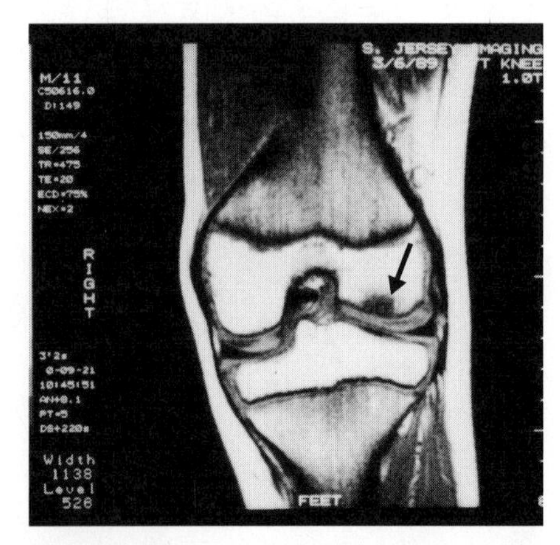

FIGURE 10-25 ■ MRI of an osteochondral defect. The arrow points to an OCD on the lateral femoral condyle.

Special Test 10-10
External Rotation Test (Dial Test) for Posterolateral Knee Instability

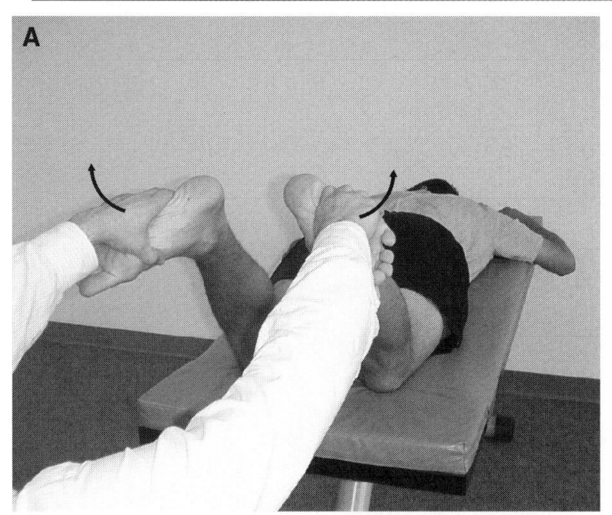

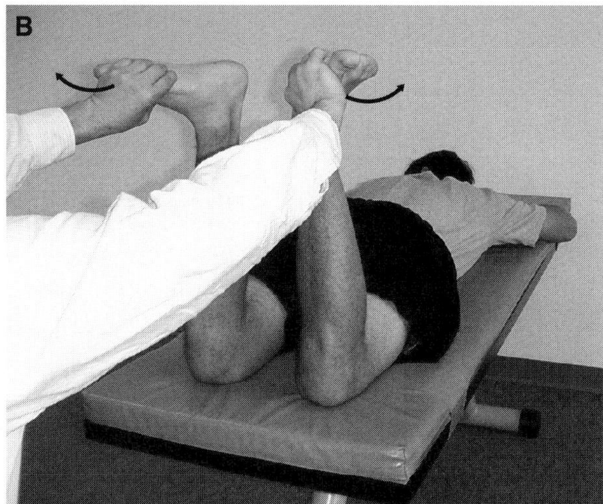

The external rotation test (Dial test) for posterolateral knee instability at 30° of the knee flexion **(A)** and at 90° of knee flexion **(B)**.

Patient Position	Prone or supine
Position of Examiner	Standing at the patient's feet
Evaluative Procedure	The knee is flexed to 30°. Using the medial border of the foot as a point of reference, the examiner forcefully externally rotates the patient's lower leg. The position of external rotation of the foot relative to the femur is assessed and compared with the opposite extremity. The knee is then flexed to 90° and the test repeated. Care must be taken to keep the knees together during the examination.[21]
Positive Test	An increase of external rotation greater than 10° compared with the opposite side[20,119]
Implications	Difference at 30° of knee flexion but not at 90°: Injury isolated to the posterolateral corner of the knee Difference at 30° and 90° of knee flexion: Trauma to the PCL, posterolateral knee structures, and the posterolateral corner Difference at 90° of knee flexion but not at 30°: Isolated PCL sprain
Modification	This test can also be performed with the patient in the supine position. A goniometer can be used to quantify the amount of external rotation.[5]
Comments	Normal variations for rotation are expected. The results of one extremity must be compared with those of the opposite leg.
Evidence	Inconclusive or absent in the literature

PCL = posterior cruciate ligament.

Special Test 10-11
External Rotation Recurvatum Test

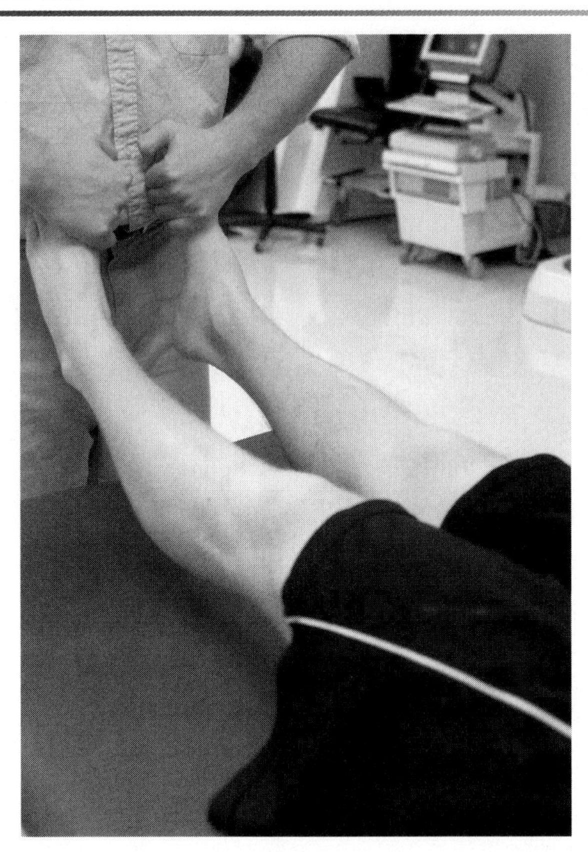

This test is a gross evaluation of the amount of external femoral rotation that occurs when the knees are hyperextended.[121]

Patient Position	Lying supine.
Position of Examiner	Standing at the patient's feet grasping the great toes/distal midfoot
Evaluative Procedure	The examiner lifts the patient's legs approximately 12 inches off the table. Observe the bilateral alignment of the two knees.
Positive Test	A marked difference in hyperextension, external femoral rotation, and varus alignment between the two knees
Implications	Posterolateral corner trauma PCL sprain Posterolateral rotatory instability
Modification	While holding the heel, the examiner flexes the knee 40°. The opposite hand grasps the posterolateral aspect of the knee. The examiner passively extends the knee while noting external rotation and hyperextension relative to the opposite extremity.
Evidence	Positive likelihood ratio Not Useful — Useful Very Small, Small, Moderate, Large 30 0 1 2 3 4 5 6 7 8 9 10 Negative likelihood ratio Not Useful — Useful Very Small, Small, Moderate, Large 1.0 0.9 0.8 0.7 0.6 0.5 0.4 0.3 0.2 0.1 0

Special Test 10-12
Posterolateral/Posteromedial Drawer Test

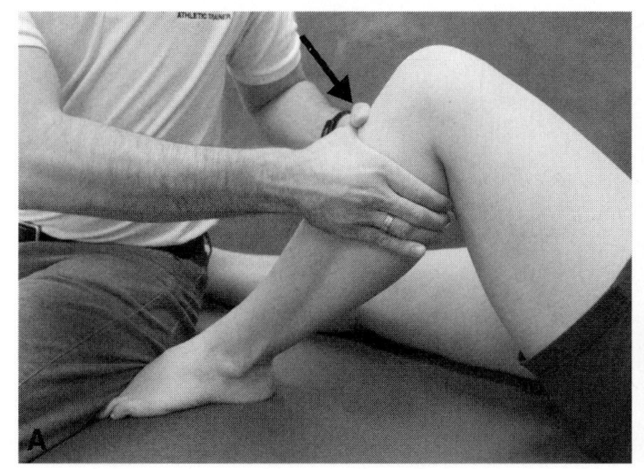

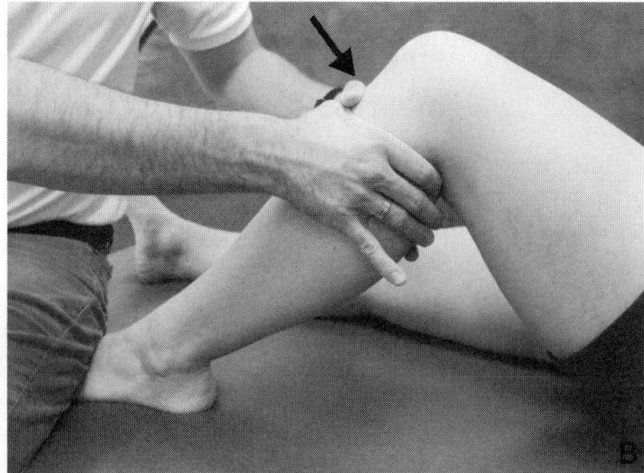

A modification of the posterior drawer test to identify lesions to the posterolateral corner of the knee.[121]

Patient Position	Supine with the hip flexed to 45° and the knee flexed to 80° **(A)** The tibia is externally rotated 15° (posterolateral test). **(B)** The tibia is internally rotated 15° (posteromedial test).
Position of Examiner	Sitting on the foot of the limb being tested. The hands grasp the proximal tibia.
Evaluative Procedure	A posterior force is applied to the proximal tibia.
Positive Test	Increased external rotation of the lateral (posterolateral) or medial (posteromedial) tibial condyle relative to the lateral femoral condyle relative to the uninvolved side
Implications	**(A)** Tibia externally rotated 15° (posterolateral test) Trauma to the posterolateral corner and PCL Possible posterolateral rotatory instability **(B)** Tibia internally rotated 15° (posteromedial test) PCL tear, oblique ligament, MCL, posteromedial capsule, semimembranosus
Modification	The posterolateral drawer test is sometimes performed with the knee flexed to 90°. This test can be performed with the patient sitting with the knees off the edge of the table.
Comments	Excessive tibial rotation can produce false-negative results, especially in the presence of a meniscal tear.
Evidence	***Posterolateral drawer test:*** Inconclusive or absent in the literature ***Posteromedial drawer test:*** Inconclusive or absent in the literature.

PCL = posterior cruciate ligament.

chondrocyte transplantation, or osteoarticular transplantation (OATs procedure). The goals of these techniques are to place newly grown articular cartilage within the defect or to transplant healthy articular cartilage from one area of the knee into the defect.[132]

After surgery, a 4- to 6-week period of protected weight-bearing activities may be necessary to reduce shearing stresses on the implant. Aquatic therapy can be used in the early active ROM period to provide ROM and strengthening while decreasing weight-bearing stresses through the joint. After the early protection phase of rehabilitation, strength, ROM, and proprioceptive exercises are advanced to restore normal function to the knee.

Iliotibial Band Friction Syndrome

Resulting from friction between the IT band and the lateral femoral epicondyle, IT band friction syndrome tends to occur in athletes who are participating in sports that require repeated knee flexion and extension, such as

Special Test 10-13
Reverse Pivot-Shift Test

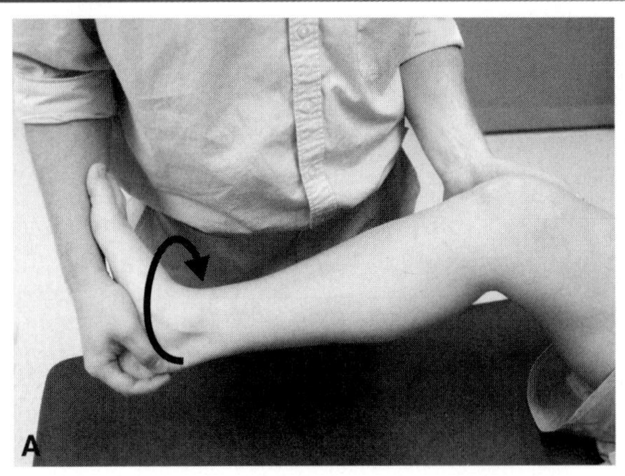

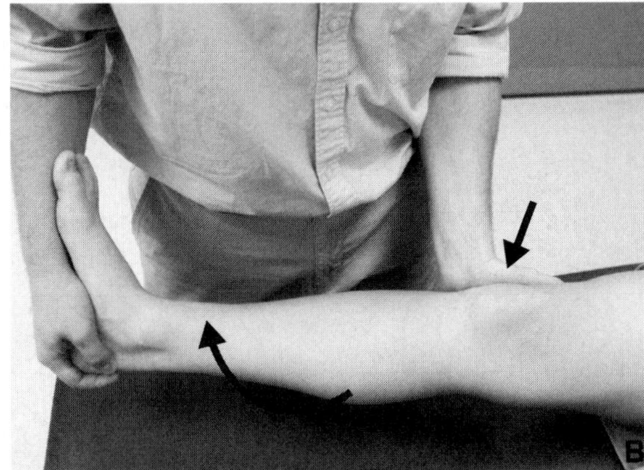

The reverse pivot-shift test is used to identify trauma to the PCL or posterolateral corner of the knee.[20]

Patient Position	Supine
Position of Examiner	Standing to the side of the involved leg
Evaluative Procedure	**(A)** The examiner flexes the knee and externally rotates the tibia of the involved leg. **(B)** The patient's knee is passively extended while a valgus stress is applied to the knee.
Positive Test	Appreciable reduction ("clunk") of the tibia on the femur
Implications	Posterolateral rotatory instability and/or trauma to the posterolateral corner
Comments	This test may be positive in 35% of knees examined under anesthesia.[6,20]
Evidence	Inconclusive or absent in the literature

running, rowing, and cycling.[134] A bursa located between the distal IT band and the lateral femoral epicondyle becomes inflamed secondary to overuse. This condition may progress to involve periostitis of the epicondyle (Examination Findings 10-8). The bursa cushioning the IT band from the lateral femoral epicondyle is not a primary bursa, but rather, a continuation of the knee joint capsule.[135,136]

Several factors may predispose IT band friction syndrome.[133,137–139] Genu varum may project the lateral femoral condyle laterally, increasing the friction as the IT band passes over it. Pronated feet, leg length differences, a lateral heel strike, and other conditions resulting in internal tibial rotation alter the angle at which the IT band approaches its attachment on Gerdy's tubercle, increasing pressure at the lateral femoral epicondyle. Activities that cause overstriding, such as running down hill may also increase tension between the distal IT band and the lateral femoral epicondyle. Finally, a large lateral femoral epicondyle may result in increased irritation of the IT band as it passes over the epicondyle.

The patient typically describes a "burning" pain over the lateral femoral condyle that may radiate distally. Point tenderness is displayed at the point where the IT band passes over the epicondyle. Pain may be described during manual muscle testing of the hamstrings or quadriceps as the knee approaches 30 degrees of flexion. However, no pain may be described during active ROM (AROM) or passive ROM (PROM) testing. The presence of IT band friction syndrome may be confirmed through the **Noble compression test** as the IT band passes over the lateral femoral condyle (Special Test 10-19). Iliotibial band tightness can be identified by the **Ober's test** (Special Test 10-20).

The initial treatment approach for IT band friction syndrome is to correct any biomechanical faults such as the use of orthotics to correct hyperpronation or alterations in training during athletic activities. The use of nonsteroidal antiinflammatory medication and local modalities to decrease the inflammation at the bursa and IT band as it passes over the lateral epicondyle are usually helpful. Stretching of the tensor fascia latae, the IT band,

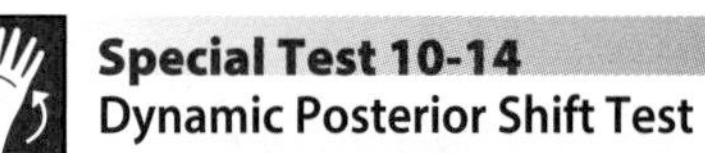

Special Test 10-14
Dynamic Posterior Shift Test

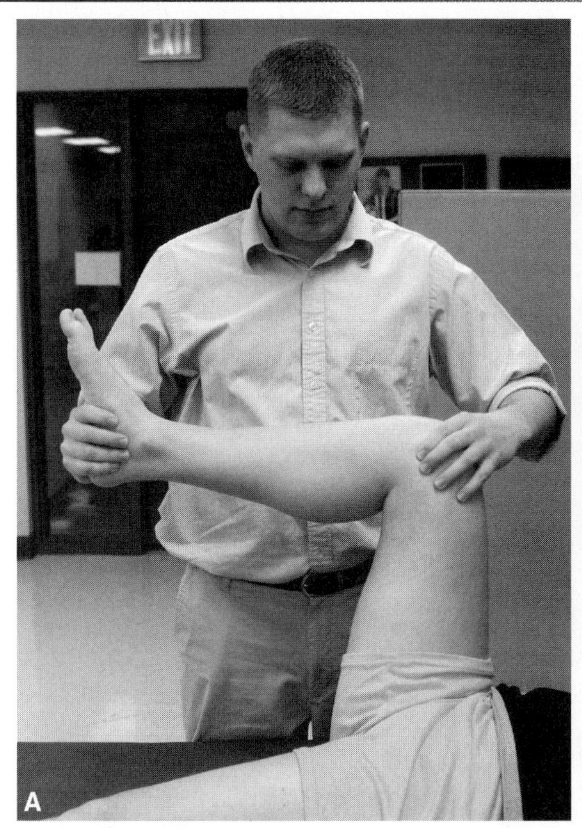

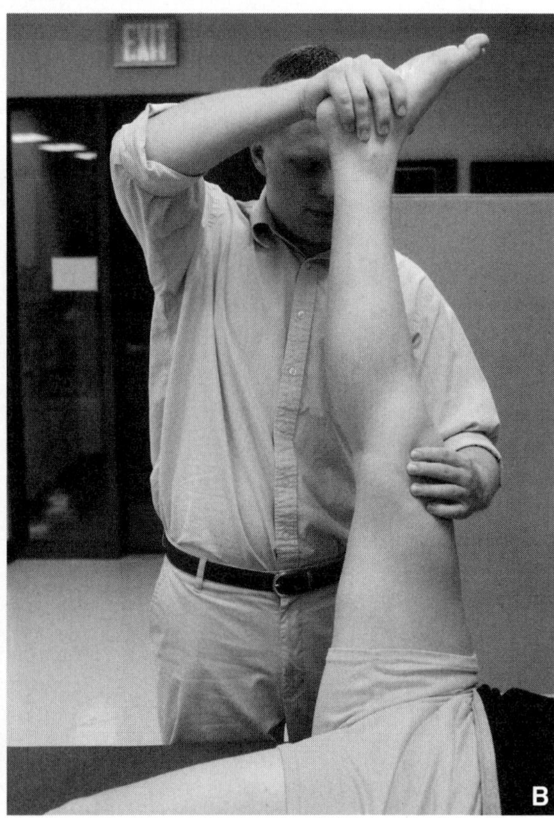

In the presence of posterolateral instability, the lateral tibial plateau is subluxed during knee flexion and reduces during knee extension.[20]

Patient Position	Supine
Position of Examiner	Standing on the side being tested
Evaluative Procedure	**(A)** The examiner passively flexes the patient's hip and knee to 90°. **(B)** The knee is then passively extended.
Positive Test	A "clunk" or "jerk" as the knee nears full extension, representing the subluxated tibia reducing on the femur
Implications	Posterolateral instability
Comments	During knee flexion, the tibia is posteriorly subluxated on the femur. Relocation is noted by an appreciable clunk during extension.[104]
Evidence	Inconclusive or absent in the literature

Special Test 10-15
McMurray's Test for Meniscal Lesions

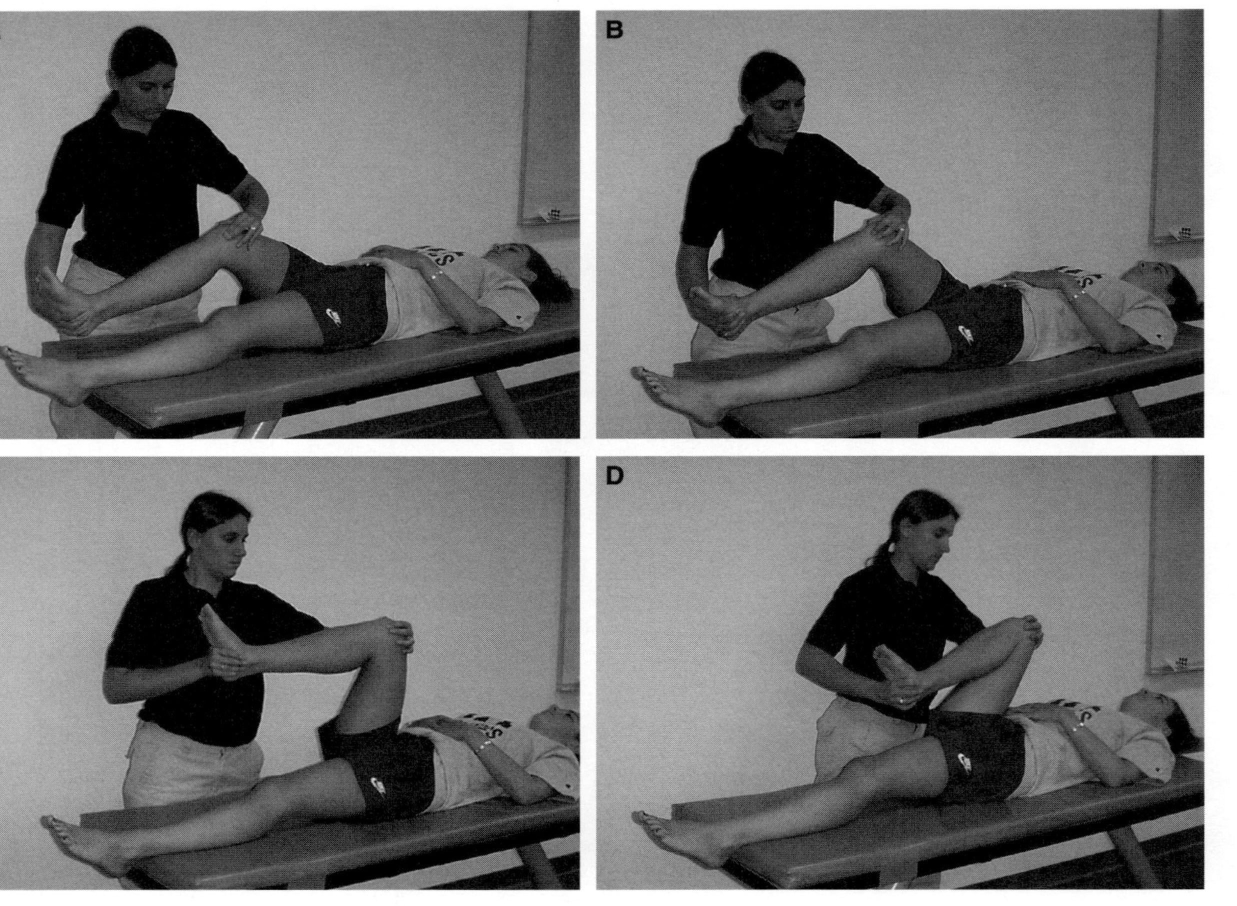

The McMurray's test aims to impinge the meniscus, especially the posterior horns, between the tibia and femur.

Patient Position	Lying supine
Position of Examiner	Standing lateral and distal to the involved knee One hand supports the lower leg while the thumb and index finger of the opposite hand is positioned in the anteromedial and anterolateral joint line on either side of the patellar tendon **(A)**.

Evaluative Procedure	**(B) Pass one:** With the tibia maintained in its neutral position, a valgus stress is applied while the knee is flexed through its available ROM. A varus stress is then applied as the knee is returned to full extension. **(C) Pass two:** The examiner internally rotates the tibia and applies a valgus stress while the knee is flexed through its available ROM. A varus stress is then applied as the knee is returned to full extension. **(D) Pass three:** With the tibia externally rotated, the examiner applies a valgus stress while the knee is flexed through its available ROM. A varus stress is then applied as the knee is returned to full extension.
Positive Test	A popping, clicking, or locking of the knee; pain emanating from the menisci; or a sensation similar to that experienced during ambulation
Implications	A meniscal tear on the side of the reported symptoms
Modification	Multiple modifications have been derived from the original test, including variations of additional varus and valgus stress and internally and externally rotating the tibia.
Comments	In acute injuries, the available ROM may not be sufficient to perform this test. Full flexion is required to isolate the posterior horns of the meniscus. Chondromalacia patellae or improper tracking of the patella may produce a click resembling that is associated with a meniscal tear, leading to false-positive results. Sensitivity is greater for lateral meniscus tears than the medial meniscus.[122] Different interpretations and methods of performing the test lead to widely varied opinions about the diagnostic usefulness of this test.
Evidence	Positive likelihood ratio 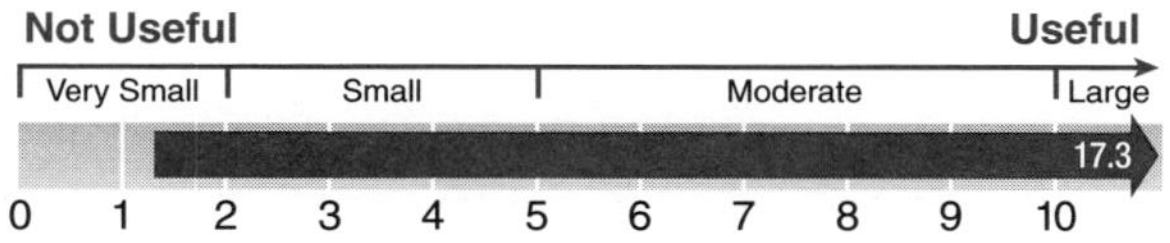 Not Useful — Useful Very Small / Small / Moderate / Large 17.3 0 1 2 3 4 5 6 7 8 9 10 Negative likelihood ratio 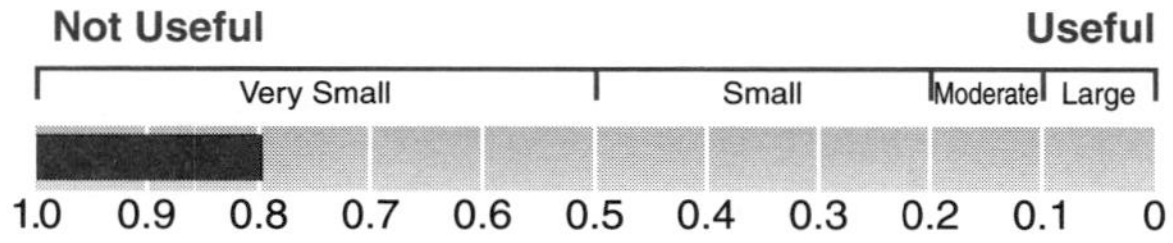 Not Useful — Useful Very Small / Small / Moderate / Large 1.0 0.9 0.8 0.7 0.6 0.5 0.4 0.3 0.2 0.1 0

ROM = range of motion.

Examination Findings 10-6
Meniscal Tears

Examination Segment	Clinical Findings
History	***Onset:*** Acute; patients with involving accumulated microtrauma often still present as having an acute onset. ***Pain characteristics:*** Along the medial or lateral joint line with possible posterior knee pain ***Other symptoms:*** The patient may report episodes of the knee "giving out." "Clicking" may be described with chronic meniscal lesions. Snapping or locking may be associated with a discoid meniscus[25,37] ***Mechanism:*** Tibial rotation, often in combination with knee flexion and/or a varus or valgus stress Hyperflexion impinges the posterior horns; hyperextension impinges the anterior horns. ***Predisposing conditions:*** Over time, repetitive motion can degrade the lateral meniscus.
Inspection	Inspection of a patient with an acutely torn meniscus may not present any conclusive initial findings. Over time, or in the case of a peripheral tear of the meniscus, swelling may be seen along the joint or in the popliteal fossa. Joint effusion may develop over 24–48 hours and may recur sporadically with irritation of the meniscus.[122] A torn meniscus may prevent the patient from fully extending the knee, thus carrying it in a flexed position.
Palpation	Possible pain and crepitus along the joint line A meniscal cyst, highly suggestive of a meniscal tear, may be palpable.[23]
Joint and Muscle Function Assessment	The ROM available may be limited owing to a mechanical block formed by a defect in the meniscus. ***AROM:*** Possible decrease in ROM A displaced longitudinal ("bucket handle") tear of the meniscus can present a mechanical block to extension.[23] Discoid menisci or other meniscal variants may cause blocks to motion and/or compensatory motion (e.g., increased external rotation) to obtain full extension or flexion.[25] Pain or locking is revealed as the torn portion of the meniscus passes beneath the femur's articular surface. ***MMT:*** Typically unremarkable. ***PROM:*** Pain is present near the extremes of flexion or extension. Apprehension may be experienced as the knee nears terminal extension if locking is caused by the meniscus' anterior horn.[37]
Joint Stability Tests	***Stress tests:*** The integrity of all the knee ligaments must be established. The presence of any ligamentous injury to the knee limits the ability to determine meniscal pathology during the clinical examination ***Joint play:*** Unremarkable
Special Tests	McMurray's Apley's compression Thessaly
Neurologic Screening	Within normal limits
Vascular Screening	Within normal limits
Functional Assessment	The patient may complain of clicking or locking during activity in the presence of a chronic tear.
Imaging Techniques	MR imaging can be used to identify the presence of a meniscal tear, but its value is debatable, showing approximately equal predictive results as the clinical examination.[23] A widened lateral joint space may be noted on radiographs in the presence of a discoid meniscus.[25]
Differential Diagnosis	Patellofemoral joint dysfunction, synovial plica irritation, osteochondral defect, instability
Comments	All suspected ACL and MCL injuries should be suspected of involving a meniscal tear until proven otherwise.

ACL = anterior cruciate ligament; AROM = active range of motion; MMT = manual muscle test; PCL = posterior cruciate ligament; PROM = passive range of motion; ROM = range of motion.

Special Test 10-16
Apley's Compression and Distraction Tests for Meniscal Lesions

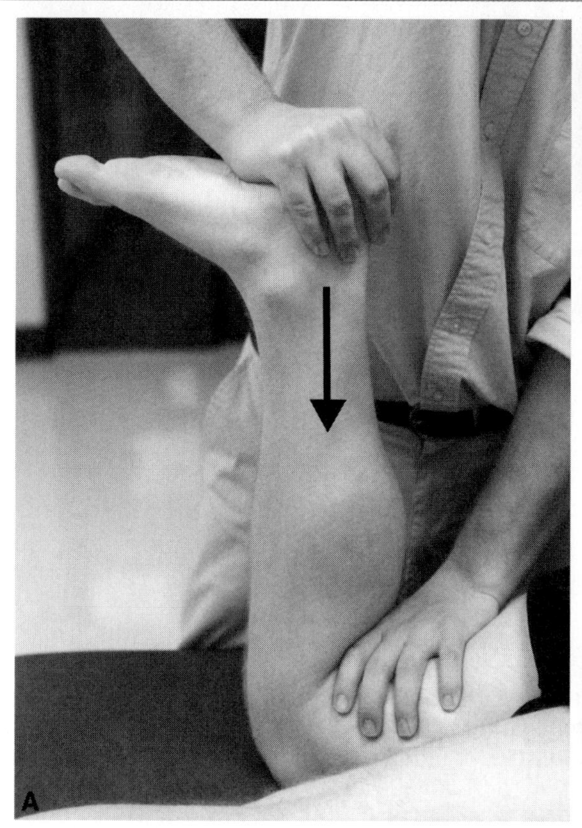

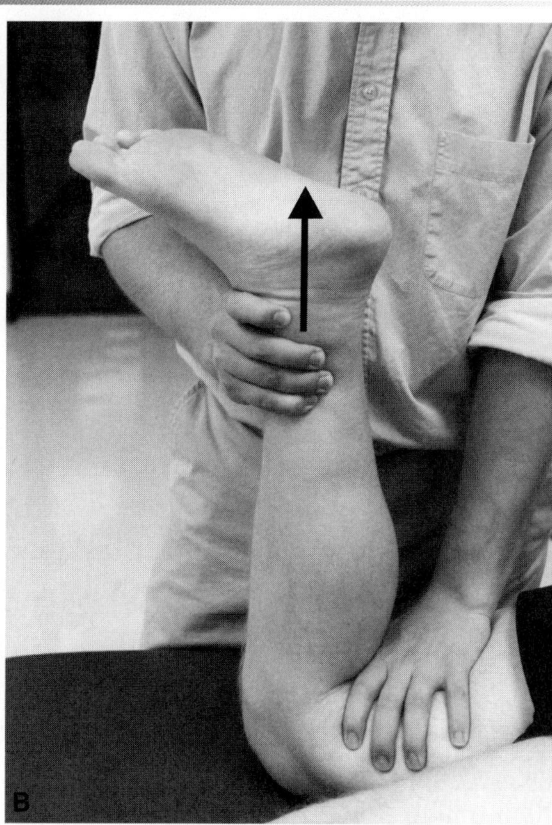

During the compression segment, pain may be caused by the menisci being caught between the tibia and femur **(A)**. During the distraction segment, the joint's ligaments are stressed **(B)**. Also, pain exhibited during compression should be reduced as the tibia is distracted from the femur.

Patient Position	Lying prone with knee flexed to 90°
Position of Examiner	Standing lateral to the involved side
Evaluative Procedure	**(A)** Compression test: The clinician applies pressure to the plantar aspect of the heel, applying an axial load to the tibia while simultaneously internally and externally rotating the tibia. **(B)** Distraction test: The clinician grasps the lower leg and stabilizes the knee proximal to the femoral condyles. The tibia is distracted away from the femur while internally and externally rotating the tibia.
Positive Test	Pain experienced during compression that is reduced or eliminated during distraction
Implications	Meniscal tear
Comments	90° of knee flexion is required to perform this test. Pain that is experienced only during distraction or during both compression and distraction may indicate trauma to the collateral ligaments, joint capsule, or cruciate ligaments.
Evidence	Positive likelihood ratio Not Useful — Useful Very Small / Small / Moderate / Large 58 0 1 2 3 4 5 6 7 8 9 10 Negative likelihood ratio Not Useful — Useful Very Small / Small / Moderate / Large 1.0 0.9 0.8 0.7 0.6 0.5 0.4 0.3 0.2 0.1 0

Special Test 10-17
Thessaly Test for Meniscal Tears

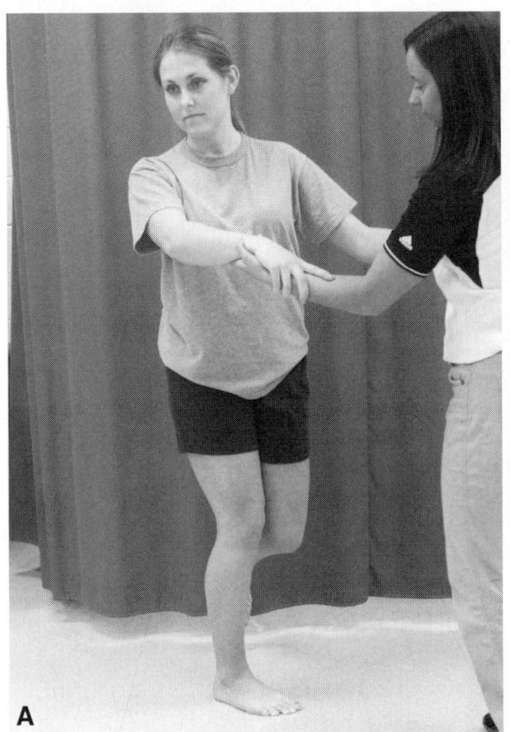

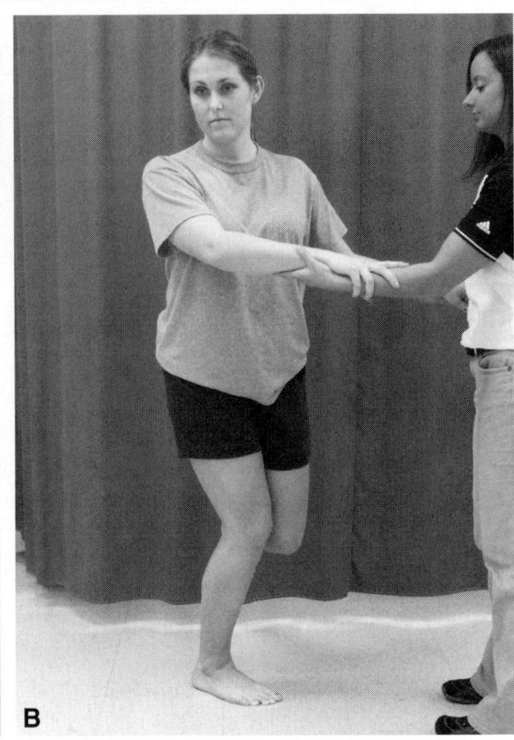

Performed weight-bearing and with femoral internal and external rotation, the Thessaly test is used to identify meniscal lesions. **(A)** The patient rotates on a fixed leg with the knee flexed to 5° and again **(B)** with the knee flexed to 20°.

Patient Position	Standing flatfooted on the involved leg The knee of the opposite leg is flexed to approximately 45°.
Position of Examiner	Standing in front of the patient, supporting the patient's arms
Evaluative Procedure	The uninvolved limb is tested first, allowing the patient to practice the maneuver. **Bout 1** The patient flexes the knee to 5°. The patient rotates the body to internally and externally rotate the femur on the tibia. Repeat three times. **Bout 2** The patient flexes the knee to 20°. The patient rotates the body to internally and externally rotate the femur on the tibia. Repeat three times.
Positive Test	Joint-line discomfort Complaints of "locking" or "catching"
Implications	A lesion of the medial or lateral meniscus, depending on the source of the pain and/or catching sensation
Evidence	Positive likelihood ratio* Not Useful — Useful Very Small / Small / Moderate / Large 22.25 – 30.67 0 1 2 3 4 5 6 7 8 9 10 Negative likelihood ratio* Not Useful — Useful Very Small / Small / Moderate / Large 1.0 0.9 0.8 0.7 0.6 0.5 0.4 0.3 0.2 0.1 0 *20° of flexion

Examination Findings 10-7
Osteochondral Lesions

Examination Segment	Clinical Findings
History	***Onset:*** Osteochondritis dissecans: Insidious Osteochondral defect: Acute or insidious ***Pain characteristics:*** Diffuse pain within the knee ***Other symptoms:*** Locking or catching may be described. Knee instability may be reported. ***Mechanism:*** Shear or rotational forces across the joint line Compressive force Osteochondritis dissecans may result from repetitive microtrauma. ***Predisposing conditions:*** Prior injury and/or repetitive stress may predispose the onset of osteochondritis dissecans; family history.
Inspection	Joint effusion may be noted. Quadriceps atrophy may be noted in chronic cases.
Palpation	Joint effusion
Joint and Muscle Function Assessment	***AROM:*** Normal range of motion for flexion and extension may be within normal limits when non–weight bearing, but decreased when weight bearing. ***MMT:*** Within normal limits Quadriceps MMT may reveal weakness in chronic cases. ***PROM:*** Within normal limits
Joint Stability Tests	***Stress tests:*** Stress tests may be positive with concurrent injury. ***Joint play:*** Not applicable
Special Tests	Wilson's test
Neurologic Screening	Within normal limits
Vascular Screening	Within normal limits
Functional Assessment	Pain is increased and strength is decreased when the involved extremity is weight bearing. Antalgic gait may be noted. Symptoms decrease with rest.
Imaging Techniques	AP and lateral radiographs of the knee and axial views of the patellofemoral joint CT or MRI can visualize the osteochondral defect.
Differential Diagnosis	Osteoarthritis, meniscal tear or cyst, patellofemoral joint dysfunction, tibial femoral epicondyle fracture
Comments	Osteochondral defects often occur concurrently to soft tissue trauma, especially ACL sprains.

ACL = anterior cruciate ligament; AP = anteroposterior; AROM = active range of motion; CT = computed tomography; MMT = manual muscle test; MRI = magnetic resonance imaging; PROM = passive range of motion.

Special Test 10-18
Wilson's Test for Osteochondral Defects of the Knee

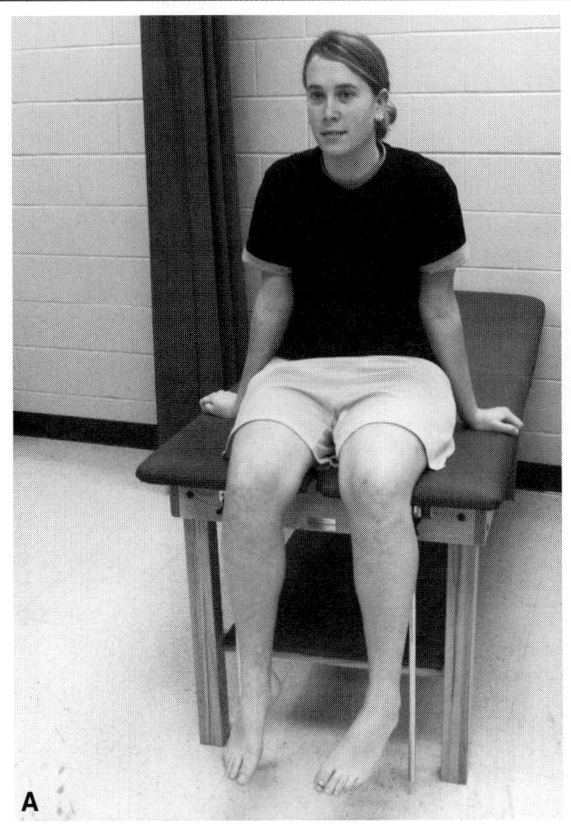

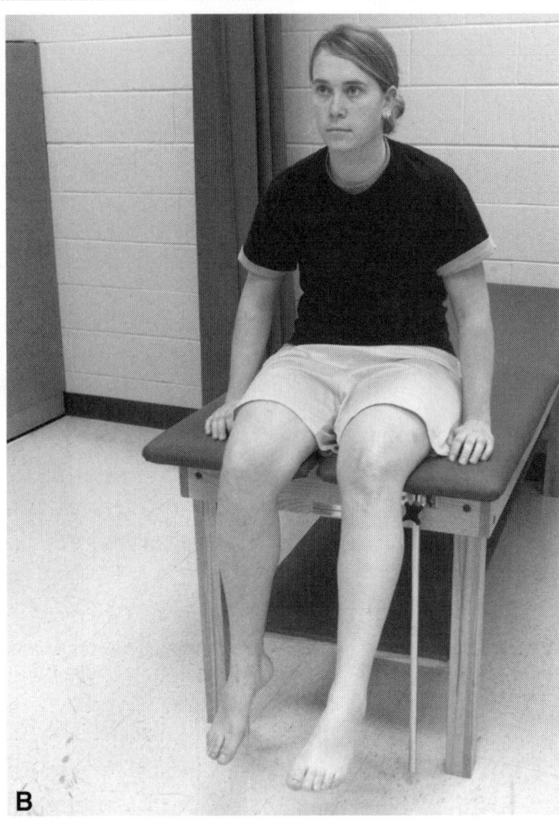

While the tibia is internally rotated, the patient extends the knee **(A)**. When pain is experienced, the patient externally rotates the tibia **(B)**. In the presence of some OCDs, pain is relieved during the external rotation.

Patient Position	Sitting with the knee flexed to 90°
Position of Examiner	In front of the patient to observe any reactions secondary to pain
Evaluative Procedure	**(A)** The patient actively extends the knee while maintaining the tibia in internal rotation. The patient is told to stop the motion and hold the knee in the position in which pain is experienced. **(B)** If pain is experienced, the patient is instructed to externally rotate the tibia while the knee is held at its present point of flexion.
Positive Test	Pain experienced during extension with internal tibial rotation that is relieved by externally rotating the tibia
Implications	OCD or osteochondritis dissecans on the intercondylar area of the medial femoral condyle
Evidence	Inconclusive or absent in the literature

OCD = osteochondral defect.

Examination Findings 10-8
Iliotibial Band Friction Syndrome

Examination Segment	Clinical Findings
History	***Onset:*** Insidious ***Pain characteristics:*** Pain over the lateral femoral condyle proximal to the joint line that may radiate distally; pain is increased when running downhill. ***Mechanism:*** Activities involving repeated knee flexion and extension ***Predisposing conditions:*** Tightness of the iliotibial band; genu varum, excessive pronation, leg-length discrepancy, excessive lateral heel strike[133]
Inspection	Genu varum Excessive pronation during gait; a lateral heel strike may be noted during observation of running and walking gait. Leg-length discrepancy
Palpation	In advanced cases, pain elicited over the lateral femoral condyle, about 2 cm above the joint line
Joint and Muscle Function Assessment	***AROM:*** Within normal limits Pain may be described as the knee passes 30° during flexion and extension (representing the point where the IT band shifts over the lateral femoral condyle). ***MMT:*** Tensor fascia latae: May be weak and/or painful (see p. 416). Often associated weakness of hip abductors/external rotators (see p. 426). ***PROM:*** Within normal limits
Joint Stability Tests	***Stress tests:*** None ***Joint play:*** Tightness of the lateral patellar restraints may be noted during medial patellar glide tests (see Joint Play 11-1 [patellar glide testing]).
Special Tests	Noble's compression test Ober's test
Neurologic Screening	Within normal limits
Vascular Screening	Within normal limits
Functional Assessment	The patient may demonstrate limited ability to control hip motion during a single leg squat. Pain or limitations may be described when decelerating gait, descending stairs, or walking down hills. Patient may avoid full knee extension during push-off phase of gait.
Imaging Techniques	Anteroposterior and lateral radiographs or CT scans may be ordered to identify enlargement of, or bony outgrowths from, the lateral femoral condyle.
Differential Diagnosis	Lateral meniscus tear; biceps femoris tendinopathy; patellofemoral dysfunction; popliteus tendinopathy
Comments	IT band tightness should be confirmed with Ober's test. IT band tightness may be noted on the opposite hip.[133]

AROM = active range of motion; IT = iliotibial; MMT = manual muscle test; PROM = passive range of motion; ROM = range of motion.

and any other tight musculature is also warranted. Proprioceptive hip and lower extremity exercises are useful in enhancing the dynamic control of foot pronation.[133] As with any lower extremity injury, the full return of strength to the leg is required to send the patient back to full pain-free activity.

Popliteus Tendinopathy

Popliteus tendinopathy arises secondary to other biomechanical changes in the knee or lower extremity or secondary to repetitive stress. The popliteus muscle is often injured in conjunction with other knee injuries.[141] Popliteus

Special Test 10-19
Noble's Compression Test for Iliotibial Band Friction Syndrome–Renne's Test

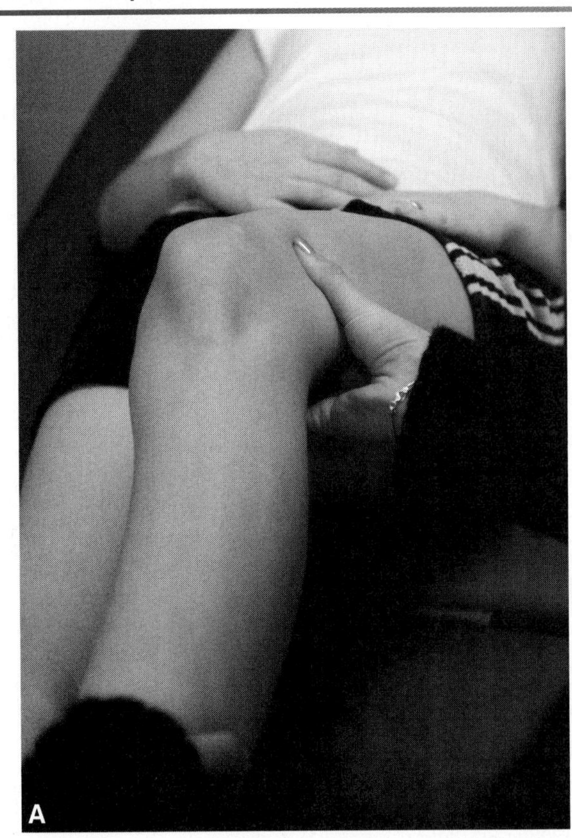

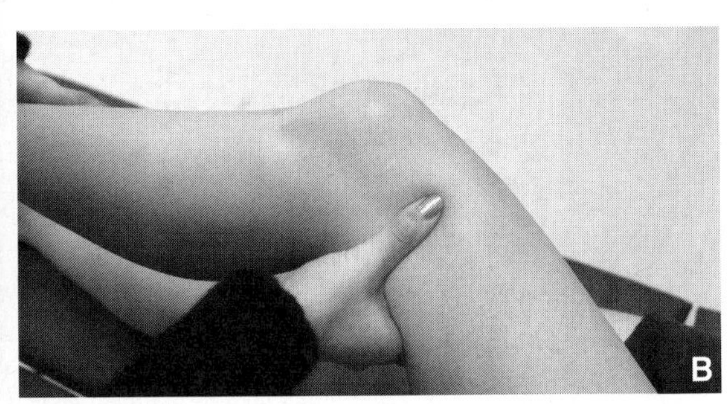

The examiner attempts to compress the distal portion of the IT band against the lateral femoral condyle during passive motion of the knee. In the presence of IT band inflammation, pain will be elicited.

Patient Position	Lying supine with the knee flexed
Position of Examiner	Standing lateral to the side being tested The knee is supported above the joint line with the thumb over or just superior to the lateral femoral condyle **(A)**. The opposite hand controls the lower leg.
Evaluative Procedure	While applying pressure over the lateral femoral condyle, the knee is passively extended and flexed **(B)**.
Positive Test	Pain under the thumb, most commonly as the knee approaches 30°
Implications	Inflammation of the IT band, its associated bursa, or inflammation of the lateral femoral condyle
Modification	**Renne's test** replicates the mechanics of the Noble compression test, but is performed with the patient standing on the involved leg and flexing the knee. No pressure is applied to the lateral femoral epicondyle.
Evidence	Inconclusive or absent in the literature

IT = iliotibial.

Special Test 10-20
Ober's Test for Iliotibial Band Tightness

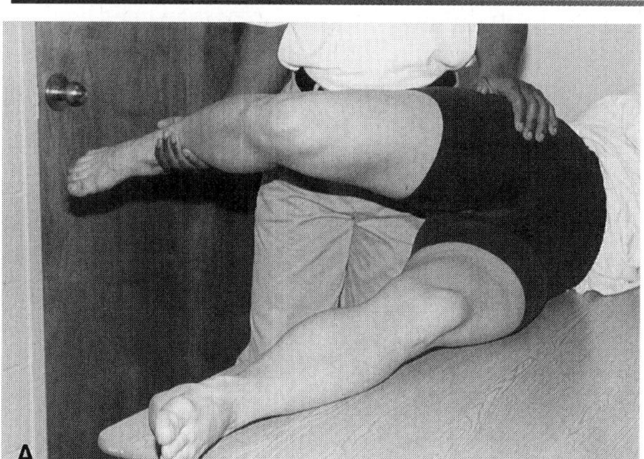

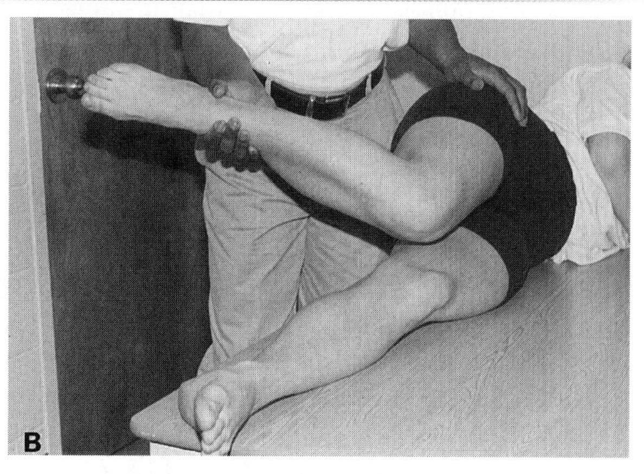

The original Ober's test. To eliminate false-positive test results, the tensor fasciae latae must first clear the greater trochanter. A positive test result occurs when the knee does not adduct past horizontal.

Patient Position

Lying on the side opposite that being tested

The opposite hip (the bottom leg) is flexed to 45° and the knee flexed to 90° to stabilize the torso and pelvis.

Ober's Test: The knee of the involved leg is flexed to 90°.

Modified Ober's Test: The knee of the involved leg is extended.

Position of Examiner

Standing behind the patient

One hand stabilizes the patient's pelvis.

The opposite hand supports the leg being tested along the medial aspect of the distal tibia.

Evaluative Procedure

Passively abduct and extend the patient's hip to allow the tensor fasciae latae to clear the greater trochanter.

The hip is then allowed to passively adduct to the table.

Positive Test

Normal: The femur adducts past horizontal.

Minimal tightness: The femur adducts to horizontal.

Maximal tightness: The leg is unable to adduct to horizontal.

Implications

Tightness of the IT band, predisposing the individual to IT band friction syndrome and/or lateral patellar malalignment

Modification

A goniometer can be used to quantify the results. The proximal arm is aligned with both ASISs and the distal arm is aligned with the midline of the thigh.

An inclinometer can be placed over the lateral femoral condyle. If the leg remaining in abduction relative to 0° it is recorded as a negative value. If the leg adducts past 0° it is recorded as a positive value.[134]

Comments

Flexing the knee to 90° can place tension on the femoral nerve (see Femoral Nerve Stretch Test in Chapter 13) and on the medial structures of the knee.

Adequate pelvic stabilization (limiting trunk lateral flexion) is important to avoid false-negative results.

The modified Ober's test produces less adduction; therefore both tests should be performed.[140]

Evidence

Ober's test

Intra-rater reliability:

Not Reliable — Very Reliable

Poor | Moderate | Good

0 0.1 0.2 0.3 0.4 0.5 0.6 0.7 0.8 0.9 1.0

Modified Ober's test

Intra-rater reliability:

Not Reliable — Very Reliable

Poor | Moderate | Good

0 0.1 0.2 0.3 0.4 0.5 0.6 0.7 0.8 0.9 1.0

IT = iliotibial.

inflammation manifests itself similarly to IT band friction syndrome. The exception is the location of the pain. Individuals suffering from popliteus tendinopathy describe pain in the proximal portion of the tendon, immediately posterior to the LCL. Similar to IT band friction syndrome, patients who excessively pronate their feet are predisposed to this condition, which worsens when running downhill (Examination Findings 10-9). The popliteus acts to prevent a posterior shift of the tibia on the femur during midstance, and running downhill places increased demand on the tendon.[142] Palpation of the popliteus tendon is most easily conducted when the foot of the involved leg is placed on the uninvolved knee in the figure-4 position, a position that may produce pain in and of itself (Fig. 10-26).

The function of the popliteus muscle changes, albeit slightly, in knees that are ACL deficient[143] and more significantly when the PCL is absent.[16] Because the popliteus helps retract the lateral meniscus during knee flexion, inhibition or dysfunction of this muscle may alter the biomechanics of the lateral meniscus, possibly resulting in an increased loading on the cartilage.[26] As with other tendinous conditions, correction of abnormal biomechanics, the use of nonsteroidal anti-inflammatory agents, and the use of local modalities to decrease inflammation are needed to return the patient to full activity.

Tibiofemoral Joint Dislocations

The potential of permanent disability or loss of the leg secondary to trauma of the neurovascular structures makes tibiofemoral dislocations a medical emergency. Several systems are used to classify and describe the dislocation, including the direction of tibial displacement, complete or partial displacement, open and closed, and if the trauma was caused by low- or high-velocity forces (athletic-related dislocations are the result of low-velocity forces), although accurate descriptions of the injury include elements from each of these classifications.[33] The nature of this injury results in profound disruption of the knee's ligaments, joint capsule, musculotendinous structures, meniscus, articular surfaces, and neurovascular elements (Examination Findings 10-10).

Most tibiofemoral dislocations are the result of uniplanar knee hyperextension, hyperextension combined with tibial rotation, or posterior displacement of the tibia with the knee flexed, but any extreme force applied across the knee joint line can result in dislocation.[144] Most dislocations occur perpendicular to the long axis of the femur, usually with the tibia displacing anterior to the femur, although posterior, medial, lateral, and rotational components or combinations of these directions can result. Anterior or posterior tibial displacement is most likely to produce an open dislocation than other directions.[33,144]

Dislocations of the tibiofemoral joint present with severe pain, muscle spasm, and obvious deformity of the joint. Unreduced gross dislocations may be marked by obvious deformity and a possible shortening of the involved limb (Fig. 10-27). Posterolateral dislocations can be clinically identified by the presence of a transverse indentation along the medial joint line caused by the capsule being displaced laterally (the dimple sign). The presence of the dimple sign usually indicates that surgical reduction of the dislocation will be required.[33]

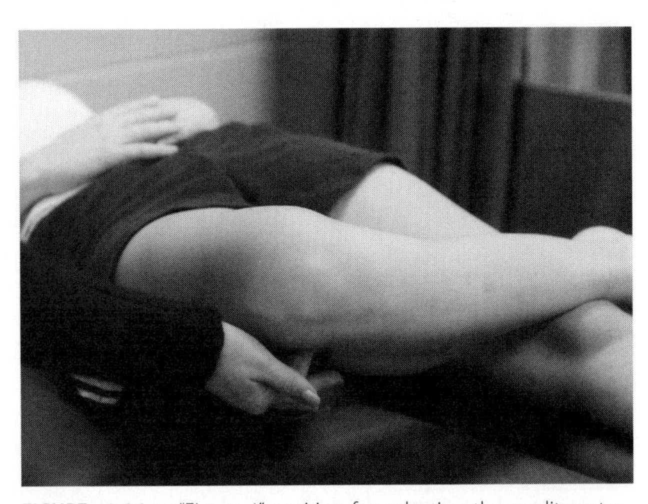

FIGURE 10-26 ■ "Figure 4" position for palpating the popliteus tendon, located just posterior to the lateral collateral ligament.

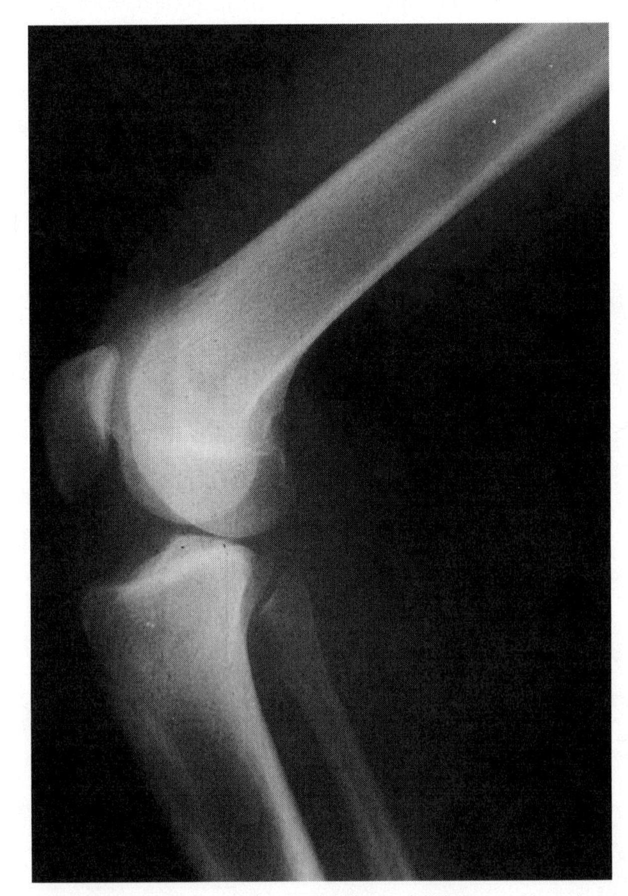

FIGURE 10-27 ■ Radiograph of a tibiofemoral dislocation. Note the anterior displacement of the tibia relative to the femur.

Examination Findings 10-9
Popliteus Tendinopathy

Examination Segment	Clinical Findings
History	***Onset:*** Insidious ***Pain characteristics:*** Pain in the popliteal fossa radiating along the length of the popliteus tendon posterior to the LCL; increased when running downhill ***Mechanism:*** Overuse ***Predisposing conditions:*** Hyperpronation during gait Posterior knee instability Running down hill
Inspection	In acute conditions, inspection is unremarkable; in chronic conditions, swelling may be noted along the lateral joint line.
Palpation	Palpation is best performed in the figure-4 position (see Fig. 10-27). Pain and crepitus elicited along the tendon anterior to the LCL
Joint and Muscle Function Assessment	***AROM:*** Within normal limits ***MMT:*** The popliteus cannot be specifically isolated but is active during testing of the hamstrings. Pain is possible during resisted flexion from full extension as the popliteus "unscrews" the tibia. ***PROM:*** Within normal limits
Joint Stability Tests	***Stress tests:*** None ***Joint play:*** Posterior glide of the tibia is assessed using the posterior drawer test.[83]
Special Tests	None
Neurologic Screening	Within normal limits
Vascular Screening	Within normal limits
Functional Assessment	Pain is increased when running down hill. Excessive and prolonged pronation during gait evaluation
Imaging Techniques	MRI can be used to rule out rupture of the popliteus tendon. Thickening of the tendon may be identified on MR images.
Differential Diagnosis	Biceps femoris tendinopathy, IT band friction syndrome, gastrocnemius strain (lateral head), lateral meniscus tear, LCL sprain, PCL sprain
Comments	The findings for popliteus tendinopathy are similar to those of IT band friction syndrome, except for the location of the pain.

AROM = active range of motion; LCL = lateral collateral ligament; MRI = magnetic resonance imaging; MMT = manual muscle test; PROM = passive range of motion; ROM = range of motion.

Examination Findings 10-10
Tibiofemoral Joint Dislocations

Examination Segment	Clinical Findings
History	***Onset:*** Acute ***Pain characteristics:*** Severe diffuse pain about the knee The patient will report "popping" and other sensations of tearing at the time of injury. ***Mechanism:*** Knee hyperextension, hyperextension and rotation, posterior tibial shear force, posterior femoral shear force, valgus stress, varus force, or any combination thereof ***Predisposing conditions:*** Significant knee instability Muscular weakness Morbid obesity
Inspection	Frank dislocations will reveal obvious deformity of the joint. Spontaneously reduced or subtly displaced dislocations may not reveal any obvious immediate deformity. Swelling and discoloration may appear soon after the injury. A transverse indentation along the medial joint line ("dimple sign") may indicate an unreduced posterolateral dislocation.
Palpation	Frank and subtle dislocations will have a palpable incongruence of the joint line.
Joint and Muscle Function Assessment	***AROM:*** Obvious dislocation: Contraindicated Spontaneously reduced or subtle dislocation: Absent or incomplete; the patient may be unwilling to perform the procedure ***MMT:*** Obvious dislocation: Contraindicated Spontaneously reduced or subtle dislocation: Flexion and extension are weak or absent; the patient may be unwilling to perform the procedure ***PROM:*** Obvious dislocation: Contraindicated Spontaneously reduced or subtle dislocation: Premature end-point; the patient may be unwilling to allow the procedure to be performed

Joint Stability Tests	***Stress tests:*** Obvious dislocation: Contraindicated Anterior drawer test Lachman's test Posterior drawer test Valgus stress test Varus stress test ***Joint play:*** Anterior glide of the tibia on the femur is assessed using anterior drawer. Posterior glide of the tibia is assessed using the posterior drawer test.[83]
Special Tests	Avoided in the presence of an obvious dislocation
Neurologic Screening	Peroneal nerve distribution (superficial and deep branches) Tibial nerve distribution
Vascular Screening	Posterior tibial artery Dorsal pedal pulse Distal capillary refill Skin color Skin temperature
Functional Assessment	The patient will be unwilling and/or unable to bear weight on the involved limb.
Imaging Techniques	Angiograms assist in determining the viability of the popliteal artery.
Differential Diagnosis	Femoral fracture, tibial fracture
Comments	A patient who presents with a mechanism of injury described above has sustained a rupture of at least three of the major ligaments (ACL, PCL, MCL, LCL) and/or and who displays distal neurovascular symptoms should be suspected of a tibiofemoral dislocation. Ligamentous and special tests should not be performed on knee that is obviously dislocated. Deep vein thrombosis may occur secondary to a tibiofemoral dislocation.[144]

ACL = anterior cruciate ligament; AROM = active range of motion; LCL = lateral collateral ligament; MCL = medial collateral ligament; MMT = manual muscle test; PCL = posterior cruciate ligament; PROM = passive range of motion.

Partial dislocations or frank dislocations that have spontaneously reduced may not reveal remarkable findings on initial inspections. A tibiofemoral joint dislocation should be suspected if distal neurovascular symptoms are present and if at least any three of the ACL, PCL, MCL, and/or LCL have been torn.[33] Swelling and discoloration may rapidly occur soon following the injury. On palpation, the joint line and surrounding structures are sensitive. Unreduced dislocations will have a palpable deformity across the joint line.

Patients suffering from a tibiofemoral dislocation will be unwilling and unable to move the joint or bear weight on the involved limb. ROM and ligamentous, special, and functional tests should not be performed on obvious dislocations.

The popliteal artery's anatomical fixation to the structures proximal and distal to the joint line makes it more predisposed to injury than the tibial artery.[33,144] Vascular injuries occur in 32% to 40% of dislocations and nerve injuries may occur in as many as 30% of the cases.[33,145]

Dislocations caused by low-velocity forces are less likely to result in neurovascular compromise than high-velocity forces.[33] The posterior tibial and dorsal pedal pulses, distal capillary refill, and skin color and temperature must be carefully bilaterally assessed in any suspected tibiofemoral dislocation.[144] The collateral circulation around the knee is not sufficient to maintain the viability of the lower extremity if the popliteal artery is obstructed.[33] The longer the popliteal artery is occluded, the greater the probability of permanent disability or loss of the leg[146] Circulation must be restored in 6 to 8 hours to minimize the risk of lower leg amputation.[33] Doppler blood flow measurements and arteriograms are used to confirm or rule out the presence of vascular trauma.[146]

Some tibiofemoral dislocations, especially those in the posterolateral direction, require surgical reduction and require surgical repair of the damaged ligaments. These repairs may require multiple surgeries.

On-Field Evaluation of Knee Injuries

The process used during the on-field evaluation of knee injuries is similar to that described for the ankle. The presence of a gross fracture or dislocation of the tibiofemoral joint or the patellofemoral joint (see Chapter 11) must be ruled out before a finite examination is performed. Question the athlete about the mechanism of injury, the fixation of the foot, and any associated sounds and sensations.

Equipment Considerations

Protective devices around the knee include both stabilizing and prophylactic braces, neoprene sleeves, and padding, all of which must be removed before evaluating the knee and patella.

Football pants

The pants worn for practice and competition in football are tight fitting but, fortunately, are elastic. Expose the knee by reaching under the anterior portion of the pant and locating the kneepad. Hold down the kneepad while the pant leg is pulled up and over the knee or the pad is removed from the pocket. Then remove the pad and flip the pouch up and out of the way (Fig. 10-28). If the pants are extraordinarily tight fitting or inelastic or if a brace is worn beneath the pants, making the preceding procedure difficult, cut the pant leg along one of the seams.

Knee brace removal

Both prophylactic and stabilizing knee braces greatly hinder the on-field evaluation of knee injuries. After the pant leg has been pulled over the brace, prophylactic knee braces can be removed by loosening the lower strap holding it in place or cutting the tape. To remove the upper support, slide a hand under the strap or tape while pulling downwardly on the brace (see Fig. 10-28).

Because of the complexity of many of the stabilizing knee braces, it is usually easiest to remove or detach all of the tibial straps first and then those on the femur. Detach the femoral ones. If the athlete does not experience pain during knee flexion, slightly flex the knee to allow the lower (tibial) portion of the brace to move away from the leg and then lift the upper portion up and downward, away from the knee.

On-Field History

- **Location of the pain:** Inquire about the location of any pain. Pain localized to the joint line can indicate meniscal tears. Diffuse pain can indicate trauma to the MCL or joint capsule. Pain described as arising from within the knee joint, from "under the knee cap," or in the posterior aspect of the knee is associated with cruciate ligament sprains.
- **Mechanism of injury:** Identify the forces exerted on the knee, keeping in mind that the injury may involve multiple forces (e.g., valgus stress with tibial rotation). To cross-reference the injury mechanism with the possible trauma, refer to Table 10-3.
- **History of injury:** Ascertain if the athlete has suffered any significant prior ligamentous injury that may influence the findings of the current examination.
- **Associated sounds and sensations:** Question the patient about any sounds or sensations. A "snap" or "pop" may be associated with a ligament rupture, most commonly associated with the ACL. True locking of the knee can be associated with an unstable meniscal tear that has lodged between the knee's articular surfaces. A snapping, popping, or giving-way sensation may also be associated with a patellar dislocation or subluxation (discussed in Chapter 11).

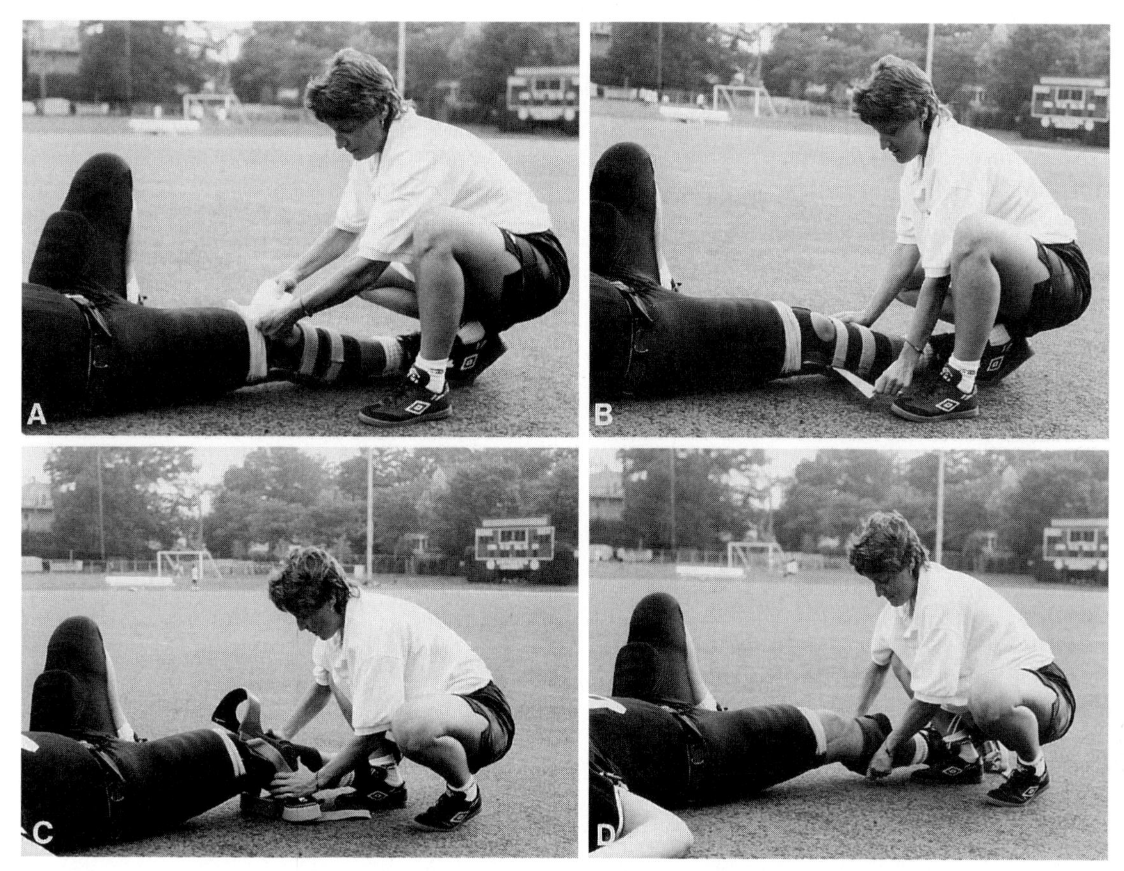

FIGURE 10-28 ■ Removing a knee brace. (A) Remove the knee pad and flip its pouch upward. (B) Remove the Velcro straps. (C) Displace the distal (tibial) portion of the brace and slide the proximal portion from beneath the pant. (D) Remove any underlying padding.

- **Associated neurologic symptoms:** Inquire about any neurologic symptoms. Reports of paresthesia distal to the knee or the inability to dorsiflex the foot indicate trauma to the common peroneal nerve. In the presence of these symptoms, suspect a dislocated tibiofemoral joint until this condition can be ruled out.

On-Field Inspection

- **Patellar position:** Ensure that the patella is properly seated within the femoral trochlea.
- **Alignment of the tibiofemoral joint:** Through concurrent inspection and palpation, identify that the tibia and femur are properly aligned. Note that a normal alignment does not preclude consideration that a tibiofemoral dislocation occurred and subsequently reduced.

On-Field Palpation

- **Extensor mechanism:** Palpate the length of the patellar tendon, patella, quadriceps tendon, and distal quadriceps for incongruity and point tenderness, noting the overall integrity of the extensor mechanism.
- **Medial collateral ligament and medial joint line:** Note any point tenderness along the joint line, indicating meniscal pathology.
- **Lateral collateral ligament and lateral joint line:** Palpate the LCL, an extracapsular structure, for areas of defect or point tenderness. As with the medial meniscus, lateral joint line pain can indicate pathology of the lateral meniscus.
- **Fibular head:** Palpate the fibular head to rule out the presence of a fracture and determine the stability of the proximal tibiofibular syndesmosis.

On-Field Range of Motion Tests

In the absence of gross deformity, suspected fracture, or joint dislocation, have the athlete actively flex and extend the knee throughout the ROM. The inability to perform this motion signifies that the patient should be transported in a non–weight-bearing manner from the field to the sideline for further evaluation. Passive ROM and manual muscle testing may not be indicated during the on-field assessment.

On-Field Ligamentous Tests

If a ligamentous injury is suspected, valgus stress testing, varus stress testing, Lachman's test, and if possible, a posterior drawer test may be carried out before moving the athlete and the onset of reflexive muscle guarding. If the athlete cannot be properly assessed on the field, transport the individual to the sideline in a non–weight-bearing position. Because of the awkward position that an examiner is placed in when performing on-field ligamentous tests, repeat these tests for accuracy when the athlete has been moved to the sideline.

On-Field Management of Knee Injuries

Tibiofemoral Joint Dislocations

Tibiofemoral dislocations must be immediately evaluated by a physician; gross dislocations must be reduced as soon as possible. Prior to transporting the patient, establish the presence of the distal pulses, immobilize the limb in the position it was found, and treat for shock. If an open dislocation has occurred then the open wound must also be cared for prior to transportation.

*** Practical Evidence**

The presence of a distal pulse following knee dislocation does not rule out severe arterial damage or blockage. Because of potential catastrophic consequences (amputation), a 79% rate of detecting arterial damage via pulse palpation is not sufficiently sensitive. Angiography is recommended after a dislocation, even with normal pulse and well-perfused limb. Angiography is not recommended if vascular injury is obvious (diminished pulse; signs of ischemia) because any delay in surgery greatly hurts the outcome.[147]

Collateral and Cruciate Ligament Sprains

While the athlete is still on the playing field or court, only uniplanar ligamentous stress tests are performed. This sequence should consist of Lachman's test for ACL deficiency, valgus and varus stress testing for the collateral ligaments, and the posterior drawer test for PCL laxity. For the basis of comparison and if the situation permits, also evaluate the uninvolved knee at this time. Laxity in the involved knee warrants the athlete's being removed from the field in a non–weight-bearing manner, such as a two-person assist.

After removing the patient to the sideline and, if significant laxity or pain is demonstrated, treat the knee with ice, compression, and elevation. Place the knee in an immobilizer and refer the athlete to a physician.

Meniscal Tears

The on-field determination of the possibility of a meniscal tear is based on the athlete's description of the injury mechanism. Until otherwise ruled out, suspect a meniscal tear in athletes who describe a "locking" or "giving way" at the time of the injury or are hesitant to move the knee. Likewise, assume any rotational mechanism or possible ACL or MCL sprain to involve the meniscus.

REFERENCES

1. Snyder-Mackler, L, and Lewek, M: The knee. In Levangie PK, Norkin CC: *Joint Structure and Function*, ed 4. Philadelphia, PA, FA Davis, 2006, p 393.
2. Moore, KL, and Dalley, AF: The lower limb. In Moore KL, Dalley AF: *Clinically Oriented Anatomy*, ed 5. Baltimore, Williams & Wilkins, 2006, p 563.
3. Moglo, KE, and Shirazi-Adl, A: On the coupling between anterior and posterior cruciate ligaments, and knee joint response under anterior femoral drawer in flexion: A finite element study. *Clin Biomech*, 18:751, 2003.
4. Rasenberg, EIJ, et al: Grading medial collateral ligament injury: Comparison of MR imaging and instrumented valgus-varus laxity testing device. A prospective double-blind patient study. *Eur J Radiol*, 21:18, 1995.
5. Davies, H, Unwin, A, and Aichroth, P: The posterolateral corner of the knee. Anatomy, biomechanics and management of injuries. *Injury, Int J Care Injured*, 35:68, 2004.
6. Chen, FS, Rokito, AS, and Pitman, MI: Acute and chronic posterolateral rotatory instability of the knee. *J Am Acad Orthop Surg*, 8:97, 2000.
7. Fu, F, et al: Biomechanics of knee ligaments. Basic concepts and clinical application. *J Bone Joint Surg Am*, 75:1716, 1993.
8. Arms, SW, et al: The biomechanics of anterior cruciate ligament rehabilitation and reconstruction. *Am J Sports Med*, 12:8, 1984.
9. Beynnon, BD, et al. Anterior cruciate ligament strain behavior during rehabilitation exercises in vivo. *Am J Sports Med*, 23:24, 1995.
10. Van Dommelen, BA, and Fowler, PJ: Anatomy of the posterior cruciate ligament. A review. *Am J Sports Med*, 17:24, 1989.
11. Harner, CD, et al: Comparative study of the size and shape of human anterior and posterior cruciate ligaments. *J Orthop Res*, 13:429, 1995.
12. Hop, J: Anatomy and pathomechanics of the posterior cruciate ligament. *Athl Ther Today*, 6:6, 2001.
13. Wind, WM, Bergfeld, JA, and Parker, RD: Evaluation and treatment of posterior cruciate ligament injuries. *Am J Sports Med*, 32:1765, 2004.
14. Margheritini, F, et al: Posterior cruciate ligament injuries in the athlete. An anatomical, biomechanical and clinical review. *Sports Med*, 32:393, 2002.
15. Race, A, and Amis, AA: Loading of the two bundles of the posterior cruciate ligament: An analysis of bundle function in a-P drawer. *J Biomech*, 29:873, 1996.
16. Harner, CD, et al: The effects of a popliteus muscle load on in situ forces in the posterior cruciate ligament and on knee kinematics. A human cadaveric study. *Am J Sports Med*, 26:669, 1998.
17. Gollenhon, DL, Torzilli, PA, and Warren, RF: The role of the posterolateral and cruciate ligaments in the stability of the human knee. A biomechanical study. *J Bone Joint Surg*, 69A:233, 1987.
18. Grood, ES, Stowers, SF, and Noyes, FR: Limits of movement in the human knee. Effect of sectioning the posterior cruciate ligament and posterolateral structures. *J Bone Joint Surg*, 70A:88, 1988.
19. Andrews, JB, et al: Surgical repair of acute and chronic lesions of the lateral capsular ligamentous complex of the knee. In Feagin JA (ed): *Injuries About the Knee*. New York: Churchill Livingstone, 1988, p 425.

20. Covey, DC: Injuries of the posterolateral corner of the knee. *J Bone Joint Surg*, 83(A):106, 2001.
21. Stannard, JP, et al: The posterolateral corner of the knee. Repair versus reconstruction. *Am J Sports Med*, 33:881, 2005.
22. Wadia, FD, et al: An anatomic study of the popliteofibular ligament. *Int Orthop*, 27:172, 2003.
23. Greis, PE, et al: Meniscal injury: I. Basic science and evaluation. *J Am Acad Orthop Surg*, 10:168, 2002.
24. Hauger, O, et al: Characterization of the "Red zone" of knee meniscus: MR imaging and histologic correlation. *Radiology*, 217:193, 2000.
25. Jordan, MR: Lateral meniscal variants: Evaluation and treatment. *J Am Acad Orthop Surg*, 4:191, 1996.
26. Jones, CD, Keene, GC, and Christie, AD: The popliteus as a retractor of the lateral meniscus of the knee. *Arthroscopy*, 11:270, 1995.
27. Tienen, TG, et al: Displacement of the medial meniscus within the passive motion characteristics of the human knee joint: An RSA study in human cadaver knees. *Knee Surg Sports Traumatol Arthroc*, 13:287, 2005.
28. Rosene, JM, and Fogarty, TD: Anterior tibial translation in collegiate athletes with normal anterior cruciate integrity. *J Athl Train*, 34:93, 1999.
29. Pandy, MG, and Shelburne, KB: Dependence of cruciate-ligament loading on muscle forces and external load. *J Biomech*, 30:1015, 1997.
30. Terry, GC, and LaPrade, RF: The biceps femoris muscle complex at the knee: Its anatomy and injury patterns associated with acute anterolateral-anteromedial rotatory instability. *Am J Sports Med*, 24:2, 1996.
31. Terry, GC, et al: How iliotibial tract injuries of the knee combine with acute anterior cruciate ligament tears to influence abnormal anterior tibial displacement. *Am J Sports Med*, 21:55, 1993.
32. Soderberg, GL: Kinesiology: *Application to Pathological Motion*. Baltimore: Williams & Wilkins, 1986, p 207.
33. Good, L, and Johnson, RJ: The dislocated knee. *J Am Acad Orthop Surg*, 3:284, 1995.
34. Smith CC: Evaluating the painful knee: A hands-on approach to acute ligamentous and mensical injuries. *Adv Stud Med*, 4:362, 2004.
35. Kempson, GE: Relationship between the tensile properties of articular cartilage from the human knee and age. *Ann Rheum*, 41:508, 1982.
36. Reid, DC: Knee ligament injuries: Anatomy, classification, and examination. In Reid, DC (ed): *Sports Injury: Assessment and Rehabilitation*. New York: Churchill Livingstone, 1992, p 449.
37. Garofalo, R, et al: Locking knee caused by subluxation of the posterior horn of the lateral meniscus. *Knee Surg Sports Traumatol Arthroc* 13:569, 2005.
38. Akima, H, and Furukawa, T: Atrophy of thigh muscles after meniscal lesions and arthroscopic partial meniscectomy. *Knee Surg Sports Traumatol Arthrosoc*, 13:632, 2005.
39. Tothill, P, and Stewart, AD: Estimation of thigh muscle and adipose tissue volume using magnetic resonance imaging and anthropometry. *J Sports Sci*, 20:563, 2002.
40. Soderberg, GL, Ballantyne, BT, and Kestel, LL: Reliability of lower extremity girth measurements after anterior cruciate ligament reconstruction. *Physiother Res Int*, 1:7, 1996.
41. Voight, M, and Weider, D: Comparative reflex response times of vastus medialis oblique and subjects with extensor mechanism dysfunction. *Am J Sports Med*, 19:131, 1991.
42. Curl, WW: Popliteal cysts: Historical background and current knowledge. *J Am Acad Orthop Surg*, 4:129, 1996.
43. Yu, WD, and Shapiro, MS: Cysts and other masses about the knee. Identifying and treating common and rare lesions. *Phys Sports Med*, 27:59, 1999.
44. Handy, JR: Popliteal cysts in adults: A review. *Semin Arthritis Rheum*, 31:108, 2001.
45. Frobell, RB, Lohmander, LS, and Roos, HP: Acute rotational trauma to the knee: poor agreement between clinical assessment and magnetic resonance imaging findings. *Scand J Med Sci Sports*, 17:109, 2007.
46. Petsche, TS, and Hutchinson, MR: Loss of extension after reconstruction of the anterior cruciate ligament. *J Am Acad Orthop Surg*, 7:119, 1999.
47. Hislop, HJ, and Montgomery, J: *Muscle Testing: Techniques of Manual Examination*. Philadelphia: W.B. Saunders, 2002, p 187.
48. Blair, DF, and Willis, RP: Rapid rehabilitation following anterior cruciate ligament reconstruction. *Athl Train J Nl Athl Train Assoc*, 26:32, 1991.
49. Johnson, BC, and Cullen, MJ: The anterior cruciate ligament: Injuries and functions in anterolateral rotatory instability. *Athl Train J Natl Athl Train Assoc*, 17:79, 1982.
50. DiStefano, VJ: The enigmatic anterior cruciate ligament. *Athl Train: J Natl Athl Train Assoc*, 16:244, 1981.
51. Girgis, FG, Marshall, JL, and Al Monajem, ARS: The cruciate ligaments of the knee joint. Anatomical, functional, and experimental analysis. *Clin Orthop*, 106:216, 1975.
52. Furman, W, Marshall, JL, and Girgis, FG: The anterior cruciate ligament: A functional analysis based on post mortem studies. *J Bone Joint Surg Am*, 58:178, 1976.
53. More, RC, et al: Hamstrings-an anterior cruciate ligament protagonist. *Am J Sports Med*, 21:231, 1993.
54. Lintner, DM, et al: Partial tears of the anterior cruciate ligament. Are they clinically detectable? *Am J Sports Med*, 23:111, 1995.
55. Jackson, JL, O'Malley, PG, and Kroenke, K: Evaluation of acute knee pain in primary care. *Ann Intern Med*, 139:575, 2003.
56. Scholten, RJPM, et al: Accuracy of physical diagnostic tests for assessing ruptures of the anterior cruciate ligament: A meta-analysis. *J Fam Pract*, 52:689, 2003.
57. Benjaminse, A, Gokeler, A, van der Schans, CP: Clinical diagnosis of an anterior cruciate ligament rupture: a meta-analysis. *J Orthop Sports Phys Ther*, 36:267, 2006.
58. Cooperman, JM, Riddle, DL, and Rothstein, JM: Reliability and validity of judgments of the integrity of the anterior cruciate ligament of the knee using the Lachman's test. *Phys Ther*, 70:225, 1990.
59. Whitehill, WR, Wright, KE, and Nelson, K: Modified Lachman test for anterior cruciate ligament instability. *J Athl Train*, 29:256, 1994.
60. Adler, GG, Hoekman, RA, and Beach, DM: Drop leg Lachman test: A new test of anterior knee laxity. *Am J Sports Med*, 23:320, 1995.
61. Harter, RA, et al: A comparison of instrumented and manual Lachman test results in anterior cruciate ligament-reconstructed knees. *Athl Train J Natl Athl Train Assoc*, 25:330, 1990.

62. Barber-Westin, SD, and Noyes, FR: The effect of rehabilitation and return to activity on anterior-posterior knee displacements after anterior cruciate ligament reconstruction. *Am J Sports Med*, 21:264, 1993.
63. Cross, MJ, et al: Acute repair of injury to the anterior cruciate ligament. A long-term followup. *Am J Sports Med*, 21:128, 1993.
64. Webright, WG, Perrin, DH, and Gansneder, BM: Effect of trunk position on anterior tibial displacement measured by the KT-1000 in uninjured subjects. *J Athl Train*, 33:233, 1998.
65. Papandreou, MG, et al: Inter-rater reliability of Rolimeter measurements between anterior cruciate ligament injured and normal contralateral knees. *Knee Surg Sports Traumatol Arthroc*, 13:592, 2005.
66. Berry, J, et al: Error estimates in novice and expert raters for the KT-1000 arthrometer. *J Orthop Sports Phys Ther*, 29:49, 1999.
67. Fleming, BC, et al: Measurement of anterior-posterior knee laxity: A comparison of three techniques. *J Orthop Res*, 20:421, 2002.
68. Draper, DO, and Schulthies, S: A test for eliminating false positive anterior cruciate ligament injury diagnoses. *J Athletic Train*, 28:355, 1993.
69. Jonsson, H, and Karrholm, J: Three-dimensional knee kinematics and stability in patients with a posterior cruciate ligament tear. *J Orthop Res*, 17:185, 1999.
70. Covey, DC, and Sapega, AA: Injuries to the posterior cruciate ligament. *J Bone Joint Surg*, 75A:1376, 1993.
71. Covey, DC, and Sapega, AA: Anatomy and function of the posterior cruciate ligament. *Clin Sports Med*, 13:509, 1994.
72. Sawant, M, Murty, AN, and Ireland, J: Valgus knee injuries: Evaluation and documentation using a simple technique of stress radiography. *Knee*, 11:25, 2004.
73. Indelicato, PA: Isolated medial collateral ligament injuries of the knee. *J Am Acad Ortho Surg*, 3:9, 1995.
74. Robbins, AJ, Newman, AP, and Burks, RT: Postoperative return of motion in anterior cruciate ligament and medial collateral ligament injuries. The effects of medial collateral ligament rupture location. *Am J Sports Med*, 21:20, 1993.
75. Veenema, KR: Valgus knee instability in an adolescent. Ligament sprain or physeal fracture? *Physician Sportsmed*, 27:62, 1999.
76. Reider, B: Medial collateral ligament injuries in athletes. *Sports Med*, 21:147, 1996.
77. Hillard-Sembell, D: Combined injuries of the anterior cruciate and medial collateral ligaments of the knee. Effect of treatment on stability and function of the joint. *J Bone Joint Surg Am*, 78:169, 1996.
78. Reider, B, et al: Treatment of isolated medial collateral ligament injuries with early functional rehabilitation: A five-year follow-up study. *Am J Sports Med*, 22:470, 1993.
79. Noyes, FR, and Barber-Westin, SD: The treatment of acute combined ruptures of the anterior cruciate and medial ligaments of the knee. *Am J Sports Med*, 23:380, 1995.
80. Krivickas, LS, and Wilbourn, AJ: Peripheral nerve injuries in athletes: A case series of over 200 injuries. *Semin Neurol*, 20:225, 2000.
81. Murakami, Y, et al: Quantitative evaluation of nutritional pathways for the posterior cruciate ligament and the lateral collateral ligament in rabbits. *Acta Physiol Scand*, 162, 447, 1998.
82. Latimer, HA, et al: Reconstruction of the lateral collateral ligament of the knee with patellar tendon allograft. Report of a new technique in combined ligament injuries. *Am J Sports Med*, 26:656, 1998.
83. Kaltenborn, FM: *Manual Mobilization of the Joints*. Oslo, Norway: Olaf Norlis Bokhandel, 2002, p 286.
84. Anderson, AF, Rennirt, GW, and Standeffer, WC: Clinical analysis of the pivot shift tests: Description of the pivot drawer test. *Am J Knee Surg*, 13:19, 2000.
85. Stanitski, CL: Anterior cruciate ligament injury in the skeletally immature patient: Diagnosis and treatment. *J Am Acad Orthop Surg*, 3:146, 1995.
86. Snyder-Mackler, L, et al: The relationship between passive joint laxity and functional outcome after anterior cruciate ligament surgery. *Am J Sports Med*, 25:191, 1997.
87. Sgaglione, NA, et al: Arthroscopically assisted anterior cruciate ligament reconstruction with the pes anserine tendons. *Am J Sports Med*, 21:249, 1993.
88. Arendt, E, and Dick, R: Knee injury patterns among men and women in collegiate basketball and soccer: NCAA data and review of literature. *Am J Sports Med*, 23:694, 1995.
89. Griffin, LY, et al: Noncontact anterior cruciate ligament injuries: Risk factors and prevention strategies. *J Am Acad Orthop Surg*, 8:141, 2000.
90. Davis, IM, and Ireland, ML: ACL injuries – The gender bias. *J Orthop Sports Phys Ther*, 33:A-1, 2003.
91. Beckett, ME, et al: Incidence of hyperpronation in the ACL injured knee: A clinical perspective. *J Athl Train*, 27:58, 1992.
92. Woodford-Rogers, B, Cyphert, L, and Denegar, CR: Risk factors for anterior cruciate ligament injury in high school and college athletes. *J Athl Train*, 29:343, 1994.
93. Loundon, JK, Jenkins, W, and Loundon, KL: The relationship between static posture and ACL injuries in female athletes. *J Orthop Sports Phys Ther*, 24:91, 1996.
94. Loudon, JK, Jenkins, W, and Loudon, KL: The relationship between static posture and ACL injury in female athletes. *J Orthop Sports Phys Ther*, 24:91, 1996.
95. Heitz, NA, et at: Hormonal changes throughout the menstrual cycle and increased anterior cruciate ligament laxity in females. *J Athl Train*, 34:144, 1999.
96. Flynn, RK, et al: The familial predisposition towards the anterior cruciate ligament. *Am J Sports Med*, 33:23, 2005.
97. Schickendantz, MS, and Weiker, GG: The predictive value of radiographs in the evaluation of unilateral and bilateral anterior cruciate injuries. *Am J Sports Med*, 21:110, 1993.
98. Shelbourne, KD, Davis, TJ, and Klootwyk, TE: The relationship between intercondylar notch width of the femur and the incidence of anterior cruciate ligament tears. *Am J Sports Med*, 26:402, 1998.
99. Ageberg, E, et al: Balance in single-limb stance in patients with anterior cruciate ligament injury: Relation to knee laxity, proprioception, muscle strength, and subjective function. *Am J Sports Med*, 33:1527, 2005.
100. Shelbourne, KD, and Nitz, P: Accelerated rehabilitation after anterior cruciate ligament reconstruction. *Am J Sports Med*, 18:292, 1990.
101. Shelbourne, KD, and Gray, T: Anterior cruciate ligament reconstruction with autogenous patellar tendon graft followed by accelerated rehabilitation: A two to nine year followup. *Am J Sports Med*, 25:786, 1997.
102. Hewett, TE, et al: Biomechanical measures of neuromuscular control and valgus loading of the knee predict anterior cruciate ligament injury risk in female athletes. *Am J Sports Med*, 33:492, 2005.

103. Slauterbeck, JR, et al: The menstrual cycle, sex hormones, and anterior cruciate ligament injury. *J Athl Train*, 37:275, 2002.
104. Cosgarea, AJ, and Jay, PR: Posterior cruciate ligament injuries: Evaluation and management. *J Am Acad Orthop Surg*, 9:297, 2001.
105. Schulz, MS, et al: Reliability of stress radiography for evaluation of posterior knee laxity. *Am J Sports Med*, 33:502, 2005.
106. Fontboté, CA, et al: Neuromuscular and biomechanical adaptations of patients with isolated deficiency of the posterior cruciate ligament. *Am J Sports Med*, 33:982, 2005.
107. Sauers, RJ: Isolated posterior cruciate tear in a college football player. *J Athl Train*, 21:248, 1986.
108. Rubinstein, RA, et al: The accuracy of the clinical examination in the setting of posterior cruciate ligament injuries. *Am J Sports Med*, 22:550, 1994.
109. Keller, PM, et al: Nonoperatively treated isolated posterior cruciate ligament injuries. *Am J Sports Med*, 21:132, 1993.
110. Shelbourne, KD, Davis, TJ, and Patel, DV: The natural history of acute, isolated, nonoperatively treated posterior cruciate ligament injuries. A prospective study. *Am J Sports Med*, 27:276, 1999.
111. Ochi, M, et al: Isolated posterior cruciate ligament insufficiency induces morphological changes of anterior cruciate ligament collagen fibrils. *Arthroscopy*, 15:292, 1999.
112. Wroble, RR, et al: The role of the lateral extraarticular restraints in the anterior cruciate ligament-deficient knee. *Am J Sports Med*, 21:257, 1993.
113. Katz, JW, and Fingeroth, RJ: The diagnostic accuracy of ruptures of the anterior cruciate ligament comparing the Lachman test, the anterior drawer sign, and the pivot shift test in acute and chronic knee injuries. *Am J Sports Med*, 14:88, 1986.
114. Ostrowski, JA. Accuracy of 3 diagnostic tests for anterior cruciate ligament tears. *J Athl Train*, 41:120, 2006.
115. Shelbourne, KD, and Nitz, PA: The O'Donoghue triad revisited. Combined knee injuries involving anterior cruciate and medial collateral ligament tears. *Am J Sports Med*, 19:474, 1991.
116. Ross, G, et al: Evaluation and treatment of acute posterolateral corner/anterior cruciate ligament injuries of the knee. *J Bone Joint Surg*, 86(A):2, 2004.
117. Cooper, DE: Tests for posterolateral instability of the knee in normal subjects. Results of examination under anesthesia. *J Bone Joint Surg*, 73(A):30, 1991.
118. Ferrari, DA, Ferrari, JD, and Coumas, J: Posterolateral instability of the knee. *J Bone Joint Surg*, 76-B:187, 1994.
119. Loomer, RL: A test for posterolateral rotatory instability. *Clin Orthop*, 235, 1995.
120. Cooper, DE: Tests for posterolateral instability of the knee in normal subjects: Results of examinations under anesthesia. *J Bone Joint Surg*, 70-A:386, 1991.
121. Hughston, JC, and Norwood, LA: The posterolateral drawer test and external rotational recurvatum test for posterolateral rotatory instability of the knee. *Clin Orthop*, 147:82, 1980.
122. Karachalios, T, et al: Diagnostic accuracy of a new clinical test (the Thessaly test) for early detection of meniscal tears. *J Bone Joint Surg*, 87A:955, 2005.
123. Krinskey, MB, et al: Incidence of lateral meniscus injury in professional basketball players. *Am J Sports Med*, 20:17, 1992.
124. Scriber, K, and Mathney, M: Knee injuries in college football: An 18 year report. *J Athl Train*, 25:233, 1990.
125. Davis, E: Clinical examination of the knee following trauma: An evidence-based perspective. *Trauma*, 4:135, 2002.
126. Clinical Inquiry: For knee pain, how predictive is physical examination for meniscal injury? *J Fam Pract*, 53:918, 2004.
127. Ellis, MR, Griffin, KW, and Meadows, S: For knee pain, how predictive is physical examination for meniscal injury? *J Fam Pract*, 53:918, 2004.
128. Greis, PE, et al: Meniscal injury: II. Management. *J Am Acad Orthop Surg*, 10:177, 2002.
129. Stone, JW: Osteochondral lesions of the talar dome. *J Am Acad Orthop Surg*, 4:63, 1996.
130. Cetik, O, Turker, M, and Uslu, M: Bilateral osteochondritis dissecans of lateral femoral condyle. *Knee Surg Sports Traumatol Arthrosc*, 13:468, 2005.
131. Ralston, BM, et al: Osteochondritis dissecans of the knee. *Physician Sportsmed*, 24:73, 1996.
132. Minas, T, and Nehrer, S: Current concepts in the treatment of articular cartilage defects. *Orthopedics*, 20:525, 1997.
133. Pettitt, R, and Dolski, A: Corrective neuromuscular approach to the treatment of iliotibial band friction syndrome: A case report. *J Athl Train*, 35:96, 2000.
134. Reese, NB, and Bandy, WD: Use of an inclinometer to measure flexibility of the iliotibial band using the Ober test and modified Ober test: Differences in the magnitude and reliability of measurements. *J Orthop Sports Phys Ther*, 33:326, 2003.
135. Muhle, C, et al: Iliotibial band friction syndrome: MR imaging findings in 16 patients and MR arthrographic study of six cadaveric knees. *Radiology*, 212:103, 1999.
136. Nemeth, WC, and Sanders, BL: The lateral synovial recess of the knee: Anatomy and role in chronic Iliotibial band friction syndrome. *Arthroscopy*, 12:574, 1996.
137. Lebsack, D, Gieck, J, and Saliba, E: Iliotibial band friction syndrome. *J Athl Train*, 25:356, 1990.
138. Lucas, CA: Iliotibial band friction syndrome exhibited in athletes. *J Athl Train*, 27:250, 1992.
139. Olsen, DW: Iliotibial band friction syndrome. *Athl Train J Natl Athl Train Assoc*, 21:32, 1986.
140. Gajdosik, RL, Sandler, MM, and Marr, HL: Influence of knee positions and gender on the Ober test for length of the iliotibial band. *Clin Biom*, 18:77, 2003.
141. Brown, TR, et al: Diagnosis of popliteus injuries with MR imaging. *Skelet Radiol*, 24:511, 1995.
142. Davis, M, Newsam, CJ and Perry, J: Electromyograph analysis of the popliteus muscle in level and downhill walking. *Clin Orthop*, Jan:211, 1995.
143. Weresh, MJ, et al: Popliteus function in ACL-deficient patients. *Scand J Med Sci Sports*, 7:14, 1997.
144. Henrichs, A: A review of knee dislocations. *J Athl Train*, 39:365, 2004.
145. Green, NE, and Allen, BL: Vascular injuries associated with dislocation of the knee. *J Bone Joint Surg*, 59(A):236, 1977.
146. Chabra, A, et al: Surgical management of knee dislocations. *J Bone Joint Surg*, 87(A) Suppl:1, 2005.
147. Barnes, CJ, Pietrobon, R, and Higgins, LD: Does the pulse examination in patients with traumatic knee dislocation predict a surgical arterial injury? A meta-analysis. *J Trauma*, 53:1109, 2002.

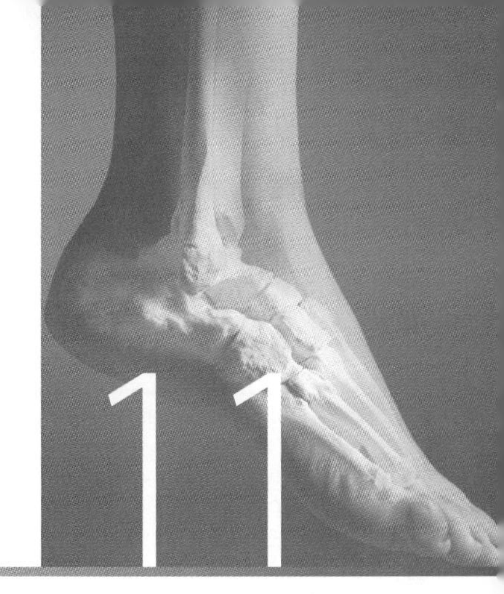

CHAPTER 11

Patellofemoral Articulation Pathologies

Although the patellofemoral (PF) articulation is an integral part of the knee, the two areas are separated in this text because of the differences in the mechanisms and onset of injury. Injury to the patellofemoral articulation is the result of overuse, congenital malalignment, structural insufficiency, or trauma. Pathology at the PF joint is influenced by the mechanics (or pathomechanics) at the foot, ankle, knee, and hip.

Examination of the patellofemoral joint is based on lower extremity, lumbar spine, and gait biomechanics. A distinct lack of research evidence fails to support (or refute) the predictive value of many of the techniques used in the examination of the patellofemoral articulation.

Clinical Anatomy

Lying within the patellar tendon, the **patella** is the largest sesamoid bone in the body. The patella's anatomical design allows for increased mechanical efficiency of the quadriceps muscle group, protection of the anterior portion of the knee joint, and the absorption and transmission of the **joint reaction forces**. In the frontal and sagittal planes the patella is triangular. In the frontal plane, the superior portion is wider than its inferior apex; in the sagittal plane, it is marked with an anterior, nonarticulating surface and a narrower posterior articulating surface (Fig. 11-1).

Joint reaction forces Forces that are transmitted through a joint's articular surfaces.

Articulations and Ligamentous Support

The patella's articular surface has three distinct facets: medial, lateral, and odd. Each facet is covered with up to a 5-mm thickness of hyaline cartilage, thicker than the femur's articular cartilage. The medial and lateral facets have superior, middle, and inferior articular surfaces. The odd facet, lying medial to the medial facet, has no articular subdivisions (Fig. 11-2).

During knee flexion and extension, the patella tracks within the femoral trochlear groove, the area between the two femoral condyles lined with articular cartilage. As the knee moves from flexion into extension, the patella tracks medially within the range of 45 to 18 degrees. The patella then tracks laterally during the final 18 degrees of extension. During flexion, the patella increases its angle of lateral tilt, which then decreases during extension.[1]

When the knee is fully extended, the patella rests just proximal to the femoral groove, leaving it vulnerable to dislocating forces. During flexion, the patella initially makes

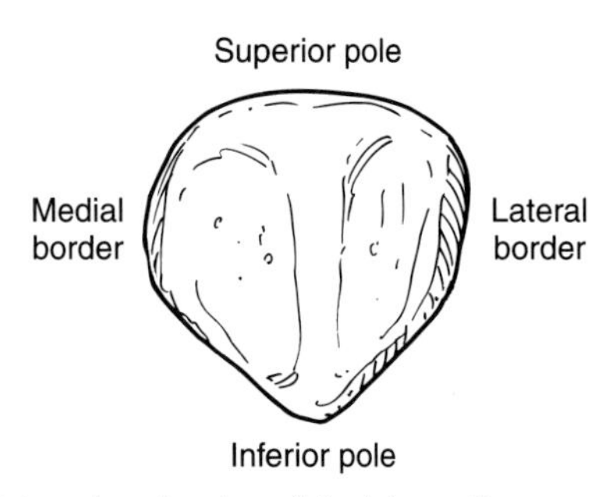

FIGURE 11-1 ■ Anterior view of the left patella.

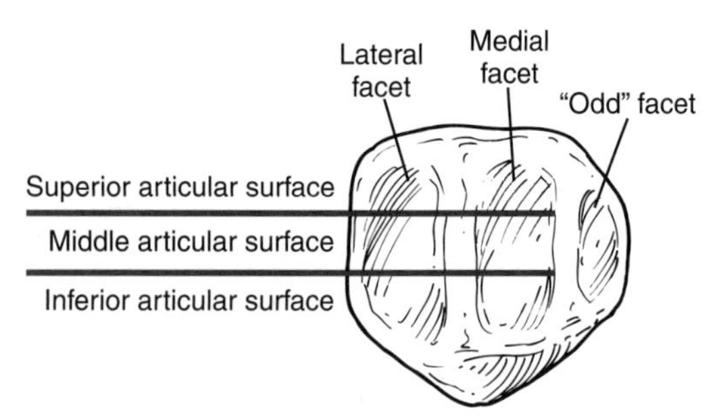

FIGURE 11-2 ■ Posterior view of the left patella. The lateral and medial facets may be conceptualized as having superior, middle, and inferior articular surfaces. The odd facet has no such subdivisions.

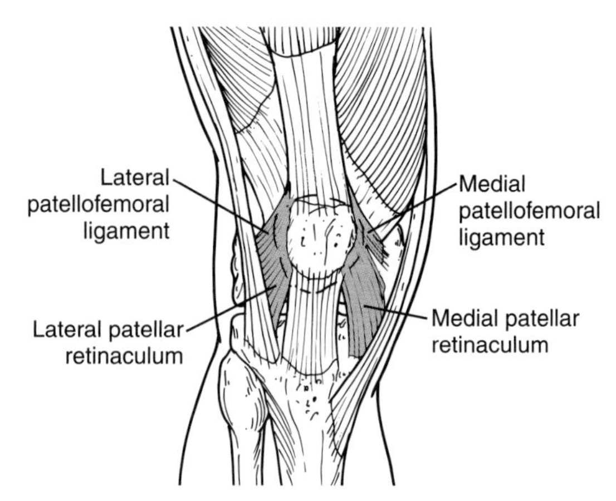

FIGURE 11-3 ■ Patellar retinaculum and medial and lateral patellofemoral ligaments (partially hidden by the quadriceps muscle).

contact with the groove at 10 to 20 degrees of flexion and becomes seated within the groove as the knee approaches 20 to 30 degrees.[2,3] At this point, the lateral border of the femoral trochlea forms a strong barrier against lateral patellar movement. Patellar tracking is improved when the leg is bearing weight, the rationale for incorporating closed-chain exercises early in patellofemoral rehabilitation programs.[3] A shallow trochlear groove is associated with an increased incidence of patellofemoral pain, as it allows increased lateral patellar tilt and displacement as the knee nears full extension.[5]

Compressive forces between the patella and femoral trochlea vary within the range of motion (ROM). These forces range from 0.5 times body weight when walking on a level surface to 3.3 times body weight when walking up and down stairs or running on hills.[6] The maximum compressive force placed on the patella occurs at 30 degrees of flexion.[7,8] The amount of patellofemoral contact area varies throughout the range of motion as well, with the greatest amount of surface area being involved between 60 and 90 degrees of flexion (Table 11-1).[7,9,10]

The patellar retinaculum and **patellofemoral ligaments** maintain the patella's position through the arc of motion (Fig. 11-3). The **lateral retinaculum** originates as an expansion off the vastus lateralis tendon and the iliotibial band to insert on the patella's lateral border.[11] The **medial retinaculum** originates from the distal portion of the vastus medialis and adductor magnus and inserts on the medial border of the patella. The superior portion of the knee's fibrous capsule thickens and inserts on the patella's superior border, forming the medial and lateral patellofemoral ligaments. With attachments on the medial portion of the upper patella, on the femoral condyle near the adductor tubercle, and on the posteromedial joint capsule, the **medial patellofemoral ligament** (MPFL) is a primary restraint against lateral patellar displacement, especially in the lateral inferior direction.[12–14]

Table 11-1 Articulation of the Patellofemoral Joint

Position (Flexion), Degrees	Patellar Facets in Contact with the Femoral Trochlear Groove
0	Patella resting on the suprapatellar fat pad on the distal femoral shaft
20	Inferior portion of facets
45	Medial and lateral facets
90	Largest contact area across the medial and lateral facets
135	Odd facet

Muscular Anatomy and Related Soft Tissues

The muscles of the quadriceps femoris specifically affect the patella's function. During flexion, the patella is pulled inferiorly by the patellar tendon's attachment to the tibial tuberosity. During extension, the quadriceps femoris and its tendon pull the patella superiorly.

Normally the length of the patellar tendon is approximately the same length as the long axis of the patella (±10%) (Fig. 11-4).[15] Abnormally long or short tendons alter the mechanics, and therefore the strength, of the extensor mechanism.

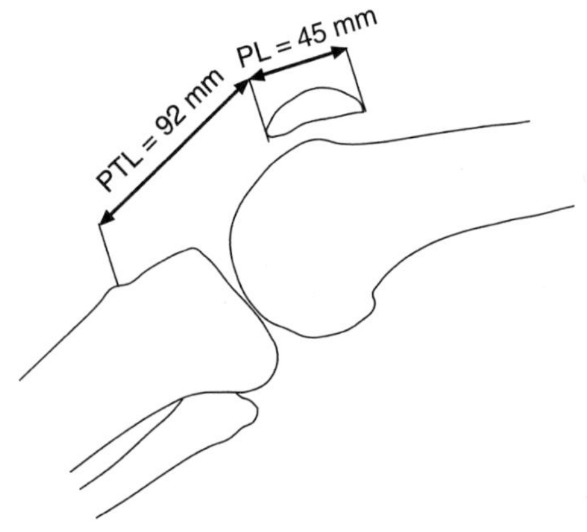

FIGURE 11-4 ■ Calculation of patellar tendon length (drawn from a radiograph) demonstrating a high-riding patella (patella alta). PTL = patellar tendon length; PL = patellar length.

The **vastus lateralis** is the primary muscle pulling the patella laterally. Further lateral tension is derived from slips arising from the iliotibial (IT) band and attaching to the lateral patellar restraints. Tightness of the IT band can accentuate the lateral tracking of the patella because of its attachment to the retinaculum, resulting in subluxations or patellar malalignment.

Medially, the **oblique fibers of the vastus medialis (VMO)** approach the patella at a 55-degree angle, guiding the patella medially and proximally, preventing lateral patellar subluxation. Wide individual differences in the orientation and medial tracking functions of the VMO have been described.[16] The adductor magnus, serving as part of the origin of the VMO and medial retinaculum, may have a secondary function in limiting the amount of lateral patellar tracking.[17,18]

Normal flexibility and strength ratios between the quadriceps, triceps surae, and hamstring muscle groups are needed to provide adequate knee range of motion and normal patellofemoral mechanics.[19] Decreased quadriceps length relative to the hamstrings increases the risk factor for developing patellofemoral pain.[20] Tightness of the gastrocnemius or soleus muscle may prohibit the 10 degrees of dorsiflexion required while walking and the 15 degrees of dorsiflexion required when running. The most common compensation for a lack of dorsiflexion is excessive foot pronation. Increased foot pronation causes internal rotation of the hip and femur which moves the patella medially. This more medial position of the patella results in an increased Q angle and increased lateral force on the patella (refer to Fig. 11-12).[21]

Bursa of the Extensor Mechanism

Anatomic differences and varying biomechanics from individual to individual result in varying numbers of bursae forming within the extensor mechanism. However, four bursae are consistently found throughout the population (Fig. 11-5). Lying deep at the distal end of the quadriceps femoris muscle group and allowing free movement over the distal femur, the **suprapatellar bursa** is an extension of the knee's joint capsule. This bursa is held in place by the articularis genus muscle. The **prepatellar bursa** overlies the anterior portion of the patella and allows the patella to move freely beneath the skin. The distal portion of the patellar tendon and tibial tuberosity receives protection against friction and blows by the **subcutaneous infrapatellar bursa**. The **deep infrapatellar bursa** is located between the tendon and the tibia.

The **infrapatellar fat pad**, one of three fat pads located in the anterior knee compartment, is intracapsular, but extrasynovial. Covered by a synovial membrane posteriorly, the infrapatellar fat pad separates the patellar tendon and the deep infrapatellar bursa from the joint capsule of the knee and extends posteriorly to fill the anterior joint line of the tibiofemoral joint.[22] The infrapatellar fat pad can be injured, inflamed, or fibrotic secondary to patellar dislocation, surgery, or synovitis.[22]

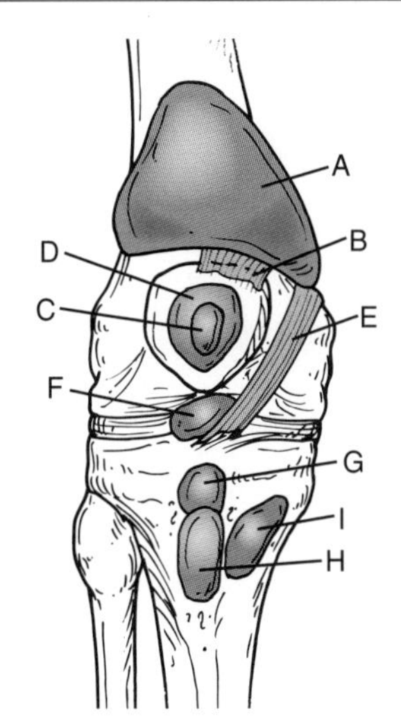

FIGURE 11-5 ■ Bursae and plicae about the knee joint (anterior view, right knee): **(A)** Suprapatellar pouch, **(B)** suprapatellar plica, **(C)** superficial prepatellar bursa, **(D)** deep prepatellar bursa, **(E)** medial plica, **(F)** infrapatellar bursa, **(G)** deep infrapatellar bursa, **(H)** superficial infrapatellar bursa, and **(I)** pes anserine bursa.

Clinical Examination of the Patellofemoral Joint

Findings of the patellofemoral joint evaluation may necessitate evaluation of the back, hip, lower leg, ankle, and foot. Dysfunction of the joints superior or inferior to the knee may result in patellofemoral pain. Pain originating from the lumbar spine can alter posture and gait mechanics, increasing or altering patellofemoral stresses. To meet this need, have the patient dress in shorts and bring his or her casual and competitive footwear to the examination.

History

Many patellofemoral joint pathologies can be the result of overuse stresses, structural abnormalities, or biomechanical deficiencies of the lower leg. However, several acute, traumatic conditions can affect the patella and the extensor mechanism.

Past medical history

Question the patient regarding a family history of patellofemoral pain or osteoarthritis. Meniscal tears, ACL tears, PCL tears, and other trauma to the knee may result in tibiofemoral osteoarthritis, but a history of these conditions may not significantly influence patellofemoral joint degeneration.[23]

- **Relevant past history:** Prior injuries to the lower leg commonly alter the biomechanics of the extensor mechanism. Question the patient and review the

Examination Map

HISTORY

Past Medical History

History of the Present Condition

INSPECTION

Functional Assessment

Patella Alignment
Normal
Patella alta
Patella baja
Squinting
"Frog eyed"

Patellar Orientation
Medial/lateral glide
Spin
Anterior/posterior tilt
Medial/lateral tilt

Lower Extremity Posture
Genu varum
Genu valgum
Genu recurvatum

Q-Angle

Patellar Tendon

Tubercle Sulcus Angle

Leg Length Difference

Foot Posture

PALPATION

Palpation of the Anterior Structures
Tibial tuberosity
Patellar tendon
Patellar bursae
- Subcutaneous infrapatellar
- Deep infrapatellar

Fat pads
Patellar articulating surface
Femoral trochlea
Suprapatellar bursa
Medial patellofemoral ligament
Medial patellar retinaculum
Synovial plica
Lateral patellar retinaculum
Pes anserine insertion
Iliotibial band

JOINT AND MUSCLE FUNCTION ASSESSMENT

Goniometry
Knee flexion
Knee extension

Active Range of Motion
Knee flexion
Knee extension
Patellar tracking

Manual Muscle Tests
Quadriceps
Hamstrings
Sartorius

Passive Range of Motion
Flexion
Extension

JOINT STABILITY TESTS

Stress Testing
Testing of the major knee ligaments may be indicated

Joint Play Assessment
Medial patellar glide
Lateral patellar glide
Patellar tilt
Patellar spin

NEUROLOGIC EXAMINATION

Lower Quarter Screen

Common Peroneal Nerve

VASCULAR EXAMINATION

Distal Capillary Refill

Distal Pulse
Posterior tibial artery
Dorsal pedal artery

PATHOLOGIES AND SPECIAL TESTS

Patellofemoral Pain with Malalignment

Patellofemoral Instability
Apprehension test

Acute Patellar Dislocation

Patellofemoral Pain without Malalignment
Patellofemoral tendinopathy
Apophysitis
Osgood–Schlatter's disease
Sinding–Larsen–Johansson disease
Patellofemoral bursitis
Synovial plica

Traumatic Conditions
Patellar fracture
Patellar tendon rupture

medical file to identify conditions such as foot pathologies, recurrent ankle sprains, Achilles tendon pathology, knee sprains, injury to the hip, osteoarthritis, or conditions involving the lumbar region. Prior injury to the opposite limb may result in compensatory motion of the currently involved knee.

- **Previous history of patellofemoral conditions:** Question the patient regarding a past history of dislocations, patellofemoral pain, and/or surgery.
- **History of injury to the knee:** Ligamentous and meniscal knee injuries can result in biomechanical changes of the patellofemoral joint. Prior knee surgery can result in inflammation, adhesion, or entrapment of the patella's restraints, resulting in painful movement and reduced ROM.[24] Use of patellar tendon grafts for ACL reconstruction can result in residual changes in patellofemoral joint mechanics.
- **History of hip injury:** Pain may also be referred to the knee secondary to **Legg–Calvé–Perthes disease** or a **slipped capital femoral epiphysis** (see Chapter 12).

Box 11-1
Chondromalacia Patella

Although often referred to and treated as a discernible ailment, chondromalacia patella (CP) is best thought of as a finding related to a more distinct pathology. Chondromalacia patella is the softening and subsequent erosion of the patella's hyaline cartilage. This malady presents itself as grinding beneath the patella and may cause related swelling and pain. It is confirmed only via visual inspection during arthroscopy. CP is nebulous in nature because it is often found incidentally in otherwise normal knees.[2,26] Likewise, many individuals describing these symptoms before surgery have no signs of CP at the time of arthroscopy.[27–29]

CP is most often, if not always, the result of biomechanical changes affecting the lower extremity. As such, chondromalacia may be treated symptomatically but the key to its remedy is determining and correcting the underlying pathology.

History of the Present Condition

Identify the duration and intensity of the pain, functional limitations, and resulting disability. Patients describing more subjective symptoms and having more functional limitations are more apt to have an associated cartilage defect.[25]

- **Mechanism and onset of injury:** Determine if the chief complaint is the result of a single traumatic episode or if it stems from a gradual progression of symptoms.
  - **Acute onset:** Contusions and fractures may result from direct blows. Strains or ruptures of the patellar tendon are caused by dynamic overload of the musculotendinous unit. A dislocated patella has an acute onset, but repeated subtle subluxations represent chronic instability.
  - **Chronic or insidious onset:** Low-energy repetitive trauma, such as that associated with walking and running, can magnify the impact of patellofemoral maltracking and also lead to tendinopathy, bursitis, fat pad syndrome (**Hoffa's disease**), or chronic patellar instability (Box 11-1).
- **When pain occurs:** For chronic conditions, questions focus on when the pain occurs throughout the day, which activities cause its onset, and how these symptoms affect the level of activity. Activities such as ascending or descending stairs or open chain knee extension exercises through the full ROM increase compressive forces of the patella on the knee.[30] Pain occurring after prolonged periods of sitting, the "movie sign" ("theater sign"), may arise from prolonged pressure being placed on one or more articular facet. Descriptions of the knee as "locking" or "giving way" require follow-up for more details to determine the underlying cause. A distinction must be made between true locking of the knee and "clicking" beneath the patella. True locking of the knee is not normally indicative of patellofemoral pathology but, rather, of meniscal tears or an intra-articular loose body. Reports of the knee's giving way may be the result of patellar subluxation, inhibition secondary to pain, or internal derangement of the knee.
- **Location of the pain:** Pain radiating medially or laterally from the patella may indicate restricted or excessive glide within the trochlea or an abnormal patellar orientation causing atypical compression of the facets. Posterior knee pain is a common complaint associated with synovitis, but the pain may radiate to any area of the knee.
- **Level of activity:** Any changes in the level of activity, a change in the surface on which the activity occurs, or any other change in physical demand (e.g., as occurs in changing from playing first base to playing catcher or from bicycling to running) must be determined. Each of these may place excessive or unaccustomed forces on the patellofemoral joint.
- **Other biomechanical changes:** Many different factors can influence patellofemoral joint mechanics and resulting compressive forces.
  - Has the patient changed type of footwear for exercising? For example, switching from a running shoe designed to control pronatory forces to a running shoe with a softer midsole may magnify the impact of excessive pronation.
  - Are the patient's running shoes too old? Excessively worn shoes can lose their orthotic capacity and alter the mechanics of the patellofemoral joint.

- Has the patient recently gained weight? Weight gain such as seen with obesity or pregnancy is a predisposing factor for secondary arthritis of the knee and increases compressive forces on the patellofemoral articular surfaces during gait.

Inspection

Examine the entire knee complex for signs of gross deformity, including patellar malalignment, dislocation, and the integrity of the patellar tendon. Patellar alignment and orientation should be examined twice, once with the quadriceps relaxed and again with the quadriceps contracted. The patellofemoral joint should also be assessed with the patient weight bearing.

✱ Practical Evidence

Approximately half of the patients describing patellofemoral pain will have normal patellar alignment when the quadriceps are relaxed but will display malalignment when the quadriceps are contracted.[31]

Functional assessment

Ask the patient to replicate those functional tasks that exacerbate the symptoms and observe for compensations, lack of hip control (particularly an inability to control adduction and internal rotation), and strategies to minimize pain. Patients with patellofemoral pain or patellar tendinopathy pain often complain of pain in the midrange of motion and with eccentric loading, such as when descending stairs, squatting, or landing from a jump.[2]

Patellar motion and function differ between open and closed kinetic chain activities, so the patient may report difference complaints when squatting than when kicking a ball. Isokinetic knee testing for patients suffering from acute patellofemoral pain may be contraindicated because of the increased compressive forces placed on the patella at slower speeds.[32]

Patellar position

- **Patellar alignment:** With the knee fully extended and the patient weight bearing, observe the patella for alignment, at approximately the center of the femur, with the inferior pole located at the upper margin of the femoral trochlea (Fig. 11-6). Observe for possible malalignment while the lower extremity is weight bearing (Inspection Findings 11-1). Clinically, patella alta—a high-riding patella—may be identified via the camel sign (Fig. 11-7). Atypical alignment or orientation of the patella can increase the rate of erosion of the patellar and/or femoral articulating surfaces.[9]
- **Patellar orientation:** Clinical examination of the resting position of the patella on the femur provides gross evidence of the patella's orientation within the trochlea and on the femur (Inspection Findings 11-2).[33] The clinical examination of static patellar orientation has questionable validity when compared to MRI findings,[34] fair to good intrarater reliability and poor inter-rater reliability.[31] More precise measurements of patellar orientation can be determined using various radiographic techniques.[34,35]

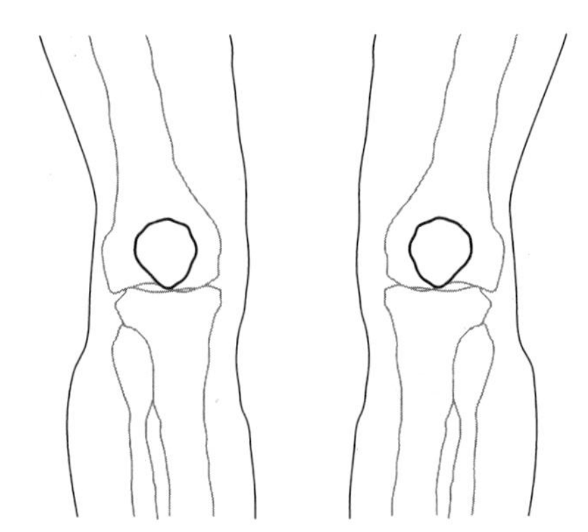

FIGURE 11-6 ■ Normal patellar alignment with the knee extended.

Inspection of the lower extremity

- **Posture of the lower extremity:** Inspect the lower extremities for the presence of the following alignments, which are also described in Chapter 6:
  - **Genu varum** places an increased compressive force on the lateral patellar facets.
  - **Genu valgum** causes excessive lateral forces, increasing the pressure on the medial and odd facets.
  - **Genu recurvatum** places additional pressure on the superior articular surfaces. The articulation may also be hypermobile as the patella distracts from the femur.[36]
  - The effects of the surrounding soft tissues on patellar position occur in three dimensions. Changing the tibiofemoral angle causes the patella to rotate

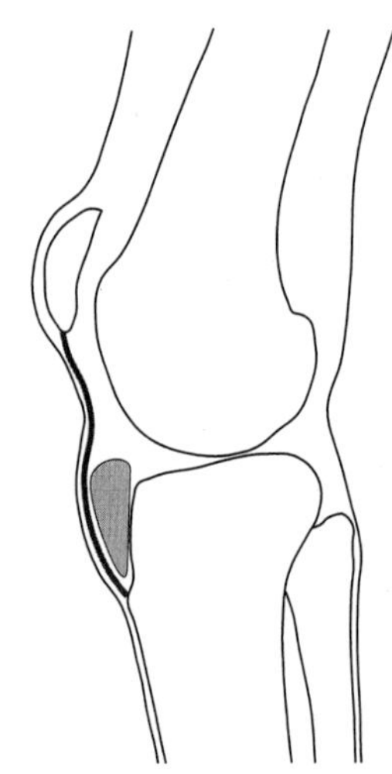

FIGURE 11-7 ■ "Camel sign," a clinical indication of patella alta. The high-riding patella exposes the fat pad, forming a "double hump" when viewed from the lateral side.

Inspection Findings 11-1
Patellar Alignment

	Patella Alta	Patella Baja	Squinting Patellae	"Frog Eyed" Patella
Description	High-riding patellae; the camel sign may be present (see Fig. 11-7)	Low-riding patellae	Patellae positioned medially	Patellae high riding and laterally
Potential Causes	Congenitally long patellar tendon	Congenitally short patellar tendon Arthrofibrosis after surgery or injury	Femoral anteversion, internal tibial rotation Arthrofibrosis after surgery or injury	Femoral retroversion, external tibial rotation
Consequences	Increased patellar mobility, decreased quadriceps strength, increased patellofemoral compressive forces when the knee is flexed	Decreased patellar glide, decreased tibiofemoral range of motion, decreased quadriceps strength, increased compressive patellofemoral forces when the knee is flexed	Increased Q-angle, tight medial retinaculum, maltracking of the patella, altered patellofemoral compressive forces Compensations include external tibial torsion.	Increased lateral patellar glide, tight lateral retinaculum, patellar maltracking decreased quadriceps strength, increased patellofemoral compressive forces when the knee is flexed

Inspection Findings 11-2
Patellar Orientation

	Medial/Lateral Patellar Glide	Patellar Rotation (Spin)	Anterior/Posterior Patellar Tilt	Medial/Lateral Patellar Tilt
Description	Position of the patella in the frontal plane.	The longitudinal (superior to inferior pole) orientation in the frontal plane	Rotation in the sagittal plane	Rotation in the transverse plane
Evaluation of Alignment	The patella should be centered between the medial and lateral patellar condyles. Displacement is described in the direction to which the patella is shifted. See Joint Play 11-1.	The long axis of the patella should be directed toward the ASIS. If the long axis is directed lateral to the ASIS then the patella is laterally rotated and vice versa.	The inferior patellar pole should be palpable when the knee is extended and the quadriceps are relaxed. The patella is anteriorly rotated if the superior pole of the patella must be depressed to make the inferior pole palpable.	See Joint Play 11-2.

ASIS = anterior superior iliac spine.

about its long axis. A varus alignment causes lateral rotation, causing increased pressure between the lateral facet and the lateral femoral trochlea. A valgus alignment causes medial rotation and increased pressure on the odd and medial facets.

- **Q-angle:** Determine the approximate tracking of the patella through the measurement of the Q-angle, the relationship between the anterior superior iliac spine, midpoint of the patella, and tibial tuberosity (Fig. 11-8). The Q-angle helps quantify the line of pull of the quadriceps and the patellar tendon and the resultant forces on the patella (Special Test 11-1). The **A angle** is the relationship between the long axis of the patella and the tibial tuberosity.[35]

The Q-angle typically decreases as the knee is flexed due to the internal tibial rotation that occurs. With the knee extended, the normal Q-angle is 13 degrees for men and 18 degrees for women. The Q-angle appears to be inversely proportional to height. Taller people have lower Q-angles than shorter people. The difference in Q-angle between sexes is therefore probably related to males having longer femurs than females.[37]

A measurement in standing, the functional Q-angle is more representative of the forces that occur in weight bearing.[2] Likewise, isometrically contracting the quadriceps muscle tends to decrease the Q-angle and more accurately reflects the biomechanics of patellar motion.[38]

Multiple factors can cause an increased Q-angle. External tibial rotation increases lateral compression of the patella in the trochlea and causes rotation of the patella in the frontal plane, increasing its susceptibility to subluxation, although evidence suggests that smaller Q-angles may also increase the risk.[39] Internal femoral rotation, resulting from femoral **anteversion**, causes more translational—as opposed to rotational forces—on the patella. Lateral compression of the patellofemoral joint is increased but the patella is pushed medially.[3] Increased Q-angles increase the forces placed on the lateral patellar facet, medial patellar retinaculum, and lateral border of the femoral trochlea secondary to an increased lateral glide of the patella. The amount of torque produced by the quadriceps muscle group decreases as the Q-angle increases.[40]

A Q-angle that is within normal limits does not necessarily mean that normal forces are present at the patellofemoral joint. The line between the anterior iliac superior spine (ASIS) and patella may not represent the line of pull of the quadriceps due to variations in timing and strength imbalances. A patella that is laterally positioned due to tight lateral structures may result in a Q-angle measurement that is within normal limits.

Anteversion A forward bending or angulation of a bone or organ.

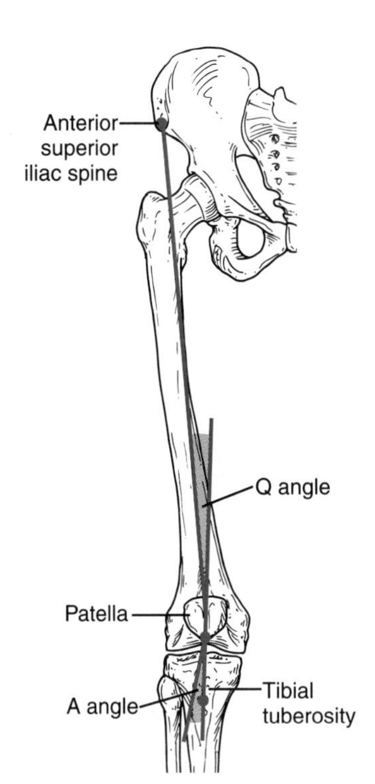

FIGURE 11-8 ■ The Q-angle describes the relationship between the long axis of the femur, measured from the anterior superior iliac spine to the center of the patella, to the long axis of the patella tendon, measured from the midpoint of the patella to the center of the tibial tuberosity. The A-angle is the relationship between the long axis of the patella and the tibial tuberosity.

*** Practical Evidence**

The majority of patients complaining of patellofemoral pain will not demonstrate patellar maltracking during closed-chain knee flexion. The absence of this finding should not rule out patellar tracking or malalignment as the cause of pain and dysfunction.[33] To determine the forces acting on the patella, Q-angle findings must be considered with other findings of the examination including patella position, glide, tilt, and kinematics.[43]

- **Patellar tendon:** Inspect the length of the patellar tendon, noting for signs of inflammation or other defects. An inflamed infrapatellar fat pad may cause bulging from beneath either side of the tendon.
- **Tubercle sulcus angle:** With the patient short sitting, observe the relationship between the tibial tuberosity and the inferior patellar pole. If the tuberosity is more than 10 degrees lateral to the inferior pole, the patient is predisposed to lateral patellar tracking (Fig. 11-9). Note that this alignment will also result in an increased Q-angle.
- **Leg-length difference:** Structural or functional leg length differences can affect the extensor mechanism and influence patellar tracking. Refer to Chapter 6 for methods of determining the presence of structural and functional leg-length differences.

Special Test 11-1
Q-Angle Measurement

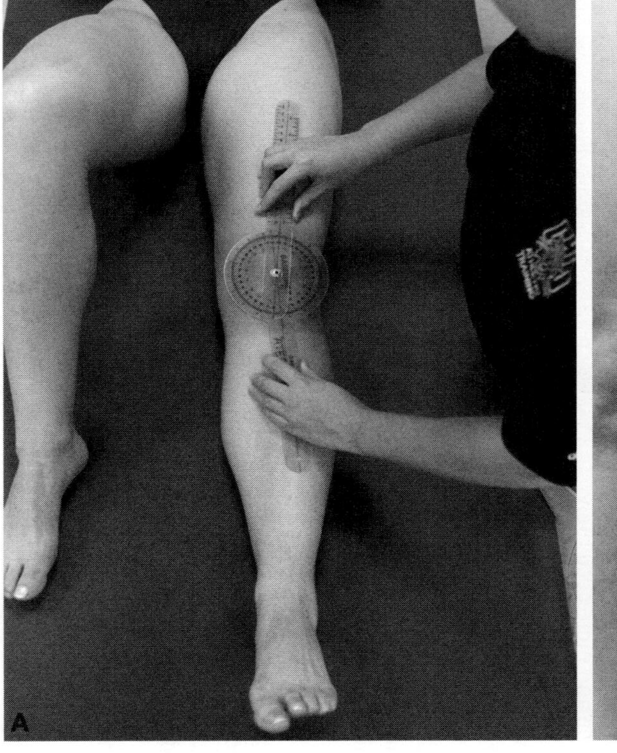

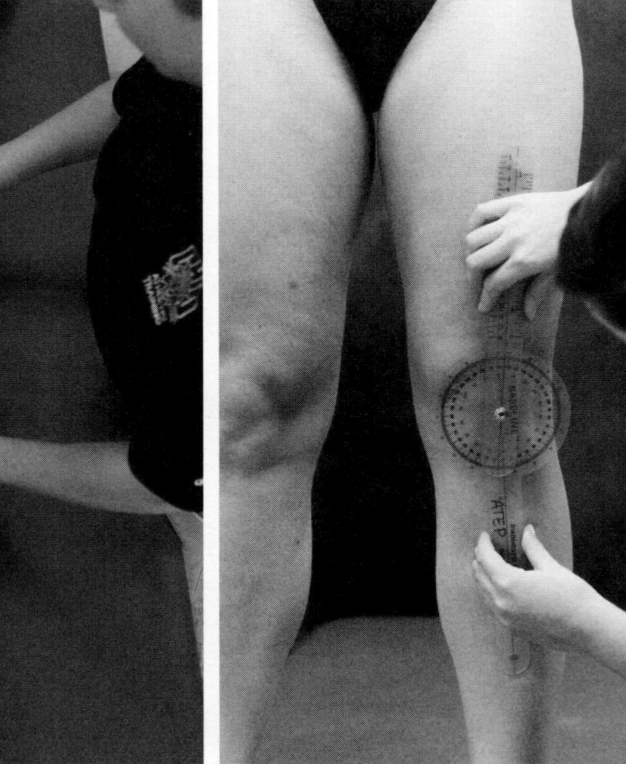

Measurement of the Q-angle with the knee extended in **(A)** a non–weight-bearing position and **(B)** weight-bearing; the anatomic landmarks of the ASIS, center of the patella, and the tibial tuberosity are used to align the goniometer.

Patient Position	**(A)** Lying supine with the knee fully extended with the ankle in neutral and the toes pointing up, replicating the standing position. Standardized foot position improves the reliability of this assessment.[41] **(B)** Standing with the feet shoulder-width apart.
Position of Examiner	Standing on the side of the limb to be measured
Evaluative Procedure	The examiner identifies and marks the ASIS, the midpoint of the patella, and the tibial tuberosity. A goniometer is placed so that the axis is located over the patellar midpoint, the center of the stationary arm is over the line from the ASIS to the patella, and the moving arm is placed over the line from the patella to the tibial tuberosity.
Positive Test	A Q-angle greater than 13° in men or 18° in women

Implications	Increased lateral forces leading to a laterally tracking patella
Modification	Re-measure the Q-angle with the quadriceps isometrically contracted. Differences between the two measures may provide insight to patellar tracking abnormalities.[38] The Q-angle may be measured with the knee in 30° of flexion, centering the patella within the femoral trochlea.
Comments	Measurement of the Q-angle in standing better replicates the functional alignment of the lower extremity. If the Q-angle is measured with the patient supine, this stance position should be replicated as indicated above. The Q-angle measured with the patient short-sitting should be smaller than measures obtained with the patient standing or long-sitting. When correlated with radiographic Q-angle measurements, clinical measurements routinely overestimate the angle.[42]
Evidence	Inter-rater reliability Not Reliable — Very Reliable Poor / Moderate / Good 0 0.1 0.2 0.3 0.4 0.5 0.6 0.7 0.8 0.9 1.0 Intra-rater reliability Not Reliable — Very Reliable Poor / Moderate / Good 0 0.1 0.2 0.3 0.4 0.5 0.6 0.7 0.8 0.9 1.0

ASIS = anterior superior iliac spine.

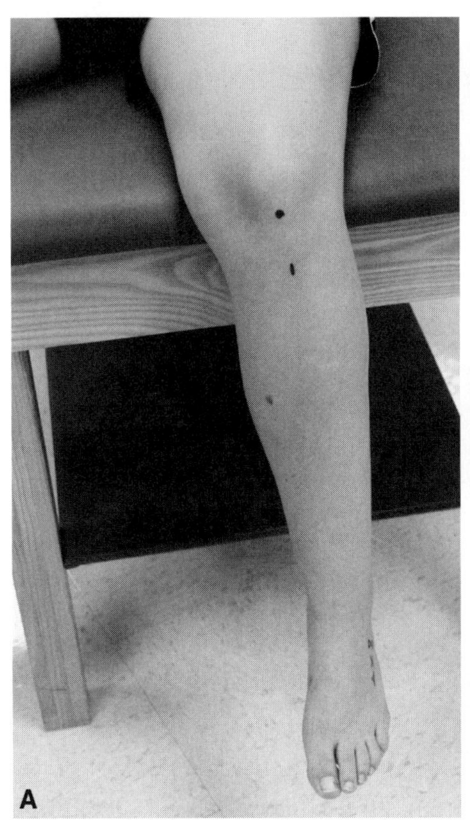

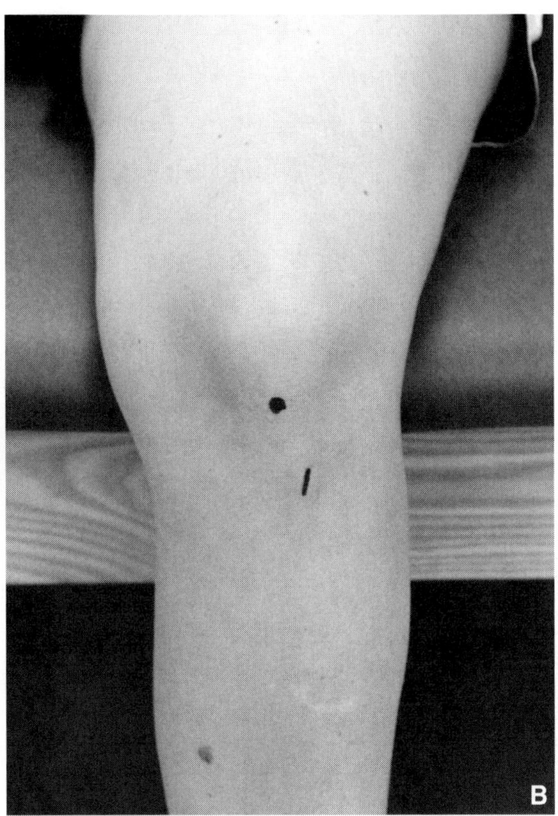

FIGURE 11-9 ■ Tubercle sulcus angle. (A) The tibial tuberosity is positioned inferior to the inferior pole of the patella, demonstrating normal alignment. (B) Laterally positioned tibial tuberosity, increasing lateral tracking of the patella.

✱ Practical Evidence

Instrumented measurement demonstrating unequal heights of the anterior superior iliac spine is 83% accurate in predicting patients who will demonstrate patellofemoral pain from those who will not and is more reliable than leg-length discrepancies identified using a tape measure.[44]

- **Foot posture:** Observe the position of the foot. While the patient is weight bearing, the foot should maintain a neutral or slightly pronated position. Excessive pronation results in internal tibial rotation, and excessive supination results in external tibial rotation. Pronation of one foot and supination of the other indicates a leg-length discrepancy, with the supinated foot representing the shorter leg. A standing leg-length difference can be confirmed if supinating the pronated foot brings the anterior superior iliac spines to an equal level (see Fig. 6-10).
- **Areas of scars, skin disruption, or skin discoloration:** Examine for any scars from previous injury such as lacerations or abrasions or prior surgeries for medial collateral ligament (MCL), lateral collateral ligament (LCL), meniscal, or cruciate ligament pathology. These areas may develop a keloid (see Fig. 1-4) or result in the formation of a neuroma, either of which may be the source of the pain. Because of its superficial location the prepatellar bursa is predisposed to infections from abrasions or other wounds.

✱ Practical Evidence

A hypomobile medial glide in the presence of restricted lateral tilt result tends to respond favorably to conservative treatment. A normal patellar tilt test result combined with a hypomobile medial glide may require the surgical release of the lateral retinacular structures to permit proper glide within the trochlea. A negative preoperative patellar tilt result has been positively correlated with a successful outcome of the release of the lateral structures.[47]

PALPATION

Caution is necessary when moving the patella, especially laterally. Patients who have a history of patellar dislocations or subluxations may become fearful or apprehensive about the patella being displaced as it is moved during the examination process. The complete palpation of the patellofemoral articulation must also include the tibiofemoral articulation.

This section describes palpation of the knee and patella only as it relates to patellar dysfunction.

1 **Tibial tuberosity:** Palpate the tibial tuberosity, identified by the insertion of the patellar tendon. The tibial tuberosity

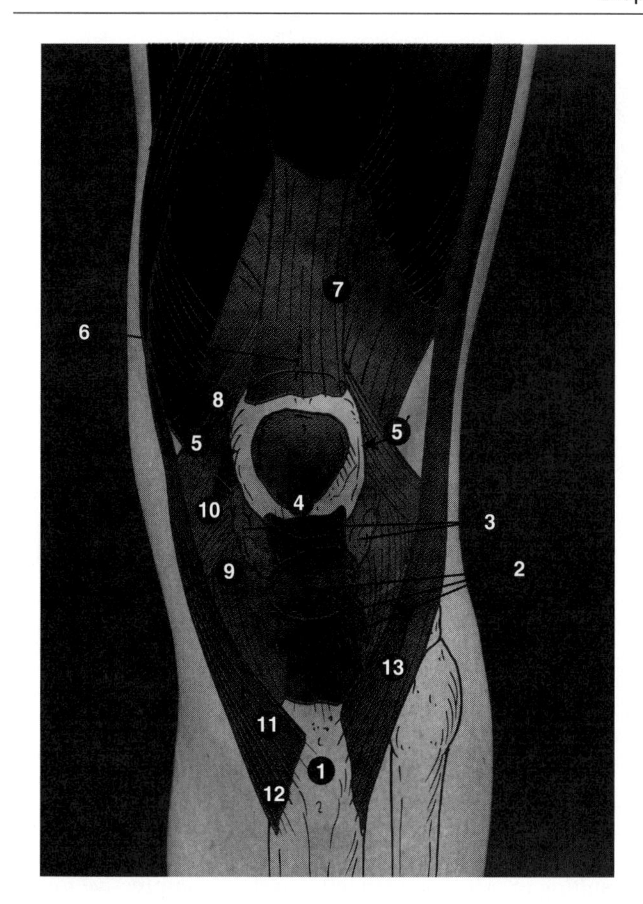

can become tender secondary to patellar tendinopathy or a contusion. Tenderness and enlargement of the tuberosity in adolescent patients may indicate Osgood–Schlatter disease.

2 Patellar tendon and bursae: Palpate the tendon at the level of the infrapatellar pole, moving distally to the tendon's midsubstance to its insertion at the tibial tuberosity. Pain or thickening detected at the infrapatellar pole through the midsubstance may indicate patellar tendinopathy; pain localized in the midsubstance may reflect a strain of this structure or tendon pathology. Palpate the **subcutaneous infrapatellar bursa** and **deep infrapatellar bursa** for tenderness, swelling, and the skin's ability to glide freely over the tibial tuberosity.

3 Fat pads: Place the knee in extension to squeeze the fat pads beneath the patellar tendon out to either side, masking the deep infrapatellar bursa from palpation. Palpate these fat pads for signs of inflammation as they exit from behind, medially, and laterally to the patellar tendon, spanning the area from the inferior patellar pole to the tibial tuberosity.[22] Because these structures are highly innervated, they are prone to hypersensitivity during inflammatory conditions and may mimic patellar tendinopathy.

4 Patella and bursae: During palpation of the patella, be alert for pain arising from the bone itself to distinguish it from pain arising from the soft tissue. Palpate the patellar body to rule out the presence of fracture, indicated by pain, roughening, discontinuity, or crepitus. Continue to palpate along the periphery of the four borders, attempting to elicit tenderness secondary to inflammatory conditions. If pain is present at the superior border, palpate up the length of the quadriceps group, noting the point at which the pain disappears. A bipartite patella, although not always identified through palpation, may be present either from previous trauma or a congenital defect (Fig. 11-10). At birth, the patella is cartilaginous, ossifying between 3 and 6 years of age. When separate ossification centers fail to join, a bipartite patella may result.[45] Regardless of the nature of its onset, a bipartite patella reduces the efficiency of the extensor mechanism.

The **prepatellar bursa** overlies the patella. Ensure that the skin over the patella moves freely and is not painful. The prepatellar bursa may become irritated and inflamed from overuse; from a contusing force to the anterior patella; or from prolonged periods of kneeling, as is seen with wrestlers. This bursa is also a common site of bacterial (i.e., staphylococcal) infection.

5 Patellar articulating surface: With the knee extended, move the patella laterally to expose the outer portion of the lateral articular facet and medially to expose the odd facet. The exposed facets are palpated for signs of tenderness. Exercise caution when moving the patella laterally, as this motion duplicates the mechanism for patellar dislocations and can create patient apprehension.

6 Femoral trochlea: In the patella's resting position on an extended knee, palpate the medial and lateral femoral trochlear borders for tenderness, keeping in mind that the lateral border is more exposed than the medial border is. Moving the patella medially and laterally exposes more of the femoral articular surface.

Grinding beneath the patella while it is compressed and moved against the femur suggests the presence of chondromalacia. Although the condition occurs in a significant portion of the population, its presence may reflect biomechanical changes in the extensor mechanism or elsewhere in the lower extremity.

7 Suprapatellar bursa: Locate the suprapatellar bursa under the quadriceps group approximately 3 inches (four-finger breadth) above the patella. With the exception of puncture wounds, the suprapatellar bursa is rarely injured by direct trauma. It may, however, become inflamed or enlarged secondary to effusion of the knee joint capsule.

8 Medial patellofemoral ligament: Palpate the length of the MPFL from the femur's adductor tubercle and MCL to the superomedial aspect of the patella. This structure will become tender after acute dislocation of the patella.

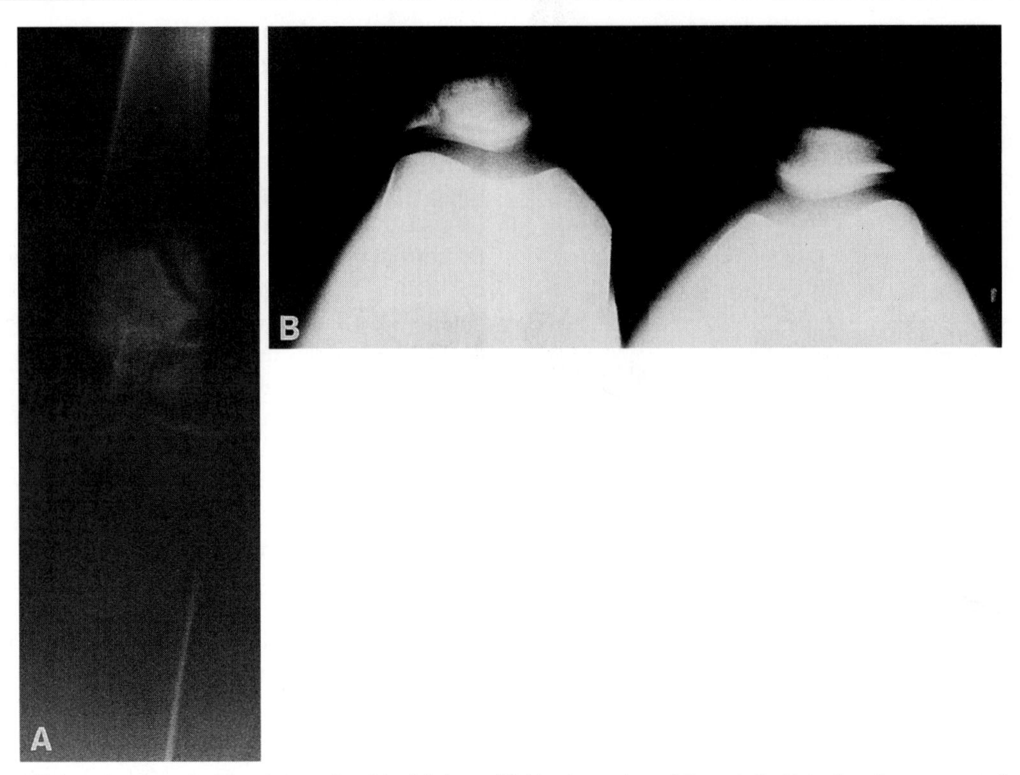

FIGURE 11-10 ■ (A) Anterior view of a bipartite patella of the left knee. (B) Merchant view of the patella. Note the discrepancy in the continuity of the left and right patellae.

9 **Retinacular and capsular structures:** Palpate the medial and lateral retinacula, patellofemoral ligaments, and capsule for pain. The retinaculum and the associated structures may become painful with patellar hypermobility.

10 **Synovial plica:** Palpate the anteromedial and anterolateral joint capsule for bands of thickened or folded tissue, denoting a synovial plica. These areas may become irritated and inflamed from being rubbed across bony structures or other tissues.

11, 12, 13. **Related structures:** The **pes anserine muscle group** and its associated bursae in the area of the medial tibial flare are common sites of inflammation (**11**). Hypersensitivity of one or more nerves can result in pain radiating through the knee and lower extremity. A neuroma, most commonly occurring from laceration of nerves during surgery involving the infrapatellar branch of the saphenous nerve, may be confirmed via a test for Tinel's sign over the medial aspect of the knee (**12**). Determine the flexibility of the IT band because tightness of this structure serves to increase the amount of lateral patellar tracking. Trigger points can be found in the IT band, causing tightness along its entire length (**13**).

Joint and Muscle Function Assessment

Unrestricted movement of the patella is required for the lower leg to achieve its full range of motion. Pain at the patella during movement may indicate a malalignment, resulting in soft tissue stretch as well as compressive forces on the articular facets, more so on the medial side. The normal and abnormal movement of the patella as the knee moves from flexion to extension is discussed here. The complete ROM testing of the knee joint is described in Chapter 10 and the hip is presented in Chapter 12.

Active range of motion

As the knee moves from flexion into extension, the patella normally glides superiorly and tracks somewhat laterally, creating the **J sign**. Tightness of the lateral structures accentuates the lateral glide and tilt of the patella. During flexion, the patella glides inferiorly and medially as it situates itself in the femoral trochlea. The **reverse J sign** is occurs when tight medial restraints pull the patella medially during terminal extension.

Manual muscle testing

Strength assessment of the quadriceps and hamstrings at the knee joint is described in Chapter 10. Weakness of the hip abductors and external rotators such as gluteus medius is frequently implicated in patellofemoral pathology, as these muscles eccentrically control the internal rotation of the lower extremity that occurs during the stance phase of gait. Weakness of these muscles results in excessive internal rotation and a resulting increase in lateral forces at the patellofemoral joint. These manual muscle tests are described in Chapter 12.

Passive range of motion

Passively assess motion at the hip, knee, and ankle for joint restrictions. Assess the muscle length of the hamstrings, quadriceps, and triceps surae (see Chapter 6). A limitation in knee flexion with the hip in neutral indicates tightness of the rectus femoris. A limitation in hip flexion with the knee extended indicates insufficient hamstring length and a limitation in ankle dorsiflexion with the knee fully extended or flexed may indicate tightness in the triceps surae. Decreased gastrocnemius and soleus length, particularly when coupled with decreased strength of the hip abductors, is associated with patellofemoral pain.[46] Decreased hamstring flexibility results in increased joint reaction forces at the patellofemoral joint secondary to the added force generated by the quadriceps group.[31]

Joint Stability Tests

The ligamentous and capsular stability of the patella is assessed using patellar tilt and glide. Glide tests are performed to assess the laxity or tightness of the retinacula by measuring how far the patella can be moved passively from its resting position in the trochlea.

Stress testing

Evaluate all major knee ligaments for normal integrity, as described in Chapter 10. Laxity of the knee joint can result in abnormal patellar tracking secondary to uniplanar or rotatory shifting of the tibia or femur, causing patellofemoral pain.

Joint play assessment

The following description of the assessment of patellar glide and tilt have been adapted from the American Academy of Orthopaedic Surgeons' guidelines.[47]

- **Resting position:** Before determining the extent of mobility, the resting position of the patella must be assessed (see Inspection Box 11-1).
- **Patellar glide:** To determine the amount of glide, visualize the patella as having four quadrants. Place the knee on a bolster so that it is flexed to 30 degrees. The patient must be fully reclined to relax the quadriceps muscles (Fig. 11-11). To ensure accuracy during the measurements, avoid tilting the patella as it is glided medially and laterally (Joint Play 11-1).
- **Patellar tilt:** The amount of patellar tilt, the rotation of the patella about its longitudinal axis, evaluates the tension within the lateral retinaculum, lateral capsule, IT band, and lateral portion of the quadriceps tendon. Patella tilt is described by the direction that the medial and lateral borders are positioned. The evaluation is performed with the patient lying supine with the knee extended and the femoral condyles parallel to the table (Joint Play 11-2).

Special tests

IT band tightness is associated with increased lateral tracking secondary to its attachment on the lateral retinaculum. The tension of the iliotibial band can be assessed via the **Ober's test** (Chapter 10). The **navicular drop test** (Chapter 8) is used to identify excessive pronation. Foot structure, including an assessment of rearfoot and forefoot position (Chapter 8), is routinely determined with patellofemoral conditions of gradual onset.

Neurologic and Vascular Testing

The assessment of the sensory, motor, and reflex function and vascular testing for the patellofemoral joint is the same as described for the knee in Chapter 10.

Hip problems such as **Legg–Calvé–Perthes disease** or a **slipped capital femoral epiphysis** may refer pain to the knee. A childhood history of these conditions warrants an examination of the hip.

Pathologies and Related Special Tests

The interrelated nature of patellofemoral pathologies makes classification difficult, at best. The nonspecific terms "patellofemoral dysfunction" and "patellofemoral pain syndrome" describe a wide range of knee and patella symptoms, but they do little to reveal the underlying cause of the symptoms.[31] Symptoms range from dull to sharp pain arising from anterior (prepatellar) or posterior (retropatellar) portions of the patella or borders. The working diagnosis of patellofemoral dysfunction

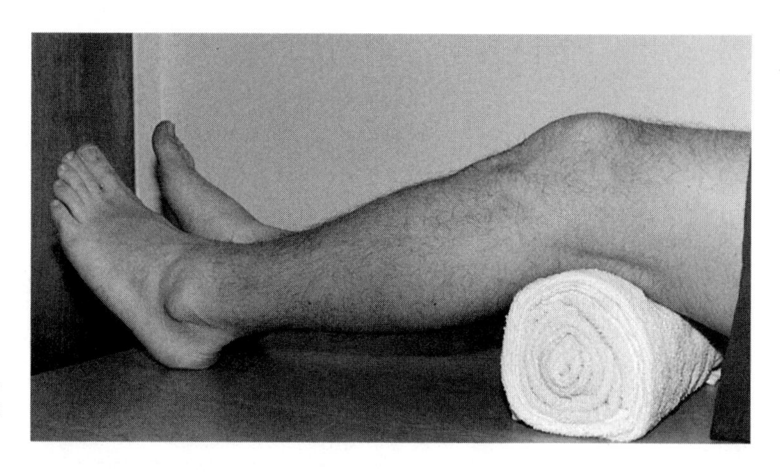

FIGURE 11-11 ■ Positioning of the patient during the patellar glide tests. The knee is flexed to 30° and the individual is encouraged to keep the quadriceps musculature relaxed.

Joint Play 11-1
Medial and Lateral Patellar Glide Test

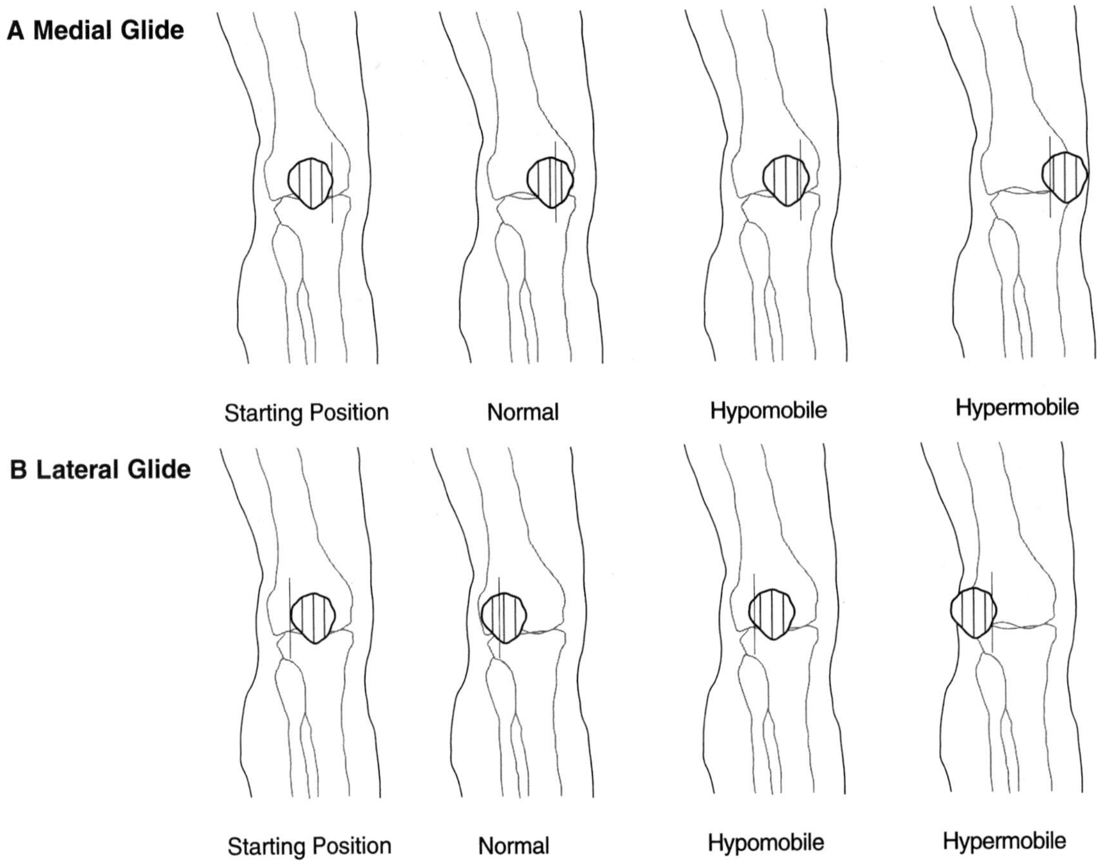

A Medial Glide

Starting Position | Normal | Hypomobile | Hypermobile

B Lateral Glide

Starting Position | Normal | Hypomobile | Hypermobile

During medial (**A**) and lateral (**B**) patellar glide tests, the patella is viewed as having four quadrants. The amount of glide is based on the movement relative to the quadrants.

Patient Position	Supine with a bolster placed under the knee so that it is flexed to 30°
Position of Examiner	Standing lateral to the patient
Evaluative Procedure	**(A)** Medial glide: Move the patella medially, placing stress on the lateral retinaculum and other soft tissue restraints. **(B)** Lateral glide: Move the patella laterally, placing stress on the medial retinaculum, VMO, and medial capsule.
Positive Test	***Medial glide:*** The patella should glide one to two quadrants (approximately half its width) medially. Movement of less than one quadrant is considered hypomobile. Movement of more than two quadrants is hypermobile medial glide. ***Lateral glide:*** Normal lateral motion is 0.5–2.0 quadrants of glide. Less than that is hypomobile lateral glide; greater than two quadrants is hypermobile lateral glide.
Implications	***Medial glide:*** Hypomobile glide: Tightness of the lateral retinaculum or IT band. Hypermobile glide: Laxity of the lateral restraints. ***Lateral glide:*** Hypomobile glide: Tightness of the medial restraints, specifically the medial patellofemoral ligament.[14] Hypermobile glide: Laxity of the medial restraints
Comments	The patient may be apprehensive during lateral glide tests, fearful that the motion could result in a patella dislocation or subluxation. Hypermobile lateral glide creates a predisposition to patellar dislocations. Hypomobile medial glide is more common than hypermobile medial glide.
Evidence	Absent or inconclusive in the literature

IT = iliotibial; VMO = oblique fibers of the vastus medialis.

Joint Play 11-2
Patellar Tilt Assessment

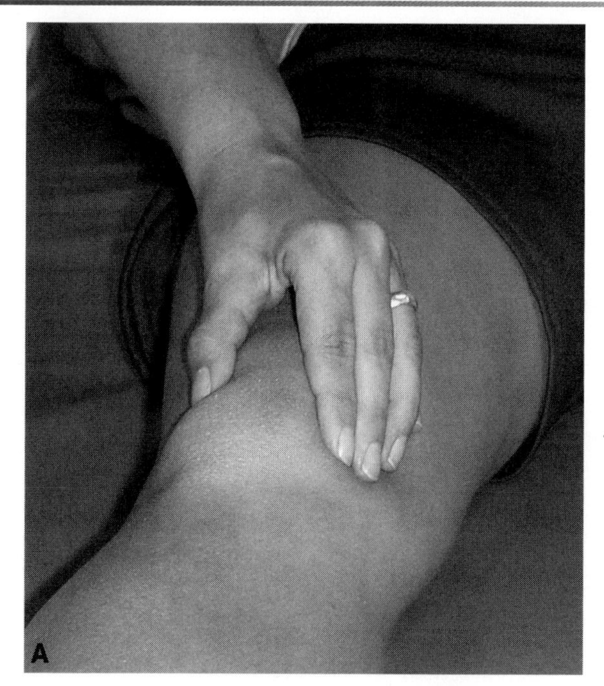

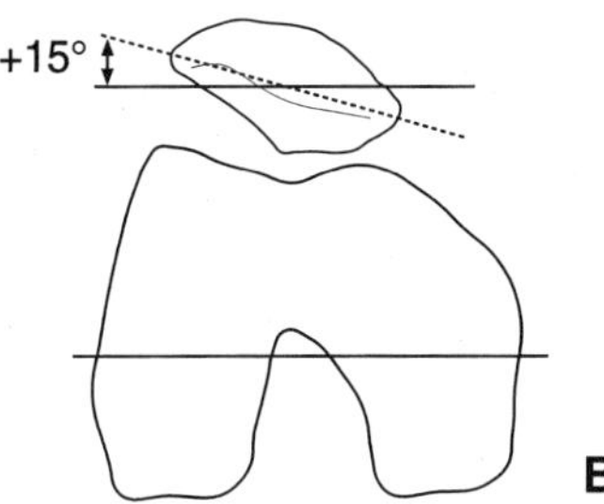

The patellar tilt test evaluates rotation of the patella around its midsagittal axis.

Patient Position	Supine with the knee extended and the femoral condyles parallel to the table
Position of Examiner	Standing lateral to the patient
Evaluative Procedure	Grasp the patella with the forefinger and thumb, elevating the lateral border and depressing the medial border.
Positive Test	A normal result is the lateral border raising between 0° and 15°. More than 15° is hypermobile lateral tilt; less than 0° is a hypomobile lateral tilt.
Implications	A tilt of less than 0° indicates tightness of the lateral restraints and often occurs in the presence of a hypomobile medial glide.[48] A tilt of more than 15° may predispose the individual to anterior knee pain
Evidence	Inter-rater reliability

Not Reliable **Very Reliable**

Poor | Moderate | Good

0 0.1 0.2 0.3 0.4 0.5 0.6 0.7 0.8 0.9 1.0

is often made for cases of unexplained pain when other more serious soft tissue and bony pathologies have been ruled out.[26]

Pain and dysfunction arising from the patellofemoral complex often mimic the symptoms of meniscal injury. Table 11-2 presents subjective findings that are used to differentiate between injuries of the two structures. Patellofemoral pain may also be the result of osteochondral defects of the femur or patellar articulating surface (see Chapters 4 and 10).

This section classifies patellofemoral joint pathology in four major categories:

- Patellofemoral pain with malalignment[31,50]
- Patellofemoral instability[31,50]
- Patellofemoral pain without malalignment[31,50]
- Traumatic conditions.

This classification system organizes the examination findings and forms the basis for developing the optimal intervention strategy. For example, treatments for patellofemoral pain

Table 11-2 Subjective Findings in the Differentiation of Meniscal and Patellar Pain

History	Meniscus	Patella
Onset	Usually acute twisting injury	Occasionally direct anterior knee blow but usually insidious related to overuse and training errors
Symptom Site	Localized medial or lateral joint line	Diffuse, most commonly anterior
Locking	Frank transient locking episodes with the knee unable to fully terminally extend	Catching without locking, stiffness after immobility, but not true locking
Weight Bearing	Pain sharp and simultaneous with loaded weight bearing	Pain possibly coming on during weight bearing but often continuing into the evening and night
Cutting Sports	Pain with loaded twisting maneuvers	Some pain possible, but not sharp and clearly related to cutting
Squatting	Pain at full squat; inability to "duck walk"	Pain when extensors used to descend or rise from a squat
Kneeling	Not painful because meniscus is not weight loaded	Pain from patellar compression
Jumping	Weight loaded without torque or twist tolerated	Extensors heavily stressed, causing pain on descent impact
Stairs or Hills	Pain often going upstairs with loaded knee flexion, causing squatlike meniscal compression	More patellar loading and pain going downstairs because gravity-assisted impact increases patellofemoral stress
Sitting	No pain	Stiffness and pain from lack of the distraction–compression effect on abnormal articular cartilage

that result from malalignment are directed at correcting the underlying cause of the tracking problem such as the use of orthotics, stretching tight tissues, or surgery. Classification of these pathologies is not mutually exclusive. Patellar tendinopathies may be influenced by malalignment, malalignment can be caused by trauma, and patellofemoral instability can be associated with malalignment.

Patellofemoral Pain with Malalignment

With malalignment of the patella in the trochlea, the patella tracks abnormally, causing atypical compressive or tensile forces on the patella and its soft tissue restraints. These forces result in pain. The onset of patellofemoral dysfunction has historically been attributed solely to an increased Q-angle. However, patellofemoral function is based on a number of individual variables, each influencing the extensor mechanism.[51,52] Normal tracking of the patella within the femoral trochlea depends on the relationships between the alignment of the femur on the tibia; the Q-angle; the integrity of the patella's soft tissue restraints; foot mechanics; and the flexibility of the triceps surae, quadriceps, hamstring muscle groups, and IT band (Table 11-3). The combined influence of joint motion acting at the tibiofemoral and patellofemoral joints is functionally more significant than static structure. For example, internal rotation of the tibia and femur create a valgus force that increases lateral tracking of the patella (Fig. 11-12).

Many of the predisposing conditions to patellar tracking disorders are congenital. However, injury to the patella or knee may cause a change in one of the variables. For example, a lateral dislocation of the patella results in tearing of the medial restraints, causing increased laxity and increased lateral migration of the patella during knee extension. Likewise, an injury to the knee can cause atrophy of the VMO, increasing the amount of lateral patellar glide with subsequent shortening of the lateral restraints. Other variables affecting the equation are increased body weight and gait mechanics.[53]

In healthy individuals, the VMO contracts simultaneously with or before vastus lateralis contraction. This contractile pattern results in normal patellar tracking. When the knee is effused, a fluid buildup of 20 to 30 mL of excess fluid neurologically inhibits the VMO. With an effusion of 50 to 60 mL, the rest of the extensor mechanism is inhibited. When the VMO is inhibited, the relatively unopposed pull from the VL can cause excessive lateral tracking and increase compressive forces on the lateral facet.[54] Contrary to prevalent belief, the activation timing between the VMO and VL is not different when comparing those with and without patellofemoral pain syndromes in the absence of effusion.[55]

Patients suffering from patellofemoral pain syndrome caused by malalignment describe a gradual onset with symptoms related to increase or change in activity. Complaints of pain are usually associated with descending stairs, sitting for long periods of time, and other activities in

Examination Findings 11-1
Patellofemoral Pain Syndrome

Examination Segment	Clinical Findings
History	***Onset:*** Gradual, with typical description of abrupt change in surface, activity level, or activity intensity. ***Pain characteristics:*** Pain arising from the peripatellar area, frequently at lateral facet and lateral trochlea secondary to increased compressive forces. ***Other symptoms:*** The patient may describe symptoms such as "clicking" or the knee "giving out." ***Mechanism:*** A discrete mechanism of injury is typically not reported. ***Predisposing conditions:*** Increased Q-angle, shallow trochlear groove, patella alta, patella baja. A change in footwear may also be implicated.
Inspection	Increased Q-angle, patella alta, patella baja, femoral anteversion, excessive tibial torsion, or pronated foot may be noted.
Palpation	Pain at medial retinaculum, odd medial facet, lateral facet, lateral femoral condyle
Joint and Muscle Function Assessment	***AROM:*** Knee extension may increase symptoms. ***MMT:*** Quadriceps pain and weakness Weakness of the hip abductors and external rotators is commonly noted (see Chapter 12). ***PROM:*** End range of knee flexion may increase symptoms due to compression of the patella. Shortened quadriceps, hamstrings, or triceps surae
Joint Stability Tests	***Stress tests:*** A full examination of the knee may be warranted to rule out chronic tibiofemoral instability. ***Joint play:*** Lateral patellar glide may be increased. Medial patellar glide may be decreased.
Special Tests	Ober's test for IT band tightness (Chapter 10) Navicular drop test for excessive foot pronation/internal tibial rotation (Chapter 8)
Neurologic Screening	Within normal limits
Vascular Screening	Within normal limits
Functional Assessment	Increased pain with sitting, descending and ascending stairs, and squatting[33]
Imaging Techniques	Skyline view radiograph
Differential Diagnosis	Meniscal tear, patellar instability, synovial plica, patellar tendinopathy
Comments	Patellofemoral problems are often related to poor neuromuscular control of the hip, which is worsened by fatigue, which increases valgus fories at the knee.

AROM = active range of motion; IT = iliotibial; MMT = manual muscle test; PROM = passive range of motion.

which the knee is flexed for prolonged periods. Patients may describe "popping" and "clicking," and palpation during active motion will reveal that this is occurring at the patellofemoral articulation. Mild swelling in the peripatellar region may be present (Examination Findings 11-1).

The functional examination may reveal increased and prolonged pronation during weight bearing and an inability to control medial rotation and adduction of the hip when accepting weight during the stance phase of gait. This aberration may become more apparent with fatigue, which associates with increased complaints of pain with a longer duration of activity. Lower extremity internal rotation is also demonstrated when the excessive valgus occurs when stepping down, such as descending stairs.[2] Both of these functional deviations result in increased lateral tracking of the patella.

Physical examination of the joint may reveal patella baja or alta, both of which contribute to atypical joint function. Patella baja increases joint compressive forces and patella alta leads to decreased patellofemoral joint stability as the patella has reduced contact with the stabilizing trochlea. At rest,

Table 11-3 Structural Abnormalities and Their Resultant Forces and Biomechanical Changes

Alignment	Resulting Forces and Biomechanical Changes
Genu Varum	Increased compressive forces on the medial tibiofemoral articulating surfaces
	Tensile forces on the lateral tibiofemoral soft tissue structures and LCL
	Quadriceps exerting medially directed forces on the patella
	Compressive forces on the lateral facet
	Stretching of the lateral patellar restraints
Genu Valgum	Increased compressive forces on the lateral tibiofemoral articulating surfaces
	Tensile forces on the medial tibiofemoral ligaments
	Quadriceps exerting laterally directed forces on the patella
	Compressive forces on the odd and medial facets
	Stretching of the medial patellar restraints
Increased Q-angle or Lax Medial Restraints	Lateral tracking of the patella
	Compressive forces on the lateral facet
	Stretching of the medial patellar restraints
Decreased Q-angle or Lax Lateral Restraints	Medial tracking of the patella
	Compressive forces on odd and medial facets
	Stretching of the lateral patellar restraints
Genu Recurvatum	Decreased compressive forces in terminal knee extension

LCL = lateral collateral ligament.

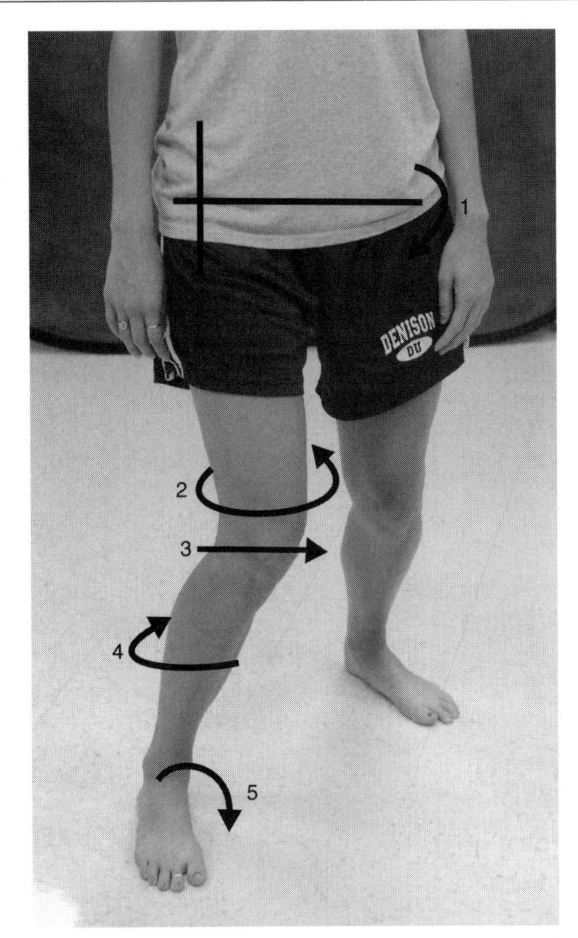

FIGURE 11-12 ■ Contributors of lower extremity segments to abnormal alignment: (1) contralateral pelvic drop, (2) internal rotation of the femur, (3) valgus knee alignment, (4) internal rotation of the tibia, and (5) foot pronation. (Adapted from Powers, CM: *J Orthop Sports Phys Ther*, 33:639, 2003.)

lateral tilt and glide of the patella may be present, signifying tight lateral restraints and/or lax medial restraints. Lateral glide may be excessive, with medial glide restricted. Tightness of the lateral retinaculum may increase the tightness of the iliotibial band and biceps femoris, also contributing to excessive lateral forces (see Joint Play Test 11-1).[56]

Examination of the ankle, foot, and hip is needed to understand fully the contributions to maltracking. An assessment of the foot and ankle in subtalar joint neutral (see p. 177) frequently reveals a forefoot varus alignment, the cause of the increased and prolonged pronation. Reduced passive extension of the great toe in a relaxed stance also signifies a pronated foot and is predictive of patellofemoral pathology.[57] Strength and endurance of the hip external rotators and abductors is frequently diminished (Fig. 11-13).

Pain is increased with active and resisted extension of the knee and during the end range of passive flexion. **Clarke's sign**, frequently described as a diagnostic tool for patellofemoral joint dysfunction, produces an unreliably high rate of false-positive results, causing pain in otherwise healthy individuals and its use is not recommended (Special Test 11-2).

Treatment of patients with patellofemoral pain resulting from malalignment usually begins by modifying activity to avoid pain and the use of nonsteroidal anti-inflammatory medications. The use of ice, especially after activity, may be helpful. If tightness is assessed in the surrounding capsule and retinacular tissues, patellar mobilization and passive stretching may be helpful. Therapeutic exercise for improving flexibility of lower extremity musculature and improving the strength and endurance of the trunk, hip, and thigh muscles to improve patellar tracking is also useful.[59]

The use of shoe orthotics as an adjunct to exercise has been shown to reduce patellofemoral pain in patients who exhibit increased pronation, lower extremity internal rotation when weight bearing, and increased Q-angle.[60] Patellar taping is useful in reducing subjective reports of pain although it is unlikely that it accomplishes this by altering

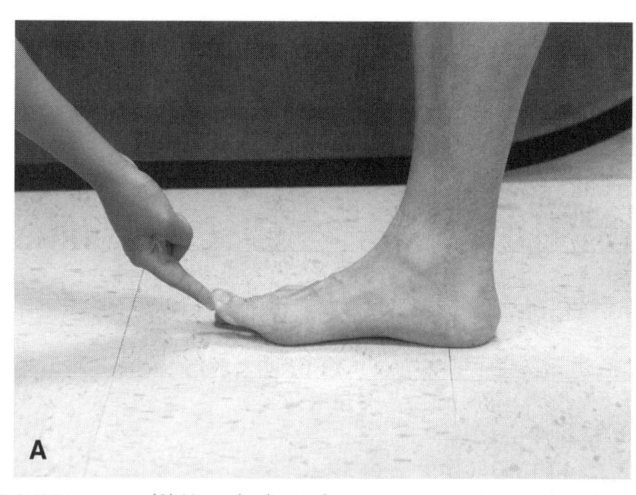

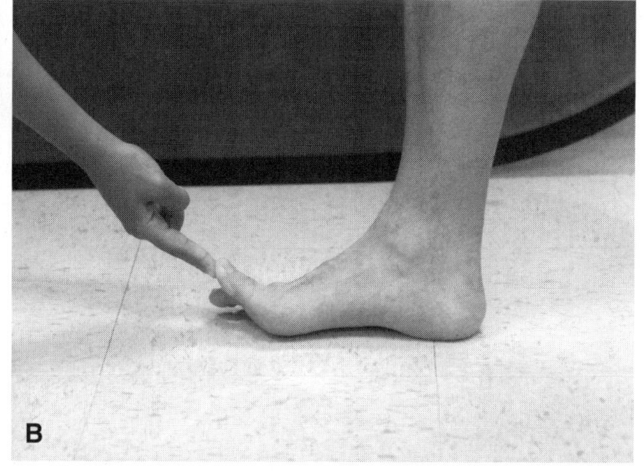

FIGURE 11-13 ■ (A) Note the limited great toe extension in relaxed stance. (B) With the patient positioned in subtalar joint neutral, the extensor hallucis longus is no longer on stretch, allowing full motion into extension.

patellar tracking kinematics.[61] Examination of the influence of patellar taping on healthy subjects revealed no change in activation patterns of the vastus medialis and vastus lateralis,[62] although it may alter the activation of these muscles in patients experiencing patellofemoral pain.[63]

Patellofemoral Instability

Patellofemoral instability can be subtle, resulting in subluxations, or dramatic, resulting in a dislocation. Resulting from laxity of the static restraints such as the medial and lateral retinacula, the patellofemoral articulation is typically unstable in the lateral direction due to the slight valgus arrangement of the knee. Medial instability is rare.

True (frank) dislocation of the patella causes it to shift laterally and lock out of place, resulting in obvious gross deformity and spasm of the quadriceps group as it guards the injury (see Acute Patellar Dislocation). Acute, chronic, or congenital laxity of the medial patellar restraints or abnormal tightness of the lateral retinaculum causes an increased lateral glide of the patella, subluxations, and dislocations. Subtle patellar subluxations may occur without the person's knowledge, producing symptoms described as the knee "giving out" during weight bearing (Examination Findings 11-2). Patients suffering from chronic patellar instability also produce a positive **apprehension test,** which should be performed before testing for patellar mobility and before performing a valgus stress test (Special Test 11-3).

The patella is most apt to dislocate or subluxate when the maximum tensile strain is placed on the lateral patellar restraints, normally within the range of 20 to 30 degrees of knee flexion, pulling the patella laterally,[64] or after a valgus blow to the knee. Dislocations caused by blunt trauma may also result in a fracture of the patella.[65] Noncontact dislocations may result in osteochondral damage, patellar bone bruises, or osteochondritis dissecans.[66,67] Multiple dislocations or subluxations may cause erosion of the articular cartilage. However, the incidence of true osteoarthritis is reduced in this population relative to those having normal tension in the patellar restraints.[68]

Several factors predispose an individual to patellar subluxations and dislocations. Those with hypomobile medial glide have an increased tendency for subluxations than persons with hypermobile lateral glide.[69] The tightness of the lateral restraints serves to pull the patella laterally during knee extension. A shallow trochlea or flattened posterior (articulating) patellar surface increases the likelihood of spontaneous (non–contact-related) patellar dislocation.[70] Factors such as external tibial rotation and hyperpronated feet increase the Q-angle, causing the patella to track laterally.[71] A family history of patellar dislocations or subluxations also increases the risk of patellofemoral instability.[72]

The use of prophylactic or rehabilitational braces has little effect on preventing the reoccurrence of patellar dislocations or subluxations.[73] Most patients with patellofemoral pain syndrome respond favorably to conservative rehabilitation that focuses on quadriceps strengthening.[74] Other forms of conservative treatment include casting, posterior splinting, and functional bracing. Of these methods, the use of posterior splints results in the lowest recurrence rate. In cases of chronic instability operative treatment frequently yields the best results.[75] The most common surgical technique involves shifting the patellar tendon attachment to correct patellar tracking problems.[76]

Acute patellar dislocation

Acute patellar dislocations result in large, bloody effusions within 24 hours after the onset of the injury (Fig. 11-14). A complete dislocation seldom occurs without tearing of the VMO from the patella or from its origin near the adductor tubercle or the adjacent intermuscular septum.[72] The insertion of the medial patellar retinaculum is often avulsed from the patella and the medial patellofemoral ligament (MPFL) is often torn.[65] Palpation of the medial patellar retinaculum, MPFL, and/or the VMO at either its origin or insertion produces pain (Examination Findings 11-3). Radiographic

Special Test 11-2
Clarke's Sign for Chondromalacia Patella

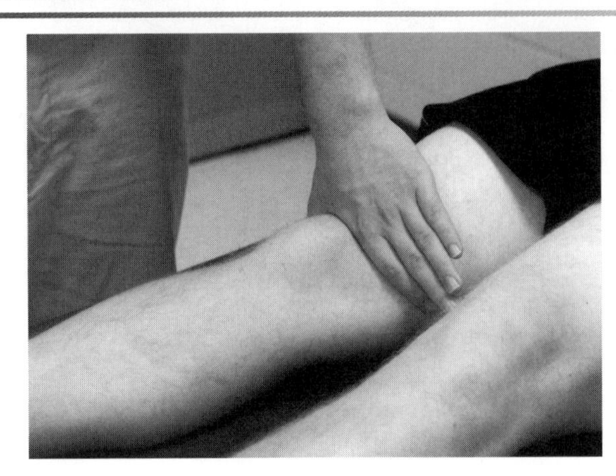

Clarke's sign for chondromalacia patella; this test elicits a great deal of pain and elicits a positive result in otherwise asymptomatic knees.

Patient Position	Lying supine with the knee extended
Position of Examiner	Standing lateral to the limb being evaluated; one hand is placed proximal to the superior patellar pole, applying a gentle downward pressure.
Evaluative Procedure	The patient is asked to contract the quadriceps muscle while pressure is maintained on the patella, pushing it into the femoral trochlea.
Positive Test	The patient experiences patellofemoral pain and the inability to hold the contraction.
Implications	Possible chondromalacia patella
Modification	The test may be performed with the knee flexed to various angles to assess different areas of patellofemoral contact.
Comments	The Clarke's sign is an unreliable test, producing false-positive results in otherwise asymptomatic knees.
Evidence	Positive likelihood ratio Not Useful — Useful Very Small / Small / Moderate / Large 0 1 2 3 4 5 6 7 8 9 10 Negative likelihood ratio Not Useful — Useful Very Small / Small / Moderate / Large 1.0 0.9 0.8 0.7 0.6 0.5 0.4 0.3 0.2 0.1 0

examination should be conducted for all dislocations or subluxations to rule out osteochondral fractures of the patella and femur. The mechanism for patellar dislocations and subluxations is similar to that of an MCL sprain, and the possibility of this injury must be ruled out.

*** Practical Evidence**

The patella most easily dislocates or subluxates when the knee is in 20°–30° of flexion.[14]

Patellofemoral Pain Without Malalignment

While patellofemoral pain caused by malalignment of the extensor mechanism can yield clinical cues including patellar position, patellar orientation, foot posture, and Q-angle deviations, patellofemoral pain without obvious malalignment can present a clinical challenge. Patellofemoral pain without malalignment can involve the patellar tendon, plica, bursa, fat pad, or soft tissue-bone interfaces and is

Examination Findings 11-2
Patellofemoral Instability: Subluxation

Examination Segment	Clinical Findings
History	***Onset:*** Recurrent ***Pain characteristics:*** Medial joint capsule, indicating trauma to the medial patellar restraints Pain beneath the patella may be described. ***Other symptoms:*** Reports of the knee "giving out," especially with change of direction maneuvers. ***Mechanism:*** During extension of the knee, change of direction, or an eccentric contraction of the quadriceps group within the last 30° of the ROM ***Predisposing conditions:*** Lateral patellar tracking; increased Q-angle; tight lateral restraints; lax medial restraints; family history of patellar dislocation/subluxation
Inspection	Increased Q-angle Patella alta
Palpation	Pain is produced over the medial retinaculum and lateral articular facet.
Joint and Muscle Function Assessment	The following assume the patella has relocated and no obvious deformity exists: ***AROM:*** Pain occurring during the first 30° of flexion or terminal extension ***MMT:*** Hip abductors and external rotators may be weak, especially with repeated testing (see Chapter 12). The quadriceps are weak and contraction may produce patellofemoral pain. Decreased strength during extension when the knee is flexed between 0° and 30° ***PROM:*** Pain may arise secondary to stretching of the retinaculum, especially as the knee enters into flexion
Joint Stability Tests	***Stress tests:*** Unremarkable unless prior history of acute knee injury ***Joint play:*** Hypermobile lateral glide usually associated with a positive patellar tilt test result. Hypomobile medial glide
Special Tests	Positive patellar apprehension test result
Neurologic Screening	Within normal limits
Vascular Screening	Within normal limits
Functional Assessment	Symptoms (pain and "giving out") described with eccentric loading of the knee, such as when descending stairs. Observation of knee flexion in standing may reveal medial rotation of the lower extremity. The patient may demonstrate a significant difference (greater than 15% deficit) during the one-legged hop test (Appendix B) and/or during isokinetic testing.[31]
Imaging Techniques	AP (standing and/or supine), lateral, Merchant axial views
Differential Diagnosis	Meniscal tear, synovial plica, patellar maltracking
Comments	Repeated subluxations of the patella may result in osteochondral fractures to the lateral femoral condyle or posterior surface of the patella.

AP = anteroposterior; AROM = active range of motion; MCL = medial collateral ligament; PROM = passive range of motion; VMO = vastus medialis oblique.

more likely to respond to nonsurgical interventions focusing on restoration of normal quadriceps length and strength.[50]

Patellofemoral tendinopathy

Common in individuals participating in jumping activities, running sports, and weight lifting, patellar tendinopathies most often have an insidious onset. Repetitive motions on a biomechanically malaligned extensor mechanism can result in unequal loads on the extensor tendon.[79,80] Anatomic or biomechanical abnormalities are not present in many patients suffering from patellofemoral pain and the onset of symptoms cannot be associated with a specific activity.[31]

Acute tendinopathy, characterized by an inflammatory response, can occur as the result of a blow to the tendon or

Special Test 11-3
Apprehension Test for a Subluxating/Dislocating Patella Fairbanks Test

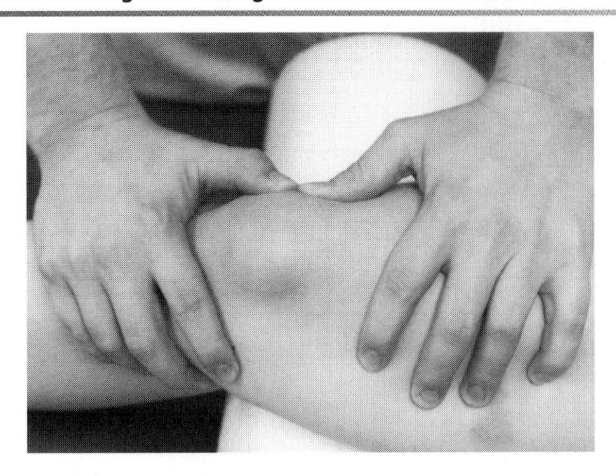

The apprehension test for patellar dislocation on a left knee. The examiner glides the patella laterally. A positive test is indicated by the patient's contracting the muscle or showing apprehension (anticipation) of an impending dislocation.

Patient Position	Lying supine with the knee extended
Position of Examiner	Standing to the patient's side
Evaluative Procedure	The examiner attempts to move the patella as far laterally as possible, taking care not to cause it to actually dislocate.
Positive Test	Forcible contraction of the quadriceps by the patient to guard against dislocation of the patella. The patient may also demonstrate apprehension verbally or through facial expression.
Implications	Laxity of the medial patellar retinaculum, predisposing the patient to patellar subluxations or dislocations
Modification	To improve the specificity of the test by isolating the medial patellofemoral ligament, move the patella distally and laterally.[12] The **Fairbanks Apprehension test** is performed with the patient's knee passively flexed to 30°. A lateral gliding force is placed on the patella while the knee is passively extended to the point where pain or apprehension is experienced.[58]
Evidence	Positive likelihood ratio Not Useful — Useful Very Small / Small / Moderate / Large 0 1 2 3 4 5 6 7 8 9 10 Negative likelihood ratio Not Useful — Useful Very Small / Small / Moderate / Large 1.0 0.9 0.8 0.7 0.6 0.5 0.4 0.3 0.2 0.1 0

a sudden increase in intensity or duration of activity. Tendinosis, a degenerative condition associated with collagen disorganization, is far more prevalent than tendinitis.

Histologic examination of tissue removed during surgery for patellar tendinopathies confirms that tendinosis is a more accurate descriptor of the chronic pathology than is tendinitis. Microtearing of the fibers results in the formation of excess connective tissues and endothelial cells, increased vascularity, and the alteration of the tendon's normal cellular structure.[80,81] The proximal portion of the posterior middle and the central thirds of the patellar tendon are the most frequently involved portions of the tendon.[80,82] Prolonged patellar tendon irritation can result in an elongation of the inferior patellar pole[82] and **morphologic** changes in the medal patellar retinaculum.[83]

Morphologic Changes in form and structure with regard to function.

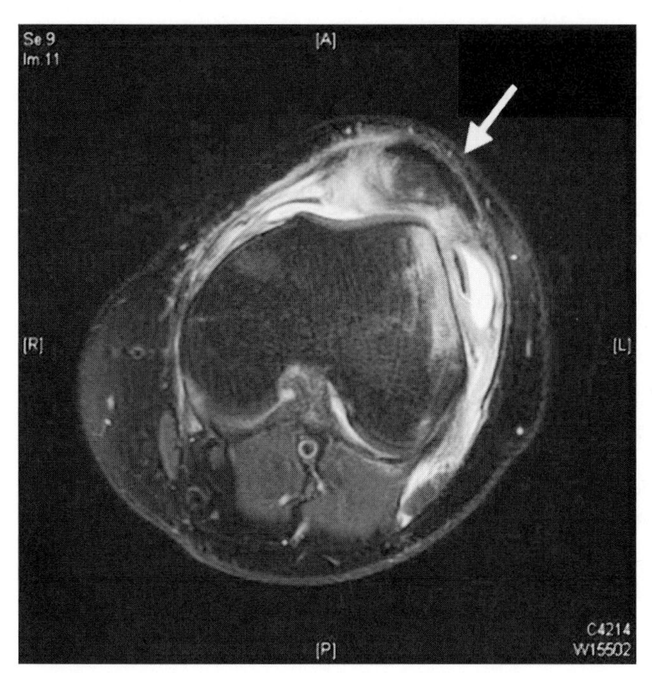

FIGURE 11-14 ■ MRI of a laterally dislocated patella. This view, obtained in the transverse plane, demonstrates the patella resting on the lateral femoral condyle.

The inferior pole of the patella is the common site of pain associated with patellar tendinopathy. Pain may also be described at the superior pole in the case of quadriceps tendinopathy (jumper's knee), in the midsubstance of the tendon, or at the tendon's attachment to the tibial tuberosity (Examination Findings 11-4). Moderate and severe pain with palpation is more predictive of patellar tendinopathy as confirmed by ultrasound than is mild pain, which is frequent in those with and without symptoms of patellar tendinopathy.[84] Resisted knee extension increases pain with a resulting decrease in strength. The end range of passive knee flexion, performed with the patient in the prone position, elicits pain in the patellar tendon and may reveal decreased quadriceps flexibility when compared to passive knee flexion with the hip flexed. Crepitus can be palpated in tendons during active or resisted movements. Magnetic resonance imaging (MRI) is useful in identifying the presence of patellar tendinopathy.[80,82,85]

Pain that is elicited from either side of the patellar tendon may be caused by infrapatellar fat pad inflammation (Hoffa's disease). This condition is marked by pain caused during knee extension that impinges the posterior (synovial) surface of the fat pad between the anterior portion of the femur and tibia and the posteroinferior part of the patella. Inflammation of the fat pat may trigger sympathetic spasm of the hamstring muscles, limiting knee range of motion to reduce compression of the infrapatellar fat pad from the patellar tendon.[22] MR images may be required for the differential diagnosis between patellofemoral bursitis, tendinopathy, and fat pad inflammation.

The treatment of patellar tendinopathy should focus on finding the patient's envelope of function and working within that range, expanding it as the patient improves.[31] The rehabilitation program should also focus on postural control with emphasis on the trunk and pelvis. On rare occasions surgical debridement of the tendon may be required if the patient fails to improve.[81]

Apophysitis

In adolescents, pain in the patellar tendon region can be associated with apophysitis, named Osgood–Schlatter or Sinding–Larsen–Johannson disease depending on the location of the pathology.

Osgood–Schlatter disease. The onset of Osgood–Schlatter disease, which occurs at the insertion of the patellar tendon on the tibial tuberosity, is traced to repeated avulsion fractures of the tendon from its attachment and is caused by rapid growth, increased strength of the quadriceps, or both. These forces result in osteochondritis of the tubercle (Fig. 11-15). The symptoms of Osgood–Schlatter disease are similar to those of patellar tendinopathies. However, differentiation is made by the patient's age (i.e., in adolescents) and the pain's being localized to the tibial tuberosity and distal portion of the patellar tendon (Examination Findings 11-5). A history of Osgood–Schlatter disease may lead to residual enlargement of the tibial tuberosity and mild exacerbation of symptoms with strenuous activity during adulthood.[87]

Osgood–Schlatter disease is managed conservatively by modifying activity to reduce antagonistic stresses on the tibial tuberosity and controlling inflammation. Surgical excision of the tibial tuberosity avulsion may be required if conservative treatment fails.[88]

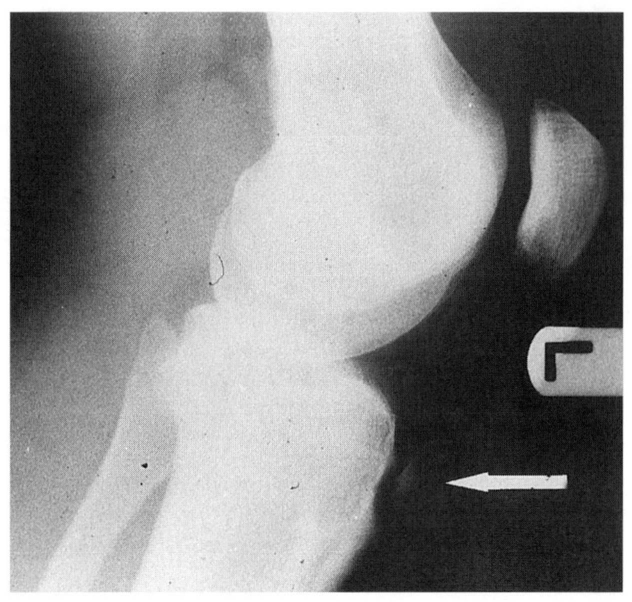

FIGURE 11-15 ■ Radiograph of Osgood–Schlatter disease showing the bony outgrowth.

Examination Findings 11-3
Patellar Dislocation

Examination Segment	Clinical Findings
History	***Onset:*** Acute ***Pain characteristics:*** Medial joint capsule, indicating trauma to the medial patellar restraints Pain in the vastus medialis, especially the oblique fibers Pain beneath the patella may be reported. ***Mechanism:*** Valgus blow to the knee; rapid change of direction with foot fixed ***Predisposing conditions:*** Patella alta, history of previous dislocations or patellofemoral instability. Low Q-angles may lead to patellar dislocation.[39]
Inspection	Obvious deformity, with patella positioned laterally and knee flexed. If examined post-reduction, a large effusion will be present. If the capsule is torn, the fluid may extravasate distally.
Palpation	Obvious deformity of displaced patella Pain at the origin of the VMO at the adductor tubercle or intermuscular septum or at its insertion on the patella Tenderness over the medial patellofemoral ligament
Joint and Muscle Function Assessment	***AROM:*** Not performed in the presence of dislocation. If examined post-reduction, extension may be limited or the patient may exhibit apprehension as full extension is approached. ***MMT:*** Not performed in the presence of a dislocation. Following reduction quadriceps strength will be decreased secondary to pain and, possibly, swelling. ***PROM:*** Not performed in the presence of a dislocation After reduction, ROM may be limited going into flexion.
Joint Stability Tests	***Stress tests:*** Not performed in the presence of a dislocation If examined post-reduction, the major ligaments of the knee should be stressed to rule out concomitant injury, especially of the MCL. ***Joint play:*** Not performed in the presence of a dislocation
Special Tests	Positive Apprehension Test post reduction. This test should not be performed if a dislocation was known to occur.
Neurologic Screening	Within normal limits
Vascular Screening	Within normal limits
Functional Assessment	The patient is unable to actively extend the knee or bear weight while the patella is still dislocated. Immediately after reduction, pain and soft tissue disruption limit strength and ROM. Significant gait alterations arise.
Imaging Techniques	AP, PA, and skyline view radiographs; ultrasound (soft tissue damage)
Differential Diagnosis	Patellar tendon rupture, fracture of posterior aspect of patella or lateral femoral condyle
Comments	With the acutely dislocated patella, knee extension is performed to reduce the dislocation. The more rapid the reduction of reduction, the less damage to soft tissue restraints. Passive knee extension will often reduce the dislocation.

AP = anteroposterior; AROM = active range of motion; MMT = manual muscle test; PA = posteroanterior; PROM = passive range of motion.

Examination Findings 11-4
Patellar Tendinopathy

Examination Segment	Clinical Findings
History	***Onset:*** Insidious onset in most cases, but inflammation is possible secondary to contusive forces to the tendon. ***Pain characteristics:*** Inferior patellar poles, midsubstance of the tendon, or the tendon's point of insertion on the tibial tuberosity ***Other symptoms:*** The patient may complain of crepitus. ***Mechanism:*** Repeated activity involving resisted knee extension (e.g., jumping) or secondary to contusive forces on the patella. Tendinitis may result from rapid increase in activity level. ***Predisposing conditions:*** Patellar maltracking; overuse
Inspection	The patellar tendon and inferior patellar pole may appear inflamed. Swelling may be localized around the patellar tendon.
Palpation	Tenderness of the patellar tendon, especially at its insertion on the infrapatellar pole Thickening of the tendon and/or crepitus may be noted
Joint and Muscle Function Assessment	***AROM:*** Pain during active knee extension is possible in advanced cases. ***MMT:*** Quadriceps: Pain and weakness ***PROM:*** Pain at the end range of knee flexion that may limit motion
Joint Stability Tests	***Stress tests:*** Not applicable ***Joint play:*** Not applicable
Special Tests	Not applicable
Neurologic Screening	Within normal limits
Vascular Screening	Within normal limits
Functional Assessment	Increased pain with eccentric loading of tendon, such as when landing from a jump or descending stairs
Imaging Techniques	Osteophytes and calcification within the tendon can be identified on AP and lateral radiographs. MRI can identify tendon lesions and bone edema within the tibial tuberosity.[77] MRI has a sensitivity of 0.78 and a specificity of 0.86.[78] Scar tissue and necrosis may be identified using diagnostic ultrasound.[77] Diagnostic ultrasound has a sensitivity of 0.58 and specificity of 0.94 for identifying thickening and calcification of the tendon. This procedure is better at ruling in tendinopathy than ruling it out.[78]
Differential Diagnosis	Fat pad impingement, meniscal tear, patellofemoral maltracking
Comments	There may be an associated tightness of the quadriceps musculature.

AROM = active range of motion; MMT = manual muscle test; MRI = magnetic resonance imaging; PROM = passive range of motion.

Sinding–Larsen–Johansson disease. Sinding–Larsen–Johansson disease is found at the attachment of the patellar tendon into the inferior patellar pole or, less commonly, at the quadriceps tendon attachment at the proximal pole of the patella.[89,90] As with Osgood–Schlatter disease, Sinding–Larsen–Johansson disease is caused by a stress fracture or avulsion because of the repetitive forces associated with running and jumping. Continued traction forces on the growth areas of the patella lead to the disruption of the epiphysis.

Sinding–Larsen–Johansson disease affects males more often than females and is most common in the 11- to 14-year age group.[91] Complaints of pain and swelling at the affected pole of the patella are usually accompanied by an antalgic gait. Physical examination reveals point tenderness at the lesion site, pain with quadriceps stretching, and pain with active and resisted quadriceps function. Radiographs typically reveal the fragmentation at the superior or inferior pole of the patella. As with Osgood–Schlatter disease, the fragmentation may cause a visible or palpable deformity at the lesion site (Examination Findings 11-6).

Treatment focuses on the underlying biomechanical changes and resulting symptoms. A rest period, followed by stretching and concentric, eccentric, and/or strengthening

Examination Findings 11-5
Osgood–Schlatter Disease

Examination Segment	Clinical Findings
History	***Onset:*** Insidious ***Pain characteristics:*** Radiating up the distal one third of the patellar tendon ***Mechanism:*** Stress placed on the growth plate of the tibial tuberosity by forceful contraction or passive tension of the extensor mechanism; onset is often associated with a rapid growth spurt or overtraining. ***Predisposing conditions:*** Rapid muscular development during adolescence
Inspection	Swelling or deformity of the tibial tuberosity
Palpation	Tenderness and perhaps crepitus over the tibial tuberosity and patellar tendon
Joint and Muscle Function Assessment	***AROM:*** Pain possibly experienced over the tibial tuberosity during active knee extension, especially when bearing weight ***MMT:*** Pain and weakness during quadriceps testing ***PROM:*** Pain over the tibial tuberosity during the end range of knee flexion secondary to strain placed on the patellar tendon
Joint Stability Tests	***Stress tests:*** Not applicable ***Joint play:*** Not applicable
Special Tests	Not applicable
Neurologic Screening	Within normal limits
Vascular Screening	Within normal limits
Functional Assessment	May describe increased pain and associated antalgic gait with increased activity.
Imaging Techniques	Standing or supine AP, lateral, and Merchant or sunrise views. In children the diagnosis is often made based on the clinical findings without the use of radiographs.[86]
Differential Diagnosis	Patellar tendinopathy, patellofemoral pain syndrome with malalignment
Comments	The signs and symptoms of Osgood–Schlatter disease may mimic those of patellar tendinopathy, but the symptoms are localized to the tibial tuberosity. These findings in postadolescent patients may indicate a history of apophysitis.

AP = anteroposterior; AROM = active range of motion; MMT = manual muscle test; PROM = passive range of motion.

of the quadriceps, is used to restore strength and muscle balance. **Palliative** treatments such as ice or iontophoresis using anti-inflammatory medications may be prescribed. On rare occasions, surgical correction of the patellofemoral alignment may be required.

Similar to patients with other growth injuries, those with Sinding–Larsen–Johansson disease may remain periodically symptomatic until skeletal maturation is reached. In this case, patients need to respect the symptoms and rest as needed from the aggravating activities such as jumping.

Palliative Serving to relieve or reduce symptoms without curing.

Patellofemoral bursitis

The extensor mechanism's bursa may be inflamed secondary to a single traumatic force, repeated low-intensity blows, overuse, or infection (e.g., with ***Staphylococcus***). The superficial prepatellar bursa and the subcutaneous infrapatellar bursa are most often injured secondary to direct trauma, resulting in localized swelling (Fig. 11-16). The suprapatellar and deep infrapatellar bursae become inflamed secondary to overuse. Pain caused by bursitis usually remains localized and the infrapatellar fat pads often become sympathetically tender (Examination Findings 11-7). Conditions with a sudden onset and no history of trauma or overuse with associated redness and warmth about the knee require referral to a

Examination Findings 11-6
Sinding-Larsen-Johansson Disease

Examination Segment	Clinical Findings
History	***Onset:*** Insidious ***Pain characteristics:*** Superior or inferior patellar pole point tenderness, beginning as activity-related pain and progressing to pain at all times ***Mechanism:*** Repetitive stresses from running and jumping ***Predisposing conditions:*** A shortened quadriceps muscle group; repetitive stress
Inspection	Antalgic gait; a deformity possibly present at the affected pole of the patella
Palpation	Point tenderness at the affected pole of the patella
Joint and Muscle Function Assessment	***AROM:*** Full, with pain experienced at the end range of flexion and with knee extension ***MMT:*** Pain and decreased knee extension strength ***PROM:*** Knee flexion limited by pain
Joint Stability Tests	***Stress tests:*** Not applicable ***Joint play:*** Not applicable
Special Tests	Not applicable
Neurologic Screening	Within normal limits
Vascular Screening	Within normal limits
Functional Assessment	May describe increased pain and associated antalgic gait with increased activity.
Imaging Techniques	AP, lateral, and Merchant views
Differential Diagnosis	Bipartite patella; patellar tendinopathy
Comments	Sinding–Larsen–Johansson disease may remain periodically symptomatic until skeletal maturation is reached.

AP = anteroposterior; AROM = active range of motion; MMT = manual muscle test; PROM = passive range of motion.

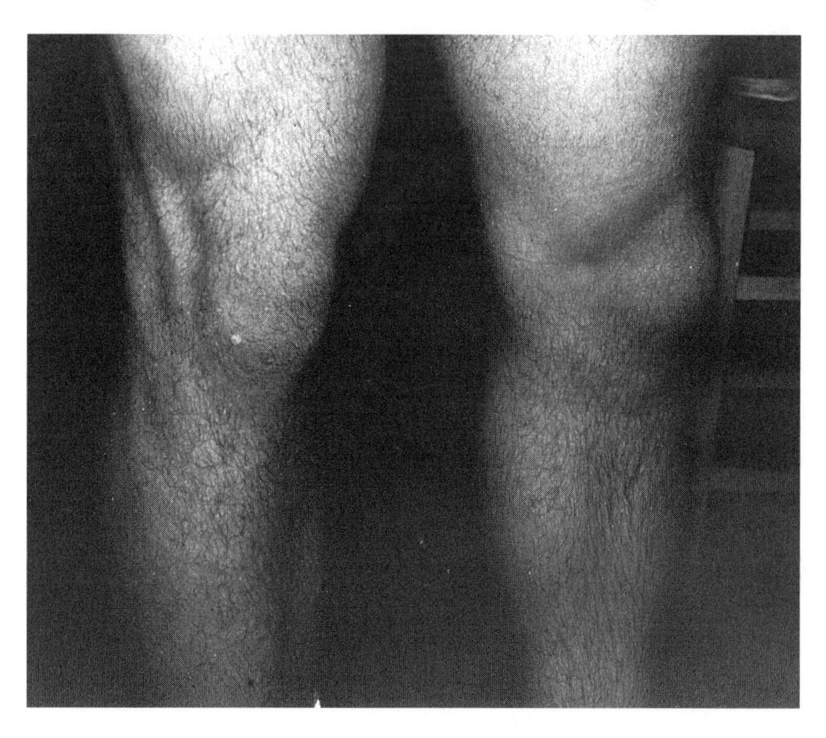

FIGURE 11-16 ■ Photograph of a visibly swollen prepatellar bursa of the left knee.

Examination Findings 11-7
Patellofemoral Bursitis

Examination Segment	Clinical Findings
History	***Onset:*** Acute or chronic ***Pain characteristics:*** Localized to a specific bursa and possibly the infrapatellar fat pads ***Mechanism:*** Direct trauma to the bursa or overuse ***Predisposing conditions:*** Other local inflammatory conditions (e.g., patellar tendinitis); weight bearing on the knees (e.g., wrestling)
Inspection	Localized extra-articular swelling
Palpation	Point tenderness when directly palpating the bursa or the area over the bursa; tenderness over the infrapatellar fat pads may also be described.
Joint and Muscle Function Assessment	***AROM:*** In chronic or severe cases, pain may be described within a specified range or throughout the entire ROM. ***MMT:*** Quadriceps: Pain and weakness ***PROM:*** Pain is experienced at a specific point in the ROM, illustrating irritation of the bursa.
Joint Stability Tests	***Stress tests:*** Not applicable ***Joint play:*** Unremarkable
Special Tests	Not applicable
Neurologic Screening	Within normal limits
Vascular Screening	Within normal limits
Functional Assessment	Increased pain with activities that compress the bursa.
Imaging Techniques	Axial MRI
Differential Diagnosis	Patellar tendinopathy; synovial plica; osteoarthritis; infection
Comments	The specific bursa involved is based on the location of pain. Patients with no relevant history for the onset of bursitis or who have superficial wounds over the bursa should be referred to a physician to rule out the possibility of infection.

AROM = active range of motion; MMT = manual muscle test; PROM = passive range of motion.

physician to rule out infection. Treatment of patellar bursitis consists of modifying activity to reduce painful stresses, padding to limit reinjury, and controlling inflammation.

Synovial plica

Forming during the embryologic stage of development, synovial plicae are normal folds of the fibrous membrane that project into the joint cavity.[92] During maturation, these folds are absorbed into the joint capsule; however, in the majority of the population, either a thickened area or a crease within the membrane remains.[93] Four plicae are found in the knee and are named relative to the patella: suprapatellar, medial patellar, infrapatellar (ligamentum mucosum), and lateral patellar.[92]

A synovial plica will remain asymptomatic until the area is traumatized by a direct blow to the capsule or becomes inflamed secondary to stretching and friction caused by the plica bow-stringing across the femoral condyle during flexion, or inflammation develops secondary to osteoarthritis.[60] Symptomatic plicae lose their normal elastic proprieties and, with time, become fibrotic, resulting in two reservoirs for synovial fluid: a suprapatellar reservoir and the cavity of the knee joint itself.[92,94,95] Although the onset of symptoms occurs most commonly in adolescents, plical syndromes may afflict patients of all ages at all stages of developmental maturity.[96] Synovial plica syndrome most commonly involves the medial joint capsule, and can involve the lateral capsule.[97]

When the plica becomes symptomatic, it loses its elastic qualities and alters the biomechanics of patellar gliding mechanism. Prolonged inflammation of the plica leads to fibrosis and chronic disturbances within the knee. The symptoms presented by synovial plica syndrome may mimic those of chondromalacia patella, meniscal tears, patellar subluxation, and patellar maltracking syndromes (Examination Findings 11-8).[95,98] Longitudinal tears of the plica can result in pseudolocking of the knee.[95] The presence of medial plica syndrome may be confirmed using either the **test for medial plica syndrome** (Special Test 11-4) or the **stutter test** (Special Test 11-5). A medial synovial plica can be confirmed via MRI.[99,100]

Initial management of a symptomatic synovial plica includes modifying activity to reduce the irritating stresses and controlling the inflammatory response. Strengthening the VMO may lessen the symptoms by reducing the tensile forces placed on the plica.[95]

Examination Findings 11-8
Synovial Plica Syndrome

Examination Segment	Clinical Findings
History	***Onset:*** Insidious ***Pain characteristics:*** Pain is located in the anterior portion of the knee; the patient may describe clicking, popping, or pseudolocking of the knee. Symptoms are often described as being worse in the morning, with a gradual decrease as the day progresses. ***Other symptoms:*** The patient may describe symptoms of the knee giving way. ***Mechanism:*** Friction caused by the plica's rubbing across a femoral condyle ***Predisposing conditions:*** Congenitally large or thickened plica; osteoarthritis[60]; the likelihood of onset decreases with increasing age.
Inspection	Joint effusion or swelling over the involved plica may be noted.[92]
Palpation	Symptomatic plica possibly felt as a thickened, bandlike structure that is tender to the touch Plicae affect the anteromedial capsule more so than the anterolateral capsule. Swelling possibly noted during palpation
Joint and Muscle Function Assessment	***AROM:*** Pain experienced as the plica crosses the femoral condyle, with possible clicking or "catching" described by the patient; a snapping heard by the examiner and felt by palpating the joint capsule A flexion contracture of 5°–10° may be noted. ***MMT:*** Quadriceps weakness secondary to pain ***PROM:*** A clicking or pseudolocking as the knee is flexed and extended over the point at which the plica rubs or catches on the femoral condyle
Joint Stability Tests	***Stress tests:*** Not applicable ***Joint play:*** Lateral patellar glide may be decreased.
Special Tests	Positive medial synovial plica test or stutter test result
Neurologic Screening	Within normal limits
Vascular Screening	Within normal limits
Functional Assessment	Weight-bearing activities, including gait, can be disrupted when the knee is within the range of motion that irritates the plica.
Imaging Techniques	Sagittal MRI
Differential Diagnosis	Meniscal tear, patellar subluxation, patellar maltracking, fat pad impingement
Comments	The symptoms of synovial plica may mimic that of a meniscal tear, subluxating patella, or chondromalacia that has been caused by biomechanical changes in the knee. Longitudinal tears within the plica can result in pseudolocking of the knee.

AROM = active range of motion; MMT = manual muscle test; MRI = magnetic resonance imaging; PROM = passive range of motion.

Special Test 11-4
Test for Medial Synovial Plica

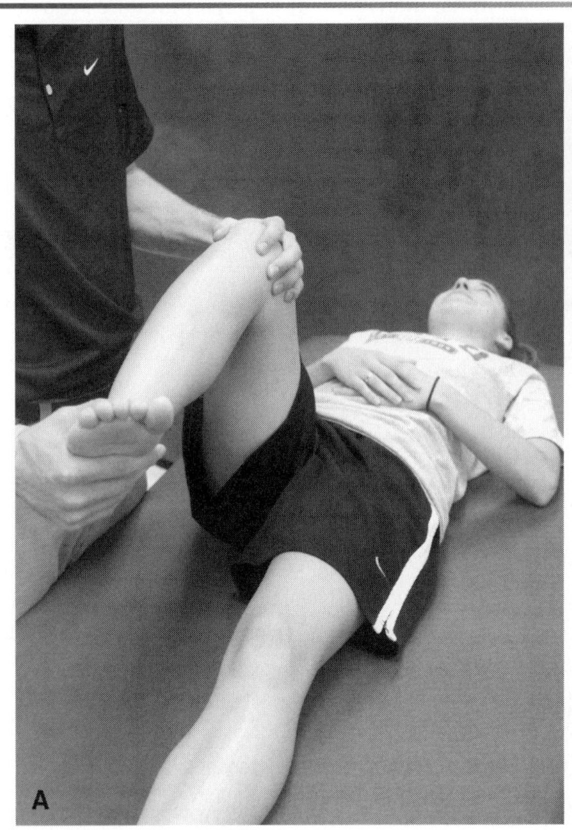

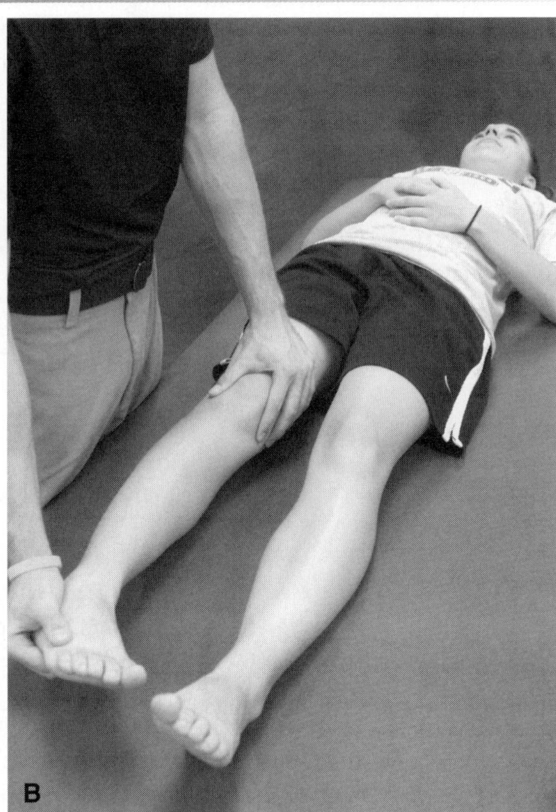

A positive test reproduces the patient's symptoms; the examiner may feel the plica as it crosses the medial femoral condyle.

Patient Position	Lying supine with the knee flexed or with the patient seated.
Position of Examiner	Standing on the side being tested.
Evaluative Procedure	**(A)** With the knee flexed to 90° and the tibia internally rotated, the examiner passively moves the patella medially while palpating the anteromedial capsule. **(B)** The knee is then extended and flexed from 90° to 0° while the tibia is internally rotated.
Positive Test	Reproduction of the symptoms is described by the patient. The clinician may feel the plica as it crosses the medial femoral condyle, especially in the range of 60°–45° of flexion.
Implications	Symptomatic medial synovial plica
Evidence	Absent or inconclusive in the literature

Traumatic Conditions

A laterally directed blow to the patella, a valgus stress, or other acute force can cause patellar dislocation, Refer to page 396 for a discussion of this condition.

Patellar fractures

Blunt trauma to the patella, such as when an ice hockey player is being driven into the boards, can result in a fracture. Fractures can also result from a rapid flexion force, such as landing from a jump. The risk of a patellar fracture may be increased if the quadriceps is contracting eccentrically at the point of impact, especially in the presence of stress fractures (Examination Findings 11-9). Palpation may reveal crepitus over the body of the patella and one or more false joints (Fig. 11-17). An associated rupture or contusion of the prepatellar bursa may cause immediate swelling and obscure the palpable findings. Active knee extension (if possible) and passive knee flexion produce severe pain.

Special Test 11-5
Stutter Test for a Medial Synovial Plica

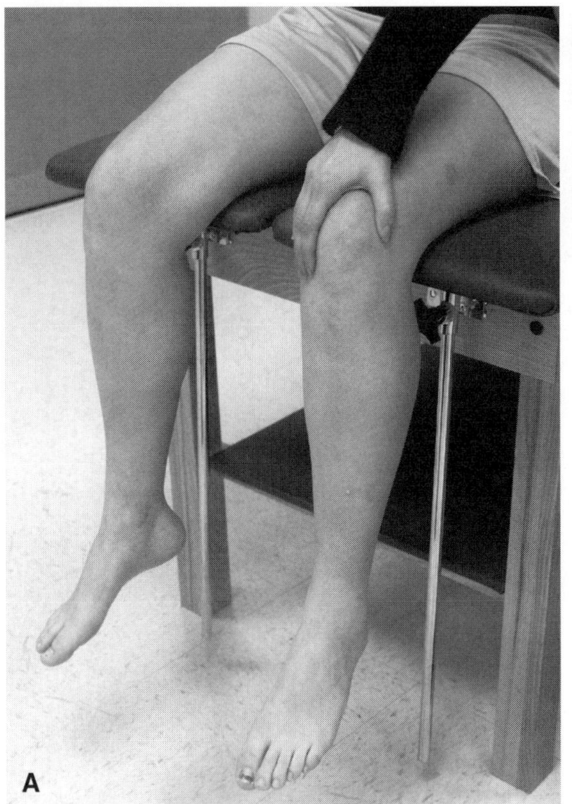

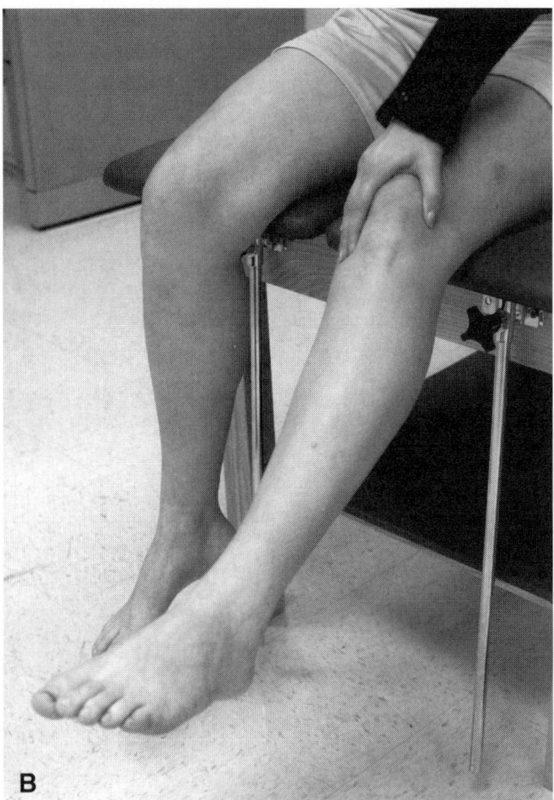

The examiner palpates the patella for irregular movement (stutter) as the patient extends the knee. When a plica snags against the medial femoral condyle, it may cause a momentary disruption in patellar motion.

Patient Position	**(A)** Sitting with the knee flexed over the edge of the table.
Position of Examiner	Standing lateral to the involved side, lightly cupping one hand over the patella, being careful not to compress the articular surfaces.
Evaluative Procedure	**(B)** The patient slowly extends the knee.
Positive Test	Irregular motion or stuttering between 40° and 60° as the plica passes over the medial condyle.
Implications	Medial synovial plica
Evidence	Absent or inconclusive in the literature.

Resistive knee extension cannot be performed because of pain secondary to the pressures placed on the fracture site.[101] Avulsion fractures (sleeve fractures) can occur at the superior or inferior pole and may mimic a patellar tendon strain or rupture.[56]

The risk of patellar fracture is increased following bone–patellar tendon–bone autograft anterior cruciate ligament reconstruction.[101,102] Children are at a decreased risk of sustaining a patellar fracture because the patella is primarily cartilaginous in children and has increased mobility relative to that of adults.[56]

Patellar tendon rupture

Sudden overloading of the extensor mechanism can result in a rupture of the patellar tendon in its midsubstance or an avulsion from its attachment on the patella's inferior pole or the tibial tuberosity. The quadriceps' attachment on the patella's superior pole is another possible site of rupture. This muscular load most commonly occurs secondary to hyperflexion of the knee or a powerful quadriceps contraction from a weight-bearing position.[105]

Mechanical failure of the patellar tendon is uncommon in otherwise healthy individuals. Diseases such as rheumatoid

Examination Findings 11-9
Patellar Fracture

Examination Segment	Clinical Findings
History	***Onset:*** Acute ***Pain characteristics:*** Pain arising from the patella ***Mechanism:*** A direct blow to the patella A history of a strong eccentric quadriceps contraction at the time of impact may increase the likelihood of a patellar fracture. ***Predisposing conditions:*** Patellar stress fractures
Inspection	Swelling over and around the patella Other deformity may be noted.
Palpation	Pain over the fracture site; a false joint may be noted
Joint and Muscle Function Assessment	***AROM:*** Extension lag of 10°–30° ***MMT:*** Decreased quadriceps strength production ***PROM:*** Flexion is limited by pain.
Joint Stability Tests	***Stress tests:*** Not applicable ***Joint play:*** Not applicable
Special Tests	Not applicable
Neurologic Screening	Within normal limits
Vascular Screening	Within normal limits
Functional Assessment	The patient is often unable to bear weight on the affected limb.
Imaging Techniques	AP and lateral radiographs
Differential Diagnosis	Patellar tendon rupture, quadriceps tendon rupture, patellar dislocation
Comments	The femoral articular surfaces may be fractured concurrently with the patella.

AP = anteroposterior; AROM = active range of motion; MMT = manual muscle test; PROM = passive range of motion.

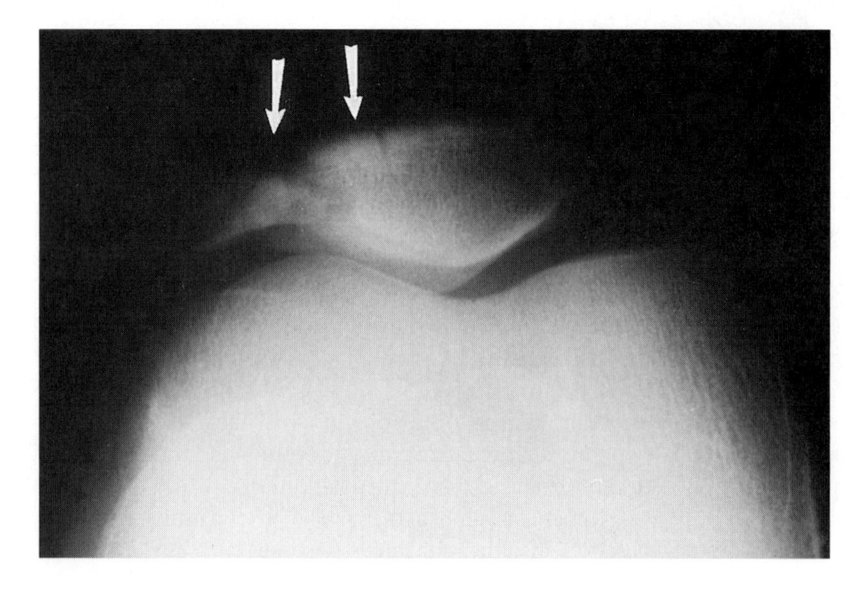

FIGURE 11-17 ■ A "sunrise" radiograph of a fractured patella.

arthritis, diabetes, **lupus**, chronic renal disease, or gout as well as chronic irritation of the patellar tendon or the use of corticosteroid medications may predispose patellar tendon ruptures.[106–108]

Patellar tendon ruptures cause immediate gross deformity as the patella is displaced proximally on the femur, exposing the condyles (Fig. 11-18). During palpation, a depression is noted in the infrapatellar region.[105] Because of the severity of the trauma, gross swelling rapidly accumulates. The ability to actively extend the knee is lost and the individual is unable to perform a straight leg raise on the affected side. However, the patient is still able to contract the quadriceps (Examination Findings 11-10). Although the ligaments of the involved knee may have been compromised at the time of injury, no ligamentous stability tests are performed before the patient is examined by a physician.

Patients suffering from patellar tendon ruptures require immediate immobilization and transportation to the hospital (see the On-field Management of Patellar Tendon Ruptures section). Surgical intervention within 7 to 10 days of the injury and appropriate rehabilitation can fully restore function to the knee. Most patients are able to progress to a full return to activity approximately 12 months after surgery.[109] Delaying surgery significantly decreases the functional outcome.[105]

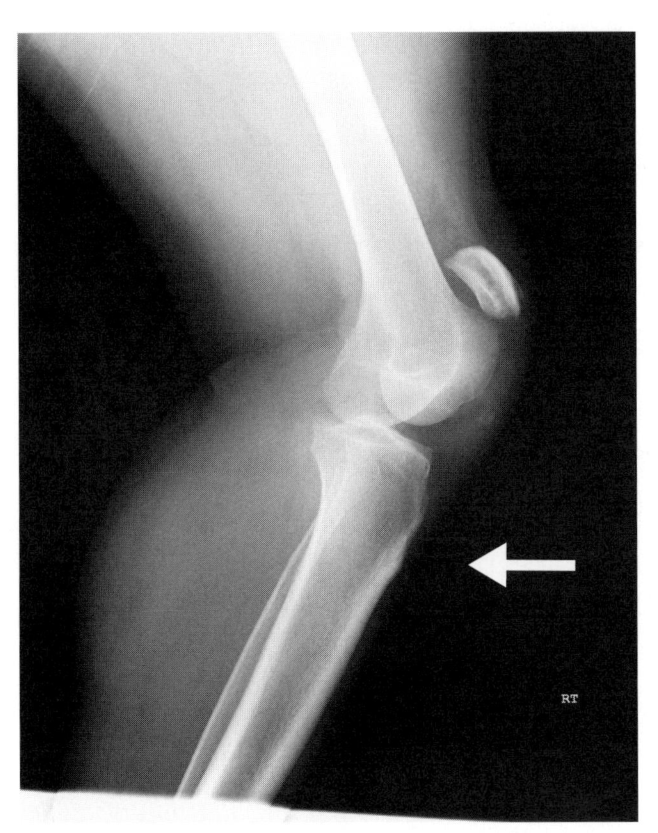

FIGURE 11-18 ■ Radiograph showing patellar displacement associated with a patellar tendon rupture.

Lupus A systemic disease affecting the internal organs, skin, and musculoskeletal system.

On-Field Evaluation of Patellofemoral Injuries

Acute, traumatic injuries of the patellofemoral articulation mainly involve the patellar tendon, tracking of the patella within the femoral trochlea, and, on rare occasions, the bone itself. This type of trauma tends to produce gross deformity and loss of knee function.

Equipment Considerations

Refer to Chapter 10 for a discussion of the removal of equipment surrounding the knee.

On-Field History

Unless the nature of the athlete's condition is obviously apparent, the location of pain, mechanism of injury, and any associated sounds or other descriptors of the injury must be established. Initially it may be difficult to differentiate trauma to the patellofemoral joint from tibiofemoral injury.

Inspect the patella to ensure that it assumes its normal position on the femur and has a normal shape. The patellar tendon should be visible as it runs from the tibial tuberosity to the infrapatellar pole. Rupture of this tendon results in violent spasm of the quadriceps muscle, causing it to "ball up" on the femur. In the event of an obvious injury, a secondary screen must be performed to rule out any less obvious injury. Confirm any suspicions of injury obtained during the history-taking or inspection process through palpation. Any indication of a patellar dislocation, fracture, or patellar tendon rupture warrants the termination of the evaluation and immediate immobilization and transportation for further medical evaluation.

On-Field Palpation

Begin by palpating the patellar tendon for tenderness, indicating a possible strain or aggravation of existing inflammation, from the tibial tuberosity to its insertion on the infrapatellar pole. Continue to palpate up the quadriceps muscles, paying close attention to the tone of muscle and tenderness over the VMO. Spasm of the quadriceps muscle may indicate a patellar dislocation, especially if the knee remains flexed. Tenderness may be elicited over the VMO secondary to tearing of the fibers during lateral dislocation of the patella.

From the VMO palpate inferiorly to locate the medial joint capsule, which is tender after a lateral patellar dislocation. Palpate the lateral joint capsule for tenderness, indicating possible medial displacement of the patella.

On-Field Functional Assessment

After the possibility of major disruption to the patellofemoral joint has been ruled out, an assessment of functional status may begin. Some of these movements may have been

Examination Findings 11-10
Patellar Tendon/Quadriceps Tendon Ruptures

Examination Segment	Clinical Findings
History	***Onset:*** Acute ***Pain characteristics:*** Patellar tendon, patella, and quadriceps muscle group ***Mechanism:*** Dynamic overload of the extensor mechanism secondary to extending the knee against resistance or a forceful eccentric contraction of the quadriceps muscle ***Predisposing conditions:*** Recurrent microtrauma, tendon degeneration, repeated corticosteroid injections, metabolic disease such as diabetes mellitus, gout, rheumatic disease[103]
Inspection	Patellar tendon rupture: Patella alta may be observed in the affected knee. Quadriceps tendon rupture: Patella baja is sometimes observed in the affected knee. Obvious anterior soft tissue swelling, possibly masking the underlying deformity
Palpation	A palpable defect may be identified in the patellar tendon or superior to the patella's superior pole. The anterior surfaces of the femoral condyles may be palpable Point tenderness will be noted over the defect. Swelling can mask the tendon defect during palpation.
Joint and Muscle Function Assessment	***AROM:*** The patient is able to contract the quadriceps but is unable to extend the knee against gravity. ***MMT:*** Not advised because further damage to the extensor mechanism may result. ***PROM:*** Pain moving into flexion An empty end-feel during flexion or a soft end-feel owing to the approximation of the hamstrings and gastrocnemius; PROM not performed acutely in the presence of an obvious tendon rupture
Joint Stability Tests	***Stress tests:*** Not performed during the initial evaluation and management of a suspected tendon rupture, although damage to the knee ligaments suspected ***Joint play:*** Not performed during the initial evaluation of a suspected tendon rupture
Special Tests	Not applicable
Neurologic Screening	Examine the lower extremity dermatomes to rule out secondary trauma to the peroneal or tibial nerve.
Vascular Screening	Within normal limits
Functional Assessment	Unwillingness to move or bear weight on the injured limb
Imaging	MRI, diagnostic ultrasound[103]
Differential Diagnosis	Tibial tuberosity avulsion fracture
Comments	Patellar tendon ruptures tend to occur in men younger than age 40 years, although any segment of the population is susceptible. Harvesting of the central one third of the patellar tendon for use as an autograft in ACL repair may increase the possibility of tendon rupture.[104]

MRI = magnetic resonance imaging; AROM = active range of motion; MMT = manual muscle test; PROM = passive range of motion.

voluntarily performed by the patient during the earlier portions of the examination.

- **Willingness to move the involved limb:** Ask the athlete to fully flex and extend the involved limb. An unwillingness or inability to complete this task is a sign that the athlete must be assisted off the field or court. If the athlete is able to complete the full ROM, break pressure may be applied with the knee near full extension and again in partial flexion to obtain a gross determination of muscular strength.
- **Willingness to bear weight:** If the preceding tests show normal or near normal results, possibly allow the athlete to bear weight by assisting the athlete to the standing position and letting him or her bear weight on the uninvolved limb. The athletic trainer then assumes a position under the involved side to help support the athlete's body weight, if needed.

Initial Management of On-Field Injuries

The primary concerns for the on-field management of patients with patellofemoral injuries involve the rupture of the patellar tendon, fractures of the patella, or an unreduced patellar dislocation. The following protocol is suggested for the initial management of patients with these conditions.

Patellar Tendon Rupture and Patellar Fracture

The management of patella fractures and patellar tendon ruptures is essentially the same. Splint the knee in extension and immediately transport the athlete for further medical attention.

*** Practical Evidence**

The **Ottawa Knee Rules** (OKR) are used to identify individuals who should be referred for radiographic examination of the knee. Following acute knee trauma, a patient who meets any of the following five criteria should be referred for radiographs: (1) age 55 or older; (2) demonstrates tenderness of the fibular head; (3) has palpable, isolated tenderness of the patella; (4) is unable to flex the knee to 90°; or (5) is unable to weight bear for four steps immediately after the trauma and/or during clinical examination. Designed to be highly sensitive, the use of these rules could reduce the need for plain knee radiographs by approximately 25%.[110–112]

Patellar Dislocation

Gross dislocation of the patella is marked by obvious deformity caused by the laterally displaced patella. Spontaneous reductions may occur if the quadriceps are relaxed and gravity causes the knee to extend, or the patient attempts to actively extend the knee. All cases of acute or traumatic patellar dislocation require referral to a physician so that fractures to the articulating surfaces of the patella and femur may be ruled out.

Reduced patellar subluxations or dislocations are splinted with the knee fully extended or slightly flexed. An unreduced dislocation must be splinted in the position in which the knee was found. This can be accomplished using a long moldable aluminum splint, bending one end to serve as a truss between the femur and lower leg or by using a vacuum splint.

REFERENCES

1. Powers, CM, Shellock, FG, and Pfaff, M: Quantification of patellar tracking using kinematic MRI. *J Magn Reson Imaging*, 8:724, 1998.
2. Powers, CM: The influence of altered lower-extremity kinematics on patellofemoral joint dysfunction: A theoretical perspective. *J Orthop Sports Phys Ther*, 33:639, 2003.
3. Lee, TQ, Morris, G, and Csintalan, RP: The influence of tibial and femoral rotation on patellofemoral contact area and pressure. *J Orthop Sports Phys Ther*, 33:686, 2003.
4. Doucette, SA, and Child, DD: The effect of open and closed chain exercise and knee joint position on patellar tracking in lateral patellar compression syndrome. *J Orthop Sport Phys Ther*, 23:104, 1996.
5. Powers, CM: Patellar kinematics, part II: The influence of the depth of the trochlear groove in subjects with and without patellofemoral pain. *Phys Ther*, 80:965, 2000.
6. Rintala, P, and Lic, P: Patellofemoral pain syndrome and its treatment in runners. *Athl Train J Natl Athl Train Assoc*, 25:107, 1990.
7. D'Agata, S, et al: An in vitro analysis of patellofemoral contact areas and pressures following procurement of the central one-third patellar tendon. *Am J Sports Med*, 21:212, 1993.
8. Reilly, DT, and Mantens, M: Experimental analysis of the quadriceps muscle force and patellofemoral joint reaction force for various activities. *Acta Orthop Scand*, 43:126, 1972.
9. Harilainen, A, et al: Patellofemoral relationships and cartilage breakdown. *Knee Surg Sports Traumatol Arthrosc*, 13:142, 2005.
10. Hubert, HH, et al: Force ratios in the quadriceps tendon and ligamentum patellae. *J Orthop Res*, 2:49, 1984.
11. Reese, NB, and Bandy, WD: Use of an inclinometer to measure flexibility of the iliotibial band using the Ober test and modified Ober test: Differences in the magnitude and reliability of measurements. *J Orthop Sports Phys Ther*, 33:326, 2003.
12. Tanner, SM, et al: A modified test for patellar instability: The biomechanical basis. *Clin J Sport Med*, 13:327, 2003.
13. Nomura, E, Inoue, M, and Osada, N: Anatomical analysis of the medial patellofemoral ligament of the knee, especially the femoral attachment. *Knee Surg Sports Traumatol Arthrosc*, 13:510, 2005.
14. Bicos, J, Fulkerson, JP, and Amis, A: Current concepts review: The medial patellofemoral ligament. *Am J Sports Med*, 35:484, 2007.
15. Insall, J, Goldberg, V, and Saluati, ER: Recurrent dislocation and the high-riding patella. *Clin Orthop*, 88:67, 1972.
16. Peeler, J, et al: Structural parameters of the vastus medialis muscle. *Clin Anat*, 18:281, 2005.

17. Brownstein, BA, Lamb, RL, and Mangine, RE: Quadriceps torque and integrated electromyography. *J Orthop Sport Phys Ther,* 6:309, 1985.
18. Hanten, WP, and Schultheis, SS: Exercise effect on electromyographic activity of the vastus medialis oblique and vastus lateralis muscles. *Phys Ther,* 70:561, 1990.
19. Devan, MR, et al: A prospective study of overuse knee injuries among female athletes with muscle imbalances and structural abnormalities. *J Athl Train,* 39:263, 2004.
20. Witvrouw, E, et al: Intrinsic risk factors for the development of anterior knee pain in an athletic population. A two-year prospective study. *Am J Sport Med,* 28:480, 2000.
21. Elias, JJ, et al: *In vitro* characterization of the relationship between the Q-angle and the lateral component of the quadriceps force. *Proc Inst Mech Engrs,* 218:63, 2004.
22. Gallagher, J, et al: The infrapatellar fat pad: Anatomy and clinical correlations. *Knee Surg Sports Traumatol Arthrosc,* 13:268, 2005.
23. Christoforakis, JJ, and Strachan, RK: Internal derangements of the knee associated with patellofemoral joint degeneration. *Knee Surg Sports Traumatol Arthrosc,* 13:581, 2005.
24. Tomaro, JE: Prevention and treatment of patellar entrapment following intra-articular ACL reconstruction. *Athl Train J Natl Athl Train Assoc,* 26:11, 1991.
25. Kettunen, JA, et al: Primary cartilage lesions and outcome among subjects with patellofemoral pain syndrome. *Knee Surg Sports Traumatol Arthrosc,* 13:131, 2005.
26. Näslund, J, et al: Comparison of symptoms and clinical findings of subgroups of individuals with patellofemoral pain. *Physiother Theor Pract,* 22:105, 2006.
27. Bentley, G, and Dowd, G: Current concepts of etiology and treatment of chondromalacia patella. *Clin Orthop,* 189:209, 1984.
28. Metcalf, R: An arthroscopic method for lateral release of the subluxating or dislocating patella. *Clin Orthop,* 167:9; 1982.
29. McGinty, J, et al: 1991 AAOS Instructional Course Lecture on Patellofemoral Pain. American Academy or Orthopaedic Surgeons, Chicago, 1991.
30. Brechter, JH, and Powers, CM: Patellofemoral joint stress during stair ascent and descent in persons with and without patellofemoral pain. *Gait Posture,* 16:115, 2002.
31. Witvrouw, E, et al: Clinical classification of patellofemoral pain syndrome: Guidelines for non-operative treatment. *Knee Surg Sports Traumatol Arthrosc,* 13:122, 2005.
32. Bennett, G, and Stauber, W: Evaluation and treatment of anterior knee pain using eccentric exercise. *Med Sci Sports Exerc,* 18:526, 1986.
33. MacIntyre, NJ, et al: Patellofemoral joint kinematics in individuals with and without patellofemoral pain syndrome. *J Bone Joint Surg,* 88(A):2596, 2007.
34. Powers, CM, et al: Criterion-related validity of a clinical measurement to determine the medial/lateral component of patellar orientation. *J Orthop Sports Phys Ther,* 29:386, 1999.
35. Ingersoll, CD: Clinical and radiological assessment of patellar position. *Athletic Therapy Today,* 5:19, 2000.
36. Snyder-Mackler, L, and Lewek, M: The Knee. In Levangie PK, Norkin CC. *Joint Structure and Function: A Comprehensive Analysis,* 4th ed. Philadelphia: FA Davis, 2005.
37. Grelsamer, RP, Dubey, A, and Weinstein, CH: Men and women have similar Q angles: A clinical and trigonometric evaluation. *J Bone Joint Surg,* 87(B):1498, 2005.
38. Guerra, JP, Arnold, MJ, and Gajdosik, RL: Q angle: Effects of isometric quadriceps contraction and body postion. *J Orthop Sport Phys Ther,* 19:200, 1992.
39. Sandridsson, J, et al: Femorotibial rotation and the Q-angle related to the dislocating patella. *Acta Radiol,* 42:218, 2001.
40. Binder, D, et al: Peak torque, total work and power values when comparing individuals with Q-angle differences. *Isokinet Exer Sci,* 9:27, 2001.
41. Livingston, LA, and Spaulding, SJ: OPTOTRAK measurement of the quadriceps angle using standardized foot positions. *J Athl Train,* 37:252, 2002.
42. Greene, CC, et al: Reliability of the quadriceps angle measurement. *Am J Knee Surg,* 14:97, 2001.
43. Post, WR, Teitge, R, and Amis, A: Patellofemoral malalignment: Looking beyond the viewbox. *Clin Sports Med,* 21:521, 2002.
44. Clarkson, M, and Wilkerson, J: Are differences in leg length predictive of patella-femoral pain? *Physiother Res Int,* 12:29, 2007.
45. Moore, KL, and Daily, AF: *Clinically Oriented Anatomy,* 5th ed. Philadelphia: Lippincott Williams & Wilkins, 2006.
46. Piva, SR, Goodnite, EA, and Childs, JD: Strength around the hip and flexibility of soft tissues in individuals with and without patellofemoral pain syndrome. *J Orthop Sports Phys Ther,* 35:793, 2005.
47. Kolowich, P, et al: Lateral release of the patella: Indications and contraindications. *Am J Sports Med,* 18:359, 1990.
48. Fulkerson, J, et al: 1991 AAOS Instructional Course Lecture on Patellofemoral Pain, American Academy of Orthopaedic Surgeons, 1991.
49. Piva, SR, et al: Reliability of measures of impairments associated with patellofemoral pain syndrome. *BMC Musculoskeletal Disorders,* 7:33, 2006.
50. Holmes, SW, and Clancy, WG: Clinical classification of patellofemoral pain and dysfunction. *J Orthop Sports Phys Ther,* 28:299, 1998.
51. Caylor, D, Fites, R, and Worrell, TW: The relationship between quadriceps angle and anterior knee pain syndrome. *J Orthop Sports Phys Ther,* 17:11, 1993.
52. Shelton, GL, and Thigpen, LK: Rehabilitation of patellofemoral dysfunction: A review of literature. *J Orthop Sports Phys Ther,* 14:234, 1991.
53. Moss, RI, DeVita, P, and Dawson, ML: A biomechanical analysis of patellofemoral stress syndrome. *J Athl Train,* 27:64, 1992.
54. Spencer, JD, Hayes, KC, and Alexander, IJ: Knee joint effusion and quadriceps reflex inhibition in man. *Arch Phys Med Rehabil,* 65:171, 1984.
55. Powers, CM, Landel, R, and Perry, J: Timing and intensity of vastus muscle activity during functional activities in subjects with and without patellofemoral pain. *Phys Ther,* 76:946, 1996.
56. Kumar, K, and Knight, DJ: Sleeve fracture of the superior pole of the patella: A case report. *Knee Surg Sports Traumatol Arthrosc,* 13:229, 2005.
57. Sutlive, TG, et al: Identification of individuals with patellofemoral pain whose symptoms improved after a combined program of foot orthosis use and modified activity: A preliminary investigation. *Phys Ther,* 84:49, 2004.
58. Nijs, J, et al: Diagnostic value of five clinical tests in patellofemoral pain syndrome. *Manual Ther,* 11:69, 2006.
59. Mascal, CL, Landel, R, and Powers, C: Management of patellofemoral pain targeting hip, pelvis, and trunk muscle function: 2 case reports. *J Orthop Sports Phys Ther,* 33:647, 2003.

60. Lyu, SR, and Hsu, CC: Medial plicae and degeneration of the medial femoral condyle. *Arthrosc,* 22:17, 2006.
61. Wilson, T, Carter, N, and Thomas, G: A multicenter, single-masked study of medial, neutral and lateral patellar taping in individuals with patellofemoral pain syndrome. *J Orthop Sports Phys Ther,* 33:437, 2003.
62. Ng, GYF: Patellar taping does not affect the onset of activities of vastus medialis obliquus and vastus lateralis before and after muscle fatigue. *Am J Phys Med Rehabil,* 84:106, 2005.
63. Gilleard, W, McConnel, J, and Parsons, D: The effect of patellar taping on the onset of vastus medialis obliquus and vastus lateralis muscle activity in persons with patellofemoral pain. *Phys Ther,* 78:25, 1998.
64. Luo, ZP, et al: Tensile stress of the lateral patellofemoral ligament during knee motion. *Am J Knee Surg,* 10:139, 1997.
65. Burks, RT, et al: Biomechanical evaluation of lateral patellar dislocations. *Am J Knee Surg,* 11:24, 1998.
66. Stanitski, CL, and Paletta, GA: Articular cartilage injury with acute patellar dislocation in adolescents. Arthroscopic and radiographic correlation. *Am J Sports Med,* 26:52, 1998.
67. Sallay, PI, et al: Acute dislocation of the patella. A correlative pathoanatomic study. *Am J Sports Med,* 24:52, 1996.
68. Maenpaa, H, and Lehto, MU: Patellofemoral osteoarthritis after patellar dislocation. *Clin Orthop,* Jun:156, 1997.
69. Stanitski, CL: Articular hypermobility and chondral injury in patients with acute patellar dislocation. *Am J Sports Med,* 23:146, 1995.
70. Maenpaa, H, Huhtala, H, and Lehto, MU: Recurrence after patellar dislocation. Redislocation in 37/75 patients followed for 6–24 years. *Acta Orthop Scand,* 68:424, 1997.
71. Cameron, JC, and Saha, S: External tibial torsion: An underrecognized cause of recurrent patellar dislocation. *Clin Orthop,* Jul:177, 1996.
72. Maenpaa, H, and Lehto, MU: Surgery in acute patellar dislocation: Evaluation of the effect of injury mechanism and family occurrence on the outcome of treatment. *Br J Sports Med,* 29:239, 1995.
73. Muhle, C, et al: Effect of a patellar realignment brace on patients with patellar subluxation and dislocation. Evaluation with kinematic magnetic resonance imaging. *Am J Sports Med,* 27:350, 1999.
74. Bolgla, L, and Malone, T: Exercise prescription and patellofemoral pain: Evidence for rehabilitation. *J Sport Rehab,* 14:72, 2005.
75. Maenpaa, H, and Lehto, MU: Patellar dislocation. The long-term results of nonoperative management in 100 patients. *Am J Sports Med,* 25:213, 1997.
76. Bellemans, J, et al: Anteromedial tibial tubercle transfer in patients with chronic anterior knee pain and a subluxation-type patellar malalignment. *Am J Sports Med,* 25:375, 1997.
77. Sarimo, J, et al: Distal patellar tendinosis: An unusual form of jumper's knee. *Knee Surg Sports Traumatol Arthrosc,* 15:54, 2007.
78. Wilson, JJ, and Best, TM: Common overuse tendon problems: A review and recommendations for treatment. *Am Fam Physician,* 72:811, 2005.
79. Verheyden, F, Geens, G and Nelen, G: Jumper's knee: Results of surgical treatment. *Acta Orthop Belg,* 63:102, 1997.
80. Yu, JS, et al: Correlation of MR imaging and pathologic findings in athletes undergoing surgery for chronic patellar tendinitis. *Am J Roentgenol,* 165:115, 1995.
81. Griffiths, GP, and Selesnick, FH: Operative treatment and arthroscopic findings in chronic patellar tenditis. *Arthroscopy,* 14:836, 1998.
82. McLoughlin, RF, et al: Patellar tendinitis: MR imaging features, with suggested pathogenesis and proposed classification. *Radiology,* 197:843, 1995.
83. Grossfeld, SL, and Engebresten, L: Patellar tendinitis—A case report of elongation and ossification of the inferior pole of the patella. *Scand J Med Sci Sports,* 5:308, 1995.
84. Cook, JL, et al: Reproducibility and clinical utility of tendon palpation to dtect patellar tendinopathy on young basketball players. *Br J Sports Med,* 35:65, 2001.
85. Popp, JE, Yu, JS, and Kaeding, CC: Recalcitrant patellar tendinitis. Magnetic resonance imaging, histologic evaluation, and surgical treatment. *Am J Sports Med,* 25:218, 1997.
86. Sarwark, JF, and Shore, RM (section eds): Pediatric Orthopaedics. In Johnson, TR, and Steinbach, LS (eds) *Essentials of Musculoskeletal Imaging.* American Academy of Orthopaedic Surgeons, Rosemont, IL, 2004, p 760.
87. Ross, MD, and Villard, D: Disability levels of college-aged men with a history of Osgood-Schlatter disease. *J Strength Condition Res,* 17:659, 2003.
88. Flowers, MJ, and Bhadreshwar, DR: Tibial tuberosity excision for symptomatic Osgood-Schlatter disease. *J Pediatr Orthop,* 15:292, 1995.
89. Medlar, RC, and Lyne, ED: Sinding-Larsen-Johansson disease. *J Bone Joint Surg,* 60A:1113, 1978.
90. Batten, J, and Menelaus, MB: Fragmentation of the proximal pole of the patella. *J Bone Joint Surg,* 67B:249, 1985.
91. Ogden, JA: *Sinding-Larsen-Johansson Disease in Skeletal Injury in the Child.* Philadelphia: WB Saunders, 1990, pp 765–768.
92. Demirag, B, Ozturk, C, and Karakayali, M: Symptomatic infrapatellar plica. *Knee Surg Sports Traumatol Arthrosc,* 14:156, 2006.
93. Hardaker, TW, Whipple, TL, and Bassett, FH: Diagnosis and treatment of the plica syndrome of the knee. *J Bone Joint Surg Am,* 62:221, 1980.
94. Amatuzzi, MM, Fazzi, A, and Varella, MH: Pathologic synovial plica of the knee. Results of conservative treatment. *Am J Sports Med,* 18:466, 1990.
95. Gerbino, PG II, and Micheli, LJ: Bucket-handle tear of the medial plica. *Clin J Sport Med,* 6:265, 1996.
96. Kim, SJ, Min, BH, and Kim, HK: Arthroscopic anatomy of the infrapatellar plica. *Arthroscopy,* 12:561, 1996.
97. Kurosaka, M, et al: Lateral synovial plica syndrome. A case report. *Am J Sports Med,* 20:92, 1992.
98. Johnson, DP, et al: Symptomatic synovial plicae of the knee. *J Bone Joint Surg Am,* 75:1485, 1993.
99. Kosarek, FJ, and Helms, CA: The MR appearance of the infrapatellar plica. *Am J Roentgenol,* 172:481, 1999.
100. Jee, WH, et al: The plica syndrome: Diagnostic value of MRI with arthroscopic correlation. *J Comput Assist Tomogr,* 22:814, 1998.
101. Exler, Y: Patellar fracture: Review of the literature and five case presentations. *J Orthop Sports Phys Ther,* 13:177, 1991.
101. Viola, R, and Vianello, R: Three cases of patella fracture in 1,320 anterior cruciate ligament reconstructions with bone-patellar tendon-bone autograft. *Arthroscopy,* 15:93, 1999.
102. Simonian, PT, Mann, FA, and Mandt, PR: Indirect forces and patellar fracture after anterior cruciate ligament reconstruction with the patellar ligament. Case Report. *Am J Knee Surg,* 8:60, 1995.

103. Heyde, CE, et al: Ultrasonography as a reliable diagnostic tool in old quadriceps tendon ruptures: A prospective multicentre study. *Knee Surg Sports Traumatol Arthroc,* 13:564, 2005.
104. Mickelsen, PL, et al: Patellar tendon rupture 3 years after anterior cruciate ligament reconstruction with a central one third bone-patellar tendon-bone graft. *Arthroscopy,* 17:648, 2001.
105. Levine, RJ: Patellar tendon rupture. The importance of timely recognition and repair. *Postgrad Med,* 100:241, 1996.
106. Podesta, L, Sherman, MF, and Bonamo, JR: Bilateral simultaneous rupture of the infrapatellar tendon in a recreational athlete. A case report. *Am J Sports Med,* 19:325, 1991.
107. Rosenberg, JM, and Whitaker, JH: Bilateral infrapatellar tendon rupture in a patient with jumper's knee. *Am J Sports Med,* 19:94, 1991.
108. Clark, SC, et al: Bilateral patellar tendon rupture secondary to repeated local steroid injection. *J Accid Emerg Med,* 12:300, 1995.
109. Enad, JG: Patellar tendon ruptures. *South Med J,* 92:563, 1999.
110. Stiell, IG, et al: Prospective validation of a decision rule for the use of radiography in acute knee injuries. *JAMA,* 275:611, 1996.
111. Emparanza, JI, and Aginaga, JR: Validation of the Ottawa Knee Rules. *Ann Emerg Med,* 38:364, 2001.
112. Bachmann, LM, et al: The accuracy of the Ottawa Knee Rule to rule out knee fractures. A systematic review. *Ann Intern Med,* 140:121, 2004.

CHAPTER 12

Pelvis and Thigh Pathologies

The pelvic girdle forms the structural base of support between the lower extremity and the trunk. A relatively immobile structure, the pelvis is formed by pairs of three fused bones joined anteriorly by the pubic symphysis. The posterior portion of the pelvis is formed by the sacrum's wedging itself between the two halves of the pelvis. The hip articulation, formed by the femoral head and the acetabulum, is the strongest and most stable of the body's joints. However, this benefit is gained at the expense of range of motion (ROM).

The hip is subject to large forces. When standing on one leg, three to four times the body weight is transmitted through the hip,[1] and when jogging up to eight times the body weight is transmitted through each joint.[2] Tolerating these forces is possible because of the sturdy bony alignment and ligamentous arrangement coupled with encompassing dynamic support.

Clinical Anatomy

The anterior and lateral portion of the pelvis is formed by two **innominate bones,** each consisting of the ilium, the ischium, and the pubis (Fig. 12-1). These bones fuse during the teenage years, but their two primary bony prominences, the ischial tuberosity and anterior superior iliac spine (ASIS), may not fuse until the third decade of life.[2] The posterior junction of the pelvic girdle is formed by its articulation with the **sacrum,** a broad, thick bone that fixates the spinal column to the pelvis. The sacrum is responsible for stabilizing the pelvic girdle.

On the lateral aspect of the pelvis, the **acetabulum,** a downwardly and outwardly directed depression, accepts the femoral head within its fossa. The superior wall of the acetabulum superior wall is formed by the ilium, the inferior wall by the ischium, and the internal (medial) wall by the pubis. A depression for the **ligamentum teres** is centered within the fossa. The **labrum,** a thick ring of fibrocartilage, lines the outer rim of the acetabulum and deepens the acetabulum by approximately 21%.[3] The labrum is thicker and stronger superiorly than inferiorly (Fig. 12-2).

The **femoral head** is globular, with an articular surface that is slightly over a 180-degree arc in diameter. Its articulating surface is thickly covered with hyaline cartilage except for a central depression that accepts the ligamentum teres. Connected to the femur's shaft by the **femoral neck,** the head is angled at approximately 125 degrees in the frontal plane (Fig. 12-3). This relationship, known as the **angle of**

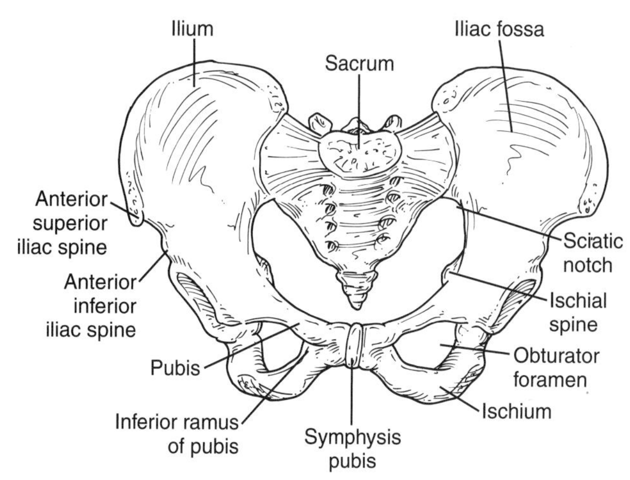

FIGURE 12-1 ■ Anterior view of the bony pelvis. A total of seven bones form the pelvis: Two ischial, two pubic, and two ilial bones form each half, and the posterior border is formed by the sacrum.

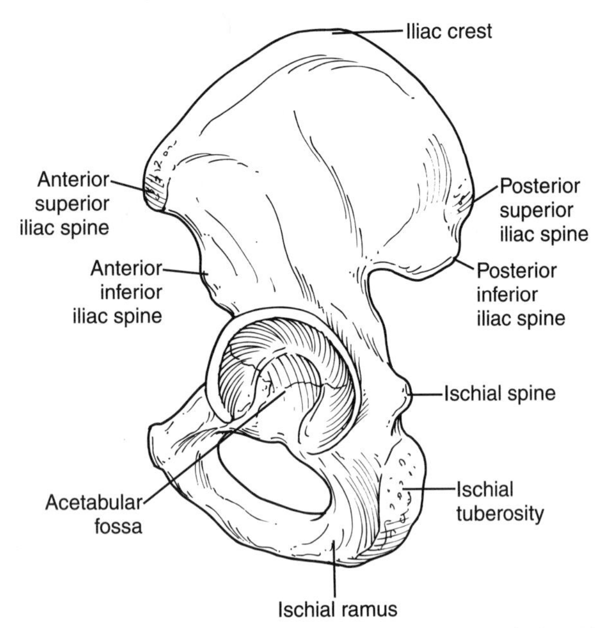

FIGURE 12-2 ■ Lateral view of the pelvis showing the acetabulum. The acetabular fossa is bordered by the fibrocartilaginous glenoid labrum.

inclination, changes as an individual grows and develops. The angle of inclination is slightly decreased in women. In the transverse plane, the relationship between the femoral head and femoral shaft is the **angle of torsion,** normally an angle of 15 to 20 degrees (Fig. 12-4).[4] The angle of torsion describes the amount of twist in the femur.

On the proximal portion of the femoral shaft, the **greater trochanter** projects laterally and the **lesser trochanter** projects medially. The trochanters are the attachment sites for many of the pelvic and hip muscles.

Articulations and Ligamentous Support

The pelvic bones articulate anteriorly at a relatively immobile joint, the **pubic symphysis** (see Fig. 12-1). Formed by the fibrocartilaginous interpubic disk, a small degree of spreading (distraction), compression, and rotation between the two halves of the pelvic girdle occurs here.

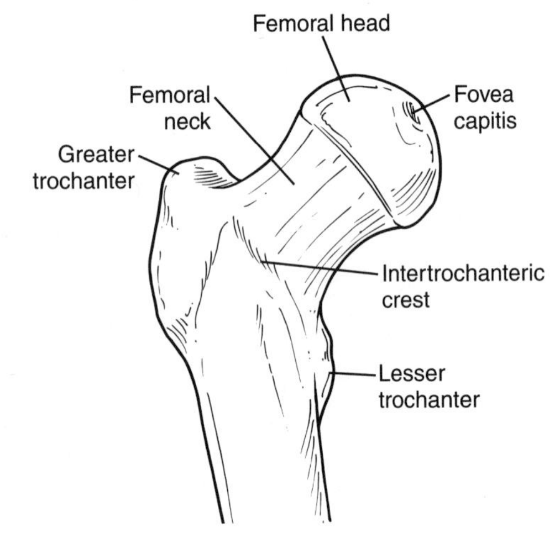

FIGURE 12-3 ■ Femoral neck and head.

Posteriorly, each ilium articulates with the sacrum at the **sacroiliac (SI) joints**. A combination of synovial and syndesmotic joints, these joints vary considerably in their shapes and sizes. The surfaces of each bone are a collection of concave and convex areas with the concavities of one bone corresponding to convexities of the opposing bone. The resulting articulation is very sturdy with limited mobility.

The hip articulation, the **coxofemoral joint,** is a ball-and-socket joint possessing three degrees of freedom of movement: flexion and extension, abduction and adduction, and internal and external rotation. The depth of the acetabulum, the relative strength of the ligaments, and the strong muscular support limit the hip's ROM in all planes (Table 12-1).

Surrounding the joint, a strong, dense synovial capsule arises from the acetabular rim and runs to the distal aspect of the femoral neck. Accessory bands, or ligaments, associated with the capsule assist in reinforcing the joint (Fig. 12-5).

The Y-shaped **iliofemoral ligament** (also referred to as the "inverted Y ligament of Bigelow") originates from the anterior inferior iliac spine. Its central fibers split, with one band inserting on the distal aspect of the anterior intertrochanteric line and the other band inserting on the proximal aspect of the anterior intertrochanteric line and the femoral neck. This strong structure reinforces the anterior portion of the joint capsule, thus limiting extension. Its superior fibers limit adduction and its inferior fibers limit abduction. The fibrous arrangement of the iliofemoral ligament allows us to stand upright with a minimal amount of muscular activity.

Also reinforcing the anterior capsule is the **pubofemoral ligament**. Emerging from the pubic **ramus** and inserting on the anterior aspect of the intertrochanteric fossa, this ligament limits abduction and hyperextension of the hip.

Posteriorly the joint is augmented by the **ischiofemoral ligament**. This triangular ligament has an origin spanning from the posterior acetabular rim with upwardly spiraling fibers attaching to the joint capsule and the inner surface of the greater trochanter. The spiraling nature of this ligament results in it limiting hip extension.

Within the joint, the **ligamentum teres** (also referred to as the "ligament of the head of the femur") serves as a conduit for the artery of the ligamentum teres and has little function in stabilizing the hip (Fig. 12-6).[5] The medial and lateral circumflex arteries provide the primary blood supply to the head of the femur. Trauma to the ligamentum teres via axial compression of the femoral head or dislocation of the joint may result in disruption of these arteries.

Ramus A division of a forked structure.

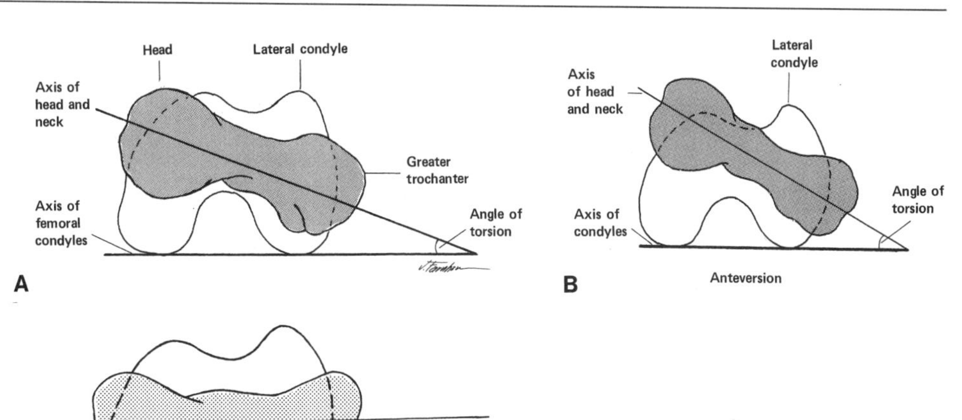

FIGURE 12-4 ■ Deviations of the hip in the transverse plane. **(A)** Normal hip angulation, 15 to 20°; **(B)** an increased angle, anteversion; **(C)** A more parallel alignment of the femoral condyles and femoral head, retroversion. (Courtesy of Norkin, CC, and Levangie, PK: *Joint Structure and Function: A Comprehensive Analysis*, ed 2. Philadelphia, FA Davis, 1992.)

Table 12-1 Ligaments Acting on the Hip

Ligament	Function/Motion Restricted
Iliofemoral Ligament	Reinforces the anterior joint capsule Anterior fibers: Hyperextension Superior fibers: Adduction Inferior Fibers: Abduction Allows standing with minimal muscular effort
Pubofemoral Ligament	Abduction Hyperextension
Ischiofemoral Ligament	Extension, extreme flexion

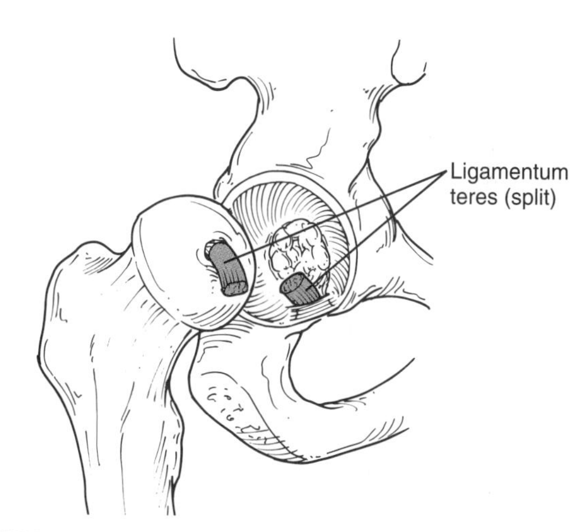

FIGURE 12-6 ■ Ligamentum teres (shown split). This structure serves little, if any, role in supporting the hip. It serves primarily as a conduit for the passage of the artery of the ligamentum teres.

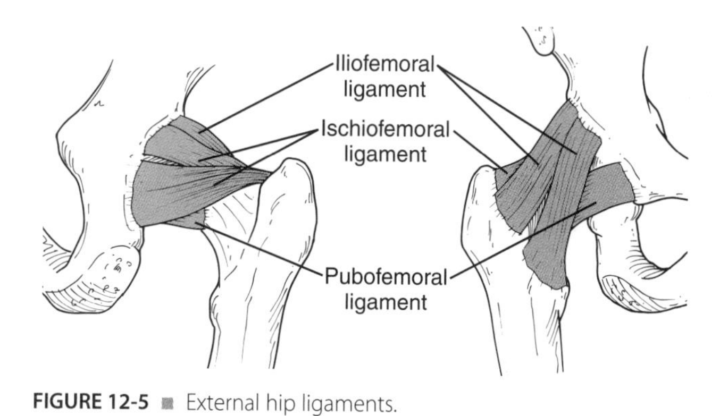

FIGURE 12-5 ■ External hip ligaments.

The **inguinal ligament** originates off the ASIS and inserts at the pubic symphysis. This ligament serves to contain the soft tissues as they course anteriorly from the trunk to the lower extremity. This structure demarcates the superior border of the femoral triangle. More detailed anatomy of the sacroiliac joint is presented in Chapter 13.

Muscular Anatomy

Movements of the hip joint are controlled by groups of large extrinsic and small intrinsic muscles. The large muscle groups act primarily to flex, extend, and internally rotate the hip. The smaller intrinsic hip muscles serve to externally rotate it. During activities such as running and cutting, the hip abductors and adductors act to stabilize the hip rather than generate mechanical power.[6] During walking and running the rectus femoris and iliopsoas muscles are active during the swing phase, and the hamstring muscles extend the hip and decelerate knee extension. Most anterior propulsion when running is derived from hip flexion and knee extension rather than from ankle plantarflexion.[2] The muscles acting on the hip, along with their origins, insertions, and innervations, are presented in Table 12-2.

Table 12-2 Muscles Acting on the Hip

Muscle	Action	Origin	Insertion	Innervation	Root
Adductor Brevis	Hip adduction Hip internal rotation	Pubic ramus	Pectineal line Medial lip of linea aspera	Obturator	L2, L3, L4
Adductor Longus	Hip adduction Hip internal rotation	Pubic symphysis	Middle one third of medial linea aspera	Obturator	L2, L3, L4
Adductor Magnus	Hip adduction Hip internal rotation	Inferior pubic ramus Ramus of ischium Ischial tuberosity	Line spanning from the gluteal tuberosity to the adductor tubercle of the medial femoral condyle	Obturator Sciatic	L2, L3, L4 L5, S1
Biceps Femoris	Hip extension Hip external rotation Knee flexion External rotation of the tibia	Long head • Ischial tuberosity • Sacrotuberous ligament Short head • Lateral lip of the linea aspera • Upper two thirds of the supracondylar line	Lateral fibular head Lateral tibial condyle	Long head • Tibial Short head • Common peroneal	Long head • S1, S2, S3 Short head • L4, L5, S1
Gemellus Inferior	Hip external rotation	Tuberosity of ischium	Greater trochanter of femur via the obturator internus tendon	Sacral plexus	L4, L5, S1
Gemellus Superior	Hip external rotation	Spine of ischium	Greater trochanter of femur via the obturator internus tendon	Sacral plexus	L4, L5, S1
Gluteus Maximus	Hip extension Hip external rotation Hip adduction (lower fibers) Hip adduction (upper fibers)	Posterior gluteal line of ilium Posterior sacrum Posterior coccyx	Gluteal tuberosity of femur Through a fibrous band to the iliotibial tract	Inferior gluteal	L5, S1, S2
Gluteus Medius	Hip abduction **Anterior fibers** Hip flexion Hip internal rotation **Posterior fibers** Hip extension Hip external rotation	External surface of superior ilium Anterior gluteal line Gluteal aponeurosis	Greater trochanter of femur	Superior gluteal	L4, L5, S1
Gluteus Minimus	Hip abduction Hip internal rotation Hip flexion	Lower portion of ilium Margin of greater sciatic notch	Greater trochanter of femur	Superior gluteal	L4, L5, S1

Gracilis	Hip adduction Knee flexion	Symphysis pubis Inferior pubic ramus	Medial tibial flare	Obturator	L3, L4
Iliacus	Hip flexion	Superior surface of the iliac fossa Internal iliac crest Sacral ala	Lateral to the psoas major, distal to the lesser trochanter	Lumbar plexus	L1, L2, L3, L4
Obturator Externus	Hip external rotation	Pubic ramus	Trochanteric fossa of femur	Obturator	L3, L4
Obturator Internus	Hip external rotation	Obturator membrane Margin of obturator foramen Pelvic surface of ischium	Greater trochanter of femur	Sacral plexus	L5, S1, S2
Pectineus	Hip adduction	Superior symphysis pubis	Pectineal line of femur	Obturator	L3, L4
Piriformis	Hip external rotation	Pelvic surface of sacrum Rim of greater sciatic foramen	Greater trochanter of femur	Sacral plexus	S1, S2
Psoas Major and Minor	Hip flexion	Transverse process of T12 and all lumbar vertebrae	Lesser trochanter of femur	Lumbar plexus	L1, L2, L3, L4
Quadratus Femoris	Hip external rotation	Tuberosity of ischium	Intertrochanteric crest of femur	Sacral plexus	L4, L5, S1
Rectus Femoris	Hip flexion Knee extension	Anterior inferior iliac spine Groove located superior to the acetabulum	To the tibial tuberosity via the patella and patellar ligament	Femoral	L2, L3, L4
Sartorius	Hip flexion Hip abduction Hip external rotation Knee flexion Internal tibial rotation	Anterior superior iliac spine	Proximal portion of the anteromedial tibial flare	Femoral	L2, L3
Semimembranosus	Hip extension Hip internal rotation Knee flexion Internal tibial rotation	Ischial tuberosity	Posteromedial portion of the medial condyle of the tibia	Tibial	L5, S1
Semitendinosus	Hip extension Hip internal rotation Knee flexion Internal tibial rotation	Ischial tuberosity	Medial portion of the tibial flare	Tibial	L5, S1, S2
Tensor Fasciae Latae	Hip flexion Hip internal rotation Hip abduction	Anterior superior iliac spine External lip of the iliac crest	Iliotibial tract	Superior gluteal	L4, L5, S1

Anterior musculature

Crossing the anterior portion of both the knee joint and the hip, the **rectus femoris,** part of the **quadriceps femoris group,** is a powerful flexor of the hip, providing the greatest contribution to hip flexion when the knee is also flexed. The **sartorius,** in addition to flexing the knee, contributes to flexion, abduction, and external rotation of the hip. The psoas major, psoas minor, and iliacus, collectively known as the **iliopsoas group,** are the primary hip flexors (Fig. 12-7).

When the leg is fixed, the rectus femoris, sartorius, and iliacus all anteriorly rotate the pelvis on the sacrum as they contract. Tightness in these muscles can cause increased stress on the sacroiliac joint, also causing the pelvis to rotate anteriorly on the sacrum.

Medial musculature

The medial hip muscles adduct and internally rotate the femur. The bulk of the inner thigh is formed by the **adductor group,** consisting of the adductor longus, adductor magnus, and adductor brevis. This muscle group's action is supplemented by the pectineus (Fig. 12-8). One additional adductor, the **gracilis,** is described in Chapter 10.

Lateral musculature

The most superficial of the lateral muscles are the **gluteus medius** and the **tensor fasciae latae** (Fig. 12-9). A prime abductor of the hip joint, the gluteus medius is also important in maintaining the horizontal position of the pelvis and the torso's upright posture during gait. For example, weakness of the right gluteus medius causes the pelvis to lower on the left side when the left leg is not bearing weight. The torso compensates for the unequal position of the pelvis by leaning to the right. This compensating movement is termed **Trendelenburg's gait pattern**. Through its insertion on the iliotibial (IT) band, the tensor fasciae latae is an abductor and internal rotator of the hip.

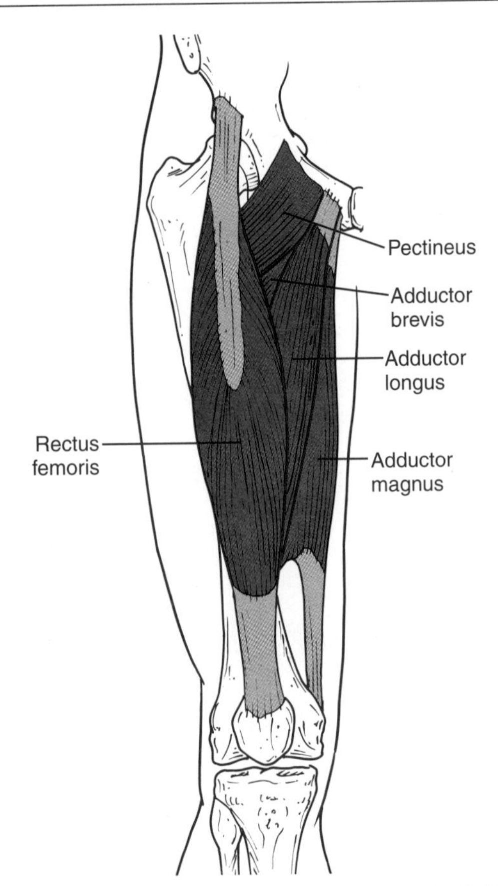

FIGURE 12-8 ■ Adductors of the hip. The only muscle of this group that is uniquely identifiable is the adductor longus, which becomes visible during resisted adduction.

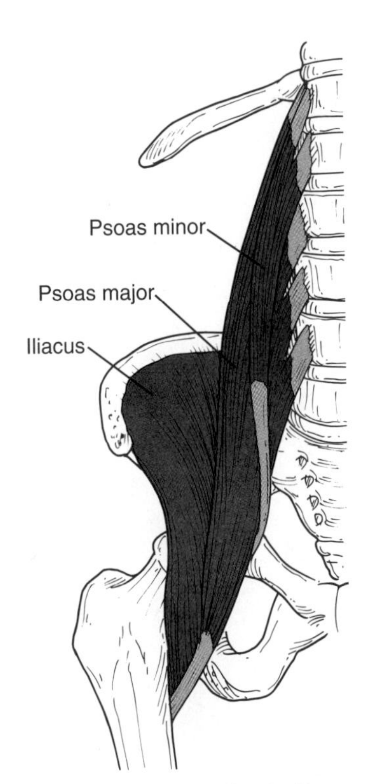

FIGURE 12-7 ■ Iliopsoas group formed by the iliacus, psoas major, and psoas minor muscles.

Although not contractile tissue, the IT band exerts biomechanical influences on the hip and provides an indirect insertion of several muscles onto the femur. The tensor fascia lata attaches directly the anterior portion of the IT band and the gluteus maximus attaches directly to the IT band on its posterior aspect. The gluteus medius attaches to the IT tract via an overlying aponeurosis. Depending on the position of the hip, these muscles exert a force on the IT band, pulling it anteriorly or posteriorly and keeping it taut as the hip moves from flexion to extension.[7] Inflammation or tightness of the IT band can cause irritation as it moves over the greater trochanter.

Six intrinsic muscles form a posterolateral cuff around the femoral head (Fig. 12-10). The **piriformis, quadratus femoris, obturator internus, obturator externus, gemellus superior,** and **gemellus inferior** all primarily function to externally rotate the hip in an open chain. During walking

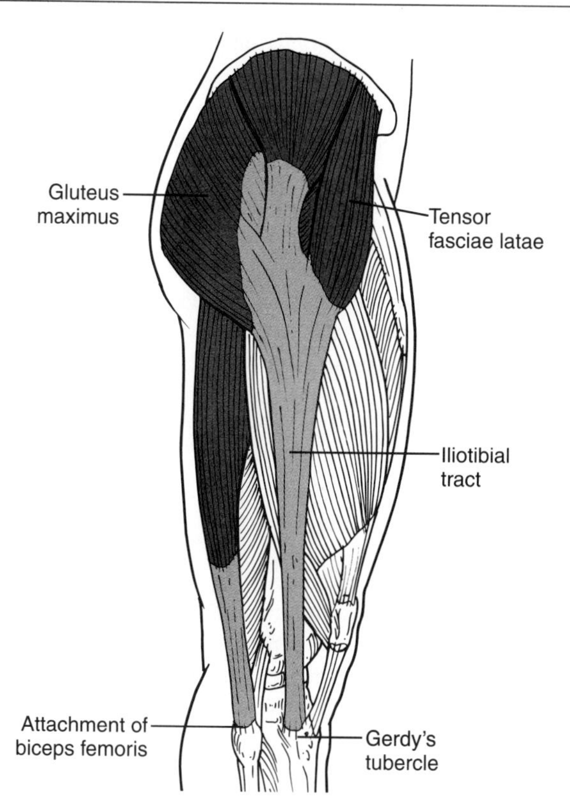

FIGURE 12-9 ■ Superficial lateral and posterior hip muscles. The tensor fasciae latae muscle attaches to Gerdy's tubercle via the iliotibial tract. The remaining lateral muscles, the gluteus medius and gluteus minimus, lie hidden beneath the gluteus maximus, tensor fasciae latae, and iliotibial tract.

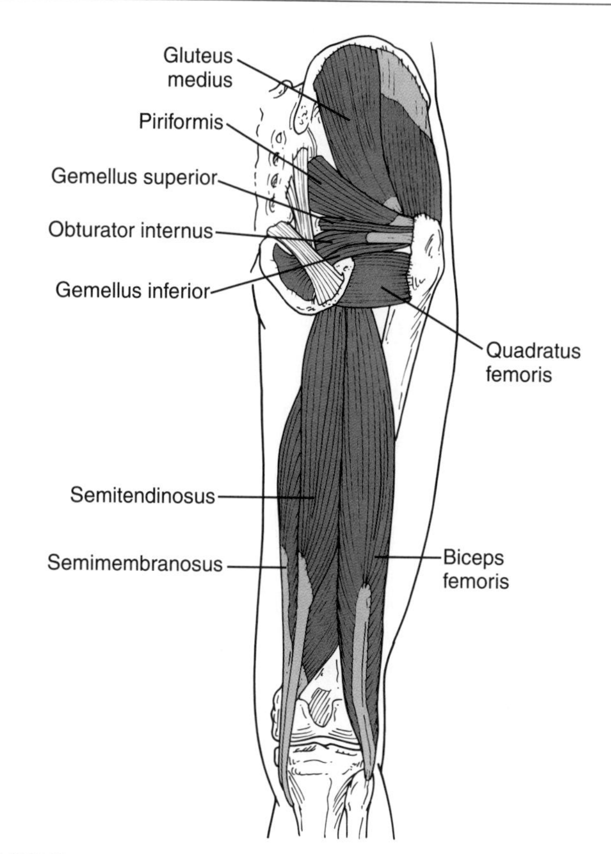

FIGURE 12-10 ■ Intrinsic hip muscles. Functionally, the intrinsic muscles serve primarily to control hip internal rotation during gait.

and running, these muscles serve a critical function to control hip internal rotation during the loading response and midstance phases of gait.

Posterior musculature

The mass of the buttocks is formed by the **gluteus maximus,** a powerful extensor of the hip, especially when the knee is flexed (see Fig. 12-9). When the knee is extended, the **hamstring muscle group** also acts as a hip extensor. In addition, the hamstring group is responsible for decelerating knee extension and hip flexion during running through an eccentric contraction. When the leg is fixed, the contraction of the hamstrings causes posterior rotation of the pelvis on the sacrum from their attachment on the ischial tuberosity.

Femoral triangle

Formed by the inguinal ligament superiorly, the sartorius laterally, and the adductor longus medially, the femoral triangle represents a clinically significant landmark (Fig. 12-11). The **femoral nerve, femoral artery,** and **femoral vein** pass through this area. The femoral pulse is palpable as it crosses the crease between the thigh and abdomen. Likewise, the triangle contains lymph nodes that may become enlarged with an infection or active inflammation in the lower extremity.

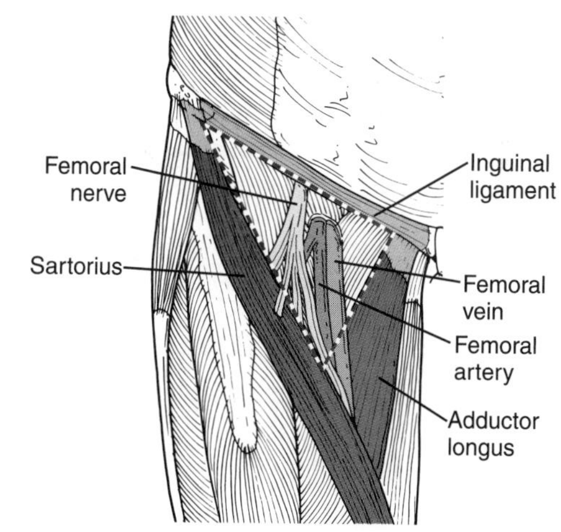

FIGURE 12-11 ■ Femoral triangle. This anatomical area is formed by the sartorius muscle laterally, the adductor longus medially, and the inguinal ligament superiorly. The femoral neurovascular bundle passes through this area.

Bursae

Four primary bursae are found in the hip and pelvic region, each serving to decrease friction between the gluteus maximus and its adjacent bony structures. The trochanteric bursa lubricates the site at which the gluteus maximus passes over the greater trochanter. The gluteofemoral bursa separates the gluteus maximus from the origin of the vastus lateralis. The ischial bursa serves as a weight-bearing structure when an individual is seated, cushioning the ischial tuberosity where it passes under the gluteus maximus. The iliopsoas bursa is the largest synovial bursa in the body, measuring up to 7 cm long and 4 cm, covering the area from the iliopectineal line, anterior inferior iliac spine, iliac fossa, and the lesser trochanter. The iliopsoas bursa frequently communicates with the hip joint.[7]

Neurologic Anatomy

The femoral and obturator nerves arise from the lumbar plexus, comprised of nerve roots from T12–L4. The motor branch of the femoral nerve innervates the hip flexors and knee extensors. The sensory distribution of the femoral nerve includes the anterior-medial thigh and the lower leg (via the saphenous nerve). The motor branches of the obturator nerve innervate the hip adductor muscles and the obturator externus, with a sensory distribution to the medial thigh.

Nerves emanating from the sacral plexus (L4–S4) converge and pass through the pelvis as the sciatic nerve via the greater sciatic foramen. Small nerves, including the nerve to the piriformis, the nerve to the obturator internus and gemellus superior, and the nerve to the quadratus femoris and gemellus inferior, innervate the muscles as named. The superior gluteal nerve innervates the gluteus medius and minimus and tensor fascia latae, with the inferior gluteal nerve innervating the gluteus maximus.

Vascular Anatomy

The blood supply of the hip joint, including the femoral head and neck, arises from the medial and lateral femoral circumflex arteries, both of which originate at the deep femoral artery from the femoral artery. The medial femoral circumflex artery runs deep to the femoral triangle and under the neck of the femur to become the primary source of blood for the femoral head. The lateral circumflex femoral artery provides the primary blood supply to the inferior femoral neck and trochanteric region. The obturator artery, originating from the internal iliac artery, sends a slip through the ligamentum teres, providing limited blood to the femoral head. In general, the labrum has a poor blood supply. Its vascularization mimics that of the knee meniscus, with the sections closer to the bone attachment more richly vascularized.[8]

The extent of vascular damage and potential for avascular necrosis associated with hip fractures depends on the location of the fracture.

Clinical Examination of The Pelvis and Thigh

Serving as the anatomic and mechanical interface between the lower extremity and spinal column, the pelvis influences and is influenced by these areas. A complete evaluation of the pelvis and thigh may also include a thorough evaluation of the lower extremity, spine, and posture.

To permit the complete examination of these areas, the patient typically is dressed in shorts and a t-shirt. Use discretion when evaluating areas around the genitalia. The evaluation should always be done in the presence of a witness.

History

The majority of pelvic girdle and hip injuries in active individuals tend to be of a chronic or overuse origin, increasing the importance of a complete and accurate history of the injury (Table 12-3).

Table 12-3 Possible Pathology Based on the Location of Pain*

	Location of Pain			
	Medial	**Anterior**	**Lateral**	**Posterior**
Soft Tissue	Adductor strain Gracilis strain	Rectus femoris strain Iliopsoas strain Sartorius strain Symphysis pubis sprain Rectus femoris or iliopsoas tendinopathy Hip sprain Labral tear Iliofemoral bursitis Lymphatic edema/infection	Trochanteric bursitis Gluteus medius strain Gluteus minimus strain Nerve compression	Ischial bursitis Hamstring strain Gluteus maximus strain Nerve compression
Bony	Adductor avulsion fracture Stress fracture	Pubic bone fracture Osteoarthritis Stress fracture	Iliac crest contusion Hip joint dysfunction Stress fracture	Sacroiliac pathology Stress fracture

*Excluding gross injury.

Examination Map

HISTORY

Past Medical History

History of the Present Condition

Mechanism of Injury

INSPECTION

Functional Assessment

Hip Angulations
Angle of inclination
Angle of torsion

Inspection of the Anterior Structures
Hip flexors

Inspection of the Medial Structures
Adductor group

Inspection of the Lateral Structures
Iliac crest
Nélaton's line

Inspection of the Posterior Structures
Posterior superior iliac spine
Gluteus maximus
Hamstring muscle group
Median sacral crests

Leg Length Discrepancy

PALPATION

Palpation of the Medial Structures
Gracilis
Adductor longus
Adductor magnus
Adductor brevis

Palpation of the Anterior Structures
Pubic bone
Inguinal ligament
Anterior superior iliac spine
Anterior inferior iliac spine
Sartorius
Rectus femoris

Palpation of the Lateral Structures
Iliac crest
Tensor fasciae late
Gluteus medius
Iliotibial band
Greater trochanter
Trochanteric bursa

Palpation of the Posterior Structures
Median sacral crests
Posterior superior iliac spine
Gluteus maximus
Ischial tuberosity
Ischial bursa
Sciatic nerve
Hamstring muscles

JOINT AND MUSCLE FUNCTION ASSESSMENT

Goniometry
Flexion
Extension
Abduction
Adduction
Internal rotation
External rotation

Active Range of Motion
Flexion
Extension
Abduction
Adduction
Internal rotation
External rotation

Manual Muscle Tests
Hip flexion (iliopsoas)
Knee extension (rectus femoris)
Hip extension
Abduction
Adduction
Internal rotation
External rotation

Passive Range of Motion
Flexion
- Thomas test
- Hip flexion contracture test
- Ely's test

Extension
Abduction
Adduction
Internal rotation
External rotation

JOINT STABILITY TESTS

Stress Testing
Not applicable

Joint Play Assessment
Passive range of motion

NEUROLOGIC EXAMINATION

Lower Quarter Screen

Sciatic Nerve

Femoral Nerve

VASCULAR EXAMINATION

Distal Capillary Refill

Distal Pulse
Posterior tibial artery
Dorsal pedal artery

PATHOLOGIES AND SPECIAL TESTS

Iliac Crest Contusions

Muscle Strains
Hamstring strain

Quadriceps Contusion

Slipped Capital Femoral Epiphysis

Iliotibial Band Friction Syndrome

Legg–Calvé–Perthes Disease

Femoral Neck Stress Fracture

Degenerative Hip Changes

Labral Tears
Hip subluxation

Athletic Pubalgia

Osteitis Pubis

Piriformis Syndrome

Snapping Hip Syndrome
Internal cause
External cause
Intra-articular cause

Bursitis
Trochanteric bursitis
Ischial bursitis
Iliopsoas bursitis

Past Medical History

- **Prior medical conditions:** Congenital or childhood abnormalities of the hip can result in altered biomechanics of the hip, knee, or ankle during adulthood. **Legg–Calvé–Perthes disease** can lead to residual flattening of the proximal femoral epiphysis, resulting in decreased hip internal rotation and abduction.[9] A **slipped capital femoral epiphysis** can lead to excessive external rotation of the hip and restricted or painful internal rotation.[10]
- **History of steroid use or alcohol abuse:** Both of these increase the risk for osteonecrosis, or avascular necrosis, of the hip.
- **Menstrual history:** Irregular or absent menses can decrease bone density, thereby increasing the risk of stress fractures. The Female Triad, consisting of disordered eating, absent menstrual periods and resulting osteoporotic changes, is further discussed in Chapter 15.

History of the Present Condition

- **Location of symptoms:** Deep hip joint pain can originate in the coxofemoral joint or be referred from the lumbar spine, sacroiliac joint, or both. A strain to the hip adductors or hip flexors causes pain in the pubic region or anterior hip, respectively. Greater trochanteric bursitis is a common hip pathology that usually results in pain in the posterior aspect of the greater trochanter. Pain and paresthesia in the upper lateral thigh, **meralgia paresthetica**, is indicative of neuropathy of the lateral femoral cutaneous nerve.
- **Onset:** Most pelvic girdle and hip pathology tend to be chronic or caused by overuse. The date of onset of the patient's symptoms must be correlated to any changes in training techniques such as surface changes, footwear, or alterations in training techniques or intensity.
- **Aggravating activities:** Question the patient regarding any increased pain with bowel movements or coughing. Anterior pain in the inguinal region coupled with pain during bowel movements or coughing may indicate the presence of a hernia.
- **Training techniques:** Recent changes in training techniques can lead to overuse injuries, including greater trochanteric bursitis or hip flexor tendinopathy, especially if the patient's running regimen includes training on a banked surface or the addition of hills. Development of stress fractures may be related to recent increases in training intensity, frequency, or duration.
- **Mechanism of injury:** A direct blow to the iliac crest may lead to a contusion (**hip pointer**). Blows to the buttocks, such as from a fall, can lead to a contusion of the coccyx or ischium or to sacroiliac pathology. A sudden pain, especially during an eccentric contraction of a muscle, usually indicates a strain of that muscle. Pain that gradually builds over time may indicate a stress fracture or tendinopathy.

The history-taking process may be expanded based on the patient's responses in the preceding categories.

Inspection

Inspection of most acute injuries is difficult because of the bony, muscular, and ligamentous arrangement of the hip and pelvis. With the exception of contusions to the iliac crest and hip dislocations, most trauma to this area does not leave visible findings. Therefore, the focus of the inspection phase is to identify secondary signs of pathology or determine the presence of conditions that may alter the biomechanics of the hip and lower extremity, predisposing the patient to injury. Patients who have inflammation of the hip joint may posture the hip in its loose-packed position of flexion, abduction, and external rotation, **Bonnet's position,** to reduce pain.

Functional assessment

Ask the patient to demonstrate the functional tasks that exacerbate the symptoms. Frequently, these are walking or running. As described in Chapter 7, observation of gait patterns can provide diagnostic information. For example, a shortened swing phase of gait is associated with a hamstring strain. Lateral hip pain coupled with a pain during the loading response and midstance of gait may indicate gluteus medius involvement. Posterior pain with pushing off during a sprint start implicates the gluteus maximus and/or hamstring.

Inspection of hip angulations

- **Angle of inclination:** The angular relationship of the femoral head and the femoral shaft may be roughly determined by observing the relationship between the femur and tibia (see Inspection Findings 10-1). Abnormalities at the epiphysis, trochanteric, or subtrochanteric regions can result in significant deviations in the angle of inclination, especially when the deformity develops during childhood (Fig. 12-12).[11,12] An increase in the angle of inclination, coxa valga, may be manifested through either genu varum or a laterally positioned patellae. Decreases in this angle, coxa vara, may lead to genu valgum or a medially positioned "squinting" patellae. In each case, the mechanical advantage of the gluteus medius is reduced by altering its line of pull on the femur. Radiographic

---

Legg–Calvé–Perthes disease Avascular necrosis occurring in children age 3 to 12 years, causing osteochondritis of the proximal femoral epiphysis and potentially decreasing the range of hip motion in adult life.

Slipped capital femoral epiphysis Displacement of the femoral shaft relative to the femoral head; common in children age 10 to 15 years and especially prevalent in boys.

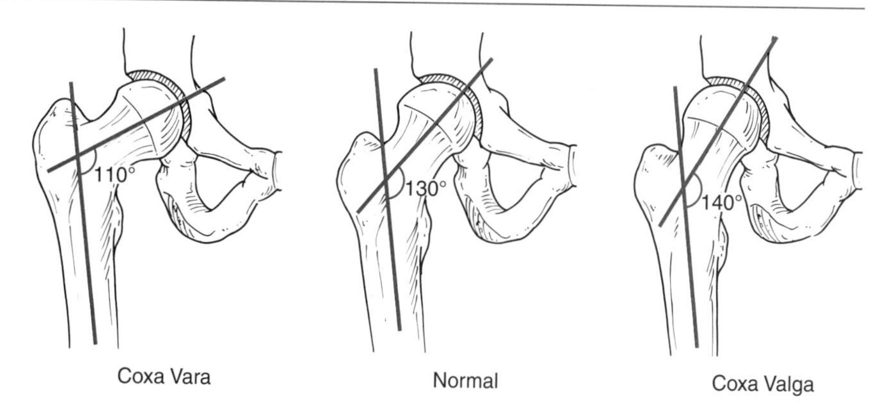

FIGURE 12-12 ■ Deviations in the angle of inclination.

examination is necessary to definitively determine the angle of inclination.

- **Angle of torsion:** Similar to the angle of inclination, the angle of torsion must be definitively measured through the use of radiographs. However, the accuracy of this method is questionable.[13,14] Special Test 12-1 presents a method for clinically estimating the angle of torsion.
  - **Anteverted femur:** Increases greater than 20 degrees in the angle of torsion, anteversion, result in internal femoral rotation, squinting patellae, and a toe-in (pigeon-toed) gait. Compensatory external tibial rotation often occurs.[4] In patients with anteverted femurs, an increase in internal femoral rotation and a decrease in external rotation occurs.
  - **Retroverted femur:** When the angle of torsion is less than 15 degrees, retroversion, the femur externally rotates, resulting in a toe-out (duck-footed) position of the feet. The patella is laterally positioned with a decrease in hip internal rotation and an increase in external rotation. The amount of retroversion demonstrated in early adolescence tends to diminish with age.[15]

Inspection of the medial structures

- **Adductor group:** Observe the area overlying the adductor muscle group for signs of swelling or ecchymosis, indicating a strain of these structures or a contusion to the area.

Inspection of the anterior structures

- **Hip flexors:** Observe the area of the hip flexors distal to the ASIS for swelling or ecchymosis, indicating a strain of these structures.

Inspection of the lateral structures

- **Iliac crest:** Inspect the iliac crest, located immediately beneath the skin. This area is vulnerable to contusions that initiate a very active inflammatory process. These contusions, or hip pointers, result in pain, disability, and discoloration (Fig. 12-13).
- **Nélaton's line:** Draw an imaginary line from the ASIS to the ischial tuberosity. Nélaton's line is a quick screen to help determine the presence of coxa vara (Fig. 12-14).[16] Location of the greater tuberosity well superior to this line indicates coxa vara.

Inspection of posterior structures

- **Posterior superior iliac spine:** If visible, compare the skin indentations bilaterally for symmetry. This should include height of the posterior superior iliac spine (PSIS) from the floor and identification of localized swelling.
- **Gluteus maximus:** Inspect the gluteals for bilateral symmetry. Atrophy of the muscle group could indicate an L5–S1 nerve root pathology.

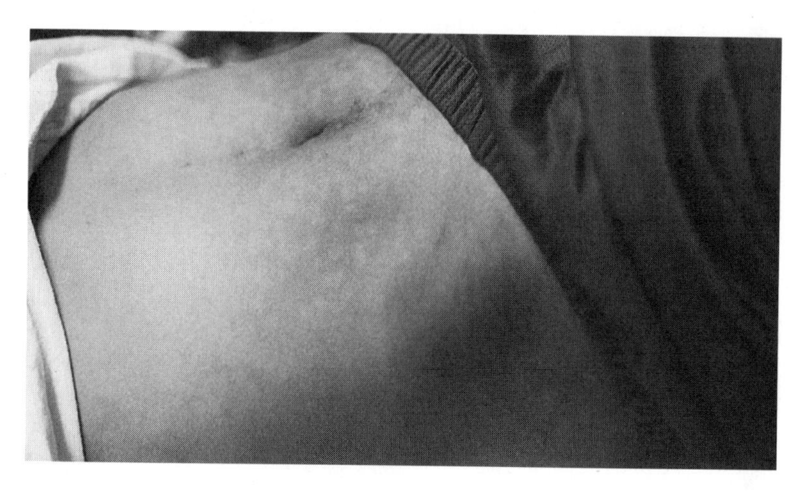

FIGURE 12-13 ■ Contusion to the iliac crest. This injury, the so-called "hip pointer," results in gross discoloration, swelling, pain, and loss of function.

Special Test 12-1
Clinical Determination of the Angle of Torsion

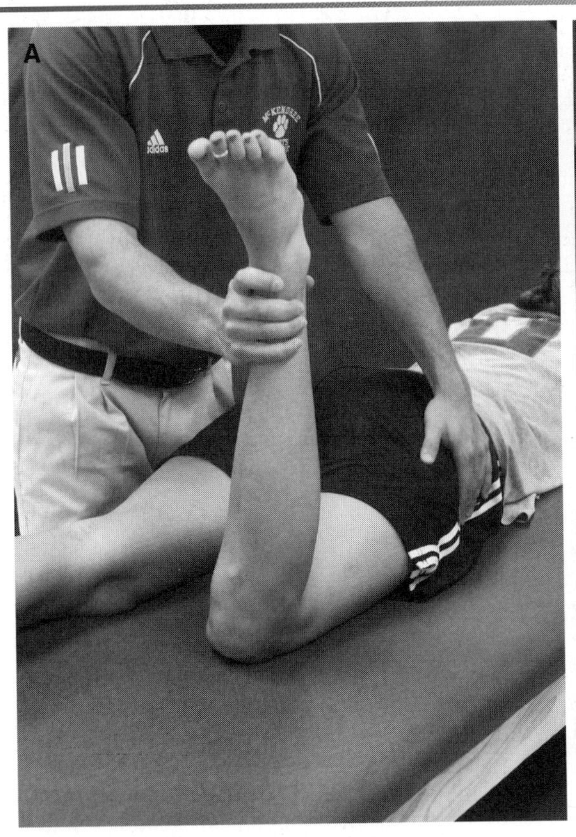

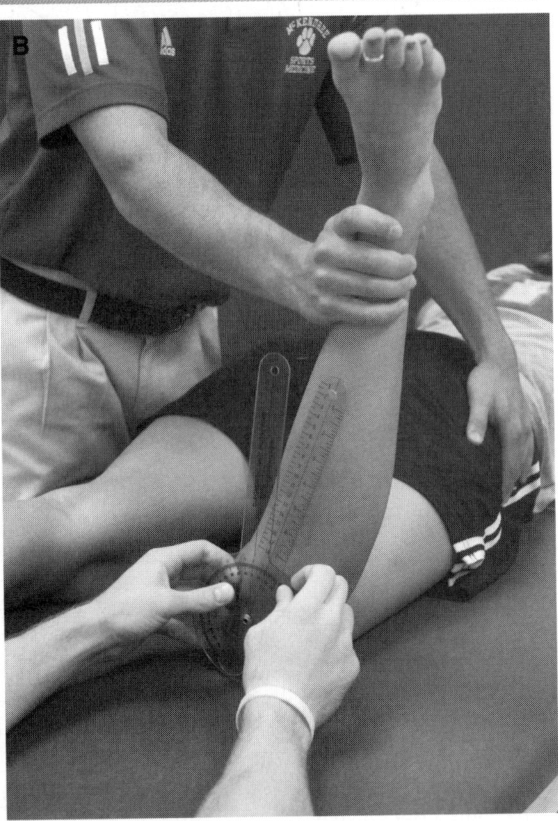

This procedure is most easily performed by two clinicians, one to manipulate the leg and the other to goniometrically measure the angle of the lower leg perpendicular to the table.

Patient Position	Prone with the knee of the leg being evaluated flexed to 90°
Position of Examiner	The use of two examiners is recommended. Examiner 1: On the contralateral side to that being tested; one hand palpates the greater trochanter and the other hand manipulates the lower extremity. Examiner 2: Holding a goniometer distal to the flexed knee with the stationary arm perpendicular to the tabletop.
Evaluative Procedure	**(A)** Examiner 1 internally rotates the femur by moving the lower leg inward and outward until the greater trochanter is maximally prominent. This represents the point at which the femoral head is parallel with the tabletop. **(B)** Examiner 2 then measures the angle formed by the lower leg while the knee remains flexed to 90°.
Positive Test	Angles less than 15° represent femoral retroversion; angles greater than 20° represent anteversion.[4]
Implications	As described in Positive Test above
Evidence	Inter-rater reliability Not Reliable — Very Reliable Poor / Moderate / Good 0 0.1 0.2 0.3 0.4 0.5 0.6 0.7 0.8 0.9 1.0 Intra-rater reliability Not Reliable — Very Reliable Poor / Moderate / Good 0 0.1 0.2 0.3 0.4 0.5 0.6 0.7 0.8 0.9 1.0

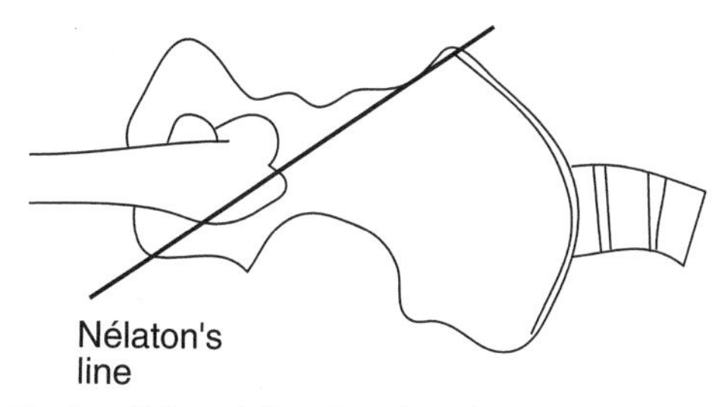

FIGURE 12-14 ■ Nélaton's line. This clinical sign is used to determine the presence of coxa vara. An imaginary line is drawn from the anterior superior iliac spine to the ischial tuberosity. If the greater tuberosity is located superior to this line, coxa vara should be suspected.

- **Hamstring muscle group:** Inspect the length of the hamstring muscles, noting for deformity or discoloration that indicates a muscular tear (Fig. 12-15).
- **Median sacral crests:** Observe the sacral area. Although injury to this area is rare, **pilonidal cysts,** an infection over the posterior aspect of the **median** sacral crests, cause severe pain and disability. As the cyst matures, it protrudes from the gluteal crease and appears violently red. Patients suspected as suffering from a pilonidal cyst require an immediate referral to a physician.

Inspection of leg-length discrepancy

Pain emanating from the foot, lower leg, knee, hip, and spine or deficits in gait may be related to leg length differences of greater than 2 cm.[17] Refer to Chapter 6 for information on the various methods of determining leg-length differences.

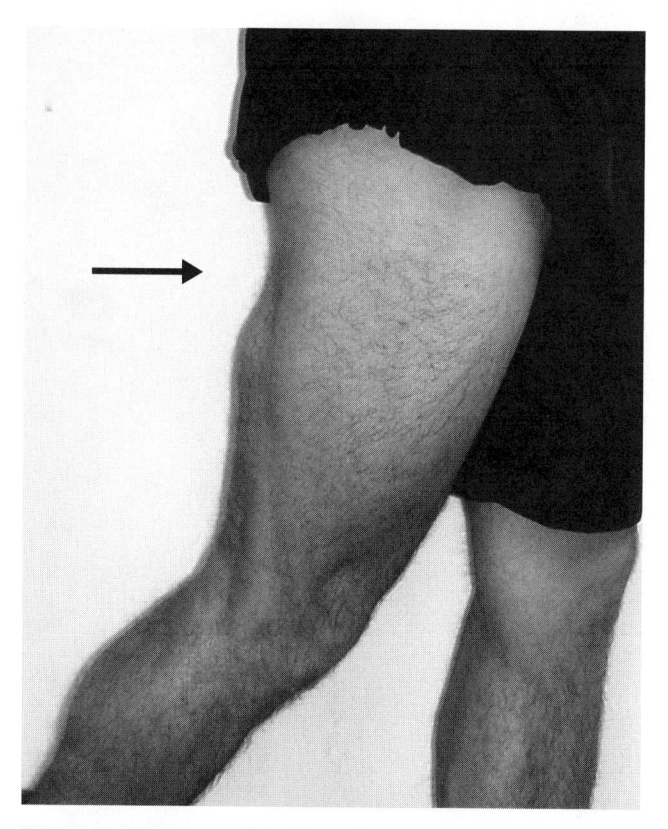

FIGURE 12-15 ■ A tear of the biceps femoris muscle. Note the indentation on the proximal portion of the posterolateral thigh.

PALPATION

The hip and thigh are characterized by areas of subcutaneous bone and other areas of large muscle mass. When performing palpation, use discretion and communicate with the patient. Respect the patient's modesty and maintain privacy at all times.

Palpation of the Medial Structures

1 Gracilis: Abduct the hip to place the adductor muscles on stretch, making the adductor longus muscle visibly prominent at the point that it arises from the symphysis pubis. Palpate the gracilis proximally from its insertion on Gerdy's tubercle.

2 Adductor longus: Using discretion, palpate close to the origin of the adductor group for any tenderness or defect indicating an avulsion fracture.

3 Adductor magnus: Locate the adductor magnus superior and lateral to the adductor longus. This muscle makes up the bulk of the inner thigh.

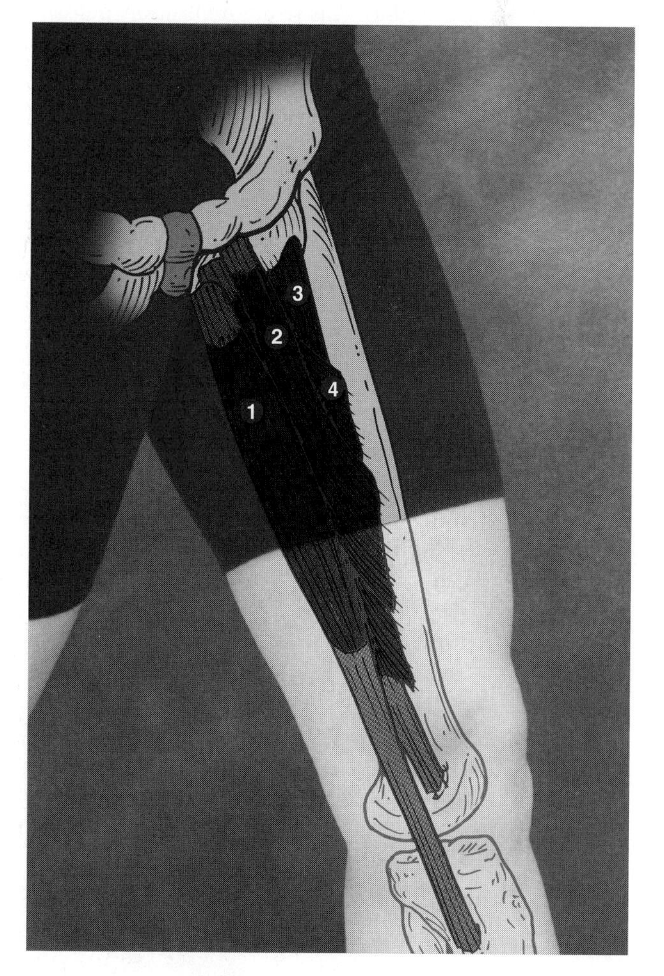

Median Along the body's midline.

4 **Adductor brevis:** Locate the bulk of the adductor brevis under the quadriceps muscle. Continue to palpate superiorly to locate the **pectineus**.

Palpation of the Anterior Structures

1 **Pubic bone:** Use discretion palpating this area. Follow the femoral creases downward toward the pubic bone, located under the pubic fat pad (mons pubis) superior to the genitalia. These bones, as well as the symphysis pubis, may be injured secondary to a blunt force such as when a gymnast strikes his or her pubic bone against the horse, balance beam, or bars. The pubic symphysis can become inflamed secondary to overuse injuries and sheer forces, leading to **osteitis pubis**.

2 **Inguinal ligament:** Palpate the inguinal ligament along its length from the ASIS to the pubic tubercle. Note any abnormal masses or tenderness that may be indicative of a hernia.

3 **Anterior superior iliac spine:** Follow the iliac crest anteriorly to locate the ASIS. This structure is easily palpable in thin patients but may become obscured in muscular or obese individuals. With the patient standing, palpate the ASIS bilaterally. These structures should be of equal height; any difference indicates a functional or true leg-length discrepancy.

4 **Anterior inferior iliac spine:** From the ASIS, continue to palpate downward to locate the anterior inferior iliac spine (AIIS). This structure is not always identifiable.

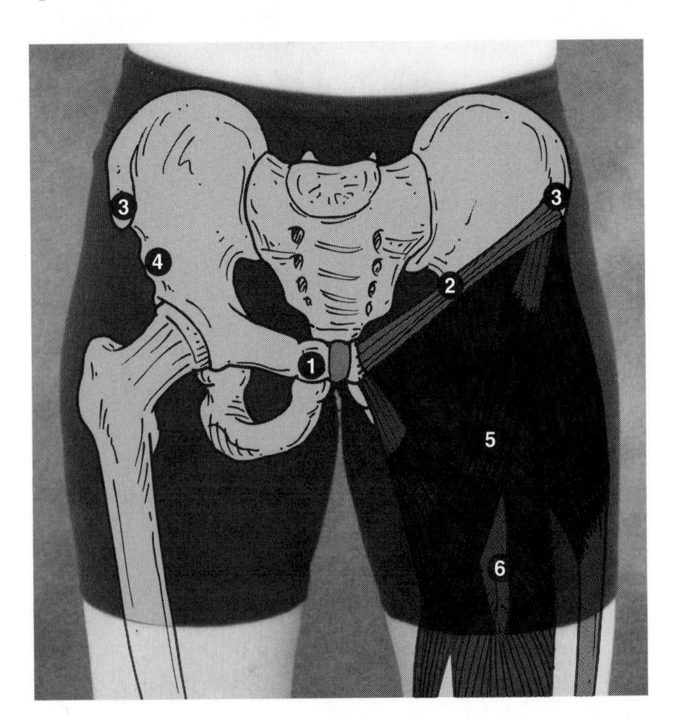

5 **Sartorius:** Palpate the sartorius from its insertion on the ASIS to where it crosses the femoral crease. In some patients, the sartorius may be palpable along its entire length.

6 **Rectus femoris:** Keep in mind that both heads of the rectus femoris lie under the sartorius and therefore are not palpable. However, when the knee is flexed and the hip forced into extension, the resulting tension may cause a strain of the rectus femoris or an avulsion of its origin. The length of the muscle belly becomes palpable just distal and lateral to the sartorius and should be palpated to its insertion on the patella.

Palpation of the Lateral Structures

1 **Iliac crest:** Find the iliac crest, usually easily located on most patients, and palpate along its length from the ASIS to the PSIS. After a contusion, the iliac crest becomes swollen and tender to the touch. Crepitus also may be present.

2 **Tensor fasciae latae:** Locate this area below the anterior third of the iliac crest. The tensor fasciae latae is not easily distinguished from the gluteus medius.

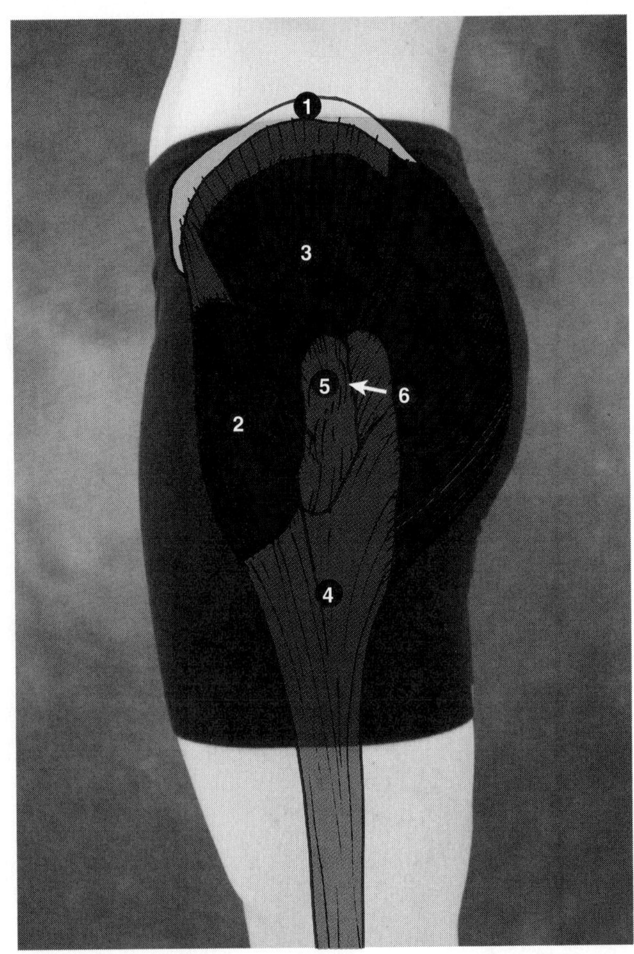

3 **Gluteus medius:** To isolate the gluteus medius, position the patient in sidelying with the upper hip actively abducted 10 to 15 degrees. The length of the muscle is palpable from its origin just inferior to the iliac crest to its insertion on the superior portion of the greater trochanter (Fig. 12-16). The inability to maintain this position during the examination may indicate gluteus medius weakness, which is then confirmed through the **Trendelenburg's test**.

4 **IT band:** Palpate the length of the IT band from its origin from the tensor fasciae latae to its insertion on Gerdy's tubercle. The IT band is a common site of trigger points and may become adhered to the underlying tissues.

5 **Greater trochanter:** Locate the greater trochanter at approximately the midline on the lateral thigh 6 to 8 inches below the iliac crest. The greater trochanter becomes more identifiable as the femur is internally and externally rotated and its posterior aspect becomes exposed. This area becomes tender secondary to bursitis, tendinopathy of the gluteus medius or IT band tightness.

6 **Trochanteric bursa:** Overlying the posterior aspect of the greater trochanter, the trochanteric bursa is not directly palpable. Inflammation of this bursa causes it to feel thick and elicits pain at the posterior aspect of the greater trochanter.

Palpation of the Posterior Structures

1 **Median sacral crests:** Palpate the fused remnants of the sacral spinous processes from below the L5 vertebra to the midportion of the gluteal crease.

2 **Posterior superior iliac spine:** Locate the PSIS at the inferior portion of the gluteal dimples. Under normal circumstances, these bony landmarks are palpable and align at the same level. Tenderness may indicate sacroiliac pathology.

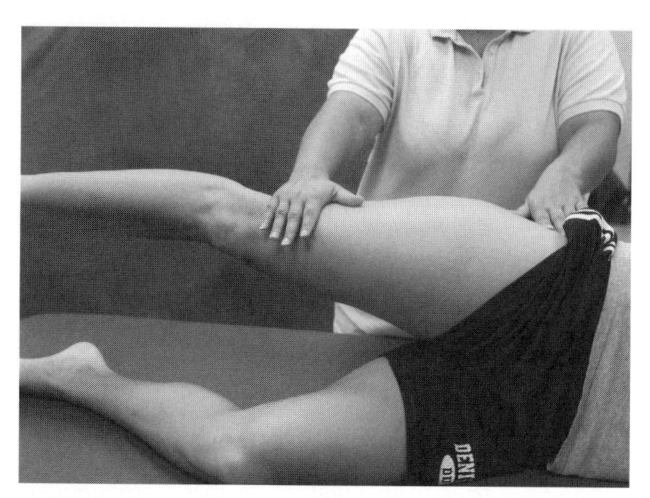

FIGURE 12-16 ■ Positioning of the patient to isolate the gluteus medius during palpation. Slightly abducting the hip makes the gluteus medius palpable.

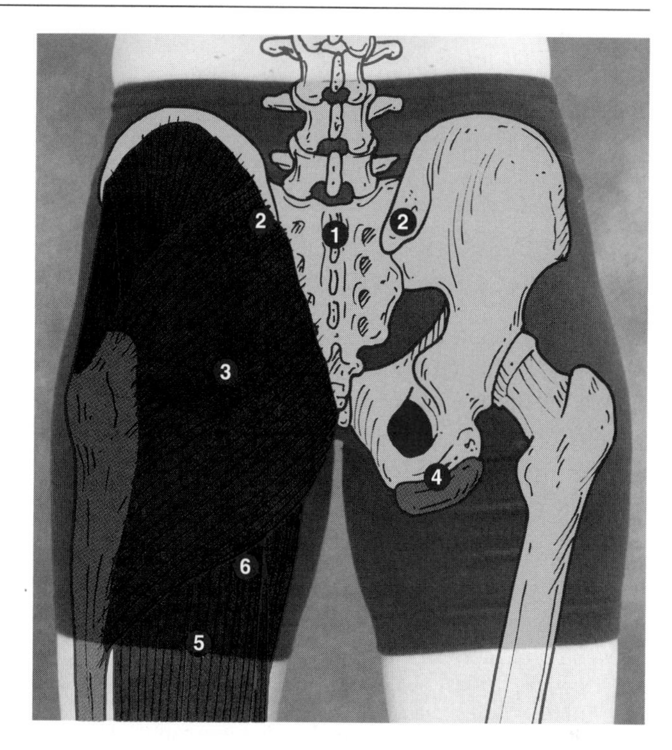

3 **Gluteus maximus:** Palpate the bulk of the gluteus maximus. This structure is easily palpable and may be made more identifiable by having the patient squeeze the buttocks together or extend the hip.

4 **Ischial tuberosity and bursa:** Position the patient in sidelying with the upper hip flexed. Identify the ischial tuberosity by locating the gluteal fold and palpating deeply at approximately the midline of the gluteal fold. Tenderness at this site may indicate an avulsion fracture or hamstring tendinopathy. Similar to the trochanteric bursa, the ischial bursa cannot be identified unless it is inflamed, at which time it is tender to the touch.

5 **Sciatic nerve:** Although the sciatic nerve is not directly palpable, attempt to palpate its approximate course for tenderness. Begin palpation of this structure by locating the ischial tuberosity and the greater trochanter. The sciatic nerve is found as a cord midway between these two structures. An irritated sciatic nerve is exquisitely tender when compared with the contralateral side.

6 **Hamstring muscles:** Position the patient prone with the knee flexed between 45 and 90 degrees. Locate the common origin of the hamstring group on the ischial tuberosity, a common site of avulsion fractures. With the exception of the short head of the biceps femoris, the hamstring tendons originate as a single mass. Approximately 5 to 10 cm distal to the tuberosity the muscles begin to diverge, with the semimembranosus the first muscle to become prominent.[18] Palpate the semitendinosus and semimembranosus down the medial side of the posterior femur. Also palpate the biceps femoris down the lateral border, noting any spasm, defects, or pain.

Joint and Muscle Function Assessment

The ROM available to the hip joint is limited by its bony and soft tissue restraints. The position of the knee also can further limit the hip's ROM and assessment of hip motion should occur with the knee flexed and extended. A fully flexed knee can limit the amount of extension at the hip because the rectus femoris is stretched to its limits. An extended knee with stretched hamstrings can limit the amount of hip flexion available. Goniometric evaluation of hip ROM is presented in Goniometry Boxes 12-1 to 12-3. The muscles acting on the hip in each of its motions are presented in Table 12-4.

Active range of motion

With three degrees of freedom, the hip has a range of motion second only to the shoulder and the carpometacarpal joint of the thumb. There is no true active range of motion (AROM) at the sacroiliac joints. Any motion is accessory in nature and is minimal in the absence of pathology.

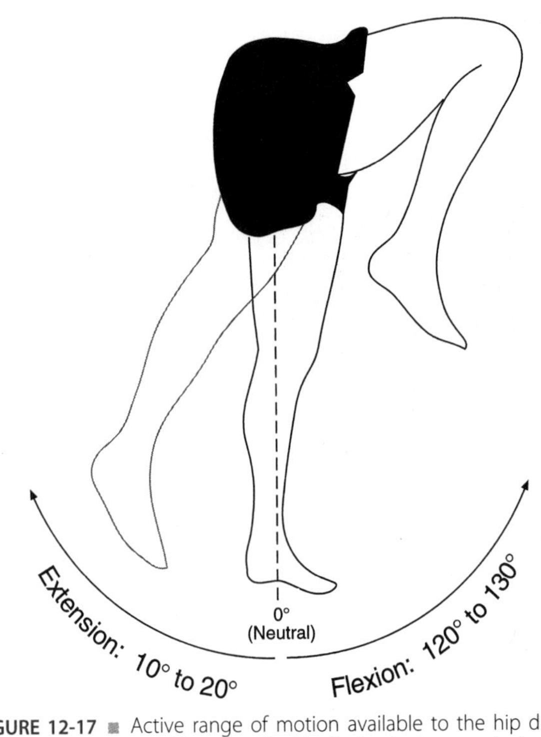

FIGURE 12-17 ■ Active range of motion available to the hip during flexion and extension. The range for hip flexion is decreased when the knee is extended secondary to tightness of the hamstring muscles and is limited during extension when the knee is flexed because of tightness of the rectus femoris.

- **Flexion and extension:** The arc of motion available to the hip with the knee flexed ranges from 130 to 150 degrees. The majority of this motion (120 degrees to 130 degrees) occurs during flexion (Fig. 12-17). Extending the knee limits the amount of flexion available to the hip by placing the hamstring muscle group on stretch.
- **Adduction and abduction:** AROM for abduction of the hip is approximately 45 degrees from the neutral position and for adduction, 20 to 30 degrees after the opposite limb is cleared from the movement (Fig. 12-18).
- **Internal and external rotation:** With the hip in the flexed position, such as when a patient is sitting with legs bent at the end of a table, external rotation ranges from 40 to 50 degrees from the neutral position. Internal rotation is slightly less, approximately 45 degrees from the neutral position (Fig. 12-19). Anteversion and retroversion of the femur influence the available range in rotation. Extending the hip reduces the ROM available in each direction.

Table 12-4 Muscles Acting on the Hip According to Motion

Flexion	Abduction	Internal Rotation
Gluteus medius (anterior fibers)	Gluteus maximus (lower fibers)	Adductor brevis
Gluteus minimus	Gluteus medius	Adductor longus
Iliacus	Gluteus minimus	Adductor magnus
Psoas major	Sartorius	Gluteus medius (anterior fibers)
Psoas minor		Gluteus minimus
Rectus femoris		
Sartorius		
Extension	**Adduction**	**External Rotation**
Biceps femoris	Adductor brevis	Gemellus inferior
Gluteus maximus	Adductor longus	Gemellus superior
Gluteus medius (posterior fibers)	Adductor magnus	Gluteus medius (posterior fibers)
Gluteus maximus	Gluteus maximus (upper fibers)	Obturator extremis
Semimembranosus	Gracilis	Obturator internus
	Pectineus	Piriformis
		Quadratus femoris
		Sartorius

Manual muscle testing

The iliopsoas muscle group is the primary flexor of the hip. The rectus femoris, a two-joint muscle crossing the hip and knee, contributes to hip flexion, especially when combined with knee extension such as when kicking a ball. Several approaches attempt to differentiate the contribution of iliopsoas and rectus femoris to hip flexion (e.g., knee flexed, knee extended). We recommend first testing hip flexion as described in Manual Muscle Test 12-1, then testing knee

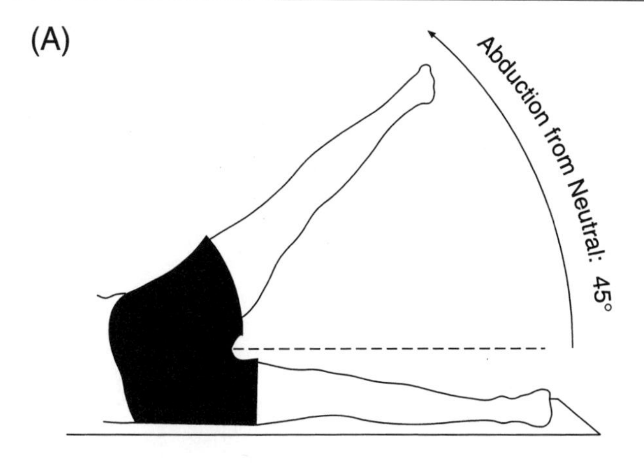

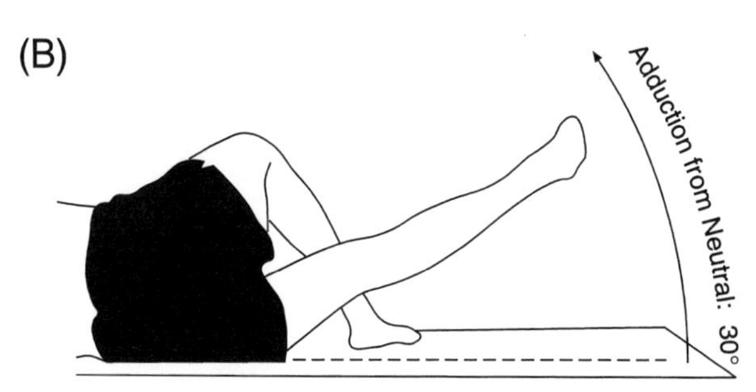

FIGURE 12-18 ■ Active hip abduction **(A)** and adduction **(B)**.

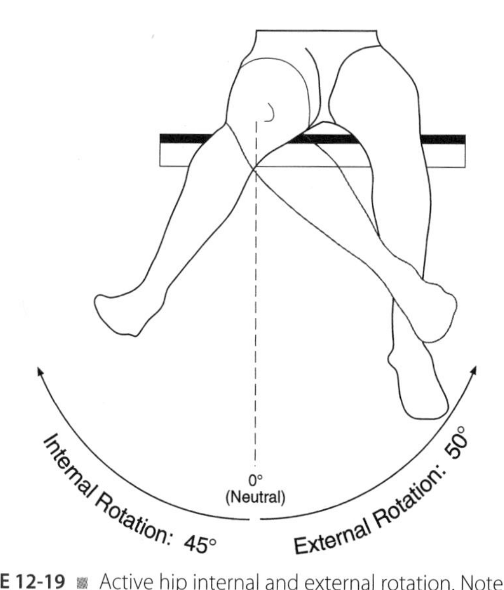

FIGURE 12-19 ■ Active hip internal and external rotation. Note that, in the seated position, the lower leg moves in a direction opposite that of the femur (e.g., during internal femoral rotation the lower leg rotates outwardly).

extension (see Manual Muscle Test 10-1). Testing of the sartorius, another two-joint muscle that acts on the hip and the knee, is described in Box 10-3.

Manual muscle tests for the other hip muscles are presented in Manual Muscle Tests 12-2 through 12-4. In addition to the standard testing of the hip muscles, the postural muscles of the pelvic girdle are assessed during gait. Patients suffering from weakness of the gluteus medius tilt the pelvis to the side opposite the insufficiency, the **Trendelenburg's test** (Special Test 12-2). Trendelenburg's gait is discussed in detail in Chapter 7.

✱ Practical Evidence

Hip abduction strength is often reduced in the presence of chronic ankle instability and recurrent ankle sprains.[19]

Passive range of motion

Hip passive range of motion most frequently results in a firm end-feel resulting from soft tissue stretch or soft tissue approximation (Table 12-5).

- **Flexion and extension:** To measure passive flexion of the hip, the patient is in the supine position. The distal hand is at the posterior thigh, just above the knee. The proximal hand is under the lumbar spine to detect pelvic rotation, which will occur at the end range of hip flexion. As the hip is flexed, the knee is allowed to flex from tension placed on the hamstring muscles and gravity. With pressure applied proximal to the knee joint (i.e., without forcing knee extension), the normal end-feel for hip flexion is soft owing to the approximation of the quadriceps group with the abdomen. When the knee is forced to remain in extension during hip flexion, the end-feel is firm because of the stretching of the hamstring muscle groups (Fig. 12-20).

Tightness of the hip flexors can result in an increased lordotic curvature of the lumbar spine. The **Thomas test** is used to differentiate between tightness of the iliopsoas muscle group and tightness of the rectus femoris muscle (Special Test 12-3). Tightness of the hip flexors can also be identified using **Ely's test** (Special Test 12-4).

During passive hip extension ROM measurements, the patient is prone and the knee is kept extended. The pelvis is stabilized to prevent it from being lifted off the table. The normal end-feel for hip extension is firm because of the stretching of the anterior joint capsule and the

Table 12-5 Hip Capsular Pattern and End-Feels

Capsular Pattern: Internal rotation, abduction, flexion, extension	
End-Feels:	
Flexion	Firm or soft: Soft tissue approximation or hamstring tension
Abduction	Firm: Stretch of the adductors
Adduction	Firm: Stretch of the abductors and joint capsule
Internal rotation	Firm: Stretch of the external rotators
External rotation	Firm: Stretch of the internal rotators
Extension	Firm: Stretch of the iliopsoas and joint capsule

Goniometry Box 12-1
Flexion and Extension

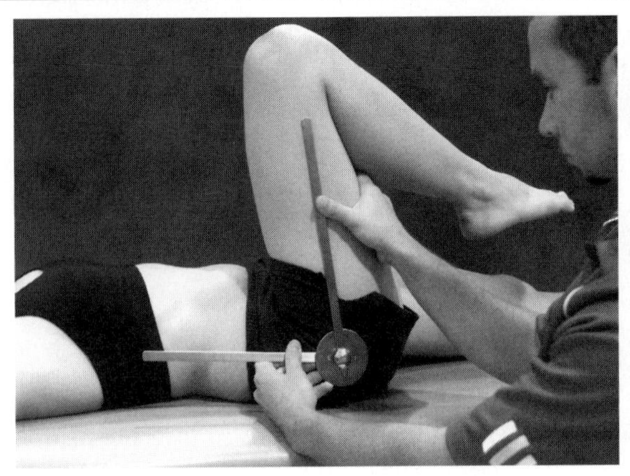

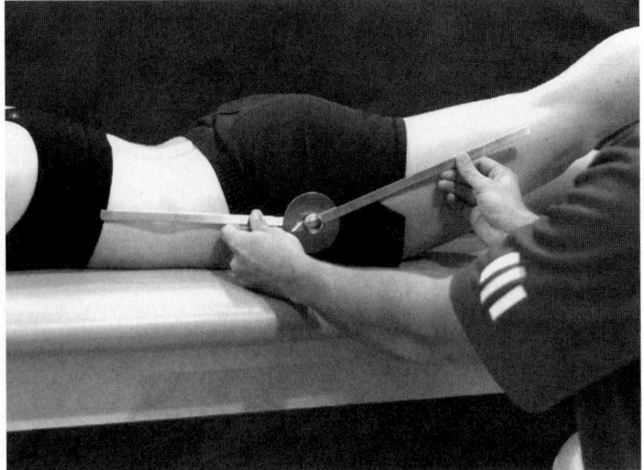

	Flexion 0°–120°	Extension 0°–30°
Patient Position	Supine	Prone
Goniometer Alignment		
Fulcrum	The axis is aligned over the greater trochanter.	
Proximal Arm	The stationary arm is aligned over the midline of the pelvis.	
Distal Arm	The movement arm is aligned over the long axis of the femur, using the lateral epicondyle as the distal reference point.	
Comments	Allow the knee to flex during the hip flexion measurement. The hip flexion measurement can also be taken with the knee extended to determine the influence of the hamstrings length. When measuring hip extension, stabilize the pelvis to avoid trunk extension. This may require help from someone. The hip extension measurement can also be taken with the knee flexed to determine the influence of the rectus femoris length.	

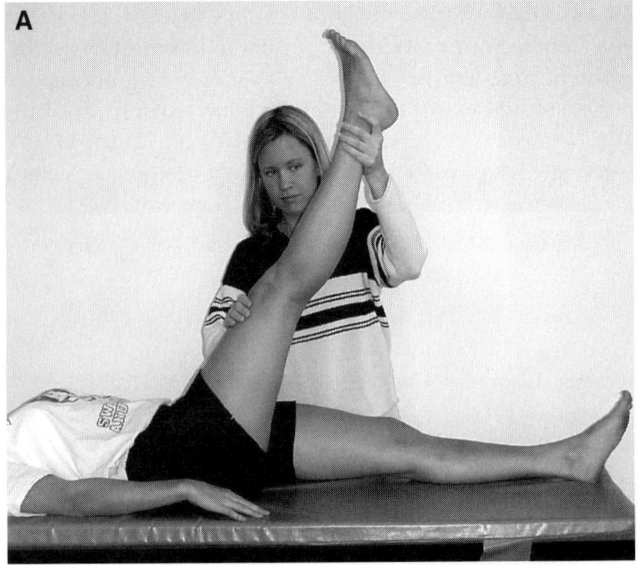

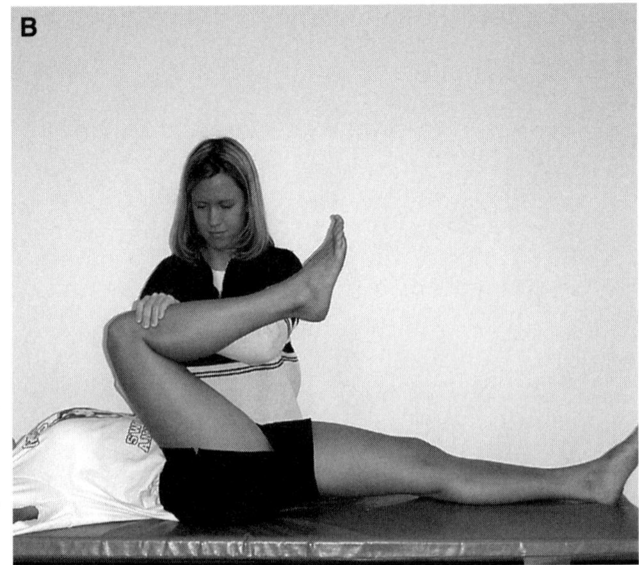

FIGURE 12-20 ■ Passive hip flexion: **(A)** knee extended; **(B)** knee flexed. The motion should also be replicated by adding pressure to the posterior distal femur. Note that hip flexion with the knee extended (shown in **A**) is the provocative phase of the straight-leg raise test and may produce sciatic nerve symptoms (see Chapter 13).

Goniometry Box 12-2
Hip Abduction and Adduction

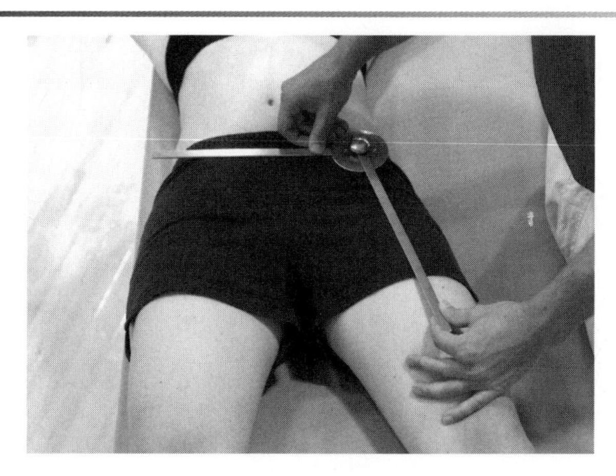

	Abduction 0°–45°	Adduction 0°–30°
Patient Position	Supine	Supine; the opposite leg is abducted.
Goniometer Alignment		
Fulcrum	The axis is aligned over the ASIS.	
Proximal Arm	The stationary arm is placed over the opposite ASIS.	
Distal Arm	The movement arm is positioned over the long axis of the femur, using the middle of the patella as the distal reference.	
Comments	Note that the start position of the goniometer is 90°, which is the baseline. Measurements are made relative to that position. The end of hip adduction is reached when the pelvis begins to laterally tilt.	

ASIS = anterior superior iliac spine.

iliofemoral, ischiofemoral, and pubofemoral ligaments. If extension is assessed with the knee flexed, a firm end-feel is obtained from tension within the rectus femoris muscle (Fig. 12-21).

- **Adduction and abduction:** The patient is in the supine position with the knee extended for the measurement of both passive adduction and abduction. The leg opposite that being tested is abducted to permit unrestricted adduction of the extremity being tested. To isolate the hip joint, the pelvis is stabilized to prevent lateral tilting during the motion (Fig. 12-22). The normal end-feel during adduction is firm owing to tension produced in the lateral joint capsule, the IT band, and the gluteus medius muscle. During abduction, a firm end-feel is obtained because of the tightness in the medial joint capsule and in the pubofemoral, ischiofemoral, and iliofemoral ligaments.
- **Internal and external rotation:** The patient is supine with the hip and knee flexed to 90 degrees. The clinician stabilizes the distal femur with one hand and maneuvers the distal lower leg to rotate the femur (Fig. 12-23).

When the knees are flexed, the lower leg rotates in the direction opposite that of the femur (e.g., when the femur is internally rotated, the lower leg rotates outwardly). The end-feel is firm in both directions. Internal femoral rotation is limited by tension in the posterior joint capsule and the intrinsic external hip rotators. External femoral rotation is limited by the anterior joint capsule and the iliofemoral and pubofemoral ligaments. Internal rotation may be increased with patients having anteverted hips and decreased in the presence of retroverted hips. External rotation may be increased in individuals with retroverted hips and decreased in those with anteverted hips.

Joint Stability Tests

Stress testing

There are no specific tests to determine the integrity of the hip ligaments. Pathology of the ligaments is determined through testing the passive movement of the joint. Extension of the hip places the iliofemoral, pubofemoral, and ischiofemoral ligaments on stretch. Adducting the hip stresses the superior fibers of the iliofemoral ligament,

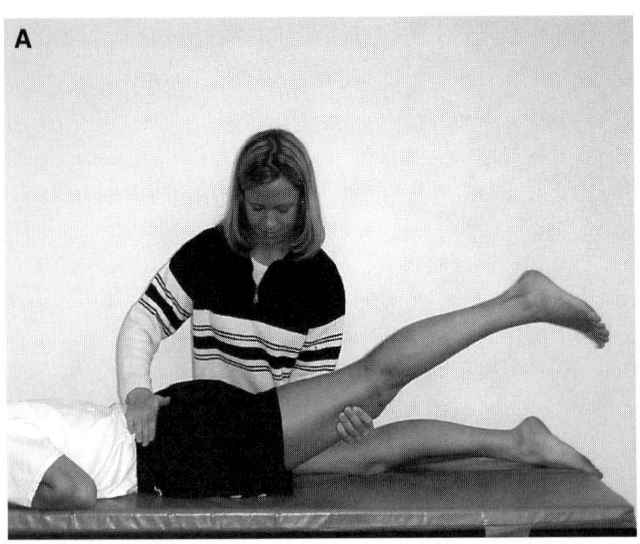

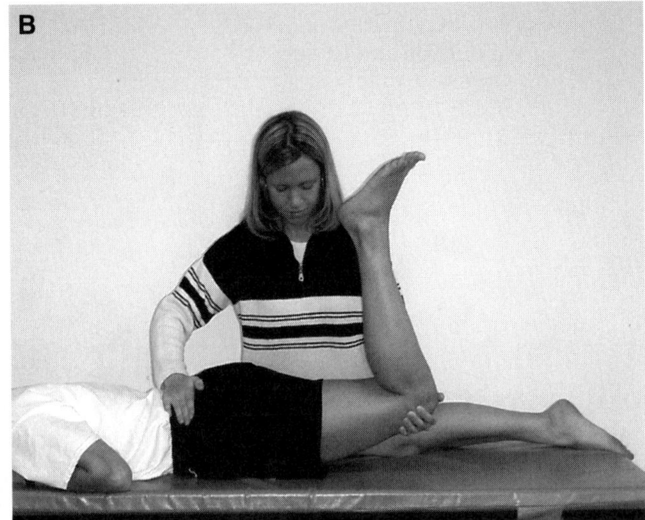

FIGURE 12-21 ■ Passive hip extension: **(A)** knee extended; **(B)** knee flexed.

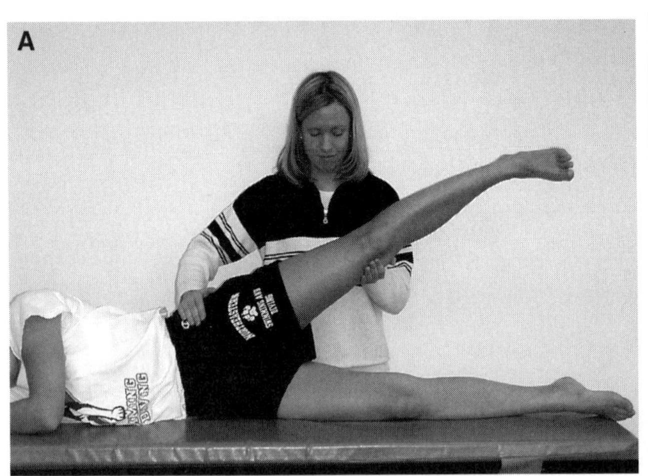

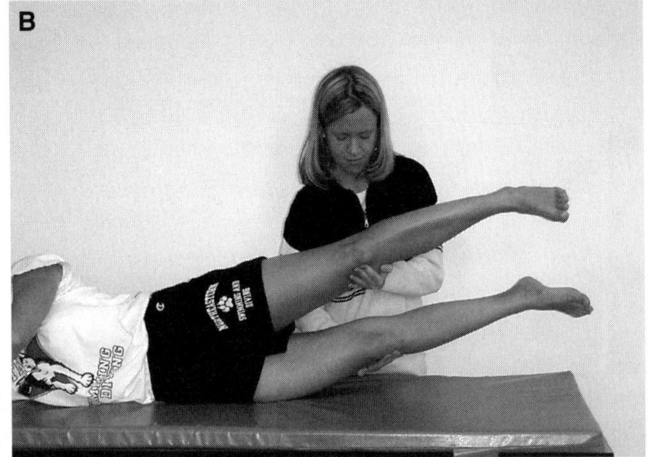

FIGURE 12-22 ■ **(A)** Passive hip abduction. **(B)** Passive hip adduction.

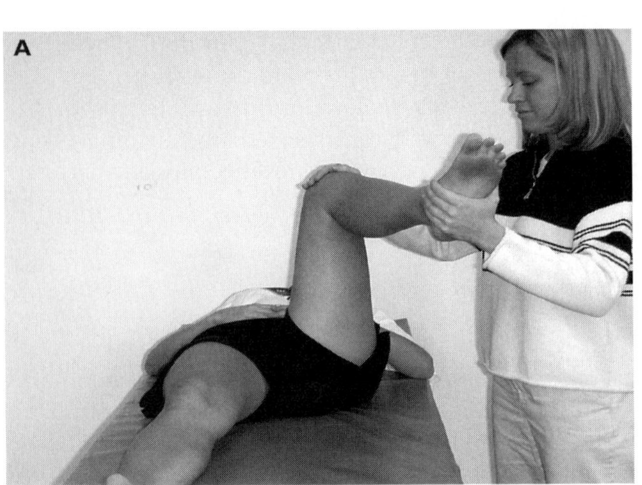

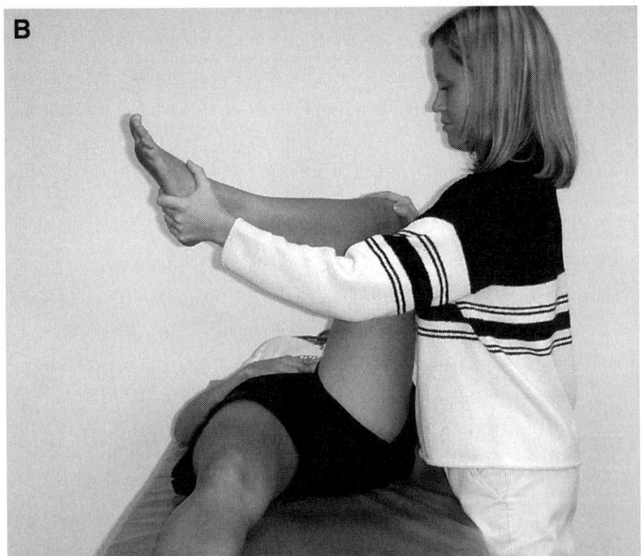

FIGURE 12-23 ■ **(A)** Passive hip internal rotation, and **(B)** passive hip external rotation.

Goniometry Box 12-3
Hip Internal and External Rotation

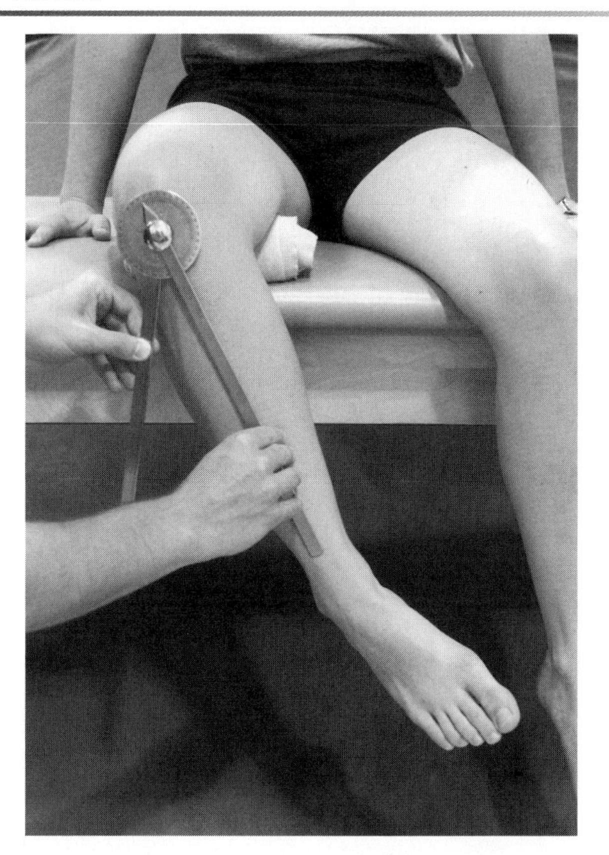

	Internal Rotation 0°–45° **External Rotation 0°–45°**
Patient Position	Seated Place a bolster under the distal femur to keep it parallel with the tabletop.
Goniometer Alignment	
Fulcrum	The axis is aligned over the center of the patella.
Proximal Arm	The stationary arm is held perpendicular to the floor.
Distal Arm	The movement arm is positioned over the long axis of the femur, using the center of the talocrural joint as the distal reference.

while abducting the hip places a strain on the pubofemoral ligament and the lower fibers of the iliofemoral ligament (see Table 12-1). The FABER test stresses the anterior joint capsule (see Stress Test 13-15).

Joint play

Assessment of joint play at the hip is not commonly performed. The large amount of soft tissue around the hip makes it difficult to maneuver the joint and to detect subtle joint motion. Restriction in joint passive ROM may identify hypomobility.

Neurologic Testing

Pain, paresthesia, and inhibition of muscular innervation may be referred through the hip and into the lower extremity from impingement of the lumbar or sacral plexus or their associated nerve roots. A complete lower quarter screen should be performed for pathology involving the femoral or sciatic nerve (see Box 1-5). Impingement of the sciatic nerve from spasm of the piriformis muscle, **piriformis syndrome,** is discussed in the Pathologies and Related Special Tests section of this chapter.

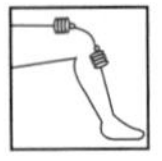

Manual Muscle Test 12-1
Iliopsoas (Hip Flexion)

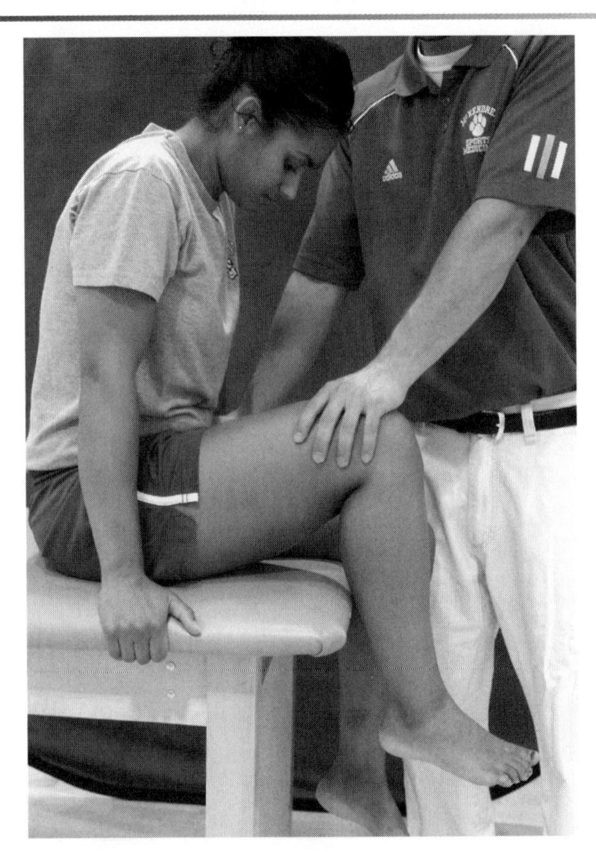

Iliopsoas

Patient Position	Seated, leaning slightly forward The patient should lightly grip the table.
Starting Position	The knee is flexed over the edge of the table.
Stabilization	Over the ASIS
Palpation	The insertion of the iliopsoas can be palpated in the inguinal crease, medial to the origin of the rectus femoris.
Resistance	Anterior aspect of the distal femur just proximal to the knee
Primary Mover(s) (Innervation)	Iliopsoas (L1, L2, L3, L4)
Secondary Mover(s) (Innervation)	Rectus femoris (L2, L3, L4) Sartorius (L2, L3)
Substitution	The patient may attempt to lean backwards to maximize the contribution of the rectus femoris.
Comments	There is no agreement on the optimal position for testing the hip flexors.

ASIS = anterior superior iliac spine.

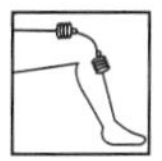

Manual Muscle Test 12-2
Hip Extension

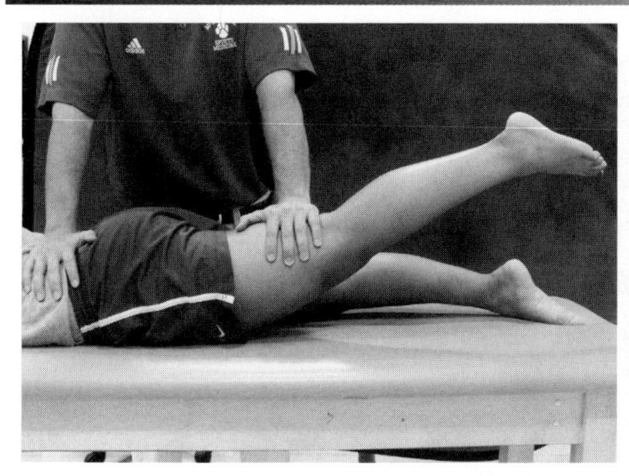

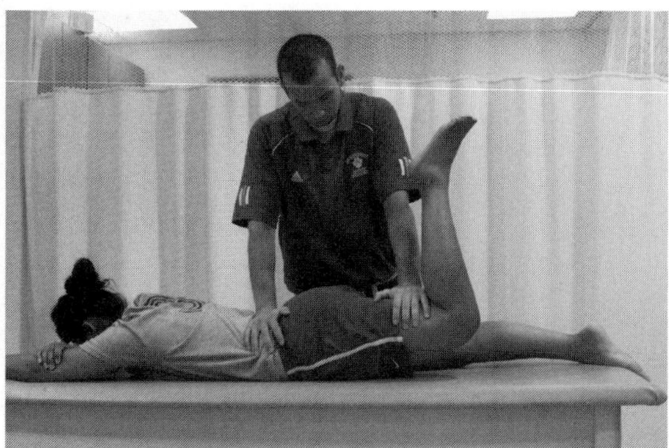

	Hamstrings and Gluteus Maximus	Gluteus Maximus
Patient Position	Prone	Prone
Starting Position	The knee is extended.	The knee is flexed to 90°.
Stabilization	Posterior pelvis	Posterior pelvis
Palpation	Posterior thigh	Buttock
Resistance	Proximal to the popliteal fossa	Posterior aspect of the distal femur
Primary Mover(s) (Innervation)	Hamstrings (L4, L5, S1, S2, S3) Gluteus maximus (L5, S1, S2)	Gluteus maximus (L5, S1, S2)
Secondary Mover(s) (Innervation)	Not applicable	Hamstrings (L4, L5, S1, S2, S3)
Substitution	Not applicable	Trunk extension
Comments	Pain with the knee extended that decreases with knee flexed implicates the hamstrings. This can be confirmed by resisting knee flexion.	Not applicable

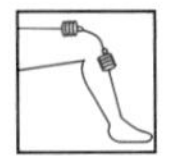

Manual Muscle Test 12-3
Hip Adduction and Abduction

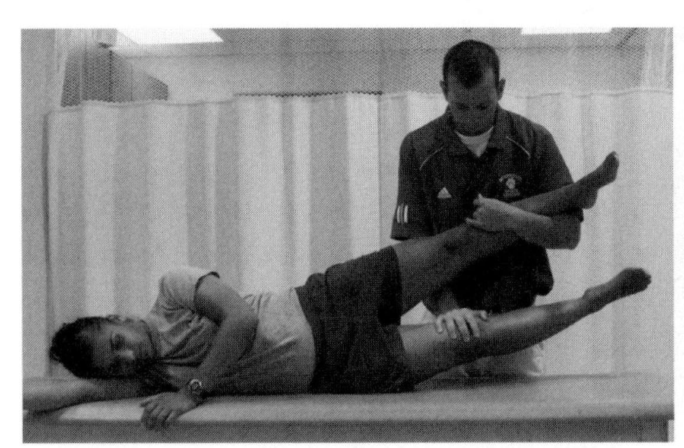

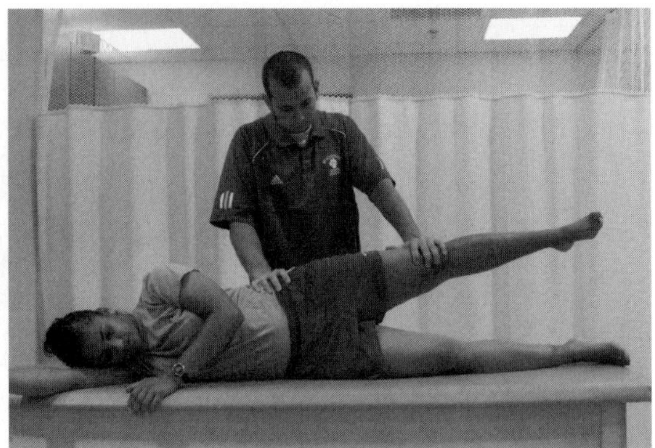

	Adduction	Abduction
Patient Position	Side-lying on the side being tested	Side-lying on the opposite side being tested
Starting Position	The knee is extended. The opposite (nontested) leg is supported by the examiner.	The knee is flexed slightly.
Stabilization	The pelvis and torso are actively stabilized by the patient.	The pelvis and torso are actively stabilized by the patient.
Palpation	Medial thigh	Proximal to greater trochanter
Resistance	Over the medial femur, proximal to the knee	Over the lateral femoral condyle
Primary Mover(s) (Innervation)	Adductor magnus (L2, L3, L4, L5, S1) Adductor longus (L2, L3, L4) Adductor brevis (L2, L3, L4) Gracilis	Gluteus medius (L4, L5, S1) Gluteus minimus (L4, L5, S1)
Secondary Mover(s) (Innervation)	Gluteus maximus (lower fibers) (L5, S1, S2) Pectineus (L3, L4)	Tensor fascia latae (L4, L5, S1) Sartorius (L2, L3)
Substitution	Not applicable	Hip flexion
Comments	The test can also be performed with the patient prone.	The tensor fascia latae is more active with slight hip flexion. The gluteus medius is more active more straight abduction.

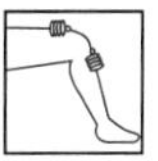

Manual Muscle Test 12-4
Hip Internal and External Rotation

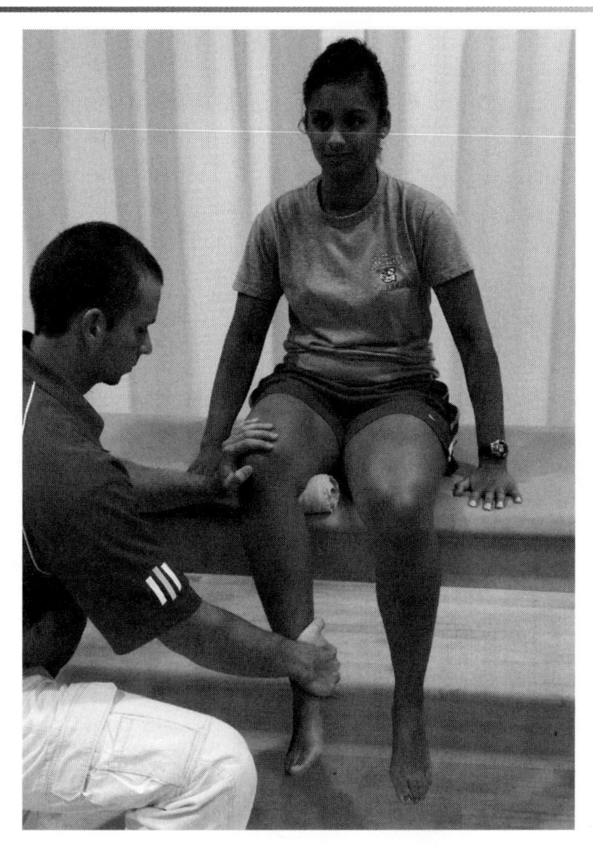

Internal Rotation and External Rotation

	Internal Rotation	External Rotation
Patient Position	Seated with the knees flexed over the edge of the table A bolster is placed under the distal femur to keep it parallel with the tabletop.	Seated with the knees flexed over the edge of the table A bolster is placed under the distal femur to keep it parallel with the tabletop.
Starting Position	Leg perpendicular to the ground	Leg perpendicular to the ground
Stabilization	The patient's arms are extended and support the torso on the table.	The patient's arms are extended and support the torso on the table.
Resistance	On the lateral aspect of the distal lower leg	On the medial aspect of the distal lower leg
Primary Mover(s) (Innervation)	Gluteus minimus (L4, L5, S1) Tensor fascia latae (L4, L5, S1) Gluteus medius (anterior fibers) (L4, L5, S1)	Obturator internus (L5, S1, S2) Obturator externus (L3, L4) Quadratus femoris (L4, L5, S1) Piriformis (S1, S2) Gemellus inferior and superior (L4, L5, S1) Gluteus maximus (L5, S1, S2)
Secondary Mover(s) (Innervation)	Adductor longus (L2, L3, L4) Adductor magnus (L2, L3, L4, L5, S1) Adductor brevis (L2, L3, L4) Semimembranosus (L5, S1) Semitendinosus (L5, S1, S2)	Sartorius (L2, L3) Biceps femoris (long head) (S1, S2, S3) Psoas major (L1, L2, L3, L4)
Substitution	Trunk lateral flexion	Knee flexion

Special Test 12-2
Trendelenburg Test for Gluteus Medius Weakness

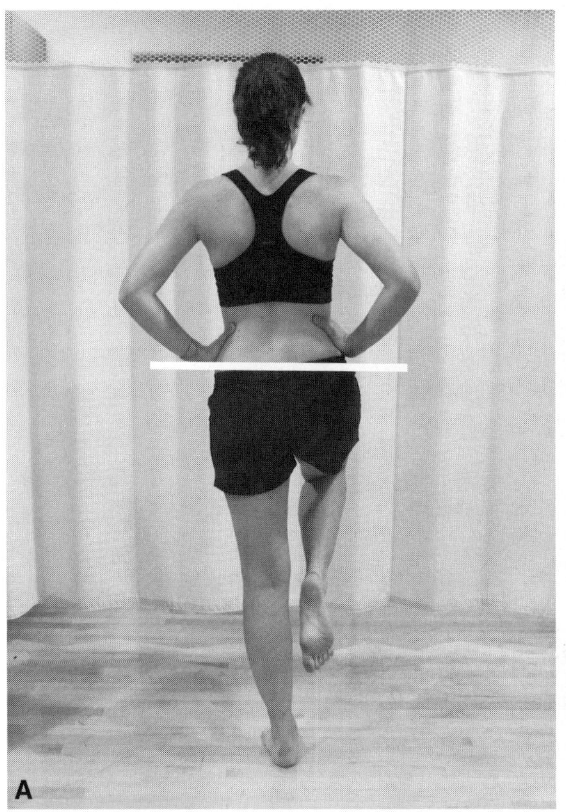

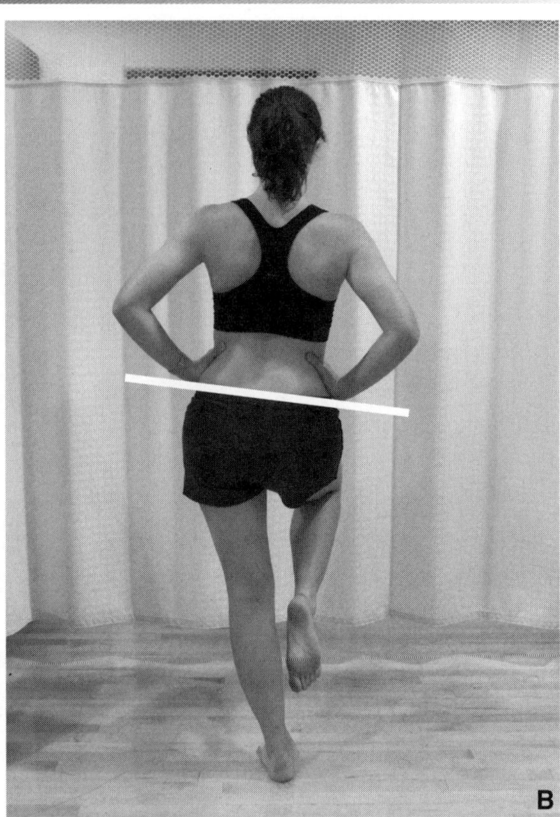

The patient is asked to stand on the affected leg **(A)**. In the presence of gluteus medius weakness, the pelvis lowers on the opposite side of the affected leg **(B)**.

Patient Position	Standing with the weight evenly distributed between both feet The patient's shorts are lowered to the point at which the iliac crests or posterior superior iliac spines are visible.
Position of Examiner	Behind the patient
Evaluative Procedure	The patient lifts the leg opposite the side being tested.
Positive Test	The pelvis lowers on the non–weight-bearing side.
Implications	Insufficiency of the gluteus medius to support the torso in an erect position, indicating weakness in the muscle
Modification	Repeated testing may be necessary, as fatigue can magnify this weakness.
Comments	Muscle weakness can result from nerve root impingement or damage to the superior gluteal nerve.
Evidence	Absent or inconclusive in the literature

Special Test 12-3
Thomas Test for Hip Flexor Tightness Rectus Femoris Contracture Test

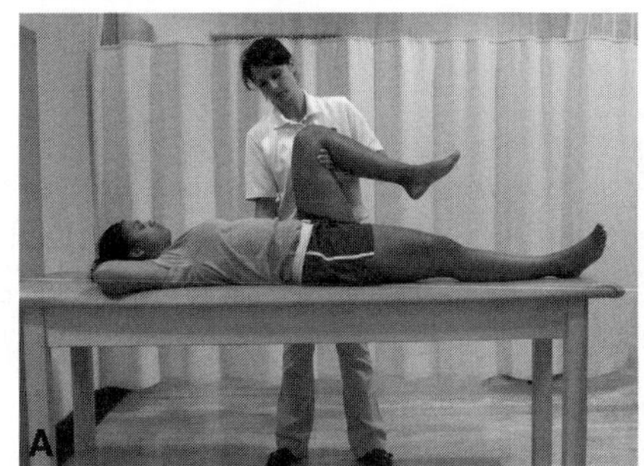

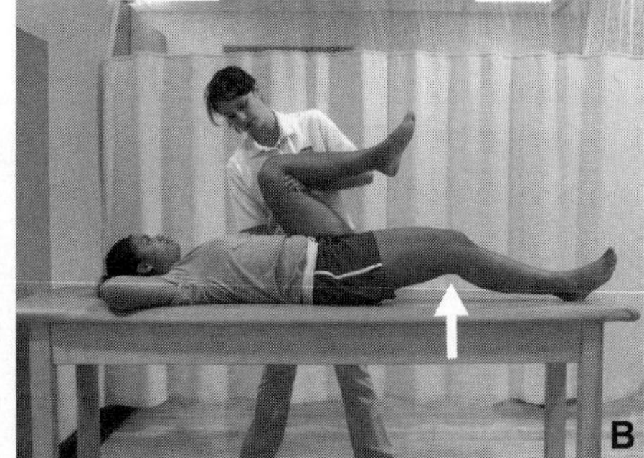

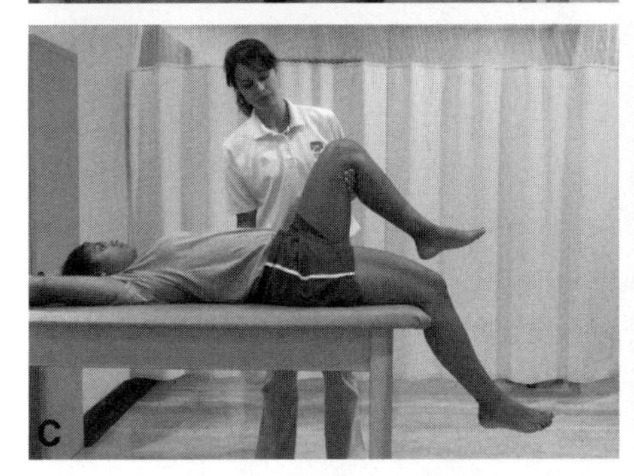

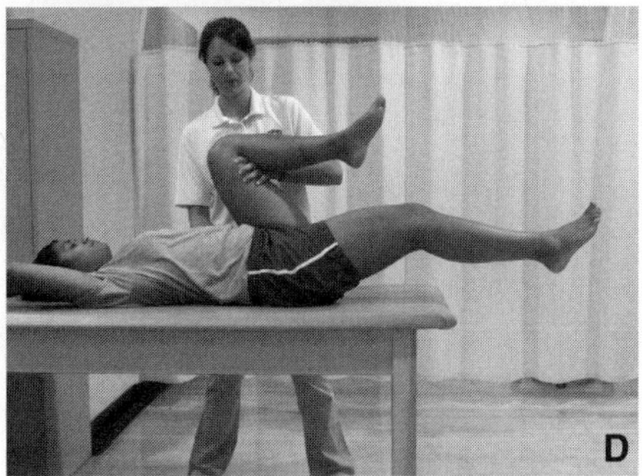

Thomas test for hip flexor tightness. The patient's left (forward) leg is tested. **(A)** Tightness of the left rectus femoris muscle; **(B)** tightness of the left iliopsoas group. Rectus femoris contracture test (a modification of the Thomas test). **(C)** A modification of the Thomas test, the patient is position so that the knee of the test leg is off the table. **(D)** Tightness of the hip flexors results in the opposite knee and hip flexing.

Patient Position	TT: Lying prone on the table RFCT: Lying supine with the knees bent at the end of the table
Position of Examiner	Standing beside the patient
Evaluative Procedure	The examiner places one hand between the lumbar lordotic curve and the tabletop. One leg is passively flexed to the patient's chest, allowing the knee to flex during the movement. The opposite leg (the leg being tested) rests flat on the table.
Positive Test	**(A)** The lower leg moves into extension. **(B)** The involved leg rises off the table.
Implications	**(A)** Tightness of the rectus femoris. **(B)** Tightness of the iliopsoas muscle group.
Modification	The patient can use the arms to passively flex the hip. The hip position may be measured goniometrically.
Comments	The patient may passively flex the hip and knee by using the arms to pull the leg to the chest.[20] The amount of lumbar flattening can be determined by placing a hand under the lumbar spine.
Evidence	***Modification***

Inter-rater reliability

Not Reliable — **Very Reliable**

Poor | Moderate | Good

0 0.1 0.2 0.3 0.4 0.5 0.6 0.7 0.8 0.9 1.0

Intra-rater reliability

Not Reliable — **Very Reliable**

Poor | Moderate | Good

0 0.1 0.2 0.3 0.4 0.5 0.6 0.7 0.8 0.9 1.0

RFCT = rectus femoris contracture test; TT = Thomas test.

Special Test 12-4
Ely's Test

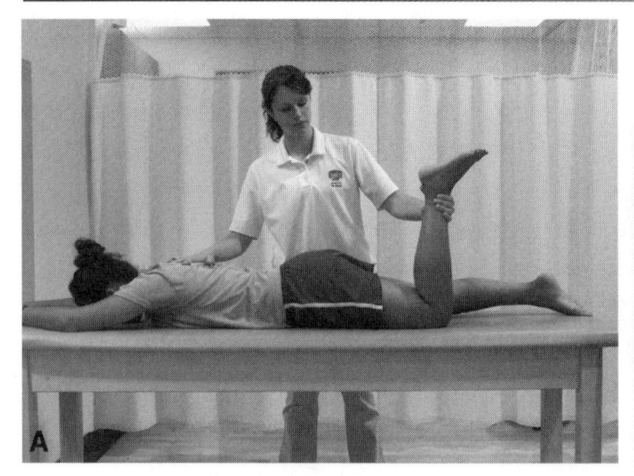

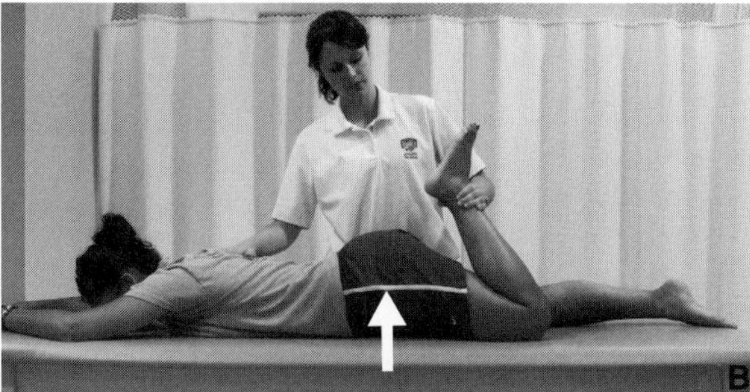

Ely's test for hip flexor tightness **(A)**. Passive flexion of the knee results in hip flexion, causing it to rise off the table **(B)**.

Patient Position	Lying prone
Position of Examiner	Standing beside the patient
Evaluative Procedure	The knee is passively flexed toward the patient's buttock.
Positive Test	The hip on the side being tested flexes, causing it to rise from the table.
Implications	Tightness of the rectus femoris
Evidence	Absent or inconclusive in the literature

Pathologies and Related Special Tests

Most often, trauma to the hip and pelvis and the related muscles results in contusions or strains. Chronic conditions often result from improper biomechanics stemming from poor posture, leg length discrepancies, or overuse syndromes. Injury to the hip joint itself is rare in athletes, but the amount of force needed to traumatize this structure acutely makes any injury to it a potential medical emergency.

Because of the magnitude of the injury and the subsequent emergent management, frank femoral fractures and hip dislocations and subluxations are presented in the On-Field Management section of this chapter.

Iliac Crest Contusion

The iliac crest is rich with multiple muscle attachments, blood vessels, and nerves. The major trunk muscles, the internal oblique, external oblique, latissimus dorsi, and paraspinals and many of the hip muscles, including the gluteus medius, gluteus minimus, the fascia of the gluteus maximus, and tensor fascia late attach to the iliac crest. Contusions to the iliac crest, "hip pointers," result in a seemingly disproportionate amount of pain, swelling, discoloration, and subsequent loss of function (see Fig. 12-14). After injury, any trunk and/or hip motions stress these muscle attachments, causing pain. The formation of a hematoma can produce pressure on the nerves, especially the femoral or lateral femoral cutaneous nerve.[2]

The key to reducing the amount of time lost because of this injury lies in the recognition of its signs and symptoms (Examination Findings 12-1) and its immediate management. Suspected iliac crest contusions require immediate removal from competition or other potential stress, treatment with ice packs, and placement on crutches to avoid weight-bearing stresses. Stretching of the affected muscles should be initiated as tolerated. Radiographs may be warranted to rule out iliac fracture.

If the injury is minor and occurs during a game situation, the athlete may be allowed to return to competition, provided that full lower extremity and torso function is demonstrated. In this case, the injured area is padded to protect against further injury. The patient must be treated immediately after the game.

Muscle Strains

Muscle strains most frequently occur secondary to a dynamic overload during an eccentric muscle contraction. Many times these injuries are typified by pain at the muscular insertion into the bone or at the musculotendinous

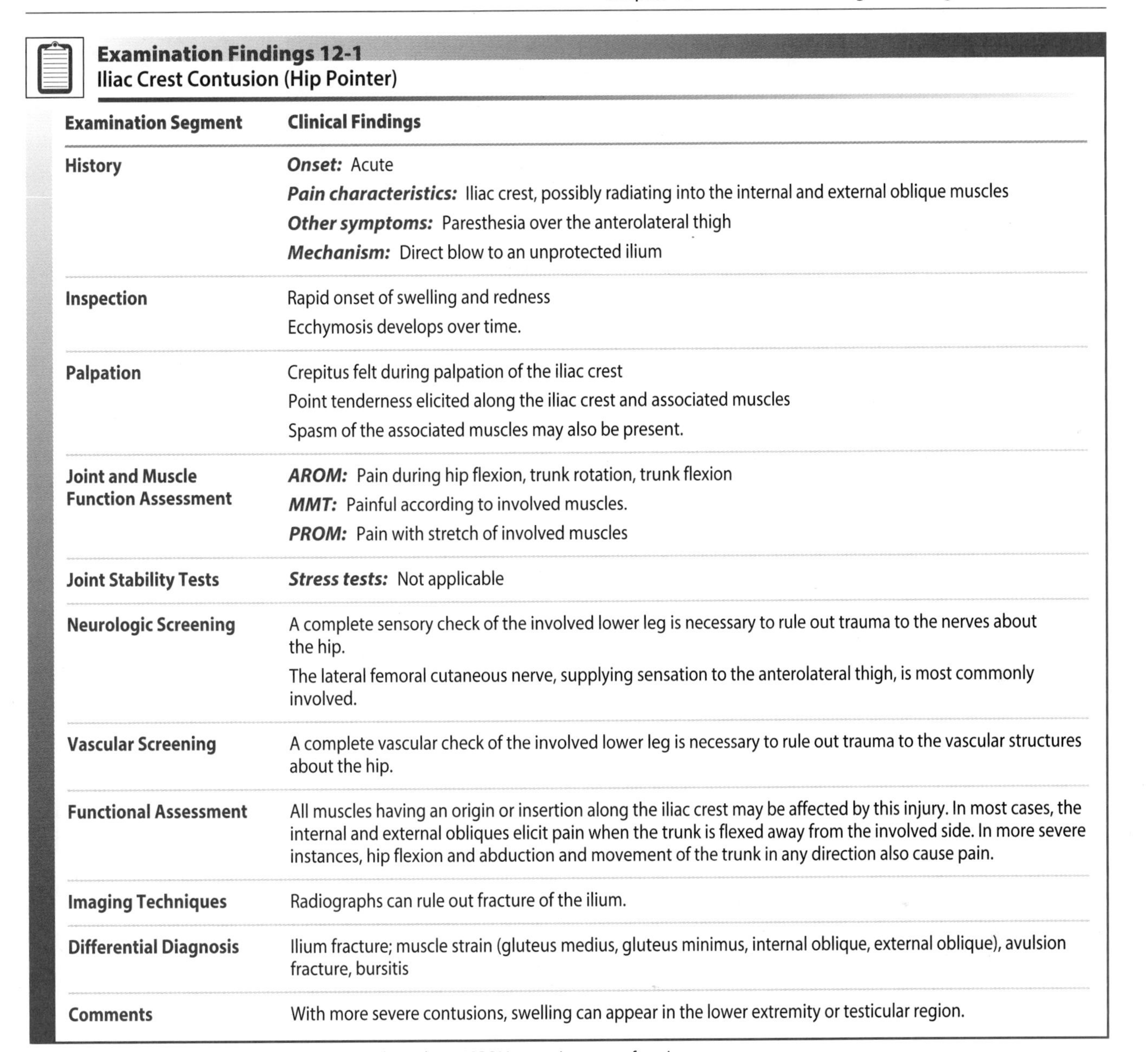

Examination Findings 12-1
Iliac Crest Contusion (Hip Pointer)

Examination Segment	Clinical Findings
History	***Onset:*** Acute ***Pain characteristics:*** Iliac crest, possibly radiating into the internal and external oblique muscles ***Other symptoms:*** Paresthesia over the anterolateral thigh ***Mechanism:*** Direct blow to an unprotected ilium
Inspection	Rapid onset of swelling and redness Ecchymosis develops over time.
Palpation	Crepitus felt during palpation of the iliac crest Point tenderness elicited along the iliac crest and associated muscles Spasm of the associated muscles may also be present.
Joint and Muscle Function Assessment	***AROM:*** Pain during hip flexion, trunk rotation, trunk flexion ***MMT:*** Painful according to involved muscles. ***PROM:*** Pain with stretch of involved muscles
Joint Stability Tests	***Stress tests:*** Not applicable
Neurologic Screening	A complete sensory check of the involved lower leg is necessary to rule out trauma to the nerves about the hip. The lateral femoral cutaneous nerve, supplying sensation to the anterolateral thigh, is most commonly involved.
Vascular Screening	A complete vascular check of the involved lower leg is necessary to rule out trauma to the vascular structures about the hip.
Functional Assessment	All muscles having an origin or insertion along the iliac crest may be affected by this injury. In most cases, the internal and external obliques elicit pain when the trunk is flexed away from the involved side. In more severe instances, hip flexion and abduction and movement of the trunk in any direction also cause pain.
Imaging Techniques	Radiographs can rule out fracture of the ilium.
Differential Diagnosis	Ilium fracture; muscle strain (gluteus medius, gluteus minimus, internal oblique, external oblique), avulsion fracture, bursitis
Comments	With more severe contusions, swelling can appear in the lower extremity or testicular region.

AROM = active range of motion; MMT = manual muscle test; PROM = passive range of motion.

junction. The iliopsoas, quadriceps, adductors, or hamstrings are commonly injured secondary to an overstretching of the fibers or dynamic overload during an eccentric contraction. Patients suffering from strains of the proximal rectus femoris may obtain relief of the pain experienced when walking up stairs by turning around and carefully walking backward. Table 12-6 presents an overview of the mechanisms and ROM deficits common to muscular strains of the hip and thigh.

In skeletally immature patients or patients with osteoporosis, eccentric muscle contractions can result in avulsion and apophyseal injuries. Clinically resembling muscle strains, these injuries tend to have pain localized to the muscle attachment. The defect can often be identified on radiographs.

In general, muscle strains present with pain during activities (or avoidance of those activities) during which the muscle is most active. For example, a quadriceps strain would result in increased pain during the loading response phase of gait, during which the quadriceps is eccentrically controlling knee flexion.

Hamstring strains

Hamstring strains, most commonly involving the long head of the biceps femoris, are common in many explosive activities, such as sprinting and soccer.[21] The risk of hamstring strains is increased if there is a bilateral strength deficit of more than 10% or if the quadriceps/hamstring ratio is less than 60%.[18] Hamstring injuries tend to recur if the strength deficits are not corrected and chance of

Table 12-6 Characteristics of Muscular Strains of the Hip and Thigh

		Pain or Deficit Elicited During Range of Motion Testing	
Muscle	**Injuring Force**	**Active**	**Passive**
Rectus Femoris	Hyperextension of the hip and flexion of the knee Dynamic overload; isometric contraction	Hip flexion, knee extension	Hip extension, knee flexion
Iliopsoas	Hyperextension of the hip Resisted hip flexion	Hip flexion	Hip extension
Quadriceps Strain (other than rectus femoris)	Hyperflexion of the knee Dynamic overload; resisted knee extension	Knee extension with a flexed hip	Knee flexion
Hamstring Strain	Dynamic overload; eccentric contraction Tensile force; overstretching the muscle	Knee flexion Hip extension with an extended knee	Knee extension Hip flexion
Gluteus Maximus	Dynamic overload; eccentric contraction; isometric contraction	Hip extension with a flexed knee	Hip flexion with a flexed knee
Adductor Group	Tensile; overstretching the muscle Dynamic overload; eccentric contraction; isometric contraction	Hip adduction	Hip abduction

reinjury increases proportionally to the size of the original injury.[21]

Patients suffering hamstring strains typically report a distinct "popping" or "snapping" sensation when initially contracting the muscle or quickly increasing running speed. In most cases, the individual cannot continue the activity. Palpation performed immediately after the injury may reveal a divot in the muscle, depending on the extent of the injury. Any defects are soon obscured by the collection of edema at the injury site. The patient will experience pain with resisted knee flexion and passive hip flexion. Ecchymosis may develop. The patient will display an antalgic gait with a shortened swing phase. Avulsion fractures should be considered if the pain is located at or close to the ischial tuberosity and the patient is not skeletally mature (an adolescent). Plain radiographs will detect avulsion fractures but MRIs are needed to detect the extent of soft tissue injury.

Hamstring strains normally require only surgical repair when the muscle's tendon has been avulsed and there is a significant amount of separation between the bone and tendon. Otherwise, rehabilitation emphasizes gradual stretching and strengthening, emphasizing eccentric control of hip flexion.[22] Factors that help predict the length of time needed to return to activity include a greater uninjured-injured difference in knee range of motion, increased firmness via palpation, a measurable difference in uninjured-injured circumference at the suprapatellar border, whether or not the patient could continue to play following injury, location of pain as ascertained by palpation, and a longer time delay before initiating treatment.[23,24]

✱ Practical Evidence

Palpating hamstring strains yields useful information. The more superior the point tenderness—the closer to the origin—the longer the time needed to return to the pre-injury level of activity.[24]

Quadriceps Contusion

Even mild contusive forces transmitted to the quadriceps group can result in the death of muscle fibers. As the severity of the impact increases, so does the proportion of muscle fiber death that occurs. Contusions to the quadriceps group result in decreased force during knee extension. Associated pain and spasm limit the amount of flexion available to the joint. The extremity is often discolored, and the traumatized area is painful to the touch. Intramuscular hematoma gives the muscle a hardened feel in the area and increases the girth of the muscle. Over time, the contour of the quadriceps group is lost secondary to atrophy. The risk of heterotopic ossification increases with effusion of the knee joint (Fig. 12-24).

The first 24 hours after the injury are critical to the long-term management and rehabilitation of quadriceps

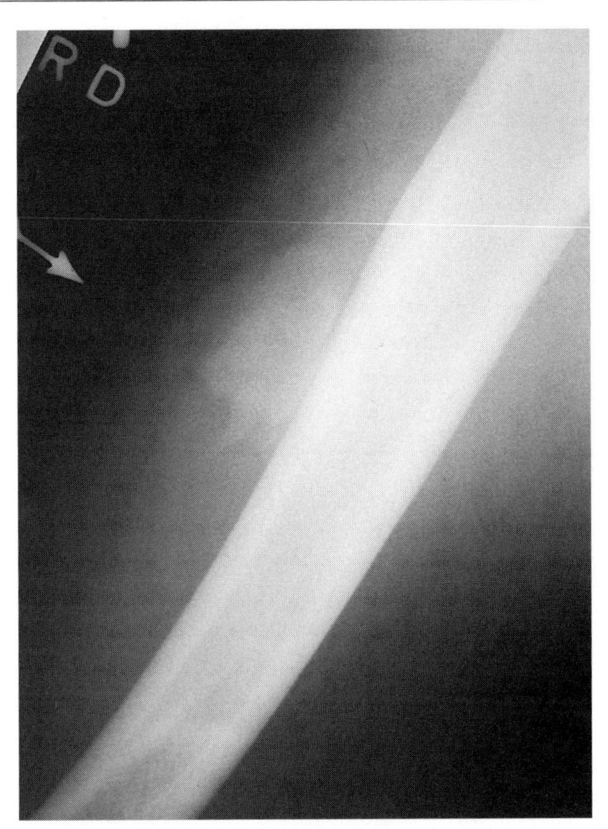

FIGURE 12-24 ■ Femoral heterotopic ossification resulting from a quadriceps contusion.

contusions. Weight bearing is restricted until control of the quadriceps muscle is regained and the patient has 90 degrees of pain-free ROM.

Athletes who describe pain during active knee or hip or knee flexion who have weakness during manual muscle testing of the involved muscles are to be removed from competition for immediate management of their injury. After the determination of the injury has been made, ice packs are applied to the area and flexion of the knee joint, as much as pain allows, is encouraged. Immobilization in 120 degrees of flexion for 24 hours has been associated with a faster return to play.[25] As the treated area becomes numb, the amount of knee flexion is gradually increased to tolerance (Fig. 12-25). Maintaining the knee's ROM decreases the possibility of heterotopic ossification.

Slipped Capital Femoral Epiphysis

Describing displacement of the femoral head relative to the femoral neck, slipped capital femoral epiphysis (SCFE) is the most common hip disorder in adolescents and more commonly affects boys than girls. The risk of acquiring a slipped capital femoral epiphysis is increased in children who are overweight and skeletally immature. This condition occurs bilaterally in 20% to 40% of the cases.[26]

The femoral head remains in the acetabulum and the femoral neck displaces anteriorly, causing the proximal femur to be retroverted. The severity of the condition is

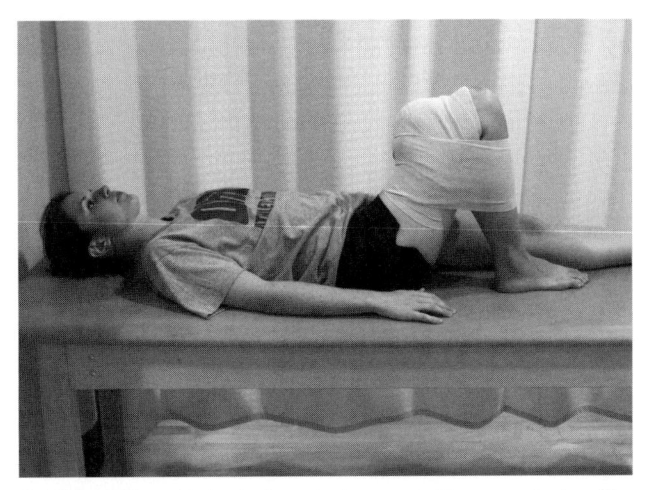

FIGURE 12-25 ■ Method of managing a quadriceps contusion. The quadriceps is flexed to the point that pain is experienced and then extended to the point that the pain disappears. Ice is applied and the process is repeated when the patient reports numbness.

based on the percentage that the femoral neck is displaced anteriorly: minimal—0% to 33%; moderate—34% to 66%; severe—67% to 100%. A stable SCFE results in a permanent retroverted deformity as the bone remodels with increased bone growth posteriorly. This retroversion results in an antalgic gait marked by external femoral rotation and toeing out. Acute trauma to a previously stable slip can result in an unstable slipped capital femoral epiphysis. When bony stability is not present, the instability of the epiphysis prevents walking, even with crutches. About half of the patients who develop an unstable slipped capital femoral epiphysis will develop avascular necrosis of the femoral head later in life.[26]

The onset of symptoms may be acute, chronic (gradual onset of symptoms over a 3-week period), or acute-on-chronic where pain has existed for several weeks or more, but is suddenly increased by a single episode that precludes walking.[26] SCFE is characterized by a limitation in internal rotation and a gait pattern with the involved extremity in external rotation. With an acute slip, the patient may be unable to bear any weight secondary to pain and will describe being more comfortable with the hip externally rotated. Occasionally, pain is referred to the knee secondary to irritation of the obturator nerve (Examination Findings 12-2). If SCFE is suspected, immediate referral is warranted.

Anteroposterior radiographs will reveal an irregular physis that is wider than normal. The epiphysis falls posterior to the anteriorly displaced femoral neck. On bilateral radiographic comparison the affected epiphysis is lower than the contralateral epiphysis.[26]

To prevent further displacement and to prevent an unstable slip, a slipped capital femoral epiphysis must be treated as soon as it is identified. Most management strategies involve surgical repair, using single-screw fixation ***in situ***, multiple

in situ In the original position or place.

Examination Findings 12-2
Slipped Capital Femoral Epiphysis

Examination Segment	Clinical Findings
History	***Onset:*** Acute, chronic, acute-on-chronic ***Pain characteristics:*** Stable: Pain in the groin or hip that increases with walking. Pain may be referred to the anterior distal quadriceps (femoral nerve), adductor area (obturator nerve), and/or buttocks and hamstrings (sciatic nerve). Unstable: Pain intense enough to prevent walking ***Mechanism:*** Gradual onset or abrupt maneuver ***Predisposing conditions:*** Obesity, skeletal immaturity, male
Inspection	A leg-length difference may be noted.
Palpation	Tenderness over the femoral head and neck
Joint and Muscle Function Assessment	***AROM:*** Decreased internal rotation; decreased hip flexion, and abduction may also be noted. ***MMT:*** Weak internal rotation In advanced cases, weakness will be noted for all hip muscles and muscle groups. ***PROM:*** Decreased internal rotation, decreased hip flexion, and abduction may also be noted.
Joint Stability Tests	***Stress tests:*** Within normal limits
Neurologic Screening	Unexplained knee and hip pain in children should raise the suspicion of a slipped capital femoral epiphysis.
Vascular Screening	Within normal limits
Functional Assessment	Stable: During gait the femur is externally rotated; the patient demonstrates an antalgic gait. Unstable: The patient is unable to bear weight and walking is not possible, including crutch walking.
Imaging Techniques	Anteroposterior and "frog-leg" pelvic radiographs are usually diagnostic. "Pistol-grip" deformity may be noted if osteoarthritis has developed
Differential Diagnosis	Strain, avulsion fracture
Comments	Long-term consequences include chronic pain and osteoarthritis.

AROM = active range of motion; MMT = manual muscle test; PROM = passive range of motion.

screw fixation *in situ*, and bone-grafting the epiphysis. Hip spica casts have also been used with good to fair results, but the cast significantly limits the patient's mobility and comfort during the treatment period.[26]

Legg–Calvé–Perthes Disease

Legg–Calvé–Perthes disease is an ischemic lesion of the femoral head that develops during the first decade of life. The degenerative process is marked by ischemia that results in resorption, collapse, and repair of the femoral head. Permanent damage to the femoral head can result in a marked decrease in hip abduction and internal rotation. The disease develops bilaterally in 10% to 20% of the cases, but each side may degenerate at different rates. If untreated, childhood Legg–Calvé–Perthes disease will lead to disabling hip arthritis by the sixth decade of life in half of the people affected.[27]

Although a necrotic process, the triggering events for Legg–Calvé–Perthes disease are not fully understood. Possible causes of the condition include single traumatic events that disrupt the blood supply, repeated or chronic blood supply disruptions, compression of the intracapsular space, and blood-borne clotting factor and/or endocrine disorders such as thyroid disease.[27]

Legg–Calvé–Perthes disease tends to develop between the ages of 4 and 10 years and is more frequent in boys than in girls. Pain may be referred to the medial thigh (obturator nerve), buttock (sciatic nerve), or suprapatellar region (femoral nerve). The child often has a painless antalgic gait and/or gluteus medius lurch. Internal hip rotation, especially when the hip is extended, and abduction are limited. Early in the degenerative process ROM is limited secondary to muscle spasm and synovitis. As the disease progresses ROM restrictions are limited by bony degeneration.[27]

Clinically, the affected leg may appear shorter than the unaffected leg secondary to a contracture, but actual bony leg-length differences rarely occur. The Trendelenburg test is often positive (see Special Test 12-2). Radiographic studies are used to confirm the presence of Legg–Calvé–Perthes disease.[27] Poor long-term prognosis is predicted when at least to of the following signs are visible on radiographs: a radiolucent "V" on the lateral epiphysis, calcification of the lateral epiphysis, lateral subluxation of the femoral head, a horizontal physis, and metaphyseal cysts, **coxa magna**, and a decreased joint space in later life.[27]

The long-term functional consequence of Legg–Calvé–Perthes disease is the result of a flattening of the femoral head, resulting in the permanent loss of abduction and rotation. The less congruent the shape of the femoral head and the acetabulum, the more severe the dysfunction and the more likely that arthritis will develop.[27]

Femoral Neck Stress Fracture

Femoral neck stress fractures are most prevalent in endurance athletes, especially female runners.[2] The weight-bearing loads and/or muscular tension place forces across the femoral neck that, over time, cause microfractures on the superior surface of the neck (tension-side fractures) or the inferior surface (compression-side fractures). Tension-side fractures tend to be more unstable than compression-side fractures and have a poorer prognosis.[2]

Fatigue-type stress fractures are the result of repeated exposure to abnormally high forces and are associated with a recent increase in volume and/or intensity of training such as an athlete in intense training. Insufficiency stress fractures are associated with individuals who have compromised bone density.

The patient will complain of a deep aching pain arising from the hip or groin that increases with the duration and intensity of activity. Night pain is often reported, especially when the patient log rolls on the involved side.[29] Initially, palpation is unremarkable, potentially delaying the identification of stress fracture as a possible cause of pain. Mature stress fractures will elicit pain when the region over femoral neck is palpated. ROM is limited and painful near the end ranges; strength may also be decreased. Axial loading of the hip joint or shear forces placed on the femoral neck, such as when standing on one leg may cause pain (Examination Findings 12-3).

Pain may be referred to the hip from the lumbar or sacral plexus or be referred proximally from the lower extremity. Concurrent examination of the both lower extremities, spine, sacrum, and gait may be required to obtained a definitive clinical diagnosis.

Only 10% of patients will demonstrate positive findings on plain radiographs taken within the first week of symptoms and fewer than 55% of patients with femoral neck stress fractures will ever have radiographic evidence of the condition.[28] With the introduction of technetium-99m methylene diphosphonate (Tc-99 MDP), the sensitivity and specificity of bone scans has significantly increased to identify possible stress fractures in asymptomatic patients.[28]

Stable compression-side femoral neck stress fractures are frequently managed conservatively, relying on avoiding aggravating activities for 4 to 6 weeks to allow the fracture to heal. Displaced stress fractures or tension-side fractures commonly require surgical fixation.[2]

Coxa magna The femoral head is at least 10% larger than normal.

Degenerative Hip Changes

Age, repetitive trauma, acute trauma, or improper bony arrangements of the hip can lead to degeneration of the articular surfaces of the femur and acetabulum. In athletes, these conditions most commonly include arthritis, osteochondritis dissecans, acetabular labrum tears, and avascular necrosis. All share the common characteristic of further degeneration if left undetected and untreated. Chronic hip degeneration occurs with age, commonly affecting people older than age 50 years (Table 12-7). Younger patients may develop degenerative hip changes secondary to acute trauma.

Osteoarthritis of the coxofemoral joint involves the degeneration of the hip's articular cartilage, fibrocartilage, bone, and synovium. **Primary osteoarthritis** results from decreased blood supply (osteonecrosis), infection (sepsis), or rheumatoid arthritis. Primary osteoarthritis is often a diagnosis of exclusion. The presence of congenital hip disease, slipped capital femoral epiphysis, or other existing anatomical abnormalities can lead to **secondary osteoarthritis**, the most common form of hip arthritis.[1]

The primary complaint associated with the early stages of hip degeneration is pain only during weight bearing. As

Table 12-7 Etiological Factors Contributing to the Development of Hip Osteoarthritis

Factor	Increased Rate of Osteoarthritis
Body Weight	Increased body weight (obesity)
	Heavier individuals may be less active, thereby decreasing the rate of OA progression.
Occupation	Lifting heavy loads
	Participation in track, field, racket sports, and soccer, especially if there is an hereditary predisposition to hip OA
Anatomic	Developmental hip dysplasia
	Acetabular abnormalities
	Femoral anteversion (inconclusive)
Hereditary	Family history of hip OA

OA = osteoarthritis.

Examination Findings 12-3
Femoral Neck Stress Fractures

Examination Segment	Clinical Findings
History	***Onset:*** Insidious ***Pain characteristics:*** Pain in the femoral triangle that occurs during activity and is relieved by rest Pain may briefly increase following the activity but subside with rest. ***Other symptoms:*** Throbbing, burning, or paresthesia may be described. ***Mechanism:*** Repetitive stress/overuse, often with a history of a rapid increase in the frequency, intensity, and/or duration of activity ***Predisposing conditions:*** A sudden increase in distance training of more than 10% per week The Female Athlete Triad (see p. 600) can predispose the onset of femoral neck stress fractures.
Inspection	Antalgic gait may be present.
Palpation	Possible point tenderness over the anterior hip
Joint and Muscle Function Assessment	***AROM:*** Limitations in the extreme ranges of hip motion ***MMT:*** Within normal limits ***PROM:*** Limitations in the extreme ranges of hip motion where torque is applied to the femoral neck
Joint Stability Tests	***Stress tests:*** Not applicable ***Joint play:*** Not applicable
Special Tests	Active straight-leg of the affected leg raise may increase pain. An axial load on the femoral head may cause pain (see Hip Scouring Test)
Neurologic Screening	Rule out the possibility of referred pain to the hip from the lumbar or sacral plexus or from the hip into the extremity.
Vascular Screening	Within normal limits
Functional Assessment	Pain is increased when standing and/or hopping on one leg. Pain may prohibit activity. Patient may describe pain when rolling over in bed (placing pressure on the involved side).
Imaging Techniques	Bone scans have .93–1.0 sensitivity and .76–.95 specificity relative to plain radiographs.[28] CT scans can be used for early identification of the fracture line. MRI can be used to differentiate between bony and soft-tissue lesions. Radiographs (anteroposterior and surgical lateral views) may produce false-negative results until the fracture lines fully develop.
Differential Diagnosis	Synovitis, labral tears, neoplasm, strains, avascular necrosis, arthritis
Comments	Percussive tests for fracture are not conclusive. Laboratory tests including CBC, erythrocyte sedimentation rate, serum calcium, and alkaline phosphatase levels are not conclusive for identifying stress fractures.[28]

AROM = active range of motion; CBC = complete blood count; MMT = manual muscle test; PROM = passive range of motion.

the degeneration continues, the pain becomes more constant. The location of this pain may lead to the suspicion of lumbar spine or sacroiliac pathology because pain may be referred to the low back and distally into the anterior thigh, knee, or adductor group.

Physical evaluation reveals a loss of motion in all of the hip's planes, with rotational motions being lost first, followed by abduction. Strength assessment with manual muscle testing may be inconclusive secondary to pain. **Hip scouring** causes the two articular surfaces to compress and rub over one another, resulting in pain (Special Test 12-5). Radiographic evaluation may provide conclusive evidence of deterioration of the hip's articular surfaces and the resulting diminished joint space.

Special Test 12-5
Hip Scouring Test (Hip Quadrant Test)

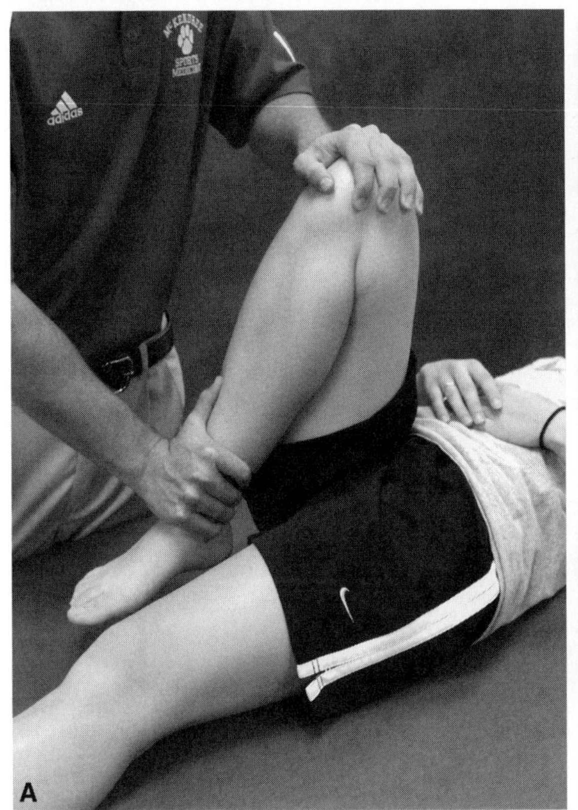

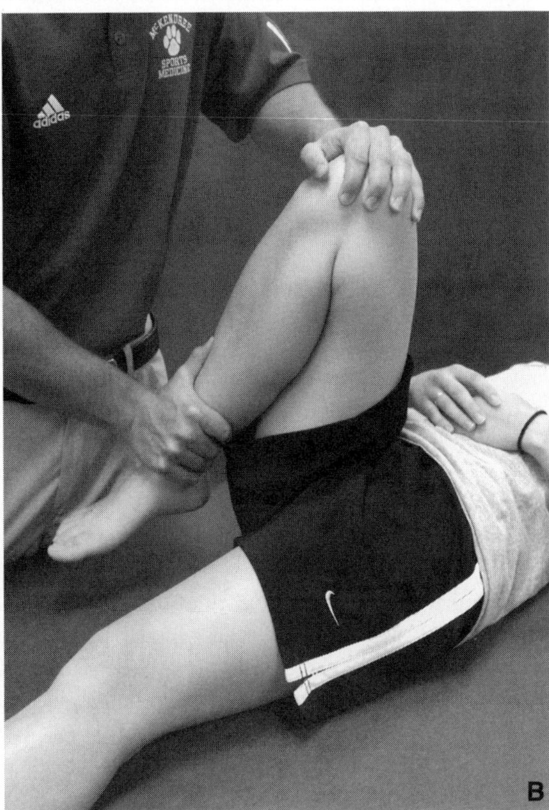

This procedure moves the hip through its range of motion while an axial load is placed on the femur. Pain within a specific location may indicate a defect of the articular surface or labral tear.

Patient Position	Supine
Position of Examiner	At the side of the patient, fully flexing the patient's hip and knee
Evaluative Procedure	The examiner applies pressure downward along the shaft of the femur to compress the joint surfaces. The femur is **(A)** internally and **(B)** externally rotated with the hip in multiple angles of flexion.
Positive Test	Pain described or symptoms in the hip is reproduced
Implications	A possible defect in the articular cartilage of the femur or acetabulum (e.g., osteochondral defects, arthritis) This test may also produce pain in the presence of a labral tear.
Evidence	Absent or inconclusive in the literature

Labral Tears

Improved imaging techniques have increased the number of labral tears diagnosed. Once thought to occur only as the result of major trauma such as hip dislocations, we now understand that labral tears can be the result of repeated subluxations, slipped capital epiphysis, acetabular **dysplasia**, or repeated athletic-related trauma.[2,30,31] Repeated impingement of the anterior femoral head and acetabulum has also been cited as a cause of labral tears.[31]

A "catching" type of pain may be described and symptoms may increase following relatively minor trauma with the location and type of complaints dependent on the location of the tear. Medically, the location of the tear is described using a clock face (e.g., tear extends from the 1:00 to 3:00 o'clock position).[32] Anterior tears produce pain and catching when the hip is moved from flexion, external rotation, and abduction to extension, internal rotation, and

Dysplasic (dysplasia) Abnormal tissue development.

adduction. Posterior labral tears are marked by pain during passive hip flexion, internal rotation while a posterior load is being applied.[2] A reported symptom of clicking during motion is highly sensitive and specific for the presence of a labral tear.[30] Patients most frequently complain of pain in the anterior hip and groin, although pain may be described in the lateral hip or buttock.[3] Pain tends to increase with activity, especially weight-bearing hip internal and external rotation (Examination Findings 12-4).[31] Hip scouring may be positive (see Special Test 12-5).

A diagnosis of a labral tear may be made by injecting a local anesthetic into the joint. If pain relief is obtained after the injection and arthrographic findings are normal, then an intra-articular defect should be assumed. MRI, especially high-resolution MRI, and magnetic resonance arthrography has improved the accuracy and specificity of identifying labral lesions and is used to rule out other possible pathologies.[30,32]

Most labral tears are surgically excised. While excision provides symptomatic relief, residual instability may result.[33] Conservative treatment of a labral lesion involves partial weight bearing for 4 weeks with corticosteroid injections being administered as needed. In cases where conservative treatment fails to resolve the symptoms or in the case of more significant tears, the torn segment can be excised via arthroscopy.[2]

Hip subluxation

Hip subluxations often have a subtle presentation and occur as the result of a fall onto a flexed knee with the hip adducted, or a jump-stop or pivot in athletics, that forces the femoral head posteriorly in the acetabulum. Subluxations are characterized by the femoral head being forced into, but not over, the posterior acetabulum, allowing the joint to spontaneously reduce.[2] In additional to stressing the joint capsule and ligaments, which may lead to chronic instability and recurrent subluxations, the mechanisms associated with hip subluxations may result in fractures or contusions of the femoral head or lead to an osteochondral defect of the articular surface.

Hip subluxations are managed by the patient non–weight bearing for up to 6 weeks. Serial MRIs are obtained to monitor possible osseous changes.

Athletic Pubalgia

Athletic pubalgia—a "sports hernia"—can be the result of increased muscular loads placed on the pubic bone and/or pubic symphysis as the result of high-speed, high-velocity twisting and turning.[2] The term pubalgia is preferred because this condition does not always result in actual tissue herniation.

Most cases of athletic pubalgia are the result of an overuse syndrome where a muscular imbalance exists between the abdominal, pelvic, and hip muscles results in contractures of the hip flexor and/or adductor muscles.[2] Isometric or eccentric contractions of the adductors while the lower extremity is in a closed kinetic chain will place a shear force across the pubic symphysis. Hip abduction, adduction, and flexion and extension and the resulting pelvic motion place a shear force across the pubic symphysis, creating a stress on the inguinal muscles perpendicular to the fascia and muscle fibers. These stresses ultimately cause a weakening or tearing of the pelvic floor muscles.[34]

The actual source of pain may be the transversalis fascia, conjoined tendons of the adductor group, the insertion of the rectus abdominis, or the avulsion of the internal oblique from the pubic tubercle (Fig. 12-26).[2] Other structures that may be involved include the aponeurosis of the external oblique, or the genital branches of the ilioinguinal or genitofemoral nerves.[2]

Clinically, the patient will describe pain on resisted contraction of the adductor group or during resisted sit-ups. Plain film radiographs may be ordered to rule out other underlying bony trauma; MRI is useful in identifying defects in the muscle or the pubic symphysis (Examination Findings 12-5).

Conservative treatment to restore muscle balance, strength, and ROM can be effective, but may require an extended course of care. Failed conservative treatment or high-level competitive athletes with an acute diagnosis of athletic pubalgia may be candidates for corrective surgery. **Herniorrhaphy** and reinforcing the abdominal wall using a mesh are the most common surgical techniques. In some cases an adductor release may be required.[2]

Osteitis pubis

The gradual ossification and widening of the public symphysis, osteitis pubis is caused by rotational, tension, or shear forces placed on the symphysis.[34] Although osteitis pubis

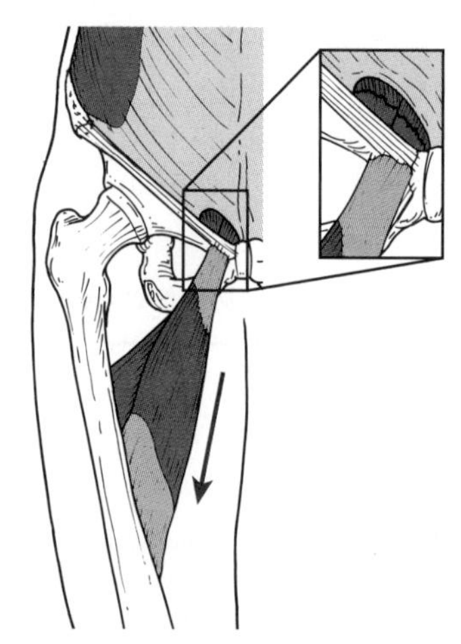

FIGURE 12-26 ■ Adductor group contributing to athletic pubalgia. A muscle imbalance exists between the strong pull of the adductor group (*arrow*) and the weak abdominal stabilizers, resulting in a stretching or avulsion of the pelvic floor.

Herniorrhaphy Surgical repair of a hernia.

Examination Findings 12-4
Labral Tears

Examination Segment	Clinical Findings
History	***Onset:*** Acute or degenerative ***Pain characteristics:*** Pain most commonly presents in the anterior or medial hip; posterior or lateral pain is reported less frequently. ***Other symptoms:*** Catching or locking may be described ***Mechanism:*** Acute: Hip dislocation or subluxation Insidious: Repeated subtle subluxations, impingement of the anterior capsule; repeated weight-bearing external rotation, hyperabduction, or hyperextension.[3] ***Predisposing conditions:*** Acetabular dysplasia Slipped capital epiphysis
Inspection	Unremarkable
Palpation	Often unremarkable; anterior tears may yield tenderness over the anterior joint capsule. Clicking or popping may be noted during joint motion.
Joint and Muscle Function Assessment	***AROM:*** Anterior tear: Pain and/or catching when the hip is moved from flexion, external rotation, and abduction to extension, internal rotation, and adduction ***MMT:*** Within normal limits ***PROM:*** Posterior tear: Pain during passive hip flexion and internal rotation while a posterior load is applied
Joint Stability Tests	***Stress tests:*** Internal rotation, flexion, and compression of the hip joint ***Joint play:*** Not applicable
Special Tests	Hip scouring test may be positive. The use of the Thomas test has been suggested to identify labral tears, but the sensitivity and specificity of this procedure is poor in detecting this condition.[30] The Trendelenburg test may be positive[31]
Neurologic Screening	Within normal limits
Vascular Screening	Within normal limits
Functional Assessment	A limp or shortened stance phase on the involved leg may be noted. Walking/running distance is often limited. Possible Trendelenburg gait
Imaging Techniques	Radiographs are used to rule out bony trauma. Magnetic resonance arthrography is more accurate in diagnosing a labral tear than MRI.[30]
Differential Diagnosis	Hernia, athletic pubalgia, osteitis pubis, adductor strain, snapping hip syndrome, osteochondral defect

AROM = active range of motion; MMT = manual muscle test; MRI = magnetic resonance imaging; PROM = passive range of motion.

may be caused by acute injury such as fracture, in the physically active population long-term activities such as running, the kicking motion in soccer, or vigorous ice skating may lead to the development of this condition. A leg-length difference may further predispose the individual to osteitis pubis.[35]

Patients complain of pain centered over the symphysis pubis, lower abdominal muscles, and adductor muscles. Spasm of the adductor muscles may also occur.[34,36] Walking, rising from seated position, or any motion that places shear forces on the symphysis pubis may also be symptomatic.[36]

Piriformis Syndrome

The sciatic nerve passes under or through the piriformis muscle as the nerve travels across the posterior pelvis. Spasm or hypertrophy of the piriformis places pressure on

Examination Findings 12-5
Athletic Pubalgia

Examination Segment	Clinical Findings
History	***Onset:*** Usually insidious, although the patient may describe a single episode that results in severe localized pain ***Pain characteristics:*** Pain is localized to the pubic bone, pubic symphysis, lower abdominal muscles, and/or genitals. Pain may be exacerbated by coughing or sneezing. ***Mechanism:*** A tensile force caused by the pull of the adductor muscle group and the lower abdominal muscles Hip abduction, adduction, flexion, and extension ***Predisposing conditions:*** Weak abdominal muscles, creating a pelvic imbalance
Inspection	No visible abnormality
Palpation	Pain over the adductor tendon, pubic tubercle, midinguinal region. A tender, dilated superficial inguinal ring may also be reported.
Joint and Muscle Function Assessment	***AROM:*** Pain may be experienced during hip adduction. Any motion in which the antagonists place tension on the public tubercle may cause pain ***MMT:*** Adductor muscle group Sartorius Trunk flexion ***PROM:*** Abduction causes pain by causing tension in the abductors.
Joint Stability Tests	***Stress tests:*** Not applicable ***Joint play:*** Not applicable
Special Tests	Pain may be reported during the Valsalva maneuver (see p. 487)
Neurologic Screening	Within normal limits
Vascular Screening	Within normal limits
Functional Assessment	Sudden movements of the hip joint may cause pain or weakness. The patient is often unable to perform a sit-up without pain. Pain may be described when coughing.
Imaging Techniques	Radiographs are used to rule out concomitant bony injury. MRI can be diagnostic of muscular lesions or trauma to the pubic symphysis.
Differential Diagnosis	Osteitis pubitis, adductor strains, arthritis, tumor
Comments	The diagnosis of athletic pubalgia can be complicated by the presence of multiple conditions and symptoms.

AROM = active range of motion; MMT = manual muscle test; PROM = passive range of motion.

the sciatic nerve, mimicking the signs and symptoms of lumbar nerve root compression or sciatica in the buttock and posterior leg.[37] The resulting symptoms, piriformis syndrome, are more common in women than in men.[38] Improved diagnostic tests for lumbar nerve root impingement and intervertebral disk disease have decreased the frequency that piriformis syndrome is diagnosed.[39]

Although the signs and symptoms of piriformis syndrome are similar to those caused by other lumbopelvic conditions, piriformis syndrome remains relatively undefined and confusing.[40] Complaints include burning, pain, numbness, or paresthesia that are increased with contraction of the piriformis or during palpation or prolonged sitting.[37] Symptoms may be heightened by the straight-leg raising test on

Examination Findings 12-6
Piriformis Syndrome

Examination Segment	Clinical Findings
History	***Onset:*** Acute Insidious can occur secondary to hypertrophy of the piriformis muscle or biomechanical changes in the hip, pelvis, or sacrum; in most cases, the time of onset is not discernible. ***Pain characteristics:*** Pain deep in the posterior aspect of the hip, radiating into the buttock and down the posterior aspect of the leg; increases on standing and often decreases with the patient lying supine and the knees flexed ***Mechanism:*** Few common traits are associated with the onset of piriformis syndrome; factors such as a blow to the buttock, hyperinternal rotation of the hip, or other trauma may cause spasm of the piriformis muscle. ***Predisposing conditions:*** Anatomic deviation in which the sciatic nerve passes through the piriformis muscle; females have an increased risk of acquiring piriformis syndrome.
Inspection	In chronic conditions, atrophy of the gluteus maximus may be noted.
Palpation	Tenderness during palpation of the sciatic notch; also, an associated increase in symptoms may be reported.
Joint and Muscle Function Assessment	***AROM:*** Pain may be experienced during external rotation owing to the piriformis muscle's contracting and placing pressure on the sciatic nerve. ***MMT:*** Pain elicited or symptoms increased during resisted external hip rotation with the patient in the seated position (see Fig. 12-27); pain also possible during resisted hip abduction. ***PROM:*** Increased symptoms with passive internal rotation of the hip while patient supine; symptoms reduced with passive external rotation
Joint Stability Tests	***Stress tests:*** Not applicable ***Joint play:*** Not applicable
Special Tests	Positive straight-leg-raise test result or resisted hip abduction in the seated position
Neurologic Screening	The L2–L4 dermatomes require evaluation for numbness or paresthesia.
Vascular Screening	Within normal limits
Functional Assessment	The patient may present with an antalgic gait, with increased pain during the loading response and midstance phases.
Imaging Techniques	MRI is used to rule out other bony or soft tissue abnormality. Hypertrophy of the piriformis may be noted.
Differential Diagnosis	Nerve root compression and many others
Comments	The signs and symptoms of piriformis syndrome closely replicate those of other lumbopelvic disorders. A definitive diagnosis by a physician is required.

AROM = active range of motion; MMT = manual muscle test; MRI = magnetic resonance imaging; PROM = passive range of motion.

the involved side, passive hip internal rotation, and resisted external rotation with the patient seated (Examination Findings 12-6). Resisted hip abduction with the patient seated may also increase the symptoms (Fig. 12-27). These symptoms may also be caused by entrapment of the sciatic nerve by the hamstring muscles, termed **hamstring syndrome**.[41]

Treatment of piriformis syndrome includes stretching, strengthening, and possible injection of the piriformis muscle. Surgical release of the piriformis muscle may be indicated in cases that do not respond to conservative care.[42]

Snapping Hip Syndrome (Coxa Saltans)

Snapping hip syndrome, coxa saltans, is characterized by a palpable and audible "snapping" within the hip as the joint flexes and extends. Although the physical sensation of snapping may be the patient's only complaint, pain may arise from the anterior or lateral aspect of the hip, especially when

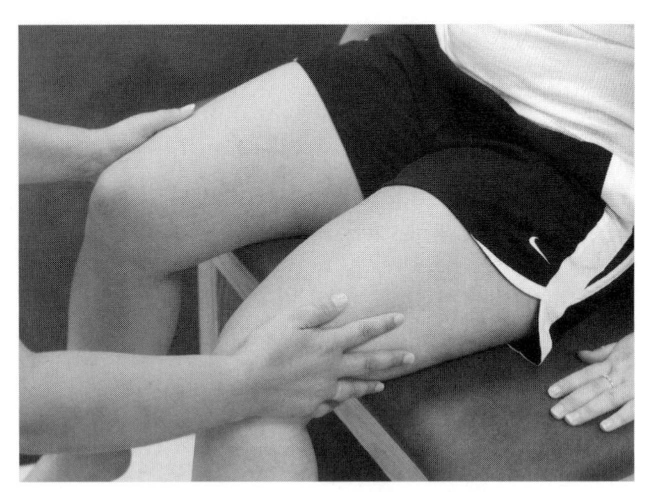

FIGURE 12-27 ■ Resisted hip abduction with the patient seated to duplicate pain caused by piriformis syndrome.

there is concurrent bursal inflammation (Examination Findings 12-7). Although there are many possible causes for this condition, snapping hip syndrome can be classified as having an internal, external, or intra-articular origin.[7,43–45]

Internal cause

The iliopsoas tendon is held in position by the inguinal ligament. When the hip is flexed, abducted, and externally rotated the tendon is positioned laterally; when the hip is extended, adducted, and internally rotated the tendon is medially position. Internal snapping hip syndrome is attributed to the iliopsoas passing over the femoral head, iliopectineal ridge, iliopsoas bursa, or bony outgrowth on the lesser trochanter as the hip moves from flexion to extension and back (Fig. 12-28).[7,45]

Clinically, internal snapping hip syndrome can be replicated by having a supine patient move the femur from a flexed, abducted, and externally rotated position into extension, adduction, and internal rotation and back. The snapping can be reduced by applying manual pressure on the iliopsoas tendon where it crosses the hip.[7]

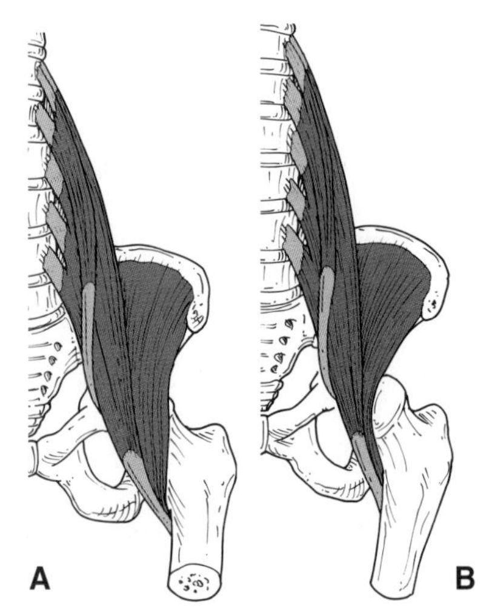

FIGURE 12-28 ■ Internal snapping hip syndrome. **(A)** During hip flexion the iliopsoas tendon shifts laterally, catching on the femoral head or other bony prominence. **(B)** During hip extension the tendon moves medially.

External cause

External causes of snapping hip syndrome are associated with the IT band sliding over the greater trochanter. When the hip is extended the IT tract is posterior to the greater trochanter. During hip flexion the band "snaps" over the trochanter. The symptoms are worsened when the posterior portion of the IT tract and/or the anterior fibers of the gluteus maximus are inflamed and thickened.[7] The maximum amount of pressure is placed on the greater trochanter when the hip is adducted with the knee extended.[2]

With the patient either lying on the unaffected side or standing, the IT band can often be felt snapping over the greater trochanter. Applying manual pressure over the trochanter and reducing the snapping sensation helps confirm the clinical diagnosis of external snapping hip syndrome.

Intra-articular cause

Intra-articular snapping hip syndrome has a unique presentation and should not be confused with the internal or external types. This type of snapping hip is frequently caused by an intra-articular lesion that intermittently lodges in the acetabulum or synovial fold. Significant pain occurs when the lesion is caused by a tear of the acetabular labrum and, infrequently, actual locking of the coxofemoral joint occurs.[7] In rare instances, recurrent congenital hip dislocations may clinically resemble snapping hip syndrome.

Most cases of internal and external snapping hip syndrome are managed conservatively, focusing on reducing inflammation, correcting biomechanical predispositions, stretching shortened tissues, and avoiding activities that cause the symptoms. Oral or injectable anti-inflammatory medications may be prescribed.[44]

On rare occasions, surgery may be required to relieve the symptoms. These procedures include excising the offending bursa, lengthening the IT band, and/or reducing the size of bony prominences that are impinging on the soft tissue structures.[7,44,45] Intra-articular causes of snapping hip syndrome frequently requires arthroscopic surgery to remove the loose body and repair labral tears.[7]

Bursitis

Resulting from increased friction between a muscle or tendon and bone, bursitis in the hip region usually is isolated to the greater trochanteric, ischial, or iliopsoas bursae. The onset of these conditions may be related to biomechanical factors, congenital influences, or environmental conditions such as prolonged periods of sitting. Septic infection has also been cited as a cause of inflammation of the hip bursae.[46] A definitive diagnosis of these conditions can be made via ultrasonic imaging, CT scans, or MRI.[46]

Examination Findings 12-7
Snapping Hip Syndrome

Examination Segment	Clinical Findings
History	***Onset:*** Internal and external types: insidious onset. Intra-articular type: Acute identifiable onset that represents a lesion to the labrum or bone, although the actual trauma may have happened years ago. ***Pain characteristics:*** Pain and discomfort associated with the snapping tends to be localized over the greater trochanter (external type) or the anterior hip (internal type). Pain is usually secondary to bursitis. ***Other symptoms:*** Intra-articular lesions tend to be described as "clicking" rather than snapping and produce more pain.[7] ***Mechanism:*** Internal snapping represents the iliopsoas tendon contacting the femoral head or other structure. External snapping is caused by the IT band catching on the greater trochanter. The motion of hip flexion and extension produces the snapping. Intra-articular snapping hip is most commonly associated with a loose body within the joint, labral tear or synovial fold. ***Predisposing conditions:*** Athletes, especially dancers, in their late teens or early 20s are at an increased risk.[7] External type: Greater trochanteric bursitis; IT band inflammation and/or tightness; reduced femoral neck angle Anterolateral knee instability (secondary to gait changes)[7] May be the result of total hip replacement surgery.
Inspection	Gross inspection is unremarkable. The patient may voluntarily demonstrate the motions that produce the snapping.
Palpation	The mechanical snapping of the tendon may be felt over the anterior hip for the internal type or over the greater trochanter for the external type.
Joint and Muscle Function Assessment	***AROM:*** Snapping may be replicated when the hip is moved from flexion to extension and back.[43] The internal type has more pronounced findings when the hip is moved from a flexed, abducted, and externally rotated position into extension, adduction, and internal rotation and back. ***MMT:*** Unremarkable. ***PROM:*** In some cases, the symptoms can be reproduced during passive hip flexion and extension.
Joint Stability Tests	***Stress tests:*** Within normal limits
Special Tests	None
Neurologic Screening	Within normal limits
Vascular Screening	Within normal limits
Functional Assessment	Pain and snapping may be experienced during running, jumping, and carioca-type cross-stepping activities.[43]
Imaging Techniques	Radiographs and MRI may be used to rule out intra-articular lesions and identify hip angulations that may cause structural impingement. **Bursography** can be used to image the size and shape of the bursae, especially the iliopsoas bursa, to identify structural involvement.
Differential Diagnosis	Trochanteric bursitis, iliopsoas bursitis, intra-articular lesion, chronic positional subluxation of the coxofemoral joint

AROM = active range of motion; MMT = manual muscle test; MRI = magnetic resonance imaging; PROM = passive range of motion.

Bursography Imaging technique that highlights the bursae.

Trochanteric bursitis

Irritation of the trochanteric bursa may result from a single blow. However, more commonly, it may be caused by friction from the IT band as it crosses over this structure during the movements of flexion, extension, internal rotation, and external rotation. A history of a rapid increase in the frequency, intensity, or duration of training is often associated with this condition. Women may be predisposed to this condition because of an increased Q-angle (Examination Findings 12-8).

Chronic inflammation of the trochanteric bursa is one of the possible causes of external **"snapping hip" syndrome,** in which an audible snap occurs as the IT band passes over the greater trochanter (see p. 449). Greater trochanteric bursitis commonly results in reduced hip ROM, especially in flexion and extension and internal and external rotation secondary to pain located directly posterior to the greater trochanter. Trochanteric bursitis can mimic or mask the signs and symptoms of a femoral neck stress fracture.[47]

Ischial Bursitis

Movement of the buttocks while the patient is weight bearing in the seated position, such as the rocking motion associated with rowing or biking, can cause friction to irritate the ischial bursa. These structures can also be traumatized secondary to a direct blow, such as a fall. Ischial bursitis can be further irritated by prolonged periods of sitting, as occurs during bus or airplane trips. Point tenderness at the ischial tuberosity is characteristic of ischial bursitis. A careful history is necessary to rule out the possibility of a hamstring strain or an avulsion of its attachment, both of which have signs and symptoms similar to those of ischial bursitis (Examination Findings 12-9). Use of an inflatable doughnut pad for sitting during prolonged periods to lessen the weight-bearing forces placed on these structures may be helpful.

Iliopsoas bursitis

Inflammation of the iliopsoas bursa, seldom occurring as an isolated event, may be associated with rheumatoid arthritis or osteoarthritis of the hip.[48] Pain in the anterior hip is often the only symptom of iliopsoas bursitis. However, a mass may be palpated in the groin or around the inguinal ligament.[48,49] The condition has also been implicated as another cause of snapping hip syndrome.[46,50–52] Strengthening the hip rotators can resolve the symptoms associated with both the inflamed bursa and snapping hip syndrome.[53]

On-Field Evaluation of Pelvis and Thigh Injuries

Trauma to the coxofemoral joint is rare in sports. The bony and muscular anatomy is normally well padded in collision sports, such as football and ice hockey, which mandate the use of protective padding over the anterior thigh, ilium, and sacrum. However, when trauma does occur, it is usually severe. More commonly, injuries to this region involve muscular strains, contusions, and sprains of the SI joint.

On arriving at the scene, note whether the athlete is moving the involved leg. If the femur is moving, a gross dislocation of the hip or fracture of the femur is less probable. However, a subluxation of the hip must still be considered. A fixed, immobile, awkwardly positioned, or noticeably shortened leg may indicate a dislocation of the hip joint or a fracture of the femoral neck. The shaft of the femur is inspected for normal contour.

The mechanism of injury and other factors surrounding the onset of the injury must be ascertained as soon as possible in the history-taking process. Relevant questions include determining the injurious force, associated sounds and sensations, and any pertinent history of injury.

After a hip dislocation or subluxation and femoral fracture have been ruled out, AROM of both the knee and the hip is initiated. This is easily performed by having the athlete flex the thigh to the chest and straightening the leg back out again. If the athlete is unable to fully bear weight, a decision needs to be made on how to remove the athlete from the playing arena. These techniques are described in Chapter 1.

Initial Evaluation and Management of On-Field Injuries

On-field management of hip and thigh injuries is needed primarily for contusions or muscle strains. However, hip dislocations and femur fractures represent medical emergencies requiring astute management to limit the scope of trauma and increase the athlete's chances for a full recovery.

Hip dislocation

Because of the hip's strong ligamentous and bony arrangement, dislocations are rare. However, their occurrence represents a medical emergency requiring immediate care. The majority of hip dislocations involve posterior displacement of the femoral head.[54] Fractures to the femoral neck or the acetabulum (or both) may also result. Most dislocations occur when the hip is in flexion and adduction and an axial force is delivered to the femur, displacing it posteriorly and causing the head to be driven through the posterior capsule.[55]

Athletes suffering from a hip dislocation complain of immediate, intense pain within the joint and buttock, possibly describing the sensation of the hip's "going out." The femur and lower leg are often positioned in flexion, internal rotation, and adduction so that the involved knee rests against the knee of the opposite side (Fig. 12-29).[2] AROM is impossible or results in severe pain. Although no attempt is made to reduce the dislocation on the field, the examiner must perform a sensory and vascular check of the involved extremity. Integrity of the motor nerves can be determined by asking the athlete to extend and flex the toes. These results

Examination Findings 12-8
Trochanteric Bursitis

Examination Segment	Clinical Findings
History	***Onset:*** Acute or insidious ***Pain characteristics:*** Over the greater trochanter, radiating posteriorly to the buttock; pain increased when the patient climbs stairs ***Other symptoms:*** Increased pain or inability to sleep on involved side ***Mechanism:*** Acute: Direct blow to the greater trochanter Chronic: Irritation from the IT band passing over the bursa ***Predisposing conditions:*** Increased Q-angles (above the norm for the patient's gender) possibly predisposing him or her to overuse forces being placed on the trochanteric bursa; leg-length discrepancy
Inspection	The area over the greater trochanter is usually unremarkable.
Palpation	Palpation reveals tenderness over the trochanteric bursa. Crepitus may also be noted during active movement of the hip.
Joint and Muscle Function Assessment	***AROM:*** Flexion and extension and internal and external rotation cause pain as the IT band passes over the greater trochanter, resulting in decreased ROM. ***MMT:*** Hip extension weak secondary to pain Hip adduction weak secondary to pain ***PROM:*** Flexion and extension and internal and external rotation cause pain as the IT band passes over the greater trochanter, resulting in decreased ROM.
Joint Stability Tests	***Stress tests:*** Not applicable
Special Tests	Ober's test for IT band tightness
Neurologic Screening	Within normal limits
Vascular Screening	Within normal limits
Functional Assessment	Increased pain during loading response and midstance phase of gait Discomfort when lying on the involved side
Imaging Techniques	Magnetic resonance imaging Diagnostic ultrasound
Differential Diagnosis	Tendinopathy, femoral neck stress fracture, contusion, gluteus medius strain, tensor fascia latae strain
Comments	Chronic trochanteric bursitis may result in external "snapping hip" syndrome. The signs and symptoms of trochanteric bursitis may mimic those of a femoral neck stress fracture. Pain may be referred from the sacroiliac joint or low back.

AROM = active range of motion; IT = iliotibial; MMT = manual muscle test; PROM = passive range of motion.

Examination Findings 12-9
Ischial Bursitis

Examination Segment	Clinical Findings
History	***Onset:*** Acute or insidious ***Pain characteristics:*** Over the ischial tuberosity in the vicinity of the gluteal fold ***Mechanism:*** Acute: Direct blow to the ischial tuberosity, such as falling on it Chronic: Repeated shifting and moving while weight bearing in the seated position (e.g., rowing) ***Predisposing conditions:*** Tightness of the hamstring muscle group, prolonged sitting and rocking, especially on a hard surface (i.e., bike seat, scull seat)
Inspection	Unremarkable
Palpation	Tenderness over the ischial tuberosity; the bursa feels thick and crepitus may be present.
Joint and Muscle Function Assessment	***AROM:*** Pain during active hip flexion ***MMT:*** Pain during resisted hip extension with the knee flexed to isolate the gluteus maximus ***PROM:*** Pain at the end of passive hip flexion
Joint Stability Tests	***Stress tests:*** Not applicable
Neurologic Screening	Prolonged irritation of the ischial bursa possibly placing pressure on the sciatic nerve, requiring the evaluation of the sensory and motor nerves of the posterior lower leg
Vascular Screening	Within normal limits
Functional Assessment	Prolonged periods of sitting may cause an increase in symptoms.
Imaging Techniques	Magnetic resonance imaging Diagnostic ultrasound
Differential Diagnosis	Hamstring avulsion fracture

AROM = active range of motion; MMT = manual muscle test; PROM = passive range of motion.

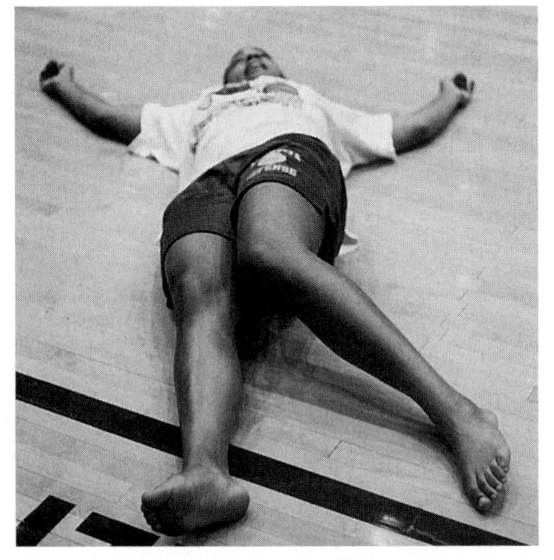

FIGURE 12-29 ■ Position of the lower leg following a posterior hip dislocation: adduction and internal rotation of the hip.

are documented for reference by the emergency room staff. Immediate transport to an emergency facility is necessary to allow rapid reduction of the dislocation with the patient under anesthesia.[54]

Closed reduction of the dislocation can often be performed with the patient sedated or anesthetized. More complex dislocations or dislocations that involve a concomitant fracture may require open reduction and/or internal fixation.

Femoral fracture

Resulting from a torsional or shear force to the shaft, femoral fractures are relatively rare in athletes. This fact is based on the "weak link" principle, in which these forces are more likely to result in trauma to the ankle, lower leg, or knee. Because they result in immediate loss of function, pain, and deformity, complete fractures of the femur are easily recognizable (Fig. 12-30).

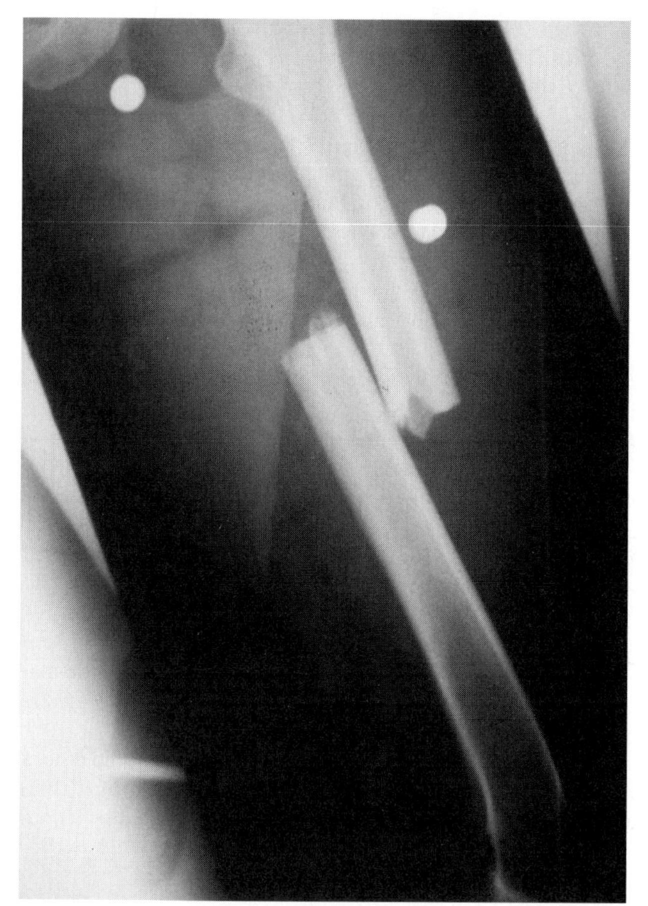

FIGURE 12-30 ■ Radiograph of a complete fracture of the femoral shaft. This type of injury results in obvious deformity of the thigh.

REFERENCES

1. Hoaglund, FT, and Steinbach, LS: Primary osteoarthritis of the hip: Etiology and epidemiology. *J Am Acad Orthop Surg*, 9:320, 2001.
2. Anderson, K, Strickland, SM, and Warren, R: Hip and groin injuries in athletes. *Am J Sports Med*, 29:521, 2001.
3. Lewis, CL, and Sahrmann, SA: Acetabular labral tears. *Phys Ther*, 86:110, 2006.
4. Tonnis, D, and Heinecke, A: Current concepts review – Acetabular and femoral anteversion: Relationship with osteoarthritis of the hip. *J Bone Jt Surg [Am]*, 81:1747, 1999.
5. Levangie, PK: The hip complex. In Levangie PK, Norkin, CC (eds): *Joint Structure and Function: A Comprehensive Analysis*, ed 4. Philadelphia, FA Davis, 2005, p 362.
6. Neptune, RR, Wright, IC, and van den Bogert, AJ: Muscle coordination and function during cutting movements. *Med Sci Sports Exerc*, 31:294, 1999.
7. Allen, WC, and Cope, R: Coxa saltans: The snapping hip revisited. *J Am Acad Orthop Surg*, 3:303, 1995.
8. Kelly, BT, et al: Vascularity of the hip labrum: A cadaveric investigation. *Arthroscopy*, 21:3, 2005.
9. Carney, BT, and Minter, C: Nonsurgical treatment to regain hip abduction motion in Perthes disease: A retrospective review. *South Med J*, 97:485, 2004.
10. Loder, RT, Starnes, T, and Dikos, G: Atypical and typical (idiopathic) slipped capital femoral epiphysis. Reconfirmation of the age-weight test and description of the height and age-height tests. *J Bone Joint Surg*, 88(A):1574, 2006.
11. Beals, RK: Coxa vara in childhood: Evaluation and management. *J Am Acad Orthop Surg*, 6:93, 1998.
12. Shim, JS, et al: Genu valgum in children with coxa vara resulting from hip disease. *J Pediatr Orthop*, 17:225, 1997.
13. Sugano, N, Noble, PC, and Kamaric, E: A comparison of alternative methods of measuring femoral anteversion. *J Comput Assist Tomogr*, 22:610, 1998.
14. Hermann, KL, and Egund, N: Measuring anteversion in the femoral neck from routine radiographs. *Acta Radiol*, 39:410, 1998.
15. Matovinovic, D, et al: Comparison in regression of femoral neck anteversion in children with normal, intoeing and outtoeing gait: Prospective study. *Coll Antropol*, 22:525, 1998.
16. Adams, MC: *Outline of Orthopaedics*. London: E and S Livingstone, 1968.
17. Brand, RA, and Yack, HJ: Effects of leg length discrepancies on the forces at the hip joint. *Clin Orthop*, Dec:172, 1996.
18. Clanion, TO, and Coupe, KJ: Hamstrings strains in athletes: Diagnosis and treatment. *J Am Acad Orthop Surg*, 6:237, 1998.
19. Friel, K, et al: Ipsilateral hip abductor weakness after inversion ankle sprain. *J Athl Train*, 41:74, 2006.
20. Winters, MV, et al: Passive versus active stretching of hip flexor muscles in subjects with limited hip extension: A randomized clinical trial. *Phys Ther*, 84:800, 2004.
21. Verrall, GM, et al: Assessment of physical examination and magnetic resonance imaging findings of hamstring injury as predictors for recurrent injury. *J Orthop Sports Phys Ther*, 36:215, 2006.
22. Brockett, CL, Morgan, DL, and Proske, U: Predicting hamstring strain injury in elite athletes. *Med Sci Sports Exer*, 36:379, 2004.
23. Alonso, A, Hekeik, P, and Adams, R: Predicting recovery time from the initial assessment of a quadriceps contusion injury. *Austral J Physiother*, 46:167, 2000.
24. Askling, CM, et al: Acute first-time hamstring strains during high speed running. A longitudinal study including clinical and magnetic resonance imaging findings. *Am J Sports Med*, 35:197, 2007.
25. Aronen, JG, et al: Quadriceps contusions: Clinical results of immediate immobilization in 120 degrees of knee flexion. *Clin J Sports Med*, 16:383, 2006.
26. Aronsson, DD, and Karol, LA: Stable slipped capital femoral epiphysis: Evaluation and management. *J Am Acad Orthop Surg*, 4:173, 1996.
27. Skaggs, DL, and Tolo, VT: Legg-Calve-Perthes disease. *J Am Acad Orthop Surg*, 4:9, 1996.
28. Shin, AY, and Gillingham, BL: Fatigue fractures of the femoral neck in athletes. *J Am Acad Orthop Surg*, 4:293, 1997.
29. Gurney, B, Boissonnault, WG, and Andrews, R: Differential diagnosis of a femoral neck/head stress fracture. *J Orthop Sports Phys Ther*, 36:80, 2006.
30. Narvani, AA, et al: A preliminary report on prevalence of acetabular labrum tears in sports patients with groin pain. *Knee Surg Sports Traumatol Arthrosc*, 11:403, 2003.
31. Burnett, SJ, et al: Clinical presentation of patients with tears of the acetabular labrum. *J Bone Joint Surg*, 88(A):1448, 2006.
32. Blankenbaker, DG, et al: Classification and localization of acetabular labral tears. *Skelet Radiol*, 36:391, 2007.

33. Petersen, W, Petersen, F, and Tillmann, B: Structure and vascularization of the acetabular labrum with regard to the pathogenesis and healing of labral lesions. *Arch Orthop Trauma Surg,* 123:283, 2003.
34. LeBlanc, KE, and LeBlanc, KA: Groin pain in athletes. *Hernia,* 7:68, 2003.
35. Morelli, V, and Smith, V: Groin injuries in athletes. *Am Fam Physician,* 64:283, 2001.
36. Mehin, R, et al: Surgery for osteitis pubis. *Can J Surg,* 49:170, 2006.
37. Parziale, JR, Hudgins, TH, and Fishman, LM: The piriformis syndrome. *Am J Orthop,* 25:819, 1996.
38. McCrory, P, and Bell, S: Nerve entrapment syndromes as a cause of pain in the hip, groin, and buttock. *Sports Med,* 27(4):261, 1999.
39. Hughes, SS, et al: Extrapelvic compression of the sciatic nerve. An unusual cause of pain about the hip: Report of five cases. *J Bone Joint Surg Am,* 74:1553, 1992.
40. Silver, JK, and Leadbetter, WB: Piriformis syndrome: Assessment of current practice and literature review. *Orthopedics,* 21:1133, 1998.
41. Woodhouse, ML: Sciatic nerve entrapment: A cause of proximal posterior thigh pain in athletes. *Athletic Training: Journal of the National Athletic Trainers Association,* 25:351, 1990.
42. Hanania, M, and Kitain, E: Perisciatic injection of steroid for the treatment of sciatica due to piriformis syndrome. *Reg Anesth Pain Med,* 23:223, 1998.
43. Keskula, DR, Lott, J, and Duncan, JB: Snapping iliopsoas tendon in a recreational athlete: A case report. *J Athl Train,* 34:382, 1999.
44. Dobbs, MB, et al: Surgical correction of the snapping iliopsoas tendon in adolescents. *J Bone Joint Surg (A),* 84:420, 2002.
45. Gruen, GS, Scioscia, TN, and Lowenstein, JE: The surgical treatment of internal snapping hip. *Am J Sports Med,* 30:607, 2002.
46. Ginesty, E, et al: Iliopsoas bursopathies. A review of twelve cases. *Rev Rhum Engl Ed,* 65:181, 1998.
47. Jones, DL, and Erhard, RE: Diagnosis of trochanteric bursitis versus femoral neck stress fracture. *Phys Ther,* 77:58, 1997.
48. Fortin, L, and Belanger, R: Bursitis of the iliopsoas: Four cases with pain as the only clinical indicator. *J Rheumatol,* 22:1971, 1995.
49. Flanagan, FL, et al: Symptomatic enlarged iliopsoas bursae in the presence of a normal plain hip radiograph. *Br J Rheumatol,* 34:365, 1995.
50. Johnston, CA, et al: Iliopsoas bursitis and tendinitis. A review. *Sports Med,* 25:271, 1998.
51. Vaccaro, JP, Sauser, DD, and Beals, RK: Iliopsoas bursa imaging: Efficacy in depicting abnormal iliopsoas tendon motion in patients with internal snapping hip syndrome. *Radiology,* 197:853, 1995.
52. Janzen, DL, et al: The snapping hip: Clinical and imaging findings in transient subluxation of the iliopsoas tendon. *Can Assoc Radiol J,* 47:202, 1996.
53. Johnston, CA, Lindsay, DM, and Wiley, JP: Treatment of iliopsoas syndrome with a hip rotation strengthening program: A retrospective case series. *J Orthop Sports Phys Ther,* 29:218, 1999.
54. Parris, HG, Sallis, RE, and Anderson, DV: Traumatic hip dislocation. Reducing complications. *Physician Sportsmed,* 21:67, 1993.
55. Stiris, MG: MR imaging after sports-induced hip dislocations. Report of three cases. *Acta Radiol,* 41:300, 2000.

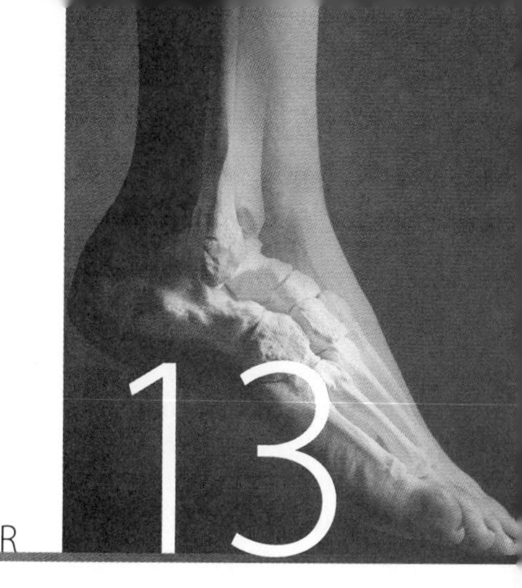

CHAPTER 13

Thoracic and Lumbar Spine Pathologies

Formed by 33 vertebral segments and divided into four distinct portions, the spinal column and its associated muscles provide postural control to the torso and skull, while also protecting the spinal cord. The conflicting needs for range of motion (ROM) versus protection of the spinal cord are met in varying degrees throughout the various regions of the spine (Fig. 13-1).

The cervical spine provides the greatest ROM, but here the spinal cord is the most vulnerable. The thoracic spine provides the greatest protection of the spinal cord but does so at the expense of ROM. The lumbar spine provides a more equal balance between protection of the spinal cord and available ROM. The sacrum and coccyx are composed of fused bones. The sacrum affixes the spinal column to the pelvis and serves as a site for muscle attachment. At this level, the spinal cord has exited the column.

Spine-related pain is a prevalent condition.[1] Seventy percent of adults will experience back or neck pain during their lives.[2] The high prevalence, the significant association of back pain to mental illnesses such as depression, and the resulting demands on the health care system make the cost of back pain exorbitant. Injury to the spine during athletic competition accounts for an estimated 10% to 15% of all spinal injuries, with 6% to 10% of these injuries resulting from trauma to the spinal cord or spinal nerve.[3] This chapter discusses conditions affecting the spine that are most likely to be evaluated away from practice and competition. On-field recognition and

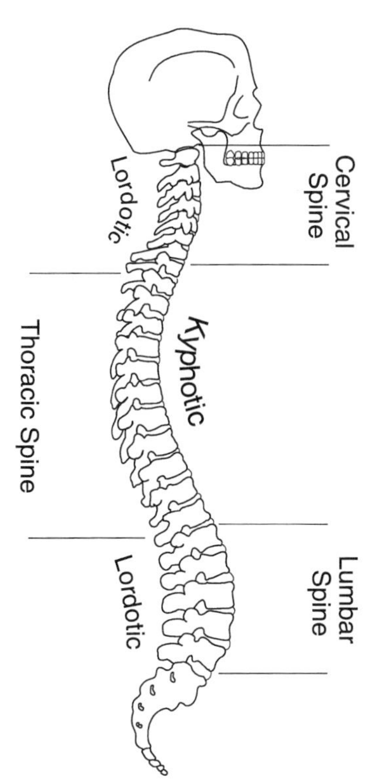

FIGURE 13-1 ■ The three segments of the mobile spinal column with their normal curvature noted.

management of cervical, thoracic, and lumbar spinal injuries are discussed in Chapter 21.

Clinical Anatomy

Figure 13-2 compares the relative sizes of the cervical ($n = 7$), thoracic ($n = 12$), and lumbar ($n = 5$) vertebrae and identifies the bony landmarks. The body's weight is transmitted primarily along the spinal column via the vertebral body, whose size is related to the amount of force it transmits. Carrying only the weight of the head, the vertebral bodies of the cervical vertebrae are much smaller than those of the lumbar vertebrae, which are required to transmit and absorb the weight of the entire torso. A segment, comprised of two adjacent vertebral bodies and the intervening disk, represents the smallest functional unit of the spine. The vertebrae of the cervical spine are included in this section for a basis of comparison. Refer to Chapter 14 for further description of the cervical spine.

Bony Anatomy

Each vertebra, with the exception of the first cervical vertebra, has a distinct body that is situated anteriorly and comprises the primary weight-bearing surface. Projecting immediately posteriorly from the body are the sturdy pedicles, forming the anterior portion of the neural arch. The posterior portion of the arch is composed of the lamina. The laterally projecting **transverse processes**, arising from the laminae, provide an attachment site for the spine's intrinsic ligaments and muscles and increase the muscles' mechanical leverage. The prominent posterior projections, the **spinous processes**, act as attachment sites for muscles and ligaments. Their angulation relative to the vertebrae below limits extension of the spine.

The **neural arch**, forming the posterior element of the spinal canal, serves as the protective tunnel through which the spinal cord passes. Lined with a continuation of the cerebral meninges (see Chapter 21), the spinal cord is normally buffered from the walls of the spinal canal by cerebrospinal fluid. Narrowing of the canal, stenosis, due to an acute, acquired, or congenital development of soft tissue or bone, leads to an increased possibility of pressure being placed on the spinal cord that results in radicular symptoms in the lower extremity.[4]

Two sets of articular processes arise from the superior and inferior surfaces of the lamina. The superior facets of the vertebrae articulate with the inferior facets of the vertebrae immediately above, forming synovial **facet joints** (zygapophyseal joints), which transmit 20% of the weight-bearing forces through the spine.[5] The bony arrangement of these joints is such that the lateral portion of the superior facet articulates with the medial portion of the inferior facet. The orientation and resulting direction of motion change throughout the spine. In the rotating upper cervical region, the facet joints have a more horizontal orientation. In the lower cervical and thoracic regions, the

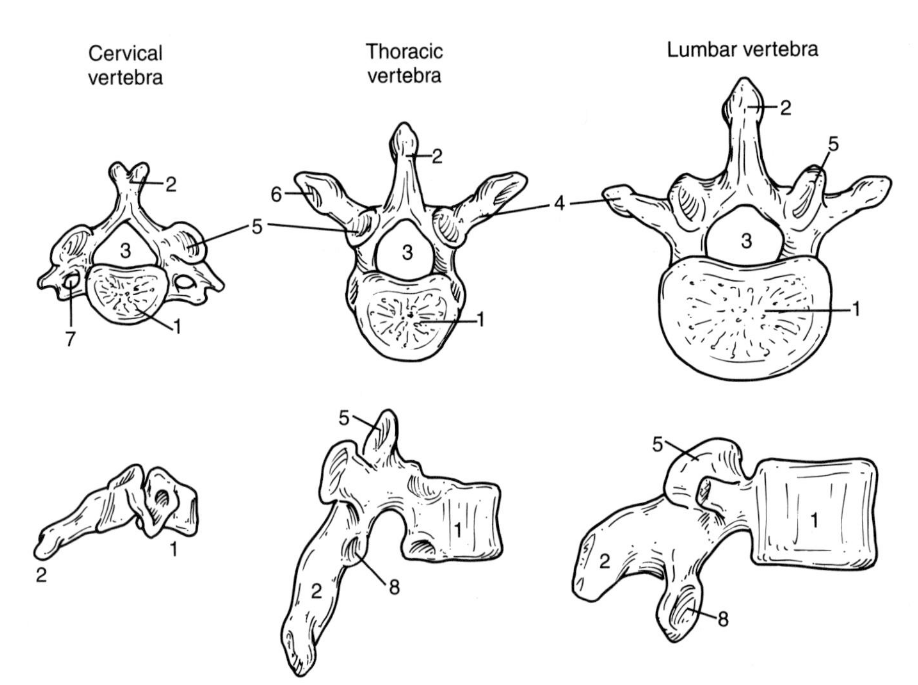

FIGURE 13-2 ■ Comparative anatomy of the cervical, thoracic, and lumbar spine. (*1*) Vertebral body, (*2*) spinous process, (*3*) vertebral foramen, (*4*) transverse process, (*5*) superior articular facet, (*6*) costotransverse facet, (*7*) transverse foramen, (*8*) inferior articular facet.

Facet joints An articulation of the facets between each contiguous part of vertebrae in the spinal column.

more frontal plane orientation allows lateral flexion but restricts rotation. In the lumbar region, the sagittal plane orientation favors flexion and extension.[6] The area between the superior and inferior facets of a vertebra, the **pars interarticularis**, is a common site of stress fractures in the lumbar spine.

The anterior portions of each pedicle contain vertebral notches, concave depressions along the inferior surfaces and superior portions of the bone. The vertebral notch on the inferior portion of one pedicle is matched with the vertebral notch on the superior portion of the pedicle below, forming the **intervertebral foramen**, the space where spinal nerve roots exit the vertebral column (Fig. 13-3).

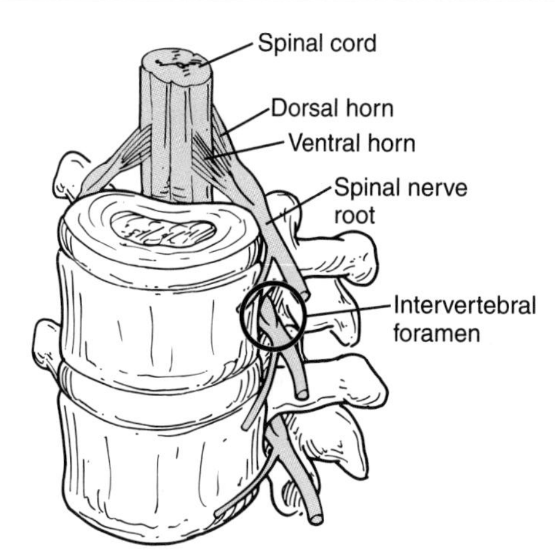

FIGURE 13-3 ■ Nerve roots exiting between the vertebrae. The pedicle of the superior and inferior vertebrae align to form the intervertebral foramen, allowing the spinal nerves to exit the vertebral column.

The relative sizes of the vertebral bodies and the transverse and spinous processes vary according to their function at each of the spinal levels (Table 13-1). The cervical spine, the most mobile of the vertebral segments, has the smallest vertebral bodies. Refer to Chapter 14 for a description of the cervical spine.

In the thoracic segment of the spinal column, the vertebral bodies begin to widen and thicken to assist in managing the weight of the torso. The spinous processes project downward to limit extension and provide a strong attachment site for the thoracic muscles and ligaments. The transverse processes thicken to articulate with the ribs, forming the **costotransverse joints** in ribs 1–10. Ribs 11 and 12 do not articulate with the transverse processes, so these joints do not exist at these levels. In addition to articulating with the transverse processes, a **costovertebral joint** is formed between each rib and the vertebral bodies. The joints formed on the T1 and T10–T12 vertebral levels articulate with a single rib on each side. The remaining ribs articulate with two vertebrae at the **superior costal** and **inferior costal facets** and the associated intervertebral disk on each side.

Table 13-1 Structural Adaptations of Vertebral Anatomy at the Different Spinal Levels

	Bony Anatomy			
Level	**Vertebral Body**	**Transverse Process**	**Spinous Process**	**Facet Joints**
Cervical	Small; view in the frontal plane is wider than in the sagittal plane Vertebral body is absent in C1; C2 body has vertical projection called dens; the remaining bodies progressively increase in size.	Short; processes contain the transverse foramen for passage of the vertebral artery.	Small and short, except for C7, which has characteristics of a thoracic vertebra.	C0 and C1: Ellipsoid joint C1 and C2: Positioned in the transverse plane C3–C7: Approximately 45° from transverse plane in the frontal plane
Thoracic	Diameter and thickness increase as the spine continues inferiorly. Demifacets are present to accept the head of the ribs.	Solid configuration allows for the attachment of muscles and costovertebral ligaments. The processes of T1–T12 have articular surfaces for the ribs.	Long and slender; their downward projections result in an overlap of spinous process of the vertebra below; the spinous processes of the lower thoracic vertebrae gradually thicken and straighten to resemble those of the lumbar vertebrae.	Oblique, but lying primarily in the frontal plane
Lumbar	Vertebral bodies are broad in both the frontal and sagittal planes.	Long for leverage; thin in the cross section.	The superior borders are posteriorly projected with a large inferior flare.	The facet joints of L1–L3 are located in the sagittal plane; the facets of L4 and L5 are frontally oriented.

Molded by five fused vertebrae, the sacrum is a broad, thick, triangular bone that fixates the spinal column to the pelvis and is responsible for stabilizing the pelvic girdle (Fig. 13-4). The weight of the torso and skull is transmitted through the **sacroiliac (SI) joints** to the lower extremity. Ground reaction forces from the lower extremities are transmitted through the SI joints up the spinal column.

The laterally projecting articular surfaces of the sacrum have an irregular shape that, when matched to the iliac's facets, form the very stable SI joint. Its anterior and posterior surfaces are roughened to permit firm attachment of muscles acting on the femur and pelvis. Four pairs of foramina perforate the bone to permit the passage of the dorsal and ventral primary divisions of the nerves of the sacral plexus from their posterior origin into the pelvic cavity. Once adulthood is reached, the amount of movement at the sacroiliac joint is minimal and it continues to decrease with age.[6]

Lumbarization occurs when the first sacral vertebra fails to unite with the remainder of the sacrum, forming a separate vertebra having characteristics similar to those of the lumbar spine, essentially becoming a sixth lumbar vertebra. **Sacralization**, on the other hand, occurs when the fifth lumbar vertebra becomes fused to the sacrum (Fig. 13-5). This may occur unilaterally or bilaterally, resulting in complete fusion of these segments. Except for radiographic diagnosis, these conditions are virtually undetectable and typically asymptomatic. However, patients may demonstrate decreased lumbar ROM.

The distal end of the spinal column is formed by the **coccyx**. Formed by the fusion of three or four rudimentary bony pieces, the coccyx provides an attachment site for some of the muscles of the pelvic floor and, sometimes, portions of the gluteus maximus.

Intervertebral Disks

Found in varying thicknesses between the cervical, thoracic, and lumbar vertebrae, intervertebral disks act to increase the total ROM available to the spinal column.

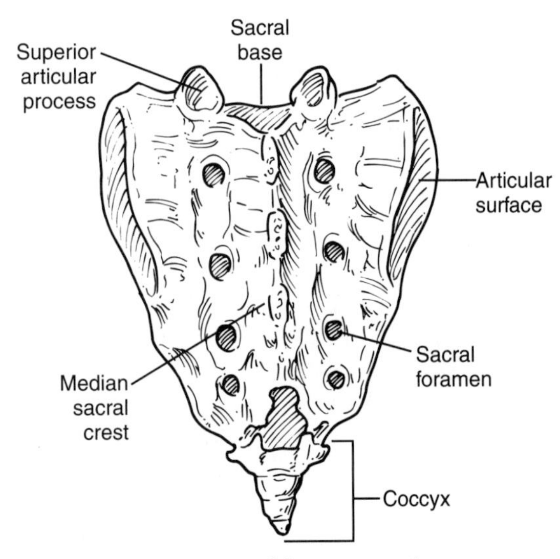

FIGURE 13-4 ■ Posterior view of the sacrum and coccyx.

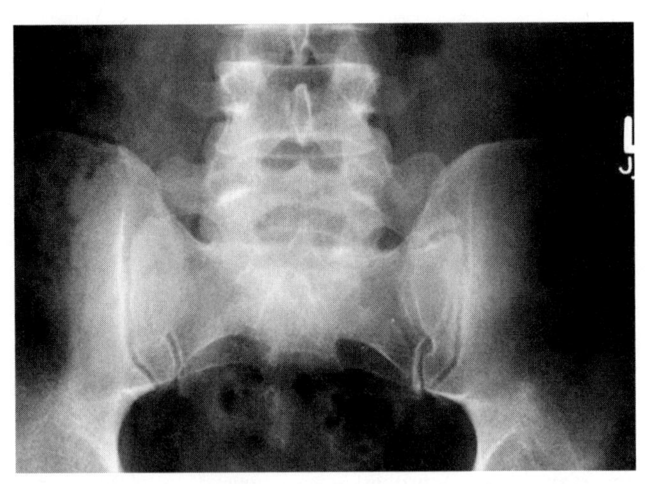

FIGURE 13-5 ■ Sacralized L5 vertebrae. The L5 and S1 vertebra are fused together.

The disks also serve as shock absorbers of longitudinal and rotational stresses placed on the column through compression. Each disk is formed by a tough, dense outer layer, the **annulus fibrosus**, surrounding a flexible inner layer, the **nucleus pulposus** (Fig. 13-6).

Twenty-three intervertebral disks are found along the spinal column. No disk is found between the skull and the first cervical vertebra (C0–C1) or between the first and second cervical vertebrae (C1–C2). Individual disks are referenced by the vertebrae between which they are found. For instance, the disk located between the fourth and fifth lumbar vertebrae is known as the L4–L5 intervertebral disk.

The annulus fibrosus consists of multilayered fibers that cross from opposite directions, forming an X pattern. This arrangement leaves some portion of the disk taut regardless of the position of the vertebral column and increases the overall strength of the tissue. When viewed in cross-section, the annulus fibrosus is thinner posteriorly than anteriorly. A vertebral endplate, an expanse of fibrocartilage from the annulus fibrosus, inserts on the vertebra above and below to secure the disk to the spinal column.

The core of the disk, the nucleus pulposus, is a highly elastic, semigelatinous substance that is 60% to 70% water.[7] The

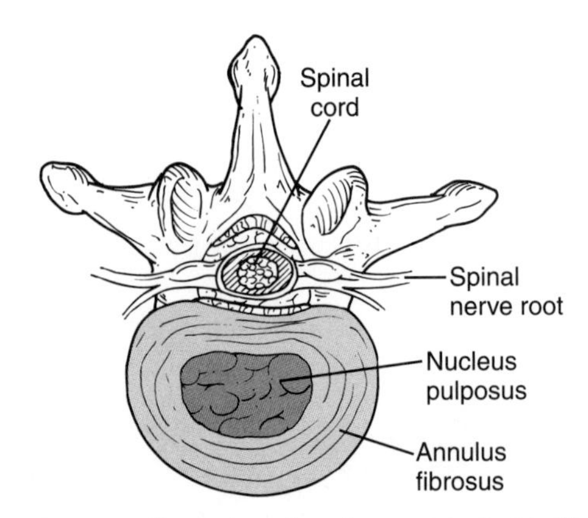

FIGURE 13-6 ■ Illustration of an intervertebral disk. The firm, outer annulus fibrosus surrounds the pliable nucleus pulposus.

high water content makes the nucleus pulposus resistant to compression while allowing it to be deformable. During the course of the day, the nucleus pulposus becomes dehydrated from the body weight placed on it, compressing water out of its core. During sleep or other long periods of reclining, the compressive forces placed on the disks are eliminated, allowing the nucleus pulposus to become rehydrated. Physical activity such as running compresses the intervertebral disks between T7–L1 and L5–S1, resulting in a decreased ROM in the lumbar spine after activity.[8]

Permanent dehydration also occurs through the aging process. Until the age of approximately 40 years, the disk is fully hydrated. After this age, dehydration begins. By age 60 years, the disks have reached their maximum state of dehydration, resulting in decreased ROM and a slight narrowing of the intervertebral foramen.[9]

The annulus fibrosus and the posterior longitudinal ligament are richly innervated by sensory nerves.[10] This nerve supply can account for much of the pain associated with disk degeneration or herniation. This type of pain is referred to as **diskogenic pain**.

The amount of stress placed on the lumbar intervertebral disks is influenced by the position of the trunk. In the supine position, the disk is under a load of approximately 75 kg of pressure. When an individual stands up, the load increases to 100 kg. When sitting and leaning forward, the total load increases to 275 kg.[11] Lateral bending, flexion, lateral shear, and compression place the largest shear loads on the disk.[12]

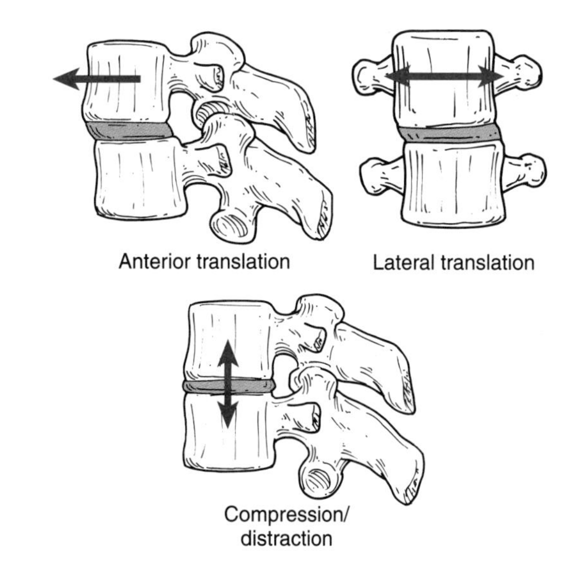

FIGURE 13-7 ■ Accessory vertebral motions. In addition to the cardinal spinal movements of flexion and extension, rotation, and lateral bending, the facet joints allow for anterior and posterior translation, lateral translation, and compression and distraction of contiguous vertebrae.

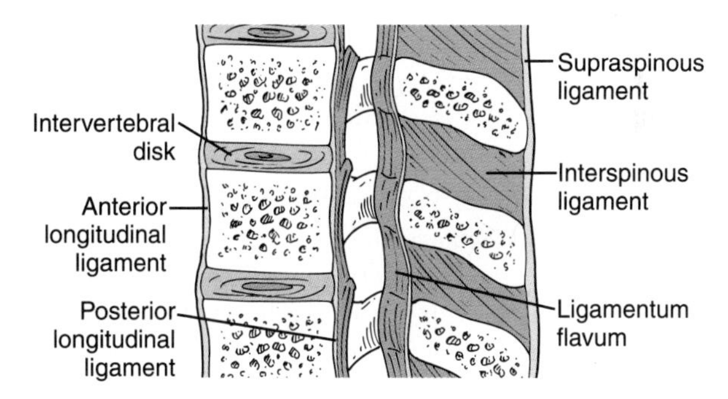

FIGURE 13-8 ■ Cross-sectional view of the ligaments of the vertebral column.

Articulations and Ligamentous Anatomy

The spinal column allows for three degrees of freedom of movement: (1) flexion and extension, (2) rotation, and (3) tilting, resulting in lateral bending. The accessory motions occurring at the facet joints allowing these physiologic motions to occur include (1) anterior and posterior glide, or flexion; (2) lateral glide, or extension; and (3) compression and distraction, or side bending and rotation (Fig. 13-7). The amount of movement between any two vertebrae is rather limited, but the sum of these motions provides a large amount of ROM for the spinal column as a whole. **Coupled motions** occur because of the varied orientations of the facet joints. For example, lateral flexion occurs concurrently with rotation and vice versa: neither is a pure, single plane movement.

The articulation between each pair of vertebrae is formed by cartilaginous and synovial joints. The union between an intervertebral disk and the superior and inferior vertebrae forms the **cartilaginous joint**, and the facet joints represent the synovial articulations. The exception to this is the joint formed between the first and second cervical vertebrae.

The entire length of the spinal column is reinforced by the **anterior and posterior longitudinal ligaments** (Fig. 13-8). The broader, thicker anterior longitudinal ligament (ALL) spans the length of the vertebral column from the occiput to the sacrum, attaching to both the vertebral bodies and the intervertebral disks. The fibrous arrangement of this ligament strengthens the anterior portion of the intervertebral disks and vertebrae, functioning to limit extension of the spine. The ALL is thinnest in the lumbar spine.

The posterior longitudinal ligament (PLL) originates from the occiput as a thick structure but gradually thins as it progresses down the vertebral column. Lining the anterior portion of the vertebral canal, the PLL fans out and thickens as it passes over the intervertebral disks, attaching to their margins only to allow the passage of blood vessels. This ligament serves primarily to limit flexion of the spine.

Traversing the length of the spinal column, the **supraspinous ligament** attaches to the posterior apex of each spinous process. In the cervical spine, the supraspinous ligament becomes the **ligamentum nuchae**. Two ligaments are intrinsic to the adjoining vertebrae. Filling the space

---

Coupled motion The concurrent and necessary association of a motion around one axis with a different motion around another axis.

Cartilaginous joint A relatively immobile joint in which two bones are fused by cartilage.

formed between the spinous processes, the **interspinous ligaments** limit flexion and rotation of the spine. The posterior margin of the vertebral canal is formed by the **ligamentum flavum**, a pair of elastic ligaments connecting the lamina of one vertebra to the lamina of the vertebra above it. The ligamentum flavum reinforces the facet joints, and its unusual elastic property assists the trunk in returning from flexion to the neutral position.

Sacroiliac joint

A series of ligaments serve to bind the sacrum to the pelvis. The **interosseous sacroiliac** ligaments are formed by strong fibers spanning the anterior portion of the ilium and the posterior portion of the sacrum, filling the void behind the articular surfaces of these bones (Fig. 13-9). The anterior and posterior surfaces of the articulation are strengthened by the **dorsal and ventral sacroiliac ligaments**. The dorsal SI ligament is made of fibers that run transversely to join the ilium to the upper portion of the sacrum and vertical fibers connecting the lower sacrum to the posterior superior iliac spine (PSIS). Lining the anterior portion of the pelvic cavity, the ventral SI ligaments attach to the anterior portion of the sacrum. Two accessory ligaments assist in maintaining the stability of the SI joint. The **sacrotuberous ligament** arises from the ischial tuberosity to blend with the inferior fibers of the dorsal SI ligaments. Indirectly supporting the sacrum, the **sacrospinous ligament** originates from the sacrum's ischial spine and attaches to the coccyx.

The SI joints are more mobile in young individuals and become less mobile with age. In **postpartum** females, the stresses of athletics can injure the structurally weakened SI joints. During pregnancy and at the time of birth, the hormone relaxin is released into the mother's system. Relaxin increases the extensibility of the ligamentous structures in and around the birth canal.[13] These hormones affect the ligaments of the SI joint, resulting in increased pelvic motion and increasing the risk of pathology at the SI joint.

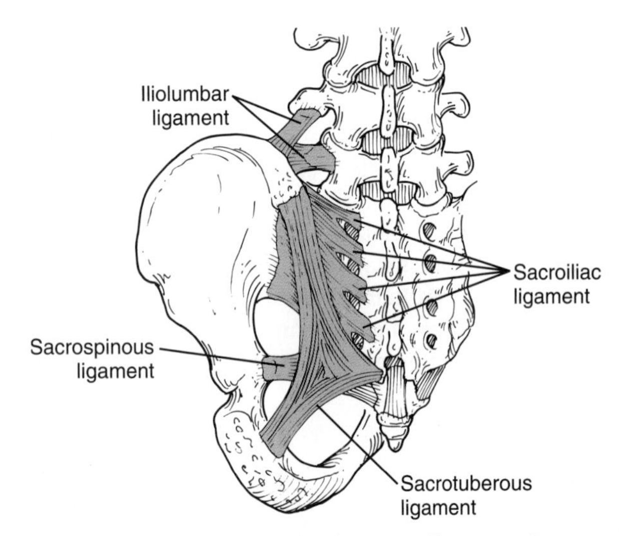

FIGURE 13-9 ■ Posterior sacroiliac ligaments. The strong ligamentous configuration of the sacroiliac joint permits only slight movement.

Neurologic Anatomy

A nerve plexus is a network formed by a consecutive series of spinal nerves. These systems are formed by both **convergent** and **divergent** pathways, causing an intermixing of sensory and motor impulses. Although the root of a plexus may be supplied by one spinal nerve, the nerves exiting the plexus contain fibers from more than one spinal nerve root.

A total of 31 pairs of nerve roots exit the spinal column (Fig 13-10). The thoracic and lumbar regions have a pair of nerves exiting below the corresponding vertebra (e.g., the T1 nerve root exits below the body of the first thoracic vertebra). There are 12 pairs of thoracic nerves and five pairs of lumbar

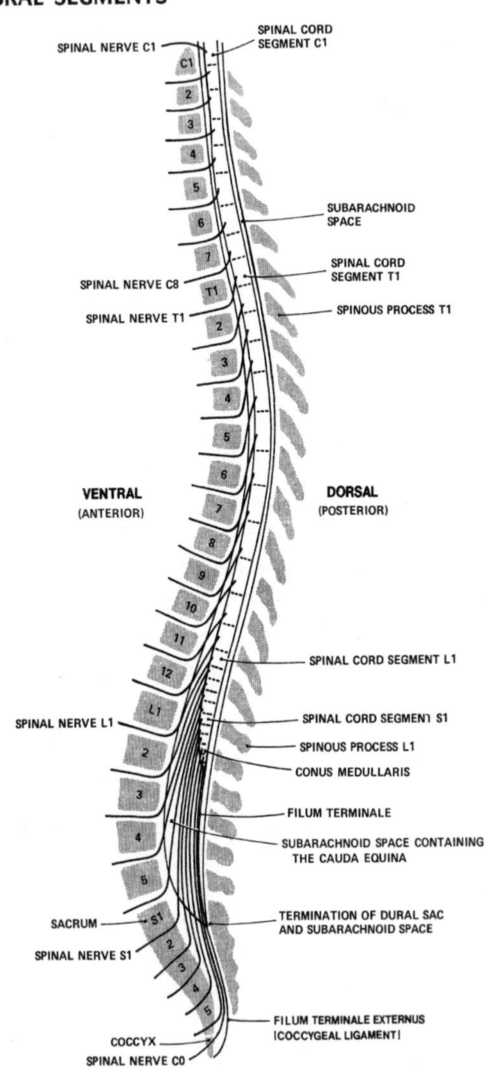

FIGURE 13-10 ■ Relationship between the vertebrae and spinal nerve roots showing anatomical relationships.

Postpartum After childbirth.

Convergent Two nerves combining together to form a single nerve.

Divergent One nerve splitting to form two individual nerves.

nerves. Although there are seven cervical vertebrae, eight pairs of nerve roots exit in this area. The first seven cervical nerves exit above the vertebrae. The "odd" cervical nerve, C8, exits below the seventh cervical vertebra (between the seventh cervical and first thoracic vertebrae).

Several pairs of nerve plexus are formed by the sacral, lumbar, thoracic, cervical, and cranial nerve roots. This chapter addresses the lumbar plexus and sacral plexus. The brachial plexus is described in Chapter 14, and the cranial plexus is presented in Chapter 21. Note that few resources agree on the actual nerve roots forming each plexus.

Lumbar plexus

Formed by the 12th thoracic nerve root and the L1–L5 nerve roots, the lumbar plexus innervates the anterior and medial muscles of the thigh and the dermatomes of the medial leg and foot. The posterior branches of the L2, L3, and L4 nerve roots converge to form the **femoral nerve**, and their anterior branches merge to form the obturator nerve (Fig. 13-11).

Sacral plexus

A portion of the L4 nerve root, the L5 nerve root, and the lumbosacral trunk courses downward to form the superior portion of the sacral plexus (Fig. 13-12). This plexus supplies the muscles of the buttocks and, via the sciatic nerve, innervates the muscles of the posterior femur and the entire lower leg. The sciatic nerve has three distinct sections: (1) the **tibial nerve**, formed by the anterior branches of the upper five nerve roots; (2) the **common peroneal nerve**, formed by the posterior branches of the upper four nerve roots; and (3) a slip of the **tibial nerve** that innervates the hamstring muscles.

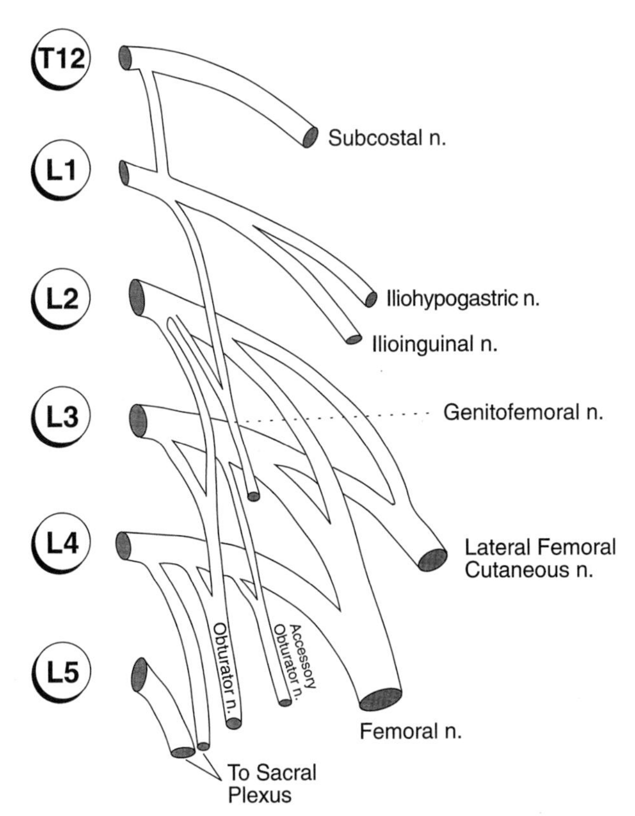

FIGURE 13-11 ■ Lumbar plexus. Note that the lower portion of the lumbar plexus merges with the upper portion of the sacral plexus.

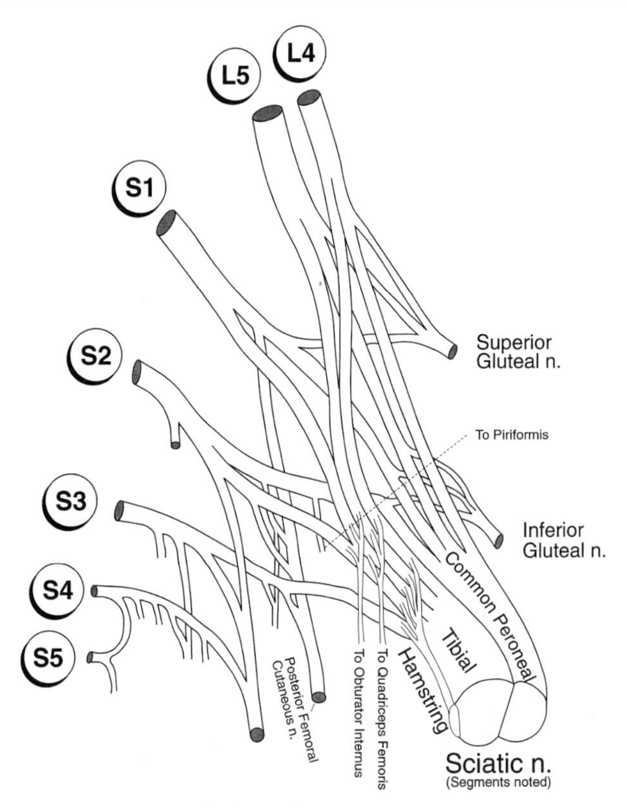

FIGURE 13-12 ■ Sacral plexus. This nerve package supplies the lower leg, ankle, and foot through the tibial and common peroneal nerves.

Muscular Anatomy

A complex network of muscles acts on the spinal column. These muscles, interwoven with the fibers of other muscles, function in an orchestrated manner to provide the static support needed for posture and the dynamic control needed for motion.

Two groups of muscles influence the movement of the spinal column. **Extrinsic muscles** primarily function to provide respiration and movement associated with the upper extremity and scapula, indirectly influencing the spinal column. **Intrinsic muscles** lie close to the spinal column and directly influence its motion.

No muscles act directly to affect the movement at the SI joint, but movement can be indirectly influenced through two means: (1) the muscles originating on the sacrum that function to control the hip joint and (2) any musculature attaching to the pelvic bones that can cause rotation of the pelvis.

Extrinsic muscles

The posterior muscles acting on the spinal column are the **latissimus dorsi**, **levator scapulae**, **rhomboid major and minor**, and **trapezius**. Serving to connect the upper extremity to the axial skeleton, these muscles primarily influence humeral and scapular motion (Table 13-2). These muscles are described in Chapter 16.

Table 13-2 Extrinsic Muscle Acting on the Spinal Column

Muscle	Action	Origin	Insertion	Innervation	Root
Rectus Abdominis	Flexion of the lumbar spine against gravity Posterior rotation of the pelvis	Pubic crest Pubic symphysis	Costal cartilage of the 5th–7th ribs Xiphoid process of sternum	Ventral rami	T5–T12
External Oblique	Bilateral contraction: Flexion of the lumbar spine Posterior rotation of the pelvis Unilateral contraction: Rotation of the lumbar spine to the opposite side Lateral bending of the lumbar spine to the same side	5th– 8th ribs (anterior fibers) 9th–12th ribs (lateral fibers)	Via an aponeurosis to the linea alba (anterior fibers) Anterior superior iliac spine, pubic tubercle, and the anterior portion of the iliac crest (lateral fibers)	Iliohypogastric Ilioinguinal Ventral rami	T1–T12
Internal Oblique	Bilateral contraction: Support of the abdominal viscera Posterior rotation of the pelvis Flexion of the lumbar spine Unilateral contraction: Rotation of the lumbar spine to the same side Lateral bending of the lumbar spine to the same side	Lateral two thirds of the inguinal ligament (lower fibers) • Anterior one third of the iliac crest (upper fibers) • Middle one third of the iliac crest (lateral fibers)	Crest of pubis, pectineal line (lower fibers) 10th–12th ribs (lateral fibers) • Linea alba (all portions)	Iliohypogastric Ilioinguinal Ventral rami	T7–T12
Latissimus Dorsi	Extension of the spine Anterior rotation of the pelvis (also see shoulder function) Stabilization of the lumbar spine via the thoracodorsal fascia	Spinous processes of T6–T12 and the lumbar vertebrae via the thoracodorsal fascia Posterior iliac crest	Intertubercular groove of the humerus	Thoracodorsal	C6, C7, C8
Trapezius (middle one third)	Retraction of scapula Fixation of thoracic spine	Lower portion of the ligamentum nuchae Spinous processes of the 7th cervical vertebra and T1–T5	Acromion process Spine of the scapula (superior, lateral border)	Accessory	Cranial nerve XI
Trapezius (lower one third)	Depression of scapula Retraction of scapula Upward rotation of the scapula Fixation of thoracic spine	Spinous processes and supraspinal ligaments of T8– T12	Spine of the scapula (medial portion)	Accessory	Cranial nerve XI
Rhomboid Major	Retraction of scapula Elevation of scapula Downward rotation of scapula Fixation of thoracic spine	Spinous processes of T2, T3, T4, and T5	Vertebral border of scapula (lower two thirds)	Dorsal scapular	C5
Rhomboid Minor	Retraction of scapula Elevation of scapula Downward rotation of scapula Fixation of thoracic spine	Inferior portion of the ligamentum nuchae Spinous processes C7 and T1	Vertebral border of scapula (upper one third and superior angle)	Dorsal scapular	C5

Anteriorly and laterally, the rectus abdominis, internal oblique, and external oblique function to flex, rotate, or laterally bend the spinal column. The primary flexor of the spine, the **rectus abdominis** also influences spinal posture by rotating the pelvis posteriorly, flattening the lumbar spine. When the **internal and external obliques** on the same side of the trunk contract, the torso bends to that side. Contraction of the internal oblique and the external oblique muscles on the opposite side of the body result in the torso's rotating toward the side of the internal oblique muscle (Table 13-3). The **transverse abdominis** assists in stabilizing the lumbar spine by acting like a corset. Individuals with low back pain have a delayed contraction of the transversus abdominis, implicating it as a result or cause of low back pain.[14]

The muscles of the hip and pelvis, as described in Chapter 12, influence the spine by anteriorly or posteriorly rotating the pelvis and create a firm foundation or support for muscle attachment.

Intrinsic muscles

The intrinsic spinal muscles are divided into superficial, intermediate, and deep layers (Fig. 13-13). The superficial layer of the lumbar and thoracic spine muscles is presented in Table 13-4. The intrinsic muscles acting on the cervical spine are discussed in Chapter 14.

Forming the intermediate layer of the intrinsic muscles, the **erector spinae** is composed of three pairs of muscles; from lateral to medial, these are the **iliocostalis**, the **longissimus**, and the **spinalis**. Each of these muscles is then divided into three individual elements: the **iliocostalis**, formed by the **lumborum**, **thoracis**, and **cervicis** portions; and the longissimus and spinalis muscles, consisting of the **thoracis**, **cervicis**, and **capitis** portions. Small bundles of muscle fibers overlap to the point that every vertebra and rib has both a muscular attachment and insertion on it. The erector spinae muscle group is the primary mover for spinal extension and, when upright, controls the rate of spinal flexion against gravity through eccentric contractions. The

Table 13-3 Motions Produced by the Internal and External Oblique Muscles

Muscle	Bilateral Contraction	Unilateral Contraction
External Oblique	Flexion of the lumbar spine	Contralateral rotation of the trunk
	Posterior pelvic rotation	Ipsilateral lateral flexion of the trunk
	Compression of the abdominal viscera	Rotation of the pelvis
	Depression of the thorax	
	Assistance in respiration	
Internal Oblique	Flexion of the lumbar spine	Ipsilateral rotation of the trunk
	Compression of the abdominal viscera	Ipsilateral lateral flexion of the trunk
	Depression of the thorax	
	Assistance in respiration	

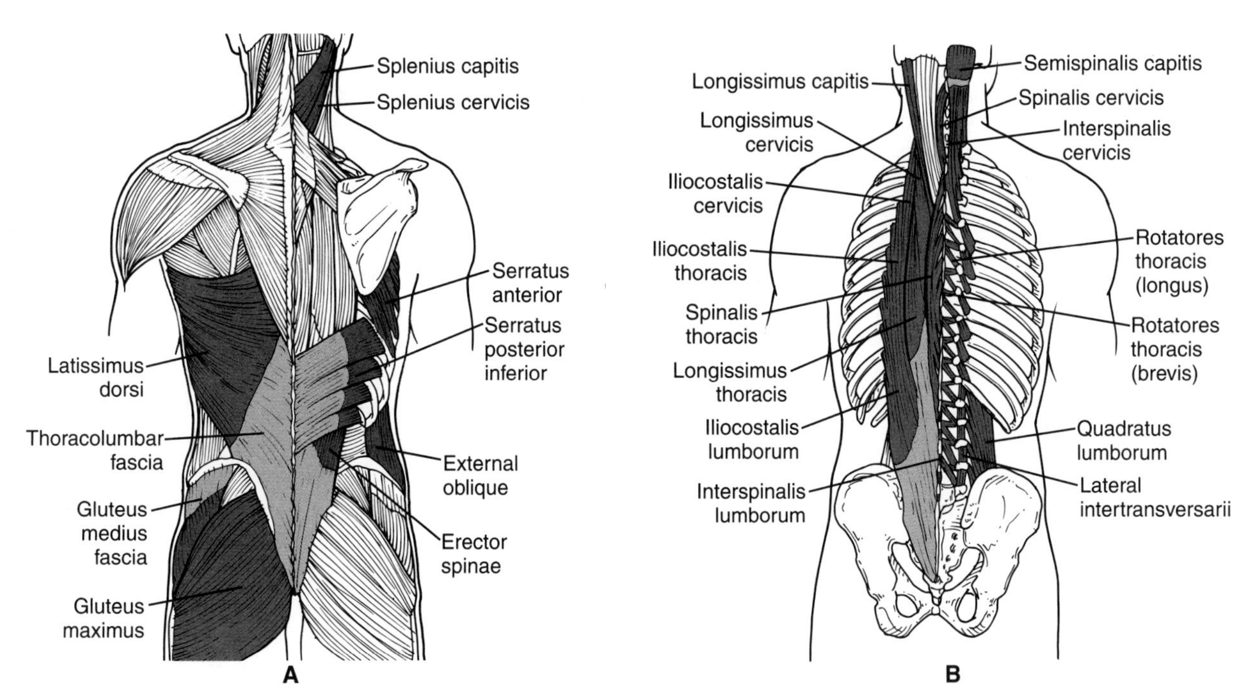

FIGURE 13-13 ■ Muscles of the spinal column: (A) superficial muscles, (B) deep muscles.

Table 13-4 Intrinsic Muscles Acting on the Spinal Column

Muscle	Action	Origin	Insertion	Innervation	Root
Iliocostalis Lumborum	Bilateral contraction: Extension of spinal column Unilateral contraction: Lateral bending of spinal column to the same side	Posterior aspect of the iliac crest	Inferior angles of ribs 6–12	Posterior primary divisions of the spinal nerves	Multiple roots, segmentally along the length of the muscle
Iliocostalis Thoracis	Bilateral contraction: Extension of spinal column Unilateral contraction: Lateral bending of spinal column to the same side	Ribs 6–12	Ribs 1–6 Transverse process of C7	Posterior primary divisions of the spinal nerves	Multiple roots, segmentally along the length of the muscle
Longissimus Thoracis	Bilateral contraction: Extension of spinal column Unilateral contraction: Lateral bending of spinal column	Common erector spinae tendon	Transverse process of T3–T21 Ribs 3–12	Posterior primary divisions of the spinal nerves	Multiple roots, segmentally along the length of the muscle
Spinalis Thoracis	Bilateral contraction: Extension of the spine Unilateral contraction: Lateral bending of the spine to the same side	Common erector spinae tendon	Spinous processes of upper thoracic spine	Posterior primary divisions of the spinal nerves	Multiple roots, segmentally along the length of the muscle
Semispinalis Thoracis	Bilateral contraction: Extension of thoracic and cervical spine Unilateral contraction: Rotation to the opposite side	Transverse process	Travel upwardly and medially to attach to a spinous process 5 or 8 vertebrae above the origin	Posterior primary divisions of the spinal nerves	Multiple roots, segmentally along the length of the muscle
Multifidus (or multifidi)	Bilateral contraction: Stabilization of vertebral column Unilateral contraction: Rotation of spine to the opposite side	Lumbar region • Superior aspect of sacrum Thoracic region • Transverse processes Cervical region • Articular processes	Spinous process	Posterior primary divisions of the spinal nerves	Multiple roots, segmentally along the length of the muscle
Rotatores	Bilateral contraction: Extension of spine Stabilization of vertebral column Unilateral contraction: Rotation of spine	Transverse process	Spinous process of the vertebra immediately above the origin	Posterior primary divisions of the spinal nerves	Multiple roots, segmentally along the length of the muscle

erector spinae group also assists in the movements of lateral flexion and rotation of the trunk.

The deep intrinsic layer is collectively known as **transversospinal** muscles because the fibers run from one transverse process to the spinous process superior to them. Individually, this group is formed by the **semispinalis**, **multifidus**, and **rotatores** muscles. The multifidii muscles play an important role in the dynamic, segmental stabilization of the lumbar spine and are active during lifting and rotational maneuvers.[15] The multifidii show atrophy, weakness, and decreased activation in individuals who experience low back pain.[16]

The semispinalis muscle is divided into thoracis, cervicis, and capitis segments. These muscles act primarily to contralaterally rotate the spinal column, especially above the lumbar level. They also contribute slightly to spinal extension and ipsilateral lateral flexion.

Clinical Examination of the Thoracic and Lumbar Spine

Examination Map

HISTORY

Past Medical History
- Mental health status

History of the Present Condition
- Location of pain
- Radicular symptoms
- Onset and severity of symptoms

INSPECTION

Functional Assessment
- Gait
- Movement and posture

General Inspection
- Frontal curvature
- Sagittal curvature
- Skin markings

Inspection of the Thoracic Spine
- Breathing patterns
- Skin folds
- Chest shape

Inspection of the Lumbar Spine
- Lordotic curve
- Standing posture
- Erector muscle tone
- Faun's beard

PALPATION

Palpation of the Thoracic Spine
- Spinous processes
- Supraspinous ligaments
- Costovertebral junction
- Trapezius
- Paravertebral muscles
- Scapular muscles

Palpation of the Lumbar Spine
- Spinous processes
  - Step-off deformity
- Paravertebral muscles

Palpation of the Sacrum and Pelvis
- Median sacral crests
- Iliac crests
- Posterior superior iliac spine
- Gluteals
- Ischial tuberosity
- Greater trochanter
- Sciatic nerve
- Pubic symphysis

JOINT AND MUSCLE FUNCTION ASSESSMENT

Goniometry
- Flexion
- Extension
- Lateral bending
- Rotation

Active Range of Motion
- Flexion
- Extension
- Lateral bending
- Rotation

Manual Muscle Tests
- Flexion
- Extension
- Rotation
- Pelvic elevation

Passive Range of Motion
- Flexion
- Extension
- Rotation
- Side gliding

JOINT STABILITY TESTS

Joint Play Assessment
- Spring test

SPECIAL TESTS

Test for Nerve Root Impingement
- Valsalva
- Milgram
- Kernig
- Straight leg raise
- Well straight leg raise
- Slump test
- Quadrant test

NEUROLOGIC EXAMINATION
- Lower quarter screen

PATHOLOGIES AND SPECIAL TESTS

Spinal Stenosis

Intervertebral Disk Lesions
- Femoral nerve stretch test
- Tension sign

Segmental Instability
- Erector spinae strain
- Facet joint dysfunction

Spondylopathies
- Spondylolysis
- Spondylolisthesis
  - Single leg stance test

Sacroiliac Dysfunction
- Fabere sign
- Patrick's test
- Gaenslen's test
- Long sit test

Because of its important role in protecting the spinal cord and spinal nerve roots, injury to the vertebrae can have catastrophic results. In acute trauma, the primary role of the initial evaluation is to rule out the presence of trauma that has, or can, jeopardize the integrity of the spinal cord or nerve roots. Chapter 21 discusses these evaluative procedures. The techniques presented in this chapter assume that significant vertebral fractures or dislocations have been ruled out.

Low back pain is multidimensional, with psychological and physiological influences. Identification of specific structures that are pathologically involved is difficult, leading to the widespread diagnosis of nonspecific low back pain. Many spinal pain syndromes are associated with or complicated by improper foot mechanics, muscular tightness of the lower extremity, and imbalances of the pelvic and abdominal muscles (see Chapter 6).

History

Pain produced during activities of daily living (ADLs) provides valuable information about the cause of the pain and other activities that may reproduce or decrease the pain (Table 13-5). These patient-described activities serve as the foundation for the functional assessment portion of the exam. Pain that occurs during certain times of the day can

Table 13-5 Ramifications of Spinal Pain Exhibited During the Activities of Daily Living

Activity	Ramifications
Bending	Pain may be initially worsened with flexion exercises.
Sitting	Pain may be initially worsened with flexion exercises.
Rising from Sitting	This motion causes changes in the interdiscal forces. Sharp pain suggests derangement of the disk.
Standing	The spine is placed in extension. Pain may be initially experienced with extension exercises.
Walking	The amount of spinal extension increases as the speed of gait increases.
Lying Prone	The spine is placed in or near full extension.
Lying Supine	When lying supine on a hard surface, the amount of extension is maintained. When lying on a soft surface, the spine falls into flexion.

indicate a postural position that irritates the involved nerve root (or roots) or other soft tissue structures.

Past Medical History

- **History of spinal injury**: Any pertinent history that may lead to structural degeneration or predispose the patient to chronic problems is important. The current symptoms may be the result of the formation of scar tissue that is impinging or restricting other structures. Low back pain tends to recur, with episodes or "flare ups" occurring sporadically.[17] Low back pain as an adolescent is a significant predictor of low back pain as an adult.[18]
- **General health**: Infection of the kidney and/or urinary track may cause back pain.
- **Changes in activity**: Changes in the level, intensity, or duration of activity or changes in running surfaces, footwear, sleeping mattress, and so on can redistribute the forces transmitted to the spinal column. (Refer to Chapters 6 and 8 for more information on how these changes can affect posture and cause pain.)
- **Mental Health Status**: The association between mental health status and onset, chronicity, and disability associated with low back pain has been studied extensively. Emotional distress, fear-avoidance behaviors, and depressed moods are all associated with an increased risk, prolonged duration, and increased severity of low back pain.[19–21]

*** Practical Evidence**

Multidimensional in nature, the pain and disability associated with low back pain is associated with psychological variables such as depression, anxiety, and distress.[19] Depression coupled with low back pain is associated with a worse outcome than low back pain alone. A positive response to either or both of the questions: (1) "During the past month, have you often been bothered by feeling down, depressed or hopeless?" or (2) "During the past month, have you often been bothered by little interest or pleasure in doing things?" warrants referral of the patient for evaluation for depression.[22]

History of the Present Condition

- **Location of the pain and referred or radicular symptoms**: Pain radiating into the extremity or peripheral paresthesia or numbness is the result of impingement or pressure on the spinal cord itself, a nerve root exiting the intervertebral foramen or dural irritation proximal to the site of pain. In addition, leg or buttock pain may be referred from structures in the low back and not related to nerve root compression. Unlike pain in other anatomical areas, the exact location and underlying cause of low back pain are often ambiguous.[23] Sacroiliac pathology usually causes pain around the PSIS of the affected side or radiating into the hip and groin. Spasm of the piriformis muscle can cause symptoms of sciatic nerve dysfunction. Having the patient complete a pain drawing by placing symbols on the body representing pain locations may provide insight as to pathology. For example, the patient might indicate symptoms along a dermatomal distribution, describing impingement of a specific nerve. Pain in the buttock and pelvis area but not in the lumbar region is consistent with sacroiliac joint pathology.[24]
- **Onset of the pain**: The patient's description of the onset of the pain, such as a description of acute, chronic, or insidious onset of pain, along with other symptoms is important. Although patients may describe a single incident that acutely initiated the pain, the injury results from an accumulation of repetitive stresses and macrotrauma developed during the episode described.
- **Severity of pain**: Several reliable pain severity scales can be used to quantify the patient's pain (see Box 1-5).
- **Mechanism of injury**: Any known mechanism of injury (e.g., flexion, extension, lateral bending, or rotation) can be used to possibly identify the involved structures. A direct blow to the lumbar or thoracic area may cause a contusion of the involved structures, the kidneys, or other internal organs. Sports (e.g., gymnastics, blocking in football, cheerleading) in which the spine is regularly placed in hyperextension place increased compressive stress on the pars interarticularis and other posterior spinal structures. Offensive linemen in football place enormous compressive and shear forces on the lumbar spine and therefore are particularly predisposed to injury.[25] Frequently, patients are unable to identify a specific episode of injury.

- **Consistency of the pain**: The frequency and consistency of the patient's pain can serve as an indication of the type of pathology that is involved.
  - **Constant pain**: Pain that is unyielding and does not increase or subside based on the position of the patient's spine is indicative of chemically induced pain, such as that resulting from inflammation of the dural sheath. Unremitting pain or pain that cannot be modified by change of position can also be a signal of another space-occupying lesion such as a tumor and warrants referral.
  - **Intermittent pain**: Symptoms that increase or decrease based on the position of the spine (e.g., flexion, extension, lateral bending) indicate pain of a mechanical origin. Placing the body in one position may cause compression or stretching of a nerve root. Likewise, relief (or a decrease in symptoms) can be obtained by moving the spine into a specific position that lessens the pressure on the involved structure, a posture that the patient will try to maintain.
- **Bowel or bladder control**: Reports of changes in bowel or bladder control, **incontinence**, urinary retention, or slow-healing wounds may indicate central stenosis, lower nerve root lesions (e.g., cauda equina syndrome) or spinal cord injury warranting immediate referral to a physician.[26]
- **Disability associated with low back pain**: Many questionnaires, such as the Oswestry Disability Index, attempt to measure the extent of disability attributed to low back pain. Objective measures of disability provide useful outcome measures, which are particularly helpful with the nonspecific origin of most low back pain. The Oswestry Disability Index has demonstrated reliability and detects clinically significant changes in patient-reported disability in the general adult population; however, it has not been validated in an athletic population.[27,28]
  - **Sleeping pattern**: Disrupted sleep or difficulty falling asleep is commonly associated with low back pain. Question the patient regarding the most comfortable sleeping position: lying on the stomach positions the trunk in extension while lying supine causes the spine to assume a relatively flexed position.

✱ Practical Evidence

Peak bone mineral density is realized between 20 and 30 years of age. Because of hormonal changes and decreased calcium intake, the risk of osteoporosis may be increased in endurance runners. Although this change is most common in females, males are also affected. After peak bone mass has been obtained, both males and females demonstrate decreased density with each cycle of remodeling. In females, this loss is accelerated in early menopause. Consequently, decreased bone mineral density increases the risk of stress fractures.[29]

Nonorganic Origin of Pain

Low back pain may be nonorganic in nature, with no structural or physiological source. **Waddell signs** are physical findings such as pain with axial loading, widespread tenderness, and an excessive show of emotion that may be present in patients with greater behavioral influences on their pain. Patients who display Waddell signs have worse outcomes than patients who do not.[30–32] Unlike malingering patients, nonorganic low back pain is not generally associated with potential secondary gain such as receiving workman's compensation or validation of not playing in the case of an athlete.

By their very nature, lumbopelvic disorders are difficult to evaluate objectively, forcing the clinician to rely on subjective information gained from the history of the injury. On occasion, a person may intentionally describe or produce symptoms for secondary gain, such as prolonging the absence from work or activity. Malingering is extremely difficult to diagnose and the label of "malingerer" should be used only in the presence of conclusive evidence. Warning signs of malingering include persistent noncompliance, inconsistency between the physical exam and stated symptoms, and referral from an insurance company or attorney.[30] The **Hoover test** (Special Test 13-1) is a classic procedure used to determine whether the individual is malingering during the performance of functional and special tests.[33–35]

Inspection

A general inspection of the entire spinal column is necessary to determine the alignment in the sagittal and frontal planes. The muscles of the spinal column and torso require inspection to determine the presence of spasm or atrophy, each indicating a possible irritation of one or more spinal nerve roots. Last, finite inspection at the level of each spinal segment may provide an indication of a malalignment of one vertebra relative to the ones above and below it. The patient's general posture, as described in Chapter 6, also must be assessed.

Functional assessment

Observing the patient performing activities or assuming positions that aggravate or alleviate the symptoms provides compelling evidence about the involved structures.

- **Gait observation**: Note the patient's gait. Spinal pain may grossly influence walking and running gait. Common gait deviations resulting from spinal pain

Incontinence A loss of bowel or bladder control.

Special Test 13-1
Hoover Test

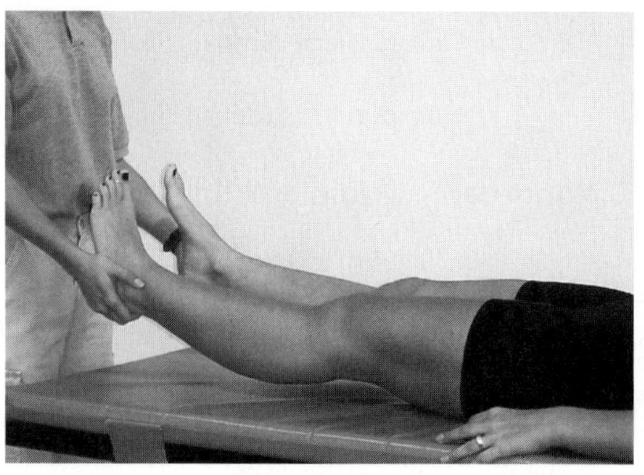

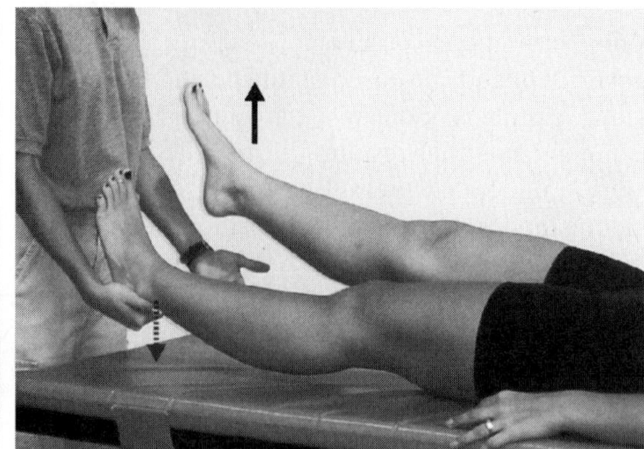

The Hoover Test is used to identify if a patient is actually exerting effort during the testing procedure. A positive test suggests that the patient is malingering.

Patient Position	Supine
Position of Examiner	At the feet of the patient with the evaluator's hands cupping the calcaneus of each leg
Evaluative Procedure	The patient attempts an active straight leg raise on the involved side
Positive Test	The patient does not attempt to lift the leg and the examiner does not sense pressure from the uninvolved leg pressing down on the hand as should instinctively happen.
Implications	The patient is not attempting to perform the test (i.e., malingering).
Evidence	Absent or inconclusive in the literature

include a slouched, shuffling, or shortened gait. Chapter 6 provides detailed discussion regarding gait analysis. In addition, a patient's unwillingness to move the body as a whole after injury to the spinal region may become evident during walking.

- **General movement and posture**: Observe the patient for poor postural movement habits such as improper standing or sitting postures and improper lifting mechanics (e.g., bending instead of squatting to lift objects). When the patient is standing, observe for the **mannequin posture**, where the involved-side leg is flexed at the hip and knee with the pelvis tilted to the involved side. This posture is associated with a disk herniation.[36]

General inspection

- **Frontal curvature**: Inspect the alignment of the lumbar, thoracic, and cervical vertebrae with the patient lying prone and while he or she is standing. Normally this alignment should be straight. Lateral curvature of the spinal column, scoliosis, generally afflicts the thoracic or lumbar spine (or both) in the frontal plane (Fig. 13-14). Scoliosis may be visible when the patient is bearing weight, not bearing weight, or both. Functional and structural scoliosis may be detected by having the patient flex the spine segmentally in a slow, controlled manner while bearing weight (Special Test 13-2). Functional scoliosis is marked by the curvature's disappearance during forward flexion; in structural scoliosis, the curve is still present in this position. Individuals who are suspected of having previously undiagnosed scoliosis need to be referred to a physician for further evaluation, although scoliosis is a common finding in adults who do not suffer any back pain.[37] Adolescents who have been previously diagnosed with scoliosis need monitoring on a regular basis for increases in the amount of curvature.

*** Practical Evidence**

With the exception of general back pain and cosmetic concerns, patients with late-onset idiopathic scoliosis who do not receive treatment fair as well as those patients who do receive treatment.[38]

- **Sagittal curvature**: From the side, observe the patient's lordotic cervical, kyphotic thoracic, lumbar lordotic, and sacral kyphotic curves. Changes in any of these curves may be causative or result from pathology. In

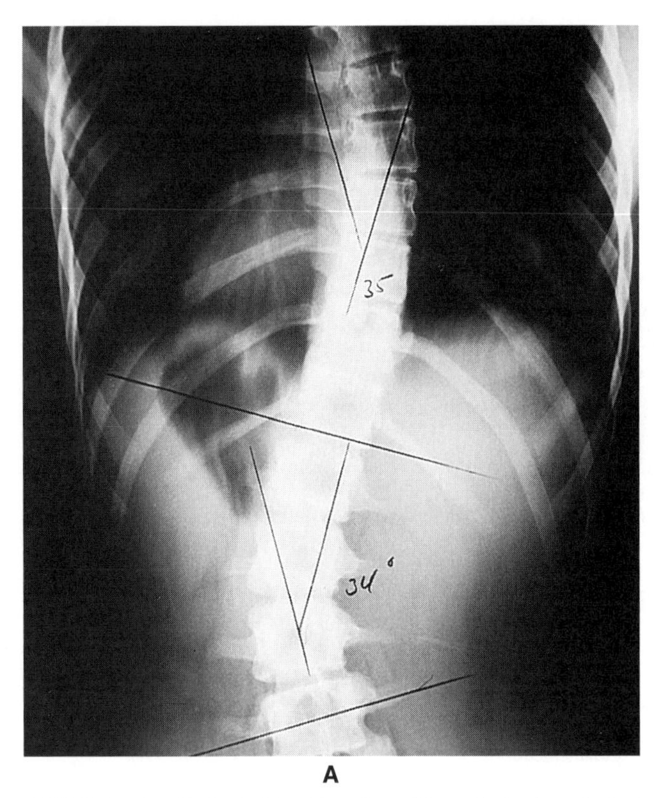

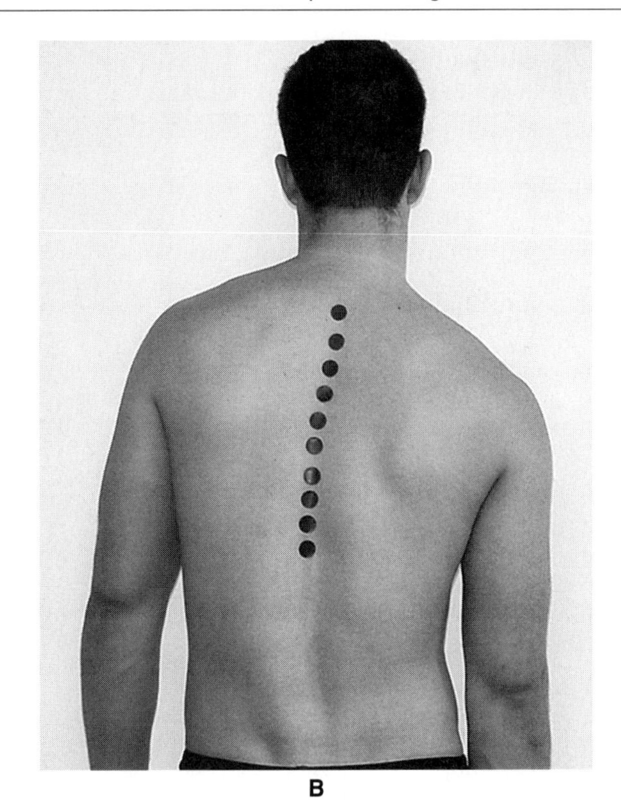

FIGURE 13-14 ■ Scoliosis, lateral bending of the spinal column in the frontal plane. (A) A radiograph of moderate to severe scoliosis. (B) Dots have been placed over the spinous processes.

either event, these changes produce abnormal stresses on spinal structures, leading to pain and dysfunction. Muscular spasm, as seen in patients with acute injuries, usually serves to flatten these curves.

- **Skin markings**: Note the presence of any darkened areas of skin pigmentation. **Café-au-lait spots** (Fig. 13-15) may be normally occurring skin discolorations or may represent collagen disease or **neurofibromatosis**.[39,40]

Inspection of the thoracic spine

- **Breathing patterns**: Injury to the thoracic vertebrae, pressure on the thoracic nerve roots, or trauma to the ribs or costal cartilage may result in pain during respiration, resulting in irregular or shallow breathing patterns.
- **Bilateral comparison of skin folds**: The natural folds of the patient's torso are compared for symmetry. Unevenness or asymmetry of these folds could be caused by a bilateral muscle imbalance, increased or decreased kyphosis, scoliosis, or disease.
- **Shape of the chest**: The chest should be shaped symmetrically from side to side. An advanced scoliosis may cause a noticeable "rib hump" as the vertebrae rotate and sidebend as the disease progresses. The vertebral rotation causes the ribs to become prominent in the posterior aspect of the spine.

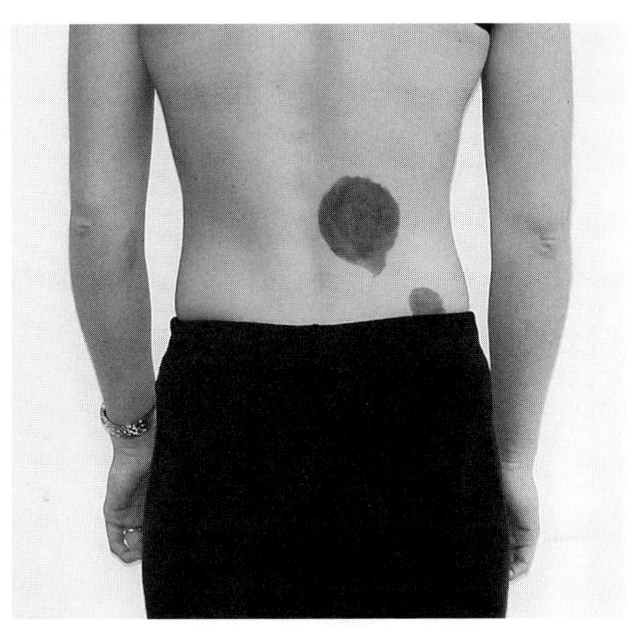

FIGURE 13-15 ■ Café-au-lait spots. These skin discolorations could potentially represent a collagen disorder, neurofibromatosis 1, or can be normally occurring.

Neurofibromatosis Increased cell growth of neural tissues; normally a benign condition; pain possible secondary to pressure on the local nerves.

Special Test 13-2
Test for Scoliosis (Adams Forward Bend Test)

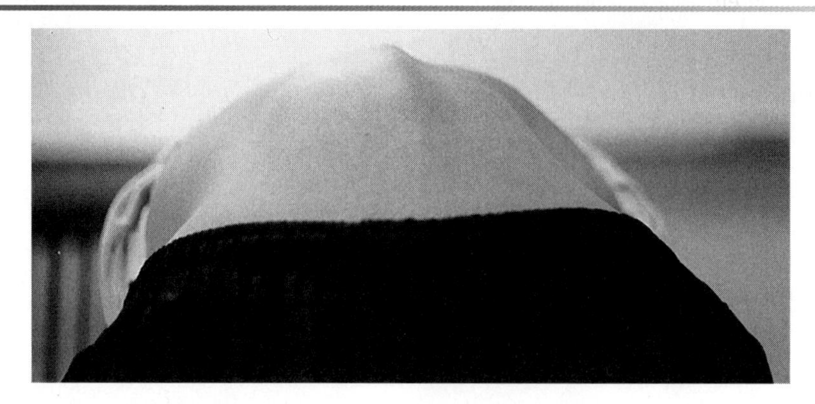

Posterior view of the spinal column while the patient flexes the spine; note the presence of a hump over the left thoracic spine, suggesting scoliosis.

Patient Position	Standing with hands held in front with the arms straight
Position of Examiner	Seated in front of or behind the patient
Evaluative Procedure	The patient bends forward, sliding the hands down the front of each leg.
Positive Test	An asymmetrical hump is observed along the lateral aspect of the thoracolumbar spine and rib cage.
Implications	If scoliosis is present but disappears during flexion, then functional scoliosis is suggested. Scoliosis that is present while the patient is standing upright and while forwardly flexed indicates structural scoliosis.

Evidence

Inter-rater reliability

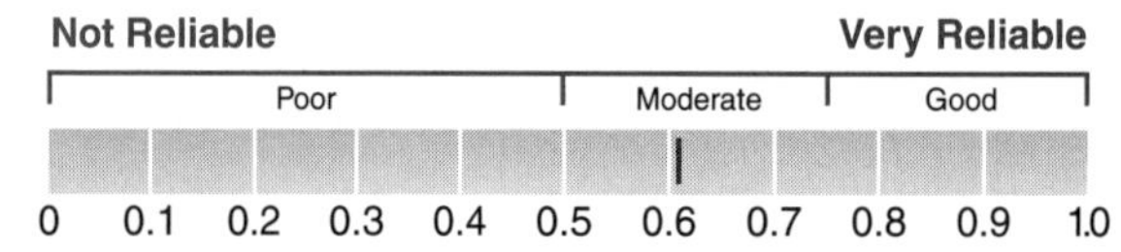

Thoracic curvature

Positive likelihood ratio

Not Useful
Useful
Very Small
Small
Moderate
Large
0 1 2 3 4 5 6 7 8 9 10

Negative likelihood ratio

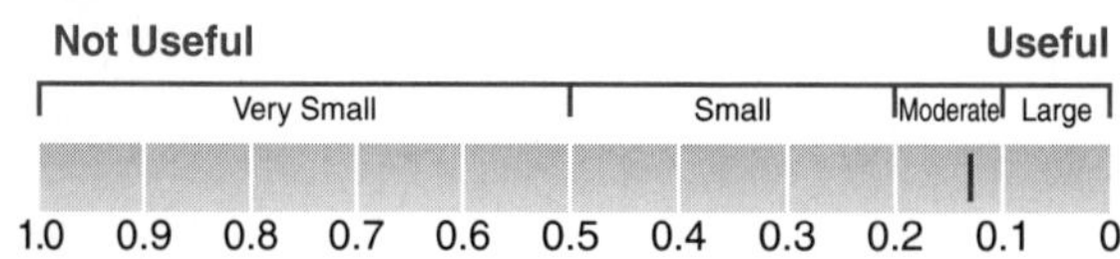

Lumbar curvature

Positive likelihood ratio

Not Useful
Useful
Very Small
Small
Moderate
Large
0 1 2 3 4 5 6 7 8 9 10

Negative likelihood ratio

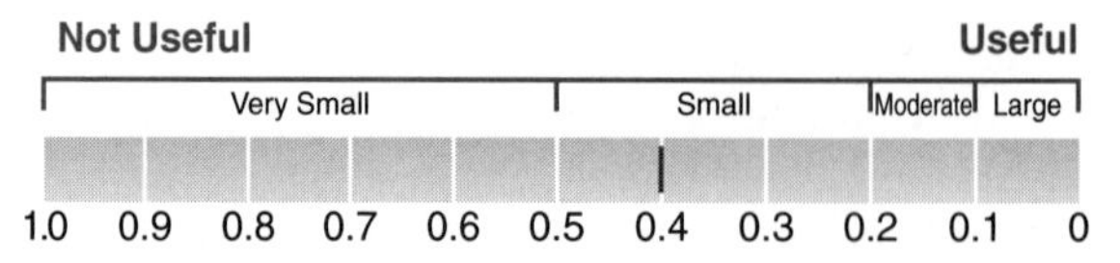

Inspection of the lumbar spine

- **Lordotic curve**: Note the patient's lordotic curve. The lordotic curve can be either accentuated or reduced in patients suffering from low back pain or trauma. Reduction of the lordotic curve may be attributed to acute pain, muscle spasm, or tightness of the hamstring muscle group. Increased lordosis may be traced to tightness in the hip flexor muscle groups or weakness in the abdominal musculature.
- **Standing posture**: While observing the patient from behind, observe for a lateral shift in the trunk and pelvis, indicating possible impingement of a nerve root. In this case, the patient instinctively shifts the upper trunk to reduce the amount of pressure on the nerve (Fig. 13-16). The shift is named for the direction the upper trunk moves relative to the patient.
- **Erector muscle tone**: Inspect the paraspinal muscles for equal tone. A unilaterally hypertrophied or atrophied muscle could indicate instability or poor or abnormal posture.
- **Faun's beard**: Observe the sacrum and lower lumbar spine for a tuft of hair, **Faun's beard**, possibly indicating **spina bifida occulta**.

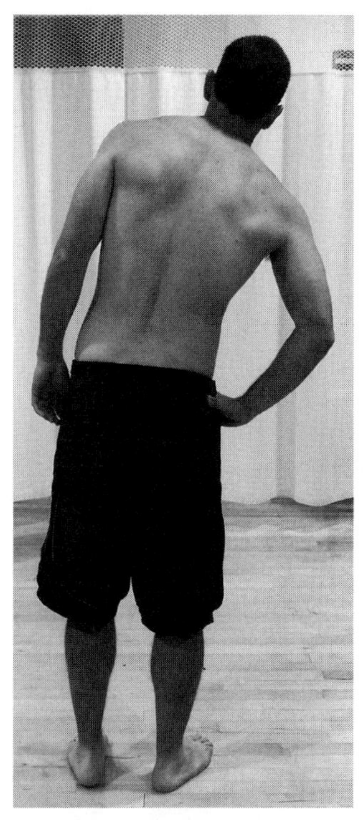

FIGURE 13-16 ■ Compensatory posture for nerve root impingement. The patient will naturally shift the body to lessen the pressure on the nerve root. The posture is labeled for the side of the patient's body. This would be a right compensatory posture.

Table 13-6 Bony Landmarks During Palpation

Structure	Landmark
Cervical Vertebral Bodies	On the same level as the spinous processes
C1 Transverse Process	One finger's breadth inferior to the mastoid process
C3–C4 Vertebrae	Posterior to the hyoid bone
C4–C5 Vertebrae	Posterior to the thyroid cartilage
C6 Vertebra	Posterior to the cricoid cartilage; moves during flexion and extension of the cervical spine
C7 Vertebra	Prominent posterior spinous process
Thoracic Spinal Bodies	Underlying the spinous processes of the superior vertebra
T1 Vertebra	Prominent protrusion inferior to the cervical spine; does not disappear during extension
T2 Vertebra	Posterior from the jugular notch of the sternum
T3 Vertebra	Even with the medial border of the scapular spine
T7 Vertebra	Even with the inferior angle of scapula
Lumbar Spinal Bodies	Upper portion of the spinous processes overlying the inferior half of the same vertebra
L3 Vertebra	In normal body build, posterior from the umbilicus
L4 Vertebra	Level with the iliac crest
L5 Vertebra	Typically demarcated by bilateral dimples, but variable from person to person
S2	At the level of the posterior superior iliac spine

Spina bifida occulta Incomplete closure of the spinal vertebrae.

PALPATION

Table 13-6 presents a list of landmarks used to orient the location of specific spinal structures. The ease of palpation of these structures depends on the patient's body mass. Identification of landmarks, including vertebral level (e.g., L4 or L5) has poor inter-rater reliability, making the validity of techniques that require known landmarks questionable from the start.[41]

Palpation of the Thoracic Spine

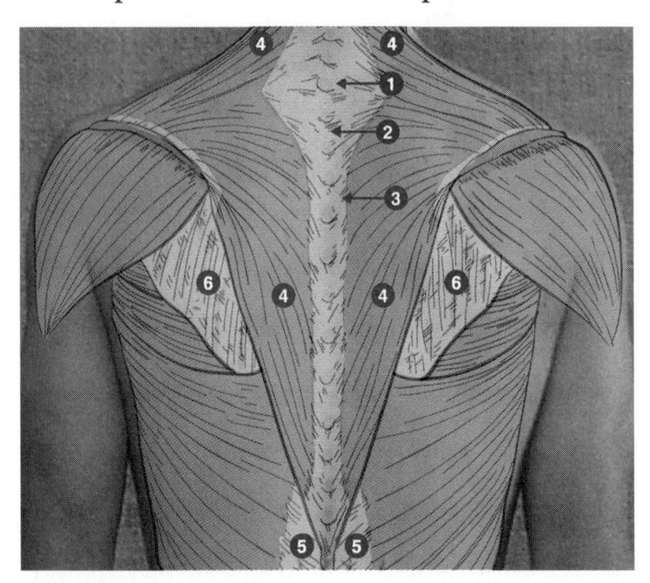

1 Spinous processes: Palpate the spinous processes along the length of the thoracic spine. The spinous process of T3 normally aligns with the medial border of the scapular spine, and T7 aligns with the inferior angle of the scapula. Use the "Rule of 3's" (Table 13-7) to help orient yourself to the spinous processes relative to the vertebral body.

2 Supraspinous ligaments: Identify the supraspinous ligament as it fills the space between the spinous processes.

Table 13-7 Relative Alignment of the Thoracic Spinous Processes (Rule of 3's)

Level	Spinous Process Alignment
T1–T3	At the same level as the transverse processes and the vertebral body
T4–T6	Midway between the transverse processes of the originating vertebra and the transverse processes of the one below
T7–T9	At the same level as the transverse processes of the inferior vertebra
T10	At the level of the T11 vertebral body
T11	Halfway between T11 and T12
T12	At the same level as the T12 vertebral body

Other ligamentous structures of the spinal column can be palpated lateral to this structure.

3 Costovertebral junction: The articulations between the ribs and thoracic vertebrae are not directly palpable when they are covered by large paravertebral muscles but can be palpated on individuals with slender to normal builds.

4 Trapezius: Palpate the middle and lower portions of both trapezius muscles from their origin on the spinous processes to their insertions on the scapular spines. The rhomboid major and minor and the levator scapulae lie underneath the middle and upper trapezius. Tenderness of these muscles, including the presence of trigger points, may be elicited during palpation.

5 Paravertebral muscles: Palpate the paravertebral muscles as they become prominent in the area of the scapula along their length to the pelvis (actual muscle group not shown in this figure).

6 Scapular muscles: Palpate the muscles acting on the scapula to identify areas of tenderness, spasm, or other abnormality.

Palpation of the Lumbar Spine

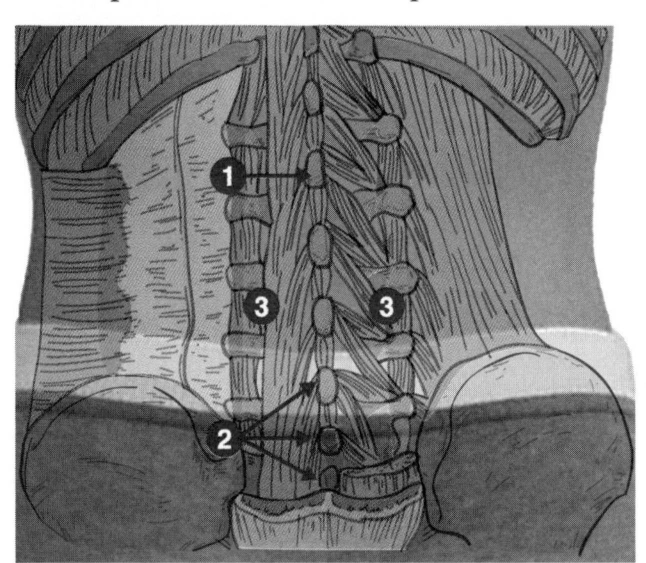

1 Spinous processes: Palpate the spinous processes along the entire length of the lumbar spine, with the L4 process at approximately the same level as the iliac crests. The L5 spinous process is relatively smaller and rounder than the other spinous processes and normally disappears when the hip is passively extended.

2 Step-off deformity: During palpation of the lumbar spinous process, note whether one process is located more anteriorly than the one below it. Step-off deformities indicate **spondylolisthesis**, which most commonly occurs between the L4 and L5 or L5 and S1 vertebrae.

3 **Paravertebral muscles**: From the thoracic spine, continue to palpate the length of the paravertebral muscles along the lumbar spine. Tightness of these muscles increases the amount of lordosis in the lumbar spine.

Palpation of the Sacrum and Pelvis

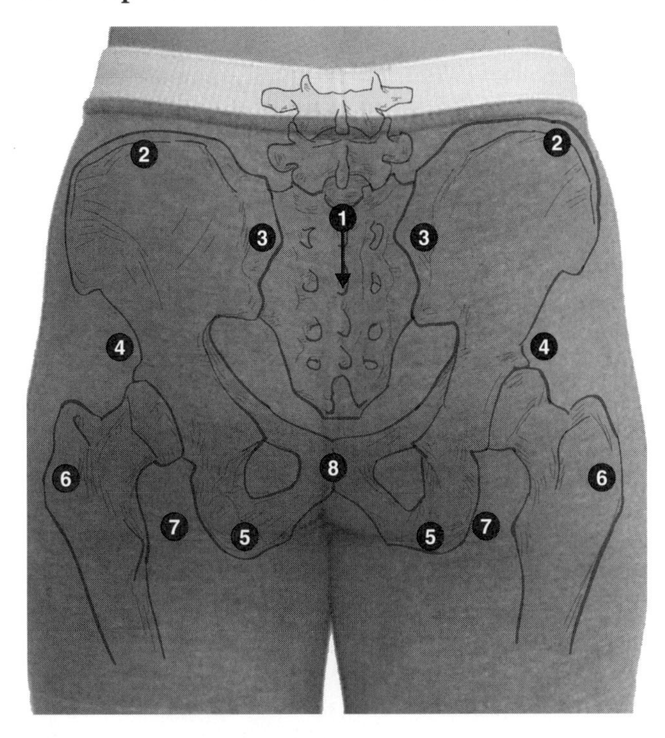

1 **Median sacral crests**: Attempt to palpate the fused remnants of the sacral spinous processes from below the L5 vertebra to the midportion of the gluteal crease.

2 **Iliac crests**: Palpate laterally from the PSIS to find the iliac crests and anteriorly to locate the anterior superior iliac spine (ASIS) and check for level and symmetry (see Fig. 3–9).

3 **Posterior superior iliac spine**: Locate the PSIS near the inferior portion of the gluteal dimples (Fig. 13-17). Under normal circumstances, these bony landmarks are palpable and align at the same level (see Fig. 6–13). Tenderness may indicate sacroiliac pathology.

4 **Gluteals**: Posteriorly, locate the gluteus maximus, the most prominent muscle mass. From this point, palpate laterally to identify the gluteus medius as it emerges from beneath the iliac crest. Atrophy of the gluteals can indicate nerve pathology.

5 **Ischial tuberosity**: Locate the ischial tuberosity at the proximal aspect of the hamstrings. The ischial tuberosity

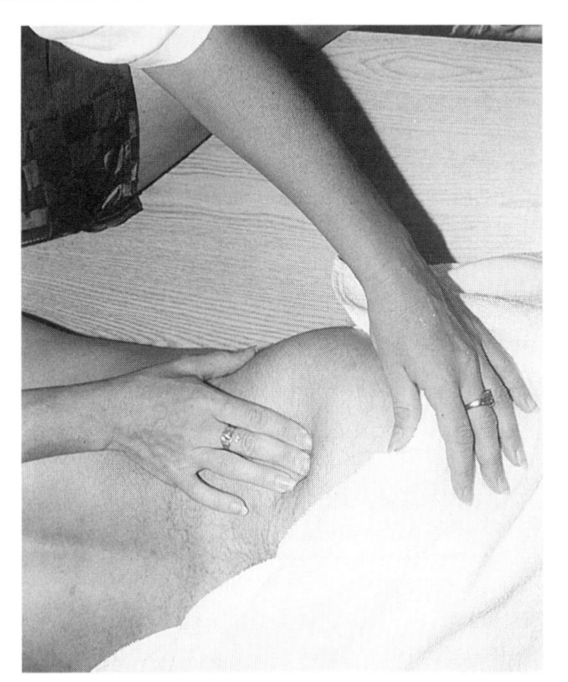

FIGURE 13-17 ■ Location of the posterior superior iliac spine.

may become irritated secondary to high hamstring strains, ischial bursitis, or contusive forces.

6 **Greater trochanter**: Palpate the lateral femur to locate the greater trochanter, which should be bilaterally level. During active or passive internal and external hip rotation, the greater trochanter can be felt as it rolls beneath the fingers. Identify localized pain that may be caused by inflammation of the gluteus medius attachment or by greater trochanteric bursitis versus referred spinal pain.

7 **Sciatic nerve**: Palpate the sciatic nerve by placing the thumb on the ischial tuberosity and the third finger on the PSIS. The second finger will fall into the sciatic notch. The nerve is at its most superficial point as it passes by the ischial tuberosity. Tenderness on one tuberosity and not on the other may indicate sciatic nerve inflammation.

8 **Pubic symphysis**: Locate the symphysis pubis on the anterior portion of the pelvis, just superior to the genitalia at the midline of the body. This structure may become subluxed secondary to a hard jarring injury such as a fall. Use discretion and appropriate draping when palpating this area.

Joint and Muscle Function Assessment

Although various forms of goniometers and protractors are available to assess the ROM available in the spine, in actual practice, gross observation of the ROM is typically used and the grade is expressed as a percentage of the total possible normal ROM. Similar to what occurs with the body's other joints, spinal ROM is graded quantitatively as well as qualitatively, noting any pain produced during or

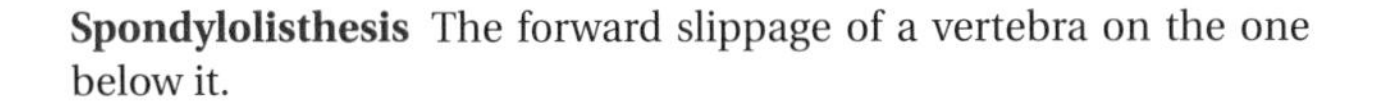

Spondylolisthesis The forward slippage of a vertebra on the one below it.

at the end of the movement. ROM fluctuates throughout the day, even in those with chronic low pain. Reliability will be improved if measurements are taken at the same time each day.[42]

A set of 10 repetitions of any particular motion can be used to determine the effect of repeated movement on the quantity and location of pain. In general, repeated movements in one direction that result in pain radiating distally are to be avoided during the rehabilitation program. Motions resulting in the centralization of pain should be incorporated in the rehabilitation program. This latter concept forms the basis of the **McKenzie exercises** and rehabilitation protocol.[43]

The total motion produced by the thoracic and lumbar spines is difficult to isolate into its individual segments. The motions of these two areas are evaluated as a single unit, the trunk. In addition, it is difficult to isolate passive motion in a gravity-dependent position, so active and passive ROM testing often occurs concurrently when the techniques described in the "Active Range of Motion" section are used.

Tape measures, inclinometers, goniometers, and specially designed devices have been used to quantify spinal ROM measurement. Goniometry Box 13-1 describes the use of a tape measure to assess trunk flexion and extension. Goniometry Box 13-2 describes the use of a goniometer to quantify lateral bending and rotation.

Goniometry Box 13-1
Trunk Flexion and Extension (Tape Measure)

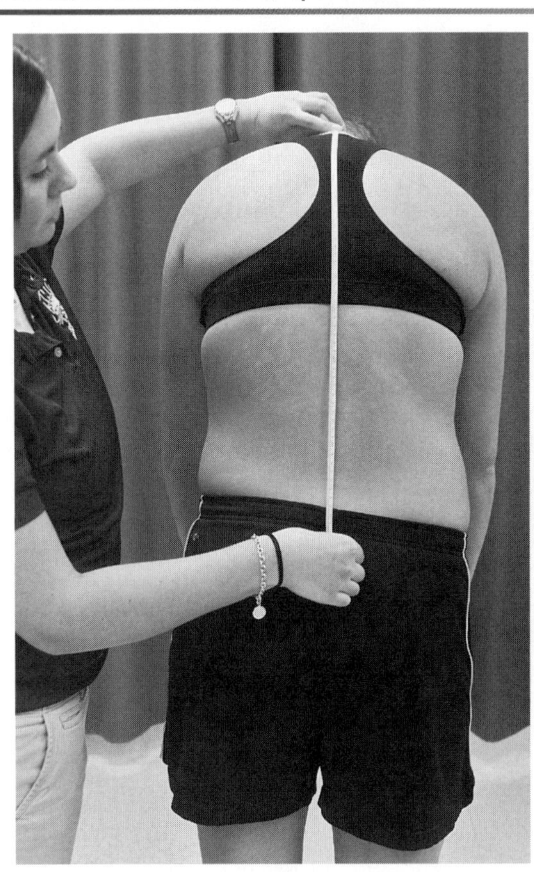

Flexion

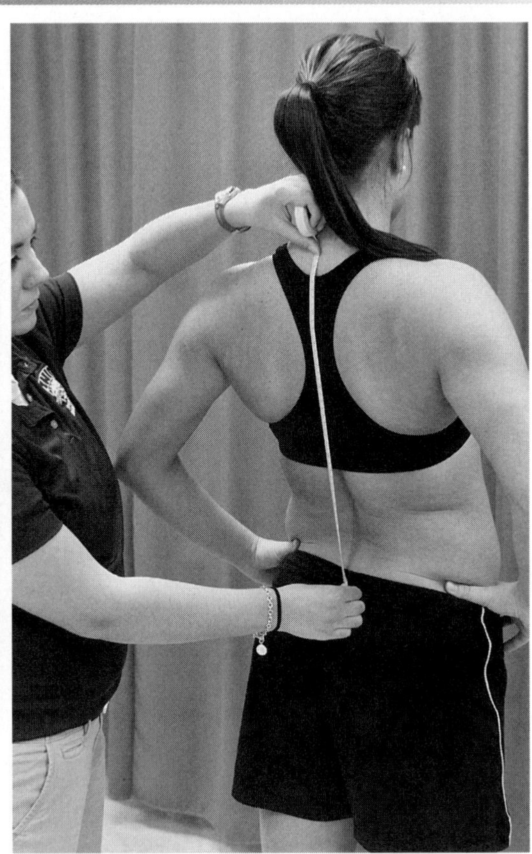

Extension

Patient Position	Standing with the knees extended, feet shoulder-width apart, and the spine in the neutral position
Procedure	
Initial Measurement	Using a tape measure, the distance (in cm) between the C7 and S1 spinous processes is determined.
Motion	The patient fully flexes or extends the trunk. Observe for pelvic rotation that is indicative of compensatory spinal motion.
Final Measurement	The distance between the C7 and S1 spinous processes is determined. The difference between the initial and final measurement is calculated and the value is recorded.

Goniometry Box 13-2
Lateral Bending and Rotation

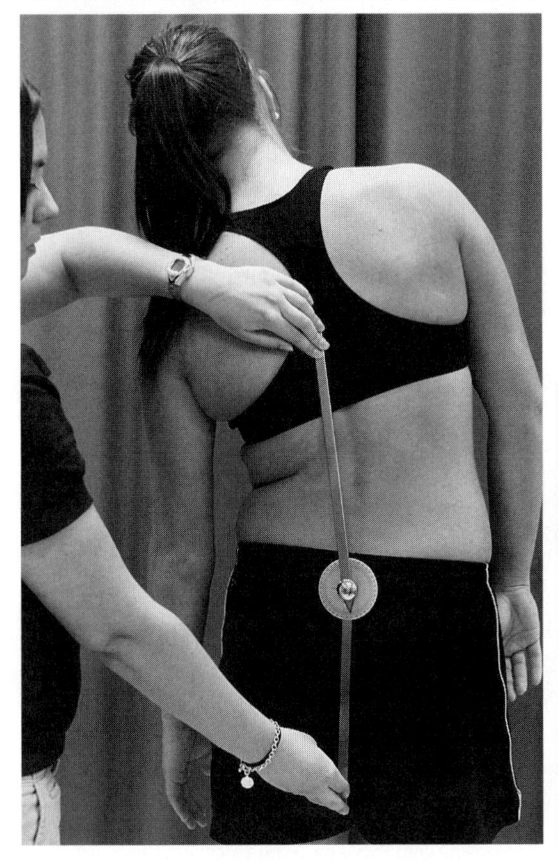

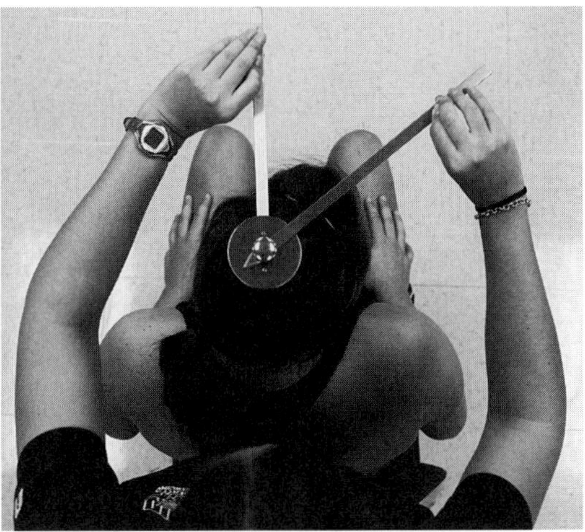

	Lateral Bending	Rotation
Patient Position	Standing with the knees extended and the spine in the neutral position	Seated The feet are placed firmly on the floor
Goniometer Alignment		
Fulcrum	The axis is aligned over the S1 spinous process	Aligned over the center of the patient's head
Proximal Arm	Aligned over the median sacral crest	Parallel to a line formed by the iliac crests
Distal Arm	Aligned with the C7 vertebrae	Parallel to the line formed by the two acromion processes.

The results of measurements taken with a goniometer correlate well to measurements obtained from MR images.[44] Goniometry Boxes 13-3, 13-4, and 13-5 present the use of an inclinometer to quantify spinal motion.

Active range of motion

Active range of motion is performed with the patient standing. ROM assessment, as described in this section, is contraindicated for patients with acute injuries until the possibility of a vertebral fracture or dislocation has been ruled out.

- **Flexion and extension**: Active trunk flexion is assessed with the patient standing. Note any pain or "catches" in the movement pattern. To aid in documenting the available motion and the progression of this motion over time, the distance from the fingertips to the floor can be measured (the accuracy of this

McKenzie exercises A protocol of exercises involving spinal flexion and extension used during the treatment and rehabilitation of back injuries, for improving range of motion and strengthening the spine.

Goniometry Box 13-3
Trunk Flexion and Extension (Inclinometer)

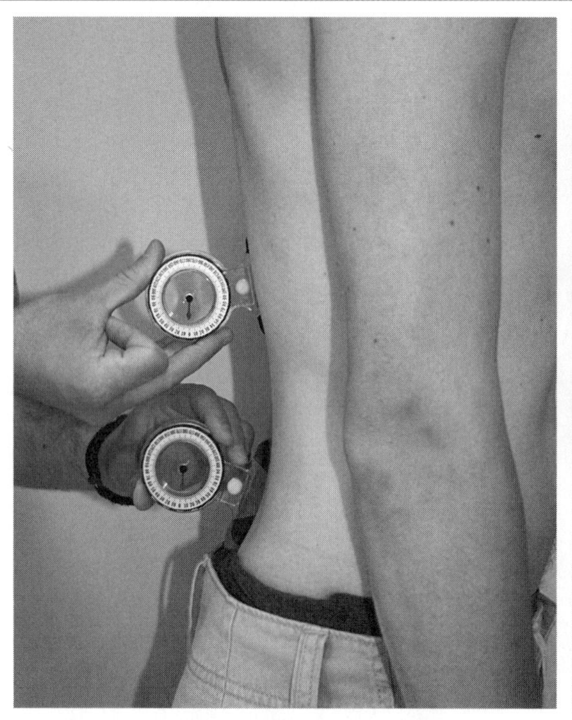

Flexion

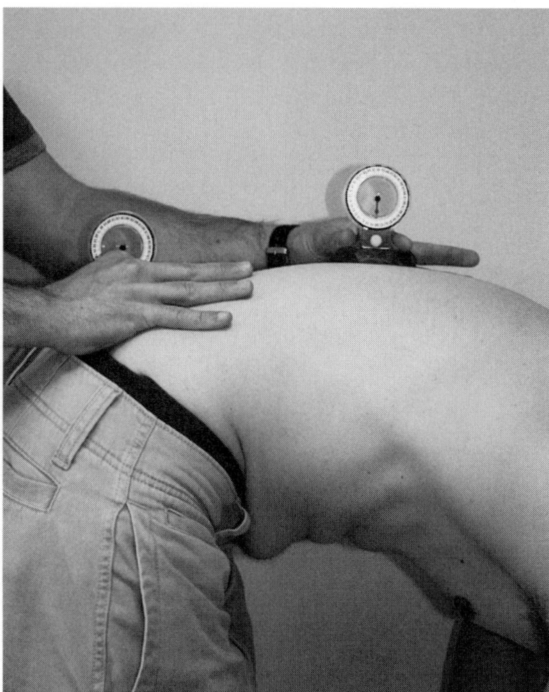

Extension

Patient Position	Standing with the feet shoulder-width apart
Procedure	Place one inclinometer at midline of spine in line with PSIS. The second inclinometer is placed 15 cm above first. Both inclinometers are set at 0°.
Measurement	
Motion	The patient forward flexes while the clinician holds the inclinometers.
Final Measurement	Flexion ROM is recorded as superior inclinometer reading minus the reading obtained from the inferior inclinometer. The reading at the superior inclinometer represents hip and spine motion; reading at the inferior inclinometer represents hip motion only.
Comments	This technique can be performed using a single inclinometer: Have the patient forward flex. Position and read the inferior goniometer, moving the inferior goniometer proximally and taking a reading. Motion measurements taken using inclinometers demonstrate a high correlation with measurements taken on MRI images.[44]

measurement is affected by tightness of the hamstrings and calf muscles, hip movement, and scapular protraction). Even though this position allows gravity to assist the movement, it is a more accurate indication of available motion than trunk flexion from the **hook-lying position**. Testing in the hook-lying position is the initial step to assess the strength of the abdominal muscles as they overcome the weight of the trunk. To avoid motion initiating at the hips and ensure that spinal flexion is being observed, forward flexion is begun by bending the patient's chin to the chest and then rolling the flexion down the vertebral column until hip flexion is seen or felt (Fig. 13-18).

Hook-lying position Lying supine with the hips and knees flexed and the feet flat on the table.

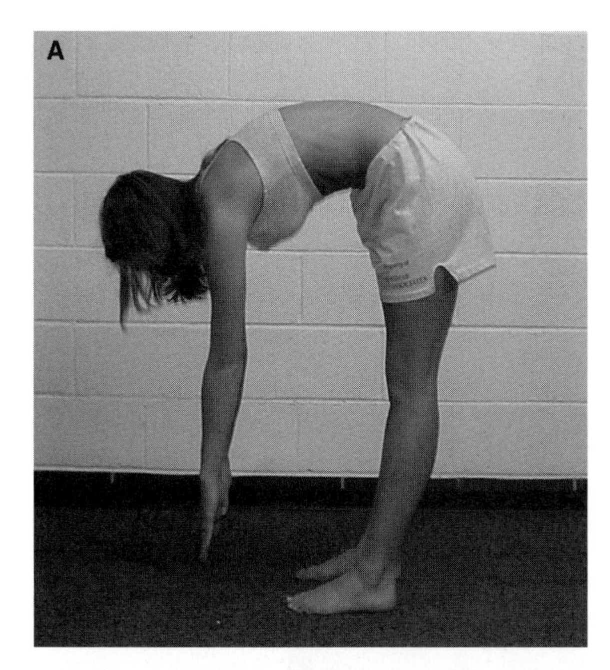

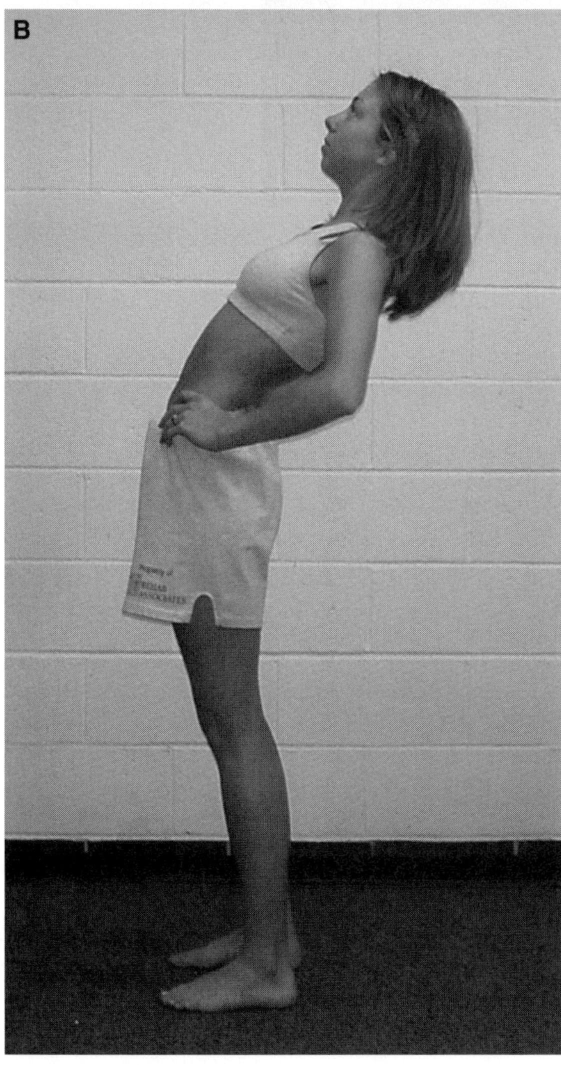

FIGURE 13-18 ■ Active trunk (A) flexion and (B) extension.

Normally, the abdominal muscles receive concurrent innervation from the T5–T12 nerve roots. **Beevor's sign** (Special Test 13-3), a modified sit-up, can indicate pathology to the lower thoracic nerve roots.

Extension is also measured with the patient standing, feet shoulder-width apart and hands on the hips, while the spine is slowly extended. The end range occurs when the hips begin to extend (see Fig. 13-18).

- **Lateral bending**: The patient stands with the feet shoulder-width apart and the hand opposite the direction of the movement resting on the ilium. The patient then bends the trunk laterally, attempting to touch the fingertips to the ground as the clinician stabilizes the pelvis to prevent lateral tilt. The distance between the ground and the fingertips can be compared bilaterally, measured, and recorded (Fig. 13-19).
- **Rotation**: The patient is placed in the sitting position to stabilize the pelvis and lower extremity. The patient then rotates the shoulder girdles and spinal column as if looking behind the back (Fig. 13-20). Rotation of the trunk occurs primarily in the thoracic spine. The amount of rotation should be equal in each direction.

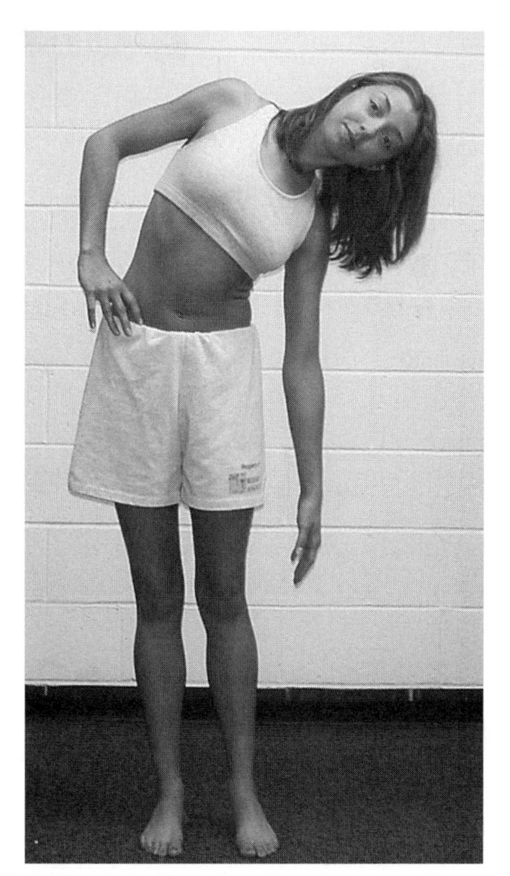

FIGURE 13-19 ■ Active lateral bending with gravity. The patient attempts to touch the fingers to the floor. Observe for normal segmental motion.

Special Test 13-3
Beevor's Sign for Thoracic Nerve Inhibition

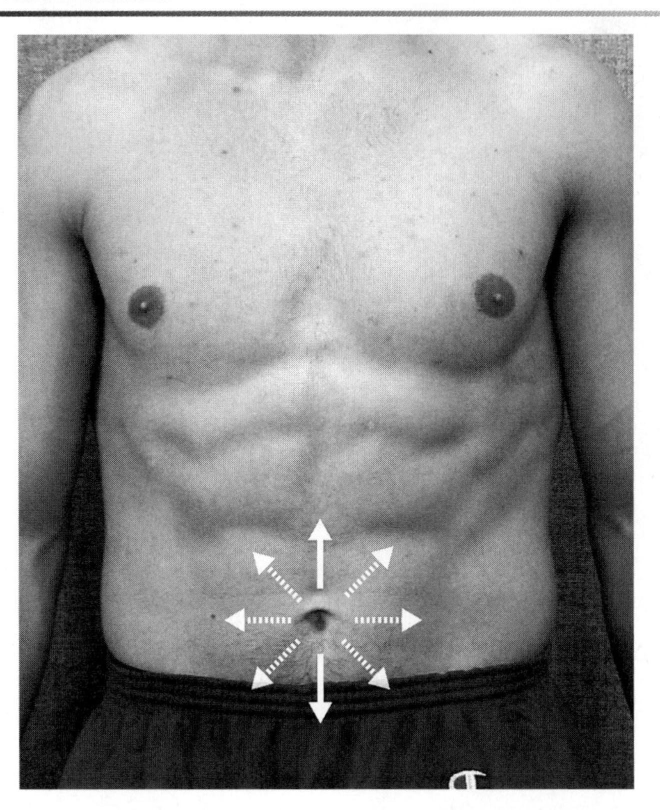

Lateral movement of the umbilicus can indicate inhibition of the thoracic nerves innervating the abdominal muscles.

Patient Position	Hook-lying
Position of Examiner	At the side of the patient
Evaluative Procedure	The patient performs an abdominal curl (partial sit-up).
Positive Test	The umbilicus moves up, down, or to one side.
Implications	Segmental involvement of the nerves innervating the rectus abdominis (T5–T12); this should draw suspicion to the paraspinal muscles innervated by the same nerve roots.
Comments	Normally the umbilicus should not move at all during this test, but will move toward the stronger muscle group in the presence of pathology.
Evidence	Absent or inconclusive in the literature

Manual muscle tests

The procedure for assessing muscle strength for muscles around the thoracic and lumbar spine is presented in Manual Muscle Testing Boxes 13-1 and 13-2. Testing of flexion and rotation also checks the strength of the muscles responsible for lateral bending. Manual Muscle Test Box 13-3 describes the procedures for relative isolation of the quadratus lumborum.

Passive range of motion

- **Flexion**: With the patient in the hook-lying position, the examiner brings the knees to the chest by lifting under the knees and thighs and flexing the hip and thoracic spine (Fig. 13-21A). Flexion in the thoracic area is limited by the rib articulations, with the exception of T11 and T12, both of which are relatively mobile.

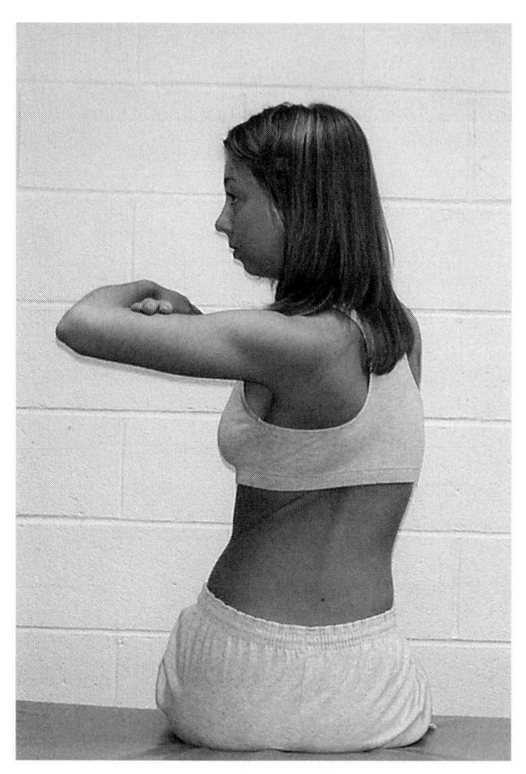

FIGURE 13-20 ■ Active trunk rotation. This motion occurs primarily in the thoracic spine.

- **Extension**: The patient is placed in the prone position with the hands flat on the table at shoulder level in a position to perform a push-up. The patient then extends the elbows, lifting the torso while the hips and legs remain flat on the table (Fig. 13–21B). This motion is limited by the spinous process' making contact with the one below it.
- **Rotation**: From the hook-lying position, the patient's legs and pelvis are rotated to bring the lateral portion of the knee toward the table while the shoulders remain flat (Fig. 13-22). The amount of motion available is compared in each direction. This movement is limited by the alignment of the facet joints. Virtually no rotation occurs between the L1 and L4 vertebrae.
- **Side gliding**: With the patient standing, the clinician braces his or her shoulder against the patient's outer portion of the upper arm. While reaching around the patient with both arms and interlocking the fingers at the iliac crest, the upper and lower trunk is glided, returning the shifted spine into a neutral position. A modification of this procedure is shown in Figure 13-23. This test is repeated on each side. Side gliding is considered significant for nerve root compression if the motion alters the quantity or location of the pain. This maneuver needs to be performed only in the presence of a laterally shifted spine or with complaints of radiating pain.

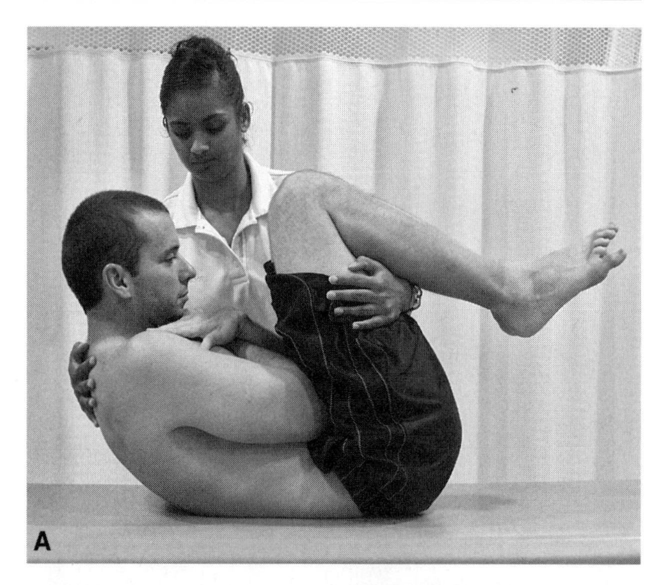

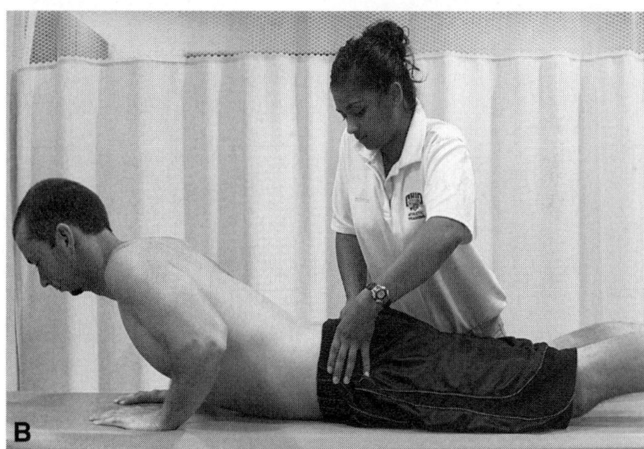

FIGURE 13-21 ■ Passive trunk (A) flexion and (B) extension.

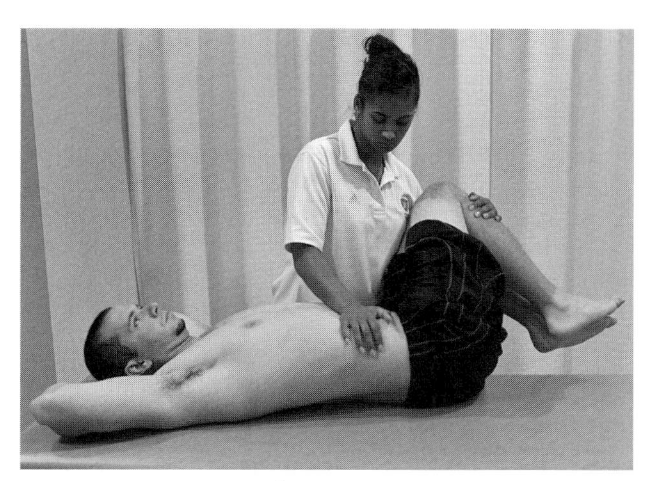

FIGURE 13-22 ■ Passive trunk rotation.

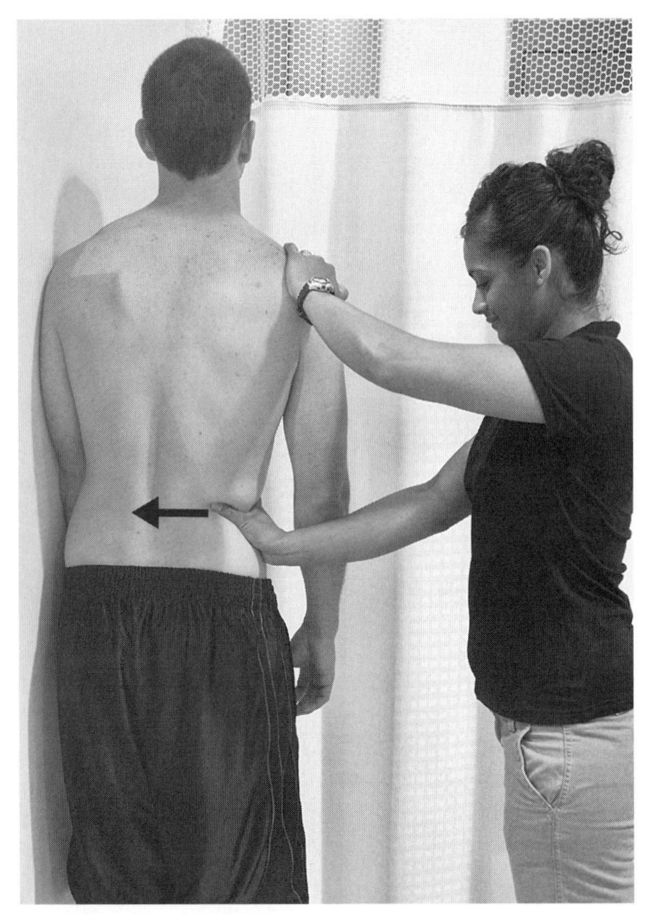

FIGURE 13-23 ■ Passive lateral glide of the trunk. The patient's shoulder is stabilized against the wall while the examiner forces the pelvis laterally.

Joint Stability Tests

There are no tests to check the integrity of single isolated ligaments. Clues as to the presence of ligamentous pathology arise during the passive testing of the spine's ROM (Table 13-8). However, these results may easily be confused with pain caused by intervertebral disk lesions or pathology to the nerve roots or peripheral nerves.

Sprains to the spinal ligaments usually occur more frequently in the cervical spine because of its increased ROM. The conclusion of a ligamentous sprain is generally derived by excluding the possibility of other pathologies. The history of a mechanism that would stress the spinal ligaments, pain along the spinal column and at the end of PROM, and static pain when the muscles are relaxed and the ligaments are acting as the only static stabilizers, can lead to the conclusion of a sprain. This assumes that all other possible pathologies have been ruled out.

Joint play tests

The total ROM available to the spinal column is equal to the sum of the motions between any two contiguous vertebrae. Although it is difficult to quantify the amount of motion that occurs at each individual spinal segment, the accessory movement of the segment can be grossly determined. Posterior–anterior joint play (Joint Play Box 13-1) is used to determine hypomobility, hypermobility or pain at a vertebral segment caused by facet joint pathologies, degenerative changes, or spondylitic defects. Hypomobility or hypermobility of the facet joints can potentially cause pain along the spinal column. Reliability of posterior–anterior testing is affected by the surface on which the patient is lying, so repeat testing should be performed on the same surface.[45]

Table 13-8 Spinal Ligaments Stressed During the End-Range of Passive Range of Motion Assessment

Motion	Ligaments Stressed
Flexion	Posterior longitudinal ligament
	Supraspinous ligament (thoracic and lumbar spine)
	Interspinous ligament
	Ligamentum flavum
Extension	Anterior longitudinal ligament
Rotation	Interspinous ligament
	Ligamentum flavum
Lateral Bending*	Interspinous ligament
	Ligamentum flavum

*Testing these motions is usually inconclusive

Special Tests

Several special tests are commonly incorporated into all spinal evaluations. They are presented in this section and the remaining special tests are described in their appropriate locations in the "Pathologies and Related Special Tests" section of this chapter.

Test for nerve root impingement

Impingement of spinal nerve roots may result from a narrowing of the intervertebral foramen caused by stenosis, facet joint degeneration, herniated intervertebral disks, or other space-occupying lesions. Increased **intrathecal** pressure can increase the patient's symptoms by forcing the annulus pulposus outward, compressing the nerve root and causing radicular pain. The **Valsalva test** (Special Test 13-4) and the **Milgram test** (Special Test 13-5) are used clinically to identify the effect of increased intrathecal pressure, but equally persuasive findings are self-reported increase in symptoms while bearing down during a bowel movement, sneezing, or while lifting weights.

Intrathecal Within the spinal canal.

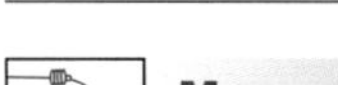

Manual Muscle Test 13-1
Trunk Flexion and Extension

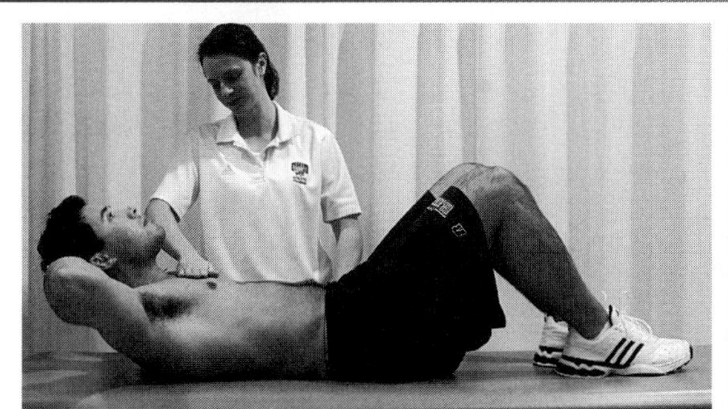

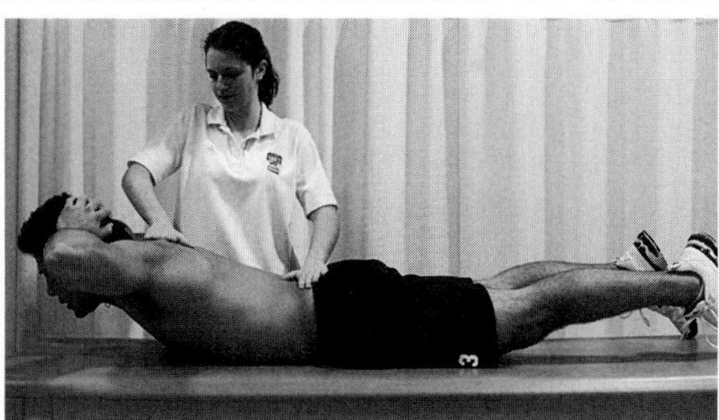

	Flexion	Extension
Patient Position	Supine	Prone
Starting Position	The knees are flexed and the feet flat on the table The patient's hands are interlocked behind the head with the elbow in line with the ears.	The elbows flexed with the hands interlocked behind the head
Stabilization	Pelvis	Pelvis
Palpation	Lateral to the abdominal midline	Lateral to the spine
Resistance	Resistance is applied to the superior sternum as the patient lifts the scapulae off the table.	Resistance is applied to the upper thoracic spine as the patient lifts the head, chest, and arms off the table.
Primary Mover(s) (Innervation)	Rectus abdominis	Iliocostalis lumborum, iliocostalis thoracis, longissimus thoracis, spinalis thoracis, semispinalis thoracis, multifidus
Secondary Mover(s) (Innervation)	Iliopsoas, rectus femoris, internal oblique and external oblique	Rotatores, latissimus dorsi, quadratus lumborum
Substitution	Reaching with shoulders/elbows, hip flexion	Hip extension
Comments	The ability to sit up with the elbow by the head constitutes a grade of 5/5. If the patient cannot do this, try again with the arms folded across the chest.	The ability to extend the trunk with the elbows by the hand constitutes a grade of 5/5. If the patient cannot do this, try again with the arms at the side and the hands behind the back.

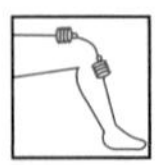

Manual Muscle Test 13-2
Trunk Rotation

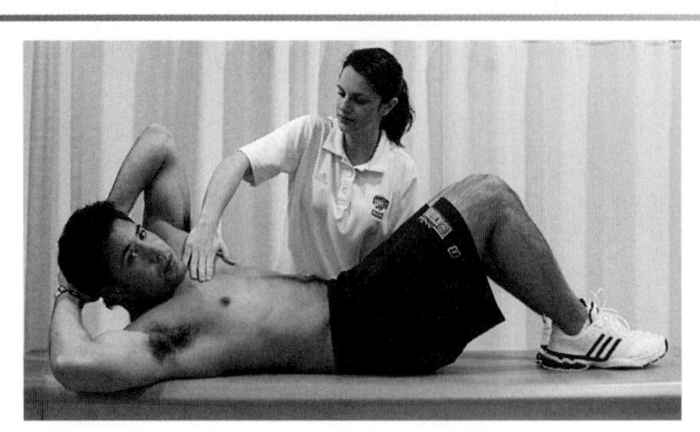

Patient Position	Supine
Starting Position	The knees are flexed and the feet flat on the table. The patient's hands are interlocked behind the head, with the elbows in line with the ears.
Stabilization	Opposite ASIS
Palpation	External oblique: Just below rib cage Internal oblique: Medial and just above anterior superior iliac spine
Resistance	Resistance is applied over the anterior aspect of the shoulder as it is rotated off the table. This procedure is repeated for the opposite side.
Primary Mover(s) (Innervation)	Internal oblique, external oblique (opposite side)
Secondary Mover(s) (Innervation)	Rotatores, multifidii (opposite side), latissimus dorsi
Substitution	Cervical flexion
Comments	The ability to sit up with the elbow by the head constitutes a grade of 5/5, even with no resistance. If the patient cannot do this, try again with the arms folded across the chest.

ASIS = anterior superior iliac spine.

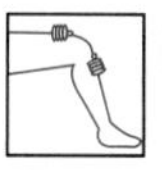

Manual Muscle Test 13-3
Pelvic Elevation

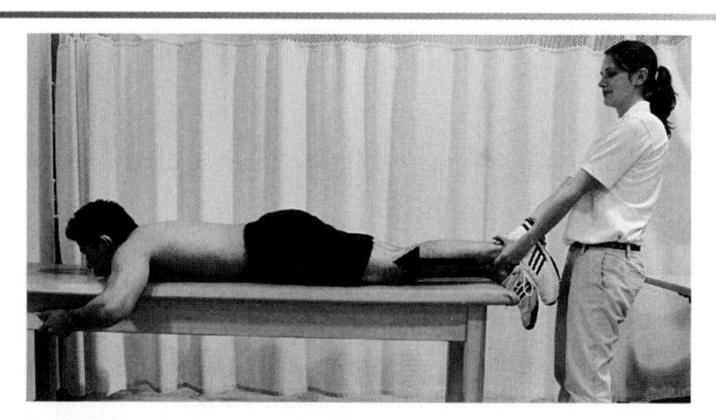

Patient Position	Supine or prone
Starting Position	The examiner grasps the patient's leg just proximal to the ankle.
Stabilization	The patient holds the edges of the table to maintain stabilization.
Palpation	Lateral lumbar spine
Resistance	The examiner distracts the leg by applying longitudinal resistance. The patient is then instructed to "hike" the pelvis, attempting to move the pelvis on the side being tested toward the rib cage.
Primary Mover(s) (Innervation)	Quadratus lumborum External oblique Internal oblique
Secondary Mover(s) (Innervation)	Latissimus dorsi (with the patient's arm's flexed) Iliocostalis lumborum
Substitution	Trunk lateral flexion (abdominals)
Comments	The test may also be performed with the patient standing on a lift and hiking the opposite leg.

Joint Play 13-1
Posterior–Anterior Vertebral Joint Play (Spring Test)

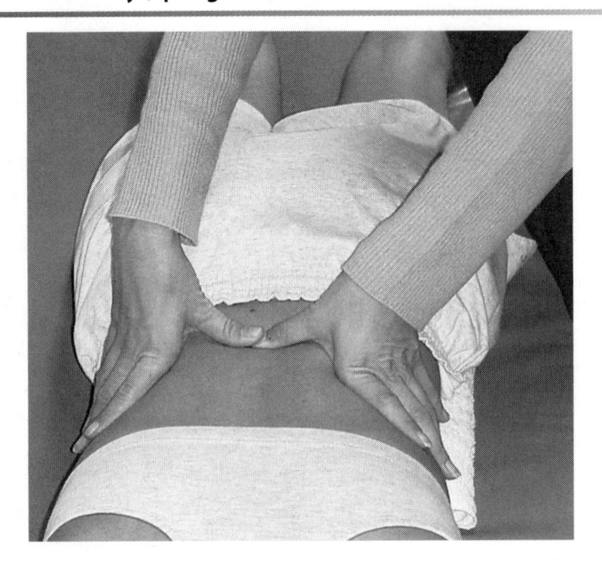

Posterior–anterior joint play is used to determine normal vertebral movement (spring).

Patient Position	Prone
Position of Examiner	Standing over the patient with the thumbs placed over the spinous process to be tested
Evaluative Procedure	The examiner carefully pushes the spinous process anteriorly, feeling for the springing of the vertebrae.
Positive Test	The vertebra does not move ("spring"), moves excessively, or pain is elicited.
Implications	Hypomobility or hypermobility of the vertebral segment
Evidence	Inter-rater reliability (pain)

Not Reliable — Very Reliable
Poor | Moderate | Good
0 0.1 0.2 0.3 0.4 0.5 0.6 0.7 0.8 0.9 1.0

Inter-rater reliability (stiffness)

Not Reliable — Very Reliable
Poor | Moderate | Good
0 0.1 0.2 0.3 0.4 0.5 0.6 0.7 0.8 0.9 1.0

Positive likelihood ratio

Not Useful — Useful
Very Small | Small | Moderate | Large
0 1 2 3 4 5 6 7 8 9 10

Negative likelihood ratio

Not Useful — Useful
Very Small | Small | Moderate | Large
1.0 0.9 0.8 0.7 0.6 0.5 0.4 0.3 0.2 0.1 0

Special Test 13-4
Valsalva Test

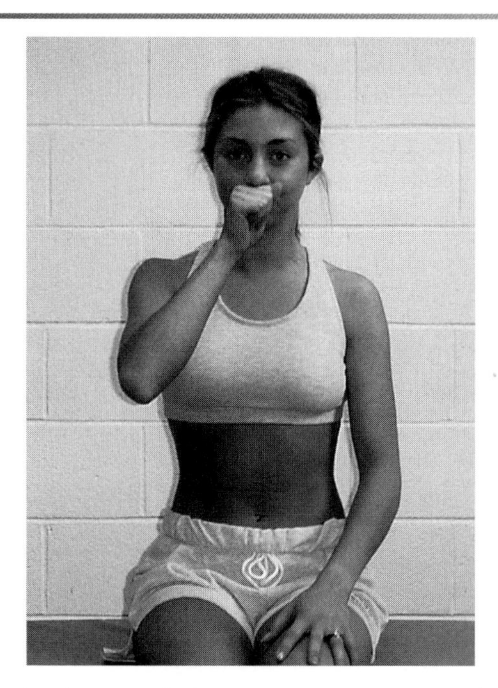

The Valsalva test attempts to increase intrathecal pressure, duplicating nerve-root pain that may be elicited while coughing or with bowel movements.

Patient Position	Sitting
Position of Examiner	Standing within arms' reach in front of the patient
Evaluative Procedure	The patient takes and holds a deep breath while bearing down similar to performing a bowel movement.
Positive Test	Increased spinal or radicular pain
Implications	Increase in intrathecal pressure causes pain secondary to a space-occupying lesion such as a herniated disk, tumor, or osteophyte anywhere along the spinal column.
Modification	If the patient is embarrassed or apprehensive about simulating a bowel movement, he or she may be instructed to blow into a closed fist as if inflating a balloon.
Comments	This can be performed for any level of the spine. The test increases intrathecal pressure, resulting in a slowing of the pulse, decreased venous return, and increased venous pressure, all of which may cause fainting.
Evidence	Inter-rater reliability

Not Reliable — Very Reliable

Poor | Moderate | Good

0 0.1 0.2 0.3 0.4 0.5 0.6 0.7 0.8 0.9 1.0

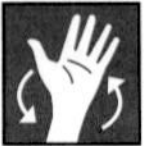

Special Test 13-5
Milgram Test

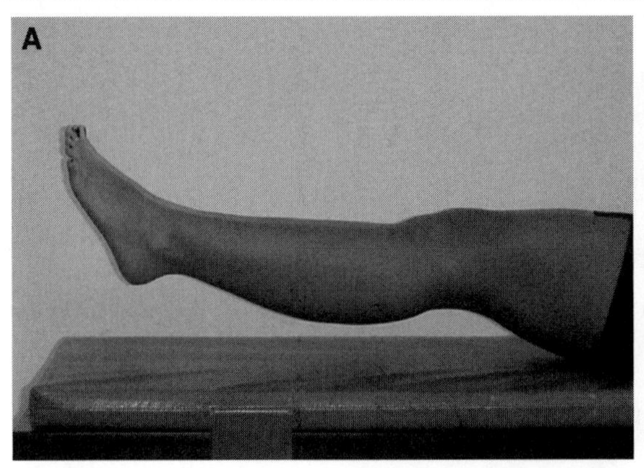

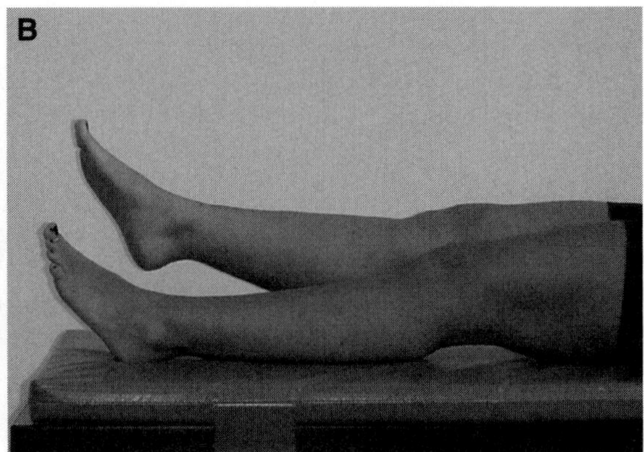

A bilateral straight leg raise is used to increase pressure on the lumbar nerve roots. In the presence of a disk lesion one or both legs will drop.

Patient Position	Supine
Position of Examiner	At the feet of the patient
Evaluative Procedure	The patient performs a bilateral straight leg raise to the height of 2–6 inches and is asked to hold the position for 30 seconds **(A)**.
Positive Test	The patient is unable to hold the position, cannot lift the leg, or experiences pain with the test **(B)**.
Implications	Intrathecal or extrathecal pressure causing an intervertebral disk to place pressure on a lumbar nerve root
Evidence	Absent or inconclusive in the literature

*** Practical Evidence**

A dermatomal distribution of pain, pain worse in the leg rather than the back, pain that worsens with coughing and sneezing, and a cold sensation in the leg are all associated with nerve root compression.[22]

Kernig's test (Special Test 13-6) is also used to identify disk pathology but also presents positive results in the presence of inflammation of the nerve or its dural sheath.

Several tests are designed to place tension on peripheral nerves, nerve roots, and the dura mater. Each of these tests involves provoking and then relieving symptoms. A positive **straight leg raise test** (Special Test 13-7) indicates either sciatic nerve irritation or a herniated intervertebral disk that is irritating the nerve root. Because many patients without disk herniations have positive findings with the straight leg raise, its usefulness in diagnosing a herniated intervertebral disk is limited. The **well or cross straight leg raise** (Special Test 13-8) can be used to discriminate between symptoms caused by sciatic neuropathy or disk herniations.[46–48] The **slump test** (Special Test 13-9), another test that assesses the effect of increasing nerve tension, can be used to identify possible compression of the lumbar nerve roots from spinal stenosis, disk herniation, or distal entrapment of a nerve. Because many patients report radicular symptoms while sitting, the slump test may be better than the straight leg raise test in reproducing symptoms.[49]

The **quadrant test** (Special Test 13-10) is used to determine dural irritation and facet joint compression.

Neurologic Testing

Because of the close involvement of the spinal column to the spinal cord and its nerve roots, many of the maladies affecting the spine may result in decreased neurologic function in the extremities as well as the trunk. Impingement of the lower spinal cord, including disk disease, or the lumbar or sacral nerve roots are likely to result in referred pain to the extremity.[52] Clinically, this involvement can be determined through the use of manual muscle tests, deep tendon reflexes, and sensory testing. Chapter 21 discusses the management of acute spinal injuries.

Special Test 13-6
Kernig's Test/Brudzinski Test

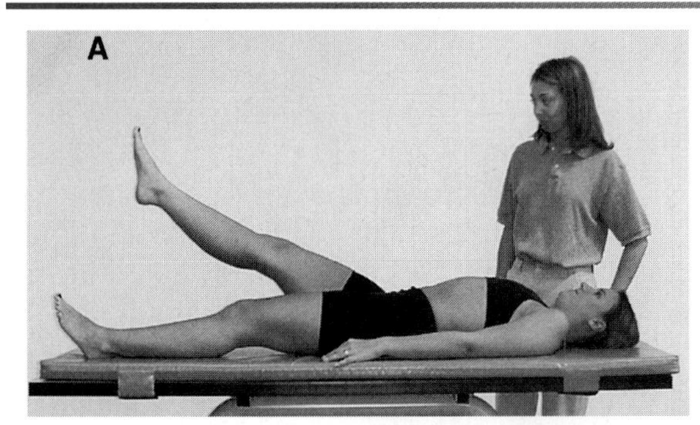

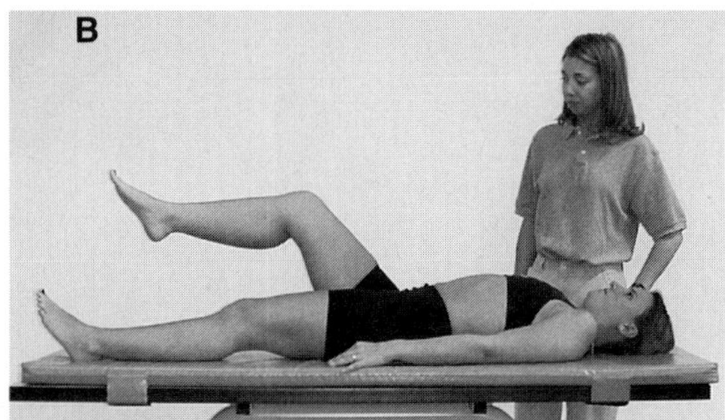

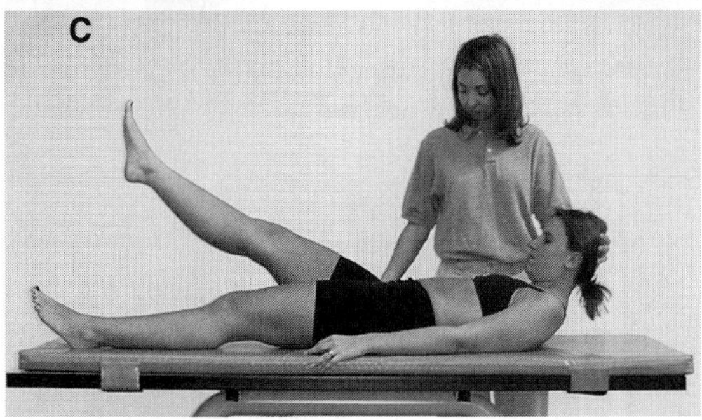

The Kernig test identifies nerve root entrapment caused by a bulging of an intervertebral disk or narrowing of the intervertebral foramen. The Brudzinski test **(C)** identifies symptoms caused by a stretching of the dural sheath.

Patient Position	Supine
Position of Examiner	At the side of the patient
Evaluative Procedure	The patient performs a unilateral active straight leg raise with the knee extended until pain occurs **(A)**. After pain occurs, the patient flexes the knee **(B)**.
Positive Test	Pain is experienced in the spine and possibly radiating into the lower extremity. This pain is relieved when the patient flexes the knee.
Implications	Nerve root impingement secondary to a bulging of the intervertebral disk or bony entrapment; irritation of the dural sheath; or irritation of the meninges.
Modification	In the absence of pain during the active straight leg raise, the examiner may further elongate the spinal cord and increase the tension on the dural sheath by passively flexing the patient's cervical spine (**Brudzinski's test**) and repeating the test **(C)**.
Evidence	Absent or inconclusive in the literature

Tests for lower motor neuron lesions

Lower motor neuron trauma to the spinal nerve roots or the peripheral nervous system results in **hyporeflexia,** flaccidity of the muscles, and denervation atrophy. This condition most often results from compression or stretching of the nerves. Temporary hyporeflexia, sensory deficit, or muscle weakness or paralysis may indicate nerve root impingement or transient quadriplegia (see Chapter 21).

Lower motor neuron injuries include neurapraxia, axonotmesis, and neurotmesis. Refer to Chapter 1 for a description of upper motor neuron lesions.

The upper and lower quarter screens provide an efficient evaluation for neurologic function in the extremities. The screens use manual muscle testing, sensory testing, and deep tendon reflexes to assess neurologic function (Neurologic Screening 13-1). Upper quarter screens are presented in Chapter 14.

Special Test 13-7
Straight Leg Raise Test (Test of Lasègue)

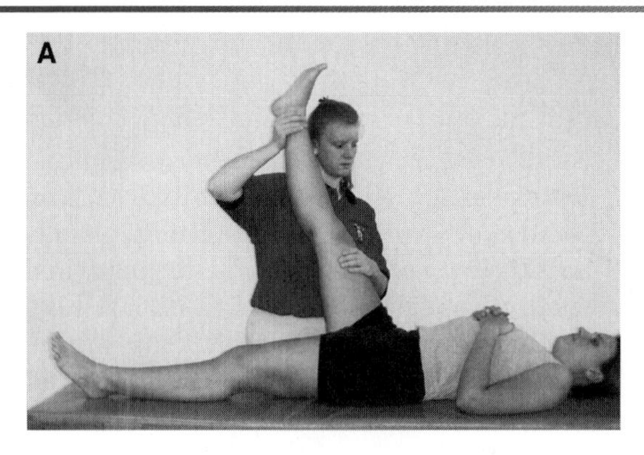

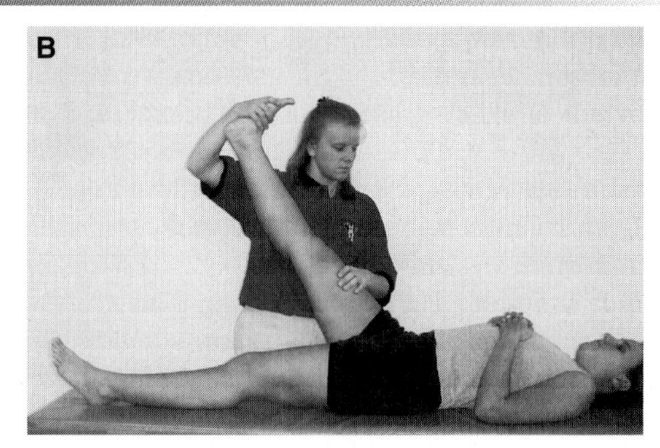

(A) The involved leg is flexed at the hip until symptoms are experienced. **(B)** The involved leg is extended approximately 10° (until symptoms subside) and the ankle is then passively dorsiflexed. A return of the symptoms indicates a stretching of the dural sheath.

Patient Position	Supine
Position of Examiner	At the side to be tested; one hand grasps under the heel while the other is placed on the anterior knee to keep it in full extension during the examination.
Evaluative Procedure	While keeping the knee in extension, the examiner raises the leg by flexing the hip until discomfort is experienced or the full ROM is obtained.
Positive Test	The patient complains of pain before the end of the normal ROM (70°). The pain may be described as radiating distally along the tested leg, usually in the posterior thigh, radiating into the calf and perhaps the foot. The findings are highly significant if they are elicited at 30° or less of hip flexion.[36]
Implications	Sciatic nerve irritation/compression Pain described before the hip reaches 70° of hip flexion may indicate disk involvement.[50]
Modification	After pain is experienced, the leg is lowered to the point at which the pain stops. The examiner passively dorsiflexes the ankle and/or has the patient flex the cervical spine. Serving to stretch the dural sheath, this flexion recreates the symptoms. If the patient's prior pain was caused by tight hamstrings, this modification does not elicit pain.
Comments	The SLR may be helpful in differentiating between tarsal tunnel syndrome and plantar fasciitis. Beginning with the foot dorsiflexed and everted additionally stresses the tibial nerve. The SLR is then performed. An increase in symptoms points to tibial nerve entrapment because strain on the plantar fascia would not further increase.[51]
Evidence	Inter-rater reliability

Inter-rater reliability

Not Reliable — Very Reliable
Poor | Moderate | Good
0 0.1 0.2 0.3 0.4 0.5 0.6 0.7 0.8 0.9 1.0

Intra-rater reliability

Not Reliable — Very Reliable
Poor | Moderate | Good
0 0.1 0.2 0.3 0.4 0.5 0.6 0.7 0.8 0.9 1.0

Positive likelihood ratio

Not Useful — Useful
Very Small | Small | Moderate | Large
0 1 2 3 4 5 6 7 8 9 10

Negative likelihood ratio

Not Useful — Useful
Very Small | Small | Moderate | Large
1.0 0.9 0.8 0.7 0.6 0.5 0.4 0.3 0.2 0.1 0

ROM = range of motion.

Special Test 13-8
Well (Cross) Straight Leg Raising Test

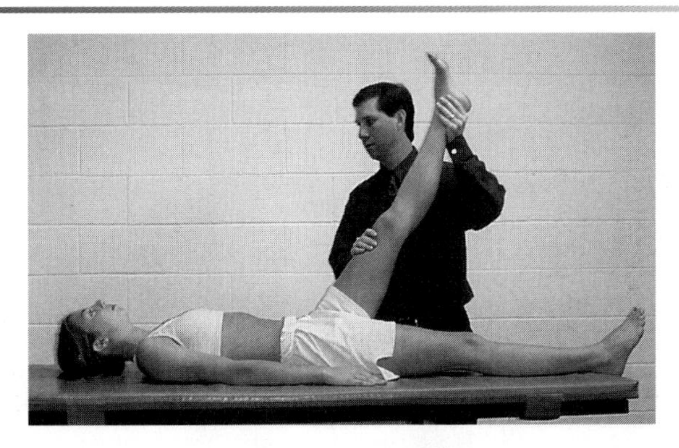

The well straight leg raise test differs from the straight leg raise test in that the unaffected leg is elevated.

Patient Position Supine

Position of Examiner At the side to be tested (the size not suffering the symptoms); one hand grasps under the heel while the other is placed on the anterior thigh just superior to the knee to maintain the leg in extension.

Evaluative Procedure Keeping the knee in extension, the examiner raises the leg by flexing the hip until symptoms are reported.

Positive Test Pain is experienced on the side opposite that being raised.

Implications A large space-occupying lesion such as a herniated intervertebral disk

Evidence Positive likelihood ratio

Not Useful Useful
Very Small | Small | Moderate | Large
0 1 2 3 4 5 6 7 8 9 10

Negative likelihood ratio

Not Useful Useful
Very Small | Small | Moderate | Large
1.0 0.9 0.8 0.7 0.6 0.5 0.4 0.3 0.2 0.1 0

Special Test 13-9
Slump Test

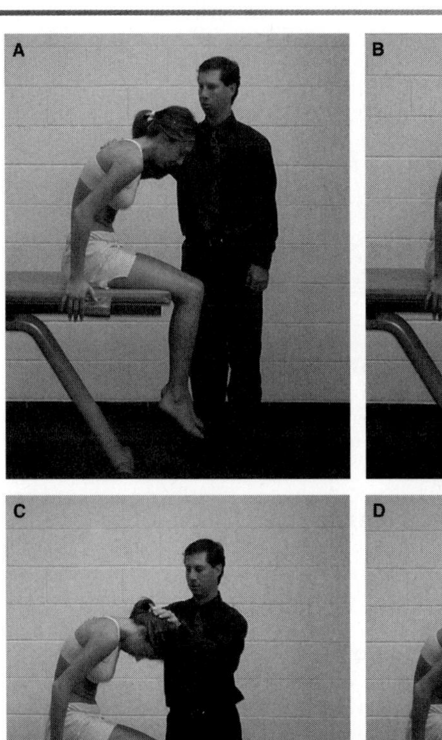
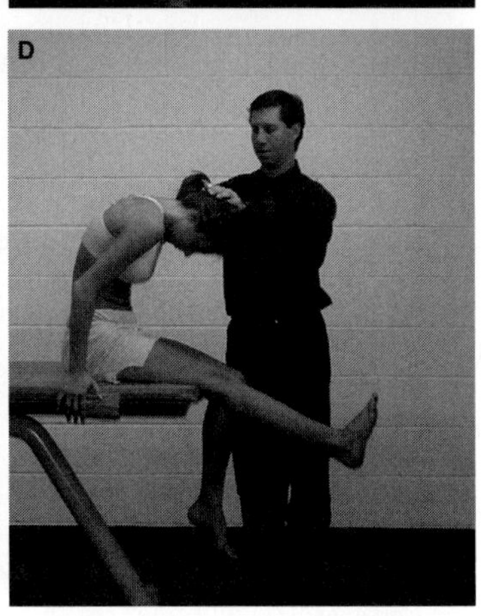

The slump test is designed to place progressively more tension on the nerve and nerve roots by changing positions and then systematically positioning the patient to provoke or alleviate symptoms.

Patient Position	Sitting over the edge of the table
Position of Examiner	At the side of the patient
Evaluative Procedure	The following sequence is followed until symptoms are provoked: 1. The patient slumps forward along the thoracolumbar spine, rounding the shoulders while keeping the cervical spine in neutral **(A)**. Overpressure to trunk flexion is then applied. 2. The patient flexes the cervical spine by bringing the chin to the chest. The clinician then holds the patient in this position **(B)**. 3. The knee is actively extended **(C)**. 4. The ankle is actively dorsiflexed **(D)**. 5. Repeat steps 2–4 on the opposite side. 6. **Alleviation maneuver**: At any step that symptoms are elicited, the provoking position is slightly relieved and tension is reduced at the other end of the nervous system. For example, if knee extension reproduces symptoms, slightly flex the patient's knee and extend the cervical spine. Extend the patient's knee again. In this example if the symptoms reappear the cause is nerve tension as opposed to hamstring pathology.
Positive Test	Sciatic pain or reproduction of other neurologic symptoms
Implications	Impingement of the dural lining, spinal cord, or nerve roots
Modification	Many modifications have been proposed, most of which describe different sequences of motions.
Evidence	Absent or inconclusive in the literature

Special Test 13-10
Quadrant Test

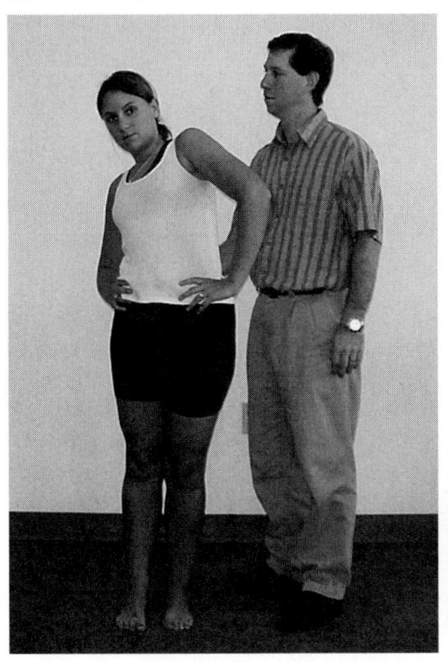

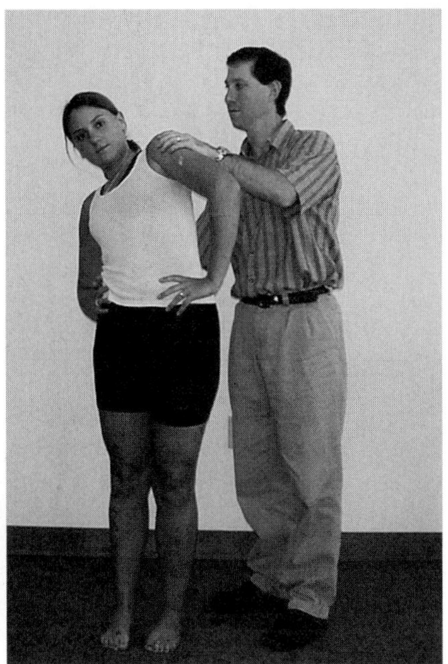

The patient moves into extension, followed by sidebending and rotation to the same side. The examiner provides overpressure to emphasize the position.

Patient Position	Standing with the feet shoulder-width apart
Position of Examiner	Standing behind the patient, grasping the patient's shoulders
Evaluative Procedure	The patient extends the spine as far as possible, then sidebends and rotates to the affected side. The examiner provides overpressure through the shoulders, supporting the patient as needed.
Positive Test	Reproduction of the patient's symptoms
Implications	Radicular pain indicates compression of the intervertebral foramina that impinges on the lumbar nerve roots. Local (nonradiating) pain indicates facet joint pathology. Symptoms isolated to the area of the PSIS; may also indicate SI joint dysfunction
Evidence	Inter-rater reliability Not Reliable — Very Reliable Poor — Moderate — Good 0 0.1 0.2 0.3 0.4 0.5 0.6 0.7 0.8 0.9 1.0

PSIS = posterior superior iliac spine; SI = sacroiliac.

Neurologic Screening Box 13-1
Lower Quarter Neurologic Screen

Nerve Root Level	Sensory Testing	Motor Testing	Reflex Testing
L1	Femoral cutaneous n.	Lumbar plexus	None
L2	Femoral cutaneous n.	Lumbar plexus	Femoral n. (partial)
L3	Femoral cutaneous n.	Femoral n.	Femoral n. (partial)
L4	Saphenous n.	Deep peroneal n.	Femoral n. (partial)
L5	Superficial peroneal n.	Deep peroneal n.	Tibial n.
S1	Posterior femoral cutaneous n. and sural n.	Superficial peroneal n.	Tibial n.
S2	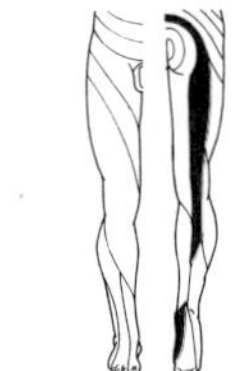 Posterior femoral cutaneous n.	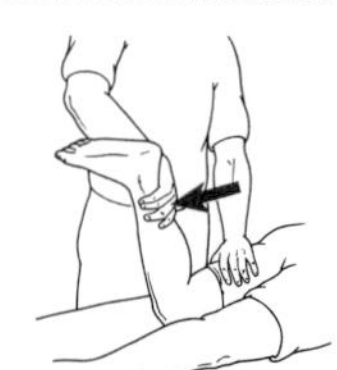 Tibial n. and common peroneal n.	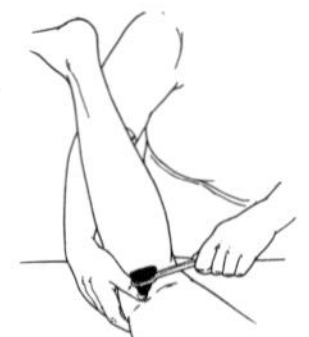 Tibial n.

Table 13-9 Classification Categories of Low Back Injury Based on the Treatment Approach[54]

Classification (Treatment Approach)	Evaluation Findings
Specific Exercise Classification	
Extension	Flexion activities such as sitting and bending increase symptoms Pain exhibited or radiating during trunk flexion ROM testing Pain decreased during extension activities such as when standing or walking Pain reduced or centralized with extension ROM testing
Flexion	Extension motions such as standing and walking increase symptoms Pain exhibited or radiating during trunk extension ROM testing Pain decreased with flexion activities such as sitting and bending Pain reduced or centralized with flexion ROM testing
Lateral Shift	Shifting of trunk laterally relative to the pelvis Unequal lateral bending ROM Symptoms improving with pelvic translocation Symptoms worsening with opposite pelvic translocation
Manipulation Classification	Recent onset of symptoms No symptoms distal to knee
Stabilization Classification	Average straight leg raise ROM greater than 90° Positive prone instability test Aberrant movement pattern (e.g., "hitch" when extending from flexed position) Age less than 40 years

ROM = range of motion.

Pathologies and Related Special Tests

The structure and function of the spinal column exposes it and its supportive structures to almost constant stress during ADLs. These stresses are increased further during heavy labor or athletic competition. In addition to the contact forces related to athletic competition, movement of the torso results in shear forces across the column. Sitting or standing upright places an axial load on these structures. Even lying down can result in dysfunction if the surface is too hard or too soft. Regardless, the spinal column displays an enormous capability to adapt to the forces placed on it. When the spinal column is unable to adapt, injury occurs. Dysfunction of the SI joint can occur acutely secondary to a dynamic overload or insidiously from an unknown cause.

The evaluation of back injuries relies on a thorough, accurate history to provide the examiner with, minimally, an understanding of the positions and movements that aggravate and alleviate the symptoms and, ideally, identification of the involved structure. Identification of the specific pathology is often difficult with chronic low back pain, leading to a general classification of nonspecific low back pain. Chronic low back pain is often idiopathic, with the patient unable to describe any instigating factor. The correlation between imaging studies such as MRI and low back pain is poor.[37] A standardized physical evaluation is used to corroborate the findings from the patient's history.

The idiopathic and inconsistent behavior of low back pain makes identifying the underlying pathology difficult. The treatment and rehabilitation implications of the pathology are equally uncertain. Classification systems have been developed that categorize low back pain by treatment approach, identified impairments, and provocation/alleviation patterns.[53] A system that classifies low back pathology based on the treatment approach has been proposed.[20,54–56] This system groups patients based on the evaluation findings to determine the treatment approach and decreases the need to implicate a specific structure and focuses on the intervention (Table 13-9). For example, patients who demonstrate pain during flexion and pain relief during extension are grouped into the "extension" category, and this motion is emphasized during the initial rehabilitation and education protocol.

Spinal Stenosis

Spinal stenosis, narrowing of the spinal canal or intervertebral foramen, most often results from degeneration associated with aging, and includes arthritic changes to disks, facet joints, and ligaments. These changes narrow the space available in the spinal canal and compress the contents within and exiting the canal. Stenosis can also result from congenital factors. Degenerative stenosis is most common in the 50- to 60-year-old person.[57]

Symptoms include pain during walking, numbness, tingling, muscle weakness, and radiating pain. These symptoms

Examination Findings 13-1
Lumbar Disk Pathology

Examination Segment	Clinical Findings
History	***Onset:*** Insidious: Degeneration Acute: Rupture ***Pain characteristics:*** Pain localized to the affected segment; compression of the spinal nerve root leading to pain in the low back and buttocks possibly radiating into the thigh, calf, heel, and foot ***Other symptoms:*** Not applicable ***Mechanism:*** Repetitive loading of the intervertebral disk over time ***Predisposing conditions:*** History of lumbar spine trauma
Inspection	Slow gait Flattened lumbar spine Changes in position are guarded and painful.
Palpation	Spasm of the musculature possible
Joint and Muscle Function Assessment	***AROM:*** Limited by pain in all directions ***MMT:*** Weakness of the abdominal muscles may be noted. The patient may be unable to maintain a neutral spine. ***PROM:*** Limited by pain in all directions
Joint Stability Tests	***Stress tests:*** Not applicable ***Joint play:*** Initially, increased P-A mobility is demonstrated. As the condition worsens the amount of play decreases.
Special Tests	Straight leg raising, well straight leg raising, Milgram test, sciatic and femoral nerve tension tests
Neurologic Screening	Lower quarter screen
Vascular Screening	Within normal limits
Functional Assessment	Determination by the examiner which activities (and associated movement patterns) increase or decreases the symptoms Motion that decreases symptoms possibly useful in the treatment of the patient
Imaging Techniques	Discography MRI can visualize the annulus fibrosus, nucleus pulposus, spinal cord, spinal nerve roots, and vertebrae and is often used to make the definitive diagnosis. Degenerative changes to the disk as assessed via MRI are often present in asymptomatic people.[58]
Differential Diagnosis	Spondylolytic change, facet joint dysfunction, spinal stenosis, piriformis syndrome, peripheral nerve entrapment
Comments	Standard lumbar spine radiographs are reliable for making a definitive diagnosis of lumbar disk degeneration. All disks tend to begin degenerating by the fourth decade of life and may be a concurrent finding with other spine pathology. Cases of lumbar disk degeneration are often first reported as complaints of a hamstring strain or knee pain.[59]

AROM = active range of motion; MMT = manual muscle test; PROM = passive range of motion.

can occur centrally, when the canal itself is narrowed, or unilaterally, when the foramen is narrowed. Patients frequently report increased leg pain with standing that is resolved by sitting, a flexed position that increases the space available in the lumbar spinal canal.

Intervertebral disk lesions

The degeneration of intervertebral disks involves the loss of water from the nucleus pulposus, decreasing the protein content and altering the chemical structure. Biochemical changes associated with the aging process further extenuate the loss of water, causing an increased stress load to be placed on the annulus fibrosus and leading to the bulging of the nucleus pulposus (Fig. 13-24). Tears of the annulus in early adulthood are likely to lead to eventual disk degeneration and herniation.[12]

Disk herniation is the extrusion of the nucleus pulposus through a weakened region in the annulus fibrosus with subsequent impingement on one or more lumbar nerve roots. A complete herniation typically results in pressure of the nerve root exiting below the affected disk (Fig. 13-25). For example, a herniation of the L4–L5 disk places pressure on the L5 nerve root. The lesion can involve any protrusion of the nuclear material into the annulus, even if it has not herniated through the entire structure. The worst-case scenario involves the nuclear material's breaking away from the rest of the disk and becoming **sequestrated**. Note that many disk protrusions remain asymptomatic.[60]

The signs and symptoms of an intervertebral disk herniation are primarily those of nerve root compression that results in pain in the lumbar spine and radicular pain aggravated by activity (Examination Findings 13-1).[50] The patient typically describes an insidious onset, but the pain may be related to a single specific episode. Often, the breakdown of the disk is related to repetitive stress, but the episode resulting in the symptoms reflects the final failure in the annulus fibrosus to contain the nucleus pulposus. Changes in body position (e.g., sitting to standing or standing to lying) are painful as the changes in disk pressure increase pressure on the structures. On inspection, the patient may be noted as having a slow, deliberate gait and, in the acute and subacute stages, a flattened lumbar spine. In an attempt to decrease the pressure on the nerve root, the patient may stand with a lateral shift, usually away from the side of the leg pain. If the patient demonstrates a leg length discrepancy, the pain usually occurs on the side of the body with the shorter leg.[61]

Question the patient to determine the exact location (or locations) of pain. Typically, the pain is in the low back and buttocks. However, it also can radiate into the posterior thigh, calf, heel, and foot, depending on the level of the nerve root irritation (Box 13-1). The pain patterns stemming from disk lesions may be inconsistent, with changes in the position of the lumbar spine reducing the pressure on the nerve root causing a decrease in symptoms. A precise neurologic evaluation is needed to determine the spinal levels that are involved. A lower quarter neurologic screen is used to evaluate strength, deep tendon reflexes, and sensation. Findings of bilateral leg pain, absent deep tendon reflexes, or changes in bowel and bladder function warrant immediate referral for evaluation of **cauda equina syndrome**.

Sequestrated Pertaining to a necrotic fragment of tissue that has become separated from the surrounding tissue.

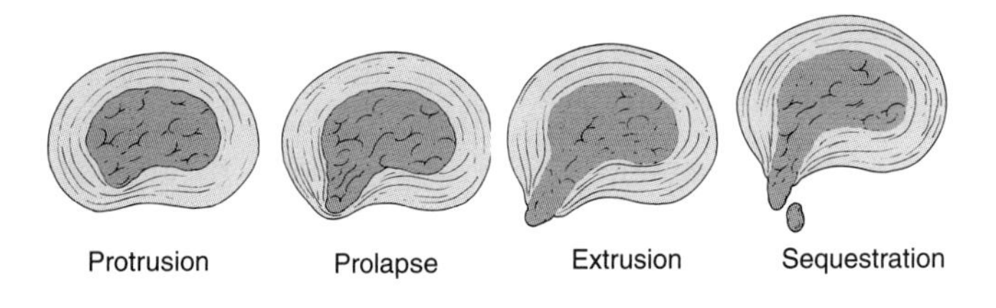

FIGURE 13-24 ■ Classifications of intervertebral disk lesions.

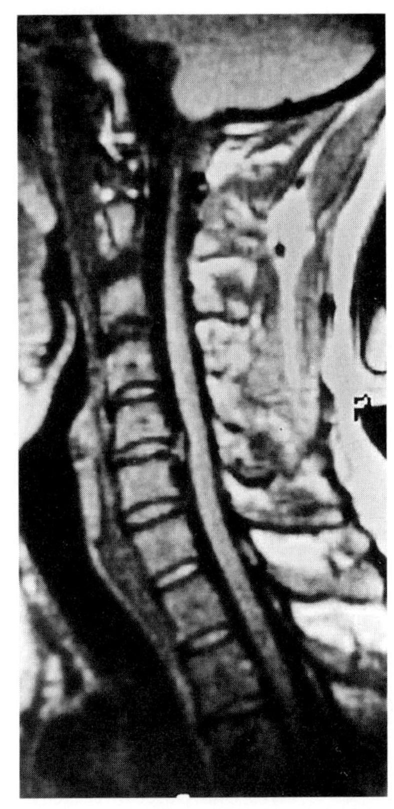

FIGURE 13-25 ■ Myelogram of a disk herniation. Notice the narrowing of the spinal canal.

Box 13-1
Sciatica: "Shin Splints" of the Spine

Sciatica, a nondescript general term for any inflammation involving the sciatic nerve, does not describe the actual condition that is insulting the nerve and causing the inflammation. Whenever possible, this term should be avoided and the source of the irritation should be determined so that an appropriate treatment plan can be developed. Causes of sciatica include lumbar disk herniation, sacroiliac joint dysfunction, piriformis muscle spasm, scar tissue formation around the nerve root, nerve root inflammation, spinal stenosis, synovial cysts, cancerous or noncancerous tumors, and other disease states.[32,63–69]

Special tests are used to confirm the findings identified during the history, inspection, and neurologic screening portions of the evaluation. The Valsalva test (see Special Test 13-4), Milgram test (see Special Test 13-5), straight leg raise (see Special Test 13-7), the well straight leg raise (see Special Test 13-8), the **femoral nerve stretch test** (Special Test 13-11), and the **tension sign** (Special Test 13-12) are commonly used to identify intervertebral disk lesions.

Standard radiographic examinations are effective only in measuring secondary changes associated with disk degeneration (i.e., a narrowing of the intervertebral space). The evaluation of disk changes through diagnostic imaging is made more effective with MRI scans. MRI has a high sensitivity in detecting those who do not have disk herniation. A negative finding is good evidence that the patient does not have disk involvement. The high number of asymptomatic individuals with apparent disk degeneration makes the determination that the disk is contributing to symptoms more difficult, and MRI findings must be coupled with examination and history for a diagnosis.[62] Discography, a contrast dye injected into disk, enhancing the ensuing CT images, is often considered to be the gold standard for diagnosing intervertebral disk lesions.

Initially, rehabilitation exercises consist of those motions that localize the pain toward the involved disk

Special Test 13-11
Femoral Nerve Stretch Test

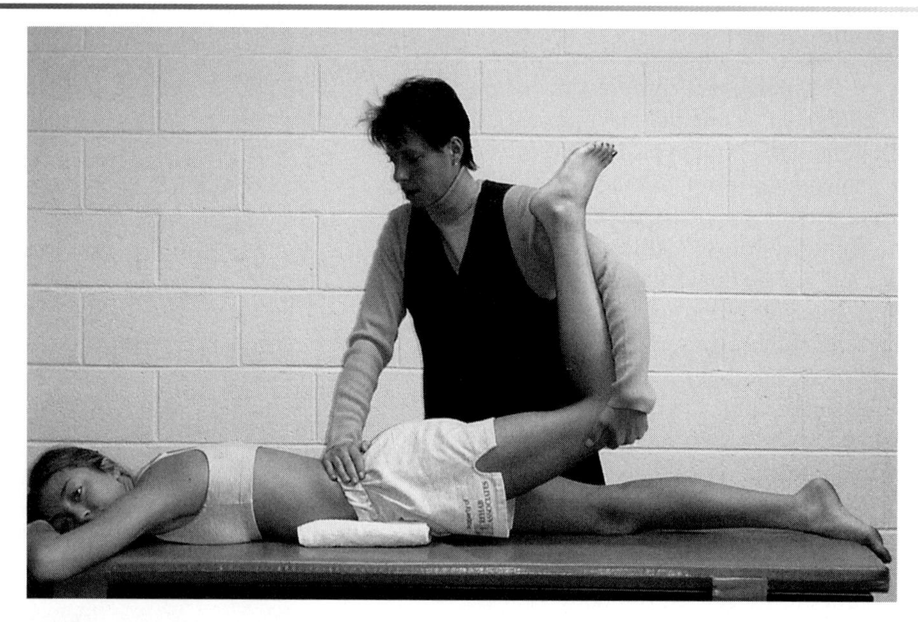

The femoral nerve (L2, L3, L4) is placed on stretch by passively flexing the patient's knee. Nerve root impingement will result in radicular pain in the anterior and/or lateral thigh.

Patient Position	Prone with a pillow under the abdomen
Position of Examiner	At the side of the patient
Evaluative Procedure	The examiner passively flexes the patient's knee.
Positive Test	Pain is elicited in the anterior and lateral thigh.
Implications	Nerve root impingement at the L2, L3, or L4 level
Modification	The femoral nerve may be further stressed by passively extending the patient's hip while maintaining knee flexion. If the patient cannot lie prone, the test can be performed in side-lying with the pelvis stabilized.
Comments	The examiner should attempt to fully flex the knee with the hip in the neutral position to determine any strain of the quadriceps muscle that may also cause pain. This test is associated with a high number of false positives due to tight or injured quadriceps.
Evidence	Absent or inconclusive in the literature

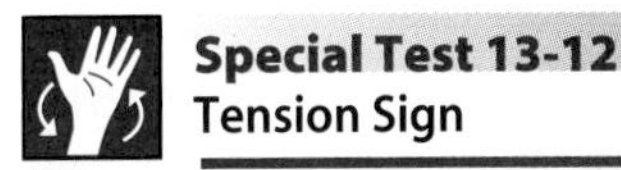

Special Test 13-12
Tension Sign

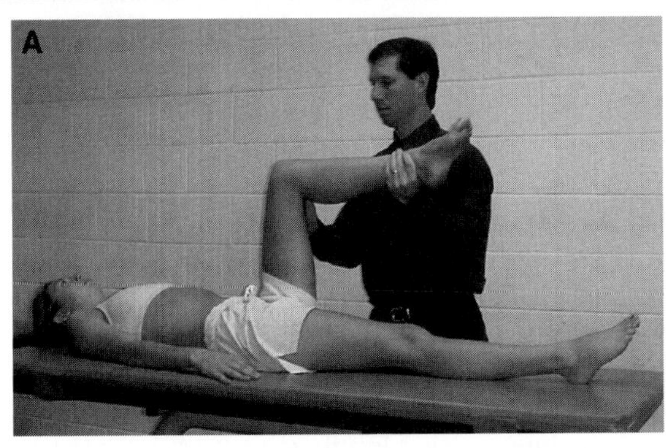

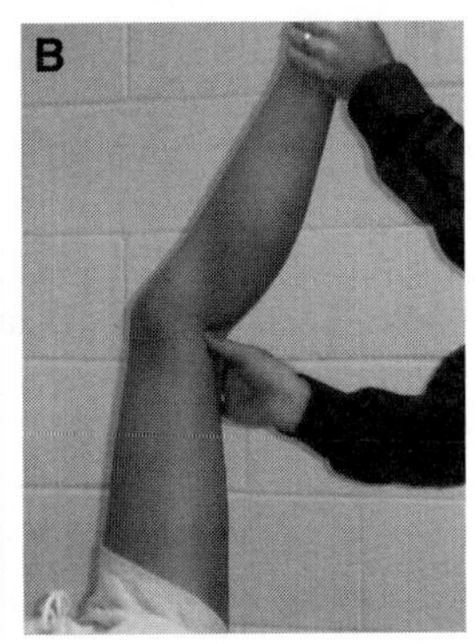

The sciatic nerve is stretched by extending the patient's knee with the hip flexed to 90° while palpating the nerve as it passes through the popliteal fossa.

Patient Position	Supine
Position of Examiner	At the patient's side that is to be tested; one hand grasps the heel while the other grasps the thigh.
Evaluative Procedure	The hip is flexed to 90°, with the knee flexed to 90°. The knee is then extended as far as possible with the examiner palpating the tibial portion of the sciatic nerve as it passes through the popliteal space **(A)**.
Positive Test	Exquisite tenderness with possible duplication of sciatic symptoms, as compared with the opposite side.
Implications	Sciatic nerve irritation
Modification	The Bowstring test is a variation of this technique **(B)**. The examiner extends the patient's knee until radiating symptoms are experienced. The knee is then flexed approximately 20° or until the symptoms are relieved. The examiner then pushes on the tibial portion of the sciatic nerve to reestablish the symptoms.
Evidence	Absent or inconclusive in the literature

(**centralization**), usually extension motions and, ultimately, core stability and pelvic stabilization exercises. Because of the stress placed on the disk during flexion and rotation of the lumbar spine, some advocate avoiding these exercises until the symptoms decrease.[50] Rehabilitation can also include the use of a support to maintain lumbar curvature while sitting and anti-inflammatory medications.[10] Disk ruptures that do not respond to conservative care may require surgery to remove the involved section of the intervertebral disk and fuse the superior and inferior vertebra.[10]

Segmental Instability

Stability of the spinal segment comes from active restraints (muscles), passive restraints (ligaments, facet joints, disks, vertebral bodies and tension from musculotendinous units) and neural control.[15] Dysfunction in any of these can result in instability. For example, spondylolisthesis results in instability as a bony restraint is disrupted. Muscle strains can result in a decreased ability to provide active stability.

Patients with segmental instability describe frequent recurrences of low back pain resulting from seemingly mild aggravating factors. They often report short-term relief from manipulation and may describe a traumatic initial event. AROM may reveal a "catch" or jerky movement, a compensatory response to a lack of stability. Increased motion with posterior-anterior stress may be present, although this technique has questionable reliability and validity (see Box 13-1).

Reduced symptoms with use of a stabilizing brace helps confirm the diagnosis. A definitive diagnosis may be made with flexion–extension radiographs, although the wide variability in a nonsymptomatic population results in many false-positive results.[15] Treatment focuses on postural control, core stability exercises, and biomechanical education.

Erector spinae muscle strain

Strains of the spinal erector muscle group may be one of the most common orthopedic conditions seen for treatment.[70,71] Although lumbar strains are common, they tend to be self-limiting conditions. Similar to sprains of the spinal ligaments, muscle strain is usually diagnosed after the exclusion of all other possible problems. Commonly, the patient presents with a history of heavy or repetitive lifting and complaints of aching pain centralized to the low back. Pain increases with passive and active flexion as well as resisted extension. Lower quarter screens show negative results.

Facet joint dysfunction

The lumbar facet joints give the spine rigidity and protect the intervertebral disks against rotational injury.[72,73] Pathology of the facet joints can account for as much as 40% of all chronic low back pain.[74] The signs and symptoms of facet joint dysfunction are vague and often resemble other low back pathologies, including strains and spasm of the paraspinal muscles, nerve root impingement, and disk degeneration.

Facet joint pathology may involve dislocation or subluxation of the facet, **facet joint syndrome** (inflammation), or degeneration of the facet itself (e.g., arthritis). Over time, the presence of one of these conditions can lead to the other. A dislocated or subluxated facet joint tends to "lock" the involved spinal segment, causing the segment to become hypomobile (see Joint Play 13-1, Spring test for vertebral mobility). The patient may report a history of extension, rotation, or lateral bending of the spine with pain that tends to be localized over the affected facet. Unlike with other spinal conditions, the patient may describe a decrease in symptoms with an increase in activity.

Facet joint syndrome occurs from repetitive stress to the facet joint through movement or loading. The pain is usually localized to the spinal level that is irritated and does not radiate unless the nerve root is secondarily involved. The pain may become more diffuse if several levels of facets are involved. Localized muscle spasm may be present in the paravertebral musculature. (Examination Findings 13-2). Any motion that loads the facet joint, especially extension, hyperextension, rotation, and side bending to the involved side, reproduces symptoms.

Examination Findings 13-2
Facet Joint Dysfunction

Examination Segment	Clinical Findings
History	***Onset:*** Insidious or acute ***Pain characteristics:*** Localized over the involved facets and the surrounding musculature ***Mechanism:*** Extension, rotation, or lateral bending of the vertebrae ***Predisposing conditions:*** Repeated motions of spinal extension, rotation, or lateral bending
Inspection	The patient may assume a posture that lessens the pressure on the affected facets.
Palpation	Possible local muscle spasm is noted in the paravertebral muscles.
Joint and Muscle Function Assessment	***AROM:*** Increased pain with extension and rotation, alleviation with flexion ***MMT:*** May have extensor weakness. ***PROM:*** Increased pain with extension
Joint Stability Tests	***Stress tests:*** Not applicable ***Joint play:*** Spring test may cause pain or reveal decreased motion.
Special Tests	Quadrant test may be positive. Tests for intervertebral disk lesions are negative.
Neurologic Screening	Within normal limits unless secondary nerve root impingement occurs. Secondary nerve root impingement warrants a lower quarter screen (see Neurologic Screening Box 13-1).
Vascular Screening	Within normal limits
Functional Assessment	Activities or motions that require extension, rotation, and/or lateral bending to the involved side all produce pain.
Imaging Techniques	Usually unremarkable
Differential Diagnosis	Herniated disk, spondylitic defect
Comments	Continued degeneration of the facet joint may reduce the size of the intervertebral foramen and result in compression of the spinal nerve root. Diagnosis is definitively made via pain relief after injection of anesthetic into joint.[62]

AROM = active range of motion; MMT = manual muscle test; PROM = passive range of motion.

Because extension and rotation also stress other surrounding soft tissues, pain with these motions is not a definitive finding.[62]

Degeneration of the facet joint has an undefined history of injury. If the degeneration is significant, the size of the intervertebral foramen will decrease, potentially impinging the associated nerve root and causing radicular pain. Nerve entrapment can be reduced by the patient's assuming a posture that decreases pressure on the nerve root, usually caused by flexion reducing the size of the intervertebral foramen. A definitive diagnosis of facet joint degeneration is made using radiographs or magnetic resonance imaging (MRI) or by a physician's injecting the facet with an anesthetic and noting the subsequent change in symptoms.[72–74] Prolonged dysfunction of the facet joint or **facetectomy** can accelerate the degeneration of the intervertebral disks or predispose the disks to injury.[72]

Initial treatment of patients with facet joint pathologies involves the use of nonsteroidal anti-inflammatory drugs (NSAIDs) to decrease joint inflammation. Instruct the patient to avoid postures and movements that irritate the facet and increase pain, especially sleeping in a prone position. Local therapeutic modalities such as moist heat, electrical stimulation, or ice may be helpful to decrease subsequent muscle spasm. The use of mobilization is helpful early on to assist in reducing pain in the area.

These patients must also be thoroughly evaluated for muscle imbalances that may be contributing to their facet joint dysfunction. The trunk and pelvic musculature must be assessed for tightness and weakness. A program of stretching and strengthening helps in decreasing pain and maintaining good health in the back. The mechanics and postures that the patient assumes should be evaluated as possible contributory causes of the facet joint pathology and corrected as needed.

Spondylopathies

Bony disorders of the posterior elements of the spinal column, spondylopathies, can afflict patients of any age and athletes in any sport, but they tend to be more prevalent in those who repeatedly hyperextend and rotate or rotate their torso against resistance during activity. Because the pars is thinner in the developing child, adolescents are more vulnerable to developing a symptomatic defect.[76–78] A genetic, congenital weakness in the pars interarticularis can predispose this structure to a stress fracture.[79] The cause may be traced to hypermobility of the spine, disease state, or acute trauma. However, a stress reaction leading to a fracture is the most prevalent bony injury to the spine in athletes.[80] These defects are caused by repetitive forced hyperextension such as that experienced by football linemen, gymnasts, and cheerleaders. Spondylopathies most commonly occur at the L5 level but may develop anywhere along the vertebral column.[77,79,81] Table 13-10 presents an encapsulated description of common spondylopathies.

Spondylolysis

Spondylolysis is a defect in the pars interarticularis, the area of the vertebral arch between the inferior and superior articular facets, usually brought on by repetitive stress. It can occur bilaterally or unilaterally (Examination Findings 13-3). Bilateral defects in the pars interarticularis result in listhesis, the posterior portion of the vertebra, the laminae, inferior articular surfaces, and spinous process separating from the vertebral body.[82] This defect, when seen on an oblique radiographic view, appears as a "collared Scotty dog" deformity, with the area of the stress fracture representing the dog's collar (Fig. 13-26). Defects in the pars are

Table 13-10 Classification of Spondylopathies

Term	Description
Spondylalgia	Pain arising from the vertebrae
Spondylitis	Inflammation of the vertebrae
Spondylizema	Downward (inferior) displacement of a vertebra caused by the degeneration of the one below it
Spondylolisthesis	Forward slippage of a vertebra on the one below it (may occur secondary to spondylolysis, in which the fracture of the pars interarticularis results in the anterior displacement of the vertebral body)
Spondylolysis	Degeneration of a vertebral structure secondary to repetitive stress, most commonly affecting the pars interarticularis but with no displacement of the vertebral body
Spondylopathy	Any disorder of the vertebrae
Spondylosis	Arthritis or osteoarthritis of the vertebrae; results in pressure being placed on the vertebral nerve roots

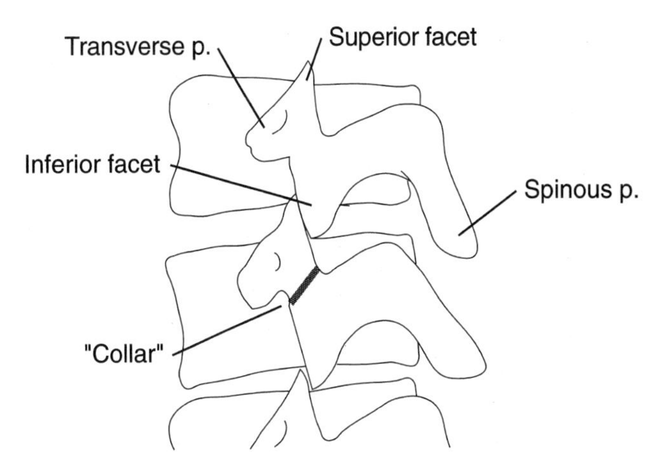

FIGURE 13-26 ■ "Collared Scotty dog" deformity. On an oblique radiograph, the presence of a collar on the Scotty dog indicates a nondisplaced stress fracture on the pars interarticularis, spondylolysis.

Facetectomy The surgical resection of a vertebral facet.

Examination Findings 13-3
Spondylolysis and Spondylolisthesis

Examination Segment	Clinical Findings
History	***Onset:*** Insidious; the pain begins as an ache and evolves to constant pain. ***Pain characteristics:*** Pain in the lumbar spine, possibly radiating into the buttocks and upper portion of the posterolateral thighs[59] The intensity of pain increases as the condition worsens. ***Mechanism:*** Repeated extension ***Predisposing conditions:*** Adolescence, when pars is thinner; imbalances in trunk muscular strength, endurance, and flexibility; activities that repetitively place the lumbar spine into hyperextension; females have a higher incidence rate of spondylolisthesis than males.
Inspection	Gross inspection of the spinal curvatures may reveal hyperlordosis in the lumbar spine. The patient may walk with a short stride and remain stiff legged. The buttocks may appear heart-shaped.[59]
Palpation	Spondylolisthesis: A palpable "step-off" deformity may be detected at the involved lumbar level. Possible spasm of the paraspinal muscles may be noted.
Joint and Muscle Function Assessment	***AROM:*** ROM during trunk flexion is restricted but pain free. Pain is described or a "catch" is experienced as the patient returns to an upright posture and during active extension of the spine. Pain may also be elicited during lumbar rotation and lateral rotation. ***MMT:*** Weakness of the spinal erector muscles ***PROM:*** Hip flexion may indicate tightness of the hamstring muscles.
Joint Stability Tests	***Stress tests:*** Not applicable ***Joint play:*** Spring test may reveal pain and/or hypermobility.
Special Tests	Single leg stance; straight leg raises may produce a pain that is worse than that normally caused by tightness of the hamstring group.
Neurologic Screening	Lower quarter screen is used to rule out involvement of one or more lumbar nerve roots. Results of this are typically negative, but the presence of positive neurologic signs can indicate that the vertebrae is slipping, requiring immediate physician referral.
Vascular Screening	Within normal limits
Functional Assessment	Activities that result in extension, such as reaching high overhead, may produce symptoms.
Imaging Techniques	Spinal instability associated with spondylolisthesis can be diagnosed using flexion and extension radiographs, although avoidance of aggravating positions may limit the usefulness.[75] CT scans: Useful to determine relative metabolic activity (old or new)[76] Radiographic examination, CT scan, or MRI is required to differentiate between spondylolysis and spondylolisthesis.
Differential Diagnosis	Disk herniation, facet joint pathology
Comments	Tightness of the hamstrings or weakness of the abdominal muscles may be noted. Refer to Chapter 6 or muscle length assessment techniques.

AROM = active range of motion; CT = computed tomography; MRI = magnetic resonance imaging; PROM = passive range of motion; ROM = range of motion.

a common radiological finding in individuals with no symptoms, so CT scans are used to determine whether or not the fracture site is metabolically active.[76,77] Radiographs may show a flattening of the inferior facet on the vertebra above the affected site.[83]

The patient presents with localized low back pain that is increased during and after activity. During observation, spinal alignment is usually normal. Those with spondylitic defects typically describe a pattern where extension (e.g., standing and walking) is aggravating and symptoms are alleviated with postures or activities that incorporate more flexion (e.g., sitting). Active ROM is normal for flexion, but pain restricts extension. Results of special tests and neurologic tests are normal. The evaluative findings of advanced spondylolysis resemble those of spondylolisthesis.

Spondylolisthesis

Spondylolysis may progress to spondylolisthesis, in which the defects in both elements of the pars interarticularis result in the separation of the vertebra into two uniquely identifiable structures and resulting spinal instability. The fixation between the affected vertebra and the one below it is lost, resulting in the superior vertebra's sliding anteriorly, and possibly inferiorly, on the one below it (Fig. 13-27). A radiographic examination of this condition reveals a "decapitated Scotty dog" deformity, in which the head of the dog, the anterior element of the vertebra, has become detached from the body, the posterior element (Fig. 13-28). The severity of the spondylolisthesis is determined by the relative amount of anterior displacement of the vertebra. After the fracture occurs, the displacement of the vertebra usually does not progress under the normal daily stresses.[81] However, the stresses of sports and other exertive activities may increase the amount of anterior displacement. True healing of the fracture site rarely occurs.[79]

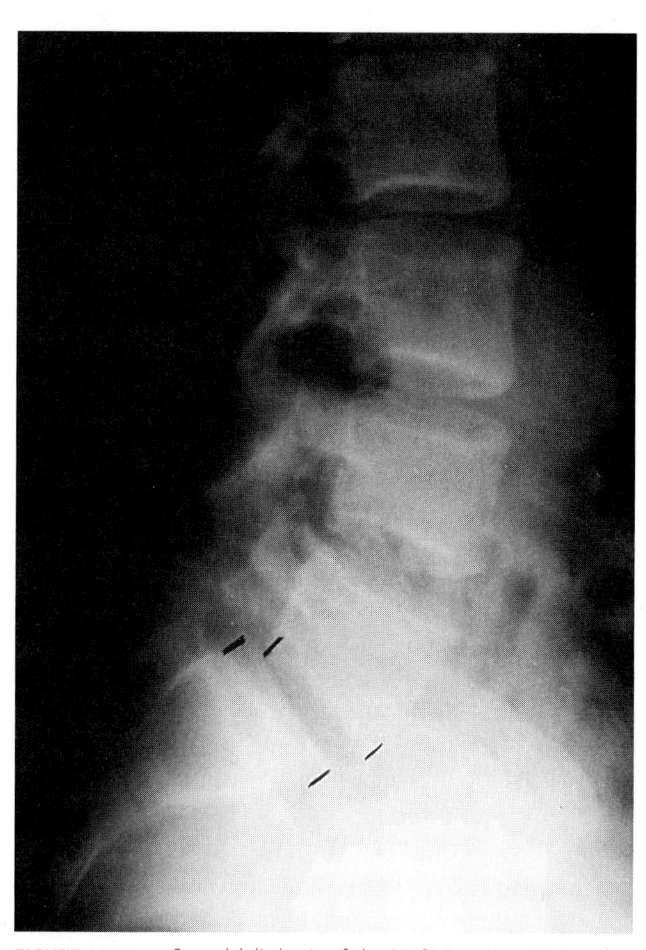

FIGURE 13-27 ■ Spondylolisthesis of the L5-S1 junction. Notice that the L5 vertebra is anteriorly displaced relative to S1.

*** Practical Evidence**

Approximately half of the individuals diagnosed with spondylolisthesis will also demonstrate thoracic kyphosis, a slouching posture, anterior wedging of the vertebrae, and intravertebral disk herniation, or **Scheuermann's disease**.[59]

Spondylolisthesis is most prevalent in adolescents and in women. Also, young gymnasts have an incidence of pars interarticularis defects four times higher than that of the average population.[84] Patients with spondylolisthesis have a history and physical presentation that is very similar to that of spondylolysis, with increased symptoms in postures that emphasize trunk extension. During AROM, the patient may reveal a "catch" when returning to upright from a flexed position.[75] The pain may be more intense and is likely to be more constant. On observation and with palpation, an actual step-off deformity may be identified, as the normal continuity of the lumbar spine is lost when the vertebra shifts forward. More severe cases of spondylolisthesis result in a flattening of the buttocks when viewed laterally and more severe limitations in ROM. Similarly to intervertebral

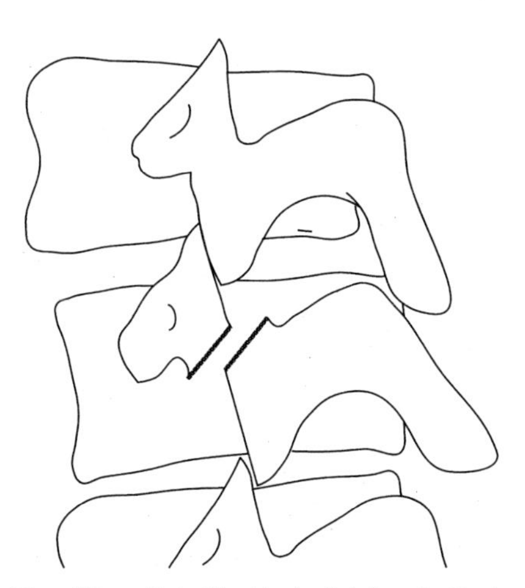

FIGURE 13-28 ■ "Decapitated Scotty dog" deformity. Further degeneration of the pars interarticularis can lead to a displaced fracture, spondylolisthesis. Here the "collared Scotty dog" loses its head as the superior vertebra slides anteriorly.

Scheuermann's disease A disease process involving the disks of the thoracic spine.

disk pathologies, pain may be described in the lumbar region when the patient returns to a standing posture.

Results of special tests and neurologic tests may become positive if the slippage of the vertebra is great enough to impinge on the neurologic structures. Pain associated with spondylolysis and early stages of spondylolisthesis tends not to radiate.[81] Although not a definitive test, a suspicion of spondylolysis or spondylolisthesis may be reinforced by the **single leg stance test** (Special Test 13-13).

The treatment of patients with spondylolysis and spondylolisthesis is primarily based on the patient's symptoms. Rehabilitation exercises should resolve muscular tightness and strength deficit problems, but extension exercises that place stress on the pars interarticularis are avoided in the early stages.[79,81] Posture awareness is emphasized. The patient is taught how to control pelvic position and instructed about ways to avoid placing the lumbar spine in extension. The most conservative form of treatment, the use of a lumbar brace, is attempted if other forms of rehabilitation fail to produce the desired results.

Sacroiliac Dysfunction

Although the SI joints are relatively immobile, a slight amount of accessory movement, rotation, or translation of the ilium on the sacrum occurs here. When these motions become extreme, the ilium rotates to the point that it subtlely subluxes on the sacrum. Injury to or degeneration of the pubic symphysis can also lead to SI dysfunction.[86] The resulting pain and dysfunction often resemble those associated with lumbar nerve root compression. Single tests for sacroiliac dysfunction are not reliable measures of the presence of pathology in this region (Examination Findings 13-4).[24,87–89] Combining the results of a series of these tests, however, may improve reliability.[90–94] Tests that attempt to provoke pain, such as Gaenslen test or Patrick test, are more reliable and valid than tests that attempt to detect differences in movement or position, such as the Gillet test. The amount of mobility at the SI joint is very small (2 mm or less), making it unlikely that displacements or changes in mobility can be detected.[24,89] Pain over the SI joint as described by the patient or during palpation may be the best criterion for a diagnosis of SI joint pathology.[24,88]

With an inflamed SI joint, compression or distraction of the two halves of the pelvis causes motion at the SI joint, resulting in a duplication of the patient's symptoms (Special Test 13-14). A positive compression or distraction test result does not indicate the nature of the pathology, but only shows that a form of pathology is present.

The **Fabere sign** (Special Test 13-15), or **Patrick's test**, is used to elicit pain in the SI joints and the hip. The term *Fabere* is used as a mnemonic describing the position of the hip during testing: **F**lexion, **AB**duction, **E**xternal **R**otation, and **E**xtension. **Gaenslen's test** (Special Test 13-16), is used to place a rotatory stress on the SI joint by forcing one hip into hyperextension.

When viewed laterally, the ilium may rotate clockwise with respect to the sacrum, producing an anterior motion. Tightness of the hip flexors may stress the ilium, causing it to rotate anteriorly. The anterior rotation is typified by the involved lower extremity's appearing to be longer than the contralateral limb with the patient supine. As the patient assumes a long sit position, the rotated ilium causes the limb to move from a relatively longer position to a shorter position. Such an occurrence is a positive **long sit test** result (Special Test 13-17), indicating an anterior rotation of the SI joint on the ipsilateral side.

Alternatively, when viewed laterally, the ilium may rotate posteriorly with respect to the sacrum, producing a posterior rotation. Tightness of the hamstrings may be a cause of this rotation. The posterior rotation is typified by the involved lower extremity's appearing to be shorter than the contralateral limb with the patient supine. As the patient assumes a long sit position, the rotated ilium causes the limb to move from a relatively shorter position to a longer one. This occurrence is a positive long sit test result, indicating a posterior rotation of the SI joint on the ipsilateral side as the leg moves from a shorter to a longer position.

Thoracic Spine

The thoracic spine is relatively well protected compared to the cervical and thoracic spinal regions. Pathology in the upper thoracic spine mimics cervical spine conditions, while lower thoracic spine pathologies behave more like lumbar spine conditions. Disk pathology is less common in the thoracic spine, probably due to the limited available motion. Thoracic spine pathology, especially with rib involvement, can affect breathing, making deep breaths painful and exercise difficult. Symptoms of many pathologies, such as cancer, gall bladder and gastroesophageal conditions, include referred pain to the thoracic or scapular region, making careful screening even more important.[95]

The articulations of the ribs with T1–T10 provide potential sites of pain. Hypomobility or hypermobility of the costovertebral articulations can result in sharp, well-localized pain that is exacerbated with rotation and radiates anteriorly to the chest. Coughing and sneezing can makes symptoms worse. Painful posterior–anterior joint play as described for the lumbar vertebrae may be painful but detecting differences in mobility is not reliable.

The intercostal and paraspinal muscles in the thoracic region are the common sites of strains and hypersensitive trigger points, generally brought on by repetitive overload mechanisms. These trigger points are palpable, defined areas or bands of point tenderness and increased tissue density.

Scheuermann's disease

Scheuermann's disease, also called juvenile kyphosis, results when the vertebral bodies wedge anteriorly, created an abnormally rounded spine. With a strong genetic component, Scheuermann's disease affects boys more than

Special Test 13-13
Single Leg Stance Test

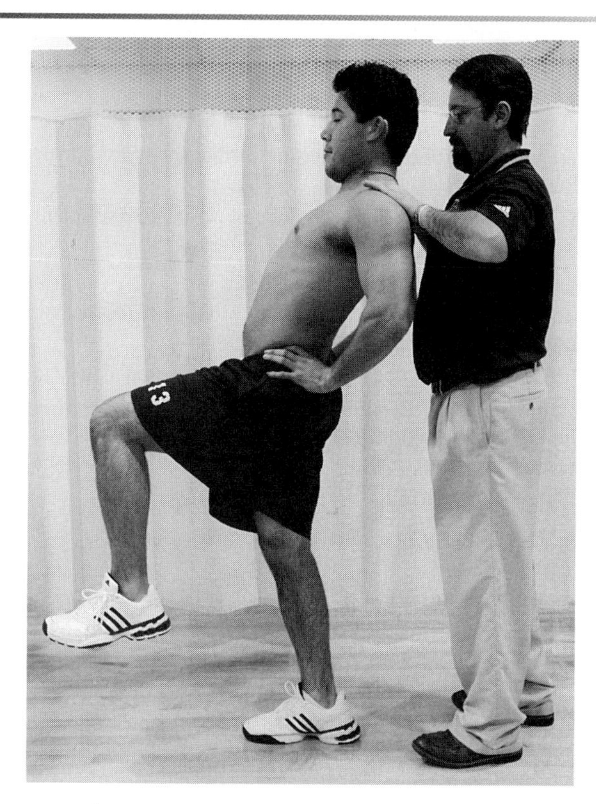

This test reproduces the positions that maximally stress the pars interarticularis by positioning the patient in extension and rotation.

Patient Position	Standing with the body weight evenly distributed between the two feet
Position of Examiner	Standing behind the patient, ready to provide support if the patient begins to fall
Evaluative Procedure	The patient lifts one leg, then places the trunk in hyperextension. The examiner may assist the patient during this motion. The procedure is then repeated for the opposite leg.
Positive Test	Pain is noted in the lumbar spine or SI area.
Implications	Shear forces are placed on the pars interarticularis by the iliopsoas pulling the vertebra anteriorly, resulting in pain.
Comments	When the lesion to the pars interarticularis is unilateral, pain is evoked when the opposite leg is raised. Bilateral pars fractures result in pain when either leg is lifted. This test may also result in pain specifically at the area of the PSIS secondary to SI joint irritation.
Evidence	Absent or inconclusive in the literature

PSIS = posterior superior iliac spine; SI = sacroiliac.

Examination Findings 13-4
Sacroiliac Dysfunction

Examination Segment	Clinical Findings
History	***Onset:*** Acute or insidious ***Pain characteristics:*** Over one or both SI joints; pain possibly radiating to the buttock, groin, or thigh. Pain does not generally go above the L5 level. The patient may complain of anterior pain at the pubis symphysis. ***Other symptoms:*** Not applicable ***Mechanism:*** No one mechanism leads to the onset of SI joint dysfunction, but it may be related to prolonged stresses placed across the sacroiliac joint by soft tissues. The patient may describe fall on the buttocks as instigating incident. ***Predisposing conditions:*** Postpartum or pregnant women may be predisposed to SI joint pathology because relaxin released prior to and following birth increases the extensibility of the ligaments surrounding the SI joints. Hormonal changes before menstrual period may increase the laxity of the SI ligaments, causing SI pain.
Inspection	The levels of the iliac crests, ASIS, and PSIS are observed for symmetry.
Palpation	Tenderness may be elicited over the SI joint and the PSIS. Palpation for asymmetry such as unequal heights of the PSIS and ASIS
Joint and Muscle Function Assessment	***AROM:*** Pain may be elicited at the extremes of trunk motion. ***MMT:*** Tests performed in mid-range generally unremarkable ***PROM:*** Hip flexion greater than 70° may produce symptoms. Restricted hip extension (tight hip flexors)
Joint Stability Tests	***Stress tests:*** Not applicable ***Joint play:*** Posterior to anterior joint play may provoke symptoms.
Special Tests	Long sit test; SI compression and distraction; straight leg raising, Fabere test; Gaenslen's test; quadrant test
Neurologic Screening	A complete lower quarter screen of the sensory, motor, and reflex distributions to rule out lumbar nerve root involvement
Vascular Screening	Within normal limits
Functional Assessment	Activities that require trunk flexion with the knees extended may cause sufficient movement of the sacrum on the ilia to cause pain.
Imaging Techniques	Axial CT scans, MRI, and AP and lateral radiographs
Differential Diagnosis	Nerve root impingement, facet joint dysfunction, pelvic stress fracture
Comments	The pain distribution may mimic lumbar nerve root involvement. A combination of findings from multiple special tests is more reliable than the results of a single test. A diagnosis can be confirmed if an intra-articular injection of an anesthetic relieves symptoms.[85]

AP = anteroposterior; AROM = active range of motion; CT = computed tomography; MMT = manual muscle test; MRI = magnetic resonance imaging; PROM = passive range of motion; ASIS = anterior superior iliac spine; PSIS = posterior superior iliac spine; SI = sacroiliac.

Special Test 13-14
Sacroiliac Joint Compression and Distraction Tests

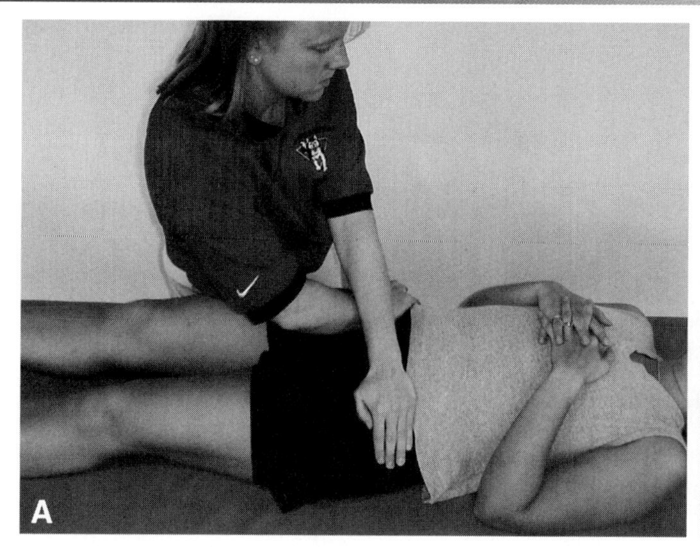

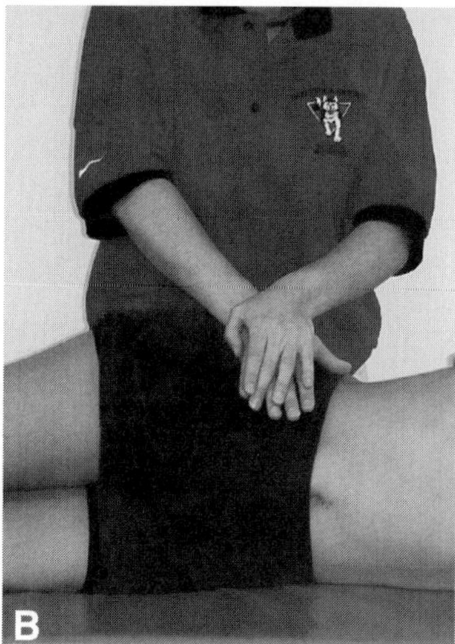

(A) Sacroiliac joint compression test. Spreading the ASIS compresses the SI joint. **(B)** Sacroiliac joint distraction test. Compressing the ASIS distracts the SI joints. The distraction test should be performed on both sides.

Patient Position	***Compression:*** Sidelying ***Distraction:*** Supine
Position of Examiner	***Compression:*** At the side of the patient with the hands placed over the opposite ASIS bilaterally ***Distraction:*** Behind the patient with both hands over the lateral aspect of the pelvis.
Evaluative Procedure	***Compression:*** The examiner applies pressure to spread the ASIS, thus compressing the SI joints. ***Distraction:*** The examiner applies pressure down through the anterior portion of the ilium, spreading the SI joints.
Positive Test	Pain arising from the SI joint
Implications	Sacroiliac pathology
Evidence	Compression inter-rater reliability Not Reliable — Very Reliable Poor — Moderate — Good 0 0.1 0.2 0.3 0.4 0.5 0.6 0.7 0.8 0.9 1.0 Distraction inter-rater reliability Not Reliable — Very Reliable Poor — Moderate — Good 0 0.1 0.2 0.3 0.4 0.5 0.6 0.7 0.8 0.9 1.0 Compression positive likelihood ratio Not Useful — Useful Very Small — Small — Moderate — Large 0 1 2 3 4 5 6 7 8 9 10 Compression negative likelihood ratio Not Useful — Useful Very Small — Small — Moderate — Large 1.0 0.9 0.8 0.7 0.6 0.5 0.4 0.3 0.2 0.1 0

ASIS = anterior superior iliac spine; PSIS = posterior superior iliac spine; SI = sacroiliac.

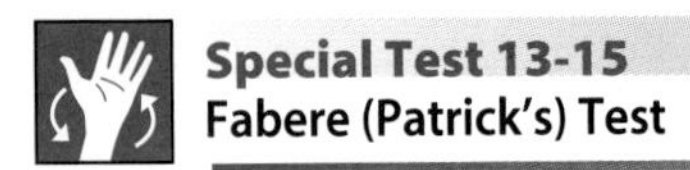

Special Test 13-15
Fabere (Patrick's) Test

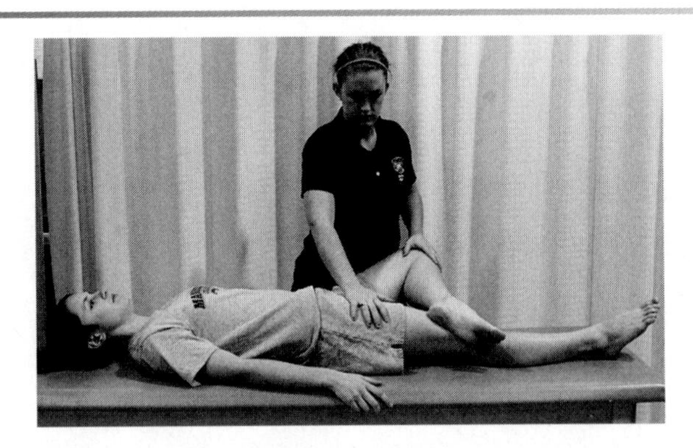

Fabere (flexion, abduction, external rotation, and extension) test for hip or sacroiliac pathology.

Position	Supine, with the foot of the involved side crossed over the opposite thigh
Position of Examiner	At the side of the patient to be tested with one hand on the opposite ASIS and the other on the medial aspect of the flexed knee
Evaluative Procedure	The extremity is allowed to rest into full external rotation followed by the examiner's applying overpressure at the knee and ASIS.
Positive Test	Reproduction of symptoms in the sacroiliac joint or hip
Implications	Pain in the inguinal area anterior to the hip may indicate hip pathology. Pain in the SI area during the application of overpressure may indicate SI joint pathology.
Evidence	Positive likelihood ratio Not Useful — Useful Very Small / Small / Moderate / Large 0 1 2 3 4 5 6 7 8 9 10 Negative likelihood ratio Not Useful — Useful Very Small / Small / Moderate / Large 1.0 0.9 0.8 0.7 0.6 0.5 0.4 0.3 0.2 0.1 0

ASIS = anterior superior iliac spine; SI = sacroiliac.

girls and generally becomes apparent during the teenage years (13 to 16 years old). The problem is attributed to osteochondrosis of the vertebral bodies and is often found in conjunction with scoliosis. The diagnosis is made with radiographs and **Schmorl's nodes** are a common associated finding.

Adolescents with Scheuermann's disease appear to have increased thoracic or, sometimes, lumbar kyphosis which is more apparent with forward flexion. These individuals describe pain or discomfort that increases with activity. Treatment of Scheuermann's disease is based on the extent and progressive nature of the curve and consists of exercise and monitoring, bracing or surgery.[96]

Schmorl's nodes Herniation of the nucleus pulposus through the vertebral endplate.

On-Field Evaluation of Thoracic and Lumbar Spine Injuries

All injuries to the spinal column requiring an on-field evaluation must be treated as being catastrophic in nature until determined otherwise. Bilateral symptoms in the upper extremities or symptoms in the lower extremities should alert the examiner to the potential of spinal cord involvement. Chapter 21 discusses the evaluation and management of potentially catastrophic spinal cord injuries.

On-Field History

- **Location of pain**: Pain that is localized to the vertebral column can indicate a disk rupture, sprain, or facet pathology. Pain running parallel to the vertebral

Special Test 13-16
Gaenslen's Test

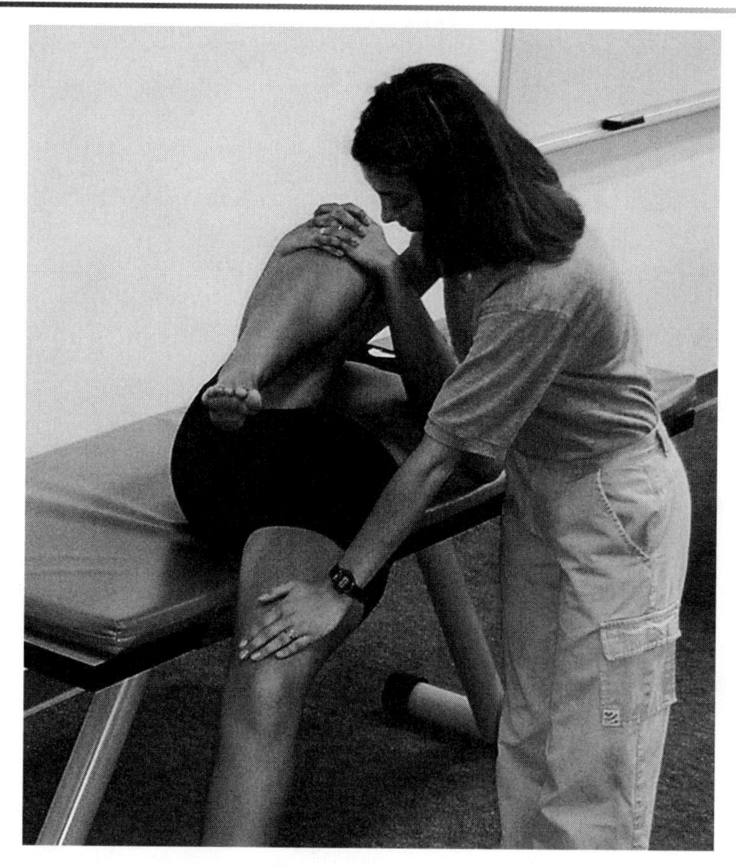

Gaenslen's test places a rotational force on the SI joints.

Patient Position	Supine, lying close to the side of the table
Position of Examiner	Standing at the side of the patient
Evaluative Procedure	The examiner slides the patient close to the edge of the table. The patient pulls the far knee up to the chest. The near leg is allowed to hang over the edge of the table. While stabilizing the patient, the examiner applies pressure to the near leg, forcing the hip into extension.
Positive Test	Pain in the SI region
Implications	SI joint dysfunction
Comments	The lumbar spine should not go into extension during this test.
Evidence	Inter-rater reliability

Positive likelihood ratio

Negative likelihood ratio

SI = sacroiliac.

Special Test 13-17
Long Sit Test

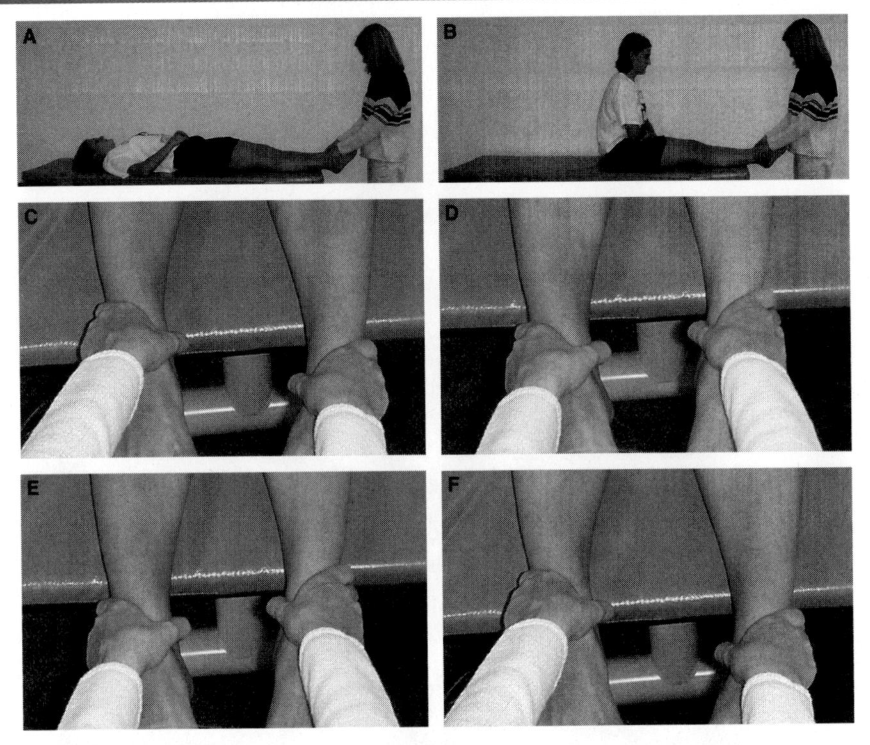

(A) Starting position. **(B)** Finishing position. **(C)** Left leg is longer when supine and becomes shorter when assuming a sitting position. **(D)** Signifying anterior rotation of the ilium. **(E)** Left leg is shorter when supine and becomes longer when assuming a sitting position. **(F)** Signifying posterior rotation of the ilium.

Patient Position	Supine with the heels off the table
Position of Examiner	Holding the feet with the thumbs placed over the medial malleoli
Evaluative Procedure	The examiner provides slight traction on the legs while the patient arches and lifts the buttocks off the table. The patient then rests supine on the table. The patient then moves from a supine to a long sit position. The examiner must pay close attention to the position of the malleoli at all times throughout the test. This test is done actively if possible, without assistance provided by the upper extremities.
Positive Test	The movement of the medial malleoli is observed. If the involved leg (painful side) goes from a longer to a shorter position, there is an anterior rotation of the ilium on that side. If the involved side goes from a shorter to a longer position, posterior rotation of the ilium on the sacrum is indicated.
Implications	Rotated ilium as noted above

Evidence

Inter-rater reliability

Not Reliable — Very Reliable

Poor | Moderate | Good

0 0.1 0.2 0.3 0.4 0.5 0.6 0.7 0.8 0.9 1.0

Positive likelihood ratio

Not Useful — Useful

Very Small | Small | Moderate | Large

0 1 2 3 4 5 6 7 8 9 10

Negative likelihood ratio

Not Useful — Useful

Very Small | Small | Moderate | Large

1.0 0.9 0.8 0.7 0.6 0.5 0.4 0.3 0.2 0.1 0

column may indicate spasm of the paravertebral muscles. Pain radiating into the extremities may indicate trauma to one or more spinal nerve roots.

- **Peripheral symptoms**: Pain, weakness, or numbness that radiates into the extremity is usually the result of nerve root impingement.
- **Mechanism of injury**: External forces that produce rotation of the spine may result in facet joint dislocation or subluxation, disk trauma, or ligamentous sprains. Eccentric contractions may result in a muscular strain.

On-Field Inspection

- **Position of the athlete**: Observe the athlete's position. Is the athlete prone or supine? If the athlete is supine and trauma to the vertebra, spinal cord, nerve roots, or spinal musculature is suspected, these structures cannot be palpated without moving the athlete. If spinal cord involvement is suspected, the athlete must be managed according to the procedures described in Chapter 21.
- **Posture**: Note the presence of abnormal posture, including flexion or extension posturing of the extremities or flaccidity of the muscles possibly indicating spinal cord involvement. The patient may also assume a posture that decreases the amount of pressure placed on the involved structure (e.g., disk, facet joints) or the posture may be influenced by muscle spasm.
- **Willingness to move**: Assume that a motionless athlete is unconscious until otherwise ruled out. Disk lesions, vertebral fractures, facet dislocations, or muscle spasm may cause the athlete to move in a guarded manner.

On-Field Neurologic Tests

If the athlete describes symptoms that radiate into the extremities, the following on-field neurologic assessments are necessary. If these tests show positive results (or if there is reason to suspect a vertebral fracture or dislocation), then the athlete must be managed as described in Chapter 21.

- **Sensory tests**: Bilaterally check the anterior, posterior, medial, and lateral aspects of the extremities to assure equal sensory function within the dermatomes. Absent or diminished sensation in one or more extremity can indicate serious spinal cord trauma.
- **Motor tests**: Ask the athlete to wiggle the feet and hands and bend the knees and elbows. An inability to perform these tasks may indicate spinal cord trauma.

On-Field Palpation

If the athlete is in the prone position, the majority of the lumbar and thoracic spine can be easily palpated, although portions of the back may be covered by protective equipment. Do not roll an athlete who is supine to perform palpation if the possibility of spinal cord involvement or vertebral fracture exists.

- **Bony palpation**: Palpate the spinous processes of the lumbar and thoracic spine (typically easily palpable [refer to Tables 13-6 and 13-7 for the approximate location of the spinous processes]). The transverse processes may be masked by the paravertebral muscles, but their location can be palpated for tenderness.
- **Paraspinal muscles**: Palpate the paraspinal muscles to identify areas of spasm. If the trauma was caused secondary to a direct blow, the area may be tender to the touch.

On-Field Management of Thoracic and Lumbar Spine Injuries

This section describes the on-field management of thoracic and lumbar spine injuries. Athletes suspected of having vertebral fractures or dislocations in these areas of the spinal column should be spine boarded as described in Chapter 21.

Thoracic Spine

Forced flexion or lateral bending of the thoracic spine places compressive forces on the anterior aspect of the vertebral bodies in the lower thoracic spine. The upper thoracic spine can be compressed by an axial load's being placed on the cervical spine.[97,98] In most instances, neurologic function is normal, leaving the on-field determination of a possible fracture to be based on the mechanism of injury and point tenderness over the affected vertebra.[99] If the fracture goes unrecognized, pain and stiffness in the thoracic region and pain during deep inspiration may be reported.[97] Although it is a rare occurrence, fractured thoracic vertebra may puncture the esophagus[100] or the aorta.[101]

Although most thoracic spine fractures are stable, athletes suspected of suffering from this pathology must be spine boarded and transported to undergo further medical evaluation.[99] Radiographs are used to confirm the presence of the fracture.

Lumbar Spine

Catastrophic injury to the lumbar spine is relatively rare because of the decreased ROM of this area and the extremely high forces needed to cause this injury. However, this fact should not allow the athletic trainer or physician to become complacent during the evaluation process. As with all spinal injuries, the evaluation of the lumbar spine must be approached as if a catastrophic injury exists until it has been ruled out.

The athlete must be questioned for a history of symptoms, including pain and paresthesia. Pain localized over a spinous process may indicate a compression or burst fracture. This alone is reason for immediate referral. Any symptoms suggesting neurologic involvement must be investigated. An athlete reporting bilateral symptoms must be treated as having a spinal cord injury, immobilized on a spine board, and properly transported to a medical facility.

Direct blows to the lumbar or thoracic region may result in trauma to the kidneys, ribs, or other internal organs. The evaluation of these conditions is discussed in Chapter 15.

REFERENCES

1. Strine, TW, and Hootman, JM: US national prevalence and correlates of low back and neck pain among adults. *Arthr Rheum*, 57:656, 2007.
2. Leboeuf-Yde, C, and Kyvik, KO: Is it possible to differentiate people with or without low-back pain on the basis of tests of lumbopelvic dysfunction? *J Manipulative and Physiol Ther.* 23:160, 2000.
3. Tall, RL, and DeVault, W: Spinal injury in sport: Epidemiologic consideration. *Clin Sports Med*, 12:441, 1993.
4. Hilibrand, AS, and Rand, N: Degenerative lumbar stenosis: Diagnosis and management. *J Am Acad Orthop Surg*, 7:239, 1999.
5. Nachemson, A, and Eifstrom, G: Intravital dynamic measurements in lumbar discs. *Scand J Rehabil Med* (suppl):1, 1960.
6. Dalton, D: The vertebral column. In Levangie PK, Norkin CC. *Joint Structure and Function*. Philadelphia: FA Davis, 2005.
7. Oegema, TR: Biochemistry of the intervertebral disc. *Clin Sports Med*, 12:419, 1993.
8. Carrigg, SY, and Hillemeyer, LE: The effect of running-induced intervertebral disc compression on thoracolumbar vertebral column mobility in young, healthy males. *J Orthop Sports Phys Ther*, 16:19, 1992.
9. Naylor, A, and Shentall, R: Biochemical aspects of intervertebral discs in aging and disease. In Jayson, M (ed): *The Lumbar Spine and Back Pain*. New York, Grune and Stratton, Inc, 1976, pp 317–326.
10. Hanley, ED, and David, SM: Lumbar arthrodesis for the treatment of back pain. *J Bone Joint Surg*, 81(A):716, 1999.
11. Nachemson, A, and Morris, JM: In vivo measurements of intradiscal pressure. *J Bone Joint Surg*, 46(A):1077, 1964.
12. Costi, JJ, et al: Direct measurement of intervertebral disc maximum shear strain in six degrees of freedom: Motions that place disc tissue at risk of injury. *J Biomech*, 40:2457, 2007.
13. MacLennan, AH: The role of the hormone relaxin in human reproduction and pelvic girdle relaxation. *Scand J Rheumatol*, 20(suppl 88):7, 1991.
14. Hodges, PW, and Richardson, CA: Inefficient muscular stabilization of the lumbar spine associated with low back pain: A motor control evaluation of transversus abdominis. *Spine*, 21:2640, 1996.
15. Fritz, JM, Erhard, RE, and Hagen, BF: Segmental instability of the lumbar spine. *Phys Ther*, 78:889, 1998.
16. Kolber, MJ, and Beekhuizen, K: Lumbar stabilization: An evidence-based approach for the athlete with low back pain. *Strength and Conditioning Journal*, 29:26, 2007.
17. Van Dillen, LR, Sahrmann, SA, and Wagner, JM: Classification, intervention, and outcomes for a person with lumbar rotation with flexion syndrome. *Phys Ther*, 85:336, 2005.
18. Hestbaek, L, et al: The course of low back pain from adolescence to adulthood. *Spine*, 31:468, 2006.
19. Linton, SJ: A review of psychological risk factors in back and neck pain. *Spine*, 25:1148, 2000.
20. George, SZ, Bialosky, JE, and Donald, DA: The centralization phenomenon and fear-avoidance beliefs as prognostic factors for acute low back pain: A preliminary investigation involving patients classified for specific exercise. *J Orthop Sports Phys Ther*, 35:580, 2005.
21. Grotle, M, Vollestad, NK, and Brox, JI: Clinical course and impact of fear-avoidance beliefs in low back pain. *Spine*, 31:1038, 2006.
22. Haggman, S, Maher, C, and Refshauge, KM: Screening for symptoms of depression by physical therapists managing low back pain. *Phys Ther*, 84:1157, 2004.
23. Boissonnault, W, and DiFabio, RP: Pain profile of patients with low back pain referred to physical therapy. *J Orthop Sport Phys Ther*, 24:180, 1996.
24. Potter, NA, and Rothstein, JM: Intertester reliability for selected clinical tests of the sacroiliac joint. *Phys Ther*, 65:1671, 1985.
25. Gatt, CJ, et al: Impact loading of the lumbar spine during football blocking. *Am J Sports Med*, 25:317, 1997.
26. Sizer, PS, Brismée, J, and Cook, C: Medical screening for red flags in the diagnosis and management of musculoskeletal spine pain. *Pain Practice*, 7:53, 2007.
27. Fairbank, JCT, and Pynsent, PB: The Oswestry Disability Index. *Spine*, 25:2940, 2000.
28. Davidson, M, and Keating, JL: A comparison of five low back disability questionnaires: Reliability and reponsiveness. *Phys Ther*, 82:8, 2002.
29. Voss, LA, Fadale, PD, and Hylstyn, MJ: Exercise-induced loss of bone density in athletes. *J Am Acad Orthop Surg*, 6:349, 1998.
30. Greer, S, and Chambliss, L: What physical exam techniques are useful to detect malingering? *J Fam Pract*, 54:719, 2005.
31. Gaines, WG, and Hegmann, KT: Effectiveness of Waddell's nonorgnic signs in predicting a delayed return to regular work in patients experience acute occupational low back pain. *Spine*, 24:396, 1999.
32. Waddell, G: *The Back Pain Revolution*. Edinburgh: Churchill Livingstone, 2004, p. 186.
33. Hoover, CF: A new sign for the detection of malingering and functional paresis of lower extremities. *JAMA*, 51:746, 1908.
34. Archibald, AC, and Wiechec, F: A reappraisal of Hoover's test. *Arch Phys Med Rehabil*, 51:234, 1970.
35. Arieff, AJ, et al: The Hoover sign: An objective sign of pain and/or weakness in the back or lower extremities. *Arch Neurol*, 5:673, 1961.
36. Westbrook, A, et al: The mannequin sign. *Spine*, 30:E115, 2005.
37. Weiner, DK, et al: Chronic low back pain in older adults: Prevalence, reliability, and validity of physical examination findings. *J Am Geriatr Soc*, 54:11, 2006.
38. Weinstein, SL, et al: Health and function of patients with untreated idiopathic scoliosis. A 50-year natural history study. *JAMA*, 289:599, 2003.
39. Landau, M, and Krafchik, BR: The diagnostic value of café-au-lait macules. *J Am Acad Dermatol*, 40:877, 1999.
40. Abeliovich, D, et al: Familial café-au-lait spots: A variant of neurofibromatosis type 1. *J Med Genet*, 32:985, 1995.
41. Binkley, J, Stratford, PW, and Gill, C: Interrater reliability of lumbar accessory motion mobility testing. *Phys Ther*, 75:786, 1995.

42. Ensink, F, et al: Lumbar range of motion: Influence of time of day and individual factors on measurements. *Spine*, 21:1339, 1996.
43. McKenzie, RA: The lumbar spine: *Mechanical Diagnosis and Therapy.* Waikanae, New Zealand, Spinal Publications, 1981.
44. Reese, NB, and Bandy, WD: *Joint Range of Motion and Muscle Length Testing.* Philadelphia: W.B Saunders Co., 2002.
45. Latimer, J, et al: Plinth padding and measures of posteroanterior lumbar stiffness. *J Manipulative and Physiol Ther*, 20:315, 1997.
46. Scham, SM, and Taylor, TKF: Tension signs in lumbar disc prolapse. *Clin Orthop*, 75:195, 1971.
47. Hudgens, WR: The crossed-straight-leg-raising test. *N Engl J Med*, 297:1127, 1977.
48. Woodhall, R, and Hayes, GJ: The well-leg-raising test of Fajersztajn in the diagnosis of ruptured lumbar intervertebral disc. *J Bone Joint Surg Am*, 32:786, 1950.
49. Johnson, EK, and Chiarello, CM: The slump test: the effects of head and lower extremity position on knee extension. *J Orthop Sports Phys Ther*, 26:310, 1997.
50. Fritz, JM: Lumbar intervertebral disc injuries in athletes. *Athletic Therapy Today*, March:27, 1999.
51. Coppieters, MW, et al: Strain and excursion of the sciatic, tibial, and plantar nerves during a modified straight leg raising test. *J Orthop Res*, 24:1883, 2006.
52. Beskin, JL: Nerve entrapment syndromes of the foot and ankle. *J Am Acad Orthop Surg*, 5:261, 1997.
53. Van Dillen, LR, et al: Reliability of physical examination items used for classification of patients with low back pain. *Phys Ther*, 78, 979, 1998.
54. Fritz, JM, Cleland, JA, and Childs, JD: Subgrouping patients with low back pain: Evolution of a classification approach to physical therapy. *J Orthop Sports Phys Ther*, 37:296, 2007.
55. Delitto, A, Erhard, RE, and Bowling, RW: A treatment-based classification approach to low back syndrome: Identifying and staging patients for conservative treatment. *Phys Ther*, 75:740, 1995.
56. Fritz, JM, Erhard, RE, and Vignovic, M: A nonsurgical treatment approach for patients with lumbar spinal stenosis. *Phys Ther*, 77:963, 1997.
57. de Graaf, I, et al: Diagnosis of lumbar spinal stenosis. *Spine*, 31:1168, 2006.
58. Luoma, K, et al: Low back pain in relation to lumbar disc degeneration. *Spine*, 25:487, 2000.
59. Ginsburg, GM, and Bassett, GS: Back pain in children and adolescents: Evaluation and differential diagnosis. *J Am Acad Orthop Surg*, 5:67, 1997.
60. Jensen, MC, et al: Magnetic imaging of the lumbar spine in people without back pain. *N Engl J Med* 331:69, 1994.
61. ten Brinke, A, et al: Is leg length discrepancy associated with the side of radiating pain in patients with a lumbar herniated disc? *Spine*, 24:684, 1999.
62. Revel, M, et al: Capacity of the clinical picture to characterize low back pain relieved by facet joint anesthesia: Proposed criteria to identify patients with painful facet joints. *Spine*, 23:1972, 1998.
63. Jonsson, B, and Stromqvist, B: Clinical characteristics of recurrent sciatica after lumbar discectomy. *Spine*, 21:500, 1996.
64. Benyahya, E, et al: Sciatica as the first manifestation of a leiomyosarcoma of the buttock. *Rev Rheum Engl Ed*, 64:135, 1997.
65. Amundsen, T, et al: Lumbar spinal stenosis. Clinical and radiological features. *Spine*, 20:1178, 1995.
66. Maheshwaran, S, et al: Sciatica in degenerative spondylolisthesis of the lumbar spine. *Ann Rheum Dis*, 54:539, 1995.
67. Spencer, DL: The anatomical basis of sciatica secondary to herniated lumbar disc: A review. *Neurol Res*, 21(suppl 1):S33, 1999.
68. Zwart, JA, Sand, T, and Unsgaard, G: Warm and cold sensory thresholds in patients with unilateral sciatica: C fibers are more severely affected than a-delta fibers. *Acta Neurol Scand*, 97:41, 1998.
69. Tomaszewski, D: Vertebral osteomyelitis in a high school hockey player: A case report. *J Athl Train*, 34:29, 1999.
70. Starkey, C: Injuries and illnesses in the National Basketball Association: A 10-year perspective. *J Athl Train*, 35:161, 2000.
71. Deitch, JR, et al: Injury risk in professional basketball players. A comparison of Women's National Basketball Association and National Basketball Association athletes. *Am J Sport Med*, 34:1077, 2006.
72. Natarajan, RN, et al: Study on effect of graded facetectomy on change in lumbar motion segment torsional flexibility using three-dimensional continuum contact representation for facet joints. *J Biomech Eng*, 121:215, 1999.
73. Boden, SD, et al: Orientation of the lumbar facet joints: association with degenerative disc disease. *J Bone Joint Surg*, 78(A):403, 1996.
74. Dreyer, SJ, and Dreyfuss, PH: Low back pain and the zygapophysial (facet) joints. *Arch Phys Med Rehabil*, 77:290, 1996.
75. Kasai, Y, et al: A new evaluation method for lumbar spinal instability: Passive lumbar extension test. *Phys Ther*, 86:1, 2006.
76. Congeni, J, McCulloch, J, and Swanson, K: Lumbar spondylolysis. A study of natural progression in athletes. *Am J Sports Med*, 25:248, 1997.
77. Soler, T, and Calderón, C: The prevalence of spondylolysis in the Spanish elite athlete. *Amer J Sports Med*, 28:57, 2000.
78. Micheli, LJ, and Wood, R: Back pain in young athletes: Significant differences from adults in causes and patterns. *Arch Pediatr Adolesc Med*, 149:15, 1995.
79. Motley, G, et al: The pars interarticularis stress reaction, spondylolysis, and spondylolisthesis progression. *J Athl Train*, 33:351, 1998.
80. Jackson, D, et al: Stress reactions involving the pars interarticularis in young athletes. *Am J Sports Med*, 9:305, 1981.
81. Pezzullo, DJ: Spondylolisthesis and spondylolysis in athletes. *Athletic Therapy Today*, March:36, 1999.
82. Moore, KL: The perineum and pelvis. In Moore, KL (ed): *Clinically Oriented Anatomy*, 5th ed. Baltimore, Williams & Wilkins, 2005, p 389.
83. Youssef, M, et al: Lumbar facet anatomy changes in spondylolysis: A comparative skeletal study. *Eur Spine J*, 16:993, 2007.
84. Tertti, M, et al: Disc degeneration in young gymnasts: A magnetic resonance imaging study. *Am J Sports Med*, 18:206, 1990.
85. Freburger, JK, and Riddle, DL: Using published evidence to guide the examination of the sacroiliac joint region. *Phys Ther*, 81:1135, 2001.
86. Major, NM, and Helms, CA: Pelvic stress injuries: the relationship between osteitis pubis (symphysis pubis stress injury) and sacroiliac abnormalities in athletes. *Skeletal Radiol*, 26:711, 1997.

87. Potter, NA, and Rothstein, JM: Intertester reliability for selected clinical tests of the sacroiliac joint. *Phys Ther,* 65:1671, 1985.
88. Maigne, JY, Aivaliklis, A, and Pfefer, F: Results of sacroiliac joint double block and value of sacroiliac pain provocation tests in 54 patients with low back pain. *Spine,* 21:1889, 1996.
89. Laslett, M, and Williams, M: The reliability of selected pain provocation tests for sacroiliac joint pathology. *Spine,* 19:1243, 1994.
90. Cibulka, MT, Delitto, A, and Koldehoff, RM: Changes in innominate tilt after manipulation of the sacroiliac joint in patients with low back pain: An experimental study. *Phys Ther,* 68:1359, 1988.
91. Broadhurst, NA, and Bond, MJ: Pain provocation tests for the assessment of sacroiliac joint dysfunction. *J Spinal Disord,* 11:341, 1998.
92. Riddle, DL, and Freburger, JK: North American Orthopaedic Rehabilitation Research Network. Evaluation of the presence of sacroiliac joint region dysfunction using a combination of tests: A multicenter intertester reliability study. *Phys Ther,* 82:772, 2002.
93. Laslett, M, et al: Diagnosis of sacroiliac joint pain: Validity of individual provocation tests and composites of tests. *Man Ther,* 10:207, 2005.
94. Cibulka, MT, and Koldehoff, R: Clinical usefulness of a cluster of sacroiliac joint tests in patients with an without low back pain. *J Orthop Sports Phys Ther,* 29:83, 1999.
95. Fruth, SJ: Differential diagnosis and treatment in a patient with posterior upper thoracic pain. *Phys Ther,* 86:254, 2006.
96. Soo, CL, Noble, PC, and Esses, SI: Scheuermann kyphosis: Long-term follow-up. *Spine,* 2:49, 2002.
97. Elattrache, N, Fadale, PD, and Fu, FH: Thoracic spine fracture in a football player. A case report. *Am J Sports Med,* 21:157, 1993.
98. Kifune, M, et al: Fracture pattern and instability of throacolumbar injuries. *Eur Spine J,* 4:98, 1995.
99. McHugh-Pierzina, VL, Zillmer, DA, and Giangarra, CE: Thoracic compression fracture in a basketball player. *J Athl Train,* 30:163, 1995.
100. Brouwers, MA, Veldhuis, EF, and Zimmerman, KW: Fracture of the thoracic spine with paralysis and esophageal perforation. *Eur Spine J,* 6:211, 1997.
101. Bakker, FC, Patka, P, and Haarman, HJ: Combined repair of a traumatic rupture of the aorta and anterior stabilization of a thoracic spine fracture: a case report. *J Trauma,* 40:128, 1996.

CHAPTER 14

Cervical Spine Pathologies

The cervical spine provides the greatest range of motion (ROM) among the segments of the spinal column. However, the spinal cord is the most vulnerable in this location of the spinal column. Because of its important role in protecting the spinal cord and spinal nerve roots, injury to the cervical vertebrae can have catastrophic results. Noncatastrophic injury to the neck region can also impact daily life. Similar to low back pain, the origin of cervical spine pain is frequently nonspecific in that the aggravating structure cannot be identified. Because approximately one-third of the population will experience cervical pain during their lives, a systematic examination that leads to specific treatment options is required for proper patient care.[1]

This chapter describes the clinical evaluation of cervical spine pathology. Chapter 21 describes the on-field evaluation and management of patients with potentially catastrophic cervical spine trauma. The procedures described in this chapter assume that the possibility of spinal fracture and dislocation have been ruled out.

Clinical Anatomy

Carrying only the weight of the head, the vertebral bodies of the cervical vertebrae are much smaller than the other sections of the spinal column. The cervical transverse processes include a **transverse foramen** through which the vertebral artery and vein pass, a structure not found in the thoracic or lumbar vertebra (Fig. 14-1). Each vertebra articulates with its adjacent vertebrae via an interbody articulation and superior and inferior facet (zygapophyseal) articulations that project from the pars interarticularis. The **uncinate processes** on the posteromedial margin of the body's endplates give the superior surface a concavity and increase the joint surface of the vertebral body.

The first two vertebrae of the cervical spine are unique. The first cervical vertebra, the **atlas**, has no vertebral body and supports the weight of the skull through two concave facet surfaces articulating with the occiput, forming the **atlanto–occipital joint**. The primary movement at the junction between the atlas and the skull (the C0–C1 articulation) is flexion and extension, such as when nodding the head "yes." A slight amount of lateral flexion also occurs at the C0–C1 articulation. At the C1 vertebrae, the transverse processes are exceptionally long and no true spinous process exists. The second cervical vertebra, the **axis**, has a small body with a superior projection, the dens. The articulation between the anterior arch of the atlas and the dens forms the **atlanto–axial joint**, providing the majority of cervical rotation, as when shaking the head "no" (Fig. 14-2). The C0–C1 and C1–C2 articulations are entirely synovial joints that are lacking the substantial bony facet joints found along the remainder of the vertebral column. These superior facet joints are oriented horizontally and lack the bony congruence found in the lower cervical region. The absence of a bony restraint increases the possibility of acute or congenital subluxations at these joints.[2]

Moving inferiorly along the remainder of the cervical vertebrae, the dimensions of the bone and intervertebral disk

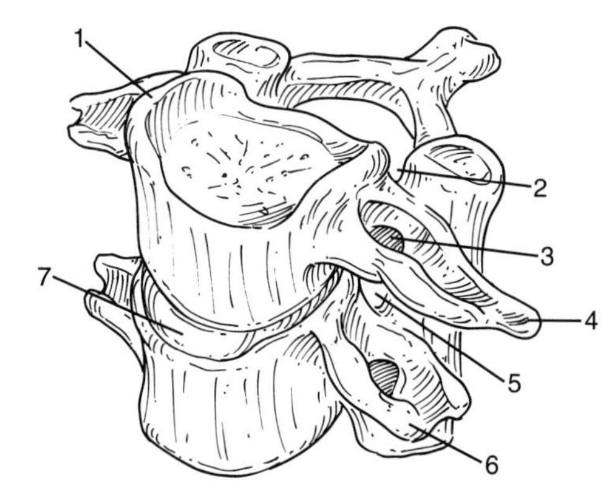

FIGURE 14-1 ■ C4 and C5 cervical vertebrae. *1*, Uncinate process; *2*, superior intervertebral notch; *3*, transverse foramen; *4*, posterior tubercle of transverse process; *5*, intervertebral foramen (spinal nerve foramen); *6*, anterior tubercle of transverse process; *7*, C4–C5 disk; *8*, spinous process.

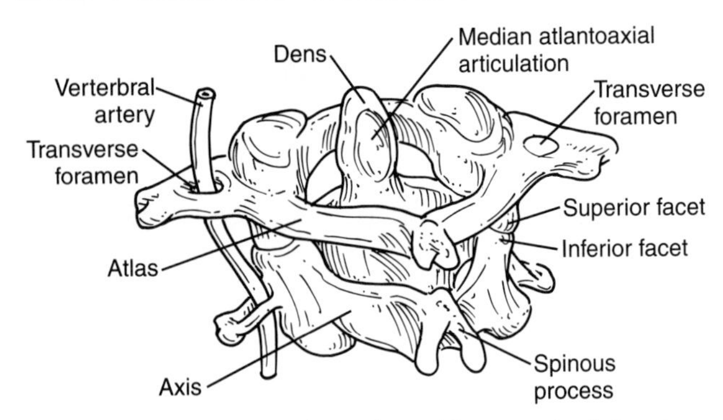

FIGURE 14-2 ■ Atlanto–axial joint formed between the first and second cervical vertebrae. The dens serves as the axis of rotation for the skull's movement on the vertebral column.

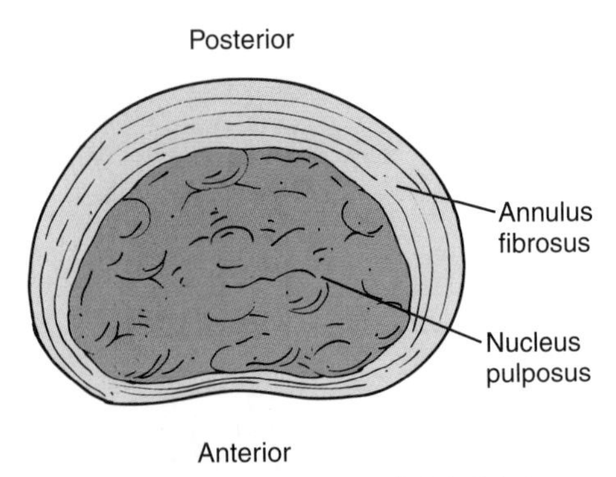

FIGURE 14-3 ■ Cross section of a cervical disk. Relative to a lumbar disk, the annulus fibrosus is significantly thinner, especially on the posterior borders and laterally. Compare this illustration to Figure 13-6.

increase to provide the stability needed to support the increasing loads and larger muscle masses attaching at these levels. As with the lumbar spine, the facet joints of the cervical spine are formed by the lateral portion of the superior facet that articulates with the medial portion of the inferior facet. Refer to Chapter 13 for more information regarding facet joints. The facet joints in the cervical region are positioned approximately 45 degrees from the frontal and horizontal planes, an orientation that favors rotation. This alignment, however, presents single plane motions from occurring in isolation and results in **coupled motions.** For example, for cervical flexion to occur, the body of the vertebrae must tilt anteriorly while it also translates anteriorly.

Spinal nerve roots pass through the intervertebral foramen. During youth the spinal nerve root occupies approximately one-third of the foramen's space. Aging and degenerative changes decrease the free space within the foramen. Space within the foramen also decreases when the cervical spine is extended, thereby increasing the potential of traumatic spinal nerve root impingement.[3]

Intervertebral Disks

The intervertebral disks in the cervical spine, as throughout the rest of the spine, are formed by the dense outer annulus fibrosus surrounding the flexible interdiscal tissue, the nucleus pulposus (see Chapter 13). Unlike the disks in the lumbar region, the annulus fibrosis does not completely encircle the nucleus pulposus. The anterior aspect of the disk is covered by a thick annulus that thins as it travels posteriorly. The lateral aspect of the disk is not covered, and the posterolateral portion of the disk receives some containment by the posterior longitudinal ligament. The posterior aspect of the disk is covered by a thin layer of annulus (Fig. 14-3).[4] In this region, the disks are smaller because they have less weight to support. Because of the unique anatomical features of the first two cervical vertebrae, intervertebral disks are not located at the C0–C1 and C1–C2 articulations.

Ligamentous Anatomy

Extending from the cervical spine to the lumbar spine, **anterior** and **posterior longitudinal ligaments** reinforce the spinal column (Fig. 14-4). The anterior longitudinal ligament runs from the sacrum to C2 and strengthens the anterior portion of the intervertebral disks and vertebrae, limiting extension of the spine. In the area between C2 and the skull, the anterior longitudinal ligament becomes the **anterior atlanto–axial** and the **atlanto–occipital** ligament.

Spanning the length of the vertebral column from the sacrum to C2, the posterior longitudinal ligament is the densest in the cervical spine, gradually thinning as it progresses down the anterior aspect of the vertebral canal. This ligament primarily limits flexion of the spine and reinforces the posterior aspect of the intervertebral disk. The posterior longitudinal ligament becomes the **tectorial membrane** as it runs from C2 to the skull.

In the cervical spine, the supraspinous ligament becomes the **ligamentum nuchae**, a triangular septum that serves as a broad area for muscle attachment. The ligamentum nuchae restricts flexion in the cervical spine (Fig. 14-5).

The **interspinous ligaments**, which occupy the space between the spinous processes, limit flexion and rotation of

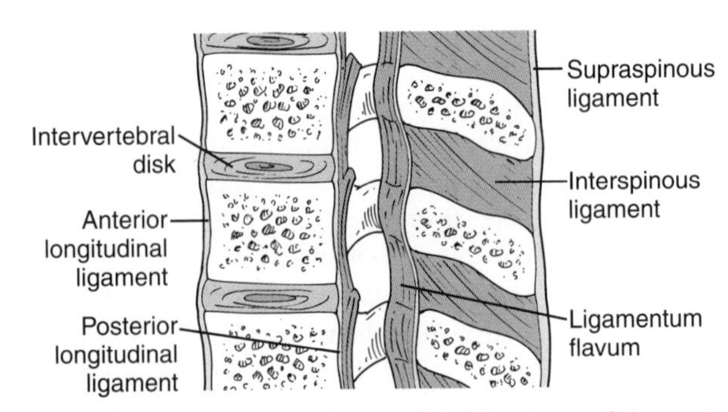

FIGURE 14-4 ■ Cross-sectional view of the ligaments of the cervical vertebral column.

Coupled motion The association of one motion about an axis with another motion around a different axis.

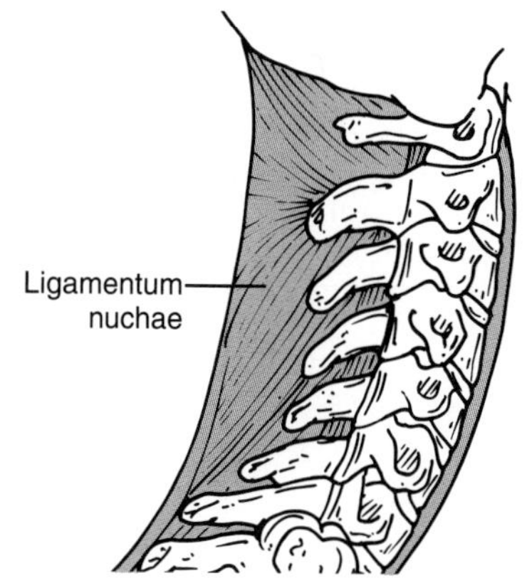

FIGURE 14-5 ■ In the cervical spine, the supraspinous ligament thickens to form the ligamentum nuchae.

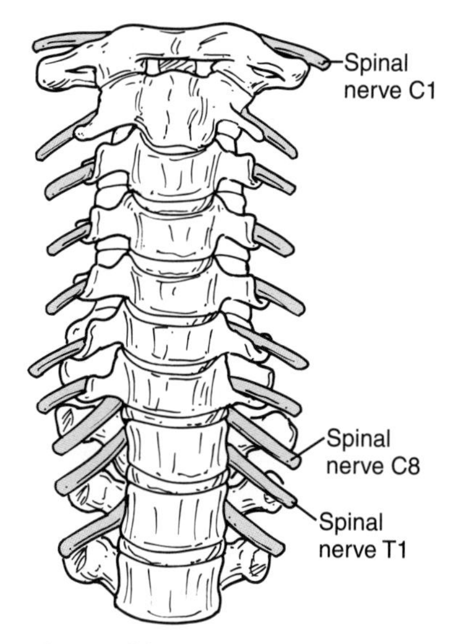

FIGURE 14-6 ■ Pairing of the cervical nerve roots.

the spine. The posterior margin of the vertebral canal is formed by the **ligamentum flavum**, a pair of elastic ligaments connecting the lamina of one vertebra to the lamina of the vertebra above it. The ligamentum flavum limits flexion and rotation of the spine.

The transverse ligament and longitudinal bands, the atlantal cruciform ligament, maintains the position of the dens in the posterior aspect of the atlas and prevent displacement of C1 on C2.

Neurological Anatomy

The brain stem exits from the foramen magnum to become the spinal cord in the upper cervical region. Cranial nerves IX (glossopharyngeal), X (vagus), and XI (accessory) exit the skull via the jugular foramen. The cranial nerves are discussed in more detail in Chapter 21.

Although there are seven cervical vertebrae, eight pairs of nerve roots exit in this area. The first seven cervical nerves exit above the corresponding vertebrae. The "odd" cervical nerve, C8, exits below the seventh cervical vertebra (between the seventh cervical and first thoracic vertebrae) (Fig. 14-6). These spinal nerves, composed of anterior (ventral) root and posterior (dorsal) roots that converge just outside of the intervertebral foramen, subsequently divide into two **rami**, a posterior (dorsal) ramus and an anterior (ventral ramus), each carrying sensory and motor information (Fig. 14-7). The posterior rami innervate the facet joints of the spine, deep muscles of the back and the overlying skin. The much larger anterior rami innervate the remaining trunk and upper extremities.[5] The accessory nerve provides motor input to the sternocleidomastoid and trapezius (see Chapter 16).

Cervical plexus

The cervical plexus is composed of the anterior rami of C1–C4. The cervical plexus provides sensory input to the occipital, supraclavicular, shoulder, and upper thoracic region. The suboccipital nerve from the dorsal ramus of C1 innervates the deep cervical flexors.

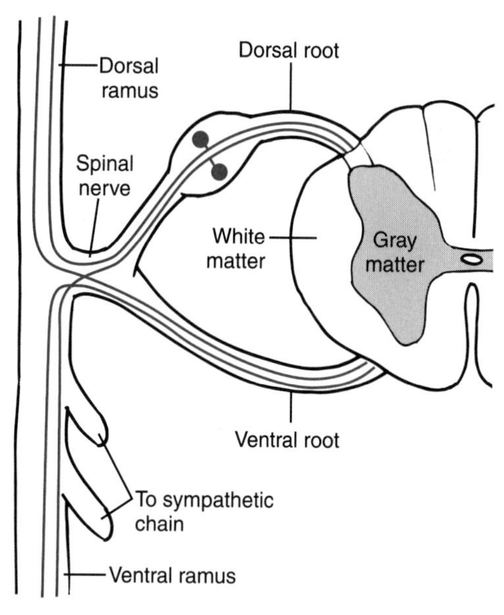

FIGURE 14-7 ■ Nerve root anatomy. The dorsal root, comprised of afferent sensory axons, and the ventral root, comprised of efferent motor axons, converge to form a single spinal nerve. This nerve then diverges into posterior (dorsal) and anterior (ventral) rami. The posterior rami provide sensory and motor innervation to the facet joints, deep muscles and overlying skin. The anterior rami of C5–T1 form the brachial plexus.

Brachial plexus

Supplying innervation to portions of the shoulder, the length of the arm, and the hand, the brachial plexus is formed by the C5 through C8 and the T1 nerve roots. The C4 or T2 nerve roots (or both) also may contribute (Fig. 14-8). The brachial plexus has five segmental areas: roots, trunks, divisions, cords, and branches. The anterior (ventral) portion of the cervical nerve roots contain the motor portion of

Ramus (pl. rami) A branch of a nerve or blood vessel.

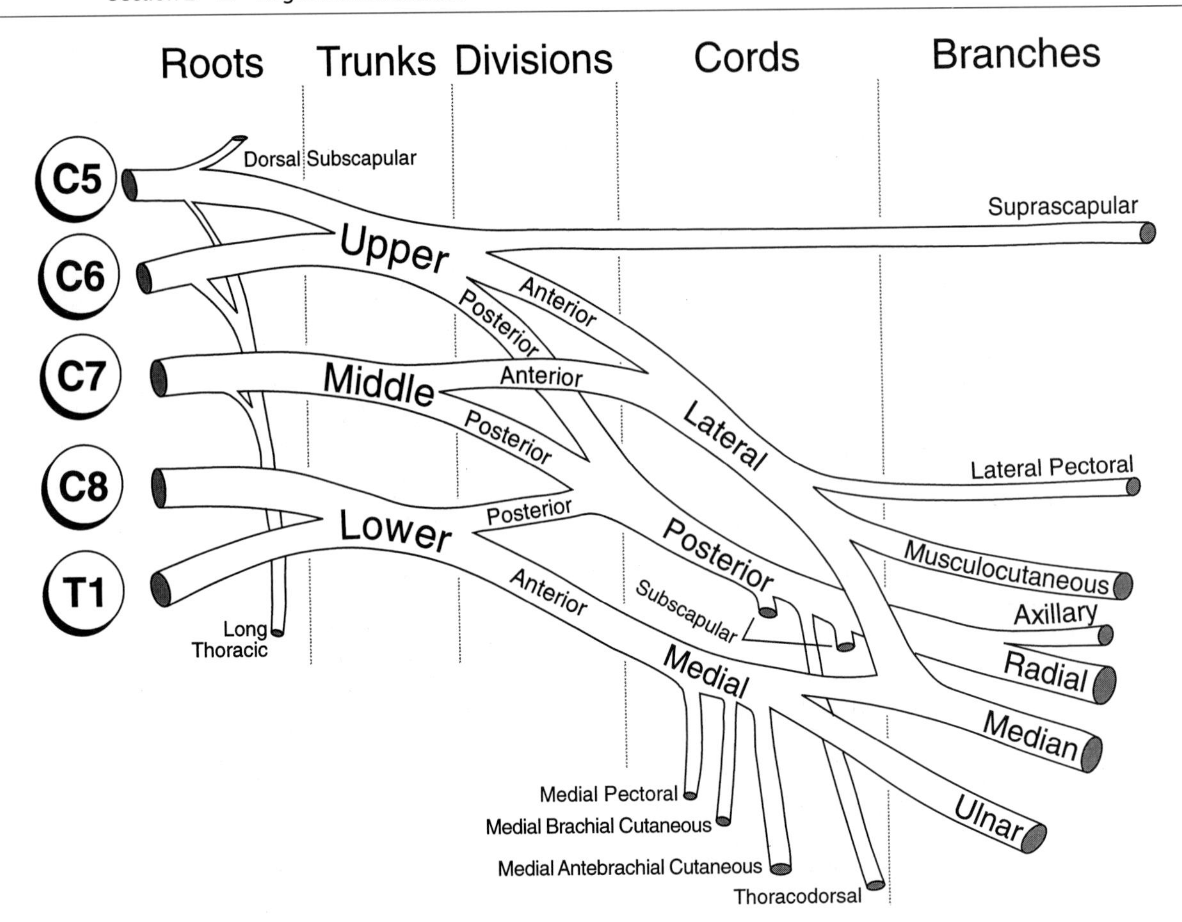

FIGURE 14-8 ■ Brachial plexus formed by the C5–C8 and T1 spinal nerve roots. Note that some texts include the C4 and/or T2 nerve roots as a part of the brachial plexus.

the nerve; the posterior (dorsal) portion transmits sensory information.[3]

The C5 and C6 nerve roots converge to form the upper trunk. The C7 nerve root forms the middle trunk. The C8 and T1 nerve roots merge to form the lower trunk. Each trunk then diverges into anterior and posterior divisions. The posterior divisions of each trunk converge to form the posterior cord; the anterior divisions of the upper and middle trunks merge to form the lateral cord, and the anterior division of the lower cord forms the medial cord.

Each cord diverges to form the terminal branches of the brachial plexus. The lateral cord diverges into the lateral pectoral nerve, the musculocutaneous nerve, and sends a branch that partially innervates the median nerve. The posterior cord splits into the axillary and radial nerves. One portion of the medial cord forms the ulnar nerve, and one portion converges with a division of the lateral cord to form the median nerve. These terminal branches innervate the arm, forearm, and hand. The nerves arising from the medial and lateral cords are routed to the pectoral muscles and the flexor muscles originating on the anterior portion of the arm (relative to the **anatomical position**). The nerves emerging from the posterior cord innervate the muscles of the shoulder itself and the extensor muscles originating on the posterior aspect of the arm. In Figure 14-8, the other nerves that arise from the brachial plexus are identified.

Muscular Anatomy

Precise control of the cervical muscles is required for maintaining the head upright so that the eyes and ears can optimally function. Many of the muscles acting on the cervical spine are superficial and, depending on the fixation of the origin or insertion, act on the shoulder, cervical spine, or head. With bilateral contraction, the cervical spine muscles extend or flex the cervical spine and head. Unilateral contractions primarily result in side bending and contribute to cervical rotation. When coupled with the contractions of other muscles contralateral to themselves, these muscles work primarily to rotate the spine.

The superficial layer of the extensor cervical musculature is formed by the large, flat **splenius capitis** and **splenius cervicis** muscles. These muscles, when acting bilaterally, extend the head and neck. When acting alone, they laterally flex and rotate the head and cervical spine to the same side as the muscle (Fig. 14-9). Just deep to the splenius muscles

Anatomical position The position that the body assumes when standing upright with the feet and palms facing anteriorly.

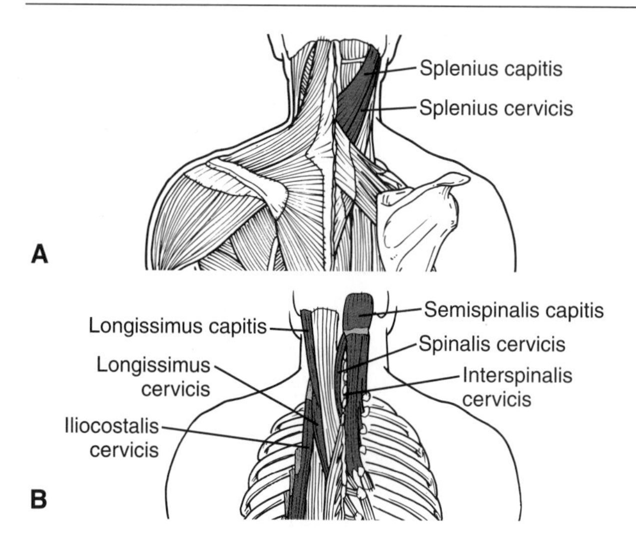

FIGURE 14-9 ■ Muscles of the spinal column: (A) superficial muscles, (B) deep muscles.

are the ropelike **semispinalis capitis** and **semispinalis cervicis**, which traverse from the thoracic transverse processes to the spinous processes of the cervical spine. Deep and lateral to the semispinalis group are the **longissimus capitis** and **longissimus cervicis**, while the suboccipital group (spanning from C2 to the occiput) is the innermost muscle layer (Table 14-1).

The **longus capitis** and **longus colli** stabilize the cervical spine anteriorly. Injury to these muscles can occur with a high-velocity "whiplash" mechanism (Table 14-2).

The extrinsic muscles (those originating away from the spinal column) are presented in Table 14-3. When its insertion on the scapula is fixed, the upper one third of the **trapezius** bilaterally acts to extend the cervical spine and skull. When the trapezius works unilaterally with other musculature, it laterally bends and rotates the cervical spine and skull.

The **sternocleidomastoid** (SCM) is responsible for rotating the skull to the opposite side and for lateral flexion of the cervical spine to the same side as the contracting muscle (Fig. 14-10). The angle of pull of the SCM extends the head on the cervical spine, but acts as a flexor of the lower cervical spine. The anterior, middle, and posterior **scalene** muscles laterally flex the cervical spine. When the cervical spine is fixated, the scalenes elevate the rib cage to assist in inspiration. The scalene group is significant because the brachial plexus passes between its anterior and middle portions. Spasm or tightness of the scalenes can place pressure on the neurovascular structures of the upper extremities, resulting in **thoracic outlet syndrome**.

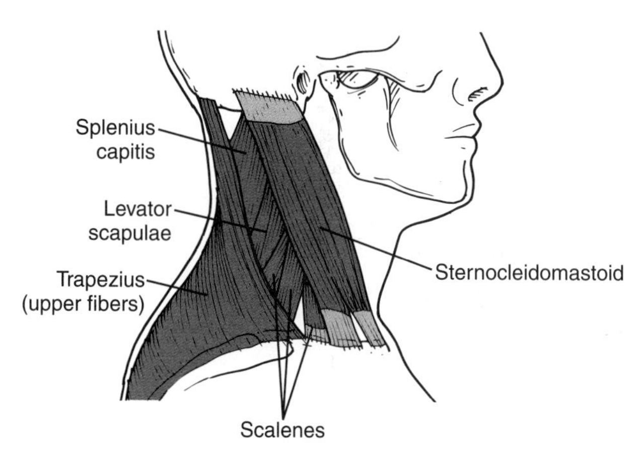

FIGURE 14-10 ■ Lateral cervical muscles.

Clinical Examination of the Cervical Spine

The spinal cord and its nerve roots are vulnerable in the cervical spine. When the magnitude of the trauma is severe, catastrophic results may ensue. This chapter describes the evaluation of patients with noncatastrophic trauma to the cervical spine and assumes that vertebral fractures and dislocations have been ruled out. Chapter 21 describes the on-field evaluation and management of patients with cervical spine injuries.

Impairment level assessment, such as determining that a patient has decreased AROM, does not help define the impact that the cervical spine pathology has on the patient's life. Increasingly, clinicians are having patients complete regional self-report forms such as the Neck Disability Index to assess the patient's current activity limitations due to pain.[6] Repeated use of these functional scales helps assess the impact of intervention, provides a standard assessment tool, and determines whether or not the patient is getting worse or improving.[7]

History

Relevant past history

- **History of spinal pathology:** Does the patient have a history of spinal injury? Identify any pertinent history that may lead to structural degeneration or predispose the patient to chronic problems. The current symptoms may be the result of scar tissue formation's impinging or restricting other structures, a previously injured disk, or the formation of osteophytes within the intervertebral foramina.[8]
- **Recurrent brachial plexus trauma**: A prior history of injury to the brachial plexus makes the tissue more susceptible to reinjury. Repetitive injury may result in permanent impairment.
- **Chest/breast pain:** Angina-like chest pain or women with breast pain who have normal cardiac workups, and who appear to be cancer-free may be experiencing radicular symptoms from the cervical spine.
- **Headaches or other head pain:** Neuropathy of the C2 or C3 nerve roots can produce complaints that include headaches, jaw and ear pain, pain in the occipital region, or superficial pain in the posterior cervical spine.[3] In addition, the greater occipital nerve pierces

Examination Map

HISTORY

Past Medical History
Mental health status

History of the Present Condition
Location of pain
Radicular symptoms
Onset and severity of symptoms
Mechanism of injury
Postural influences

INSPECTION

Functional Assessment
Movement and posture

Inspection of the Lateral Structures
Cervical curvature
Forward head posture

Inspection of the Anterior Structures
Level of the shoulders
Position of the head

Inspection of the Posterior Structures
Bilateral soft tissue comparison

PALPATION

Palpation of the Anterior Structures
Hyoid
Thyroid cartilage
Cricoid cartilage
Sternocleidomastoid
Scalenes
Carotid artery
Lymph nodes

Palpation of the Posterior and Lateral Spine
Occiput and superior nuchal line
Transverse processes
Spinous processes
Trapezius
Levator scapulae

JOINT AND MUSCLE FUNCTION ASSESSMENT

Goniometry
Flexion
Extension
Lateral bending
Rotation

Active Range of Motion
Flexion
Extension
Lateral bending
Rotation

Manual Muscle Tests
Flexion
Extension
Lateral bending
Rotation

Passive Range of Motion
Flexion
Extension
Lateral bending
Rotation

JOINT STABILITY TESTS

Joint Play Assessment
Spring test
Mobility of the first rib

NEUROLOGIC EXAMINATION

Upper Quarter Screen

Upper Limb Nerve Tension Test

Upper Motor Neuron Lesions
Babinski test
Oppenheim test

PATHOLOGIES AND SPECIAL TESTS

Cervical Radiculopathy
Cervical compression test
Spurling test
Cervical distraction test
Vertebral artery test

Intervertebral Disk Lesions
Shoulder abduction test
Valsalva maneuver

Degenerative Joint and Disk Disease

Cervical Instability

Facet Joint Dysfunction

Brachial Plexus Pathology
Brachial plexus traction test

Thoracic Outlet Syndrome
Adson's test
Allen test
Costoclavicular syndrome test
Roos test

Table 14-1 Intrinsic Muscles that Extend the Cervical Spine and Head

Muscle	Action	Origin	Insertion	Innervation	Root
Iliocostalis Cervicis	Extension of spinal column Lateral bending of spinal column	Ribs 3–6	Transverse processes of C4–C6	Posterior rami of spinal nerves	C4–C8
Longissimus Capitis	Extension of skull and cervical spine Rotation of the face toward the same side	Articular processes of C5– C7	Mastoid process of skull	Posterior rami of spinal nerves	C4–C8
Longissimus Cervicis	Extension of spinal column Lateral bending of spinal column	Transverse processes of T1– T5	Transverse processes of C2–C6	Posterior rami of spinal nerves	C4–C8
Longissimus Thoracis	Extension of spinal column Lateral bending of spinal column	Common erector spinae tendon	Transverse process of T3–T12 Ribs 3–12	Posterior rami of spinal nerves	C4–C8
Multifidus (or Multifidi)	Rotation of spine to the opposite side Stabilization of vertebral column	Articular processes	Spinous process	Posterior rami of spinal nerves	C4–C8
Semispinalis Capitis	Extension of neck and head Rotation to the opposite side	Transverse process	Travel upwardly and medially to attach to a spinous process 5 or 8 vertebrae above the origin	Posterior rami of spinal nerves	C4–C8
Semispinalis Cervicis	Extension of thoracic and cervical spine	Transverse process	Travel upwardly and medially to attach to a spinous process 5 or 8 vertebrae above the origin	Posterior rami of spinal nerves	C4–C8
Semispinalis Thoracis	Extension of thoracic and cervical spine Rotation to the opposite side	Transverse process	Travel upwardly and medially to attach to a spinous process 5 or 8 vertebrae above the origin	Posterior rami of spinal nerves	C4–C8
Spinalis Capitis	Extension of the spine Lateral bending of the spine	Upper thoracic and lower cervical spinous processes	Ligamentum nuchae	Posterior rami of spinal nerves	C4–C8
Spinalis Cervicis	Extension of the spine Lateral bending of the spine	Upper thoracic and lower cervical spinous processes	Ligamentum nuchae	Posterior rami of spinal nerves	C4–C8
Splenius Capitis	Lateral bending of the cervical spine	Lower half of the ligamentum nuchae	Mastoid process of the temporal bone and adjacent occipital bone (capitis portion)	Posterior rami of middle cervical spinal nerves.	C4–C8
Splenius Cervicis	Rotation of the head toward the same side Extension of the cervical spine	Spinous processes of C7–T6 vertebrae	Transverse processes of C2–C4 vertebrae (cervicis portion)	Posterior rami of spinal nerves	C4–C8

Table 14-2 Intrinsic Muscles Acting on the Head (atlanto-occipital flexion and extension)

Muscle	Action	Origin	Insertion	Innervation	Root
Longus Capitis	Flex head (atlanto–occipital motion)	Base of occiput	Anterior tubercles of C3–C6 transverse processes	Anterior rami of C1–C3 spinal nerves	C1, C2, C3
Longus Colli	Cervical flexion with rotation to opposite if unilateral.	Anterior tubercle of C1; bodies of C1–C3 and transverse processes of C3–C6	Bodies of C5–T3 vertebrae; transverse processes of C3–C5 vertebrae	Anterior rami of spinal nerves	C2, C3, C4, C5, C6
Obliquus Capitis Inferior	Unilateral: ipsilateral rotation	Lateral surface of spinous process of axis	Inferior surface of transverse process of C1 (atlas)	Suboccipital nerve	C1
Obliquus Capitis Superior	Bilateral: Extension of head on atlas. Unilateral: Ipsilateral rotation	Transverse process of atlas	Occipital bone	Suboccipital nerve	C1
Rectus Capitis Anterior	Flex head (atlanto–occipital motion)	Base of skull, anterior to occipital condyle	Anterior surface of lateral portion of C1 (atlas)	Branches from C1 and C2 spinal nerves	C1, C2
Rectus Capitis Lateralis	Flex (atlanto-occipital motion) and stabilize head	Jugular process of occiput	Transverse process of C1 (atlas)	Branches from C1 and C2 spinal nerves.	C1, C2
Rectus Capitis Posterior Major	Bilateral: Extension of head on atlas Unilateral: Ipsilateral rotation	Posterior edge of spinous process of axis	Inferior nuchal line on occipital bone	Suboccipital nerve	C1
Rectus Capitis Posterior Minor	Bilateral: Extension of head on atlas Unilateral: Ipsilateral rotation	Posterior tubercle of axis	Inferior nuchal line on occipital bone (medial aspect)	Suboccipital nerve	C1

Table 14-3 Extrinsic Muscles Acting on the Cervical Spinal Column

Muscle	Action	Origin	Insertion	Innervation	Root
Trapezius (upper one-third)	Cervical extension Cervical side bending Elevation of scapula Upward rotation of scapula Rotation of the cervical spine to the opposite side	Occipital protuberance Nuchal line of the occipital bone Upper portion of the ligamentum nuchae	Lateral one third of clavicle Acromion process	Spinal accessory	CN XI
Levator Scapulae	Elevation of the scapula Downward rotation of the scapula Extension of cervical spine	Spinous process of C7 Transverse processes of cervical vertebrae C1 through C4	Superior medial border of scapula	Dorsal subscapular	C3, C4, C5
Sternocleidomastoid	Flexion of the cervical spine Rotation of the skull to the opposite side Lateral bending of the cervical spine Elevation of the clavicle and sternum	Medial clavicular head Superior sternum	Mastoid process of the skull	Spinal accessory	CN XI C2, C3
Scalene, Anterior	Lateral bending of the cervical spine Elevation of the rib cage	Anterior portion of the transverse processes of C3 to C6	Sternal attachment of the 1st rib	Cervical spinal nerves	C4, C5, C6
Scalene, Middle	Lateral bending of the cervical spine Elevation of the rib cage	Anterior portion of the transverse processes of C2–C7	Lateral to the insertion of the anterior scalene on the1st rib	Anterior rami of cervical spinal nerves	C3, C4, C5, C6, C7, C8
Scalene, Posterior	Lateral bending of the cervical spine Elevation of the rib cage	Anterior portion of the transverse processes C5 and C6	Medial portion of the 2nd rib	Anterior rami of cervical spinal nerves	C7, C8

the semispinalis capitis, and spasm of this muscle can cause an occipital headache.

- **Eye examination:** Does the patient wear corrective lenses? If so, has the prescription recently changed? If not, when was the patient's last eye examination? Poor vision can result in postural changes that produce cervical headaches and neck pain.
- **Psychosocial factors:** Psychosocial behaviors such as **fear-avoidance** beliefs and depression are related to pain and disability associated with acute and chronic neck and back pain.[9,10] Patients who express high fear-avoidance beliefs avoid activities in the anticipation of pain, leading to further deconditioning and weakening of supporting and involved structures.

History of the present condition

The onset and identification of functional activities causing the symptoms assist in determining the underlying pathology.[11] Although usually mechanical in origin, cervical pain can arise from pathological sources such as tumors. A high index of suspicion of serious pathology is warranted if the patient describes unremitting pain, night pain, bowel and bladder dysfunction, or **hyperreflexia** (Table 14-4).[12]

- **Location of the pain:** Is the pain localized or does it radiate? Pain that is localized to the cervical spine may indicate a strain, sprain, vertebral fracture or dislocation, or facet syndrome. Radicular symptoms are a strong indication that trauma has occurred to the cervical nerve root or spinal cord. Table 14-5 presents common symptoms relative to the involved nerve root.
- **Mechanism and onset of injury:** Although acute injuries usually are related to specific mechanisms of injury, chronic and insidious onsets typically occur with mechanisms related to overuse and postural considerations:
    - **Insidious onset:** Symptoms that occur with a gradual or insidious onset usually warrant a thorough postural evaluation to determine a cause-and-effect relationship.
    - **Acute onset:** When an acute onset of injury is described, the mechanism of injury can provide clues to the trauma (Table 14-6). When the patient reports an axial load being placed on the cervical spine, a possible vertebral fracture must be considered until ruled out with radiographic examination. A whiplash mechanism, rapid extension followed by flexion, may be described following an automobile accident or fall.
- **Pattern of the pain:** Is the pain constant or intermittent? Chemically induced pain, such as that relating to inflammation, is more constant with no change in symptoms as the cervical spine changes position. Mechanical pain, caused by compression of a nerve root, tends to vary in intensity, and relief (or a decrease in

Table 14-4 Key Signs and Symptoms Associated with Serious Pathological Cervical Spine Conditions

Cervical Myelopathy	Neoplastic Conditions	Upper Cervical Ligamentous Instability	Vertebral Artery Insufficiency	Inflammatory or Systemic Disease
Sensory disturbance of the hands	Age older than 50	Occipital headache and numbness	Drop attacks	Temperature > 37°C
Muscle wasting of hand intrinsic muscles	Previous history of cancer	Severe limitation during neck active range of motion in all directions	Dizziness or lightheadedness related to neck movement	BP > 160/95 mm Hg
Unsteady gait	Unexplained weight loss	Signs of cervical **myelopathy**	**Dysphasia**	Resting pulse >100 bpm
Hyperreflexia	Constant pain; no relief with bed rest		**Dysarthria**	Fatigue
Bowel/bladder disturbance	Night pain		Double vision	
Multisegmental weakness and/or sensory changes			Positive cranial nerve signs	

Fear-avoidance Refraining from tasks or movements because of the potential pain or instability.

Hyperreflexia Increased action of the reflexes.

Dysarthria Speech impairment caused by dysfunction of the muscles and joints associated with speech.

Dysphasia Speech impairment caused by a brain lesion.

Myelopathy Diseases that affect the spinal cord.

Table 14-5 Overview of Cervical Spinal Nerve Root Dysfunction[3]

Cervical Nerve Root	Sensory Complaints	Motor/Functional Deficit
C2	Jaw Occipital headaches	None
C3	Headache Posterior cervical spine pain Occipital pain Ear	None
C4	Cervical spine pain Trapezius pain Superior/proximal shoulder	No skeletal muscle deficits Diaphragmatic dysfunction possible
C5	Superior aspect of the shoulder Lateral aspect of the upper arm	Deltoid muscle group weakness Biceps brachii weakness Impingement tests may be negative
C6	Cervical spine Area over the biceps brachii Dorsal hand between thumb and index fingers	Weak wrist extension Weak elbow extension Weak thumb extension
C7	Posterior aspect of arm Posterolateral forearm Middle finger	Triceps brachii weakness Wrist extensor weakness Finger extensor weakness Wrist pronator weakness
C8	Fourth or fifth finger	Weak interossei

Table 14-6 Possible Pathology Based on the Mechanism of Injury

Mechanism	Pathology
Flexion	Compression of the anterior vertebral body and intervertebral disk Sprain of the supraspinous, interspinous, and posterior longitudinal ligaments and ligamentum flavum Sprain of the facet joints Strain of the posterior cervical musculature
Extension	Sprain of the anterior longitudinal ligament Compression of the posterior vertebral body and intervertebral disk Compression of the facet joints Fracture of the spinous processes
Lateral Bending	On the side toward the bending: Compression of the cervical nerve roots Compression of the vertebral bodies and intervertebral disk Compression of the facet joints On the side opposite the bending: Stretching of the cervical nerve roots Sprain of the lateral ligaments Sprain of the facet joints Strain of the cervical musculature
Rotation	Disk trauma Ligament sprain Facet sprain or dislocation Vertebral dislocation
Axial Load	Compression fracture of the vertebral body Compression of the intervertebral disk
Whiplash	Cervical instability Cervical muscle strain Facet joint dysfunction

symptoms) can be obtained by moving the spine into a specific position, such as tilting the head away from the involved side, which lessens the pressure on the involved structure.

- **Postural influences:** Patients may describe symptoms that appear or disappear depending on the position of the cervical spine.[3] Patients with acute cervical disk compression may describe pain relief by limiting cervical motion. Extension and lateral flexion of the cervical spine may increase pain secondary to compression on the associated nerve roots.
- **Other symptoms:** Complaints of visual disturbances, dizziness, lightheadedness, and headaches may be associated with decreased blood flow to the brain due to insufficiency of the vertebrobasilar artery.[13,14] Patients with these findings should be referred to a physician for further diagnostic testing. Often, patients who sustain flexion–extension, or whiplash, injuries may also experience dizziness due to altered proprioceptive input to the vestibular system.[15]

Inspection

A general inspection of the entire body is necessary to determine proper posture in the sagittal and frontal planes. Also see Postural Evaluation, Chapter 6.

Functional assessment

Ask the patient to describe or reproduce those motions and activities that increase the symptoms. Acute cervical spine pathology may dramatically limit active ROM, making such daily tasks as driving, reaching up and reading difficult and painful. Increased pain and other symptoms with positions that require cervical flexion are often associated with cervical disk disease. The patient's work environment may aggravate neck symptoms. Frequently, chronic cervical pain is associated with sustained positioning associated with working at a desk or a computer.

Ask the patient to look up at the ceiling (extension) and down at the floor (flexion). Limitations in cervical extension will result in compensatory trunk extension or knee flexion, while limitations in cervical flexion will result in compensation through trunk flexion. Compensation for limited or painful cervical rotation occurs through increased trunk rotation.

Inspection of the lateral structures

- **Cervical curvature:** Observe for the presence of a lordotic curve, typical of the cervical spine. A flattening of the cervical curvature or lateral bending may indicate posturing to decrease pressure on the nerve roots (usually on the side away from the bend). An increased lordotic curve can lead to a forward head posture. Flattening of the lordotic curve or tilting to one side can indicate spasm of the cervical muscles.
- A forward head posture can be caused by long-standing postural changes in chronic conditions, muscle spasm, or weakness. Excessive extension of the head on the neck will produce a forward head posture, which is accompanied by excessive flexion of the cervical spine (see Chapter 6).

Inspection of the anterior structures

- **Level of the shoulders:** Standing in front of the patient, observe the level of the patient's shoulders. The height of the acromioclavicular joints, the deltoid, and clavicles should be level; the dominant shoulder is often slightly depressed relative to the nondominant shoulder.
- **Position of the head on the shoulders:** The head should be seated symmetrically on the cervical spine with the shoulders held in an upright position. Unilateral spasm of the cervical muscles results in lateral flexion of the head toward the involved side. The rotation of the chin opposite the side of the tilt may indicate torticollis ("wry neck"), a congenital or acquired spasm of the SCM muscle.

Inspection of the posterior structures

- **Bilateral soft tissue comparison:** Inspect the contour and tone of the trapezius and the other cervical musculature for equality of mass, tone, and texture. The trapezius of the dominant side may be hypertrophied relative to the opposite side. The posterior scapular muscles and the deltoids are inspected for normal muscle mass, tone, and texture. Atrophy of these muscles may result from impingement of a cervical nerve root or from brachial plexus trauma.

Table 14-7 Bony Landmarks for Palpation

Structure	Landmark
Cervical Vertebral Bodies	On the same level as the spinous processes
C1 Transverse Process	One finger breadth inferior to the mastoid process
C3–C4 Vertebrae	Posterior to the hyoid bone
C4–C5 Vertebra	Posterior to the thyroid cartilage
C6 Vertebra	Posterior to the cricoid cartilage; movement during flexion and extension of the cervical spine
C7 Vertebra	Prominent posterior spinous process

PALPATION

Table 14-7 presents a list of landmarks to assist in locating specific cervical spine structures.

Palpation of the Anterior Cervical Spine Structures

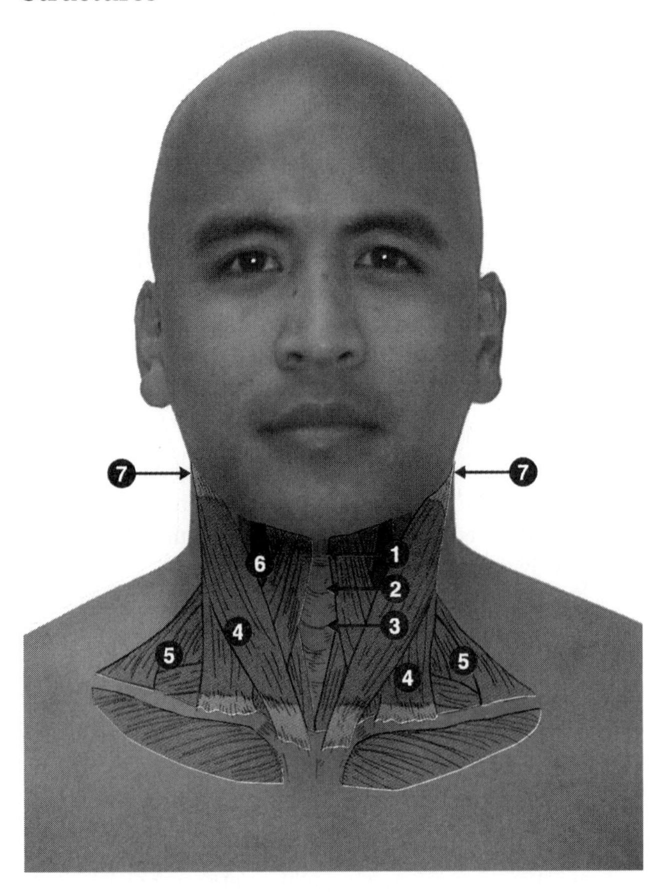

1 **Hyoid bone:** Located across from the C3 vertebra, palpate the hyoid bone for tenderness. While gently palpating this structure, request that the patient swallow, noting the superior and inferior movement of the hyoid bone.

2 **Thyroid cartilage:** Locate the thyroid cartilage, found at the level of the fourth and fifth cervical vertebrae. The thyroid cartilage is a fibrous shield protecting the anterior surface of the larynx. This structure gently shifts laterally and, similar to the hyoid bone, raises and lowers during the act of swallowing. Swelling in this region may be associated with thyroid gland enlargement.

3 **Cricoid cartilage:** Identify the cricoid cartilage, which lies at the level of the sixth cervical vertebra. The cricoid cartilage demarcates the location where the pharynx joins the esophagus and the larynx joins the trachea. The cartilage is identified by the thickened rings that can be palpated along its anterior surface.

4 **Sternocleidomastoid:** Palpate the cordlike SCM along its length from its origin on the mastoid process and superior nuchal line to its insertion on the sternum and clavicle. Rotating the head causes the SCM on the side opposite the movement to become more prominent.

5 **Scalenes:** Palpate the scalene muscles just posterior to the SCM muscle at about the C3 to C6 level. Tightness or spasm of this muscle group may cause abnormal cervical posture or lead to thoracic outlet syndrome.

6 **Carotid artery:** Palpate the carotid pulse between the thyroid cartilage and the SCM.

7 **Lymph nodes:** Near the upper trapezius and beneath the mandible, palpate the lymph nodes lying near the origin of the SCM. Lymph nodes become enlarged secondary to infection or illness.

Palpation of the Posterior and Lateral Spine Structures

1 **Occiput and superior nuchal line:** The occipital bone, the most posterior aspect of the skull, is located at the apex of the cervical spine. Palpate this area for tenderness because it is the site of attachment for many cervical muscles.

2 **Transverse processes:** Located approximately one finger breadth inferior to the mastoid processes, the transverse processes of C1 are the only processes of the cervical spine that are palpable. The areas overlying the remaining transverse processes are palpated at the same level as the spinous processes for tenderness.

3 **Spinous processes:** The spinous processes are more easily palpated when the cervical spine is slightly flexed.

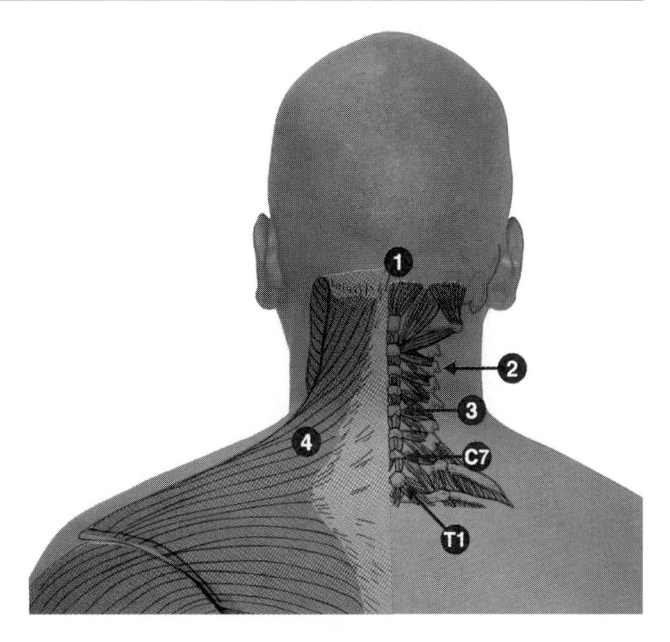

Locate the area where the cervical and thoracic spines meet slightly above the superior angle of the scapula. Here two spinous processes are more prominent than the rest. The lower protrusion is the spinous process of T1, and the superior protrusion is the C7 spinous process. From here, palpate the spinous processes of C6, C5, and, possibly, C4 and C3. Above the C5 level, the spinous processes begin to be masked by the soft tissue but the area overlying the remaining processes should be palpated for tenderness. Each of these processes should be aligned immediately superior to the one below it.

4 **Trapezius:** Beginning at the occiput and superior nuchal line, the upper portion of the trapezius is palpated inferiorly to its insertion on the lateral clavicle, acromion process, and spine of the scapula. The thickness of this muscle is easily palpated as it spans from the cervical spine to the acromion process. Most of the remaining cervical musculature lies beneath the trapezius and is not directly palpable. The upper trapezius is a common site for trigger points.

4 **Levator scapulae:** Although deep to the trapezius, the levator may be discernible as a long, vertically oriented muscle at its origin on the medial superior scapula.

Joint and Muscle Function Assessment

During ROM assessment, monitor the patient for symptoms, such as nystagmus, dizziness, and lightheadedness, that may signal decreased blood supply to the brain. Should this occur, the patient should be referred for further diagnostic testing and no further joint motions should be assessed. The vertebral artery test, described on page 551 should be performed following single-plane passive ROM assessment; however, the diagnostic accuracy of the vertebral artery test is questionable, and negative findings do not conclusively rule out vascular compromise.[16]

Active and passive ROM can be subjectively classified as "limited" or "not limited" or quantified measurements using visual estimates, inclinometers, goniometers, or tape measures (Fig. 14-11). Goniometric and visual estimates of cervical range of motion are highly inaccurate and have poor inter-rater reliability (Goniometry Boxes 14-1, 14-2, and 14-3). Better reliability is obtained using inclinometers such as the Cervical Range of Motion (CROM) device because the need to use bony landmarks is eliminated (Fig. 14-12).[17–19]

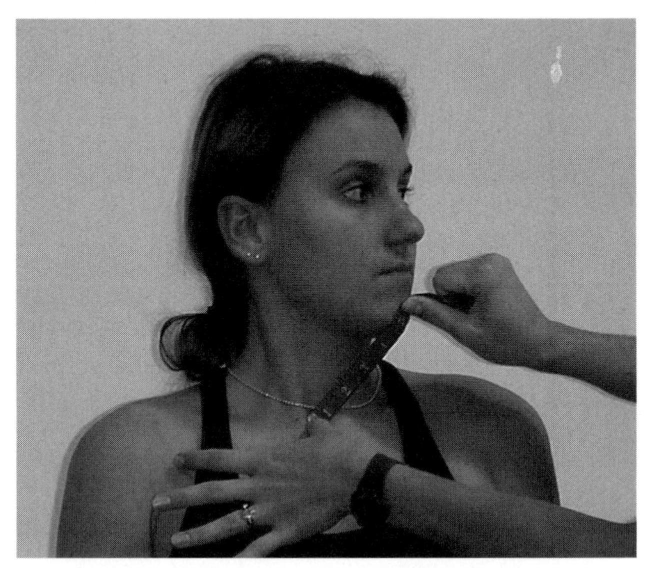

FIGURE 14-11 ■ Measuring cervical range of motion with a tape measure. The distance from the jugular notch on the sternum to the point of the chin is measured and recorded for each motion. Cervical rotation is demonstrated in this photograph.

Active range of motion

Active range of motion (AROM) is used to assess the upper and lower cervical regions. When the patient gets to the end of the voluntary range, apply slight passive pressure to assess for exacerbation of pain, tissue extensibility and available range.[17] People who have sustained whiplash-type injuries may have significantly limited AROM in the acute and chronic stages.[20]

The amount of cervical spine motion is measured at the end range of active range of motion rather than passive range of motion.

- **Flexion and extension:** Test for flexion and extension while the patient is seated. Most of the flexion and extension motion that occurs in the cervical spine takes place at the atlanto-occipital joint (capital flexion and extension) (Fig. 14-13A). Flexion of the head is achieved by asking the patient to "make a double chin." Cervical spine flexion is assessed by asking the patient to touch the chin to the chest, noting for rotation of the skull that indicates substitution by the SCM on the side opposite to the rotation. Extension is

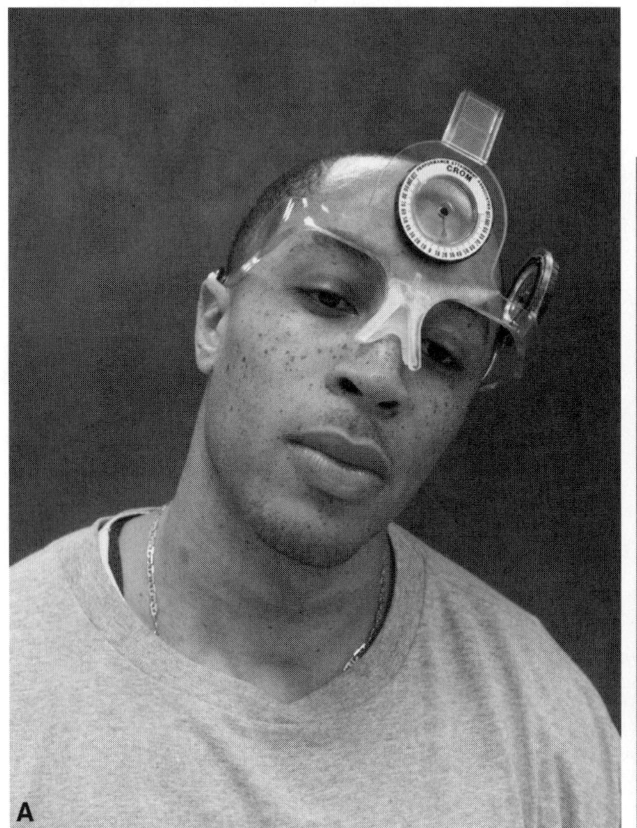

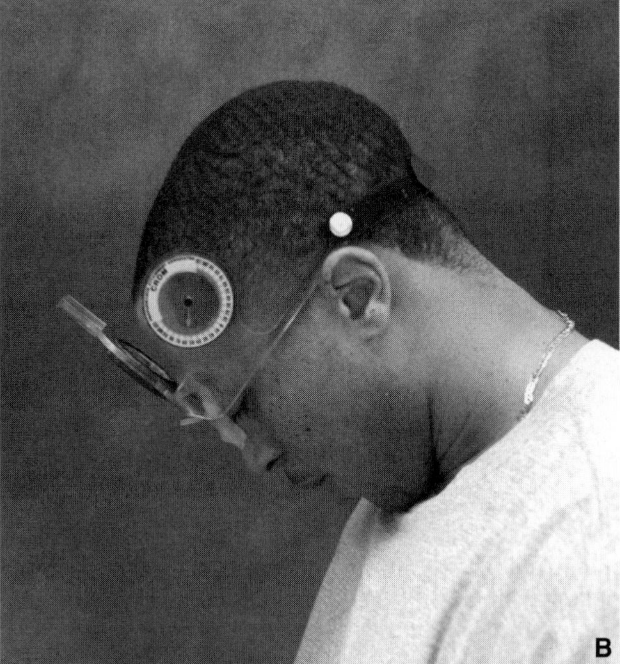

FIGURE 14-12 ■ Inclinometer. The use of an inclinometer provides improved interrater reliability for determining cervical range of motion than traditional goniometric measurements.

Goniometry Box 14-1
Cervical Flexion and Extension

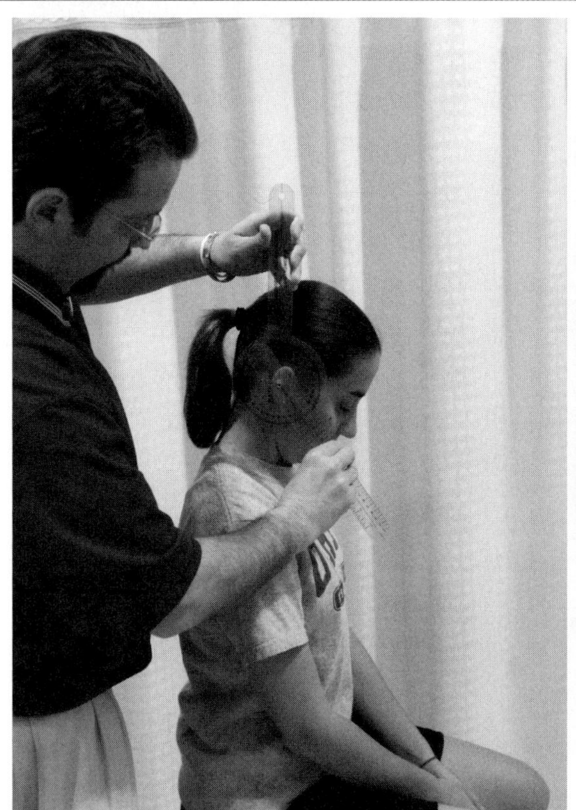

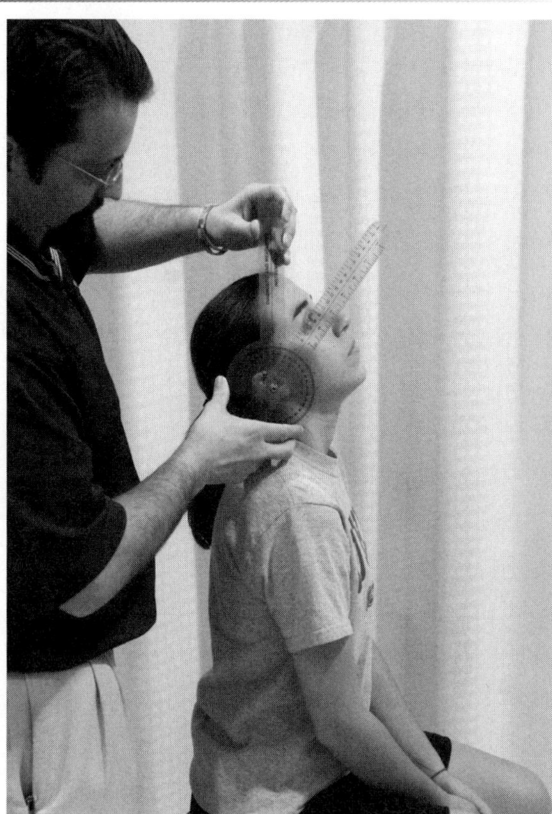

Flexion: 0 to 40–70° **Extension: 0 to 60 to 80°**

Patient Position	Seated
Goniometer Alignment	
Fulcrum	The axis is positioned over the external auditory meatus.
Proximal Arm	The stationary arm is positioned parallel with base of nasal openings.
Distal Arm	The movement arm is held perpendicular to the floor.
Comments	Start and end positions should be noted. Cervical flexion and extension can also be assessed using a tape measure to measure the distance between the chin and the suprasternal notch. Avoid trunk flexion/extension during testing

Goniometry Box 14-2
Cervical Rotation

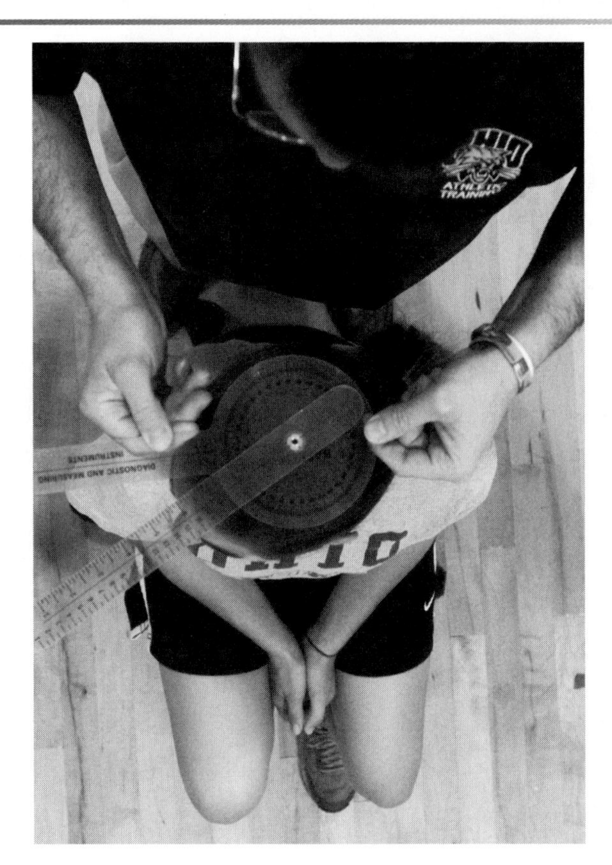

Rotation: 0 to 70° to 90° (each direction)

Patient Position	Seated with trunk supported
Goniometer Alignment	
Fulcrum	The axis is positioned over the center of patient's head.
Proximal Arm	The stationary arm is aligned with an imaginary line between the patient's acromion processes.
Distal Arm	The movement arm is positioned so that it bisects the patient's nose.
Comments	***Inter-rater Reliability:***

Not Reliable — Very Reliable

Poor | Moderate | Good

0 0.1 0.2 0.3 0.4 0.5 0.6 0.7 0.8 0.9 1.0

Goniometry Box 14-3
Cervical Lateral Flexion (Side-bending)

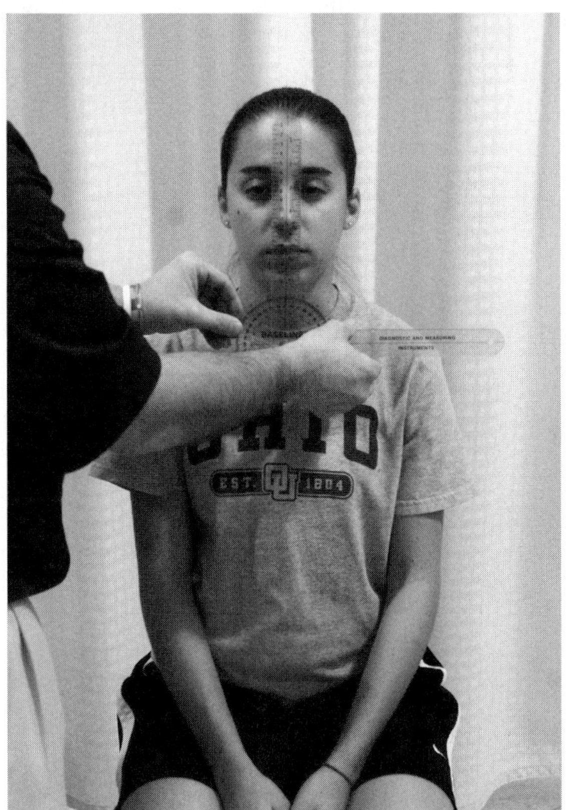

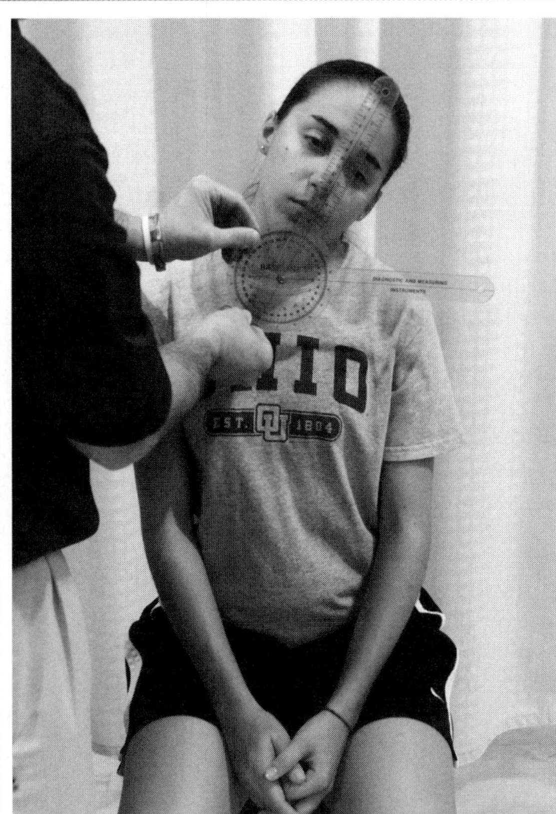

Lateral Flexion 40–50° (each direction)

Patient Position	Seated with the trunk supported
Goniometer Alignment	
Fulcrum	The axis is centered on the patient's sternal notch.
Proximal Arm	The stationary arm is aligned parallel to an imaginary line between patient's acromion processes.
Distal Arm	The movement arm is positioned so that it bisects the patient's nose.

tested by having the patient look up toward the ceiling (Fig. 14-13B). When the patient reaches the end of the range, apply passive overpressure to assess for any increase in symptoms and the quality of the end-feel.

- **Lateral flexion:** With the patient seated, determine if the ROM of the head toward each shoulder is equal and pain free (Fig. 14-14). This motion occurs primarily in the upper vertebrae, producing approximately 45 degrees of motion in each direction.
- **Rotation:** With the patient seated and the head held upright and facing forward, observe for symmetry in the amount of rotation as the patient attempts to look over each shoulder (Fig. 14-15). This motion, occurring primarily at the atlanto–axial joint, should be equal and pain free in each direction.

Manual muscle testing

Manual muscle testing of the cervical muscles is presented in Manual Muscle Tests 14-1 to 14-4.

Passive range of motion

During assessment of passive range of motion (PROM), carefully note the quality of the end-feel and any limitations in range. Positions or movements that provoke symptoms should also be determined. In addition to PROM, wherein the patient is supine with the head supported and moved by the examiner, end-feels can also be assessed at the end of AROM.

- **Flexion:** With the patient in the supine position and the head off the table to about the T2 level, grasp the patient's head under the occiput. First assess motion at the upper cervical region by flexing only the head and bringing the chin to the chest. Next repeat the motion, allowing the lower cervical spine to flex (Fig. 14-16A). The normal end-feel for this movement is firm owing to the chin striking the chest. Spasm in the posterior cervical muscles results in an early firm end-feel with complaints of "tightness"; mechanical blockage of the atlanto–occipital joint or the vertebrae causes a premature, hard end-feel.
- **Extension:** Assess PROM with the patient supine so that the head is off the end of the table and the neck is allowed to move into extension (Fig. 14-16B). First assess capitocervical extension by stabilizing the lower cervical spine and extending the head. Follow this with extension of the lower cervical spine. The normal end-feel for this motion is hard as the occiput makes contact with the rest of the cervical spine. Isolated extension may cause impingement on the vertebral artery, and resulting dizziness or nystagmus, in the presence of cervical instability or stenosis.

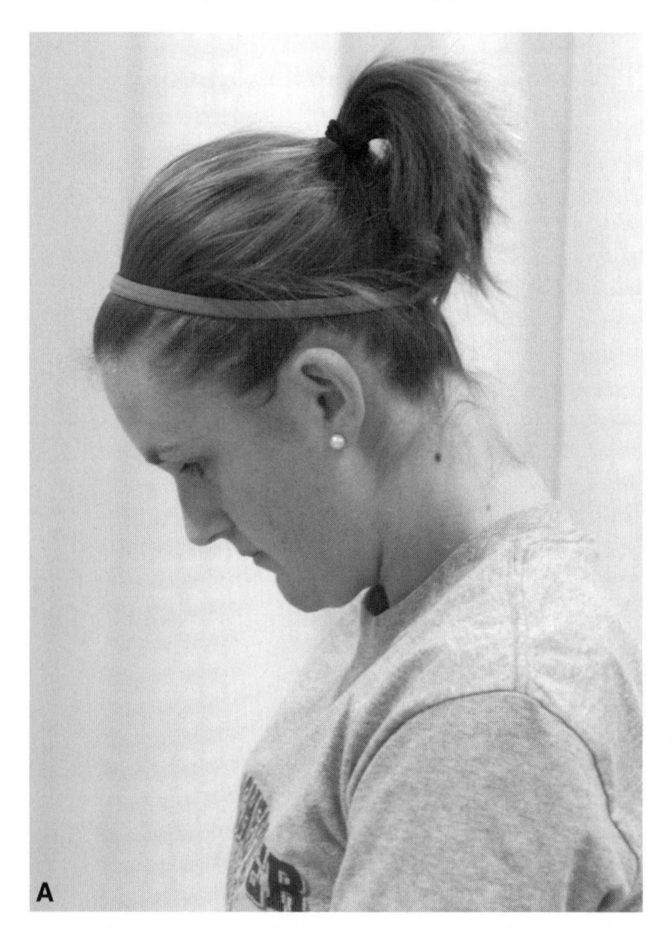

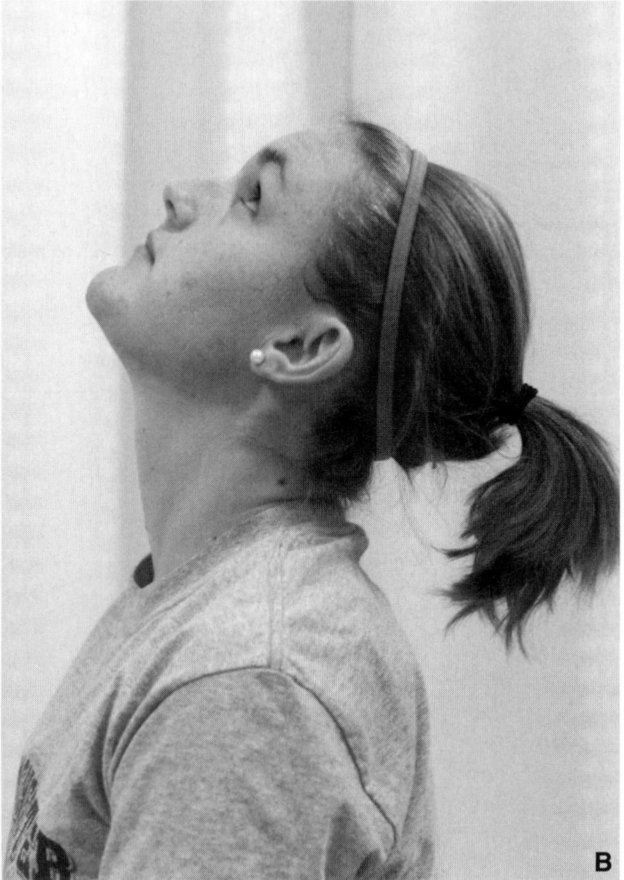

FIGURE 14-13 ■ Active (A) flexion and (B) extension of the cervical spine. The patient may attempt to compensate for a lack of cervical flexion by rounding the shoulders and compensate for a lack of extension by retracting the scapulae.

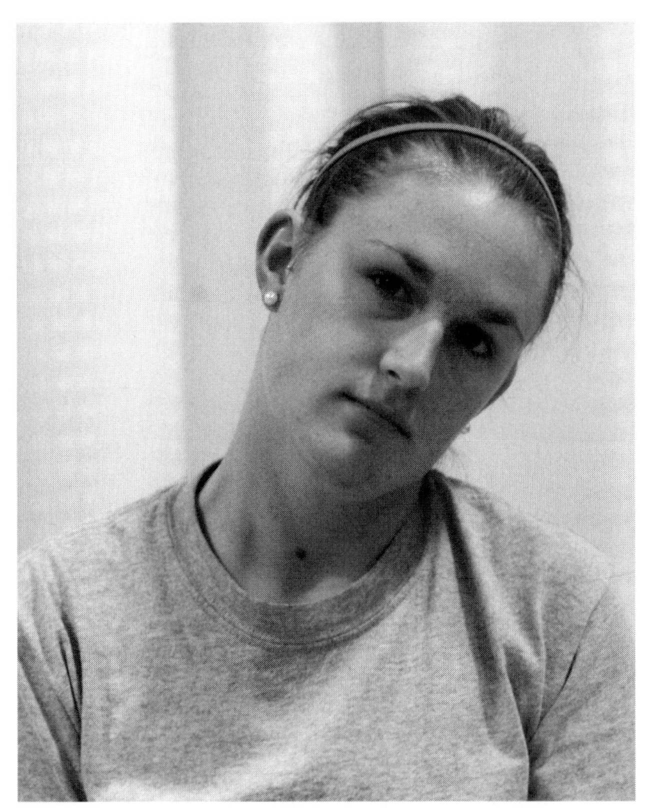

FIGURE 14-14 ■ Active left lateral bending of the cervical spine. The patient may attempt to compensate for decreased cervical ROM by elevating the shoulder girdle.

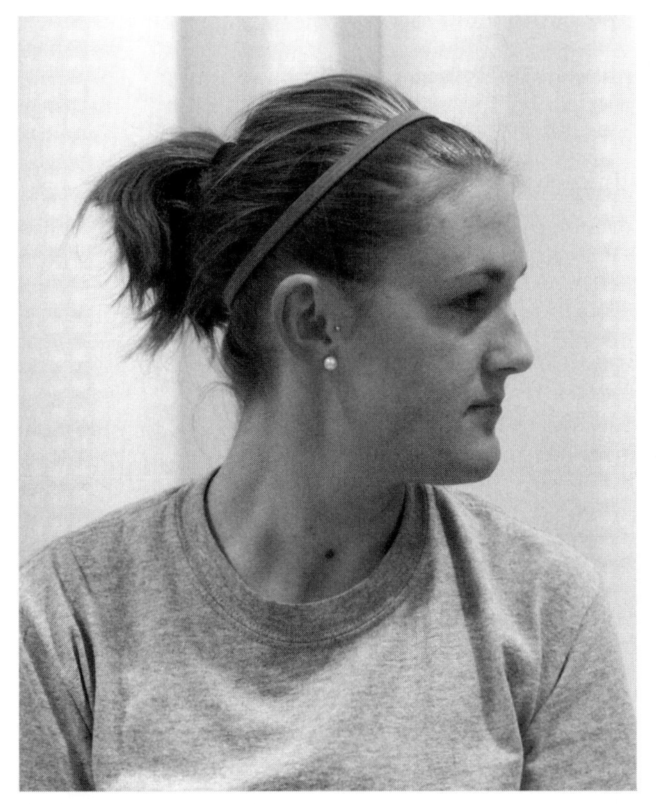

FIGURE 14-15 ■ Active left rotation of the cervical spine. The patient may compensate for a lack of cervical rotation by rotating the torso in the direction opposite that of the cervical movement.

- **Lateral flexion:** Continuing in the supine position, keep the patient's cervical spine in the neutral position between flexion and extension. Using one hand under the occiput, tilt the head and neck to bring the ear toward the shoulder (Fig. 14-17). Stabilize the contralateral shoulder with the opposite hand if needed. The normal end-feel for lateral flexion is firm owing to soft tissue stretch.
- **Rotation:** With the patient supine, grasp the patient's forehead and occiput to maintain the cervical spine in

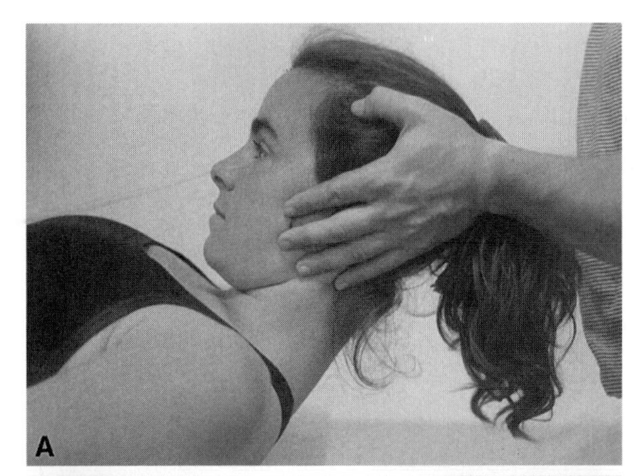

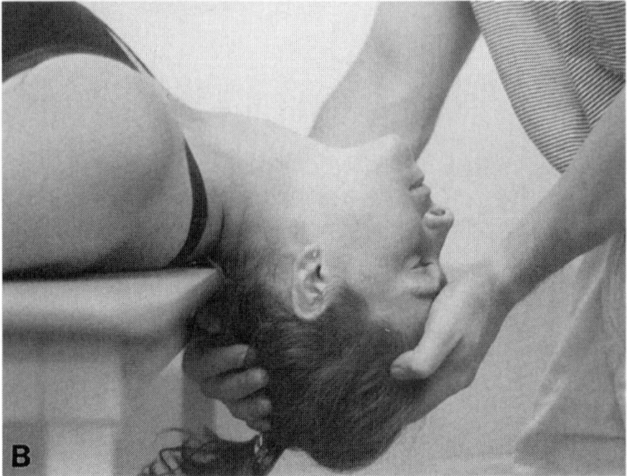

FIGURE 14-16 ■ Passive (A) flexion and (B) extension of the cervical spine.

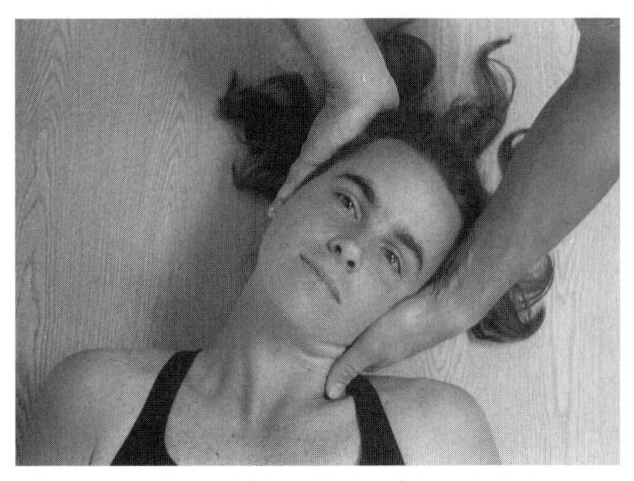

FIGURE 14-17 ■ Passive left lateral flexion of the cervical spine.

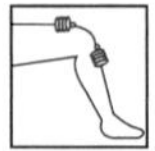

Manual Muscle Test 14-1
Flexion

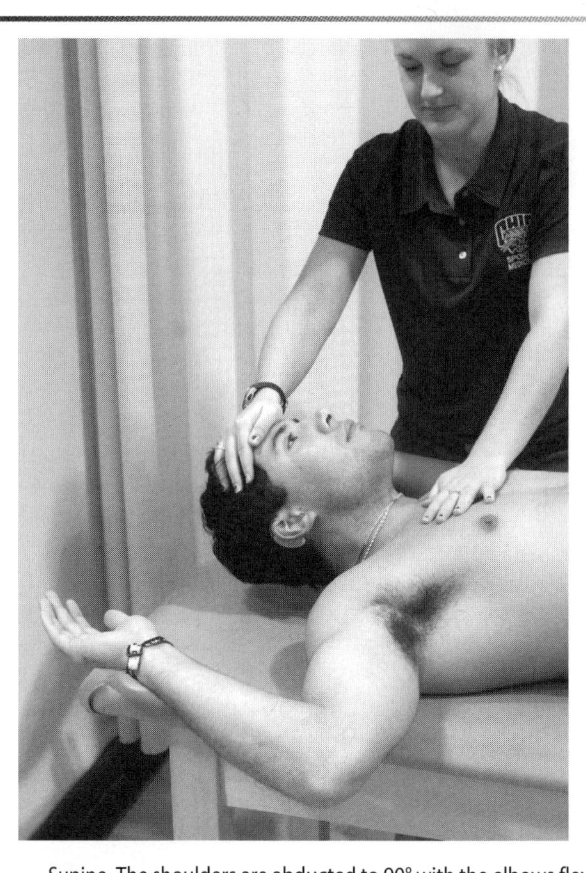

Patient Position	Supine. The shoulders are abducted to 90° with the elbows flexed to 90°.
Starting Position	The cervical spine and head are in the neutral position.
Stabilization	Over the superior aspect of the sternum if patient is unable to self-stabilize trunk
Palpation	Sternocleidomastoid at anterolateral neck and anterior scalene just posterior to sternocleidomastoid. Others are too deep to palpate.
Resistance	To the forehead
Prime Mover(s) (innervation)	Sternocleidomastoid (spinal accessory: CN XI, C2, C3) Anterior scalene (dorsal rami: C4, C5, C6) Longus capitis (branches of CN C4, C5, C6, C7, C8) Longus colli (anterior rami, C2, C3, C4, C5, C6) Rectus capitis anterior (suboccipital nerve: C1) Anterior scalene (C4, C5, C6)
Secondary Mover(s) (innervation)	Middle scalene Posterior scalene Suprahyoid Infrahyoid Rectus capitis lateralis
Substitutions	Inability to keep the chin tucked during the movement signals weakness of the deep cervical flexors and overreliance on the sternocleidomastoid.[21]
Comments	Instruct the patient to first tuck the chin and then continue flexing the neck. Weakness with upper cervical motion (tucking the chin) is a common impairment associated with chronic, nonspecific cervical pain.[22]

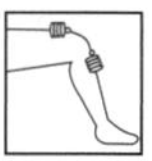

Manual Muscle Test 14-2
Extension

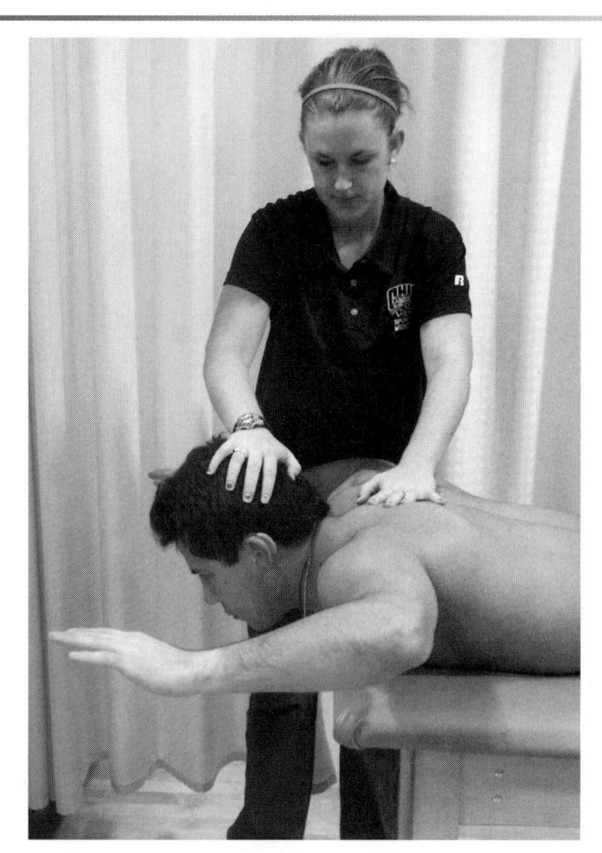

Patient Position	Prone. The shoulders are abducted to 90° and the elbows flexed to 90°.
Starting Position	The cervical spine and head are in the neutral position.
Stabilization	Superior aspect of the thoracic spine (e.g., T2–T9)
Palpation	Posterior cervical region
Resistance	To the skull over the occiput
Prime Mover(s) (innervation)	Trapezius (upper one third) (spinal accessory: CN XI) Levator scapulae (dorsal subscapular: C3, C4, C5) Cervical extensor muscles (see Table 14-1)
Secondary Mover(s) (innervation)	None
Substitutions	Lumbar and thoracic paraspinals

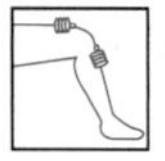

Manual Muscle Test 14-3
Lateral Flexion

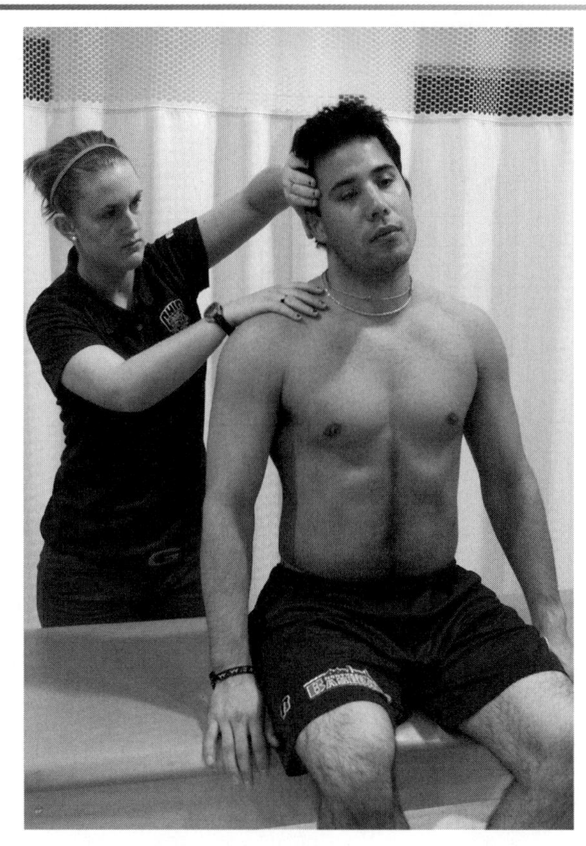

Starting Position	Seated with the cervical spine and head in the neutral position
Stabilization	Over the acromioclavicular joint on the side toward the motion
Resistance	Over the temporal and parietal bones on the side toward the motion
Prime Movers (innervation)	Sternocleidomastoid (spinal accessory: CN XI, C2, C3) Scalenes (dorsal rami: C3–C8) Paraspinal muscles on the side being tested
Secondary Mover(s) (innervation)	None
Substitutions	Cervical flexors
Comments	The muscles tested during lateral flexion are redundant with those tested for cervical rotation, flexion, and extension.

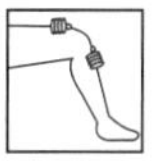

Manual Muscle Test 14-4
Rotation and Flexion

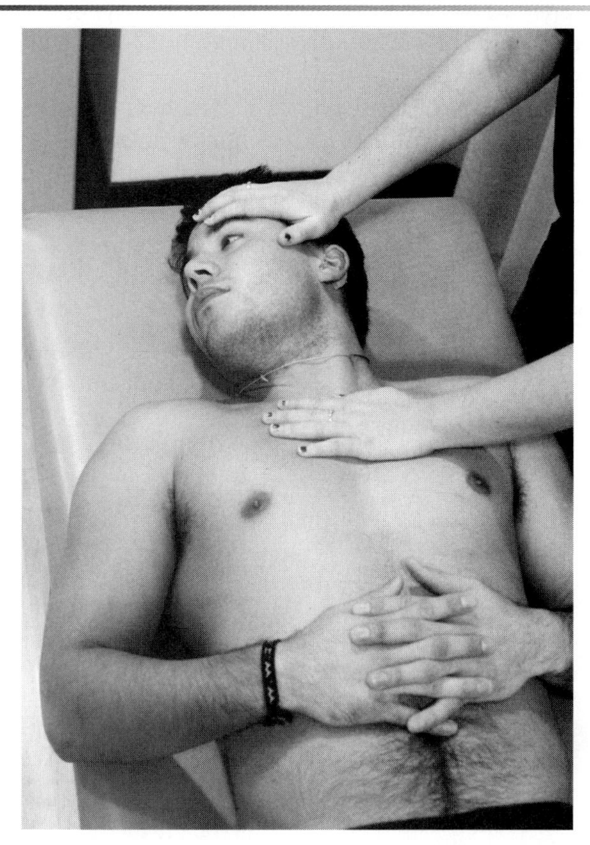

Patient Position	Supine. The shoulders are abducted to 90° and the elbows flexed to 90°.
Starting Position	The head is rotated to the side opposite that being tested.
Stabilization	Over the sternum
Resistance	Over the temporal bone on the side toward the motion
Prime Movers (innervation)	Sternocleidomastoid (accessory nerve CN XI, C2, C3)
Secondary Mover(s) (innervation)	Cervical flexors on same side
Substitutions	Uniplanar cervical flexion

its neutral position. Then apply pressure to rotate the skull and neck (Fig. 14-18). The skull and spine should be rotated together. A firm end-feel is expected from stretching of the SCM muscle and intrinsic neck ligaments. Fully flexing the neck before rotating the head better isolates the atlantoaxial joints by restricting motion in the lower cervical region.

Joint Stability Tests

Patient reports of dizziness, syncope, or nystagmus during vertebral joint stability tests warrant stopping the tests and further diagnostic testing by a physician.

Stress testing

There are no specific ligamentous tests for the cervical spine. The end range of PROM testing stresses the spinal ligaments, assuming the motion is not limited by muscular tightness or contractures (Table 14-8).

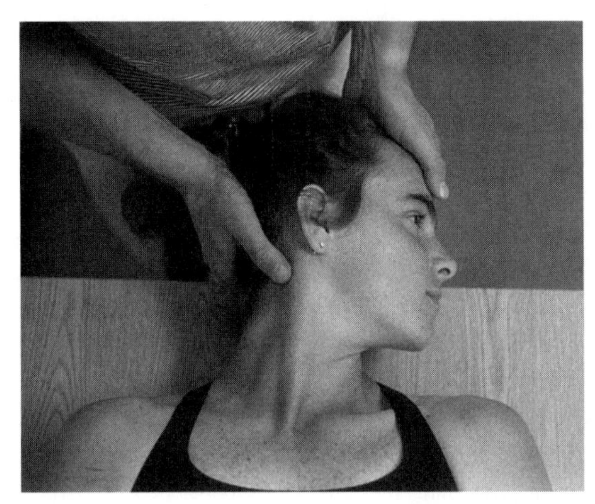

FIGURE 14-18 ■ Passive left rotation of the cervical spine.

Table 14-8 Cervical Spine Ligaments Stressed During Passive Range of Motion Testing

Motion	Ligaments Stressed
Flexion	Posterior longitudinal ligament Ligamentum nuchae Interspinous ligament Ligamentum flavum
Extension	Anterior longitudinal ligament
Rotation	Interspinous ligament Ligamentum flavum
*Lateral Bending**	Interspinous ligament Ligamentum flavum

*These assessments are usually inconclusive.

Joint play

Accessory intervertebral motion and associated pain are assessed using joint play techniques (Joint Play 14-1). Theoretically, hypomobility at one segment may result in compensatory hypermobility at the segments above and below, although the small magnitude of the available range makes differences difficult to detect clinically, and the interrater reliability of these techniques is low.[9] Hypomobility of the first rib can result in cervical pain (Joint Play 14-2).

Neurologic Testing

Because of the mobility and relative lack of protection of the cervical spine, lower motor neuron lesions in this area are common. An upper quarter neurological screen is used to determine pathology of the C5 through T1 nerve roots. The possibility of spinal cord involvement also requires a lower quarter screen (see Box 1-5). PROM may also provoke neurological symptoms such as aching, throbbing, or burning as the nerve root is compressed or placed on stretch. Common referred pain patterns for the cervical spine are presented in Figure 14-19.

Sometimes referred to as the "straight leg test of the upper extremity," the **upper limb nerve tension tests** (also known as the upper limb neurodynamic tests) assess the impact of changing nerve tension on provoking symptoms (Special Test 14-1).[14] The upper limb tension tests (ULTT) involve placing the patient in sequential positions that gradually increase tension on a specific peripheral nerve.[14] While tests that theoretically stretch the median, ulnar, and radial nerves have been described, research suggests that the ulnar and radial nerves are not selectively isolated and that only the ULTT for the median nerve demonstrates adequate specificity.[14] This ULTT commonly provokes responses such as pain or paresthesia in normal subjects as the nerve is progressively stretched. Therefore, a positive

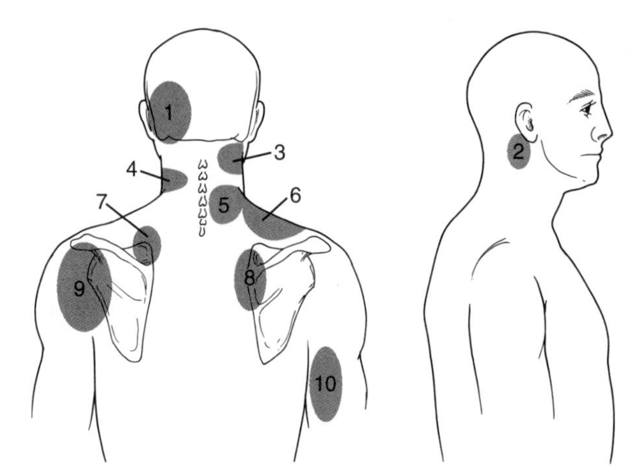

FIGURE 14-19 ■ Referred pain patterns from the cervical spine. *1*, Occipital region; *2*, upper posterolateral cervical region; *3*, upper posterior cervical region; *4*, middle posterior cervical region; *5*, lower posterior cervical region; *6*, suprascapular region; *7*, superior angle of the scapula; *8*, midscapular region; *9*, shoulder joint; *10*, upper arm.

Joint Play 14-1
Cervical Vertebral Joint Play

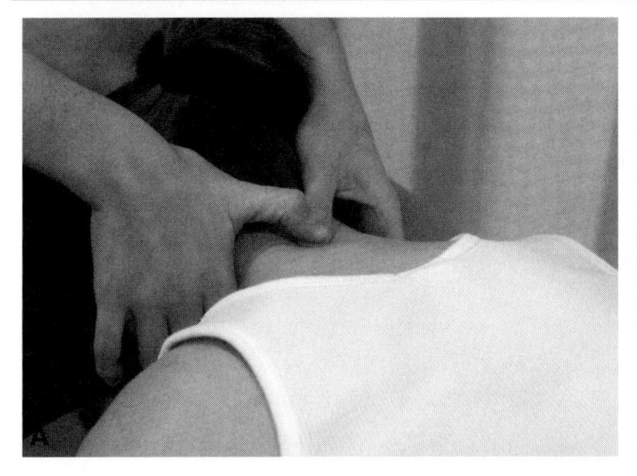

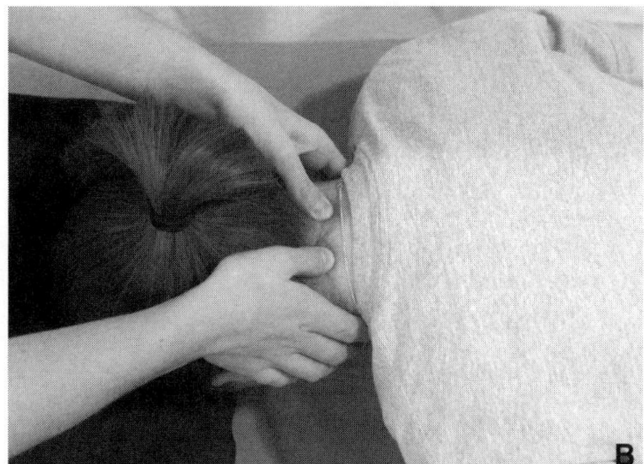

Joint play of the cervical spine. **(A)** Central posterior–anterior (CPA) and **(B)** unilateral posterior anterior (UPA)

Patient Position	Supine; the head is in a neutral position.
Position of Examiner	Standing at the head of the patient
Evaluative Procedure	**CPA:** Palpate the target spinous process using the tips of the thumbs. Apply a gradual anteriorly directed force until an end-feel is determined. Repeat at each level, noting any differences. **UPA:** Palpate the target spinous process and move laterally approximately one thumb breadth to the raised area, the articular pillar. Apply an anteriorly directed force. Repeat at each level, and then assess the opposite side.
Positive Test	Hyper- or hypomobility compared to the segment above and below
Implications	**Hypermobility:** Insufficiency of the passive supporting structures (e.g., ligaments). **Hypomobility:** Restriction of the passive supporting structures
Evidence	***Inter-rater Reliability:*** Not Reliable — Very Reliable Poor — Moderate — Good 0 0.1 0.2 0.3 0.4 0.5 0.6 0.7 0.8 0.9 1.0

CPA = central posterior-anterior; UPA = unilateral posterior–anterior.

response is considered reproduction of the patient's specified symptoms and motion limitation.[23] Like other nerve tensioning techniques such as the slump test and straight leg raise (see Chapter 13), the response is confirmed when symptoms reduce when the exacerbating position is eliminated. Once a positive response is elicited, no further components are added to the test.

Upper quarter neurologic screen

Neurologic Screen 14-1 highlights the areas of an upper quarter neurologic screen.

Upper motor neuron lesions

Trauma to the brain or spinal cord can result in hyperreflexia, spasticity, and hypertonicity of muscles; weakness of the muscles innervated distal to the lesion; loss of sensation; and ataxia. These findings are consistent with damage to the upper motor neurons, which connect the brain with the spinal cord and provide descending input to the muscles. Other findings of this condition include muscle tremor and uncontrollable involuntary movement. In addition, the loss of bowel and bladder control can be a sign of upper motor neuron lesions. The **Babinski test** (Special Test 14-2) and the **Oppenheim test** (Special Test 14-3) are used to evaluate for an upper motor neuron lesion.[24] Note that these tests are rarely needed with acute trauma: if an upper motor neuron lesion is present; other signs and symptoms will be readily apparent.

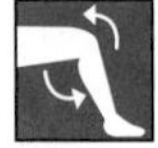

Joint Play 14-2
Mobility of the First Rib

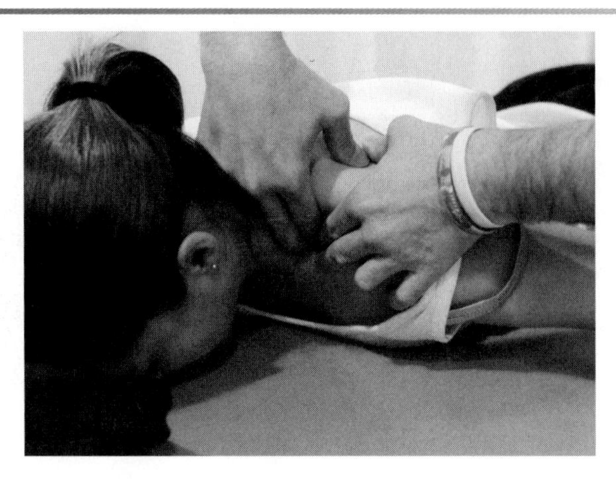

The first rib is manipulated to determine the amount of motion at the costovertebral junction.

Patient Position	Prone
Position of Examiner	Standing at the head of the patient
Evaluative Procedure	Palpate the posterior aspect of the first rib just anterior to the upper trapezius just above the vertebral border of the scapula. Provide an inferior gliding force to the rib.
Positive Test	Hypomobility and/or pain
Implications	Restricted mobility of the first costovertebral joint
Modification	There are several techniques for evaluating the mobility of the first rib.
Evidence	Absent or inconclusive in the literature

CPA = central posterior–anterior; UPA = unilateral posterior–anterior.

Pathologies and Related Special Tests

Acute injuries to the cervical spine occur in contact and collision sports when the spine is compressed or forced past its normal ROM. The whiplash type of injury occurs as the head is moving in one direction and the cervical muscles eccentrically contract to counter this motion. Chronic conditions develop from poor postural habits, repetitive movements, decreased flexibility, and muscular insufficiency. These conditions worsen with time secondary to the adaptive shortening of tissues, resulting in increased pain and spasm. Certain disease states such as viral infections (e.g., meningitis), allergic reactions to medication, and other diseases may mimic the symptoms of traumatic injury to the cervical spine, especially if they create swelling and pain of surrounding lymph glands.[25]

The first step when evaluating cervical pathologies is to rule out the presence of any potentially catastrophic injuries. Examiners must be thorough in evaluating the local cervical structures and determining any effect that the pathology may be causing distally through the radiation of signs and symptoms.

Multiple structures are usually involved with acute and chronic neck pain. For example, degenerative joint disease is commonly associated with osteophyte formation and subsequent nerve root compression. Whiplash-associated disorder (WAD) incorporates the muscle and facet joint damage that occurs following this mechanism.[20] Because of the close functional relationships among the structures of the spine, identifying one anatomical source is usually not possible.

Cervical Radiculopathy

Degenerative disk changes, acute disk trauma, a degenerated facet joint, a unilaterally dislocated cervical facet joint, osteophytes, or inflammation may result in pressure on one or more cervical nerve roots.[27,28] The resulting pressure produces pain and spasm in the cervical region with

Neurologic Screening Box 14-1
Upper Quarter Neurologic Screen

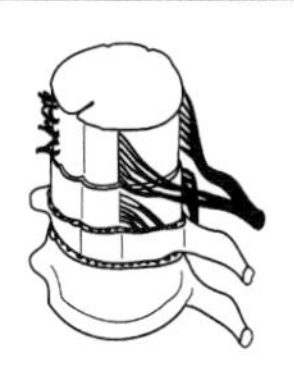 **Nerve Root Level**	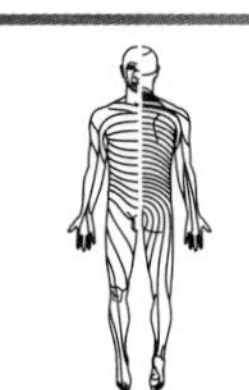 **Sensory Testing**	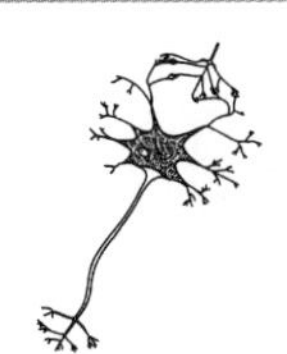 **Motor Testing**	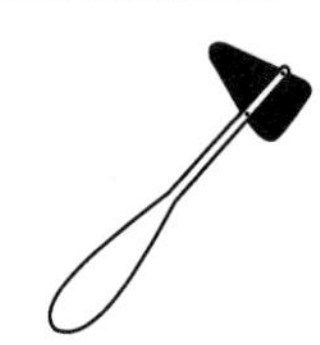 **Reflex Testing**
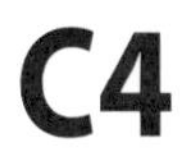 **C4**	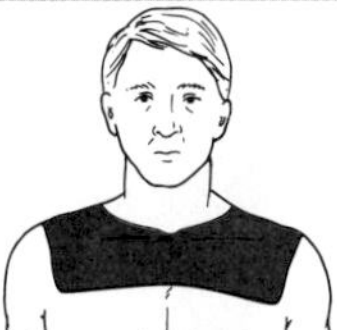 Supraclavicular n.	Shoulder shrug 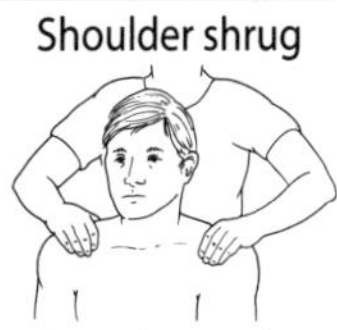 Dorsal scapular	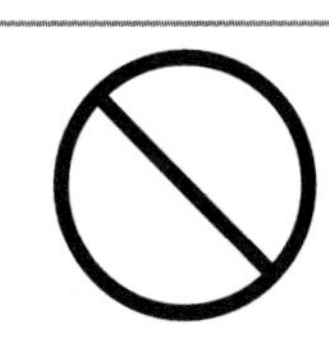 None
C5	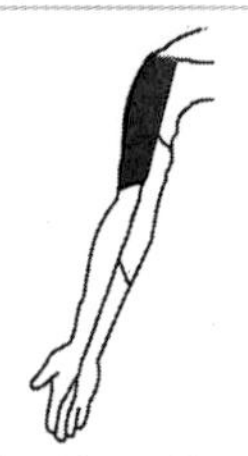 Proximal lateral brachial cutaneous n.	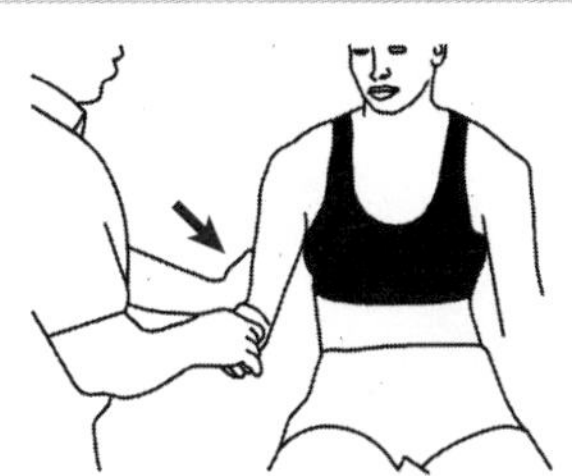 Axillary n.	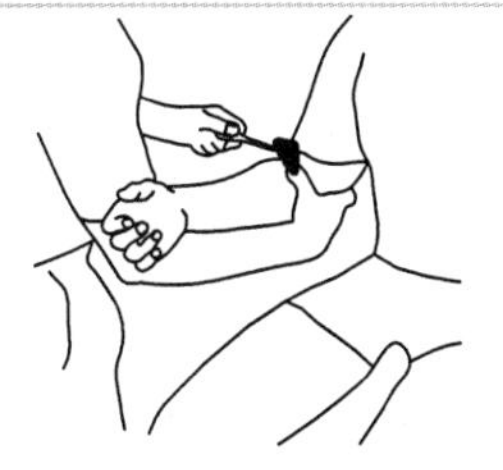 Musculocutaneous n.
C6	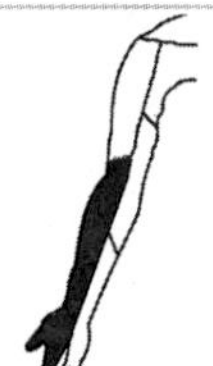 Lateral antebrachial cutaneous n.	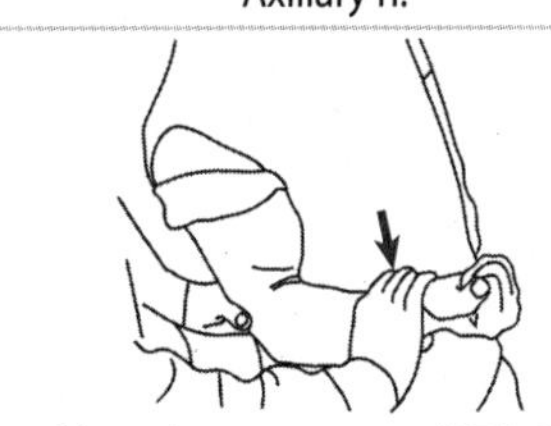 Musculocutaneous n. (C5 & C6)	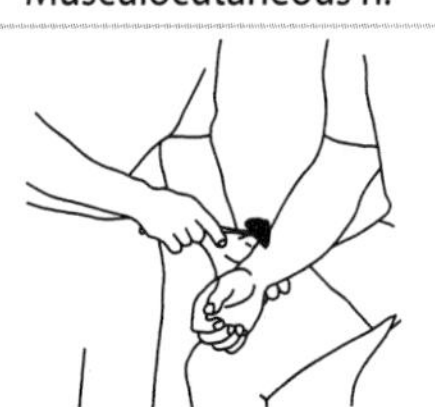 Musculocutaneous n.
C7	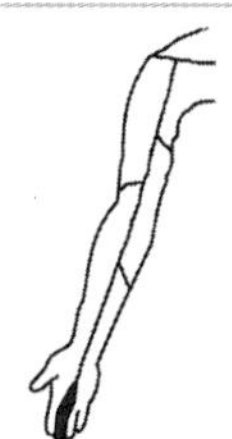 Radial n.	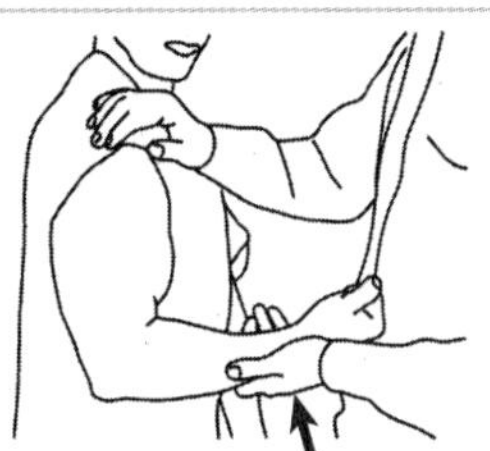 Radial n.	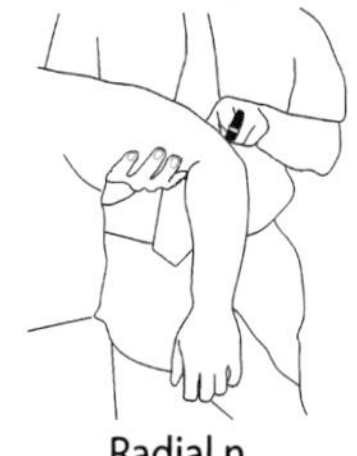 Radial n.
C8	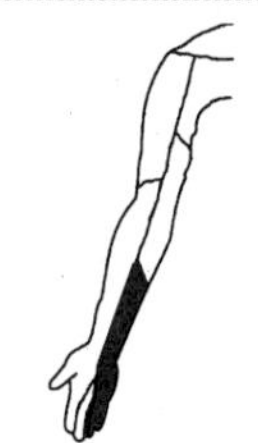 Ulnar n. (mixed)	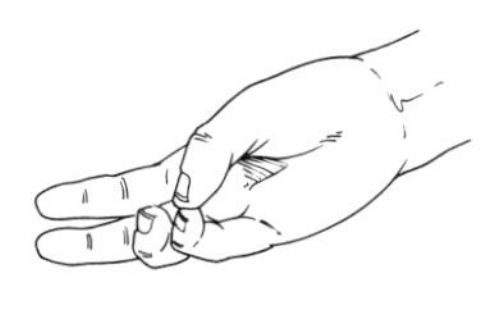 Median n.	 None
T1	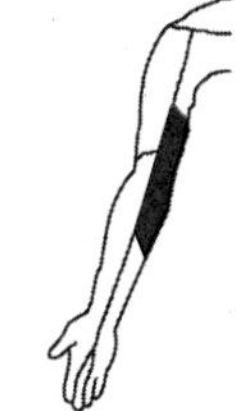 Med. brachial cutaneous n.	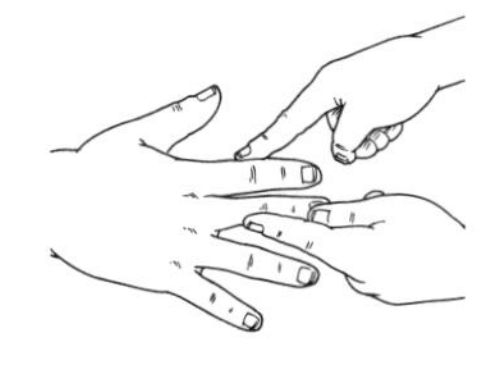 Med. brachial cutaneous n.	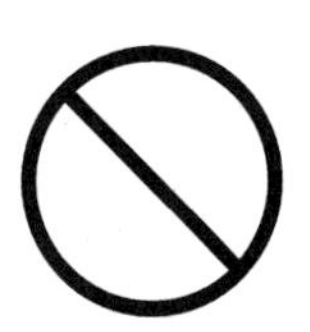 None

Special Test 14-1
Upper Limb Tension Test (ULTT)

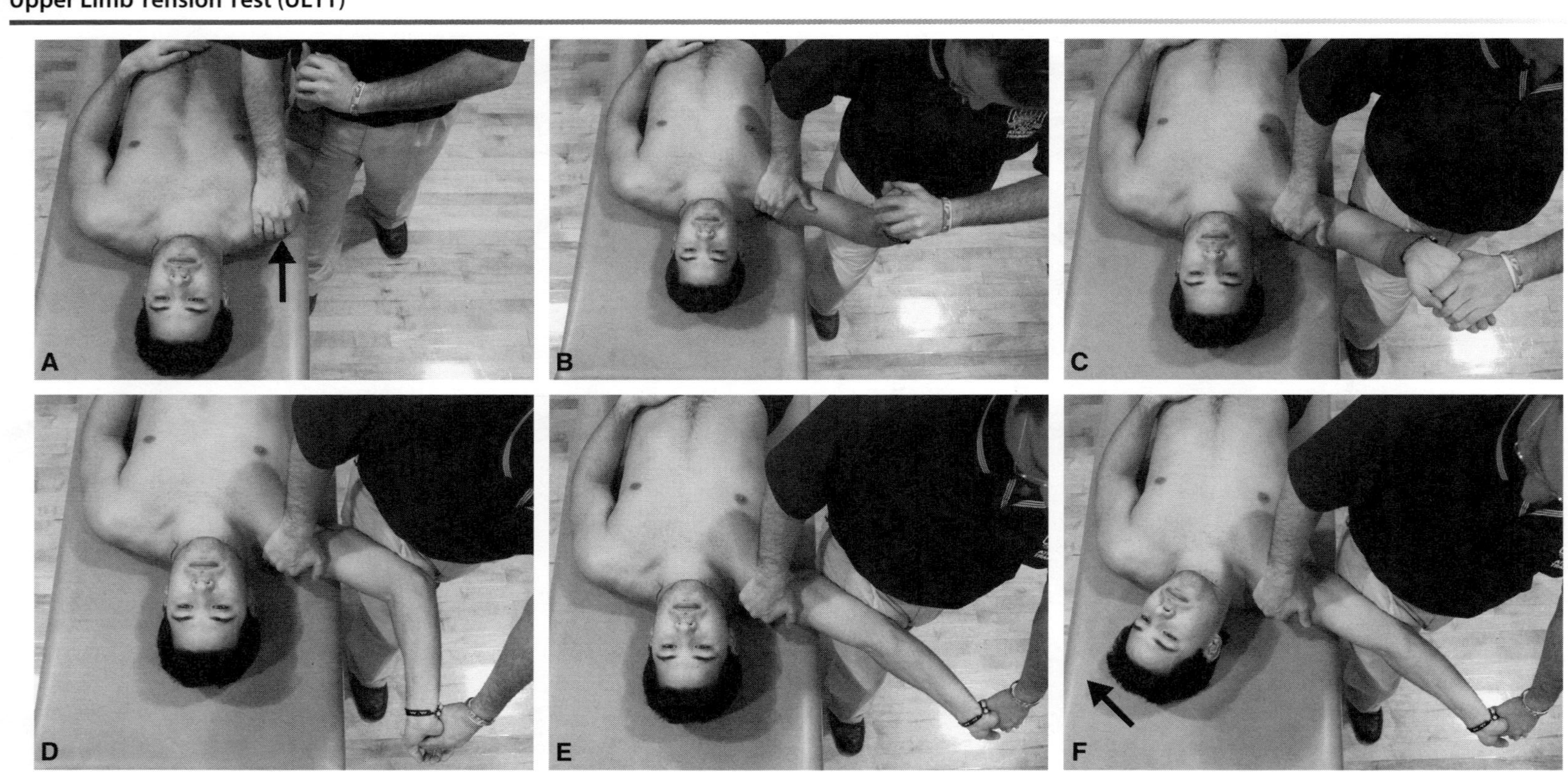

The patient's limb is sequentially positioned, pausing after each step to elicit symptoms.

Patient Position	Supine The glenohumeral joint is adducted to the side, the wrist and fingers are relaxed, the forearm is pronated, and the elbow is flexed.
Position of Examiner	On the test side

Evaluative Procedure	Hold each position for 6 seconds after the addition of each sequential position: **(A)** Depress the shoulder girdle on the same side. Maintain this force throughout the remaining steps. **(B)** Abduct the glenohumeral joint to 110°. **(C)** Supinate the forearm and extend the wrist and fingers. **(D)** Externally rotate the glenohumeral joint. Note: Avoid over-rotating the glenohumeral joint if the patient has a history of glenohumeral instability. **(E)** Extend the elbow. **(F)** Add neck lateral flexion. Lateral flexion to the opposite side will increase symptoms, while lateral flexion to the same side will decrease symptoms. The test is discontinued at whatever position evokes positive findings.
Positive Test	Provocation of stated symptoms and restricted range of motion
Implications	Hyperirritability of the peripheral nerve due to adaptive shortening, entrapment or impingement (e.g., cervical disk herniation)[23]
Evidence	***Inter-rater Reliability:*** Not Reliable — Very Reliable Poor / Moderate / Good 0 0.1 0.2 0.3 0.4 0.5 0.6 0.7 0.8 0.9 1.0 Positive likelihood ratio Not Useful — Useful Very Small / Small / Moderate / Large 0 1 2 3 4 5 6 7 8 9 10 Negative likelihood ratio Not Useful — Useful Very Small / Small / Moderate / Large 1.0 0.9 0.8 0.7 0.6 0.5 0.4 0.3 0.2 0.1 0

Special Test 14-2
Babinski Test for Upper Motor Neuron Lesions

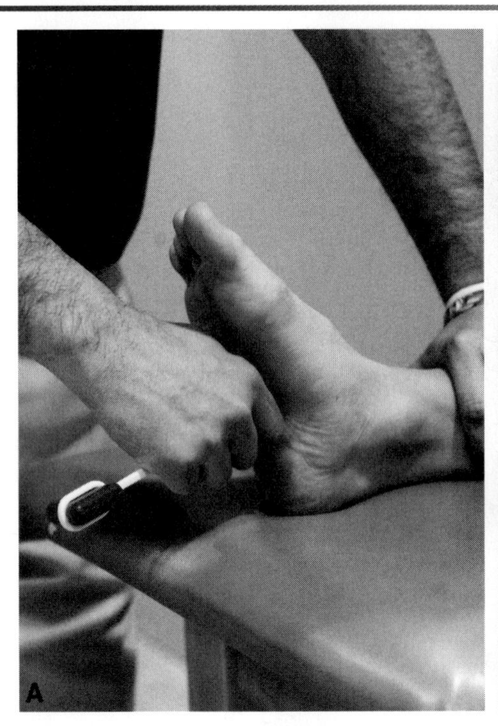

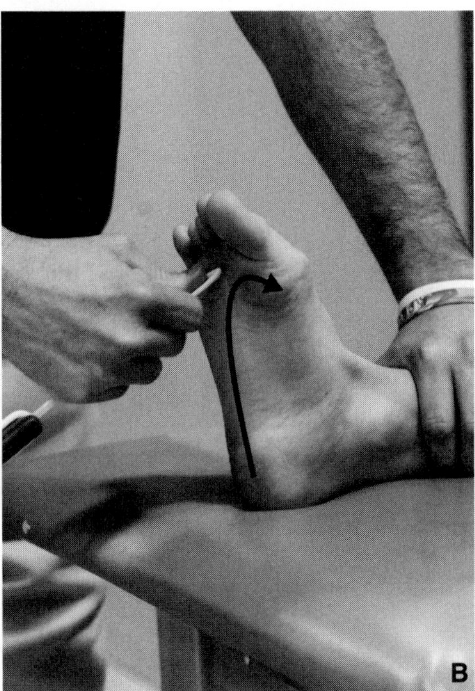

In adults, the Babinski test may be performed during the evaluation of an acute head or cervical spine injury to determine the presence of an upper motor neuron lesion.

Patient Position	Supine
Position of Examiner	At the foot of the patient; a blunt device, such as the handle of a reflex hammer or the handle of a pair of scissors, is needed.
Evaluative Procedure	The examiner runs the device up the plantar aspect of the foot, making an arc from the calcaneus medially to the ball of the great toe **(A)**. In the presence of normal innervation the toes should curl **(B)**.
Positive Test	The great toe extends and the other toes splay.
Implications	Upper motor neuron lesion, especially in the pyramidal tract, caused by brain or spinal cord trauma or pathology
Comments	The Babinski reflex occurs normally in newborns and should spontaneously disappear shortly after birth.
Evidence	***Inter-rater Reliability:***

Not Reliable — **Very Reliable**

Poor | Moderate | Good

0 0.1 0.2 0.3 0.4 0.5 0.6 0.7 0.8 0.9 1.0

Positive likelihood ratio

Not Useful — **Useful**

Very Small | Small | Moderate | Large

0 1 2 3 4 5 6 7 8 9 10

Negative likelihood ratio

Not Useful — **Useful**

Very Small | Small | Moderate | Large

1.0 0.9 0.8 0.7 0.6 0.5 0.4 0.3 0.2 0.1 0

Special Test 14-3
Oppenheim Test for Upper Motor Neuron Lesions

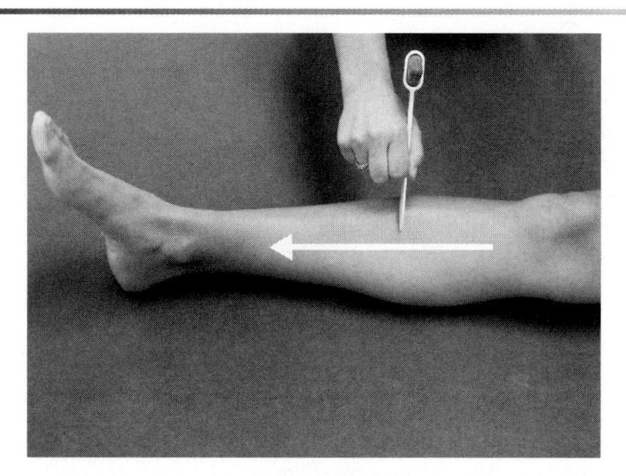

The Oppenheim test may be performed during the evaluation of a patient with acute head or cervical spine injury to determine the presence of an upper may be motor neuron lesion.

Patient Position	Supine
Position of Examiner	At the patient's side
Evaluative Procedure	A blunt object or the examiner's fingernail is run along the crest of the anteromedial tibia.
Positive Test	The great toe extends and the other toes splay or the patient reports hypersensitivity to the test.
Implications	Upper motor neuron lesion caused by brain or spinal cord trauma or pathology
Evidence	Absent or inconclusive in the literature

possible pain and paresthesia in the affected dermatome, muscular weakness, altered reflexes, and atrophy in the region supplied by the involved root (Examination Findings 14-1). The most common causes of cervical radiculopathy are disk **herniations** and osteophyte formation associated with degenerative joint and disk disease (spondylosis).[28]

The signs and symptoms of cervical nerve root impingement may closely mimic those of distal neuropathies such as radial tunnel or carpal tunnel syndrome. The upper quarter screen may be positive for altered sensation, decreased strength, or diminished reflexes. A diminished or absent biceps reflex is strongly suggestive of cervical radiculopathy.[14]

Narrowing of the intervertebral foramen secondary to exostosis of the vertebrae, enlargement or irritation of the dural sheath surrounding the cervical nerve root, and degeneration of the facet joints can be confirmed with the **cervical compression test** (Special Test 14-4). The **Spurling test** (Special Test 14-5) is a modification of the cervical compression test that increases the compression of the cervical nerve root by unilaterally decreasing the size of the foramen.[30]

The **upper limb tension tests** (see Special Test 14-1) may reproduce symptoms. Negative findings (reproduction of symptoms, involved/uninvolved differences in elbow motion or increased symptoms with contralateral neck side-bending and/or decreased symptoms with side-bending to the same side) with ULTT greatly reduce the probability that the patient has cervical radiculopathy.[14]

*** Practical Evidence**

Positive findings on the following four examination techniques increases the probability of a diagnosis of cervical radiculopathy to 90%: Upper limb traction test, active cervical rotation less than 60%, and Spurling test and cervical distraction. Positive findings on 3 of these techniques increases the probability of radiculopathy to 65%.[26]

The **cervical distraction test** may help determine the underlying cause of pain (Special Test 14-6). Manual traction to the skull separates the cervical vertebrae, relieving any pressure placed on the nerve roots. This indicates that the pain is caused by mechanical pressure arising from entrapment of the nerve root or pressure caused by a disk

Herniation The protrusion of a tissue through the wall that normally contains it.

Examination Findings 14-1
Cervical Nerve Root Compression

Examination Segment	Clinical Findings
History	***Onset:*** Acute or chronic ***Pain characteristics:*** Commonly the lower cervical roots (C4–C7); symptoms possibly radiating into the trapezius, scapula, shoulder, arm, wrist, and hand Increased symptoms as day progresses. ***Other symptoms:*** Paresthesia along distribution of involved nerve root ***Mechanism:*** Compression or irritation of the associated nerve root (or roots) ***Predisposing conditions:*** Disk pathology, narrowing of the intervertebral foramen, facet degeneration, prior trauma to the cervical spine Most common in 30- to 40-year-olds.[14,26]
Inspection	The head and cervical spine are postured to relieve pressure on the involved nerve root.
Palpation	Point tenderness may be noted at the involved vertebral level.
Joint and Muscle Function Assessment	***AROM:*** Pain experienced during extension, lateral bending toward the involved side, and rotation. Rotation to the involved side of less than 60 degrees is particularly suggestive of cervical radiculopathy.[14] ***MMT:*** Pain and weakness possible for all muscles tested ***PROM:*** Pain is experienced during extension, lateral bending toward the involved side, and rotation.
Joint Stability Tests	***Stress tests:*** Not applicable ***Joint play:*** Hypo- or hypermobility may be noted
Special Tests	Cervical compression test (increases symptoms), cervical distraction tests (decreases symptoms), Spurling test, vertebral artery test, shoulder abduction test
Neurologic Screening	Upper quarter screen may reveal muscle weakness, paresthesia, and diminished reflexes specific to the involved nerve root. C6 and C7 nerve roots are most commonly involved.[26]
Vascular Screening	Adson, Allen, and military brace position are used to assess for thoracic outlet syndrome.
Functional Assessment	The patient will often demonstrate limitations or compensations during those tasks that require full cervical rotation.
Imaging Techniques	Radiographs are used to identify structural or degenerative changes to the vertebra and/or decreased intervertebral space caused by disk degeneration. T1- and T2-weighted MR images are used to image the spinal cord, cervical nerve root, and intervertebral disks.
Differential Diagnosis	Cervical strain, cervical spondylolysis, degenerative disk disease, facet joint dysfunction, disk herniation or rupture, thoracic outlet syndrome, clinical cervical instability, tumor
Comments	Needle EMG is the most accurate diagnostic tool for cervical neuropathy.[14] Nerve conduction studies may also be used.[14] Suspect a cervical fracture, dislocation, or sprain with acute symptoms following a traumatic force.

AROM = active range of motion; MMT = manual muscle test; MR = magnetic resonance; PROM = passive range of motion.

Special Test 14-4
Cervical Compression Test

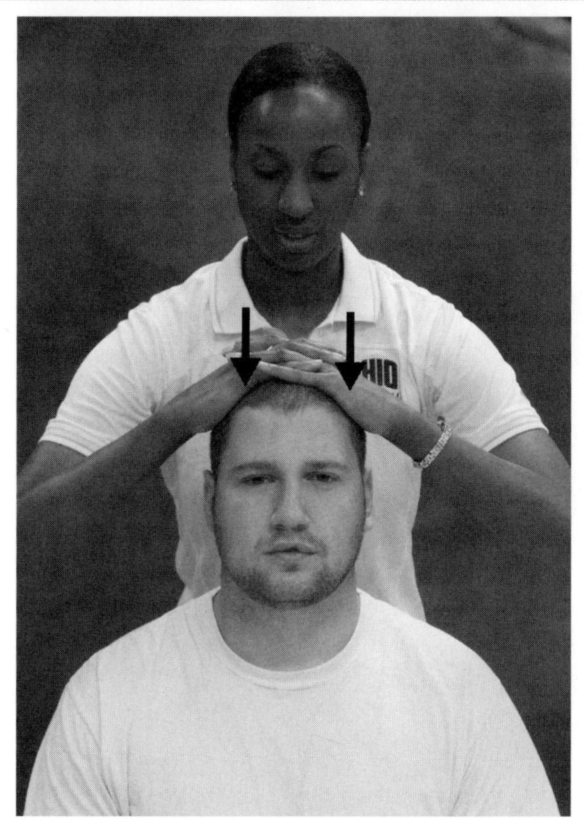

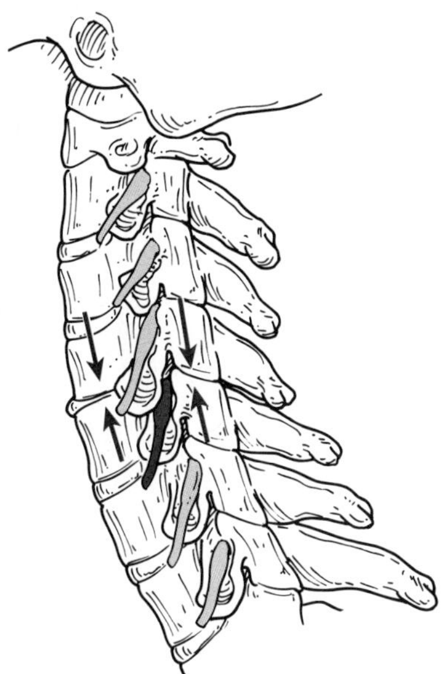

The cervical compression test attempts to duplicate the patient's symptoms by increasing pressure on the cervical nerve roots.

Patient Position	Sitting
Position of Examiner	Standing behind the patient with hands interlocked over the top of the patient's head
Evaluative Procedure	The examiner presses down on the crown of the patient's head.
Positive Test	The patient experiences pain or reproduction of symptoms in the upper cervical spine, upper extremity, or both.
Implications	Compression of the facet joints and narrowing of the intervertebral foramen resulting in pain
Comments	This test should not be performed until the possibility of a cervical fracture or instability has been ruled out.
Evidence	Absent or inconclusive in the literature

Special Test 14-5
Spurling Test

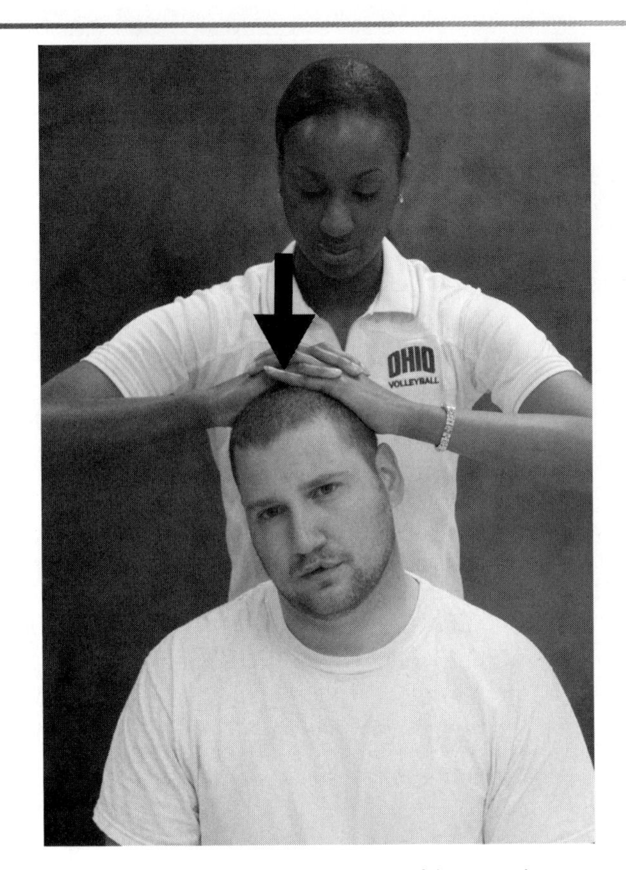

Similar to the cervical compression test, Spurling's test attempts to compress one of the cervical nerve roots.

Patient Position	Seated
Position of Examiner	Standing behind the patient with the hands interlocked over the crown of the patient's head
Evaluative Procedure	The patient laterally flexes the cervical spine. A compressive force is then placed along the cervical spine.
Positive Test	Pain or reproduction of symptoms radiating down the patient's arm
Implications	Nerve root impingement by narrowing of the neural foramina
Modification	The cervical spine may be extended and/or rotated.[14,29]
Comments	This test should not be performed until the possibility of a cervical fracture or dislocation has been ruled out.
Evidence	***Inter-rater Reliability:***

Not Reliable — **Very Reliable**

Poor | Moderate | Good

0 0.1 0.2 0.3 0.4 0.5 0.6 0.7 0.8 0.9 1.0

Positive likelihood ratio

Not Useful — **Useful**

Very Small | Small | Moderate | Large

0 1 2 3 4 5 6 7 8 9 10

Negative likelihood ratio

Not Useful — **Useful**

Very Small | Small | Moderate | Large

1.0 0.9 0.8 0.7 0.6 0.5 0.4 0.3 0.2 0.1 0

Special Test 14-6
Cervical Distraction Test

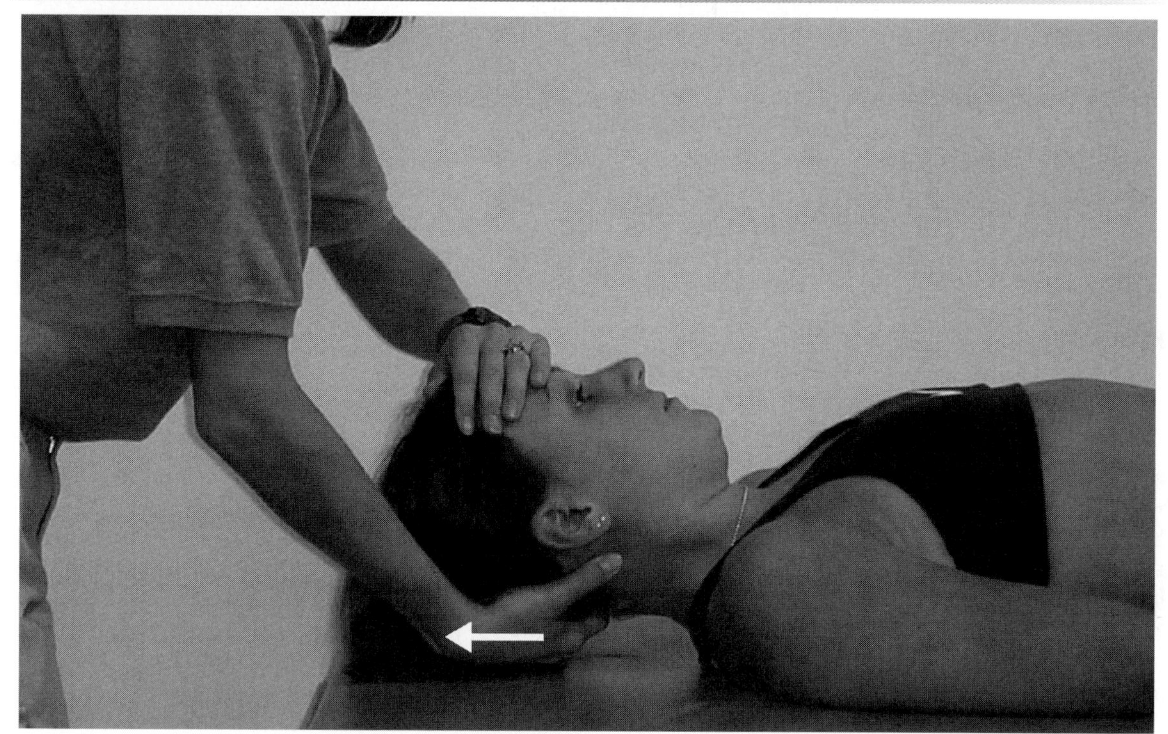

The cervical distraction test attempts to relieve the patient's symptoms by decreasing pressure on the cervical nerve roots.

Patient Position	Supine to relax the cervical spine postural muscles
Position of Examiner	At the head of the patient with one hand under the occiput and the other on top of the forehead, stabilizing the head
Evaluative Procedure	The examiner flexes the patient's cervical spine to a position of comfort.[14] A traction force is applied to the skull, producing distraction of the cervical spine.
Positive Test	The patient's symptoms are relieved or reduced.
Implications	Compression of the cervical facet joints and/or stenosis of the neural foramina
Modification	Not applicable
Comments	This test should not be performed until the possibility of a cervical fracture or dislocation has been ruled out.

Evidence

Inter-rater Reliability:

Not Reliable — Very Reliable

Poor | Moderate | Good

0 0.1 0.2 0.3 0.4 0.5 0.6 0.7 0.8 0.9 1.0

Positive likelihood ratio

Not Useful — Useful

Very Small | Small | Moderate | Large

0 1 2 3 4 5 6 7 8 9 10

Negative likelihood ratio

Not Useful — Useful

Very Small | Small | Moderate | Large

1.0 0.9 0.8 0.7 0.6 0.5 0.4 0.3 0.2 0.1 0

herniation. The distraction test is also a gross determinant of an individual's response to traction therapy.

The same mechanisms that produce cervical nerve root symptoms may also impinge the vertebral artery. A test for **patency** of the vertebral artery, the **vertebral artery test** (Special Test 14-7) determines whether there is the potential for claudication and interruption of the blood flow to the brain. Dizziness, confusion, or **nystagmus** are signs and symptoms of an impingement of the vertebral arteries.[31] A positive test result precludes further evaluation and treatment of the cervical spine until the patient is evaluated by a physician for occlusion of the vertebral arteries.

Disk pathology

In the presence of disk herniations and vertebral impingement, the patient's pain is often influenced by the position of the head and cervical spine. Because the annulus fibrosis is barely present in the lateral region of the disk, pain arising from cervical disk pathology likely results from tension on the lateral aspect of the posterior longitudinal ligaments (Fig. 14-20).[4]

Unyielding pain may signify an intervertebral disk rupture or the presence of a tumor.[32] Pain that does not subside during treatment or has an unknown cause requires a physician's examination. In the case of tumor, symptoms increase as the size of the tumor increases, possibly leading to paraplegia, quadriplegia, or death.

Many of the examination techniques described in this section must not be performed if the possibility of a cervical fracture, cervical dislocation, or other vertebral instability exists.

The majority of cervical disk herniations involve the C5–C6 or C6–C7 intervertebral disks and the C6 or C7 nerve roots.[26,33] The patient describes pain when the cervical spine is placed in a position that forces the disk's nucleus pulposus outwardly toward the involved nerve root. The **shoulder abduction test** is a clinical test used for the presence of a herniated disk and may be a position that the patient describes using to decrease the symptoms (Special Test 14-8).[34] The patient may also complain of pain during the Valsalva maneuver, when making a bowel movement, sneezing, or other activities that increase intrathecal pressure (see Valsalva Test, p. 487).

The presence of disk herniations is confirmed via magnetic resonance imaging (MRI) or myelogram (Fig. 14-21).[33–35] Conservative therapy consisting of cervical traction, muscular strengthening, patient education, and anti-inflammatory medications can produce satisfactory relief of the symptoms.[37,38] Conservative care is most effective when the protrusion is less than 4 mm and does not place pressure on the spinal cord.[37] The patient's level of activity is dictated by symptoms.

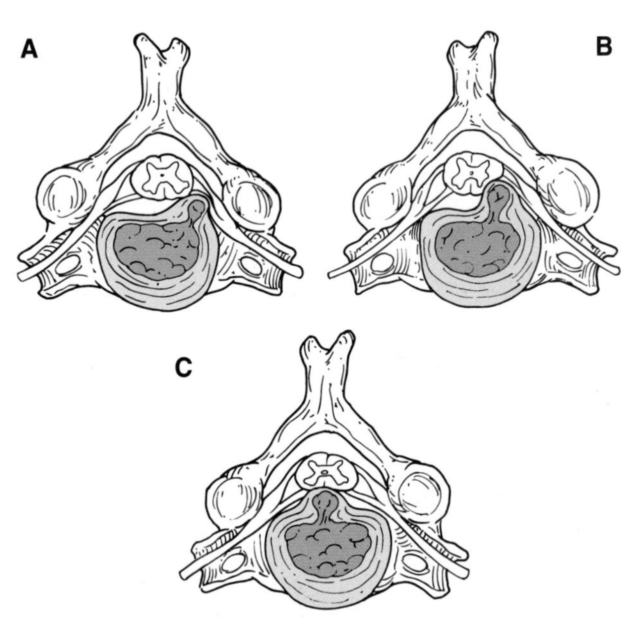

FIGURE 14-20 ■ Location of herniation influences the resulting dysfunction[3]: (A) Intraforaminal—Radicular symptoms within a discrete dermatomal pattern. (B) Posterolateral—Motor deficits, atrophy. (C) Midline—Anterior spinal cord compression that may result in bowel and bladder changes, sexual dysfunction, gait disturbance, and decreased fine motor skills

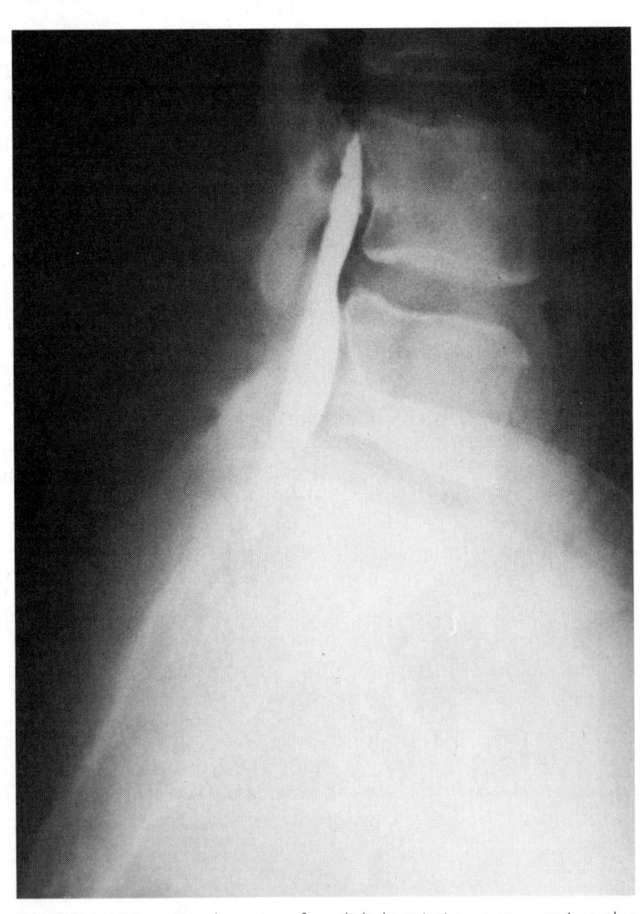

FIGURE 14-21 ■ Myelogram of a disk herniation compressing the spinal cord and associated nerve roots.

Patency Freely open.

Nystagmus An uncontrolled side-to-side movement of the eyes.

Special Test 14-7
Vertebral Artery Test

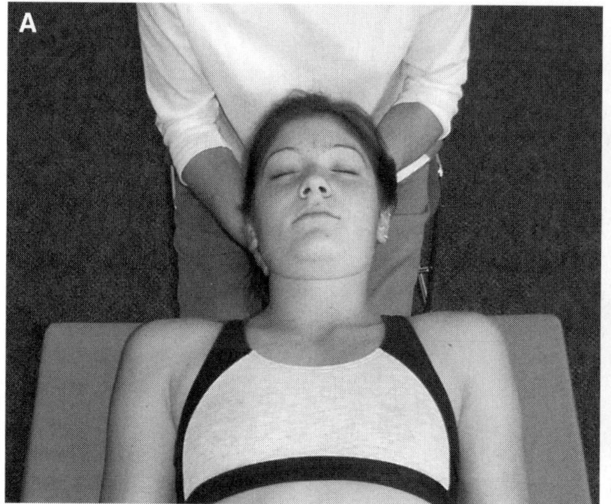

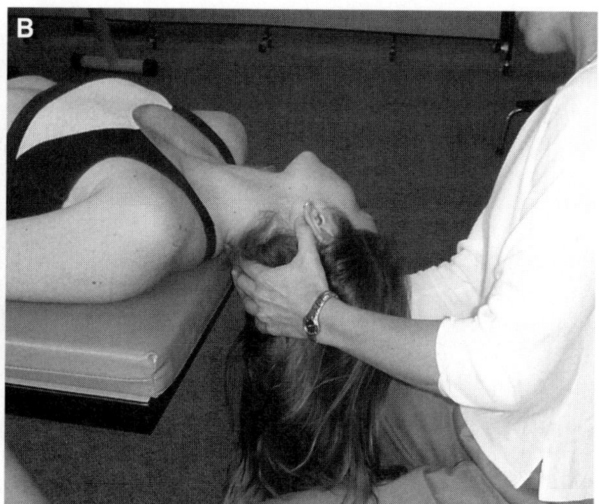

The vertebral artery test is performed to assess the competency of the vertebral artery before initiating treatment or rehabilitation techniques that may compromise a partially occluded artery. This test should not be performed until the presence of a cervical fracture, dislocation, or instability has been ruled out.

Patient Position	Supine
Position of Examiner	Seated at the head of the patient with the hands placed under the occiput to stabilize the head
Evaluative Procedure	The examiner passively extends the cervical spine **(A)**. The head is then rotated to one side and held for 30 s **(B)**. Repeat the procedure for the opposite side. During this procedure, the examiner must monitor the patient's pupillary activity.
Positive Test	Dizziness, confusion, nystagmus, unilateral pupil changes, nausea
Implications	Occlusion of the cervical vertebral arteries.
Comments	Patients with a positive test result should be referred to a physician before any other evaluative tests are performed or a rehabilitation plan is implemented and before being allowed to return to competition.
Evidence	Positive likelihood ratio: Not Useful — Useful Very Small · Small · Moderate · Large 0 1 2 3 4 5 6 7 8 9 10 Negative likelihood ratio Not Useful — Useful Very Small · Small · Moderate · Large 1.0 0.9 0.8 0.7 0.6 0.5 0.4 0.3 0.2 0.1 0

Special Test 14-8
Shoulder Abduction Test

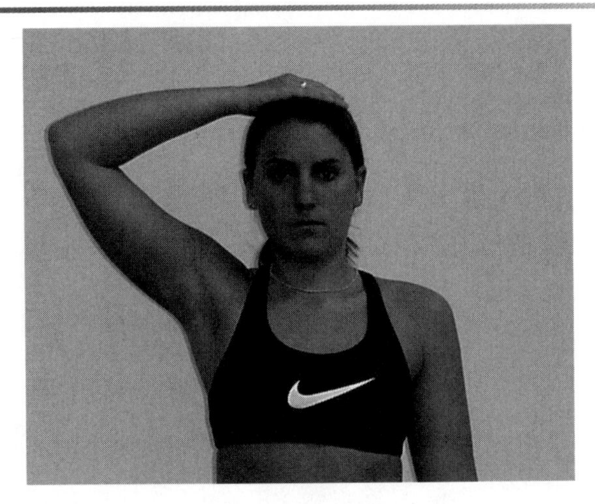

Because of its pain relieving qualities, the patient may assume this posture on his or her own.

Patient Position	Seated or standing
Position of Examiner	Standing in front of the patient
Evaluative Procedure	The patient actively abducts the arm so that the hand is resting on top of the head and maintains this position for 30 seconds.
Positive Test	Decrease in the patient's symptoms secondary to decreased tension on the involved nerve root
Implications	Herniated disk or nerve root compression
Evidence	Positive likelihood ratio

Not Useful — Useful
Very Small | Small | Moderate | Large
0 1 2 3 4 5 6 7 8 9 10

Negative likelihood ratio

Not Useful — Useful
Very Small | Small | Moderate | Large
1.0 0.9 0.8 0.7 0.6 0.5 0.4 0.3 0.2 0.1 0

Degenerative joint and disk disease

Degenerative joint and disk disease (cervical spondylosis) may be a normal consequence of aging that starts with disk degeneration or may be the result of repetitive stresses or trauma. The collapse of the disk results in segmental hypermobility. Osteophyte formation and bony hypertrophy occur to compensate for this hypermobility. This cluster of pathologies can ultimately result in pressure on the spinal cord (myelopathy).[39] Some age-related degeneration of the spine is expected and is not necessarily symptomatic. Radiologic evidence of degeneration such as osteophyte formation and a decreased disk space is often present even though the patient is asymptomatic. Likewise, patients may display signs and symptoms of degenerative disease in the absence of radiographic evidence.

Patients with degenerative joint and disk disease describe a history of joint aggravation with episodes of joint pain and cervical stiffness. Questioning may reveal an acute neck injury or an occupation or activity that repetitively stresses the neck. Suboccipital pain and headaches may also occur. Radicular symptoms may occur as a result of encroachment on the nerve roots as the intervertebral foramen becomes narrowed. These most often involve the C6 and C7 nerve roots.

AROM and PROM may be limited secondary to pain and stiffness. Joint play may reveal hypomobility at one segment with compensatory hypermobility at the segments above and below. When radicular symptoms are present, palpation of affected muscles may detect atrophy before it becomes notable on inspection.

Clinical Cervical Instability

Clinical cervical instability differs from gross instability caused by dislocations or acute fractures. Cervical stabilization is obtained through input from neurologic, active, and passive structures. Alterations in neural input, muscle activity, or bony and ligamentous restraint can result in subtle cervical instability. In large joints, noticeable instability often occurs with damage to the passive restraints, such as ligaments. In the cervical spine, the passive restraints may be intact even when clinical cervical instability is present, representing dysfunction of the active and neurologic stabilizers.[40]

Causes of clinical cervical instability include degenerative changes secondary to poor posture, repetitive movements, muscular weakness, and damage to the passive restraints such as occurs during acute trauma.

Patients with clinical cervical instability may describe relief of symptoms with external stabilization, such as a cervical collar or simply holding the neck with the hands. Pain or intolerance with sustained postures (such as working at a computer) is common, as are complaints of muscle tightness and referred pain to the shoulder and parascapular region. Occipital, frontal or retro-orbital headaches may also occur. Patients typically describe pain, weakness, or a "catching" sensation in the mid-range of motion, consistent with disruption to the active and neurologic stabilizers. Radiculopathy may or may not be present.

Poor control or uneven motion in the mid-range of active movements are characteristic examination findings.[40,41] Palpation reveals general tenderness in the cervical region, along with notable increased paraspinal muscle density due to spasm. Findings from intervertebral joint play, although having poor reliability, may include hypermobility in the cervical region that is often coincident with hypomobility in the upper thoracic region.

Facet Joint Dysfunction

A subset of clinical cervical instability, facet joint dysfunction is the result of acute trauma including whiplash mechanisms or repetitive motion, is characterized by posterior neck pain during extension and rotation of the cervical spine that load the facet joints. Patients may also complain of clicking or catching, and radicular symptoms are uncommon. Facet joint pathology is associated with a characteristic pattern of referred pain (Fig. 14-22).[42]

Examination findings include well-localized pain in the paraspinal region, just lateral to the spinous process of the involved segment. PROM and AROM may provoke symptoms, especially with extension and rotation. The upper quarter screen and upper limb tension tests are normal. Central and unilateral posterior–anterior joint play (see Joint Play 14-1) may increase symptoms and reveal hypermobility or hypomobility. Facet joint involvement is often diagnosed when symptoms are relieved after an injection of anesthetic into the joint.

Brachial Plexus Pathology

Acute trauma to the brachial plexus, often referred to as a "burner" or "stinger," is common in contact sports. The onset of this injury may be caused by a traction force placed on the brachial plexus (brachial plexus stretch) or an impingement of the cervical nerve roots (brachial plexus compression) through extension and lateral flexion to the same side. In football players, the brachial plexus may be traumatized by compression of the brachial plexus between the shoulder pad and the superior medial scapula and is more common in defensive players.[43,44] This site, **Erb's point** (Fig. 14-23), is located 2 to 3 cm above the clavicle in front

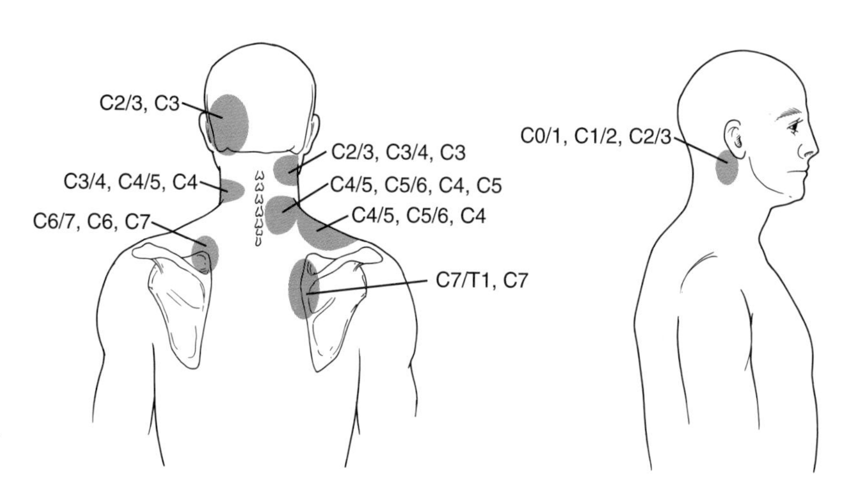

FIGURE 14-22 ■ Referred pain patterns from cervical facet joints.

Examination Findings 14-2
Brachial Plexus Trauma

Examination Segment	Clinical Findings
History	***Onset:*** Acute ***Pain characteristics:*** Pain in the trapezius and deltoid, radiating into the arm ***Other symptoms:*** Paresthesia along distribution of involved nerve. ***Mechanism:*** **Brachial plexus stretch:** Lateral bending of the cervical spine and depression of the opposite shoulder, resulting in tension on the brachial plexus; symptoms occur on the side **opposite** the lateral bend **Brachial plexus compression:** Extension and lateral bending of the cervical spine, resulting in the entrapment of the cervical nerve roots; symptoms occur on the side **toward** the lateral bend ***Predisposing conditions:*** History of repeated brachial plexus trauma; stenosis of the intervertebral foramen; degenerative changes in the cervical spine.
Inspection	The involved arm hangs limply at the patient's side, but resolves with time.
Palpation	Palpation of the cervical spine is necessary to rule out the possibility of a vertebral fracture or dislocation. Possible tenderness over Erb's point
Joint Function and Strength Assessment	***AROM:*** Initially, AROM of the cervical spine and affected limb are diminished. Return of motor function usually begins minutes after the onset of injury. ***MMT:*** Muscles innervated by the involved nerve are weak (grade 3/5 or lower). Strength typically returns quickly. ***PROM:*** Pain is increased with lateral flexion (brachial plexus stretch test).
Joint Stability Tests	***Stress tests:*** Not applicable ***Joint play:*** Not applicable
Special Tests	Brachial plexus stretch tests, cervical compression and distraction tests, and Spurling test
Neurologic Screening	A complete upper quarter screen is necessary to identify the involved cervical nerve roots or peripheral nerves.
Vascular Screening	Within normal limits
Functional Assessment	Grip strength may be diminished and, initially, the patient will not voluntarily move the involved arm.
Imaging Techniques	Plain film radiographs, CT, or MR images may be obtained to rule out stenosis of the intervertebral foramen.
Differential Diagnosis	Cervical spine fracture, herniated disk, cervical spine instability, transient quadriplegia, rotator cuff tear, AC joint pathology, thoracic outlet syndrome, injury to another peripheral nerve (e.g., long thoracic), scapular fracture, proximal humerus fracture[43]
Comments	The presence of a cervical fracture or dislocation must be ruled out before initiating the tests for brachial plexus pathology. All sensory, motor, and reflex test results must be normal and equal before allowing athletes to return to competition.

AROM = active range of motion; CT = computed tomography; MMT = manual muscle test; MR = magnetic resonance; PROM = passive range of motion.

of the transverse process of the sixth cervical vertebra and represents the most superficial passage of the brachial plexus.

Stretching of the brachial plexus occurs when the head is forced laterally while the opposite shoulder is depressed, such as when tackling in football (Fig. 14-24). The resulting force places traction on the nerves on the side opposite the lateral bending of the neck. Any of the cervical nerve roots may be affected by a traction mechanism, but the lateral and posterior cords that are innervated by the C5 and C6 nerve roots (suprascapular, lateral pectoral, musculocutaneous, and axillary nerves) are most commonly involved when the mechanism involves side bending of the head and depression of the shoulder (see Fig. 14-8).[45] Forced

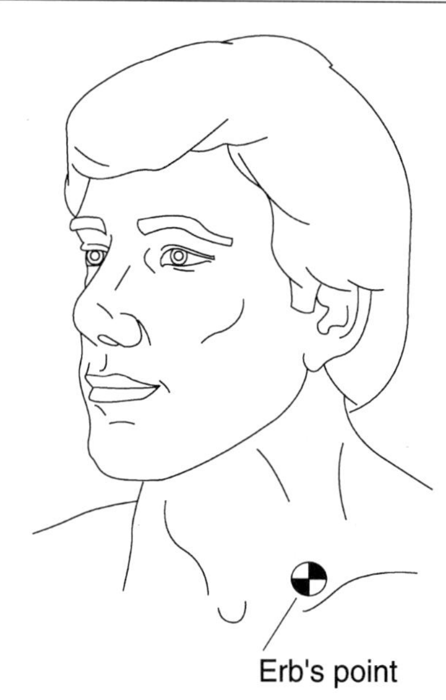

FIGURE 14-23 ■ Erb's point, representing the most superficial passage of the brachial plexus. Pressure to this area can result in pain and paresthesia radiating into the upper extremity.

abduction of the arm can involve the C8 and T1 nerve roots. Repeated low-intensity traction of the brachial plexus can hinder the local microcirculation of the plexus and cause ischemic changes in the nerves.[46] Cervical nerve root injury that quickly resolves without further consequence is associated with a traction mechanism. Recurrent and chronic nerve root injuries are associated with extension and ipsilateral side-bending mechanisms, functionally reproducing Spurling's sign. Individuals with chronic pathology are more likely to have degenerative changes in the cervical spine, disk disease, and spinal stenosis.[47]

A brachial plexus compression occurs on the side toward the bending of the neck when the nerve roots are impinged between the vertebrae. The likelihood of the impingement mechanism is increased by the narrowing of the intervertebral foramen (spinal stenosis).[48] A positive Spurling test result (described earlier in this chapter) is evidence of a mechanical narrowing of the intervertebral foramen by spinal stenosis, degenerative disk disease, or an asymmetric disk bulge (Examination Findings 14-2).[49]

The signs and symptoms of any type of brachial plexus pathology are similar. Immediate pain, often reported as "burning" or "an electrical shock" radiating through the upper extremity, is typically described, but the symptoms are not always limited to the involved dermatome(s).[3]

Characteristically, the involved arm is found dangling limply at the side or the person may be shaking the hand and arm in an attempt to regain feeling. Neck pain is not typically associated with this condition.[43] Manual muscle testing often reveals decreased strength for the muscles innervated by the involved nerve with associated paresthesia. Upper quarter reflexes may be altered, especially in chronic cases.[3] These signs and symptoms normally subside within minutes.[45] Repeated or severe brachial plexus injuries may produce signs and symptoms that diminish much more slowly.

Athletes must not be allowed to return to competition until all symptoms have cleared; they must have full ROM, a full return of sensation, and normal strength throughout the affected extremity. Athletes suffering from chronic brachial plexus pathology display a dropped shoulder and atrophy of the shoulder and cervical musculature on the involved side and note a decrease in bench press weight.[44]

Despite the presence of a common set of symptoms, examiners must not become complacent to the possibility of more severe cervical trauma. A thorough examination of the cervical spine must be undertaken to rule out the presence of a cervical fracture or dislocation. After these conditions have been ruled out, the **brachial plexus traction test,** which is fundamentally PROM in side-bending, may be used to duplicate the mechanism of injury and reproduce the patient's symptoms (Special Test 14-9). Many of the special tests described in the section on cervical nerve root impingement also produce positive results in the presence of brachial plexus pathology. Computed tomography (CT) scans, MRIs, and electromyographic (EMG) analysis can be used to identify local trauma to the nerves or nerve roots.[50]

The treatment and management of patients with brachial plexus trauma is discussed in the section on on-field management in this chapter. Rehabilitation of patients with brachial plexus trauma includes strengthening of the cervical musculature, biofeedback exercises, functional exercise programs, and cervical ROM exercises and re-educating the upper extremity muscles that may have been affected.[51] This set of exercises should also be used to prevent the onset of brachial plexus trauma and other cervical spine injuries.

Thoracic Outlet Syndrome

Thoracic outlet syndrome is caused by pressure on the trunks and medial cord of the brachial plexus, the subclavian artery, or the subclavian vein (collectively known as the neurovascular bundle). There are three types of thoracic outlet syndrome: vascular (arterial or venous), neurogenic, and nonspecific.[53] The diagnosis of thoracic outlet syndrome is one of exclusion. Cervical disk herniation, carpal tunnel syndrome, cubital tunnel syndrome, vascular occlusive disease, malignant tumors, multiple sclerosis, fibromyalgia, Raynaud disease, complex regional pain syndrome, and angina must be ruled out (Examination Findings 14-3).[43,53] Vascular TOS is the least common, with neurogenic and the vague nonspecific types having greater prevalence. Women are affected more often than men.[53]

The etiology of thoracic outlet syndrome may be linked to the presence of a cervical rib, pressure placed on the neurovascular bundle as it is impinged between the clavicle and the first rib, compression between the pectoralis minor

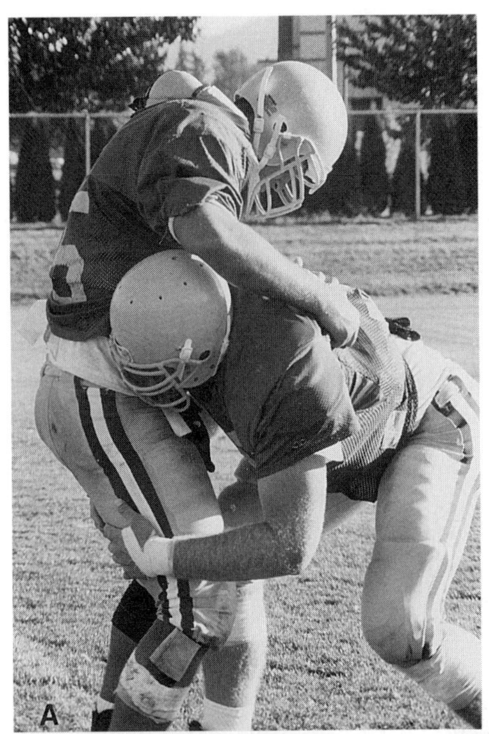

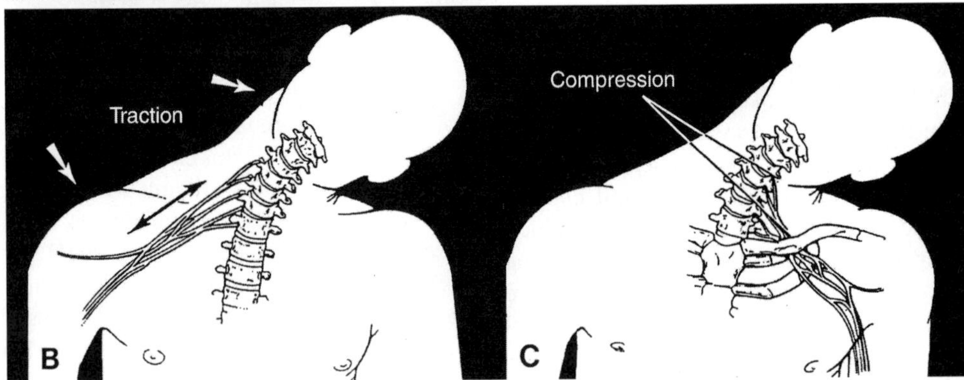

FIGURE 14-24 ■ Mechanism for a brachial plexus injury. (A) The cervical spine is forced laterally and the opposite shoulder is depressed, resulting in elongation of the trapezius and brachial plexus. (B) Elongation of the trapezius muscle with concurrent depression of the shoulder can result in a traction injury to the brachial plexus. (C) Compression (impingement) of the brachial plexus can result on the side toward which the head is tilted.

and rib cage, or tightness of the anterior and middle scalene muscles. Present in a small percentage of the population, the cervical rib is a congenital outgrowth of the seventh cervical vertebra. This structure places pressure on the neurovascular bundle, especially when the shoulder complex is pulled inferiorly, such as when carrying a heavy bag in the hand. The presence of a cervical rib is not necessarily a predisposition to thoracic outlet syndrome. Of all individuals possessing cervical ribs, less than 10% display the clinical signs and symptoms of thoracic outlet syndrome.[54]

The neurovascular bundle passes between the clavicle and the first thoracic rib and is therefore susceptible to pressure on its anterior surface. Poor posture, drooping shoulders that depress the clavicles, forward shoulder posture, prolonged pressure on the upper surfaces of the first rib such as wearing a backpack, or acute trauma may lead to the onset of thoracic outlet syndrome. The incidence of thoracic outlet syndrome is increased in athletes who perform repetitive overhead movements such as throwing or swimming.

Complaints and clinical findings associated with TOS range from dramatic vascular engorgement to mild, intermittent symptoms associated with sustained postures (functional TOS).[55] The signs and symptoms of thoracic outlet syndrome may be neurologic or vascular in nature but the nonspecific type is the most common. Neurologic symptoms commonly occur along the distribution of the medial cord of the brachial plexus (C8 and T1) because of its proximity to the first thoracic rib. Generally, clinical symptoms are produced along the distribution of the ulnar nerve; decreased function along the median nerve may also be noted.

Vascular signs and symptoms reflect the specific structure being obstructed. Occlusion of the subclavian artery presents signs and symptoms typical of decreased blood

Special Test 14-9
Brachial Plexus Traction Test

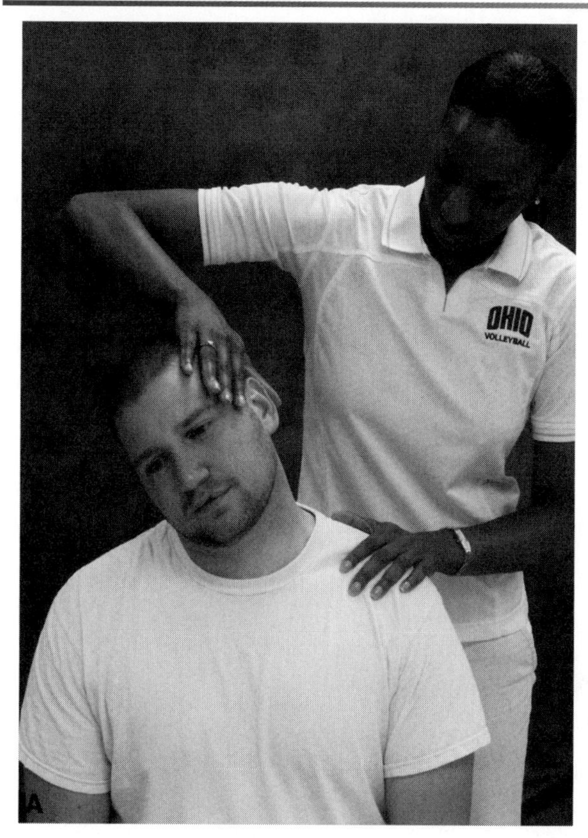

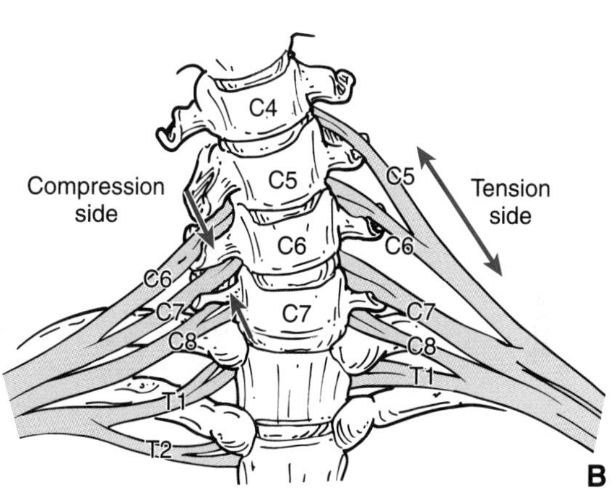

The examiner duplicates the mechanism of injury and replicate the patient's symptoms **(A)**. Pain radiates down the patient's left shoulder when a traction injury exists and down the patient's right shoulder when a compression injury exists **(B)**. This test should be duplicated in each direction

Patient Position	Seated or standing
Position of Examiner	Standing behind the patient
Evaluative Procedure	One hand is placed on the side of the patient's head; the other hand is placed over the acromioclavicular joint, stabilizing the trunk. The cervical spine is laterally bent and the opposite shoulder depressed.
Positive Test	Reproduction of pain and/or paresthesia symptoms throughout the involved upper extremity.
Implications	Brachial plexus neurapraxia **Radiating pain on the side opposite the lateral bending:** Tension (stretching) of the brachial plexus **Radiating pain on the side toward the lateral bending:** Compression of the cervical nerve roots between two vertebrae
Comments	This test should not be performed until the possibility of a cervical fracture or dislocation has been ruled out.
Evidence	Absent or inconclusive in the literature

Examination Findings 14-3
Thoracic Outlet Syndrome

Examination Segment	Clinical Findings
History	***Onset:*** Gradual. May be exacerbated by sustained positioning or compression (such as when wearing a backpack) ***Pain characteristics:*** **Neurogenic:** Achy pain may be described in the lateral cervical spine, shoulder, axillary, periscapular region, and arm. **Nonspecific:** Diffuse pain in arm and periscapular region ***Other symptoms:*** **Neurologic:** Parethesia along involved nerves of brachial plexus ***Mechanism:*** Prolonged compression of neurovascular bundle Acute neck injury (e.g., whiplash mechanism) **Vascular:** Arterial insufficiency and/or venous obstruction ***Predisposing conditions:*** Cervical rib Use of a backpack Participation in activities that require repetitive overhead movements. Tightness of pectoralis minor
Inspection	**Vascular (arterial):** Pallor and/or cyanosis in the involved arm **Vascular (venous):** Pooling edema, distended veins in the shoulder and chest. **Neurogenic:** Atrophy of thenar eminence (Gilliatt-Sumner hand). Forward head posture is common.
Palpation	Confirmation of the inspection findings of pooling edema and/or distended veins Decreased skin temperature may be noted.
Joint and Muscle Function Assessment	***AROM:*** **Nonspecific:** Symptoms may be provoked during overhead motions. **Neurologic:** Cervical rotation to opposite site may provoke symptoms [52] ***MMT:*** **Neurologic:** Weakness of the intrinsic muscles of the hand. **Nonspecific:** General weakness secondary to pain. ***PROM:*** **Nonspecific:** Symptoms may be provoked during overhead motions.
Joint Stability Tests	***Stress tests:*** Not applicable ***Joint play:*** Not applicable
Special Tests	Adson, Allen, Military Brace, Roos
Neurologic Screening	**Neurogenic:** Sensory loss along the ulnar and, possibly, the median nerve distribution **Nonspecific:** Tinel sign over the supraclavicular fossa may be positive.
Vascular Screening	**Vascular (arterial):** Diminished or absent pulse in the involved arm; >20 mm Hg decrease in arterial blood pressure relative to the uninvolved side.
Functional Assessment	**Nonspecific:** Increased complaints of symptoms during overhead motions.
Imaging Techniques	Radiographs will confirm or rule out the presence or rule out the presence of a cervical rib. Ultrasonography to identify arterial or vascular insufficiency
Differential Diagnosis	Cervical disk herniation, carpal tunnel syndrome, cubital tunnel syndrome, vascular occlusive disease, malignant tumors, multiple sclerosis, fibromyalgia, Raynaud disease, complex regional pain syndrome, and angina
Comments	Patients who present with vascular symptoms should be immediately referred to a physician. Special test findings yield a high rate of false-positive results.

AROM = active range of motion; MMT = manual muscle test; PROM = passive range of motion.

Special Test 14-10
Adson's Test for Thoracic Outlet Syndrome

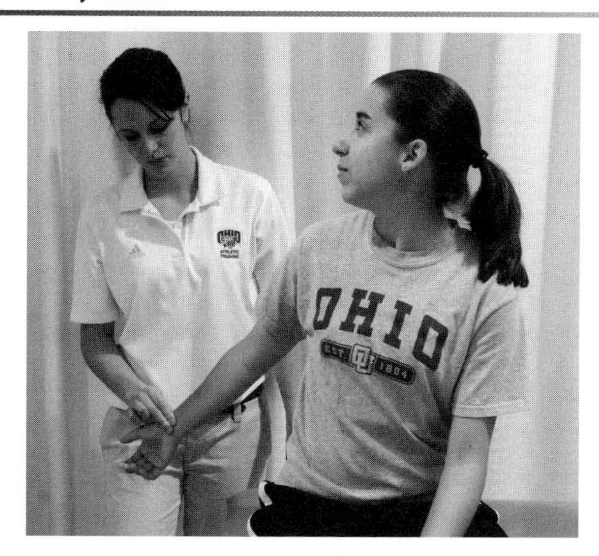

Identifies possible occlusion of the medial cord of the brachial plexus, subclavian artery, and subclavian vein secondary to entrapment of the anterior scalene.

Patient Position	Sitting The shoulder abducted to 30° The elbow extended with the thumb pointing upward The humerus externally rotated
Position of Examiner	Standing behind the patient One hand positioned so that the radial pulse is palpable
Evaluative Procedure	While still maintaining a feel for the radial pulse, the examiner externally rotates and extends the patient's shoulder while the face is rotated toward the involved side and extends the neck. The patient is instructed to inhale deeply and hold the breath.
Positive Test	The radial pulse disappears or markedly diminishes as compared to the opposite side.
Implications	The subclavian artery is being occluded between the anterior and middle scalene muscles and the pectoralis minor.
Evidence	Positive likelihood ratio Not Useful — Useful Very Small (0–2) · Small (2–5) · Moderate (5–10) · Large (10+) 0 1 2 3 4 5 6 7 8 9 10 Negative likelihood ratio Not Useful — Useful Very Small (1.0–0.5) · Small (0.5–0.2) · Moderate (0.2–0.1) · Large (0.1–0) 1.0 0.9 0.8 0.7 0.6 0.5 0.4 0.3 0.2 0.1 0

flow. Blockage of the subclavian vein is characterized by edema in the distal upper extremity and, if untreated, may result in thrombophlebitis.

The underlying principle for thoracic outlet syndrome tests is related to provoking symptoms by placing pressure on the neurovascular bundle. **Adson's test** attempts to depress the shoulder complex and place the medial cord of the brachial plexus, the subclavian artery, and the subclavian vein on stretch while simultaneously placing pressure on the bundle from the anterior scalene muscle (Special Test 14-10). Thoracic outlet syndrome caused by the pectoralis minor muscle may be detected via the **Allen test**

Special Test 14-11
Allen Test for Thoracic Outlet Syndrome

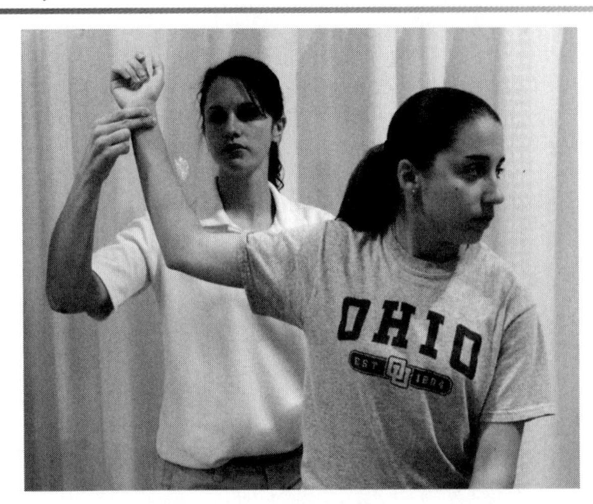

Identifies possible occlusion of the subclavian artery and vein caused by compression from the pectoralis minor.

Patient Position	Sitting The head facing forward
Position of Examiner	Standing behind the patient One hand positioned so that radial pulse is felt
Evaluative Procedure	The elbow is flexed to 90° while the clinician abducts the shoulder to 90°. The shoulder is then passively horizontally abducted and placed into external rotation. The patient then rotates the head toward the opposite shoulder.
Positive Test	The radial pulse disappears or reproduction of neurologic symptoms.
Implications	The pectoralis minor muscle is compressing the neurovascular bundle.
Evidence	Absent or inconclusive in the literature

(Special Test 14-11). Costoclavicular etiology is tested via the **costoclavicular syndrome test (military brace position)** (Special Test 14-12). The **Roos test** has demonstrated accuracy in identifying the presence of thoracic outlet syndrome resulting from either neurologic or vascular abnormalities (Special Test 14-13). Each of these tests can be positive by virtue of a diminishing radial pulse or reproduction of neurologic symptoms. The usefulness of these is limited because of the high rate of false–positive results, with asymptomatic individuals displaying a diminished pulse when placed in these positions. In addition, the upper limb tension test (see Special Test 14-1) may also reproduce neurologic symptoms.[52]

Positive test results for thoracic outlet syndromes are not necessarily definitive of any underlying pathology. Patients who test positive for thoracic outlet syndrome need to be referred to a physician for further evaluation.

Management of thoracic outlet syndrome focuses on correcting postural causes and muscle tightness that are compressing the neurovascular bundle. Postural awareness training and the use of ergonomically correct positioning, especially while driving, using a computer, or any repetitive activity, is indicated. The use of ***nerve gliding*** is also proposed to maintain the brachial plexus' moving freely from compression throughout its course.

On-Field Evaluation and Management of Cervical Spine Injuries

All injuries to the spinal column requiring an on-field evaluation must be treated as possibly life threatening until spinal cord involvement and serious injury have been ruled out. Bilateral symptoms in the upper extremities or symptoms in the lower extremities should alert the examiner to the potential of spinal cord involvement. Chapter 21 discusses the evaluation and management of patients with potentially catastrophic spinal cord injuries.

Special Test 14-12
Military Brace Position for Thoracic Outlet Syndrome

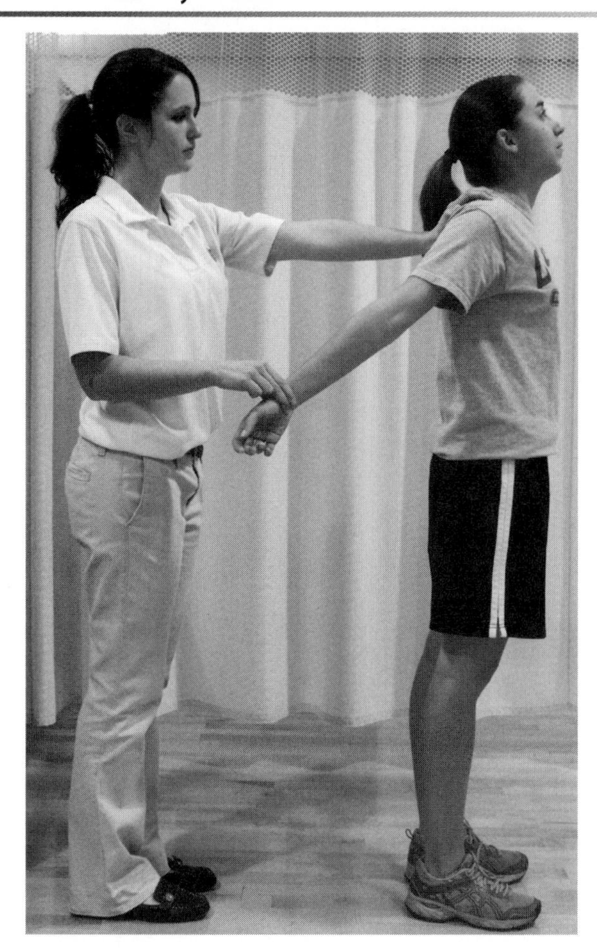

Identifies occlusion of the subclavian artery by the shoulder's costoclavicular structures.

Patient Position	Standing The shoulders in a relaxed posture The head looking forward
Position of Examiner	Standing behind the patient One hand positioned to locate the radial pulse on the involved extremity
Evaluative Procedure	The patient retracts and depresses the shoulders as if coming to military attention. The humerus is extended and abducted to 30°. The neck and head are hyperextended.
Positive Test	The radial pulse disappears.
Implications	The subclavian artery is being blocked by the costoclavicular structures of the shoulder.
Evidence	Absent or inconclusive in the literature

Special Test 14-13
Roos Test (or EAST–Elevated Arm Stress Test) for Thoracic Outlet Syndrome

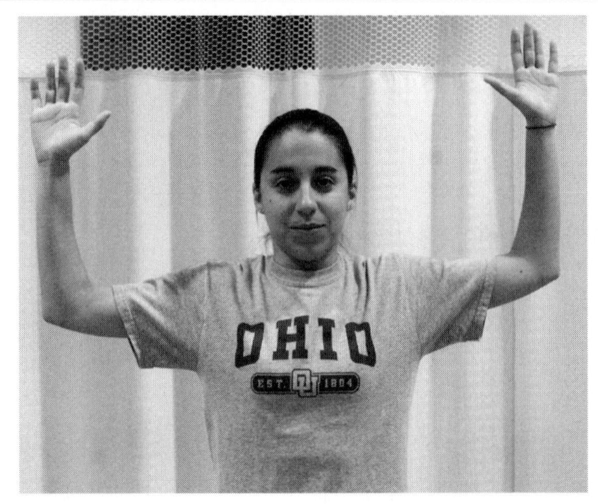

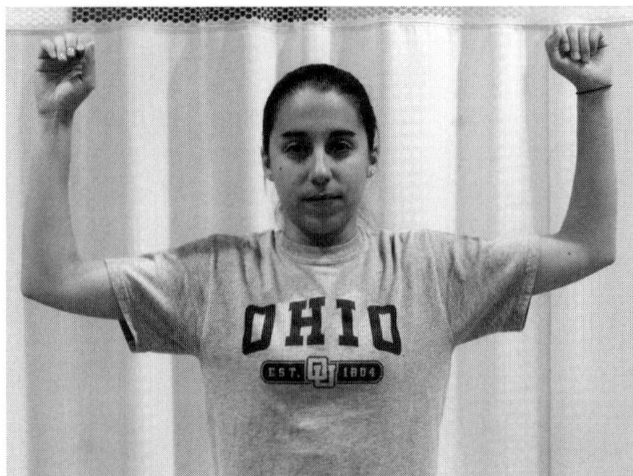

The Roos test identifies the presence thoracic outlet syndrome of neurologic or vascular etiology.

Patient Position	Sitting or standing The shoulders are abducted to 90° and the humerus is externally rotated. The elbows are flexed to 90°.
Position of Examiner	Standing in front of the patient
Evaluative Procedure	The patient rapidly opens and closes both hands for 3 minutes.
Positive Test	Inability to maintain the testing position Replication of sensory and/or motor symptoms in the extremity.
Implications	Thoracic outlet syndrome of neurologic and/or origin.
Evidence	Positive likelihood ratio Not Useful — Useful Very Small / Small / Moderate / Large 0 1 2 3 4 5 6 7 8 9 10 Negative likelihood ratio Not Useful — Useful Very Small / Small / Moderate / Large 1.0 0.9 0.8 0.7 0.6 0.5 0.4 0.3 0.2 0.1 0

Brachial Plexus Injury

Typically, athletes with a brachial plexus injury leave the field of play under their own power, with the involved arm dangling limp at the side. The head may be held in a position to relieve any stress placed on the brachial plexus as the result of spasm of the trapezius muscle. The athlete's signs and symptoms (see Examination Findings 14-2) are usually transient in nature. After a thorough evaluation to rule out the possibility of trauma to the cervical vertebrae, the cervical spine should be treated with ice packs to decrease pain and spasm.

The athlete should demonstrate a normal neurologic examination without weakness and with full pain-free ROM before returning to activity. Any continuation of the signs and symptoms precludes further participation until the athlete is cleared to return to play by a physician. Repeated episodes of brachial plexus trauma may result in scar tissue formation over one or more nerve roots. Also, a pathological narrowing of the foramen may occur.

REFERENCES

1. Olson, S, et al: Tender point sensitivity, range of motion and perceived disability in subjects with neck pain. *J Orthop Sports Phys Ther*, 30:13, 2000.
2. Monsey, RD: Rheumatoid arthritis of the cervical spine. *J Am Acad Orthop Surg*, 5:240, 1997.
3. Levine, MJ, Albert, TJ, and Smith, MD: Cervical radiculopathy: Diagnosis and nonoperative treatment. *J Am Acad Orthop Surg*, 4:305, 1996.
4. Mercer, S, and Bogduk, N: The ligaments and annulus fibrosus of human adult cervical intervertebral discs. *Spine*, 24:619, 1999.
5. Moore, KL, and Dalley, AF: Summary of cranial nerves. In *Clinically Oriented Anatomy* (ed 5). Philadelphia, Lippincott Williams & Wilkins, 2006, pp 1124–1155.
6. Cook, CE: *Orthopedic Manual Therapy. An Evidence-Based Approach*. Upper Saddle River, NJ: Pearson Prentice Hall, 2007, pp 93–142.
7. Pietrobon, R, et al: Standard scales for measurement of functional outcome for cervical pain or dysfunction. A systematic review. *Spine*, 27:515, 2002.
8. Sizer, PS, Brismée, J, and Cook, C: Medical screening for red flags in the diagnosis and management of musculoskeletal spine pain. *Pain Practice*, 7:53, 2007.
9. Fjelhner, A, et al: Interexaminer reliability in physical examination of the cervical spine. *J Manipulat Physiol Ther*, 22:511, 1999.
10. Vlaeyen, JWS, and Linton, SJ: Fear-avoidance and its consequences in chronic musculoskeletal pain: A state of the art. *Pain*, 85:317, 2000.
11. Bertilson, BC, Brunnesjö, DN, and Strender, L: Reliability of clinical tests in the assessment of patients with neck/shoulder problems – Impact of history. *Spine*, 28:2222, 2003.
12. Childs, JD, et al: Screening for vertebrobasilar insufficiency in patients with neck pain: Manual therapy decision-making in the presence of uncertainty. *J Orthop Sports Phys Ther*, 35:300, 2005.
13. Asavasopon, S, Jankoski, J, and Godges, JJ: Clinical diagnosis of vertebrobasilar insufficiency: Resident's case problem. *J Orthop Sports Phys Ther*, 35:645, 2005.
14. Wainer, RS, et al: Reliability and diagnostic accuracy of the clinical examination and patient self-report measures for cervical radiculopathy. *Spine*, 28:52, 2003.
15. Wrisley, DM, et al: Cervicogenic dizziness: A review of diagnosis and treatment. *J Orthop Sports Phys Ther*, 30:755, 2000.
16. Richter, RR, and Reinking, MF: How does evidence on the diagnostic accuracy of the vertebral artery test influence teaching of the test in a professional physical therapist education program? *Phys Ther*, 85:589, 2005.
17. Pool, JJ, et al: The interexaminer reproducibility of physical examination of the cervical spine. *J Manipulat Physiol Ther*, 27:84, 2004.
18. Youdas, JW, Carey, JR, and Garrett, TR: Reliability of measurements of cervical spine range of motion: Comparison of three methods. *Phys Ther*, 71:98, 1991.
19. Cleland, JA, et al: Interrater reliability of the history and physical examination in patients with mechanical neck pain. *Arch Phys Med Rehabil*, 87:1388, 2006.
20. Dall-Alba, PT, et al: Cervical range of motion discriminates between asymptomatic persons and those with whiplash. *Spine*, 26:2090, 2001.
21. Reese, NB: *Muscle and Sensory Testing*. St. Louis, MO: Elsevier Saunders, 2005, p 203.
22. Chiu, TTW, Law, EYH, and Chiu, THF: Performance of craniocervical flexion test in subjects with and without chronic neck pain. *J Orthop Sports Phys Ther*, 35:567, 2005.
23. Walsh, MT: Upper limb neural tension testing and mobilization: Fact, fiction, and a practical approach. *J Hand Ther*, 18:241, 2005.
24. Miller, TM, and Johnston, SC: Should the Babinski sign be part of the routine neurologic examination? *Neurology*, 65:1165, 2005.
25. Yang, SS, and Hershman, EB: Idiopathic brachial plexus neuropathy: A review. *Crit Rev Musculoskel Med*, 5:193, 1993.
26. Wainer, RS, and Gill, H: Diagnosis and nonoperative management of cervical radiculopathy. *J Orthop Sports Phys Ther*. 30:728, 2000.
27. Shapiro, S, et al: Outcome of 51 cases of unilateral locked cervical facets: Interspinous braided cable for lateral mass plate fusion with interspinous wire with iliac crests. *J Neuorsurg*, 91:19, 1999.
28. Waldrop, MA: Diagnosis and treatment of cervical radiculopathy using a clinical prediction rule and a multimodal intervention approach: A case series. *J Orthop Sports Phys Ther*, 36:152, 2006.
29. Tong, HC, Haig, AJ, and Yamakawa, K: The Spurling Test and cervical radiculopathy. *Spine*, 27:156, 2002.
30. Viikari-Junura, E: Interexaminer reliability of observations in physical examinations of the neck. *Phys Ther*, 67:1526, 1987.
31. Maitland, GD: *Vertebral Manipulation*. Butterworths, London, 1973.
32. D'Haen, B, et al: Chordoma of the lower cervical spine. *Clin Neurol Neurosurg*, 97:245, 1995.
33. Bucciero, A, Vizioli, L, and Cerillo, A: Soft cervical disc herniation. An analysis of 187 cases. *J Neurosurg Sci*, 42:125, 1998.
34. Davidson, RI, Dunn, EJ, and Metzmaker, JN: The shoulder abduction test in the diagnosis of radicular pain in cervical extradural compressive monoradiculopathies. *Spine*, 6:441, 1981.
35. van de Kelft, E, and van Vyve, M: Diagnostic imaging algorithm for cervical soft disc herniation. *Acta Chir Belg*, 95:152, 1995.
36. Dailey, AT, et al: Magnetic resonance neurography for cervical radiculopathy: A preliminary report. *Neurosurgery*, 38:488, 1996.
37. Saal, JS, Saal, JA, and Yurth, EF: Nonoperative management of herniated cervical intervertebral disc with radiculopathy. *Spine*, 21:1877, 1996.
38. Humphreys, SC, et al: Flexion and traction effect on C5-C6 foraminal space. *Arch Phys Med Rehabil*, 79:1105, 1998.
39. Emery, SE: Cervical spondylitic myelopathy: Diagnosis and treatment. *J Am Acad Orthop Surg*, 9:376, 2001.
40. Cook, C, et al: Identifiers suggestive of clinical cervical spine instability: A Delphi study of physical therapists. *Phys Ther*, 85:895, 2005.
41. Olson, KA, and Joder, D: Diagnosis and treatment of cervical spine clinical instability. *J Orthop Sports Phys Ther*, 31:194, 2001.
42. Fukui, S, et al: Referred pain distribution of the cervical zygapophyseal joints and cervical dorsal rami. *Pain*, 68:79, 1996.
43. Safran, MR: Nerve injury about the shoulder in athletes, part 2. Long thoracic nerve, spinal accessory nerve, burners/stingers, thoracic outlet syndrome. *Am J Sports Med*, 32:1063, 2004.

44. Markey, KL, Di Benedetto, M, and Curl, WW: Upper trunk brachial plexopathy: The stinger syndrome. *Am J Sports Med,* 21:650, 1993.
45. Speer, KP, and Bassett, FH: The prolonged burner syndrome. *Am J Sports Med,* 18:591, 1990.
46. Kitamura, T, et al: Brachial plexus stretching injuries: Microcirculation of the brachial plexus. *J Shoulder Elbow Surg,* 4:118, 1995.
47. Levitz, CL, Reilly, PJ, and Torg, JS: The pathomechanics of chronic, recurrent cervical nerve root neurapraxia. The chronic burner syndrome. *Am J Sports Med,* 25:73, 1997.
48. Meyer, SA, et al: Cervical spinal stenosis and stingers on collegiate football players. *Am J Sports Med,* 22:158, 1994.
49. Reilly, PJ, and Torg, JS: Athletic injury to the cervical nerve roots and brachial plexus. *Operat Tech Sports Med,* 1:231, 1993.
50. Walker, AT, et al: Detection of nerve rootlet avulsion on CT myelography in patients with birth palsy and brachial plexus injury after trauma. *Am J Roentgenol,* 167:1283, 1996.
51. Bajuk, S, Jelnikar, T, and Ortar, M: Rehabilitation of patient with brachial plexus lesion and break in axillary artery. Case study. *J Hand Ther,* 9:399, 1996.
52. Sanders, RJ, Hammond, SL, and Rao, NM: Diagnosis of thoracic outlet syndrome. *J Vasc Surg,* 46:601, 2007.
53. Huang, JH, and Zager, EL: Thoracic outlet syndrome. *Neurosurgery,* 55:897, 2004.
54. Baker, CL, and Liu, SH: Neurovascular injuries to the shoulder. *J Orthop Sports Phys Ther,* 18:360, 1993.
55. Gillard, J, et al: Diagnosing thoracic outlet syndrome: Contribution of provocative tests, ultrasonography, electrophysiology, and helical computer tomography in 48 patients. *Joint Bone Spine,* 68:416, 2001.

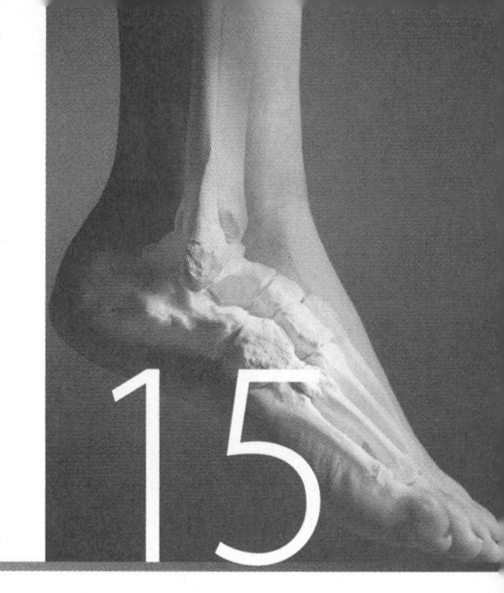

CHAPTER 15

Thoracic, Abdominal, and Cardiopulmonary Pathologies

The heart and lungs, responsible for maintaining the body's homeostasis, lie well protected within the thoracic cavity. However, extraordinary forces or subtle abnormalities can result in damage to these structures, endangering the individual's life. Although less well protected than the organs in the thorax, the abdominal organs, including the liver, spleen, digestive system, and urinary tract and reproductive organs tract, are more resilient to trauma because they are less firmly attached to the skeleton, increasing their ability to absorb shock. With the exception of the liver, the abdominal organs tend to be hollow, thus providing additional shock-absorbing capabilities.

Injury to the body's **visceral** organs can range from the mundane to the catastrophic. A keen awareness of the internal systems of the body, the factors predisposing these organs to injury, and the signs and symptoms of trauma are needed for proper recognition and management of these conditions. The progressive nature of the symptoms emphasizes the need for early identification and repeated examination and evaluation of the involved system.

Advances in the evaluation and medical management of cardiopulmonary conditions allow individuals who would have once been required to be sedentary to participate in physical activity. Even people who have had heart transplants are participating in sports. The medical community has embraced exercise as a vital component in the prevention and rehabilitation of these conditions.

Visceral Pertaining to the internal organs contained within the thorax and abdomen.

Clinical Anatomy

With the sternum anteriorly, the vertebrae posteriorly, and the ribs connecting the two, the thorax forms a protective shell around the torso's upper internal organs (Fig. 15-1). The **sternum** consists of three sections: the **manubrium** superiorly, the central **body**, and the inferiorly projecting **xiphoid process**. The sternal body and the manubrium are

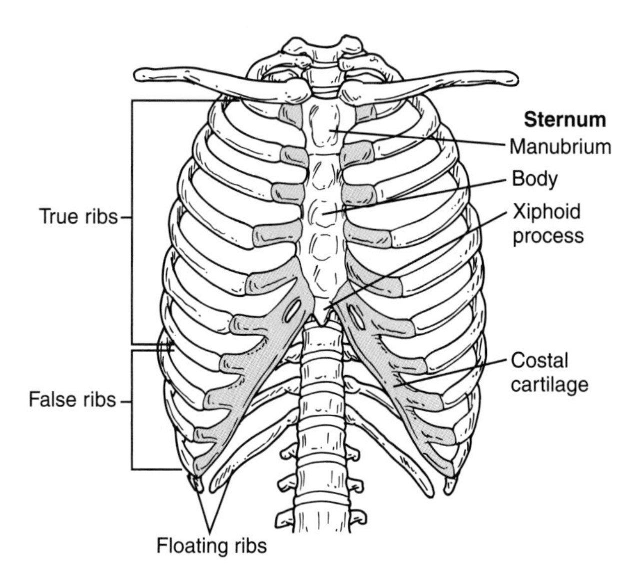

FIGURE 15-1 ■ The thorax. The rib cage formed by the true ribs (1–7), false ribs (8–10), and floating ribs (11 and 12); the sternum (manubrium, body, and xiphoid process); and the costal cartilage. The posterior margin of the thorax is formed by the thoracic vertebrae.

connected by a fibrocartilaginous joint that fuses during adolescence to form a single, solid bone.

The upper seven ribs are classified as **true ribs** because they articulate with the sternum through their own **costal cartilages**. Ribs 8–10 articulate with the sternum through a conjoined costal cartilage. Thus, they are termed **false ribs**. Ribs 11 and 12, the **floating ribs**, do not have an anterior articulation. An anomalous **cervical rib** may project off the seventh cervical vertebra. Although this structure is often benign, it can be a source of compression on the brachial plexus, the subclavian artery, or the subclavian vein, predisposing the individual to **thoracic outlet syndrome** (see Chapter 14).

The abdominal region has no anterior or lateral bony protection and receives only slight protection on its posterior surface from the thoracic and lumbar vertebrae and the floating ribs. The inferior portion of the abdomen is protected by the sacrum posteriorly and the ilium laterally.

Located within the thorax and abdomen are numerous internal organs. Many of the internal organs come in pairs. Reference to these organs is relative to the patient; thus, the right kidney is on the examiner's left side when facing the patient from the front.

Muscular Anatomy

Many of the muscles acting on the thorax and abdomen have been previously discussed and are only referenced in this chapter. In addition, the muscles arising from the thorax to act on the scapula and humerus also influence the thorax (these muscles are discussed in Chapters 14 and 16).

Muscles of inspiration

The **diaphragm** is a muscular membrane that separates the thoracic cavity from the abdominal cavity. Innervated by the **phrenic nerve**, as the diaphragm contracts, it moves downward, creating a vacuum in the thorax pulling air into the lungs. The diaphragm is interrupted at several points by portals through which the major vessels pass into the torso and lower legs.

The rib cage's intrinsic skeletal muscles are collectively referred to as the **intercostal muscles**. Spanning from rib to rib, these muscles assist in the respiratory process. Inspiration is also assisted by the **scalene muscles** that serve as secondary muscles of inspiration by elevating the first and second ribs. The sternocleidomastoid, trapezius, serratus anterior, pectoralis major and minor, and latissimus dorsi all function as secondary muscles of inspiration, used when breathing becomes difficult.

Muscles of expiration

The abdominal muscles—the **rectus abdominis**, **internal oblique**, and **external oblique**—are supported across the abdomen by the **transverse abdominis**. In addition to flexing and rotating the lumbar and thoracic spine, the contraction of these muscles creates a positive pressure gradient across the diaphragm, resulting in the expiration of air.

Respiratory Tract

The **trachea**, connecting the larynx to the bronchioles, is a membranous tube formed by muscle and connective tissue. Its anterior border is protected from crushing forces by a series of cartilaginous semicircular rings. The trachea diverges into two principal **bronchi**. The left bronchus divides into two **segmental bronchi**, and three segmental bronchi are formed on the right side, each matching the number of lobes on the corresponding lung (Fig. 15-2). Each segmental bronchus then subdivides into the **bronchioles**.

In the lungs, carbon dioxide is exchanged for oxygen. The right lung has three lobes—upper, middle, and lower—while the left lung has only an upper and lower lobe, each matching with a segmental bronchus. The thoracic cavity is encased with pleural linings. The **parietal pleura** lines the thoracic wall, and the **visceral pleura** surrounds the lungs, forming a **pleural cavity** between the two. As the chest cavity expands during inspiration, a negative pressure is formed within the pleural cavity, causing an expansion of the lungs and the subsequent inflow of air for breathing.

The actual exchange of gases occurs at the level of the **alveoli**, the terminal branches of the bronchioles. The alveolar walls contain a capillary system, which receives deoxygenated blood from the right side of the heart via the **pulmonary arteries**. After the exchange of gases, the oxygenated blood returns to the left side of the heart via the **pulmonary veins**.

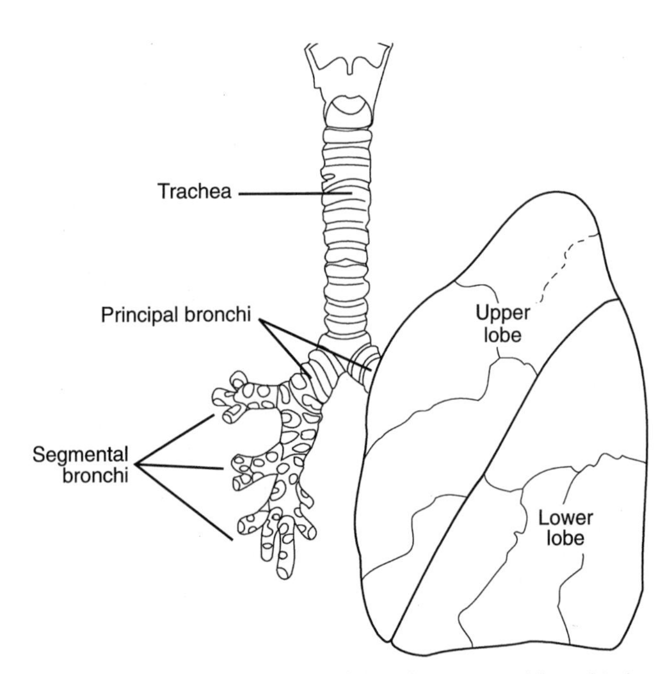

FIGURE 15-2 ■ Respiratory tract. The trachea, principal bronchi, the segmental bronchi, and the left lung (relative to the patient). The right lung has been removed to view the bronchial segments. The left lung is formed by two lobes, whereas the right lung has a third, or middle, lobe between the upper and lower ones.

The trachea and its conducting airways are lined with **mucosal cells**. Mucus, formed in the submucosa by glands, is excreted to the mucosal lining. Here, the mucus acts as a filtration system, working like millions of little sponges absorbing airborne pollutants, dust, and other unwanted substances. Normally the contaminated mucus is routed upward by **ciliary cells** to the pharynx, where it is unconsciously swallowed. When an excess demand is placed on the mucosal system, the mucus is routed up, through, and out the nasal passage.

The upper portions of the respiratory system—the nose, mouth, larynx, and pharynx—are discussed in Chapter 20.

Cardiovascular Anatomy

The heart and major vessels of the cardiovascular system lie within the mediastinum, between the lungs, from the first rib superiorly to the diaphragm inferiorly. The heart is lined by the fibrous and serous pericardium. The **fibrous pericardium** is the tough fibrous outer layer supporting the inner pericardial layer and the heart. The **serous pericardium** is divided into a **parietal layer** lining the fibrous pericardium and a visceral layer that sits tightly against the heart. The serous pericardium allows the heart to move freely within the chest and buffers forces to the heart.

The heart is divided into four chambers, with the right-side chambers handling deoxygenated blood and the left-side chambers handling oxygenated blood (Table 15-1). In the bloodstream, oxygen is exchanged for carbon dioxide, which is then returned to the lungs, where it is subsequently exhaled. The contraction of the cardiac musculature is controlled by an electrical system within the walls of the heart's chambers. This system allows for the synchronous contraction of the atria and ventricles, ensuring a smooth flow of blood through the cardiovascular system. Any disruption of the normal pattern of the heart's electrical stimulus can cause failure of the heart, potentially leading to death.

Table 15-1 The Chambers of the Heart

Heart Chamber	Function
Right Atrium	Receives deoxygenated blood via: • Superior vena cava from the head, neck, and upper extremities • Inferior vena cava from the trunk and lower extremities Delivers blood to the right ventricle through the right atrioventricular (tricuspid) valve
Right Ventricle	Receives deoxygenated blood from the right atrium Delivers blood through the semilunar valve (pulmonic valve) to the lungs via the left and right pulmonary arteries
Left Atrium	Receives oxygenated blood from the lungs via the right and left pulmonary veins Delivers blood to the left ventricle through the left atrioventicular (mitral) valve
Left Ventricle	Delivers oxygenated blood through the semilunar valve (aortic valve) to the ascending aorta

The valves of the heart all function as one-way valves (Fig. 15-3). The tricuspid and mitral valves are held tightly shut against the backflow of blood by the **chordinae tendinae,** which are attached to **papillary muscles**. The muscles and chordinae tendinae mechanically prevent the valve from opening in the wrong direction. The semilunar valves contain no papillary muscles, relying on their mechanical shape to prevent reflux of blood. The backflow of blood causes the valves to form pockets that fill and shut tightly together.

The **right atrium** of the heart receives deoxygenated blood from the head, neck, and upper extremities via the **superior vena cava**. The **inferior vena cava** delivers the deoxygenated blood from the trunk and lower extremities. As the right atrium contracts, the blood passes through the **tricuspid valve** and into the **right ventricle**. Contraction of the right ventricle causes the blood to pass through the **semilunar valves** into the **pulmonary arteries** and to the lungs, where it is oxygenated.

The newly oxygenated blood returns via the **pulmonary veins** into the **left atrium**. From the left atrium, the blood is passed through the **mitral valve** into the **left ventricle**, which contracts to distribute the blood to the body. The left ventricle contains the greatest amount of cardiac muscle because it must provide the force needed to propel the blood throughout the body. As the left ventricle contracts, the blood is pushed out through the **semilunar valves** and into the aorta.

The **aorta** exits the heart, carrying oxygenated blood to the body. Soon after leaving the heart, the aorta takes a sharp bend inferiorly, forming the **aortic arch**. From this arch, many other arteries diverge from the aorta, including the **brachiocephalic trunk**, the **left common carotid artery**, and the **left subclavian artery**. The brachiocephalic branches into the **right subclavian** and **right common**

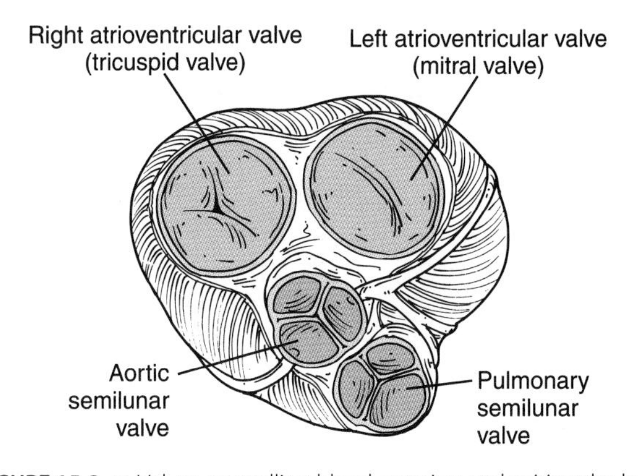

FIGURE 15-3 ■ Valves controlling blood entering and exiting the heart.

carotid arteries; it delivers blood to the right upper extremity, the brain, and the head. Continuing **caudally** from its arch, the aorta forms the **descending thoracic aorta** and when passing through the diaphragm, becomes the **abdominal aorta**, supplying blood to the torso and lower extremity (Fig. 15-4).

In addition to supplying the rest of the body with oxygenated blood, the heart must also pump blood to itself through the right and left **coronary arteries**. The right coronary artery branches into the right marginal artery and the posterior interventricular artery. The left coronary artery branches into the anterior interventricular artery and the circumflex artery, which then leads to the left marginal artery.

Under normal circumstances, the heart beats at a rate that equals the metabolic needs of the body, delivering oxygen and nutrients to the body's tissues. As the tissues' demands for these nutrients increase, so does the heart rate.

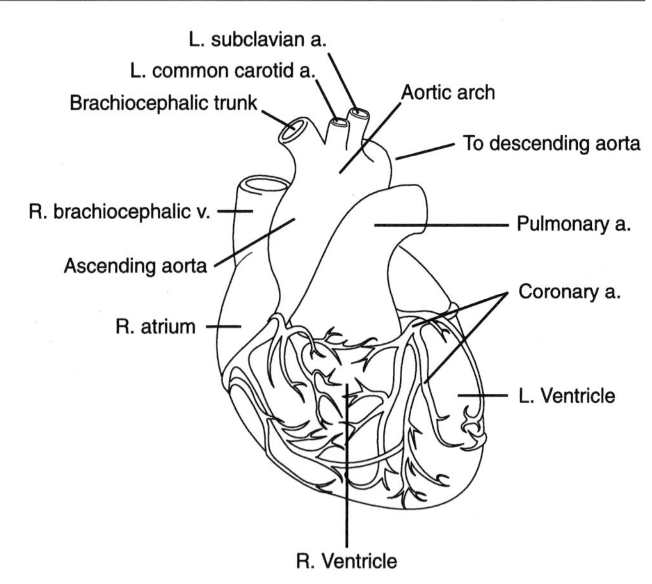

FIGURE 15-4 ■ Anterior view of the heart. Blood supply to the body is delivered through the aorta. The left atrium is hidden in this view.

Digestive Tract

Solids and liquids enter the digestive tract through the mouth and travel through the **esophagus** to enter the stomach. After they reach the stomach, the ingested food substances form a **bolus**, which is routed into the **small intestine** through the **pylorus**. The small intestine is divided into the **duodenum**, **jejunum**, and **ileum**. After passing through the small intestine, the bolus enters the **large intestine** (colon), proceeding through the **cecum**, **ascending colon**, **transverse colon**, **descending colon**, **sigmoid**, and **rectum** to its exit from the body via the **anus** (Fig. 15-5). The **appendix** projects off the cecum. Its mucus membrane lining can become inflamed or infected, leading to **appendicitis**.

The **liver**, the largest organ in the body, takes up the entire right side of the torso inferior to the diaphragm and is protected by the lower ribs and the costal arch of the false ribs (Fig. 15-6). Through its connection with the **gallbladder** and common **bile duct**, the liver introduces **bile** into the stomach to assist in the digestion of fats. The liver also acts as a warehouse for storing glucose, the body's immediate fuel system, and is a repository for the metabolism of intrinsic and extrinsic chemical substances. The many tasks of the liver require a large blood supply. Injury to this organ results in the loss of massive amounts of blood into the abdominal cavity.

In addition to its function as a digestive organ, the liver also filters toxins and wastes out of the blood and produces mediators for blood clotting.

Lymphatic Organ

Located on the left side of the body at the level of the ninth through eleventh ribs, the **spleen** is a solid, fragile organ that is supported by ligaments attaching it to the kidney, colon, stomach, and diaphragm (Fig. 15-7). The largest of

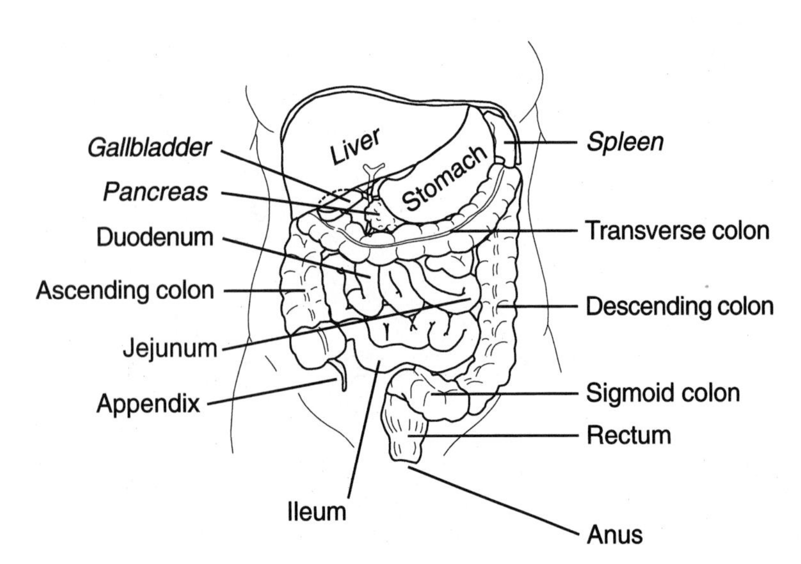

FIGURE 15-5 ■ Stomach and intestine. The liver, gallbladder, pancreas, and spleen are presented for reference purposes.

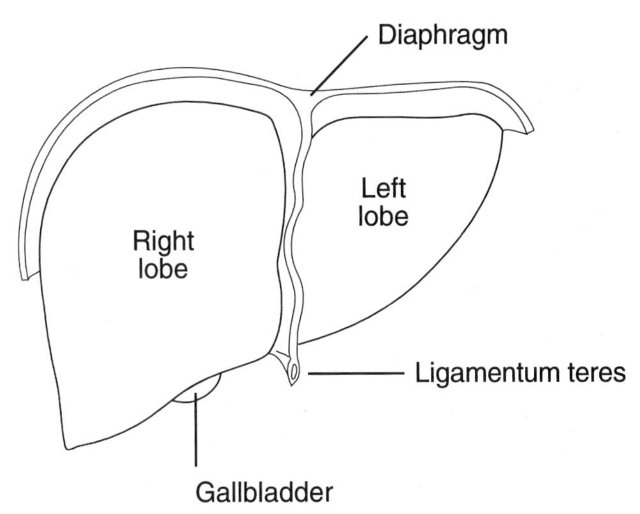

FIGURE 15-6 ■ Anterior view of the liver. This structure is supported by ligaments arising from the inferior surface of the diaphragm.

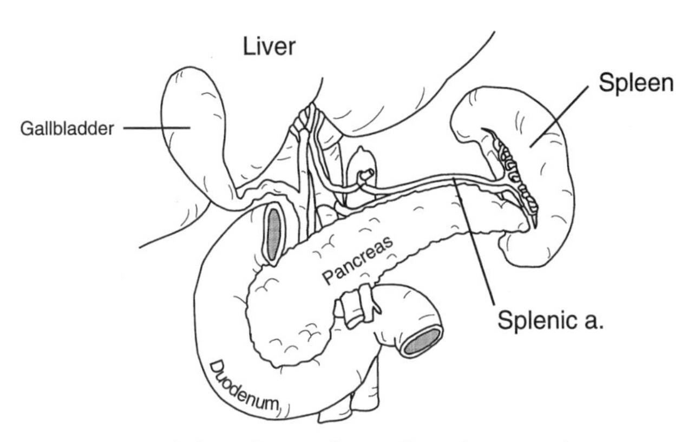

FIGURE 15-7 ■ Spleen. During illness, the spleen may become enlarged, causing it to become vulnerable to injury.

the lymphatic organs, its primary function is to produce and destroy blood cells during times of systemic infection. During certain disease states, such as **mononucleosis**, the spleen becomes engorged with blood, causing it to protrude below the ribs' protective bony cover, increasing the risk of injury. When the spleen is traumatized, surgical removal may be necessary. If the spleen is removed, its functions are assumed by the liver and bone marrow.

Urinary Tract

The kidneys, also responsible for filtering toxins from the blood, regulate the body's **electrolyte** levels by maintaining the balance of water, sodium, and potassium. The kidneys lie on each side of the vertebral column at the level of the T12–L3 vertebrae, with the right kidney lying slightly lower than the left (Fig. 15-8). The lower portion of each kidney is unprotected by the ribs, thus increasing the susceptibility to trauma secondary to direct blows to the low back.

The kidney's filtrate, **urine**, exits through small, muscular tubes, the **ureters**. Well protected by the posterior wall of the abdomen, these structures are rarely injured. Both ureters deposit their contents into a central **urinary bladder**, located posterior to the pubic symphysis, within the pelvic cavity. As the bladder fills, the smooth muscle reacts to parasympathetic stimuli, triggering the urge to urinate. From the bladder, urine exits the body through the **urethra**.

Reproductive Tract

In both men and women, the essential organs of reproduction are located in the lower abdomen. The male **testes** have the dual function of producing sperm and the male sex hormone, testosterone. The **epididymis**, a coiled tube on the posterior aspect of the testes, stores sperm (Fig. 15-9). The external location of the male reproductive organs increases the incidence of injury, most often occurring secondary to a direct blow.

The female organs of reproduction, the paired **ovaries** and **fallopian tubes** and a singular hollow **uterus**, are attached by ligaments to the pelvic wall and sit relatively well protected (Fig. 15-10). The ovaries, endocrine glands, are the source of estrogen and progesterone, the female sex hormones. They also house the reproductive eggs that are

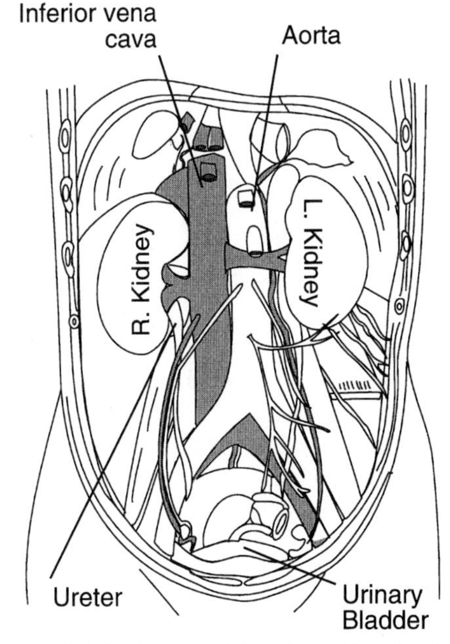

FIGURE 15-8 ■ Relative location of the kidneys. Note that the right kidney is located inferior to the left kidney, exposing its inferior border to direct trauma from blows to the posterolateral thorax.

Caudal (caudally) Moving inferiorly (toward the tail).

Mononucleosis A disease state caused by an abnormally high number of mononuclear leukocytes in the blood stream.

Electrolyte Ionized salts, including sodium, potassium, and chloride, found in blood, tissue fluids, and cells.

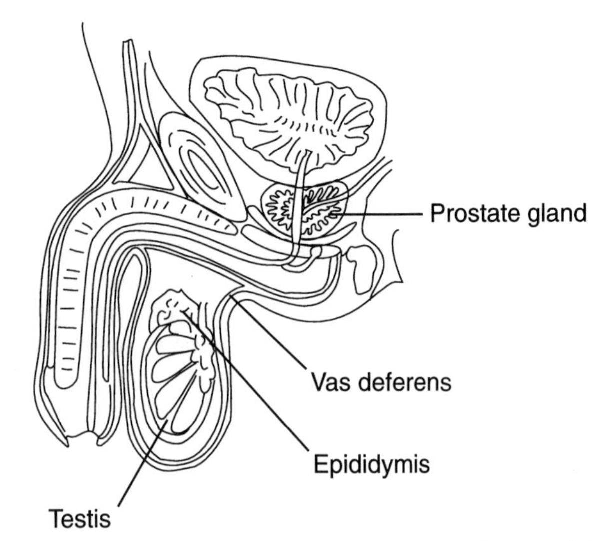

FIGURE 15-9 ■ Male reproductive system. The external location of the testicles predisposes them to injury from direct blows.

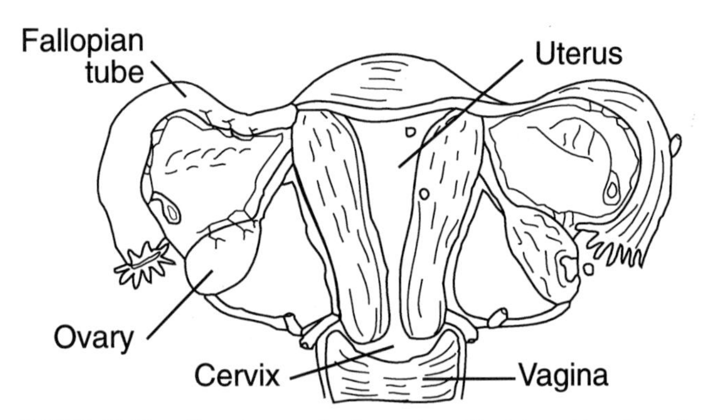

FIGURE 15-10 ■ Female reproductive system. The internal location of these organs provides excellent protection against most traumatic forces.

released for fertilization in the fallopian tubes and then implanted into the uterus.

Clinical Examination of Thoracic, Abdominal, and Cardiopulmonary Pathologies

Injuries to the internal organs and ribs usually follow a high-velocity blow to the affected area, resulting in trauma to the area beneath the impact. Structures on the side opposite of the impact may also be injured as they rebound off bony structures, a *contrecoup* injury. These conditions may not be evident immediately after the injury but can quickly progress to life-threatening conditions, thereby necessitating frequent re-examination.

The thoracoabdominal region is referenced on a quadrant system, dividing the torso into left and right upper and lower quadrants relative to the umbilicus (Fig. 15-11). The evaluation process is simplified by the clinician's knowledge

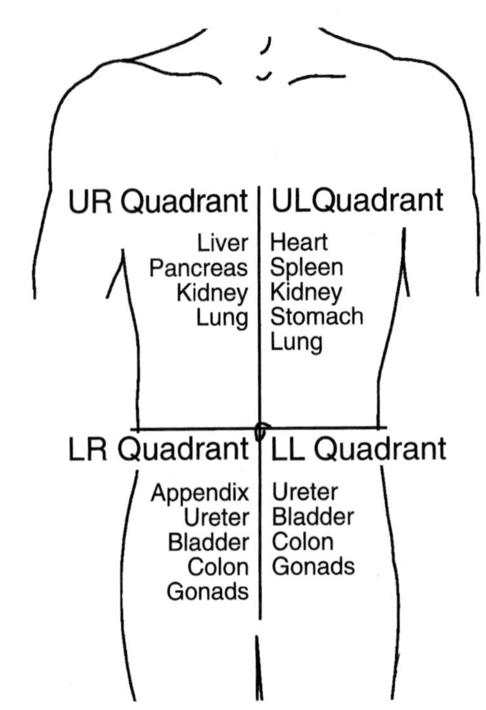

FIGURE 15-11 ■ Abdominal quadrant reference system. The sagittal quadrants are relative to the patient. Therefore, the right kidney is on the person's right-hand side.

of the organs housed in each of these quadrants and their normal functions. Pain of visceral origin may be referred to the body's periphery (see Neurologic Testing, p. 585).

History

Acute pain in the thoracoabdominal region can be attributed to trauma or a new or ongoing medical condition. For example, kidney pain can result from a blow to the low back or an infection.

Past medical history

- **General medical history**: With certain asthmatic conditions, a history of disease may be documented, but individuals with **exercise-induced asthma** may not have been previously diagnosed. Other illnesses may predispose specific internal organs to acute internal injury. For example, mononucleosis can enlarge the spleen and expose it to an increased incidence of injury. Viral **pericarditis** can cause chest pains or predispose an individual to cardiac arrest.

Individuals who are at risk of suffering catastrophic cardiovascular events may have an unrecognized or unreported history of previous symptoms or a family history cardiovascular disease. Careful preparticipation can increase the awareness of symptoms. Table 15-2 contains the

Exercise-induced asthma Bronchospasm caused by exercise.
Pericarditis Inflammation of the lining surrounding the heart.

Examination Map

HISTORY

Past Medical History
General medical history
Family history
History of drug/alcohol use
Mental health status

History of the Present Condition
Location of pain
Mechanism of injury
Onset and severity of symptoms

INSPECTION

General Assessment
Sweating
Throat
Muscle tone
Skin features

PALPATION

Palpation of the Thorax
Sternum
Costal cartilage and ribs
Spleen
Kidneys

Palpation of the Abdomen
McBurney's point
Quadrant analysis

REVIEW OF SYSTEMS

Cardiovascular
Heart rate
Blood pressure
Heart auscultation
Capillary refill

Respiratory
Breath sounds
Respiratory rate and pattern
Respiratory flow

Gastrointestinal
Vomiting
Abdominal auscultation

Genitourinary
Urinalysis

Neurologic

PATHOLOGIES AND SPECIAL TESTS

Thorax
Rib fractures
Rib compression test
Costochondral injury
Pneumothorax
Hemothorax

Abdominal and Urinary
Splenic injury
Kidney pathologies
Urinary tract infection
Appendicitis/appendix rupture
Hollow organ rupture

Reproductive Organs
Testicular contusion
Testicular torsion
Testicular dysfunction
Testicular cancer
Menstrual irregularities
Female athlete triad
Pelvic inflammatory disease

Cardiopulmonary
Commotio cordis
Cardiac contusions
Syncope
Hypertrophic cardiomyopathy
Athlete's heart
Myocardial infarction
Arrhythmia
Tachycardia
Mitral valve prolapse
Hypertension
Asthma
Hyperventilation

Table 15-2 Cardiopulmonary Checklist for the Athlete's Medical File

Family History	Personal History	General Information	Orthopedic Conditions
Episodes of syncope, dyspnea, or chest pain	Episodes of syncope or near syncope, dyspnea, or chest pain	Height	Elongated appendages
Premature **atherosclerosis**	Excessive, unexplained shortness of breath or fatigue with exercise	Weight	Severe kyphoscoliosis
Seizures	History of heart murmur of hypertension	Vital signs	Unsteady or irregular gait
Sudden death of a family member who was younger than age 50 years	Premature atherosclerosis	Heart examination	Abnormal joint laxity
Occurrence in family of hypertrophic cardiomyopathy, dilated myopathy, long QT syndrome or Marfan syndrome	Seizures	Lung examination	Club-shaped fingernails
		Dislocation of the optic lens	

Atherosclerosis The buildup of fatty tissues on the inner arterial walls.

pertinent information to identify potentially high-risk candidates for cardiopulmonary distress.[1]

- **Family Medical History**: A family history of cardiac abnormalities and cardiac-related sudden death are strong predictors for **hypertrophic cardiomyopathy**, myocardial infarction, and other heart-related conditions.[2–5] The strongest indicator of an athlete's predisposition to sudden death is a family history of cardiovascular-related sudden death. The preparticipation examination's medical history questionnaire must identify any family history of cardiac-related sudden death and any such history warrants full examination by a cardiologist.
- **Medication and drug use**: If appropriate, identify recent use of prescription medications, drug, alcohol, and tobacco use. Each of these may alter normal cardiovascular and/or respiratory function.[5]
- **General medical health**: The use of medications and other medical treatments now allows individuals to compete with conditions that once would have excluded them from competition. Conditions such as **cystic fibrosis**, asthma, HIV, spastic colitis, **Crohn's disease**, renal disease, hypertension, and undescended testicles may not preclude strenuous physical activity. A prudent evaluation involves questions regarding the existence of any underlying medical conditions and review of any existing medical records.

History of the present condition

- **Location of pain**: The location of the pain must be determined as closely as possible. Musculoskeletal injuries to the ribs, costal cartilage, or abdominal muscles are usually tender at the site of the injury. Injury to the internal organs may result in a more diffuse pain at rest. However, these areas can be more specifically localized as the patient moves or the area is palpated. Blows to the low back may result in a kidney contusion, especially on the patient's right side (see Fig. 15-8). Pain in the thorax, abdomen, shoulder, or arm can be referred from the visceral organs. Pain in the upper left quadrant and shoulder, **Kehr's sign**, may indicate a ruptured spleen that is irritating the diaphragm.

  Cardiac dysfunction results in intense pain, tightness, or squeezing in the center of the chest. Another sign of cardiac tissue ischemia is referred pain into the left shoulder, arm, jaw, or epigastric area.

  Pulmonary problems include difficulty with respiration, or pain, or both. The difficulty in breathing may cause the patient to panic. Although pain may occur secondary to pulmonary obstruction, these problems are typically recognized by the shear labor required for breathing. Excruciating, deep thoracic pain that develops in the middle and upper back is the most distinctive early sign of developing an aortic aneurysm, the typical cause of death associated with **Marfan syndrome** (Box 15-1).[4]
- **Mechanism of injury**: Injury to the thoracic, abdominal, and pelvic organs usually results from a direct blow to the area, such as being hit by a competitor or colliding with a piece of equipment or the ground. Suspicion of trauma to the ribs or internal organs is increased when the blow is received to an unprotected area.
- **Onset of symptoms**: With an internal injury to an abdominal organ, the onset of pain may be gradual, taking hours to develop as internal bleeding accumulates within the cavity. When the rib cage or abdominal muscles are injured, pain may be provoked by breathing, coughing, or sneezing. Distance runners may be affected by stomach or abdominal cramping during competition. Causes of this condition may be irregular breathing patterns, gastrointestinal upset, bloating, gas, nausea, heartburn, dehydration, constipation, or **dysmenorrhea**.

  Cardiopulmonary illness tends to be congenital or acquired gradually over time, usually manifested as previously unrecognized conditions resulting in an acute climax of cardiopulmonary distress. Certain **arrhythmias** may be caused by a traumatic incident.
- **Complaints**: The chief complaints may include pain or difficulty breathing, diffuse abdominal pain, nausea, or dizziness (Table 15-3). The patient should also be questioned regarding the presence of blood in the urine or stool. Because of the associated metabolic changes, injury to the abdominal organs increases the individual's thirst beyond that which is expected after competition. Symptoms of cardiac disorders that may be reported include shortness of breath, lightheadedness, and fatigue.
  - **Syncope**: Syncope, a sudden transient loss of consciousness, is commonly related to a cardiac arrhythmia, often occurring with previously mentioned symptoms of cardiac distress. Neurogenic (formerly called vasovagal) syncope can also result from a sudden decrease in blood pressure which results in

---

Hypertrophic cardiomyopathy Congenital thickening of the ventricular septum and left ventricular wall that results in decreased cardiac output.

Cystic fibrosis A congenital condition of the exocrine glands that affects the pancreas, respiratory system, and other systems.

Crohn's disease An inflammatory disease of the gastrointestinal tract.

Dysmenorrhea Pain during menstruation.

Arrhythmia Loss of the normal heart rhythm; an irregular heart rate.

Box 15-1
Marfan Syndrome

Clinical Findings	Other Findings
Musculoskeletal Examination	**Ophthalmologic**
Arm span greater than the person's height	Dislocation of the eye lens
Elongated metacarpal and metatarsal bones, causing the hands and feet to appear disproportionately large	Myopia
Thoracic kyphosis	**Cardiovascular**
Scoliosis	Dilated aortic root
Systemic joint laxity	Aortic regurgitation
Pectus excavatum ("sunken chest" or depression of the sternum)	Mitral valve prolapse
High arched palate	Aortic insufficiency murmur

An inherited condition, Marfan syndrome is characterized by cardiovascular, musculoskeletal, and ocular abnormalities observed during physical inspection. Although Marfan syndrome is a disease of the body's connective tissue, failure of the cardiac system usually leads to death. The connective tissue providing strength to the aorta is decreased, leading to weakness of this tissue and the development of an aneurysm. Even when the syndrome is recognized and the individual is removed from strenuous activity, the person can suffer rupture of an aortic aneurysm, causing immediate death.[4,6]

Cardiac testing may produce various abnormalities, the most common being an abnormal aorta and multivalvular deformities, leading to prolapse of the valves and aortic valve regurgitation. The decreased amount of connective tissue in the aortic wall makes it susceptible to rupture because of the high pressure exerted on the weakened wall as blood is pumped from the left ventricle. Aortic root dilation also is a prominent abnormality that eventually leads to dissecting aortic aneurysm. Signs of an aneurysm are the most common finding on echocardiography.

Suspicion of Marfan syndrome warrants a full medical examination. Although medical clearance is determined on a case-by-case basis, individuals who have Marfan syndrome are restricted from participating in vigorous physical activity. An absolute disqualifying condition is an enlarged aortic root, a predisposition to aortic rupture.[6,7]

Table 15-3 Signs and Symptoms of Cardiovascular and Pulmonary Conditions

Cardiovascular	Both	Pulmonary
Panic	Chest pain	Congestion
Dizziness	Respiratory distress	Wheezing
Nausea	Pain in mid and upper posterior thorax	Fatigue
Vomiting		Anxiety
Sweating		Tingling in fingers and toes
Decreased blood pressure		Spasm in fingers and toes
Distended jugular vein		Periorbital numbness
Pallor		Deviated trachea
Clutching at chest		
Shoulder pain		
Epigastric pain		

insufficient blood to the brain. This insufficiency first triggers dizziness and then a brief loss of consciousness. A common trigger is prolonged standing coupled with dehydration.

- **Palpitations**: Disorders of the heart's electrical system may cause the sensation of the heart's skipping beats or racing abnormally fast (tachycardia). Palpitations, rapid and/or forceful heartbeats that occur at rest and subside during exercise, are likely to be a benign vagal reaction. Palpitations that occur during exercises are of particular concern and should be evaluated by a cardiologist.[6]
- **Respiratory**: Complaints related to pulmonary problems include chest congestion, fatigue, and minor difficulty in breathing before the onset of the traumatic respiratory problem. Otherwise, labored breathing, characterized by a quick wheezing breathing pattern, often accompanied by unusual sounds is exhibited.
- **Chest pain**: Nontraumatic pain in the chest may be indicative of cardiovascular or respiratory disorders.

Inspection

The inspection process begins with observation of the patient's overall posture. Leaning of the thorax to one side may indicate that the patient is stretching a cramping muscle; flexing of the trunk may indicate cramping or difficulty breathing. The individual may also be splinting the painful area by grasping the torso or abdomen. A person suffering from a significant internal injury is often unwilling to move, preferring to remain in the fetal position or lie supine with the knees flexed.

- **Sweating**: Profuse sweating is a typical sign of cardiac arrest. This sign may be difficult to assess in an individual who has been performing vigorous physical activity.

- **Throat**: Observe the trachea and larynx for their normal positions through the midline of the cervical spine. Deviations from this position could indicate trauma to these structures or the presence of a **pneumothorax**.
- **Muscle tone**: Observe the contour of the abdominal muscles. As time progresses, the injured area may become distended secondary to bleeding.
- **Skin features**: Note the location of any contusions, wounds, or abrasions. These discolorations serve to warn of possible injury to the underlying internal organs.

PALPATION

The findings of the history-taking process are reinforced and supplemented by the findings obtained during the palpation phase. Because there are few special tests for assessing thoracic and abdominal injuries, knowledge of the underlying anatomy is needed so that a specific palpation assessment may be performed.

1–3 Sternum: Begin palpating the rib cage at the manubrium, continuing inferiorly to include the sternal body **(2)** and xiphoid process **(3)** and noting for tenderness and deformity. Injury to the upper sternum may involve the sternoclavicular joint (see Chapter 11).

4 Costal cartilage and rib: Palpate the costal cartilage and rib from anterior to posterior, noting any pain, crepitus, and deformity. Stress fractures of the ribs result in focal point tenderness. Any suspicion of a rib fracture requires full evaluation by a physician.

5 Spleen: Palpate for an enlarged or tender spleen under the left rib cage. Having the patient raise the arms above the head will make the spleen more prominent and more easily palpated.

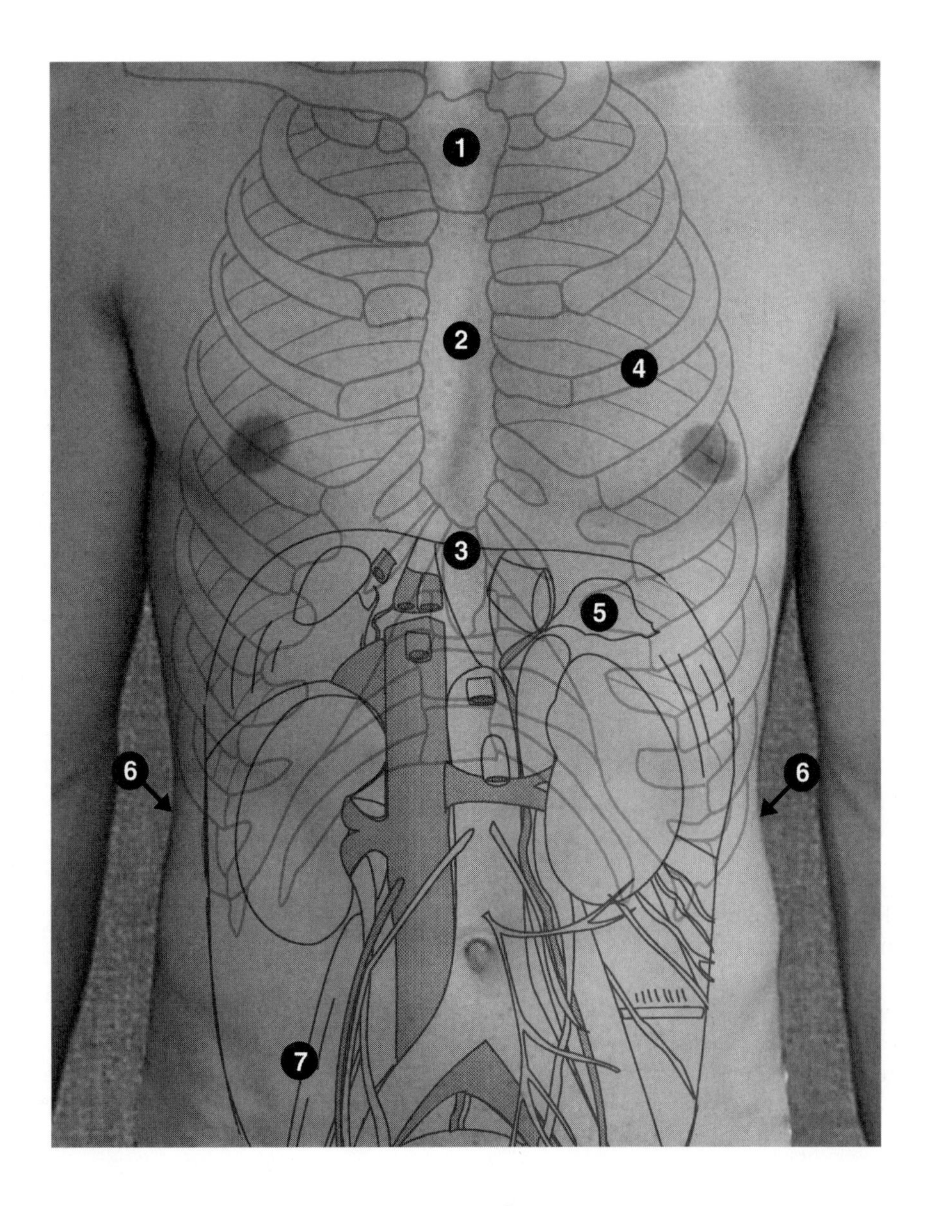

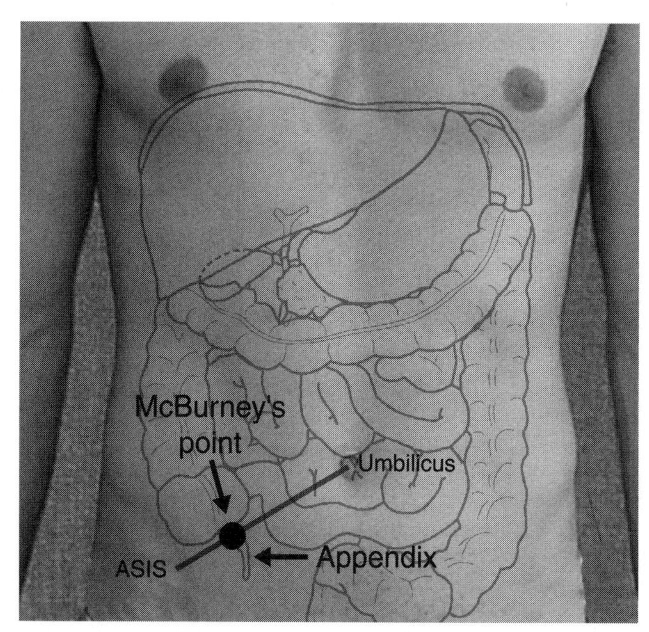

FIGURE 15-12 ■ McBurney's point, located approximately one-third of the way between the ASIS and the umbilicus. This point becomes tender in the presence of appendicitis.

6 **Kidneys**: Locate the kidneys under the posterolateral portion of the rib cage. The left kidney is relatively well protected within the rib cage. The right kidney rests more inferiorly.

7 **McBurney's point**: Note any tenderness at McBurney's point, located one third of the way between the right anterior superior iliac spine and the navel, possibly indicating acute appendicitis (Fig. 15-12).

Palpation of the abdomen

The patient should be in the hook-lying position to relax the abdominal muscles (Fig. 15-13). The abdomen is palpated relative to the four quadrants depicted in Figure 15-11.

- **Rigidity**: Abdominal rigidity may occur secondary to muscle guarding or with blood accumulating in the abdomen. The presence of guarding alone indicates internal injury, which necessitates further evaluation by a physician.
- **Areas of pain**: Pain caused by palpation is another cause of concern. An awareness of the approximate location of the organs within the abdomen assists in detecting possible injury.
- **Rebound tenderness**: An inflamed peritoneum is sensitive to stretching. Pressure applied over the injured site gradually stretches the peritoneum in a relatively pain-free manner. However, pain experienced when the pressure is suddenly released indicates inflammation of the peritoneum.
- **Tissue density**: Percussing over specific organs can be used to determine the density of the underlying tissues (Special Test 15-1).[8] Internal bleeding may fill the abdominal cavity, causing the abdomen to feel and sound solid.
- **Quadrant analysis**: The abdomen is palpated in the quadrant format as presented in Figure 15-11. Correlate quadrant tenderness and/or rigidity to the possible pathology:

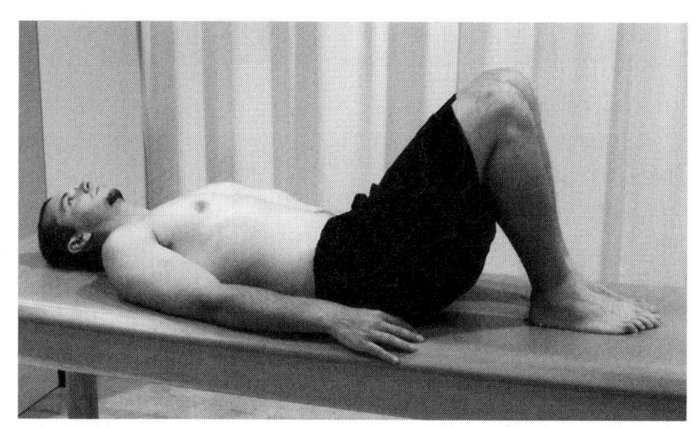

FIGURE 15-13 ■ Positioning of the patient during palpation of the abdomen. The hook-lying position relaxes the abdominal muscles, easing palpation of the underlying structures.

Quadrant segment (relative to the patient)

	Right	Left
Upper	**Liver**: Pain is associated with **cholecystitis** or liver laceration. **Gallbladder**: Pain without the history of trauma indicates gallbladder disease.	**Spleen**: Rigidity under the last several ribs indicates trauma to the spleen.
Lower	**Appendix**: Rebound tenderness indicates appendicitis. **Colon**: Colitis or diverticulitis may cause pain. Pelvic inflammation results in diffuse tenderness.	**Colon**: Colitis or diverticulitis may cause pain. Pelvic inflammation results in diffuse tenderness.

Other less specific symptoms include pain in the upper abdomen arising from the pancreas, heart, diaphragm, or esophagus or pain in the lower middle abdomen in the area of the femoral creases from bladder or **gonad** pathology. The low back may be painful and have increased tenderness with palpation owing to kidney contusions, **kidney stones**, or infection.

Review of Systems

This chapter uses the vital signs and the function of other major systems, a review of systems, to assess the integrity of the internal abdominal and thoracic organs. This

Cholecystitis Inflammation of the gallbladder.

Gonad An organ producing gender-based reproductive cells; the ovaries or testicles.

Kidney stones A crystal mass formed in the kidney that is passed through the urinary tract.

Special Test 15-1
Abdominal Percussion

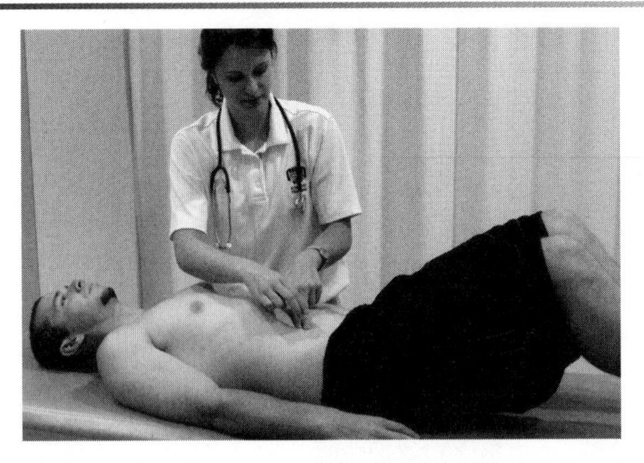

The abdominal quadrants are percussed by a quick tap of the finger tips lying gently on the abdomen. The resulting sound provides context to the density of the underlying tissues. Solid (or fluid-filled) areas produce a dull thud; hollow areas yield a more resonant sound.

Patient Position	Hook lying
Position of Examiner	Standing to the patient's side The examiner lightly places one hand palm down over the area to be assessed. The index and middle fingers of the opposite hand tap the DIP joints of the hand placed over the patient's abdomen.
Evaluative Procedure	The fingertips of the top hand quickly strike the middle phalanges of the bottom hand in a tapping motion. The sound of the echo within the abdomen is noted. Areas over solid organs have a dull thump associated with them. Hollow organs make a crisper, more **resonant** sound.
Positive Test	A hard, solid sounding echo over areas that should normally sound hollow.
Implications	Internal bleeding filling the abdominal cavity.
Evidence	***Inter-rater reliability***

DIP = distal interphalangeal.

assessment is important for any injury, especially in case of internal injury or shock (Table 15-4). During the evaluation and management of a patient with an injury or illness, the values obtained for each of these tests are recorded and regularly reevaluated to identify trends in the vital signs.

Table 15-4 Signs and Symptoms of Shock
Rapid, weak pulse
Decreased blood pressure
Rapid, shallow breathing
Excessive thirst
Nausea and vomiting
Pale, bluish skin
Restlessness or irritability
Drowsiness or loss of consciousness

Cardiovascular

Heart Rate: The heart rate is determined by palpating the carotid, radial, femoral, or brachial pulse (Special Test 15-2). An athlete's resting heart rate typically ranges from 60 to 100 beats per minute (BPM). Highly conditioned athletes have lower heart rates. Older or recreational athletes have heart rates at the higher end of the scale. When assessing the

Resonant Producing a vibrating sound or percussion.

Special Test 15-2
Determination of Heart Rate Using the Carotid Pulse

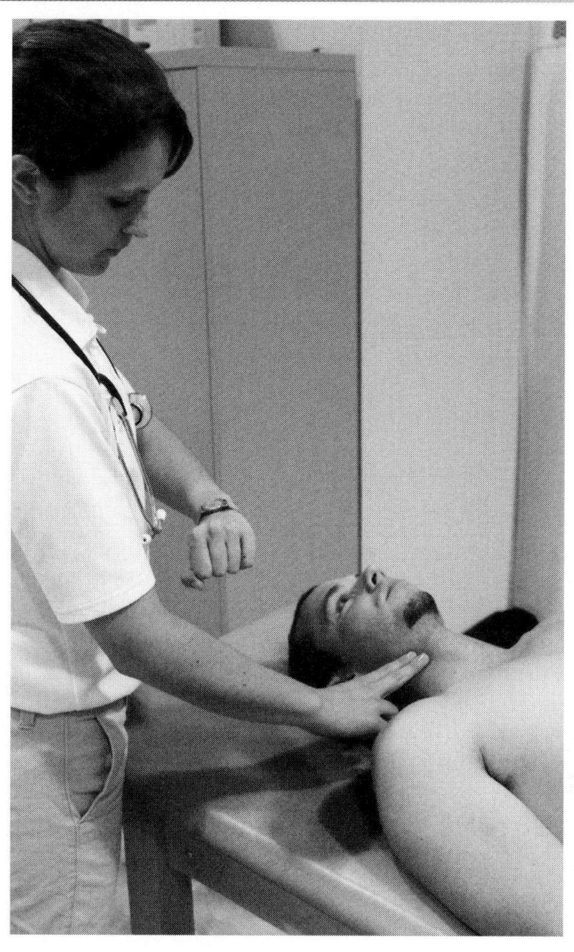

The carotid artery, palpated between the thyroid cartilage and sternocleidomastoid, is used to determine the frequency, quality, and rhythm of the pulse.

Patient Position	Seated or supine
Position of Examiner	Using the index and middle fingers to locate the thyroid cartilage, move the fingers laterally in either direction to find the common carotid artery between the thyroid cartilage and the sternocleidomastoid muscle.
Evaluative Procedure	Count the number of pulses in a 15-s interval and multiply that number by 4 to determine the number of beats per minute. The examiner also attempts to determine the quality of the pulse: strong (bounding) or weak.
Positive Test	Not applicable
Implications	The quality and quantity of the heart rate established. Normal (general population): 60–100 bpm Well-trained athletes: 40–60 bpm Tachycardia: Greater than 100 bpm Bradycardia: Less than 60 bpm
Comments	The baseline heart rate should be recorded and rechecked at regular intervals. Note the rhythm of the beats for symmetry and strength.
Evidence	Absent or inconclusive in the literature

heart rate of an athlete who has just stopped exercising, an increased heart rate caused by the demands of exercise should be considered.

Palpable pulses should have a consistent rhythm with a smooth, quick upstroke, consistent summit, and a gradual downstroke. An abnormal rate or irregular rhythm is indicative of an arrhythmia. A rapidly rising, large amplitude pulse (water-hammer pulse) suggests hypertropic cardiomyopathy, or aortic or mitral valve regurgitation; a slowly rising, small-amplitude pulse suggests aortic stenosis or heart failure.[7]

Simultaneous palpation of the radial and femoral pulses can identify narrowing (coarctation) of the aorta. A delay of the femoral pulse relative to the radial pulse warrants further cardiovascular examination.[7]

Abnormal pulses are classified by the heart's rate and rhythm:

Type	Characteristics	Implication
Accelerated	Pulse >150 beats per minute (bpm) (>170 bpm usually has fatal results).	Pressure on the base of the brain; shock
Bounding	Pulse that quickly reaches a higher intensity than normal, then quickly disappears	Ventricular systole and reduced peripheral pressure
Deficit	Pulse in which the number of beats counted at the radial pulse is less than that counted over the heart itself	Cardiac arrhythmia
High Tension	Pulse in which the force of the beat is increased; an increased amount of pressure is required to inhibit the radial pulse.	Cerebral trauma
Low Tension	Short, fast, faint pulse having a rapid decline	Heart failure; shock

Blood Pressure: A measurement of the pressure exerted by the blood on the arterial walls, blood pressure is affected by a decrease in blood volume (severe bleeding or dehydration), a decreased capacity of the vessels, shock, or a decreased ability of the heart to pump blood (cardiac arrest). Decreased blood pressure indicates a decreased ability to deliver blood, with its nutrients and oxygen, to the organs of the body. Organs are highly susceptible to **anoxia** and can be severely damaged secondary to a decrease in blood pressure.

High blood pressure, or hypertension, is commonly seen in the general population. A dangerous precursor to cardiovascular problems, high blood pressure can exert extreme pressure on the blood vessels, particularly in the smaller vasculature of the brain. Excessive pressure causes these vessels to rupture, resulting in a **cerebrovascular** accident (CVA) or stroke.[11] The presence of high blood pressure warrants referral to a physician for further evaluation (Special Test 15-3).

✱ Practical Evidence

Talking, acute exposure to cold, recent ingestion of alcohol, incorrect arm position, and incorrect cuff size can cause an error of more than ±5 mm Hg in diastolic or systolic blood pressure readings.[9]

Heart Auscultation: Auscultation of the heart should be performed with the patient supine and standing (Special Test 15-4).[5] Normally the heart makes "lub" and "dub" sounds as the valves close. The "lub" (or S_1) represents the closing of the mitral and tricuspid valves—between the atria and the ventricles—as the ventricles begin to contract to push blood out through the aorta and pulmonary artery. The "dub" (or S_2) occurs as the aortic and pulmonary valves close as the ventricles finish pushing out the blood and begin to relax.[12] Any reflux of blood through a faulty or leaking valve causes a decrease in the heart's ability to efficiently deliver the needed metabolites to the tissues of the body and alters the characteristic heart sounds (Table 15-5).

Capillary Refill: Observe for normal capillary refill in the nail beds. Disruption of the cardiac or pulmonary systems would result in cyanosis of the nail beds, fingers, and toes (see Box 1-2).

Respiratory

Intense exercise dramatically changes the respiratory rate and pattern. In the event of abnormal changes, the individual will be anxious and may have trouble speaking. Any **sputum** that may be produced as the person coughs should be checked for the presence of blood. Pink or bloody sputum indicates internal bleeding requiring emergency treatment.

Breath Sounds: Auscultate breath sounds over all the lobes of each lung, noting the pitch, intensity, quality and duration of inspirations and exhalations (Special Test 15-5).[8] Inhalation typically reveals a dry, smooth, unobstructed sound that is equal throughout each lobe. The absence of breath sounds may indicate a collapsed lung associated with a pneumothorax. Pneumonia or other buildup of fluid within the lungs may produce rhonchi, a localized moist sounding movement of air.[14]

Respiratory Rate and Pattern: At rest, normal respiration ranges from 12 to 20 breaths per minute, with well-conditioned athletes falling on the lower end of the range.

Anoxia The absence of oxygen in the blood or tissues.

Sputum A substance formed by mucus, blood, or pus expelled by coughing or clearing the throat.

Table 15-5 Examples of Heart Sounds

Sound	Status	Possible Interpretation
"Lub"	Normal systole	Closure of the mitral and mitral and tricuspid valves
"Dub"	Normal diastole	Closure of the aortic and pulmonary valves
Soft, blowing "lub"	Abnormal systole	Associated with anemia or other changes in blood constituents
Loud, booming "lub"	Abnormal systole	Aneurysm
Sloshing "dub"	Abnormal diastole	Incomplete closure of the valves; blood heard regurgitating backward
Friction sound	Abnormal	Inflammation of the heart's pericardial lining; pericarditis

Abnormal breathing patterns and the possible causes of their onset include:

- **Rapid, shallow breaths**: Internal injury; shock
- **Deep, quick breaths**: Pulmonary obstruction; asthma
- **Noisy, raspy breaths**: Airway obstruction

Note any abnormalities in the breathing pattern. Difficulty in breathing, or stridor, may have many causes that include asthma, allergies, cardiac contusion, injury to the ribs or costal cartilage, lung trauma (e.g., pneumothorax, hemothorax, or pulmonary contusion), or other injury to the internal organs. Observe respirations for rate, depth, and quality. Internal injuries can cause breathing to become rapid and shallow because deep breaths may cause pain. Observe the chest wall movement in persons having trouble breathing. The ribs should rise and fall in a symmetrical pattern; any deviations in this pattern could be the result of fractured ribs or a pneumothorax. Subcutaneous emphysema may indicate lung trauma. Atypical prominence of the secondary inspiration muscles (e.g., scalenes, sternomastoid) indicates that the patient is having difficulty breathing.

Abnormal breathing patterns are further classified based on the tempo and relationship between inspirations and exhalations:

Type	Characteristics	Implications
Apneustic	Prolonged inspirations unrelieved by attempts to exhale	Trauma to the pons
Biot's	Periods of apnea followed by hyperapnea	Increased intracranial pressure
Cheyne-Stokes	Periods of apnea followed by breaths of increasing depth and frequency	Frontal lobe or brain stem trauma
Slow	Respiration consisting of fewer than 12 breaths per minute	CNS disruption
Thoracic	Respiration in which the diaphragm is inactive and breathing occurs only through expansion of the chest; normal abdominal movement is absent	Disruption of the phrenic nerve or its nerve roots

Respiratory Flow: Peak flow meters (PFMs) may be used to assist in diagnosing and monitoring asthma by determining the peak expiratory flow rate (PEFR) (Special Test 15-6). The PEFR represents the maximum velocity of air that can be forced from the lungs after taking a deep breath.[15] This is directly affected by changes in the airways such as those found with increases or decreases in secretion buildup or bronchospasm.

Gastrointestinal

Vomiting: Observe the patient for and question about any vomiting after injury. Blood in the vomitus may also signify injury to the stomach, esophagus, pulmonary trauma, or chronic conditions such as ulcers.

Auscultation of the Abdomen: Perform auscultation, listening to sounds with a stethoscope, to help establish the presence of internal injury (Special Test 15-7). The abdomen typically makes an occasional "gurgling" sound as **peristalsis** occurs. After injury, the peristaltic mechanism may be inhibited or may sympathetically shut down. In either case, the bowel sounds are absent. The exact placement of the stethoscope over specific portions of the bowel is not crucial because these sounds resound throughout the cavity. Auscultate the abdomen before palpating it. Manipulation of the abdomen during palpation may falsely produce normal bowel sounds.

Genitourinary

Question the patient regarding a history of painful, frequent, and/or urgent urination. A history of kidney stones or urinary tract infections should also be determined.

Urinalysis: Obtain a urine sample from the patient, if possible, and note its appearance. Also question the patient about the presence of blood in the urine, or hematuria. This symptom denotes significant injury to the kidneys and warrants immediate referral to a physician. Any patient suspected of having an internal injury must be instructed to

Peristalsis A progressive smooth muscle contraction producing a wavelike motion that moves matter through the intestines.

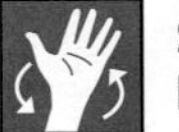

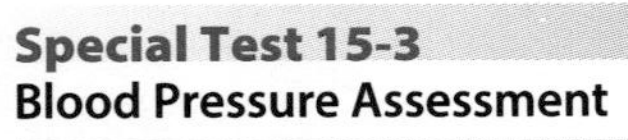

Special Test 15-3
Blood Pressure Assessment

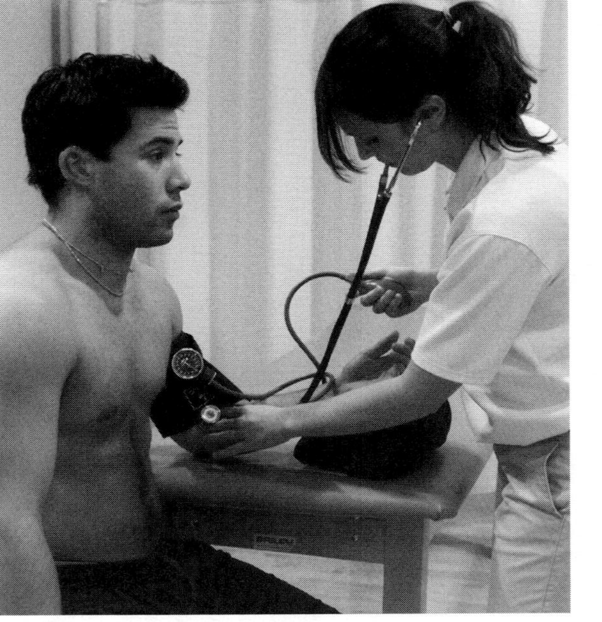

Blood pressure assessment at the brachial artery. Based on the findings of the systolic and diastolic pressures the patient's blood pressure is categorized as hypertensive, prehypertensive, normal, or hypotensive.

Patient Position	If possible, the patient should be seated; support the arm so that the middle section of the upper arm is at heart level.
Position of Examiner	In front of or beside the patient in a position to read the gauge on the BP cuff
Evaluative Procedure	The cuff is secured over the upper arm, with the lower edge of the bladder approximately 1 inch above the antecubital fossa. Many cuffs have an arrow that must be aligned with the brachial artery. The stethoscope is placed over the brachial artery. The cuff is inflated to 180 to 200 mm Hg. The air is slowly released from the cuff at a rate of 2 mm per second until the initial beat is heard.[9] While reading the gauge, note the point at which the first pulse sound, the systolic pressure, is heard. Continuing to slowly release the air from the cuff (approximately 2 mm Hg per second), note the value at which the last pulse, the diastolic value, is heard. Record to the nearest 2 mm Hg.

Positive Test	***Hypertension:*** Systolic pressure greater than 140 mm Hg Diastolic pressure greater than 90 mm Hg ***Prehypertension:*** Systolic pressure 120–139 mm Hg Diastolic pressure 80–89 mm Hg ***Normal:*** Systolic pressure 90–119 mm Hg Diastolic pressure 60–79 mm Hg ***Hypotension:*** Systolic pressure less than 90 mm Hg Diastolic pressure less than 60 mm Hg
Implications	Low BP may indicate shock or internal hemorrhage. High BP indicates hypertension.
Comments	Athlete's baseline BP should be obtained annually during the preparticipation physical examination and should be compared with the current readings. Larger patients may require the use of a larger BP cuff. A cuff that is too small erroneously increases the BP. The cuff's bladder should surround 80% of the arm.[9] Minimally, the blood pressure cuff must be 66% as wide as the upper arm from the top of the shoulder to the olecranon and encircle the arm completely.[10] The same arm should be used each time repeated measures are taken from the same patient. Multiple high readings on different days are needed for a diagnosis of hypertension.
Evidence	***Inter-rater reliability*** Not Reliable — Very Reliable Poor — Moderate — Good 0 0.1 0.2 0.3 0.4 0.5 0.6 0.7 0.8 0.9 1.0

BP = blood pressure.

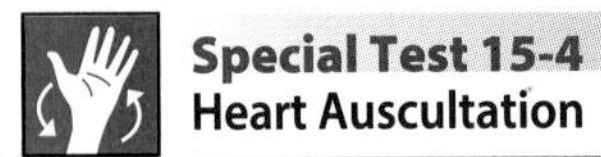

Special Test 15-4
Heart Auscultation

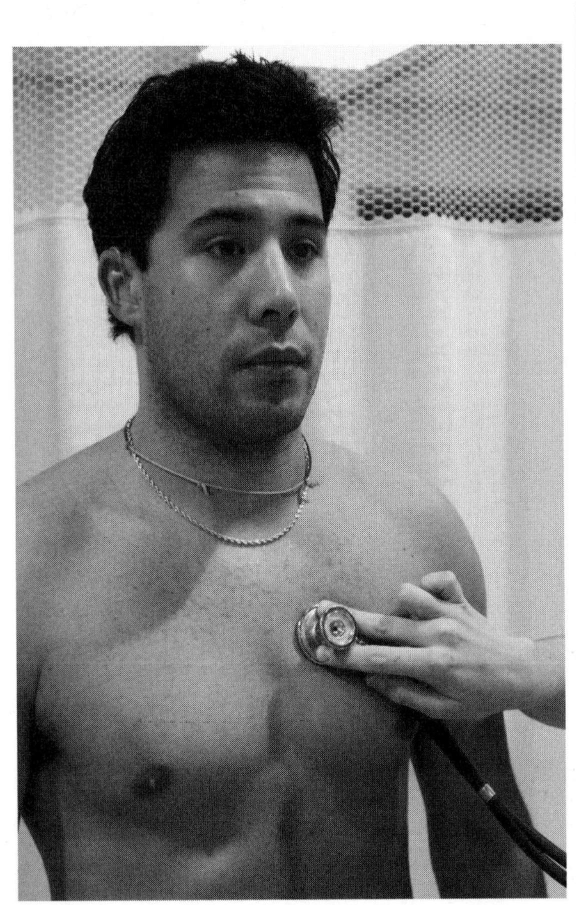

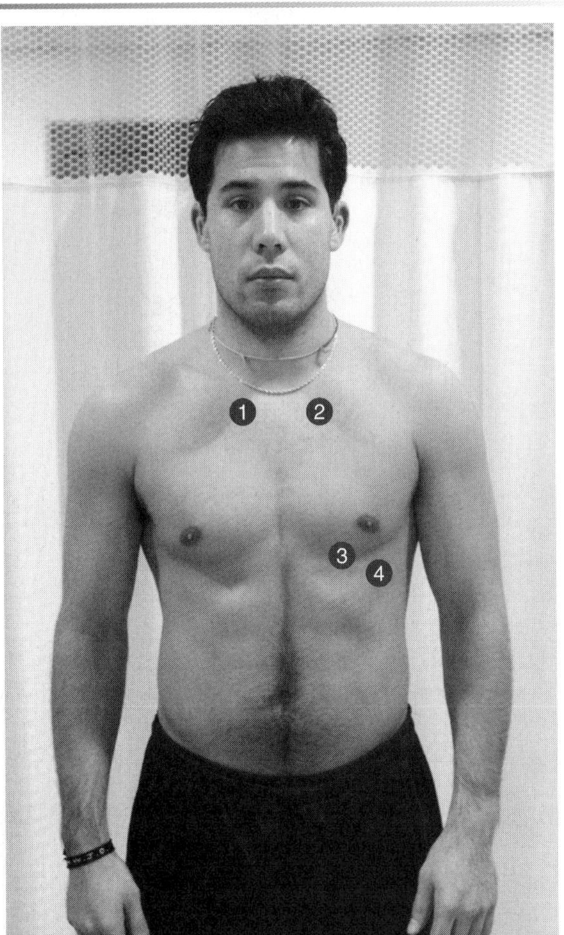

Heart auscultation identifies the presence or absence of abnormal heart sounds.

Patient Position	Sitting and/or standing
Position of Examiner	Stand facing the patient's right side
Evaluative Procedure	Listen at four locations: 1. Right sternal border between ribs 2 and 3: Aortic area 2. Left sternal border between ribs 2 and 3: Pulmonary area 3. Left sternal border between ribs 5 and 6: Tricuspid area 4. Left mid clavicle line between ribs 5 and 6: Mitral area
Positive Test	Any deviation from typical "lub" "dub" warrants referral to a physician. For examples, see Table 15-5.
Implications	A range of cardiac conditions
Comments	Do not auscultate over clothing.
Evidence	Absent or inconclusive in the literature

Special Test 15-5
Lung Auscultation

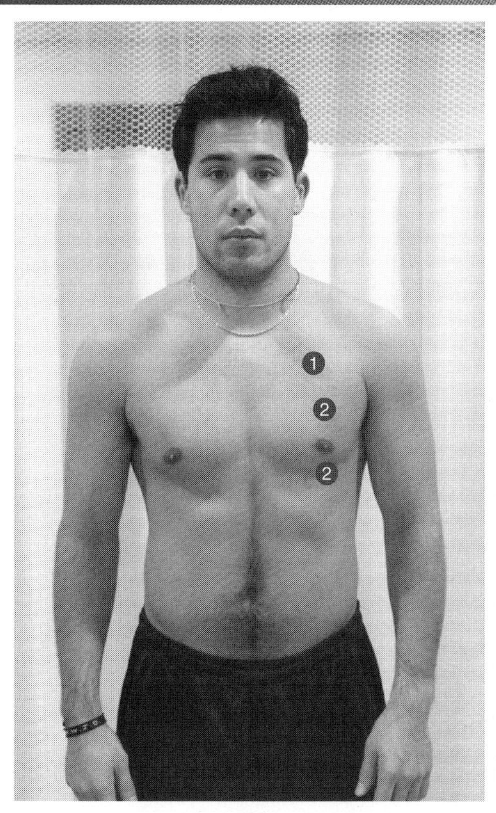

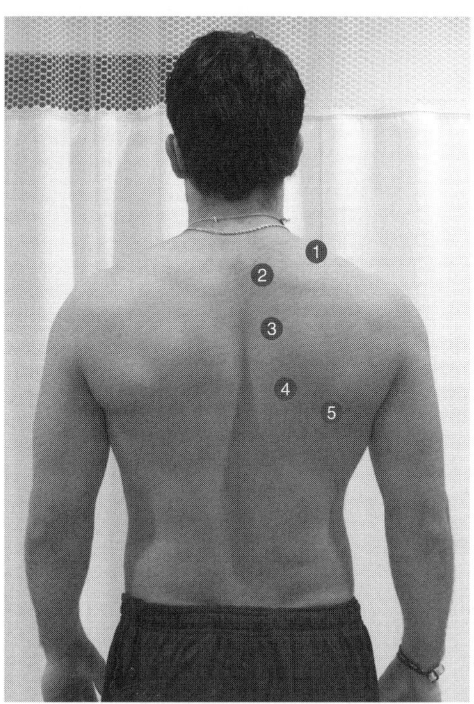

Lung sounds are obtained from the anterior and posterior thorax to determine the quality and quantity of respirations, noting for abnormal sounds.

Patient Position	Sitting
Position of Examiner	Standing on side of patient ideally with the ability to move behind
Evaluative Procedure	Instruct the patient to breathe slowly and deeply through the mouth. Listen left then right at each level ***Anterior:*** **1.** Midclavicle line just below clavicle **2.** Above and below the nipple line under breast tissue if present ***Posterior:*** Five spots each side, taking care to not listen over the scapula **1.** Above the spine of scapula **2.** At the level of scapula spine **3.** Midscapula **4.** Distal scapula **5.** Below the inferior angle
Positive Test	Absence of sound: Collapsed lung Hyper-resonance: Fluid in lung Crackles: Representing small airways "popping open" Wheeze: Narrowed airway (high pitch) Rhonchi: Secretions in larger airway (lower pitch); gurgling[13]
Comments	Do not auscultate over clothing.
Evidence	***Inter-rater reliability*** **Not Reliable** — **Very Reliable** Poor — Moderate — Good 0 0.1 0.2 0.3 0.4 0.5 0.6 0.7 0.8 0.9 1.0

Special Test 15-6
Peak Flow Meter (Spirometer)

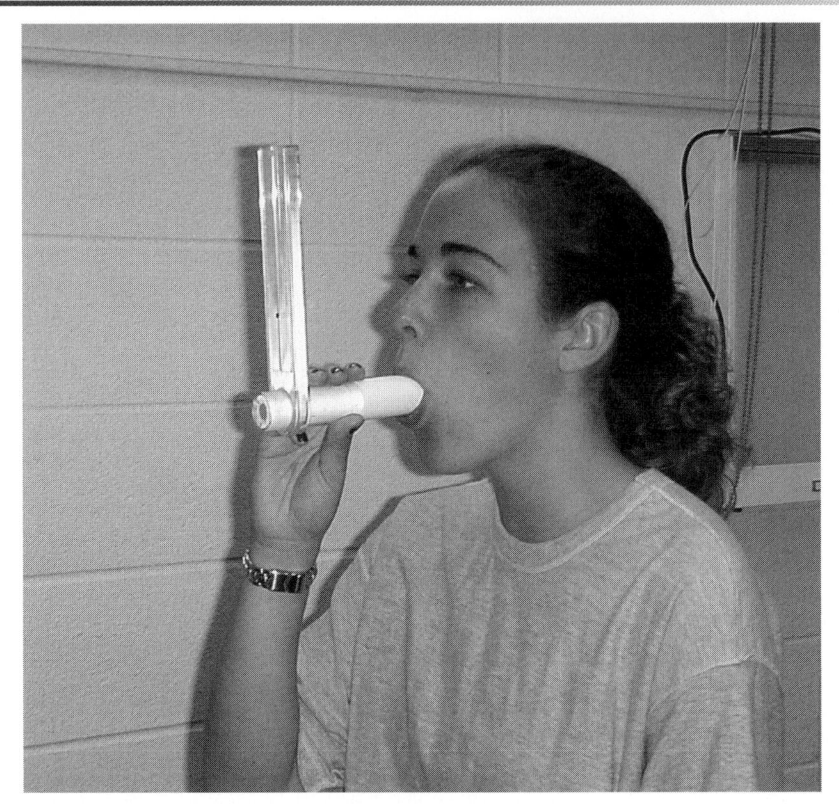

A spirometer measures the volume of air that can be displaced from the lungs.

Patient Position	Standing
Position of Examiner	Standing in front of the patient
Evaluative Procedure	The patient takes as deep a breath as possible. The mouth is placed around the mouthpiece of the peak flow meter. The patient blows as hard and as fast as possible into the device.
Positive Test	1. **Diagnostic**: Decreases greater or equal to a 15% decrease in peak expiratory flow rate from preexercise to postexercise 2. **Monitoring**: Daily percentage readings of 50%–80% of personal best or less than 50% of personal best
Implications	1. Exercise-induced asthma 2. Asthma attack requiring caution, possibly a temporary increase in bronchodilator dosage or immediate administration of bronchodilators and notification of the treating physician if levels do not return to at least 50% of personal best after medication administration
Comments	The patient must be careful not to block the mouthpiece opening with the tongue while performing the test.
Evidence	Positive likelihood ratio Not Useful / Useful Very Small / Small / Moderate / Large 0 1 2 3 4 5 6 7 8 9 10 Negative likelihood ratio Not Useful / Useful Very Small / Small / Moderate / Large 1.0 0.9 0.8 0.7 0.6 0.5 0.4 0.3 0.2 0.1 0

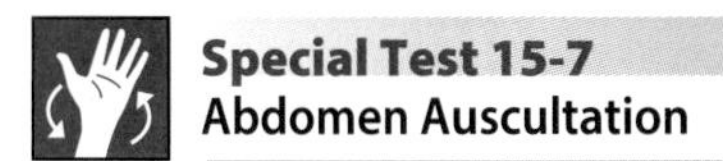

Special Test 15-7
Abdomen Auscultation

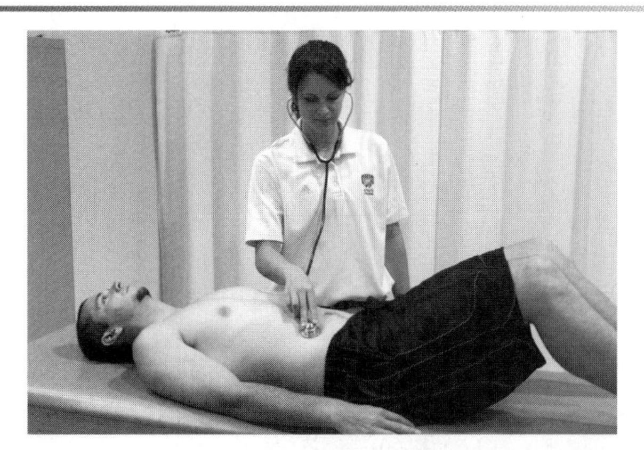

Auscultation of the abdomen. The integrity of the abdomen, the hollow organs, lungs, and descending blood vessels can be assessed through listening to the bowel sounds. Although the abdomen typically makes a gurgling sound, abdominal trauma reduces or eliminates this noise.

Patient Position	Supine; hook lying
Position of Examiner	Standing at the side of the patient
Evaluative Procedure	Examine the patient with empty bladder if possible. Bowel sounds: Place diaphragm of stethoscope gently over the lower right quadrant for 30 seconds. Medium pitched gurgles every 5–10 seconds is normal. If absent, listen in all other quadrants. Listen for bruits (the sound of turbulent air rushing past an obstruction) at the top border of the right and left upper quadrants and the lower border of the right and left lower quadrants.
Positive Test	Bowel sounds that are high pitched or tinkle indicate possible partial obstruction or early complete bowel obstruction. Absent sounds indicate bowel paralysis possibly secondary to complete obstruction or **peritonitis**. To be sure that bowel sounds are truly absent, listen for 5 minutes. Bruits at top border of upper quadrate indicates renal artery stenosis
Implications	Bowel obstruction, peritonitis, internal injury
Comments	Auscultate before palpation. Palpation can stimulate the bowel and give a false impression.
Evidence	***Inter-rater reliability***

Not Reliable — Very Reliable
Poor | Moderate | Good
0 0.1 0.2 0.3 0.4 0.5 0.6 0.7 0.8 0.9 1.0

observe the color of the urine upon the next voiding. Immediately after the injury, blood may not be visible to the unaided eye but can be detected using a microscope or chemically with specially formulated strips dipped into the urine (Special Test 15-8). Note that hematuria may normally be present after certain athletic events such as long-distance running or when menstruating.

Peritonitis Inflammation of the peritoneum as the result of infection, injury, or disease.

Excessive protein (proteinuria) or evidence of a urinary tract infection (elevated blood, protein and nitrite or leukocyte esterase levels) may also be detected using a dipstick. The dipstick is far more useful at ruling out urine abnormalities rather than ruling them in.[16]

Neurologic

Illness and trauma to the internal organs often manifest as symptoms radiating to the upper extremity, chest, and low back. These patterns of referred pain from the viscera tend to radiate to the part of the body served by the somatic

Special Test 15-8
"Clean Catch" Dipstick Urinalysis

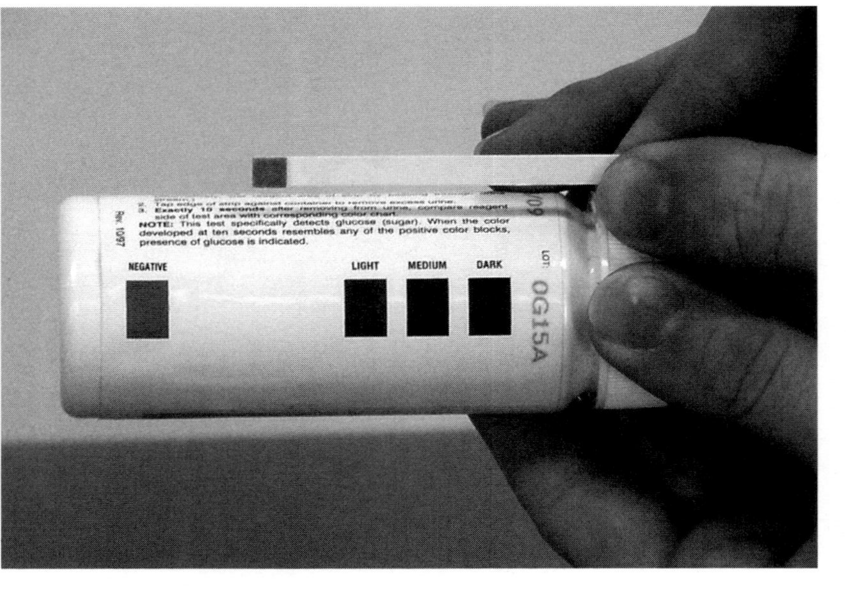

Dipstick urinalysis provides information regarding the patient's health and relative hydration level.

Evaluative Procedure

The external urethra and surrounding area is cleansed using soap and water and then rinsed.
To clear the urethra, the initial flow of urine is into a toilet bowl or "dirty" collection container.
One to 2 oz. of urine is then collected in a clean specimen cup.
The dipstick is then immersed into the specimen cup.
Follow the manufacturer's recommendations for immersion and interpretation times.

Test Results

The colors produced on the dipstick are matched to the values provided by the manufacturer.

Implications

Element	Normal	Interpretation
Specific Gravity:	1.006–1.030	Low reading: Diabetes mellitus, excessive hydration, renal failure High reading: Dehydration; heart or renal failure
pH:	4.6–8.0	Low reading: Chronic obstructive pulmonary disease, diabetic ketoacidosis High reading: Renal failure, urinary tract infection
Glucose, glucose dehydrogenase:	<0.5	Diabetes mellitus, stress
Ketones:	0	Anorexia, poor nutrition, alcoholism, diabetes mellitus
Protein:	0	Congestive heart failure, polycystic kidney disease
Hemoglobin:	0	Urinary tract infection, kidney disease or trauma
RBC:	0	Kidney disease or trauma, kidney stones, bladder infection, urinary tract infection

Comments	The above interpretations are partial lists. High or low readings should be interpreted by a physician. Factors such as diet and the level of exercise can alter the urinalysis readings.
Evidence	***Hematuria*** Positive likelihood ratio Negative likelihood ratio ***Proteinuria*** Positive likelihood ratio Negative likelihood ratio

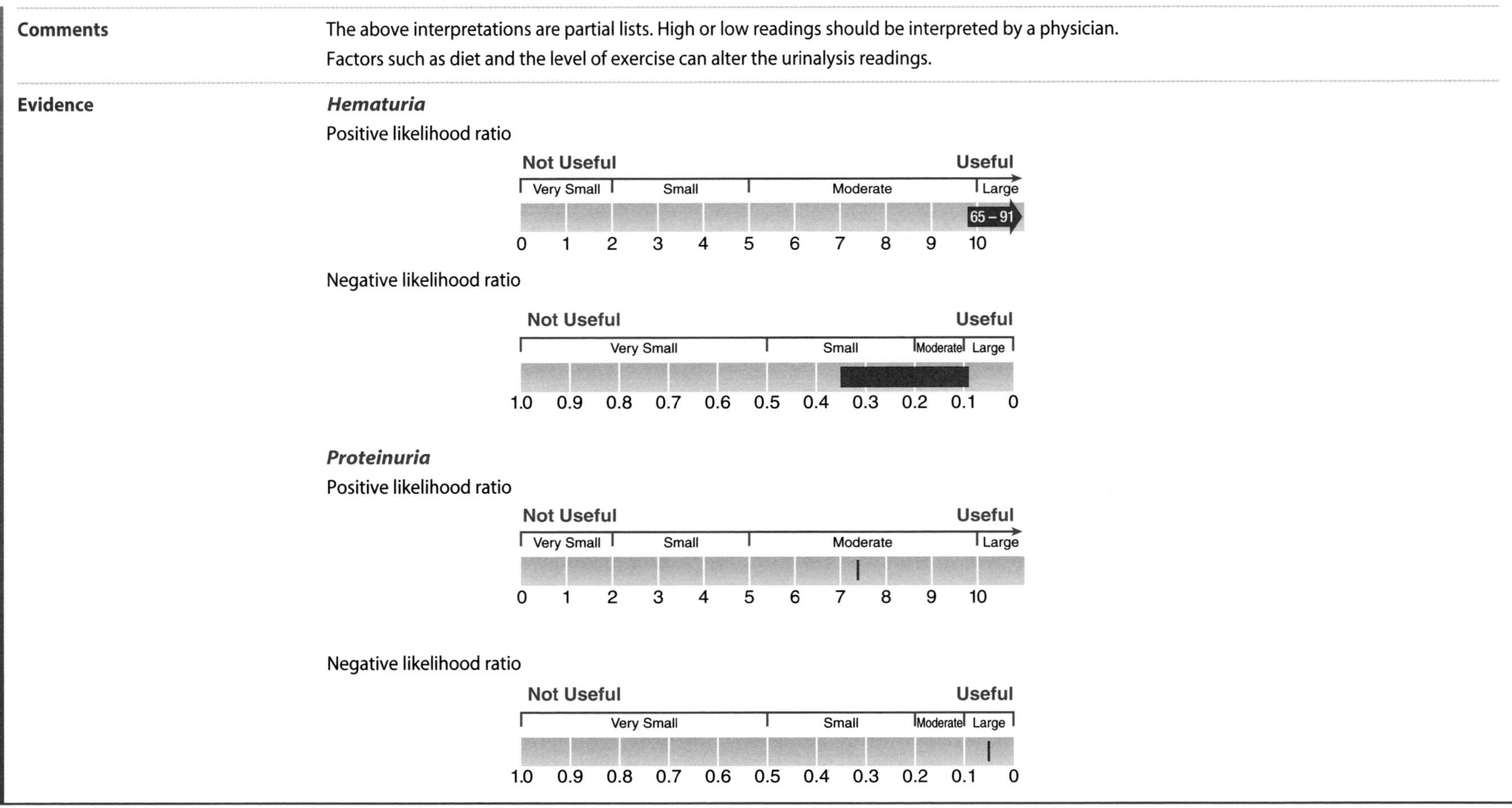

RBC = red blood cell.

sensory fibers associated with the segment of the spinal cord receiving sensory information (Fig. 15-14).

Pathologies of the Thoracic and Abdominal Regions and Related Special Tests

Almost all injuries to the thorax and abdomen have an acute onset, but an underlying disease state or illness may predispose an organ to trauma. Many of these conditions have no visible signs or symptoms, causing the assessment, management, and referral to be based on the findings obtained during the history and palpation section of the examination. When the nature of the condition is in doubt, err on the side of safety and refer the patient to a physician.

Injuries to the Thorax

The mechanism of injury of the thorax may involve the superficial tissues, ribs, heart, or lungs. Likewise, the signs and symptoms of injury to the superficial tissues may mask trauma to the underlying structures.

Rib fractures

The lateral and anterior portions of ribs 5–9 are most commonly fractured. The upper two ribs are protected by the clavicle and the mass of the pectoralis major muscle. The upper six or seven ribs are protected on their posterior aspect by the scapula, lessening the incidence of rib trauma in these areas, although fractures of the upper ribs can occur.[17] The floating ribs have only a posterior attachment on the vertebrae, allowing them to bend and absorb the force of an impact. In sports such as football, the upper ribs are protected by shoulder pads and the lower ribs by a "flak jacket" type of padding. Most rib fractures are the result of a single traumatic blow, but repetitive stresses and explosive muscle contractions may lead to a stress fracture of a rib.[18]

In cases of a rib fracture, the chief complaint is pain directly at the fracture site that worsens and radiates with deep inspirations, coughing, sneezing, and movement of the torso. The patient may assume a comfortable posture by leaning toward the side of the fracture and may actively splint the fracture site by holding the painful area to limit the amount of chest wall movement during inspiration. Respirations are usually shallow and rapid to minimize chest movement. Palpation of the area produces pain over the site of the injury, and deformity of the bone or crepitus may also be noted (Examination Findings 15-1). The suspicion of a rib fracture can be confirmed through the **rib compression test** (Special Test 15-9). This test should not be performed if a fracture is evident via simple palpation.

A blow in the anteroposterior direction usually results in an outward dispersion of forces along the ribs, forcing the fractured rib segments outward as well. Blows to the lateral rib cage have a higher incidence of inwardly projecting fractures, possibly leading to a pneumothorax or hemothorax.[1] Fractures of the first and second ribs, often associated with cervical trauma, may occlude the underlying vasculature.[1] Unrecognized rib fractures can result in a

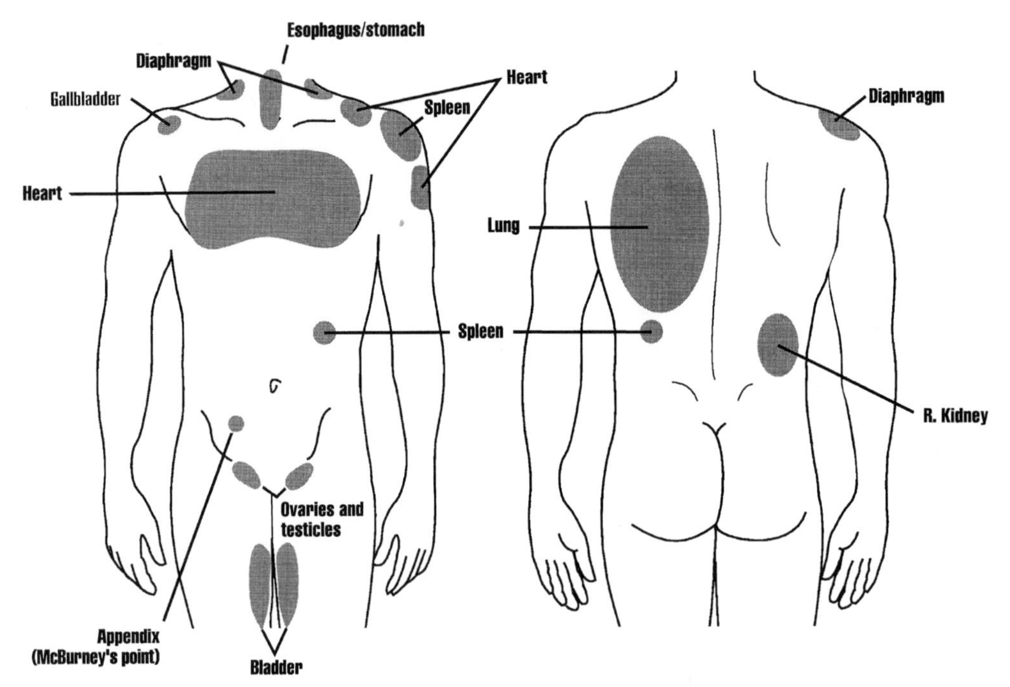

FIGURE 15-14 ■ Referred pain patterns from the viscera. Pain from the internal organs tends to radiate along the corresponding somatic sensory fibers.

Examination Findings 15-1
Acute Rib Fractures

Examination Segment	Clinical Findings
History	***Onset:*** Acute ***Pain characteristics:*** Over a discrete area of the ribs ***Other symptoms:*** Difficulty breathing; if applicable the signs of a pneumothorax or hemothorax may also be present. ***Mechanism:*** Direct blow; when the force occurs in the anteroposterior direction, the fracture has the tendency to displace outwardly. A blow from the lateral side results in the fractured ribs being displaced inwardly, threatening the lungs and other internal organs.
Review of Systems	***Cardiovascular:*** Within normal limits ***Respiratory:*** Respirations are shallow and rapid to minimize chest movement. Auscultate the chest to assess lung function. ***Gastrointestinal:*** Within normal limits ***Genitourinary:*** Rib fractures may traumatize a kidney, resulting in hematuria. ***Neurologic:*** Within normal limits
Inspection	Initial inspection should rule out an open fracture. Possible splinting posture; the patient holds the injured area or leans toward the injured side. Discoloration and swelling may be visible over the injury site.
Palpation	Point tenderness over the area of impact Deeper palpation may reveal crepitus or identification of the fracture.
Joint and Muscle Function Assessment	***AROM:*** Pain is elicited with trunk motion. ***MMT:*** Pain is elicited during testing of muscles attached to the ribs. ***PROM:*** Pain is elicited when stress is placed on the involved ribs.
Joint Stability Tests	***Stress tests:*** Not applicable ***Joint play:*** Not applicable
Special Tests	Rib compression test (contraindicated in the presence of an obvious fracture or lung trauma)
Neurologic Screening	Within normal limits
Vascular Screening	Within normal limits
Functional Assessment	Movement of the torso—either through active motion or from deep respiration, coughing, or sneezing—produces pain along the fracture site; also possible limited torso movement.
Imaging Techniques	Plain radiographs are usually sufficient to identify acute rib fractures. Stress fracture may be identified using a bone scan. MR or CT images may be used to rule out concurrent injury to the lungs or other organs.
Differential Diagnosis	Costochondral injury, erector spinae strain (for stress fractures), pneumothorax, hemothorax
Comments	Bony fragments that are displaced inward may jeopardize the integrity of the lungs and other internal organs.

AROM = active range of motion; CT = computed tomography; MMT = manual muscle test; MR = magnetic resonance; PROM = passive range of motion.

Special Test 15-9
Compression Test for Rib Fractures

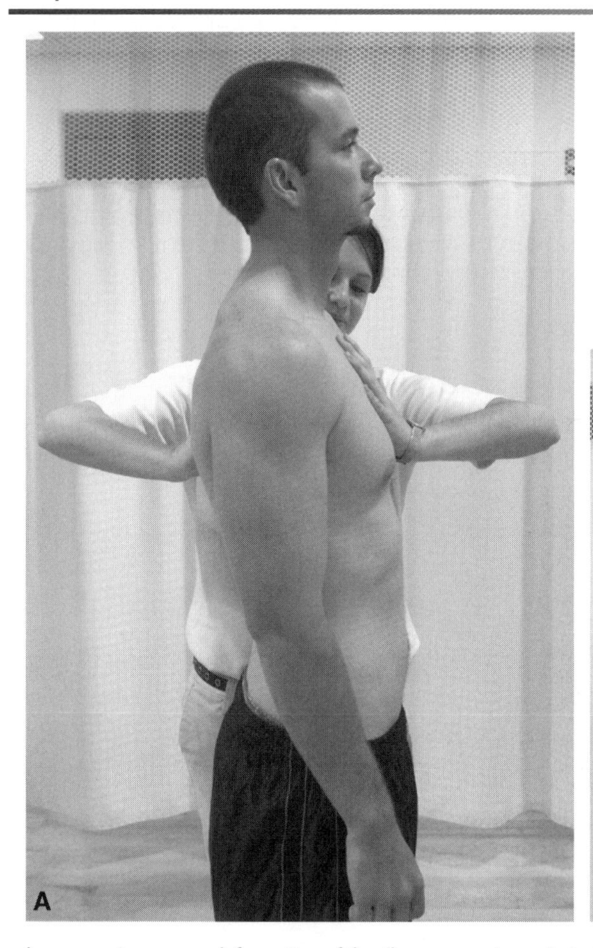

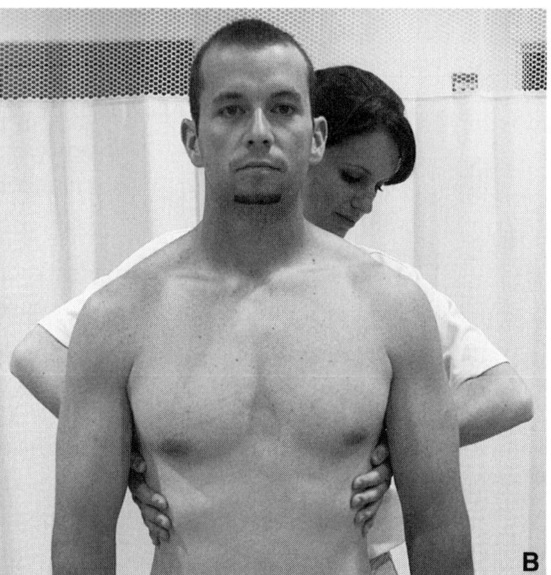

Manual compression causes deformation of the rib cage, causing pain in the presence of a rib fracture. **(A)** Anterior–posterior compression; **(B)** lateral compression. Costochondral injury may produce a false-positive result.

Patient Position	Seated or standing
Position of Examiner	Standing in front of the patient with the hands on opposite sides of the rib cage
Evaluative Procedure	The examiner compresses the rib cage in an anterior-posterior direction and quickly releases the pressure. The rib cage is then compressed from the patient's side and the pressure is quickly released.
Positive Test	Pain in the rib cage isolated to the fracture site
Implications	Damage to the rib cage, including the possibility of a fracture, contusion, or costochondral separation
Comments	Do not perform this test in the presence of palpable rib deformity or crepitus.
Evidence	Absent or inconclusive in the literature

nonunion, seriously impairing the patient's ability to move the trunk.[19]

The possible complications warrant that all patients with suspected rib fractures be referred to a physician for further evaluation and a definitive diagnosis. Rib fractures are managed by controlling the inflammatory response. Pain may be addressed with ice, medication, or both. A rib belt can be used to limit the amount of rib and chest motion that accompanies breathing and other activities of daily living. If deep breathing has been impaired, rehabilitation may involve the use of a spirometer to improve lung function (see Review of Systems).[1]

The ribs are also subject to stress fractures, especially in sports such as rowing, swimming, and golf.[20–24] Most commonly occurring in the first rib (where the anterior scalene inserts) or in the posterolateral portion of ribs 4–9 at the origin of the serratus anterior, stress fractures are the result of sudden increases in training, improper biomechanics, or change in equipment.[25] The signs and symptoms of rib stress fractures cause them to be misidentified as strains of the erector spinae or intercostal muscles or ostochondritis.[23,25] Stress fractures typically begin with vague discomfort in the thoracic region. They progress to sharp, localized pain that is often posterior and may worsen with deep breaths. Treatment includes avoidance of aggravating activities and a gradual increase in activity intensity as symptoms abate.

Costochondral injury

A costochondral injury is usually caused by overstretching the costochondral junction as the arm is forced into hyperflexion and horizontal abduction, potentially separating the costocartilage from the ribs. The signs of costochondral injury are similar to those of rib fractures, but the pain is anteriorly located at the costal–cartilage junction (see Examination Findings 15-1). The patient has immediate pain at the injury site and may report hearing a "snap" or "pop" at the time of injury. Pain is increased with deep breathing, coughing, sneezing, and movement. As with rib fractures, the patient guards the area through body positioning and splinting with the hands. Swelling is often present and palpation reveals point tenderness over the site of the trauma as well as deformity if the rib has separated from the cartilage.

Patients with costochondral injuries are managed similarly to those with rib fractures, with the protocol focused on decreasing pain, controlling inflammation, and eliminating unnecessary movement of the rib cage.

Pneumothorax

A pneumothorax is the accumulation of air in the pleural cavity that disrupts the lung's ability to expand and draw in oxygen. The decrease in inspired oxygen decreases the amount of oxygen absorbed into the bloodstream, resulting in hypoxia and the development of respiratory distress.

A pneumothorax can be either open or closed. A **spontaneous pneumothorax** occurs when **blebs** rupture and allow air to leak into the pleural cavity. It also may result from inflammatory changes in the distal airways.[26] A spontaneous pneumothorax can result secondary to a blow to the rib cage or a penetrating rib cage injury; occur without a history of mechanical force; or arise after surgery.[17,27,28] Improper breathing patterns during strenuous activities such as weightlifting may also lead to a spontaneous pneumothorax.[29]

When a spontaneous pneumothorax fails to spontaneously close or blunt or penetrating trauma occurs to the chest, a **tension pneumothorax** develops. A tension pneumothorax is created when air enters into the pleural cavity but cannot exit. A one-way valve is created. In this case, the air within the pleural cavity continues to build up, placing pressure on the lung and causing it to collapse. If this condition goes unchecked, the subsequent pressure quickly affects the opposite lung, the heart, and the major arteries, leading to death.

Respiratory distress is a common finding in patients with a tension pneumothorax. The patient may complain of pain and shortness of breath or may be unable to speak, appearing agitated or anxious. Labored and shallow respirations accompany a rapidly decreasing blood pressure. Breath sounds, as assessed during auscultation, may be decreased or completely absent on the affected side. The skin may appear to be **cyanotic** and the patient will become hypotensive and tachycardic. In extreme cases, the tissues between the ribs and clavicle are distended (Examination Findings 15-2). The trachea deviates away from the side of the trauma.

Immediate activation of the emergency system is needed for a tension pneumothorax. One hundred percent oxygen should be administered and decompression often occurs before transport to the hospital. Decompression is performed by inserting a long (3 to 6 cm) large-bore needle into the intercostal space between the second and third ribs, approximately 1 to 2 cm from the sternal edge.

Penetrating wounds through the chest wall and into the pleural cavity from a foreign object or a rib fracture result in an open pneumothorax. Air is allowed to leak in and out of the pleural cavity, disabling the normal respiratory mechanism. This injury is also referred to as a "sucking chest wound" because of the sound made when the patient inhales. Refer to the "On-Field Management" section of this chapter for a description of the initial care of patients with this condition.

Bleb A large sac filled with air or fluid having the potential to rupture.

Cyanotic Dark blue or purple tint to the skin and mucous membranes caused by a decreased oxygen supply.

Examination Findings 15-2
Pneumothorax

Examination Segment	Clinical Findings
History	***Onset:*** Acute or insidious ***Pain characteristics:*** Upper left or right quadrant; diaphragm ***Other symptoms:*** In some cases, the patient is unable or unwilling to speak. ***Mechanism:*** Rupture of a bleb, causing air to enter the pleural cavity or an object or rib puncturing the pleural cavity Tension pneumothorax: blunt or penetrating trauma ***Predisposing conditions:*** The presence of a fragile bleb within the lung
Inspection	A guarding posture possibly with the patient clutching the chest and ribs In an acute spontaneous pneumothorax, no visible signs are present over the rib cage. In the case of an acute traumatic pneumothorax, trauma may be visible at the point of impact. Possible cyanosis Progression of a traumatic pneumothorax to the point that the tissue between the clavicle and ribs and the neck veins becomes distended Possible tracheal deviation away from the side of the injury
Palpation	When resulting from a traumatic onset, the affected area is tender secondary to a contusion, fracture, or costal cartilage separation
Review of Systems	***Cardiovascular:*** Blood pressure dropping rapidly Heart rate increases with time ***Respiratory:*** Difficulty breathing; Respiration is labored and shallow. Auscultation of the involved lung revealing absent breath sounds Percussion of the affected side of the chest producing a hollow sound when compared with the opposite lung ***Gastrointestinal:*** Within normal limits ***Genitourinary:*** Within normal limits ***Neurologic:*** Within normal limits
Special Tests	Not applicable
Functional Assessment	Reluctant to move
Imaging Techniques	CT images
Differential Diagnosis	Rib fracture; hemothorax; pneumomediastinum
Comments	An open pneumothorax is characterized by a penetrating wound into the chest cavity. Air can be heard rushing in and out of the wound during respiration. Needle decompression between the 2nd and 3rd ribs is needed to equalize pressure in the plural cavity. Oxygen must be administered to decrease the amount of respiratory distress.

CT = computed tomography.

Hemothorax

A hemothorax is similar to—and often occurs concurrently with—a pneumothorax. In a hemothorax, respiratory distress is caused by a collection of blood in the pleural cavity. Bleeding occurs from an internal chest wound (e.g., a fractured rib lacerating a lung) or from the rupture of a blood vessel within the chest cavity. The signs and symptoms of a hemothorax are very similar, if not identical, to those of a pneumothorax. However, with a hemothorax, the person may cough up bloody sputum, hemoptysis (see Examination Findings 15-2). Refer to the "On-Field Management" section of this chapter for a description of the initial care of patients with this condition.

Pathologies of the Abdominal and Urinary Organs

Most of the abdominal organs lie relatively unprotected inferior to the ribs, but their ability to absorb mechanical blows is enhanced by their hollow structure. The lymphatic organs tend to be more solid in nature but are somewhat protected by the lower portion of the rib cage.

Splenic injury

The spleen may be injured when the abdomen receives a blunt blow such as when a person falls on a ball or other object. The subsequent force delivered to the spleen can result in possible contusion or laceration. An inflamed spleen, which can occur in patients with mononucleosis, pneumonia, or other systemic infections, is predisposed to injury because of the organ's increased mass and decreased elasticity.[30] In patients with advanced disease states, such as mononucleosis, the spleen may spontaneously rupture without a history of blunt force.[31] Likewise, the time between physical trauma to the spleen and the onset of symptoms may be delayed for weeks, days, or years.[32]

The signs and symptoms of shock soon develop after acute spleen trauma. The telltale indicator of a ruptured spleen is the **Kehr's sign**, pain in the upper left quadrant and left shoulder. These symptoms are aggravated by movement, and the patient may vomit or describe being nauseated (Examination Findings 15-3). The vital signs are key indicators of **hemodynamic** changes.

If the patient vomits, attempt to observe the discharge to determine if it is undigested food, red from blood, or greenish from bile. Advise the patient with abdominal injury not to eat or drink because doing so may worsen the symptoms or complicate any surgical procedure that may need to be performed. Various imaging techniques, such as magnetic resonance imaging and computed tomography (CT) scans, are used to identify splenic trauma.[33] Patients suspected of a splenic injury require referral to a physician for immediate evaluation, observation, and treatment.

Hemodynamic The process of blood circulating through the body.

✱ Practical Evidence

Determining return to play status for contact-sport athletes with mononucleosis should not rely on whether or not the spleen is palpable. Splenomegaly is palpable in only about 20% of persons who actually have the condition.[34]

Kidney Pathologies

The kidneys sit well protected behind the lower ribs and spinal musculature. Forces of sufficient magnitude to traumatize the kidneys are often associated with concurrent injury to the lower ribs, lower thoracic vertebrae, upper lumbar vertebrae, or other internal organs. Any penetrating wounds most likely involve some of these structures as well.

Patients suffering from kidney trauma have a history of blunt trauma to the upper lumbar and lower thoracic region. The only outward signs of a kidney contusion or laceration may be bruising or bleeding over the area of contact. The patient may complain of rib pain that increases in intensity during deep inspiration. Cases of severe internal bleeding also produce the signs and symptoms of shock. Palpation of the area generally reveals diffuse tenderness unless a rib is concurrently injured, at which time a more focused pain and crepitus are demonstrated (Fig. 15-15). With severe bleeding, guarding of the abdomen may reflexively occur because of pain (Examination Findings 15-4).

Hematuria is a diagnostic sign associated with an injured kidney. Except in the case of severe bleeding within

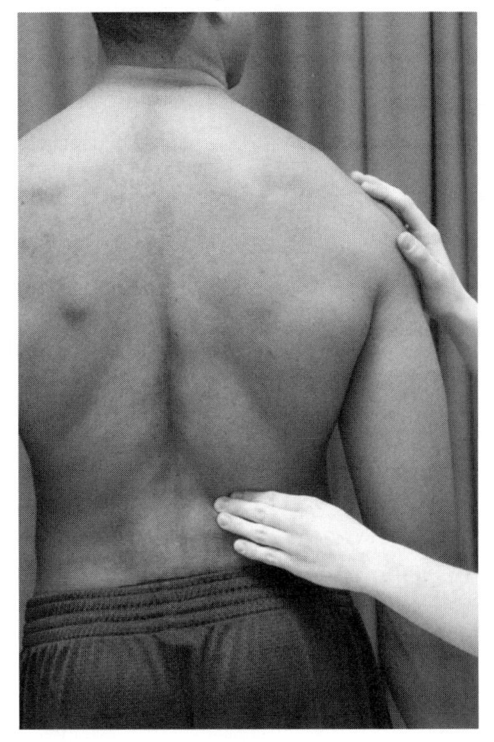

FIGURE 15-15 ■ Palpation of the right kidney. After an injury, the area overlying the kidneys may become tender to the touch or reveal crepitus secondary to a rib fracture.

Examination Findings 15-3
Splenic Injury

Examination Segment	Clinical Findings
History	***Onset:*** Acute, although the onset of symptoms may take hours ***Pain characteristics:*** Pressure experienced in the upper left quadrant, discrete area of referred pain in the anterior and posterior portions of the lower left quadrant, and the upper left shoulder (**Kehr's sign**) ***Other symptoms:*** Feeling of "fullness" in the upper left quadrant and stomach. ***Mechanism:*** Blow to the abdomen or thorax, compressing or jarring the spleen ***Predisposing conditions:*** Mononucleosis, systemic infection
Inspection	The impact site possibly showing signs of a contusion or rib fracture
Palpation	Cold and clammy skin with the onset of shock Tenderness in area over the impact site Distention of upper left quadrant
Review of Systems	***Cardiovascular:*** Low blood pressure Increased heart rate ***Respiratory:*** Increased respiratory rate if in shock. ***Gastrointestinal:*** Nausea and vomiting possible Abdominal rigidity ***Genitourinary:*** Within normal limits ***Neurologic:*** Kehr's sign
Special Tests	Not applicable
Functional Assessment	Pain in the upper left quadrant and shoulder aggravated by movement. General unwillingness to move.
Imaging Techniques	MR or CT scan Diagnostic ultrasound
Differential Diagnosis	Liver trauma; kidney injury; rib fracture
Comments	Patients suffering from mononucleosis or other systemic infections are predisposed to spleen injury secondary to the enlargement and hardening of this organ. Concurrent injury to the left kidney must be ruled out. Symptoms of mononucleosis include fever, fatigue, swollen lymph nodes (adenopathy), tonsil/throat exudate, and sore throat.

CT = computed tomography; MR = magnetic resonance.

Examination Findings 15-4
Contused or Lacerated Kidney

Examination Segment	Clinical Findings
History	***Onset:*** Acute ***Pain characteristics:*** Posterolateral portion of the upper lumbar and lower thoracic region ***Mechanism:*** Blunt trauma or penetrating injury to the kidney (e.g., contusive forces, fractured rib impaling the kidney)
Inspection	Contusion or laceration in the impacted area may be present.
Palpation	Tenderness over the impact site Abdominal rigidity may occur.
Review of Systems	***Cardiovascular:*** Hypotension ***Respiratory:*** May become rapid. ***Genitourinary:*** Macroscopic or microscopic blood may be present in the urine. ***Neurologic:*** Within normal limits
Special Tests	Not applicable
Functional Assessment	Signs and symptoms of shock may be present. Pain possible during urination
Imaging Techniques	Contrast CT scan
Differential Diagnosis	Rib fracture; muscle strain or contusion; urinary tract infection
Comments	The traumatic forces may also result in a rib fracture or costochondral injury. Trauma to the spleen must be ruled out with injury to the left kidney; liver trauma must be ruled out with injury to the right kidney. Patients suspected of suffering from a kidney injury should immediately be referred to a physician.

CT = computed tomography.

the kidney, the urine may not seem noticeably discolored to the unaided eye, and bleeding can be detected only via laboratory analysis. Urine for further analysis must be collected from a patient suspected of suffering a kidney injury. The absence of blood in the urine immediately after an injury does not rule out kidney trauma. The use of CT scans or contrast imaging of the urinary tract may be required for a definitive diagnosis. The potential loss of a kidney warrants that individuals demonstrating any of these signs and symptoms be immediately referred to a physician.

Kidney stones

Kidney stones are the result of a collection of incomplete kidney filtration. Formed by crystals of uric acid, struvite, or calcium, these stones may measure less than 1 mm to more than 2.5 cm (1 in.). A family history of kidney stones,[35] stressful life events,[36] and hypertension[37] may trigger symptomatic kidney stones. The onset of this condition can also be associated with the intake of large amounts of dietary protein and salts[35,38] and other foodstuffs such as apple or grapefruit juice.[39] Ingesting foods and drinks such as caffeinated or decaffeinated coffee, beer, and wine,[39] and increasing the intake of calcium, tea, tomatoes, and other potassium-rich foods, and fluids[40] may decrease the possibility of kidney stones (Fig. 15-16).

The first sign of a kidney stone is pain in the left or right side, and bladder discomfort may be experienced during urination. Larger stones may be felt as they progress down the ureter to the bladder, producing pain. The most excruciating pain may be experienced as the stone is passed from the urinary bladder through the urethra. When the obstruction occurs in the lower right quadrant, the signs and symptoms of a kidney stone can mimic those of appendicitis.

Patients who are suspected of having kidney stones require a referral to a physician for further evaluation. Mild to moderate kidney stones may be treated via medication and diet modification. Shock-wave lithotripsy can be used to break down small to moderate sized stones; larger stones may require surgical removal.[41]

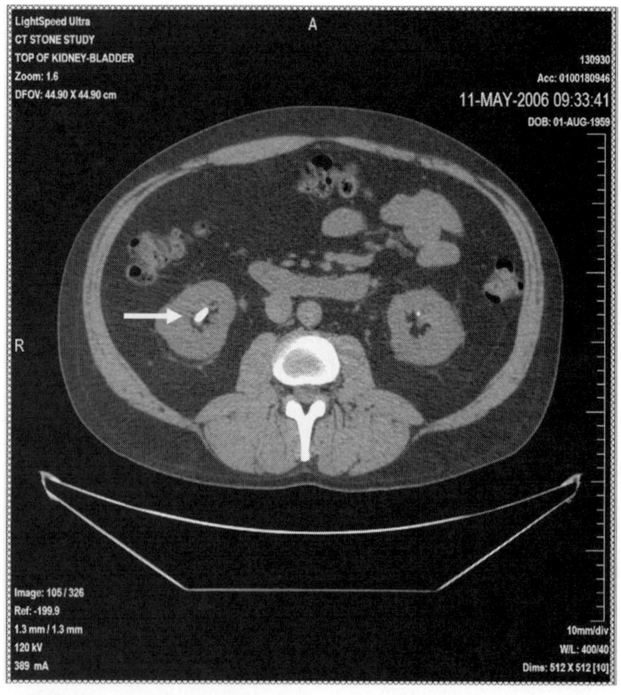

FIGURE 15-16 ■ A superior–inferior view of the thorax demonstrating a stone located within the left kidney (arrow). The stone is approximately 14 mm (0.55 in.) long.

Urinary tract infection

Urinary tract infections (UTIs) are caused by bacterial infections of the bladder or urethra and can present as acute low back pain. The ureter and kidney may also be involved. Inflammation of just the bladder, **cystitis**, may also occur. Urinary tract infections may mimic the signs and symptoms of kidney stones. The patient complains of **dysuria**, the frequent need to urinate, and describes pain in the lower abdominal region. The patient may also describe an abnormal urine color, possibly representing hematuria. Urine containing infection may have a strong, foul odor. Widespread infection leads to fever, nausea, and vomiting.

Inflammation of the urethra, **urethritis**, may have an onset linked to a specific organism such as gonococcus in the urinary tract; may be attributed to ***Chlamydia***, gonorrhea, or syphilis; or may have a nonspecific etiology. The onset of urethritis is more frequent in males than in females. Urethritis is marked by dysuria, enlarged inguinal lymph nodes, penile discharge, testicular enlargement, and blood in the urine.

Patients suspected of suffering from UTIs or urethritis must be referred to a physician for possible antibiotic therapy and tests for associated sexually transmitted diseases (STDs). These patients should refrain from sexual activity while the symptoms are present. The patient may also be advised to increase water intake and urinate frequently to flush the infecting agent out of the system.

Appendicitis and Appendix Rupture

Although the onset of appendicitis is rarely attributed to athletic competition, blows to the lower right quadrant may accelerate an existing inflammatory process or cause the inflamed appendix to rupture. Acute appendicitis, commonly occurring in patients who are 15 to 25 years old, is more common in men than in women. The outward symptoms of lower abdominal tenderness—fever, nausea, and vomiting—occur approximately 2 days after the initial inflammation of

---

Dysuria Painful urination.

Chlamydia A family of microorganisms that produce infection in the genitals and is sexually transmitted.

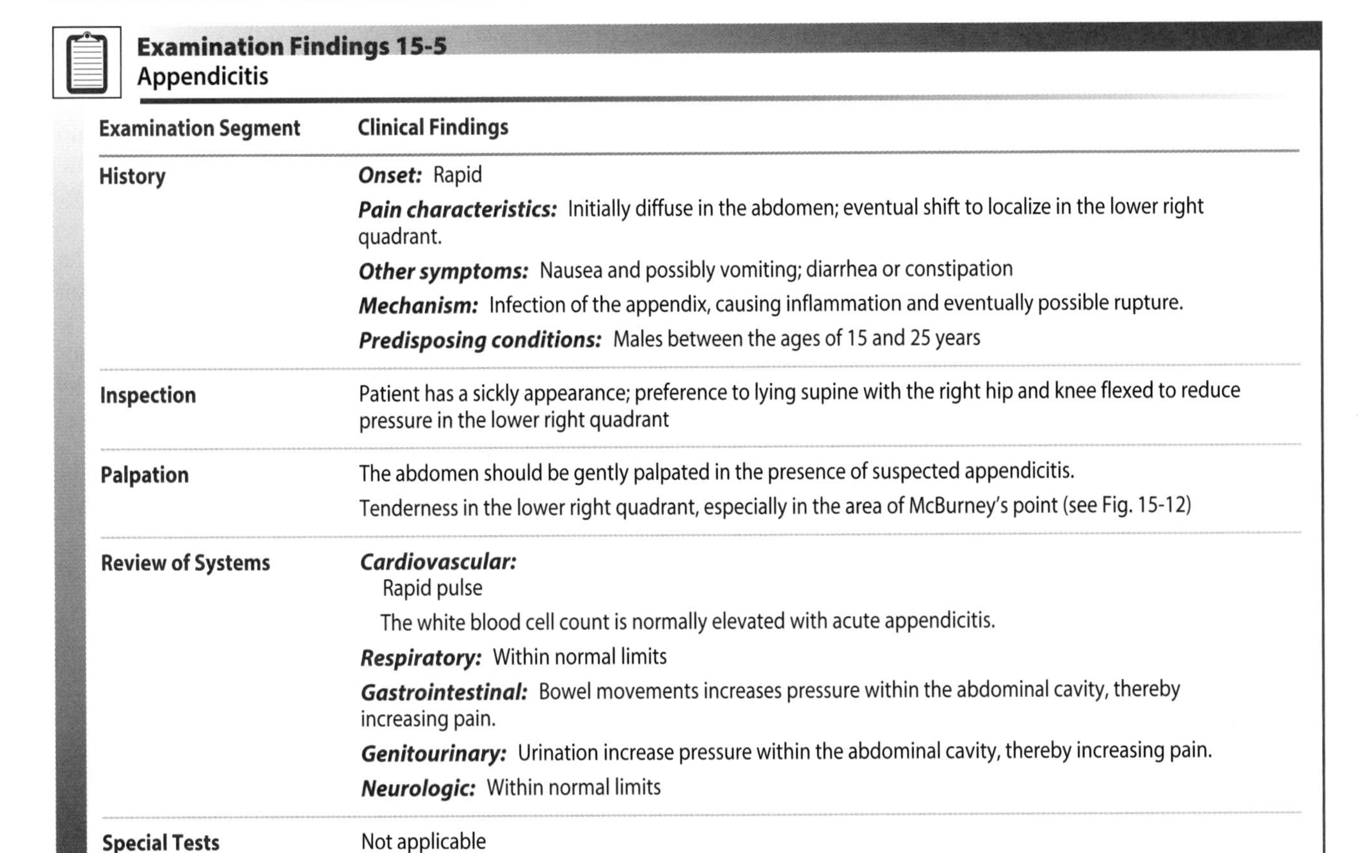

Examination Findings 15-5
Appendicitis

Examination Segment	Clinical Findings
History	***Onset:*** Rapid ***Pain characteristics:*** Initially diffuse in the abdomen; eventual shift to localize in the lower right quadrant. ***Other symptoms:*** Nausea and possibly vomiting; diarrhea or constipation ***Mechanism:*** Infection of the appendix, causing inflammation and eventually possible rupture. ***Predisposing conditions:*** Males between the ages of 15 and 25 years
Inspection	Patient has a sickly appearance; preference to lying supine with the right hip and knee flexed to reduce pressure in the lower right quadrant
Palpation	The abdomen should be gently palpated in the presence of suspected appendicitis. Tenderness in the lower right quadrant, especially in the area of McBurney's point (see Fig. 15-12)
Review of Systems	***Cardiovascular:*** Rapid pulse The white blood cell count is normally elevated with acute appendicitis. ***Respiratory:*** Within normal limits ***Gastrointestinal:*** Bowel movements increases pressure within the abdominal cavity, thereby increasing pain. ***Genitourinary:*** Urination increase pressure within the abdominal cavity, thereby increasing pain. ***Neurologic:*** Within normal limits
Special Tests	Not applicable
Functional Assessment	As the appendicitis progresses, a fever of at least 99°–101°F. High fever may not occur in young children. Pain with movement
Imaging Techniques	CT, diagnostic ultrasound
Differential Diagnosis	Urinary tract infection, constipation In female patients: pelvic inflammatory disease, ruptured **ectopic pregnancy**, ruptured ovarian cyst, and painful ovulation.
Comments	Patients suspected of suffering from appendicitis must immediately be transported to an emergency room.

CT = computed tomography.

the appendix. Pain may be referred to the right side of the chest wall as well as the right upper trapezius area. A pus-filled abscess forms 1 to 3 days after the onset of the symptoms. Patients suffering from appendicitis prefer lying supine with the right leg flexed at the hip and knee to lessen the amount of pressure on the lower right quadrant (Examination Findings 15-5). CT is commonly used to diagnose appendicitis. Patients suspected of suffering from appendicitis must be immediately referred to a physician. Also, the intake of food and liquids must be curtailed until permission to resume eating is given by a physician.

Ectopic pregnancy The formation of a fetus outside of the uterine cavity.

*** Practical Evidence**

With a sensitivity of 98.1%, the absence of three findings—(1) an elevated absolute neutrophil count, (2) nausea, and (3) maximal tenderness in the right lower quadrant—highly suggests that appendicitis is not present and may reduce the need for CT.[42] In adults, right lower quadrant pain is a much stronger predictor of appendicitis than in children.[43]

Hollow Organ Rupture

Hollow organs are able to absorb the forces from blows to the abdomen, deforming and returning to their initial shape without permanent injury. When a hollow organ is ruptured, the outcome is potentially fatal secondary to hemorrhage, peritoneal contamination, or both.

After a rupture of a hollow organ, the patient describes a history of a blow to the abdomen as well as pain and possible nausea. On further evaluation, guarding, abdominal rigidity and tenderness, and the signs and symptoms of shock may be noted. Bowel sounds are absent on auscultation.[44]

Because the onset of symptoms associated with hollow organ trauma is gradual, the symptoms may resemble those of a contusion, costal-cartilage sprain, or similar injury. Although the liver is not a hollow organ, its location and relative rigidity predispose it to injury as well. Patients with a seemingly benign abdominal injury must be cautioned to report any increase in symptoms. Patients also need to visually inspect the stool for blood because hemorrhage may leak into the feces. As with all internal organ injuries, patients with suspected ruptures of a hollow organ need to be referred for evaluation at an appropriate medical facility. Because of the possibility of surgery, individuals who have suffered significant trauma to the abdominal organs must refrain from eating or drinking until cleared to do so by a physician.

Pathology of the Reproductive Organs

Because of their external location, male reproductive organs are injured more frequently than female reproductive organs. In a direct impact to the genitals, the resulting contusion or lacerations are often embarrassing, especially for younger patients. These conditions must be professionally managed, not only to comfort the patient but also to preserve the integrity of the organs.

Male reproductive system pathologies

Trauma to—and disease of—the testicles is potentially a serious medical condition that may lead to infertility and/or hormonal changes.

Testicular contusion: Direct blows to the testicles result in immediate pain, often at an intensity sufficient to cause vomiting, speech inhibition, and breathing restriction. The priority in managing this condition is to calm the individual by instructing him to inhale deeply and slowly through the nose and exhale through the mouth. Lifting the patient's belt and waistband may reduce the feeling of pressure on the testicles and lower abdomen. The efficacy of other anecdotal techniques, such as lifting and dropping the patient on his buttocks, has never been established.

After the pain has been controlled, the patient is instructed to inspect the testicles for normal size and consistency. The trauma may cause the testicle to rupture, giving it a relatively soft, inconsistent texture. Swelling may occur within the testicles, possibly involving the collection of fluids within the scrotum. Either condition warrants immediate follow-up examination by a physician.

Testicular torsion: Torsion of the spermatic cord occurs as the testicle and spermatic cord is twisted within the scrotal sac. Testicular torsion (also referred to as spermatic cord torsion) is more common in individuals having an undescended testicle. Unsupported, the testicle and spermatic cord are susceptible to injury from a direct blow or from the simple jarring movements that occur with athletic activity. The use of an athletic supporter decreases the risk of testicular torsion.

Typically, the onset is nontraumatic and occurs in those younger than the age of 25. An onset caused by acute trauma, accounting for only 10% of all cases, is associated with intense testicular pain, nausea, and possible vomiting.[45] Symptoms of spermatic cord torsion may have an acute onset of testicular pain caused by the obstruction of the spermatic artery and vein. Inspection reveals a localized swelling of the testicle, a higher testicle on the involved side, and, possibly, a mass in the scrotum. Testicular tenderness may be elicited during palpation. The patient requires immediate referral for further evaluation and possible surgery because delayed treatment could lead to loss of the testicle. Treatment, which can include manual detorsion or surgery, within 6 hours of the onset of symptoms is associated with a high success rate.[45]

*** Practical Evidence**

An absent cremasteric reflex, where the testicle moves when the medial thigh is stroked, is 99% sensitive in detecting testicular torsion. Stated otherwise, if a cremasteric reflex is present, the probability of testicular torsion is remote.[45]

Testicular dysfunction: During fetal development, a channel is formed between the abdomen and scrotum that allows the testicles to fall into the scrotum. As physical maturity develops, the tract normally closes. Incomplete closure can allow fluids from the peritoneum to seep into the scrotum, forming a **hydrocele**, a fluid-filled sac along the spermatic cord. Hydroceles can also be caused by trauma or inflammation of the testicle, epididymis, or secondary to blockage of the spermatic cord's blood supply or the formation of a mass within the serous membrane surrounding the anterior and lateral portion of the testicle (tunica vaginalis). Inguinal hernias may also lead to the onset of a hydrocele.[46] Although the scrotum or testicle (or both) may enlarge, a hydrocele is a painless, benign condition. Other than the outward swelling, the only other symptom is an enlarged testicle that feels like a fluid-filled sack (often described as feeling like a "water balloon"). If the size of the fluid accumulation becomes problematic, the physician may choose to aspirate the hydrocele and close the portal between the scrotum and abdomen. Hydroceles associated with an inguinal hernia require immediate evaluation by a physician.

The formation of **varicose veins** within the scrotum, a **varicocele**, is the result of the obstruction of normal blood flow of the involved veins. In older men, a varicocele can develop secondary to a kidney tumor, altering blood flow from the renal vein through the spermatic vein. The veins within the scrotum may become visible, and the scrotum may appear enlarged. Upon palpation, a painless lump may be felt. The characteristic sign of a varicocele is the scrotum and spermatic cord's feeling like a "bag of worms" during palpation.[30] Varicoceles are a frequent cause of male infertility. Patients suspected of suffering from a varicocele need a referral to a physician for additional examination.

The outward signs of a varicocele are similar to those associated with **epididymitis**, or inflammation of the epididymis. Often associated with UTIs, epididymitis is caused by a bacterial infection and may be linked to STDs. Similarly to hydroceles and varicoceles, the scrotum and testicle (or testicles) are enlarged. However, epididymitis is characterized by these structures' being painful to the touch. Pain may also be described during urination, ejaculation, and bowel movements. Blood in the semen may be noted. As the infection spreads, the patient may develop a fever and swollen inguinal lymph nodes.

Testicular cancer: Although unrelated to the acute trauma, testicular cancer is often discovered after testicular injury. Testicular cancer is the most common form of cancer in college-aged male athletes. The risk of onset is greatest between ages 20 and 35 years. A history of undescended testicles (cryptorchidism), **orchitis**, and inguinal hernias increase the risk of developing testicular cancer.[47,48] The patient notices an enlarging and hardening of the involved testicle, and a painless nodule may be noted. Although testicular pain is not always present, pain may be referred to the low back, inguinal region, and abdomen. Pain may also radiate into the adductor muscle group and appear as an adductor strain. As the disease progresses, blood may be noted in the semen. In the later stages, enlargement of the breasts may occur.

With early detection, the prognosis for most types of testicular cancer is excellent. All men should conduct a testicular self-examination on a monthly basis. Definitive diagnosis of testicular cancer is based on tissue biopsies, ultrasonic imaging, and CT scans.

Female reproductive system pathologies

The female reproductive organs are well protected within the abdominal cavity. The signs and symptoms of pathology to these organs tend to duplicate those of appendicitis or trauma to the hollow organs. However, the signs and symptoms may be accompanied by untimely, irregular, or increased menstrual flow. (Injury to the pubic symphysis is discussed in Chapter 12.)

Menstrual irregularities associated with physical activity: The physical and emotional stresses that accompany many forms of athletics can disrupt or alter female athletes' menstrual cycles. External pressures such as body image, unrealistic target weights, and societal pressures may further disrupt the menstrual cycle.

The absence of the onset of normal **menstruation** by the age of 16 years, **primary amenorrhea**, or the cessation of menstruation for 6 months or more, **secondary amenorrhea**, may have a diverse range of causes (Table 15-6). Exercise, weight loss, and the resulting decrease in luteinizing hormone, stress, and anxiety may cause irregular menstrual cycles, or **oligomenorrhea**. Because of the association with disease states and nutritional factors, patients experiencing menstrual irregularities need a referral to a gynecologist. Often when the underlying cause of the menstrual irregularity is addressed, regular menstruation resumes. Because of the relationship of amenorrhea to the **female athlete triad**, athletes should be carefully monitored.

Although not normally the result of athletic participation, dysmenorrhea can significantly affect an athlete's performance. Dysmenorrhea is characterized by pain or cramping (or both) in the lower abdomen and pelvis starting 1 to 2 days before menstruation. Nausea, vomiting, diarrhea or constipation, and bloating may occur. Patients suffering from dysmenorrhea need referral to a gynecologist because this condition may also be related to **pelvic inflammatory disease** (PID), endometriosis, or other

Table 15-6 Factors Leading to the Onset of Amenorrhea
Weight reduction (may be the result of anorexia nervosa or bulimia)
Obesity
Malnutrition
Hypoglycemia
Cystic fibrosis
Heart disease
Hyperthyroidism
Ovarian disease
Prolonged exercise or overexercising (anorexia athletica)
Pregnancy
Anxiety*
Early menopause*
Pelvic inflammatory disease*

*Secondary amenorrhea only; the remaining factors can be associated with either primary or secondary amenorrhea.

Varicose veins Enlargement of the superficial veins.

Orchitis Inflammation of the testicle.

Pelvic inflammatory disease An infection of the vagina that spreads to the cervix, uterus, fallopian tubes, and broad ligaments.

Hypoglycemia The state of decreased levels of sugar in the blood, resulting in fatigue, restlessness, and irritability; commonly associated with diabetes.

medical conditions. Hormones, anti-inflammatory, analgesic, or muscle relaxant medication may be prescribed. Further decrease in symptoms may be accomplished using a moist heat pack placed over the pelvis and abdomen.

The female athlete triad: The female athlete triad syndrome consists of three related components: disordered eating, amenorrhea, and osteoporosis.[49–51] While the actual prevalence of all three parts of the triad in female athletes is relatively low, the number of women who meet the criteria for at least two of the components (generally disordered eating and menstrual dysfunction) is higher in athletes than in the general population.[52] The American College of Sports Medicine recommends that female athletes who present with one component of the female athlete triad also be screened for the presence of the remaining two components.[50] Table 15-7 lists athletes who are considered as being at risk of acquiring the female athlete triad syndrome.

Individually, any of the components of the female athlete triad poses a significant risk to the health and well-being of the athlete. For example, amenorrhea predisposes the patient to stress fractures. Any signs or symptoms of any component of the triad need to be thoroughly evaluated. If left unrecognized or unmanaged, the female athlete triad can lead to a fatal sequence of events.

Currently the best treatment of the female athlete triad is the prevention of the disorder. Athletes should be screened for each of the three components during the preparticipation examination. Athlete, coaches, parents, and health care providers must be educated regarding the predisposing conditions and the signs, symptoms, and potential consequences of the female athlete triad. After a thorough assessment and diagnosis, treatment involves a team approach to address the physical and psychological ramifications of the problem.

Pelvic inflammatory disease: Pelvic inflammatory disease is a general term used to describe inflammation or infection of the uterus, ovaries, or fallopian tubes. The etiology of PID is closely linked to the same bacteria that cause STDs. An awareness of PID in orthopedics is needed because one symptom is low back pain. Other signs and symptoms include vaginal discharge, amenorrhea, dysmenorrhea, or oligomenorrhea, fever, abdominal pain, dysuria, and frequent urination. The inguinal lymph nodes may be enlarged, and the abdomen may be tender to the touch. A referral to a gynecologist is necessary for a definitive diagnosis. The usual course of treatment includes antibiotic medications and, in severe cases, possibly surgery. Prolonged PID can result in infertility.

Table 15-7 Athletes at Risk of Developing One or More Components of the Female Athlete Triad

Category	Example
Subjectively scored sports	Dance, figure skating, diving, gymnastics
Endurance sports that emphasize a low body weight	Distance running, cycling
Sports that require contour-revealing clothing	Gymnastics, volleyball, swimming, cheerleading
Sports using weight categories	Horse racing, rowing, wrestling
Sports that rely on a prepubertal body type	Figure skating, gymnastics, diving

Cardiopulmonary Pathologies

Unfortunately, many of the conditions that predispose cardiopulmonary distress go unnoticed or unreported until an acute episode occurs. Early identification and intervention provide the best opportunity for athletes suffering from cardiopulmonary conditions to safely participate in athletics as well as perform the activities of daily living.

*** Practical Evidence**

The American College of Cardiology's Bethesda Conference Guidelines are a collection of position statements of Best Practices that make recommendations on the disqualifying conditions and return-to-play guidelines for individuals suffering from a wide range of cardiovascular conditions. The Bethesda Guidelines, now in their 36th edition, are considered by many to be a definitive source for making these medical judgments. The document can be accessed online at: http://www.acc.org/qualityandscience/clinical/bethesda/beth36/index.pdf

Commotio cordis

Commotio cordis, a "cardiac concussion," is an instantaneous cardiac arrest caused by a nonpenetrating blow to the chest in an otherwise healthy heart that does not result in injury of the overlying structures.[53–55] The most frequent cause of commotio cordis is being struck in the chest by a projectile such as a ball or a puck, followed by automobile accidents and domestic (child) abuse.[53,56] The pliability of the chest during childhood more easily transmits the force to the heart, but individuals of any age my be affected.

The onset of commotio cordis is influenced by the type, location, force, and the timing of the impact.[53] Of these factors, the timing of the impact is most crucial to its onset. A precordial impact delivered within 30 and 15 milliseconds before the peak of the T wave can trigger ventricular fibrillation (Fig. 15-17).[53,57]

The vulnerable area of the chest wall is a silhouette of the cardiac profile directly anterior to the heart.[54,57] The force of the blow is believed to activate mechanosensitive ion channels by triggering mechanoelectrical coupling. While high-velocity forces such as being struck by a lacrosse ball or hockey puck can trigger the cardiac arrhythmia, commotio

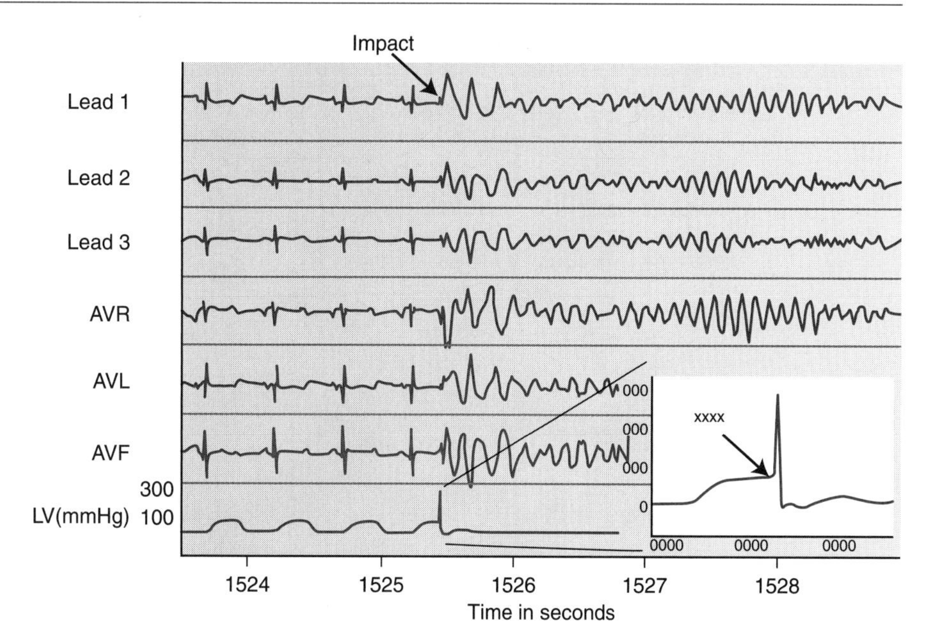

FIGURE 15-17 ■ Electrocardiogram demonstrating ventricular fibrillation caused by a blunt impact to the chest wall during vulnerable zone of repolarization (10–30 ms before the T-wave peak). (From Madias, C, et al. Commotio cordis—sudden cardiac death with chest wall impact. *J Cardiovasc Electrophysiol,* 18:115, 2007.)

cordis can also be the result of relatively low-velocity forces such as a thrown baseball. The incidence of occurrence is greater when using solid-core objects than those that are air-filled (e.g., soccer ball, football).[54]

The signs and symptoms of commotio cordis—that of cardiac arrest—occur immediately after the blow or may be delayed by several seconds, followed by cardiac arrhythmia, most frequently ventricular fibrillation.[53,55,58] Although the survival rate for commotio cordis is only about 15%, successful resuscitation and subsequent survival using on-site CPR and an automated external defibrillator has been documented.[54,56,57,59] When CPR, including defibrillation, is initiated within 3 minutes after the trauma the survival rate is 25%; when initiating CPR is delayed for more than 3 minutes the survival rate drops to 3%.[54]

The poor survivability and limited management options have led to emphasis being placed on the prevention of commotio cordis, especially in young athletes. Many youth leagues have changed to using softer balls and require that batters and those at other at-risk positions wear chest protectors. However, cases of commotio cordis have still occurred with these preventive measures in place, primarily because the chest protector was not properly fitted.[54]

Cardiac contusions

Although the heart is well protected, it may be traumatized by a direct, forceful blow to the sternum or compression of the sternum and anterior rib cage. This force can result in contusions of the pericardial lining, ventricular contusion, or aortic ruptures.[6,60] Within 24 hours after the injury, the subsequent hemorrhage can affect the electrical signals to the heart, causing an irregular heart rhythm.[1]

Symptoms include chest pain, engorgement of the neck vessels (**dyspnea**) and decreased blood pressure. The most severe ramification of cardiac contusions is cardiac arrest. In this event, emergency cardiac care procedures must be immediately initiated. Patients with suspected cardiac contusions must be immediately referred to a physician.

Syncope

Depending on its underlying cause, syncope can be an ominous sign of underlying cardiac abnormality, a symptom of heat illness, or simply a benign occurrence.[61] Initially, syncope may not be reported. However, when syncope does occur, it should always be considered a sign warranting further examination, particularly when it occurs during activity (exertional syncope).[7] The five potential mechanisms of this event (Table 15-8) are common in athletes during practice and competition. After the cause of the episode is determined, appropriate management and preventive measures against future episodes are indicated.

Hypertrophic cardiomyopathy

Sudden death is a rare occurrence among athletes.[6] When an apparently healthy person is stricken, the results are especially devastating. The most common cause of sudden death in young athletes is hypertrophic cardiomyopathy, a condition that may not display any prior physical signs or symptoms.[4] A family history of hypertrophic cardiomyopathy is a strong predictor of the occurrence of this condition. Chromosome abnormalities also contribute to the development of this disease process.[6]

Hypertrophic cardiomyopathy involves the enlargement of the heart muscles without an increase in size of the heart's chambers. The left ventricular septum is most often affected, thickening 15 to 60 mm. The left atrium and right

---

Dyspnea Air hunger marked by labored or difficult breathing; may be a normal occurrence after exertion or an abnormal occurrence indicating cardiac or respiratory distress.

Table 15-8 Syncope in Athletes

	Neurogenic Reactions	Decreased Blood Volume	Metabolic Conditions	Cardiac Disorders	Drug Reactions
Cause	Venous dilation, increased vagal tone, and bradycardia after an anxiety-provoking event	Dehydration and electrolyte imbalance such as in heat illness Vomiting Diarrhea Prolonged fasting Hemorrhage	Hypoglycemia associated with diabetes	Arrhythmias associated with hypertrophic cardiomyopathy, atherosclerosis, or anomalous coronary arteries Wolff–Parkinson–White syndrome	Stimulant abuse; possibly masquerading as arrhythmia, dehydration, or vasovagal reactions
Signs and Symptoms	Lightheadedness Dizziness Profuse sweating Nausea	Lightheadedness Dizziness Nausea Visual disturbances	Fatigue Headache Profuse sweating Trembling Slurred speech Poor coordination	Palpitations Irregular heartbeat	As associated with arrhythmia, dehydration, or vasovagal reactions

ventricle may also be involved. The enlarged muscles place an increased amount of force on an unchanged blood volume (the blood contained within the chambers), increasing the pressure on the interventricular septum and aorta. A prominent Q wave, increased amplitude (voltage) of the R wave, and a deeply inverted (negative) T wave are characteristic EMG findings of hypertrophic cardiomyopathy. Acute failure may produce syncope, cardiac arrhythmia, or, in the most profound cases, a rupture of the septum or aorta, resulting in death.

A significant heart murmur or characteristics of Marfan syndrome (see Box 15-1) may be present. In many cases of sudden death, evidence of previous arrhythmias has been documented in the medical history.[3,4] Associated congenital anomalous coronary circulation may also be discovered after the sudden death of a young person.

Acute signs and symptoms include excessive fatigue, exertional syncope, dizziness, dyspnea, or the sensation of chest pain and arrhythmias while exercising (Examination Findings 15-6). The symptoms of hypertrophic cardiomyopathy are more likely to occur during exercise than during rest. Occasionally, these episodes occur after bouts of vigorous activity or during stoppage in play.

Definitive diagnosis of this condition is complex because of the varying presence and inconsistent reporting of significant symptoms, extensive range of testing procedures, and their subsequent interpretation by cardiologists. The 36th Bethesda Conference on cardiovascular abnormalities established guidelines for competition eligibility that are often used when a physician needs to make safe participation decisions (Table 15-9). Patients displaying any of the previous symptoms should be referred to a physician for a complete medical work-up.

Table 15-9 Recommendations for Eligibility for Exercise with those Cardiovascular Diseases

Conditions Contraindicating Vigorous Exercise	Acute myocarditis Congenital coronary artery anomalies Congestive heart failure Hypertrophic cardiomyopathy Left ventricle hypertrophy (idiopathic) Marfan syndrome Pulmonary hypertension Right ventricular cardiomyopathy Uncontrolled arrhythmias or valvular heart disease
Conditions Requiring Modified Activity or Continuous Monitoring	Uncontrolled hypertension Uncontrolled atrial arrhythmias Aortic insufficiency Mitral stenosis Mitral regurgitation

Myocardial infarction

The chance of survival after a myocardial infaction (MI) ("heart attack") during exercise is better than that for hypertrophic cardiomyopathy. The onset of MI is caused by blockage of the heart's coronary arteries, causing a depletion of oxygen to the cardiac muscle, eventually resulting in necrosis.

Knowledge of the **prodromal** symptoms of heart attack risk, including chest pain, fatigue, and syncope allows for

Prodromal Pertaining to the interval between the initial disease rate and the onset of outward symptoms.

Examination Findings 15-6
Hypertrophic Cardiomyopathy

Examination Segment	Clinical Findings
History	***Onset:*** Congenital or acquired ***Pain characteristics:*** Pain resembling that of a myocardial infarction ***Other symptoms:*** Syncope, dizziness, shortness of breath ***Mechanism:*** Hypertrophy of the heart's chambers, especially the left ventricle, increasing pressure on the interventricular septum and aorta ***Predisposing conditions:*** Family history of cardiac sudden death. Significant heart murmur or arrhythmia; anomalous coronary circulation
Inspection	Fatigue, dizziness, or exertional syncope
Review of Systems	***Cardiovascular:*** Arrhythmia during exercise Palpitations ***Respiratory:*** The patient may describe shortness of breath. ***Gastrointestinal:*** Within normal limits ***Genitourinary:*** Within normal limits ***Neurologic:*** Possible referred pain to the left arm
Special Tests	Complete cardiovascular examination: Electrocardiogram, ultrasound imaging, and so on
Functional Assessment	A conscious individual will feel fatigued and possibly experience shortness of breath when lying down.
Imaging Techniques	Echocardiogram
Differential Diagnosis	Aortic stenosis, glycogen storage disease, cardiomyopathy
Comments	Individuals with hypertrophic cardiomyopathy are usually asymptomatic.

preemptive screening and referral for coronary disease. The individual usually has a history of previous symptoms. A strong family history of heart disease, hypertension, **hypercholesterolemia**, a history of smoking, excessive body weight, or a history of coronary artery disease are risk factors for heart attack.

Clinically, quick recognition of an acute attack and a rapid response provide the patient with the best chance of survival. After a living heart attack victim enters a hospital, the chance of survival increases 50%. Individuals suffering from a MI complain of intense pain in the chest, often radiating to the jaw, left shoulder, and arm. A typical finding of MI is profuse sweating, but this may be an unreliable finding in an athlete involved in vigorous physical activity. The lips and fingernails may appear cyanotic. Nausea or vomiting may be experienced. The pulse may be abnormally high and irregular for some time after exercise has been discontinued, and respirations may be quick and shallow. Evaluation of the blood pressure reveals hypotension because the ailing heart is not able to produce sufficient output.

Hypercholesterolemia A high blood cholesterol level caused by a high intake of saturated fats.

Examination Findings 15-7
Myocardial Infarction

Examination Segment	Clinical Findings
History	***Onset:*** Acute ***Pain characteristics:*** Intense chest pain, possibly radiating to the jaw, left shoulder, and arm ***Other symptoms:*** Possible sweating; difficulty breathing; anxiety ***Mechanism:*** Ischemia of the cardiac muscles ***Predisposing conditions:*** Family history of cardiac disease, hypertension, high blood cholesterol level, being overweight or obese, smoking, known atherosclerosis
Inspection	The patient may sweat profusely, even in the absence of vigorous activity.
Palpation	Sweat may be noted
Review of Systems	***Cardiovascular:*** Cyanosis is present. Rapid, irregular pulse is found. Blood pressure testing reveals hypotension. ***Respiratory:*** Shallow, rapid respirations are present. ***Gastrointestinal:*** Nausea and vomiting may occur. ***Genitourinary:*** Within normal limits ***Neurologic:*** Referred pain to left shoulder and arm
Functional Assessment	General reluctance to move
Imaging Techniques	Not applicable
Differential Diagnosis	Intercostal strain, shoulder injury, asthma, gastric reflux
Comments	Activate EMS. Continue to monitor the symptoms. If cardiac arrest occurs, initiate emergency cardiac care procedures. Treat the patient for shock.

The symptoms presented in Examination Findings 15-7 indicate the need to immediately transport the athlete for further assessment and treatment. These symptoms may become progressively more severe and result in death quite rapidly.

Arrhythmias

Arrhythmias, or irregular heart rhythms, can be relatively common in the athletic population. Although many causes of arrhythmia are benign or can be controlled through the use of medications, others are potentially fatal. Any reported arrhythmia or those discovered during a physical examination requires further evaluation by a cardiologist to prescribe the appropriate management and determine the patient's appropriate activity level.

Tachycardia

Tachycardia, an increased heart rate, can be characterized as a normal response to a stressful circumstance. Other causes of tachycardia can result in sudden death. Clinically, individuals with tachycardia may become excessively fatigued, describe exertional syncope, and experience a sensation of the heart's "racing." Evaluation of the pulse can reveal sustained heart rates in excess of

200 bpm. The inefficient pumping action of the heart results in a decreased blood pressure.

An athlete suspected to be suffering from tachycardia and presenting with a normal **sinus rhythm** should be withheld from activity and referred for further evaluation by a physician. Sustained tachycardia indicates that the patient be transported to a medical facility by trained personnel because this condition can degenerate into ventricular fibrillation and result in sudden death.

Athlete's heart

The increased cardiac pressures associated with isometric or repetitive and intense exercise can result in physiologic and anatomic changes in the heart.[2,6] Dilation of the left ventricle, enlargement of the cardiac chambers, increased thickness of the ventricular walls, and a reduced heart rate are the most common findings associated with athlete's heart syndrome.[6] During a physical examination, these can appear as cardiac abnormalities, with EKGs showing sinus bradycardia, early repolarization, and possible left ventricular hypertrophy.[4]

Athlete's heart syndrome often mimics (or may mask) other significant cardiovascular conditions such as myocardial ischemia, hypertrophic cardiomyopathy (the most common cause of sudden cardiac death), dilated cardiomyopathy, and pericarditis.[2] Doppler cardiac imaging is often required to make a differential diagnosis among these conditions.[62]

The changes associated with athlete's heart syndrome are reversible by decreasing the intensity, frequency, and duration of exercise.[6,63] It is unclear if this condition is a precursor to sudden death.

Mitral valve prolapse

Approximately 5% of the population suffers from mitral valve prolapse (MVP).[38,39] Prolapse occurs after the valve has closed. The subsequent pressure from the backflow of blood causes the valve to collapse, resulting in the regurgitation of blood back into the ventricle. Many athletes with MVP are able to participate in vigorous activity. Athletes with documented arrhythmogenic syncope, family history of sudden death associated with MVP, experience tachycardia or ventricular arrhythmia with exercise, have documented moderate or marked mitral regurgitation, or have had a previous embolic event should be restricted to low-intensity athletic activities.

Hypertension

High blood pressure, the most common cardiovascular abnormality affecting athletes, is more prevalent in the African-American population than in other groups.[64] In addition, hypertension is the most common cardiovascular condition in competitive athletes.[10] Increased peripheral vascular resistance to blood flow secondary to vasoconstriction increases the pressure required to force blood through the vessels.

Although systolic pressures greater than 140 mm Hg and diastolic pressures greater than 90 mm Hg are the clinical benchmarks for hypertension, the patient's average blood pressure should be compared with the normative data reflecting the patient's gender, age, height, and weight. Because of the prevalence of hypertension and its multiple health consequences, pre-hypertension values of 120 to 139 mm Hg for systolic and 80 to 89 mm Hg for diastolic may warrant intervention.

Many variables influence blood pressure, including the possible anxiety associated with the procedure itself. Elevated readings must be produced on several separate occasions for a diagnosis of hypertension to be made.

After the presence of hypertension has been established, its cause must be identified so that appropriate intervention can take place. Unregulated hypertension can result in MI, stroke, kidney failure, and disturbances in vision. Most people with controlled hypertension can safely participate in sports, assuming that no other associated organ damage has occurred and there is no evidence of concomitant cardiac disease. Individuals with unregulated hypertension should be limited to low-intensity activities and be closely monitored. Those with significant hypertension should have their blood pressure measured at least every 2 months to monitor the effects of exercise or medications on the disease.

Respiratory Pathologies

Asthma

Asthma is caused by a narrowing of the bronchial tree, resulting in difficulty breathing. This narrowing results from an increase in mucosal secretions, bronchospasm, or both. Asthma can be divided into two groups—extrinsic or intrinsic—as determined by the predisposing cause of the condition. **Extrinsic asthma** is caused by allergens such as hay fever, insect stings, pollen, animal **dander**, or foods. The cause of **intrinsic asthma** is less well defined, but the most common type in athletes is triggered by exercise.

Asthma is characterized by dry wheezing during respiration, an event that may be frightening to the person affected and the bystanders (Examination Findings 15-8). During an acute episode, chest tightness is associated with experienced during inspiration, but the primary limitation is associated with expiration. If a partial obstruction occurs high in the airway, as withlaryngeal injury, inspiration is commonly more difficult than expiration. It is common for asthmatic athletes to experience repeated dry coughing during the asthma attack.

Sinus rhythm Rhythm of the heart, regulated by the Sinoatrial node.

Dander Small scales from animal hair or feathers that cause allergic reactions in some individuals.

Examination Findings 15-8
Asthma

Examination Segment	Clinical Findings
History	***Onset:*** Congenital or acquired disease; acute attacks ***Pain characteristics:*** Chest pain ***Other symptoms:*** Anxiety ***Mechanism:*** Bronchospasm caused by inflammatory triggers such as allergens or exercise ***Predisposing conditions:*** Poor air quality or exposure to allergens or other irritants such as tobacco smoke, perfumes, cold air, or exercise. Upper respiratory illnesses
Inspection	In pronounced attacks, the individual may use secondary muscles of inspiration (e.g., scalenes).
Review of Systems	***Cardiovascular:*** Increased heart rate ***Respiratory:*** In the chest, breathing is difficult, more so during expiration than inspiration. Wheezing, chest tightness, breathlessness, cough Peak flow meter indicates decreased expiratory volume. ***Gastrointestinal:*** Within normal limits ***Genitourinary:*** Within normal limits ***Neurologic:*** May experience tingling in extremities.
Special Tests	Allergy testing may be performed to determine triggers. Pulmonary function testing is used to monitor baseline levels.
Functional Assessment	Disruption in breathing makes physical activity impractical.
Imaging Techniques	Not applicable
Differential Diagnosis	Myocardial infarction, cystic fibrosis, foreign body in airway, upper respiratory infection
Comments	Many acute asthma attacks can be controlled quickly with the use of a short-acting bronchodilator such as albuterol. Correct use of the inhaler, including the use of a spacer, is critical to effective dosing and reversal of the bronchospasm. Maintenance drugs, such as inhaled corticosteroids or cromolyn are used to reduce the frequency and severity of asthma attacks and improve respiratory function. Peak flow meter is used to measure pulmonary function and is used in the diagnosis of asthma.

Extrinsic asthma attacks are precipitated by contact with one of the allergens. Exercise-induced asthma is most commonly caused by exercise in a cold, dry climate, as the cool air triggers the bronchospasm. Those with exercise-induced asthma usually have fewer symptoms during activities with brief periods of intense work; with exercise in a relatively warm, humid environment; and with improvement in their aerobic condition.

Individuals with asthma often have knowledge of their condition before participating in organized sports. Athletes often use preparticipation medication and carry inhalers with rescue drugs that reverse bronchospasm.

Table 15-10 Peak Expiratory Flow Rate Grading

Color	Zone	Meaning
Green	80%–100% of personal best	All clear. No asthma symptoms are present. Routine treatment plan can be followed. For patients who use medications on a daily basis, consistent measurements in the green zone may allow them to reduce their medications under their physician's guidance.
Yellow	50%–80% of personal best	**Caution:** An acute attack may be present. Temporary increase in medications may be needed. Consistent readings in this zone may indicate that the condition is not being managed with the current dosage of medications and may need to be increased.
Red	Below 50% of personal best	Medical alert. Immediate use of bronchodilators is indicated. If levels do not return immediately to the yellow or green zone after use of the medication, the physician should be notified.

This information should be included in the athlete's medical record, and may necessitate carrying medication for the athlete in case of emergency.

The peak expiratory flow rate (PEFR) should remain steady or increase after an episode of exercise. After exercise, PEFR decreases of 15%[65,66] and 10%[67] or greater from pre-exercise levels may indicate exercise-induced asthma. Unrecognized, this condition leads to increased fatigue and decreased performance (Table 15-10).

In athletes with diagnosed asthma, routine measurements are compared with a baseline to monitor the condition. The baseline is a personal best measurement that represents the highest measurement the patient has attained over a 2- to 3-week period. After establishing the personal best, the goal is to reach this baseline every day. Guidelines for management of asthma have been developed under the National Asthma Education Guidelines for the Diagnosis and Management of Asthma. These guidelines are color coded as green, yellow, and red, similar to a traffic light so they are easier to remember.

Hyperventilation

Conditions such as asthma, **metabolic acidosis**, **pulmonary edema**, and anxiety can increase the minute volume ventilation rate by increasing the respiratory rate. Subsequently, the body's oxygen and carbon dioxide levels are skewed by decreasing the level of carbon dioxide and increasing the level of oxygen. This imbalance results in dizziness, tracheal spasm, an increased heart rate, and, eventually, fainting. As soon as the oxygen and carbon dioxide levels are stabilized, the symptoms quickly subside.

On-Field Examination of Thoracic, Abdominal, and Cardiopulmonary Pathologies

The athlete suffering from cardiopulmonary problems undergoes inspection while being questioned about his or her complaints. In the case of an unconscious athlete, the examiner must always follow standard first-responder procedures, checking the airway, breathing, and circulation before any other assessment. In either case, the examiner must be prepared to perform lifesaving procedures if the athlete's condition warrants it. A quick, precise, and prudent decision-making process is needed to give the athlete the optimum chance of survival (Fig. 15-18).

A standardized emergency cardiac care response is essential to the recovery from a cardiac event.[68] Because a cardiopulmonary condition must be quickly assessed, the inspection and pertinent palpation that goes along with the inspection are covered together, just as they are carried out together during this type of evaluation. In the event that a person is unconscious the emergency medical system must be activated immediately.

Examination of the Unconscious Athlete

- **Airway:** The first area to be inspected in the unconscious athlete is the integrity of the airway. Before checking the airway, however, stabilize the cervical spine in a neutral position if there is any possibility of head or neck injury (see Chapter 21). If the athlete is wearing a mouthpiece, it must be removed. The examiner then looks, listens, and feels for air being expired and observes for the rise and fall of the chest (see Fig. 2-2).
- **Breathing**: From the position used to inspect for a functional airway, the examiner assesses the breathing pattern and rate. A rate of fewer than 10 (**bradypnea**) or greater than 30 breaths per minute (**tachypnea**) requires assisted ventilation by properly trained personnel.[21] A labored, quick breathing pattern (**dyspnea**) is usually associated with some type of airway obstruction. Athletes with underlying pulmonary disease

Metabolic acidosis Decreased blood pH caused by an increase in blood acids or a decrease in blood bases.

Pulmonary edema Swelling of the lung and its tissues.

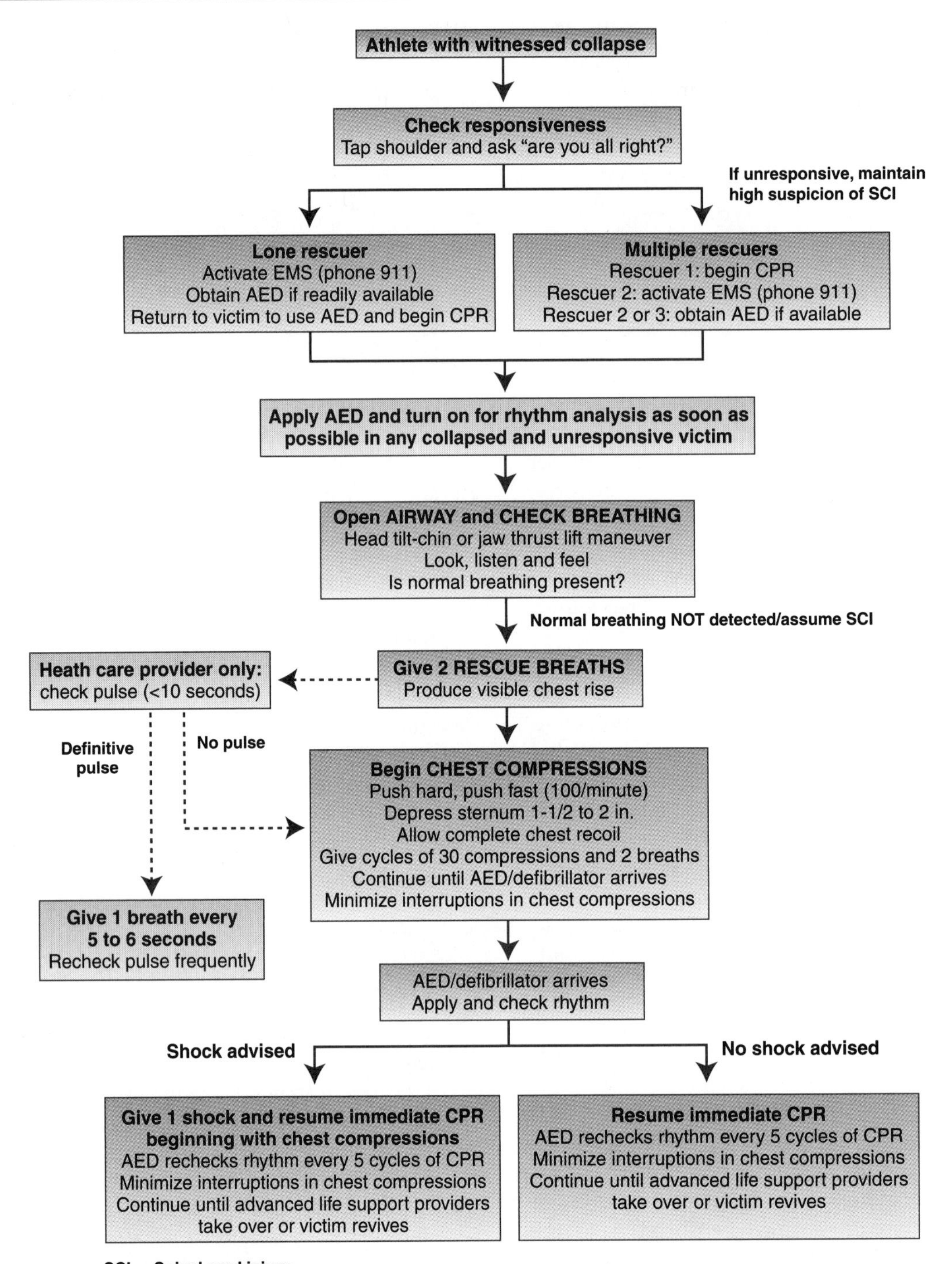

FIGURE 15-18 ■ Management of sudden cardiac arrest. AED = automated external defibrillator; CPR = cardiopulmonary resuscitation; EMS = emergency medical services; SCA = sudden cardiac arrest; SCI = spinal cord injury. (From Drezner, JA, et al. Inter-association task force recommendations on emergency preparedness and management of sudden cardiac arrest in high school and college athletic programs: A consensus statement. *J Athl Train*, 42:143, 2007.)

such as asthma or cystic fibrosis have labored breathing from obstruction by bronchospasm or excessive mucus formation. Athletes suffering from cardiac conditions may have difficulty breathing because of pain, but breathing is usually not as labored in these athletes as it is in those with pulmonary disorders.

- **Circulation**: The status of the circulation and thus the heart rate is assessed primarily by taking the pulse. While checking the airway and breathing, the examiner palpates for the carotid pulse.

Inspection and Palpation of the Conscious Athlete

- **Position of the athlete:** The athlete with cardiac problems will most likely be clutching the chest, possibly bending over in pain. The athlete with a pulmonary problem may be bent over with hands on the knees so that the secondary muscles of respiration may be used to aid breathing. By putting the hands in a closed chain position, the sternocleidomastoid and pectoral muscles can aid in expanding the chest wall. In labored breathing, these muscles may be observed to be contracting forcefully. The athlete may recruit the secondary muscles of respiration by sitting with the elbows on the knees and the head hanging between the legs.
- **Skin color**: The color of the athlete's skin is normally flushed because of exercise. Cardiopulmonary distress results in pale or ashen skin. First appearing in the lips, the discoloration progresses to cyanosis as the skin's tissues are deprived of oxygen. An unexpected change in skin tone or color from that which is normally associated with exercise should be a "red flag" for the examiner.
- **Airway**: The fact that an athlete is conscious does not rule out an airway obstruction, but the athlete's ability to speak indicates a viable airway. It should be established that the athlete has not swallowed any part of the mouthpiece, food, or other material, by direct inspection and by simply asking the athlete if he or she has swallowed anything.
- **Breathing**: The breathing pattern is established for the conscious athlete suspected of having a cardiopulmonary problem. The method of establishing the rate and pattern of respiration is described on page 578.
- **Circulation**: Although it is obvious that the conscious athlete's heart is beating, the pulse must be assessed for rate and quality at the carotid artery. The pulse should be frequently monitored and should return to normal levels within 5 minutes after cessation of the activity. A pulse rate that remains elevated may indicate underlying cardiac pathology.
- **Sweating**: Anyone suffering from cardiac problems may perspire profusely. However, the athlete involved in vigorous physical activity normally exhibits perspiration as a result of the activity. In the absence of physical activity, complaints of chest pain and profuse sweating are classic symptoms of cardiac distress.
- **Responsiveness**: In general, the athlete suffering from a cardiac condition becomes lethargic and weak. Many conditions of the heart decrease left ventricular outflow, resulting in a decreased cardiac output and depriving the tissues of oxygen.[22] The athlete may also suffer from syncope, the causes of which are discussed earlier in this chapter.
- **Nausea and vomiting**: Acute myocardial infarction (MI) often brings about nausea and vomiting.[23]

During the assessment of a conscious athlete with symptoms of cardiopulmonary distress, deterioration in vital signs warrants immediate activation of an emergency medical system.

On-Field Management of Thoracic, Abdominal, and Cardiopulmonary Pathologies

The most important aspects of the management of a patient with suspected cardiopulmonary injury or illness are the basic ABCs of first aid. The examiner must establish that the athlete has an airway, breathing is occurring, and circulation is present. Unfortunately for some of these athletes, such as those suffering from hypertrophic cardiomyopathy, illnesses not identified before participation may be fatal despite the most heroic lifesaving measures.

For other cardiac conditions in which breathing and a pulse have been established, the most important task of the athletic trainer is to initiate the emergency management system. Beyond this, the athletic trainer must take control of the situation and keep the athlete and bystanders as calm as possible. Vital signs should be continually monitored and documented until assistance arrives.

All coaches, facilities coordinators, and other individuals who supervise athletic activities should maintain certification in cardiopulmonary resuscitation (CPR). An emergency action plan as described in Chapter 2 should be developed and rehearsed at least annually.[68]

Because trauma to the thorax and abdomen is most often the result of acute, high-velocity impact, the need for on-field evaluation of these conditions is commonplace. At first, injuries to the internal organs may produce only the signs and symptoms of a contusion overlying the impact area. As blood collects within the viscera, outward symptoms of the underlying condition are produced.

Rib Fractures

Typically, athletes suffering a rib cage injury leave the area of athletic activity under their own power. In the case of a frank rib fracture or multiple rib fractures, the athlete may not be able to move and must be evaluated on the field. If the presence of a rib fracture is established, further evaluation must be performed to rule out the presence of a pneumothorax or hemothorax. In the absence of these conditions, the athlete is calmed and the area is stabilized before the athlete can be assisted from the field. The area may be stabilized by the use of a rib belt or, more commonly, by wrapping the ipsilateral arm to the side of the athlete with a swathe (Fig. 15-19). The athlete can then be assisted off the field and transported to a medical facility for further evaluation.

Pneumothorax and Hemothorax

Patients suspected of having a pneumothorax or hemothorax require continuous vital sign monitoring, treatment for shock, and placement on the affected side in a semireclined position, if possible. Oxygen is provided, if available. The immediate and potentially life-saving management of a tension pneumothorax includes insertion of a large-bore needle into the space between the second and third ribs. Prepare to assist with respiration if needed and activate the emergency medical system.

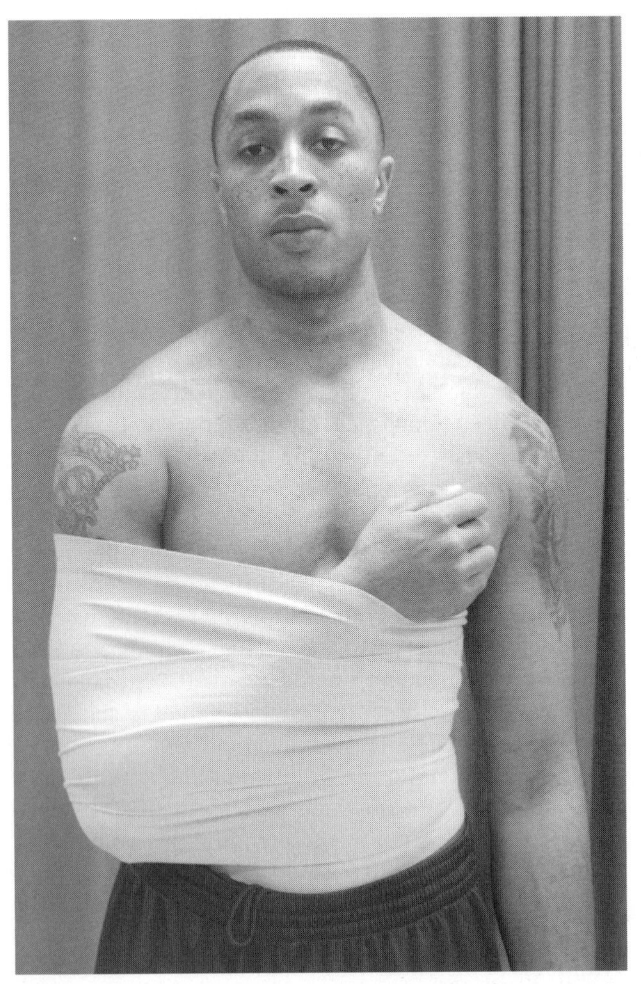

FIGURE 15-19 ■ Immobilization of the rib cage through the use of a swath. The arm of the involved side may be immobilized to reduce pain that is secondary to movement of the shoulder.

Open Pneumothorax

An open pneumothorax can result from an open rib fracture that also pierces the pleural cavity or from a puncture by an external object (e.g., javelin). An open pneumothorax is characterized by a sucking sound as the athlete attempts to inhale air.

Do not attempt to remove an object that has impaled the athlete. Cover the opening with a sterile dressing and seal it with a nonporous material (e.g., a plastic bag) to prevent the passage of air through the opening (Fig. 15-20). Oxygen may be administered to decrease the amount of respiratory distress.

Hollow Organ Injuries

Suspected injury to a hollow organ is viewed as a medical emergency. Treat the athlete for shock. For comfort, place the athlete's legs in a hook-lying position and cover him or her with a blanket to maintain body temperature. Continuously monitor and record vital signs, including the time they are taken. These readings should be given to the medical transport team to be delivered with the athlete to the medical facility.

Under no circumstances should the athlete be given anything by mouth. Oral ingestion of solids or liquids may induce vomiting, further injuring the athlete, or may complicate the task of anesthetizing the athlete for any surgical procedure that may be needed.

Solar Plexus Injury

The solar plexus (celiac plexus) is injured when an athlete suffers a direct blow to the abdomen or falls on an object, causing transitory paralysis of the diaphragm. The ensuing spasm results in the inability to inhale or, in layman's terms, "have the wind knocked out of you." The athlete is found in apparent respiratory distress, attempting to inspire and unable to communicate. The inability to breathe accompanied by the inability to communicate often leads to panic in the athlete, a condition that warrants treatment equal to that of the injury itself.

Unlike an athlete with an obstruction to the airway who grasps at the throat, this athlete tends to hold the abdomen where the insulting blow was received. Regardless, the examiner must immediately rule out that the airway has been obstructed such as by the athlete's mouthpiece, tooth, or gum.

Although the spasm is a self-limiting condition, the examiner must take actions to hasten the recovery process by reassuring the athlete and using a firm, confident voice.

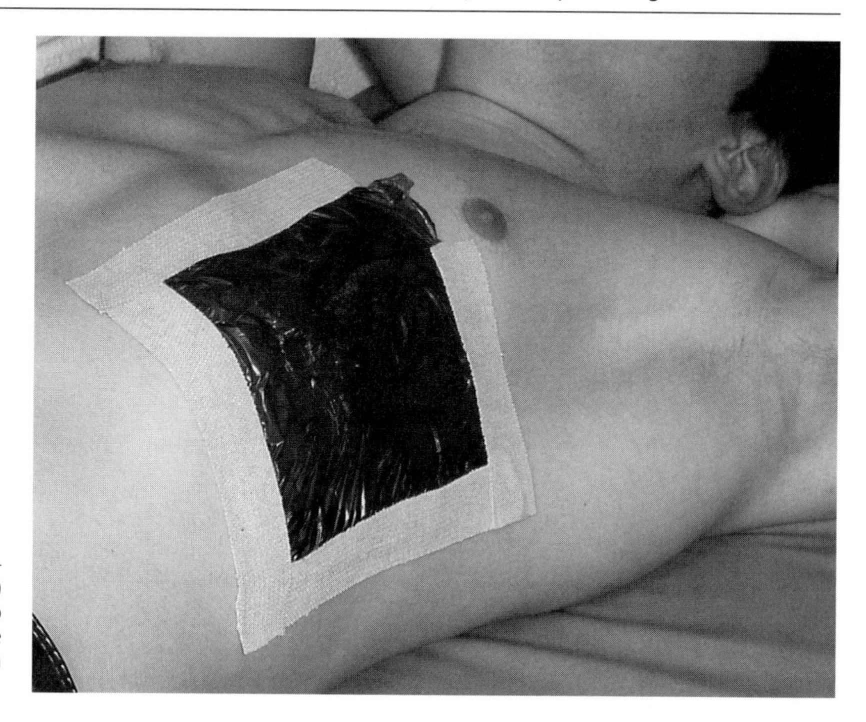

FIGURE 15-20 ■ Management of an open pneumothorax. A one-way valve (upper left-hand corner) is created over the open wound that allows air to escape during exhalation. During inhalation, the valve seals, forcing air to enter the lungs through the trachea.

Loosening the athlete's clothes is helpful in lessening the perception of pressure on the abdomen. Instruct the athlete to breathe using long inspirations and short expirations. Also, instructions for the athlete to "pant like a dog" assists in relaxing the diaphragm. Reassuring the athlete further aids in relaxing the spasm. As the athlete's breathing is controlled, obtain a history from the athlete and rule out further internal injury through palpation of the abdomen and monitoring of the athlete's condition, including assessing vital signs as necessary.

Asthma

Athletes with asthma can usually manage their own condition and may or may not require the athletic trainer's direct assistance. Proper management of these conditions includes having the athletes' medications on hand and marked as belonging to them and by making them quickly available to the athlete. These athletes are usually well versed in use of and capable of dispensing their own medication but should be assisted as needed.

Under ideal circumstances, athletes suffering from asthma have been assessed and placed on a nonpharmacologic and pharmacologic treatment program as needed to control their disease.[67] Nonpharmacologic treatment includes patient and family education and cardiovascular fitness evaluation. Pharmacologic treatments include the use of drugs to decrease airway inflammation and inhaled bronchodilators 15 minutes before exercise.

All athletes who have been previously identified as having asthma should carry an inhaler to administer a short-acting bronchodilator. The inhaler should be used with a spacer between the device and the athlete's mouth so that the medication is sufficiently aerated for inhalation. In circumstances requiring the use of an inhaler, the athletic trainer should assist the athlete by ensuring that he or she is using the inhaler and is moved to the sidelines until the breathing becomes controlled.

If the athlete does not have an inhaler available, the situation must be managed as a pulmonary emergency. Because the primary problem is in exhaling rather than inhaling, the athlete should attempt to perform controlled diaphragmatic breathing, using the abdominal muscles to slowly, yet forcefully, push the air from the lungs. Placing the athlete in a sitting position with the arms resting on the knees assists in expiration.

Typically, the athlete suffering from an exercise-induced asthma attack experiences the symptoms approximately 10 minutes after beginning exercise. Managed with inhalers and cessation of exercise, the athlete's symptoms usually cease after 30 minutes. In some cases, the symptoms worsen before they clear.[69] More than half of athletes with exercise-induced asthma experience a refractory period after asthma attacks. During this 2-hour period, the athlete seems resistant to a recurrence of the symptoms while performing similar activities.[70]

Hyperventilation

Athletes who are hyperventilating can be managed by controlling the rate at which carbon dioxide is lost from the body. The traditional method involves having the athlete breathe into a paper bag (not a plastic bag) held tightly around the mouth and nose (Fig. 15-21). An alternative method involves having the athlete breathe through only one nostril by holding the opposite nostril closed.

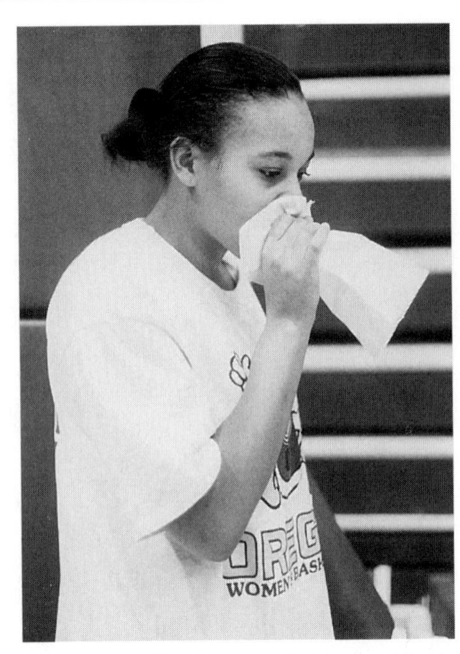

FIGURE 15-21 ■ Controlling hyperventilation. Breathing into a paper bag recirculates carbon dioxide in the respiratory system and reestablishes the body's oxygen–carbon dioxide balance.

Sudden Cardiac Arrest

Sudden cardiac arrest must be managed using a standardized approach that is emphasized in all emergency cardiac care courses. Key features of managing cardiac arrest include early activation of the emergency medical system and early defibrillation. For every 1 minute that defibrillation is delayed, the chance of survival decreases by 10%.

REFERENCES

1. Amaral, JF: Thoracoabdominal injuries in the athlete. *Clin Sports Med*, 16:739, 1997.
2. O'Brien, DL, and Rogers, IR: Athlete's heart syndrome: A diagnostic dilemma in the emergency department. *Emerg Med*, 11:277, 1999.
3. Sen-Chowdhry, S, and McKenna, WJ: Sudden cardiac death in the young: A strategy for prevention by targeted evaluation. *Cardiology*, 105:196, 2006.
4. Leski, M: Sudden cardiac death in athletes. *South Med J*, 97:861, 2004.
5. Lyznicki, JM, Nielsen, NH, and Schneider, JF: Cardiovascular screening of student athletes. *Am Fam Phys*, 62:765, 2000.
6. Lorvidhaya, P, and Huang, SKS: Sudden cardiac death in athletes. *Cardiology*, 100:186, 2003.
7. Giese, EA, et al: The athletic preparticipation evaluation: Cardiovascular assessment. *Am Fam Physician*, 75:1008, 2007.
8. Yen, K, et al: Interexaminer reliability in physical examination of pediatric patients with abdominal pain. *Arch Pediatr Adolesc Med*, 159:373, 2005.
9. McAlister, FA, and Straus, SE: Measurement of blood pressure: An evidence based review. *BMJ*, 322:908, 2001.
10. Kaplan, NM, Deveraux, RB, and Miller, HS: Task force 4: systemic hypertension. *J Am Coll Cardiol*, 24:885, 1994.
11. Edmonds, ZV, et al: The reliability of vital sign measurements. *Ann Emerg Med*, 39:233, 2002.
12. Karnath, B, and Thornton, W: Auscultation of the heart. *Hosp Physician*, 39, 2002.
13. Karnath, G, and Boyars, MC: Pulmonary auscultation. *Hosp Physician*, 22, 2002.
14. Brooks, D, and Thomas, J: Interrater reliability of auscultation of breath sounds among physical therapists. *Phys Ther*, 75:1082, 1995.
15. Aaron, SD, Dales, RE, and Cardinal, P: How accurate is spirometry at predicting restrictive pulmonary impairment? *Chest*, 115:869, 1999.
16. Simerville, JA, Maxted, WC, and Pahira, JJ: Urinalysis: A comprehensive review. *Am Fam Physician*, 71:1153, 2005.
17. Colosimo, AJ, et al: Acute traumatic first-rib fracture in the contact athlete. *Am J Sports Med*, 32:1310, 2004.
18. O'Kane, J, O'Kane, E, and Marquet, J: Delayed complication of a rib fracture. *Am J Sports Med*, 26:69, 1998.
19. Proffer, DS, Patton, JJ, and Jackson, DW: Nonunion of a first rib fracture in a gymnast. *Am J Sports Med*, 19:198, 1991.
20. Wasik, M, and McFarland, M: Rib stress fractures: An overview (poster presentation). *J Athl Train*, 27:156, 1992.
21. Brukner, P, and Khan, K: Stress fracture of the neck of the seventh and eighth ribs: A case report. *Clin J Sport Med*, 6:204, 1996.
22. Taimela, S, Kujala, UM, and Orava, S: Two consecutive rib stress fractures in a female competitive swimmer. *Clin J Sport Med*, 5:254, 1995.
23. Lord, MJ, Ha, KI, and Song, KS: Stress fractures of the ribs in golfers. *Am J Sports Med*, 24:118, 1996.
24. Christiansen, E, and Kanstrup, IL: Increased risk of stress fractures of the ribs in elite rowers. *Scand J Med Sci Sports*, 7:49, 1997.
25. Gregory, PL, Biswas, AC, and Batt ME: Musculoskeletal problems of the chest wall in athletes. *Sports Med*, 32:235, 2002.
26. Schramel, FM, Postmus, PE, and Vanderschueren, RG: Current aspects of spontaneous pneumothorax. *Eur Respir J*, 10:1372, 1997.
27. Partridge, RA, et al: Sports-related pneumothorax. *Ann Emerg Med*, 30:539. 1997.
28. Dietzel, DP, and Ciullo, JV: Spontaneous pneumothorax after shoulder arthroscopy: A report of four cases. *Arthroscopy*, 12:99, 1996.
29. Marnejon, T, Sarac, S, and Cropp, AJ: Spontaneous pneumothorax in weightlifters. *J Sports Med Phys Fitness*, 35:124, 1995.
30. Domingo, P, et al: Spontaneous rupture of the spleen associated with pneumonia. *Eur J Clin Microbiol Infect Dis*, 15:733, 1996.
31. Lippstone, MB, et al: Spontaneous splenic rupture and infectious mononucleosis in a forensic setting. *Del Med J*, 70:433, 1998.
32. Fernandes, CM: Splenic rupture manifesting two years after diagnosis of injury. *Acad Emerg Med*, 3:946, 1996.
33. Lawson, DE, et al: Splenic trauma: Value of follow-up CT. *Radiology*, 194:97, 1995.
34. Waninger, KN, and Harcke, HT: Determination of safe return to play for athletes recovering from infectious mononucleosis. *Clin J Sport Med*, 15:410, 2005.
35. Curhan, GC, et al: Family history and risk of kidney stones. *J Am Soc Nephrol*, 8:1568, 1997.

36. Najem, GR, et al: Stressful life events and risk of symptomatic kidney stones. *Int J Epidemiol,* 26:1017, 1997.
37. Cupisti, A, et al: Hypertension in kidney stone patients. *Nephron,* 73:569, 1996.
38. Massey, LK, and Whiting, SJ: Dietary salt, urinary calcium, and kidney stone risk. *Nutr Rev,* 53:131, 1995.
39. Curhan, CG, et al: Prospective study of beverage use and the risk of kidney stones. *Am J Epidemiol,* 143:240, 1996.
40. Hirvonen, T, et al: Nutrient intake and use of beverages and the risk of kidney stones among male smokers. *Am J Epidemiol,* 150:187, 1999.
41. Rutz-Danielczak, A, Pupek-Musialik, D, and Raszeja-Wanic, B: Effects of extracorporeal shock wave lithotripsy on renal function in patients with kidney stone disease. *Nephron,* 79:162, 1998.
42. Kharbanda, AB, et al: A clinical decision rule to identify children at low risk for appendicitis. *Pediatrics,* 116:709, 2005.
43. Bundy, DG, et al: Does this child have appendicitis? *JAMA,* 298:438, 2007.
44. Baker, B: Jejunal perforation occurring in contact sports. *Am J Sports Med,* 6:403, 1978.
45. Ringdahl, E, and Teague, L: Testicular torsion. *Am Fam Physician,* 74:1739, 2006.
46. Tanyel, FC, et al: Inguinal hernia revisited through comparative evaluation of peritoneum, processus vaginalis, and sacs obtained from children with hernia, hydrocele, and undescended testis. *J Pediatr Surg,* 34:552, 1999.
47. Pinczowski, D, et al: Occurrence of testicular cancer in patients operated on for cryptorchidism and inguinal hernia. *J Urol,* 146:1291, 1991.
48. Gallagher, RP, et al: Physical activity, medical history, and risk of testicular cancer. *Cancer Causes Control,* 6:398, 1995.
49. West, RV: The female athlete. The triad of disordered eating, amenorrhea, and osteoporosis. *Sports Med,* 26:63, 1998.
50. Otis, CL, et al: American College of Sports Medicine position stand. The female athlete triad. *Med Sci Sports Exerc,* 29:i, 1997.
51. Nattiv, A, et al: The female athlete triad. The inter-relatedness of disordered eating, amenorrhea, and osteoporosis. *Clin Sports Med,* 13:405, 1994.
52. Beals, KA, and Meyer, NL: Female athlete triad update. *Clin Sports Med,* 26:69, 2007.
53. McCroy, P: Commotio cordis: Instantaneous cardiac arrest caused by a blow to the chest depends on the timing of the blow relative to the cardiac cycle. *Br J Sports Med,* 36:236, 2002.
54. Madias, C, et al: Commotio cordis—sudden cardiac death with chest wall impact. *J Cardiovasc Electrophysiol,* 18:115, 2007.
55. Bode, F, et al: Ventricular fibrillation induced by stretch pulse: Implications for sudden death due to commotio cordis. *J Cardiovasc Electrophysiol,* 17:1011, 2006.
56. Salib, EA, et al: Efficacy of bystander cardiopulmonary resuscitation and out-of-hospital automated external defibrillation as life-saving therapy in commotio cordis. *J Pediatr,* 147:863, 2005.
57. Maron, BJ, Estes, NAM, and Link, MS: Task Force 11: Commotio Cordis. *JACC,* 45:1371, 2005.
58. Valani, R, Mikrogianakis, A, and Goldman, RD: Cardiac concussion (commotio cordis). *Can J Emerg Med,* 6:428, 2004.
59. Maron, BJ, et al: Death in a young athlete due to commotio cordis despite prompt external defibrillation. *Heart Rhythm,* 2:991, 2005.
60. Weiss, RL, et al: The usefulness of transesophageal echocardiography in diagnosing cardiac contusions. *Chest,* 109:73, 1996.
61. Verma, S, et al: Syncope in athletes: A guide to getting them back on their feet. *J Fam Pract,* 56:545, 2007.
62. D'Andrea, A, et al: The usefulness of Doppler myocardial imaging in the student of the athlete's heart and in the differential diagnosis between physiological and pathological ventricular hypertrophy. *Echocardiography,* 23:149, 2006.
63. Biffi, A, et al: Impact of physical deconditioning on ventricular tachyarrhythmias in trained athletes. *J Am Coll Cardiol,* 44:1053, 2004.
64. Strong, WB, and Steed, D: Cardiovascular evaluation of the young athlete. *Pediatr Clin North Am,* 29:1325, 1982.
65. Kukafka, DS, et al: Exercise-induced bronchospasm in high school athletes via a free running test: incidence and epidemiology. *Chest,* 114:1613, 1998.
66. Feinstein, RA, et al: Screening adolescent athletes for exercise-induced asthma. *Clin J Sports Med,* 6:119, 1996.
67. Kyle, JM, et al: Exercise-induced asthma in the young athlete: guidelines for routine screening and initial management. *Med Sci Sports Exerc,* 24:856, 1992.
68. Drezner, JA, et al: Inter-association task force recommendations on emergency preparedness and management of sudden cardiac arrest in high school and college athletic programs: A consensus statement. *J Athl Train,* 42:143, 2007.
69. McFadden, ER: Exercise-induced asthma. Assessment of current etiologic concepts. *Chest,* 91:151, 1987.
70. Schoeffel, RE, et al: Multiple exercise and histamine challenges in asthmatic patients. *Thorax,* 35:164, 1989.

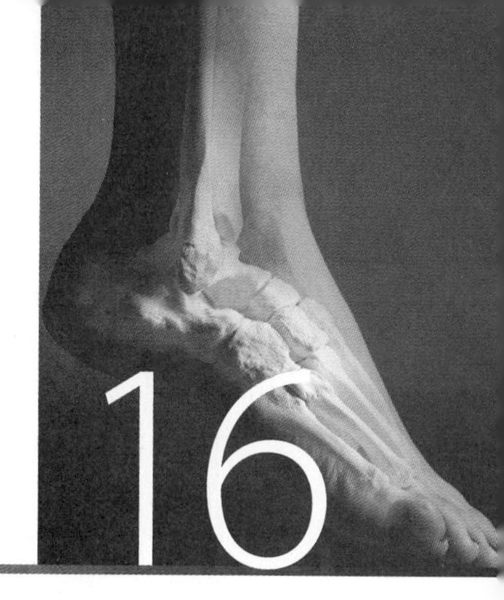

CHAPTER 16

Shoulder and Upper Arm Pathologies

The shoulder complex is perhaps the most complicated of the body's articulations because it must provide extensive yet precise range of motion (ROM) in all anatomical planes. The relationship between the glenohumeral (GH) joint and the scapula allows the humerus to be placed in 16,000 positions that can be differentiated in 1-degree increments.[1]

The shoulder complex lacks the intrinsic bony and ligamentous stabilizers that occur in other joints. Relying on its musculature to provide most of its stability, the shoulder complex in general, and specifically the GH joint, is inherently unstable. The GH joint, because of its poor bony stability and weak capsular structures, depends more on the proprioceptive and stabilizing function of its musculature than any other joint in the body.[2] Injury to the shoulder complex may occur from a direct force or secondary to forces transmitted proximally along the upper extremity. The shoulder complex also is predisposed to overuse conditions, especially in individuals participating in activities that require repeated overhead movements.

Clinical Anatomy

The upper extremity's only attachment to the axial skeleton is at the sternoclavicular (SC) joint. This configuration results in a mechanism whereby the arm is suspended from the torso by muscular attachments. The motions provided by the upper extremity arise from the intricate interactions of the four bones forming the shoulder girdle and the four articulations providing movement. Elevation describes the integrated movement of the glenohumeral, sternoclavicular, acromioclavicular, and scapulothoracic articulations as the arm is raised. Elevation can occur in the sagittal plane (flexion), frontal plane (abduction), and anywhere in between them.[3] The large ROM provided by the shoulder complex, especially the GH joint, is achieved at the expense of joint stability. Unlike the hip joint, which gains its stability through a deep ball-and-socket joint and strong ligamentous support (at the expense of mobility), the GH joint is characterized by shallow articular surfaces, inconsistent ligamentous support, and an increased reliance on dynamic support through muscle activity.

Bony Anatomy

The shoulder complex, formed by the sternum, clavicle, scapula, and humerus, may be likened to a series of hinges, pulleys, and levers working in unison to choreograph intricate motions in many anatomical planes (Fig. 16-1). A precise degree of ROM, strength, and coordination must be maintained between these bones to ensure efficient biomechanics.

The **manubrium** of the sternum serves as the site of attachment for each clavicle. Projecting above the body of the sternum, the superior surface of the manubrium is indented by the **jugular (suprasternal) notch**. Projecting off each side of the jugular notch is the **clavicular notch**, which accepts the medial head of the clavicle (Fig. 16-2).

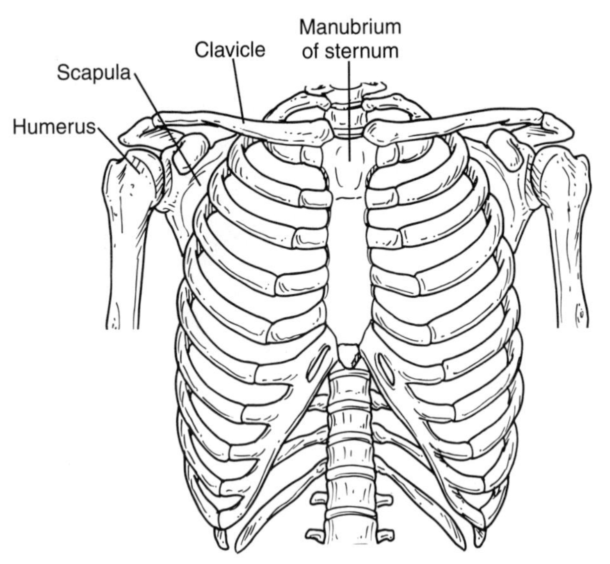

FIGURE 16-1 ■ Bones of the shoulder complex and glenohumeral joint.

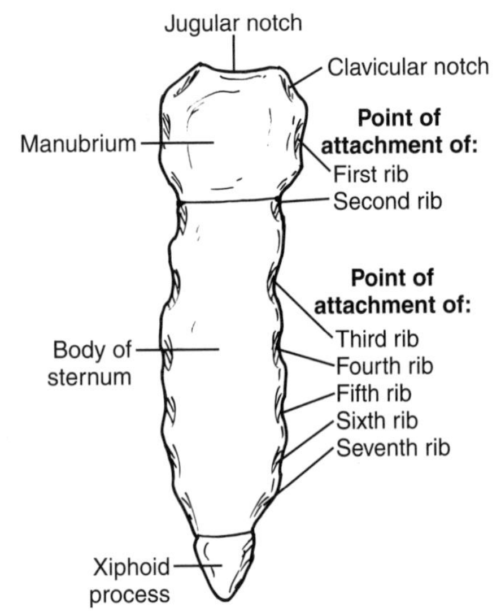

FIGURE 16-2 ■ The sternum, formed by the manubrium, body, and xiphoid process. In preadolescents, the junction between the manubrium and sternal body is pliable, but it fuses with age.

Serving as a strut between the sternum and scapula, the **clavicle** elevates and rotates to maintain the alignment of the scapula, allowing for additional motion when the arm is raised and preventing excessive anterior displacement of the scapula. The proximal two thirds of the clavicle is characterized by an anteriorly convex bend. The distal one third begins to flatten while curving concavely to meet with the scapula (Fig. 16-3). The point at which the clavicle begins to transition from a convex to a concave bend, approximately two thirds of the way along its shaft, is relatively weak and is a common site for fractures. The superior surface of the clavicle is not protected by muscle mass, making the bone susceptible to injury. The medial clavicular epiphysis is the

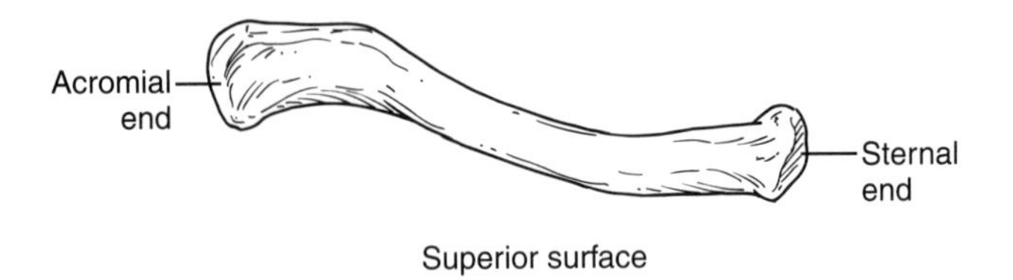

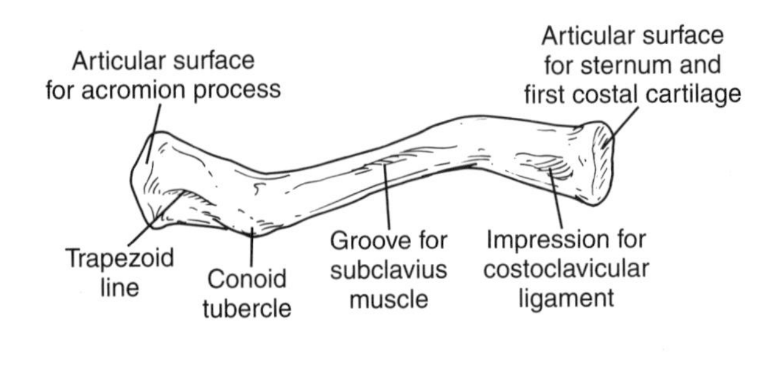

FIGURE 16-3 ■ Clavicle, superior and inferior views.

last growth plate in the body to ossify and does not fully fuse until approximately the age of 25.[4]

Having no direct bony or ligamentous attachment to the axial skeleton, the **scapula** gains its attachment to the torso by way of the clavicle. Its anterior surface is held against the torso by atmospheric pressure and muscle attachments. The scapula's unique form gives rise to its unique function of serving as both a lever and a pulley.

Thin and triangular, the scapula's anterior costal surface is concave, forming the **subscapular fossa**. The **vertebral (medial) border** is marked by the **inferior** and **superior angles**. The posterior surface is distinguished by the horizontal **scapular spine**, which divides the scapula into the large **infraspinous fossa** below and the smaller **supraspinous fossa** above. On the lateral end of the scapular spine is the anteriorly projecting **acromion process,** which articulates with the clavicle. Projecting inferiorly and anteriorly to the acromion is the beak-shaped **coracoid process**. The infraspinous, supraspinous, and subscapular fossae merge on the axial border to form the glenoid fossa. Located below the acromion, this fossa articulates with the humeral head (Fig. 16-4).

When the scapula is placed in its anatomical position, the glenoid fossa angles 30 degrees from the frontal plane and its face assumes a downward direction (Fig. 16-5).[5] The angle assumed by the face of the glenoid fossa, the **plane of the scapula**, provides a more functional arc for motion than the cardinal sagittal or frontal planes. This angle, in conjunction with the position of the scapula, places the rotator cuff muscles in their optimal length–tension relationship. For example, when reaching for an item on an overhead shelf, it is more natural to lift the arm in the plane of the scapula rather than lifting the arm through the sagittal or frontal planes.

The proximal end of the **humerus** is characterized by the medially projecting **humeral head** from the **anatomical neck** (Fig. 16-6). Bisecting the upper quarter of the

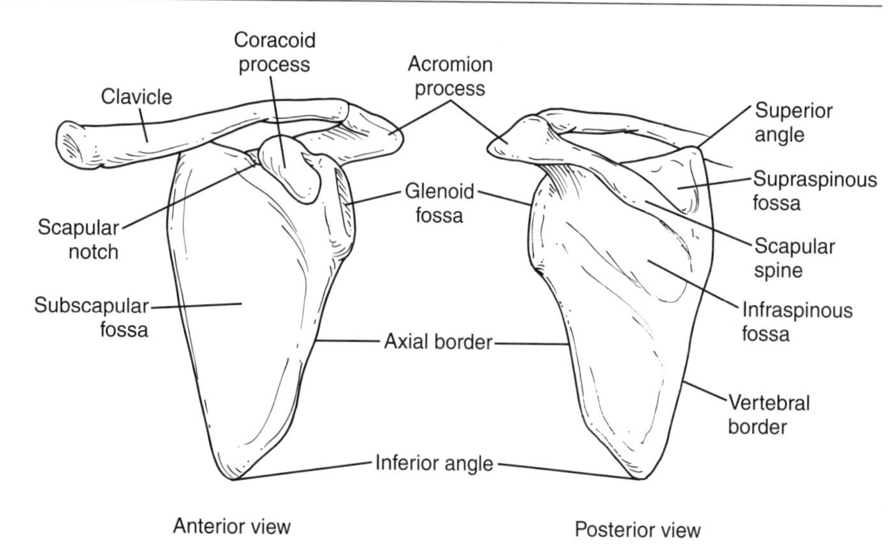

FIGURE 16-4 ■ Bony anatomy of the scapula, anterior (costal), and posterior (dorsal) views, showing the relationship with the clavicle.

anterior surface of the humerus, the **bicipital groove** (intertubercular groove) forms a canal through which the long head of the biceps tendon passes. The lateral edge of the groove is formed by the **greater tuberosity**. The medial border is formed by the **lesser tuberosity**. The inferior borders of the greater and lesser tuberosities mark the **surgical neck**, a name derived because fractures at this location generally require surgical intervention. Laterally and slightly above the midshaft is the insertion site for the deltoid muscle group, the **deltoid tuberosity**. The distal structures of the humerus are covered in Chapter 17.

The **angle of inclination** is the relationship between the shaft of the humerus and the humeral head in the frontal plane, normally 130 to 150 degrees. In the transverse plane, the relationship between the shaft of the humerus and the humeral head is the **angle of torsion**, which varies greatly from individual to individual (Fig. 16-7).[3] The humeral head is retroverted (twisted posteriorly from the frontal plane) approximately 30 degrees to permit optimal function in the plane of the scapula.[6] Decreased retroversion, which may be naturally occurring or an adaptive change to repetitive throwing, may be associated with internal rotator cuff impingement.[7]

Joints of the Shoulder Complex

The motion of the GH joint is augmented by the SC and **acromioclavicular (AC)** joints and the movement between the scapula and the thorax. A change in the mobility or function at any of these associated joints decreases the function at the GH joint.

Sternoclavicular joint

At the SC joint, the proximal portion of the clavicle meets the manubrium of the sternum and a portion of the first costal cartilage to form a gliding joint that allows 3 degrees

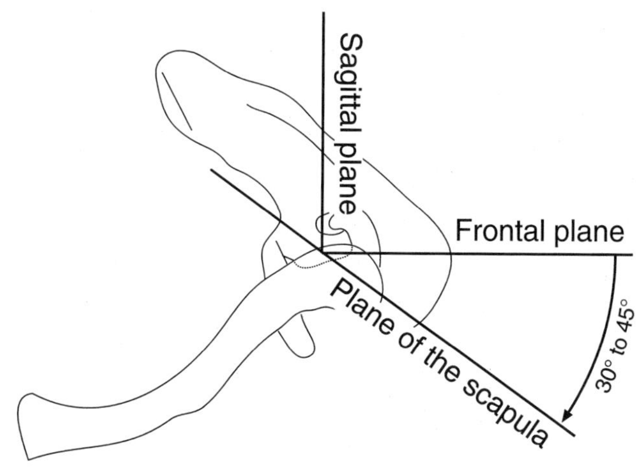

FIGURE 16-5 ■ Plane of the scapula. The face of the glenoid fossa sits at a 30° angle of horizontal adduction in the frontal plane. Movements within the plane of the scapula are more "natural" than movements in the cardinal plane.

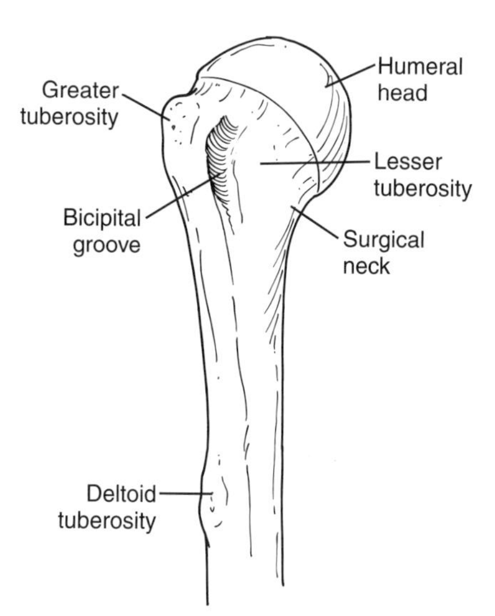

FIGURE 16-6 ■ Upper humerus, showing the prominent bony landmarks.

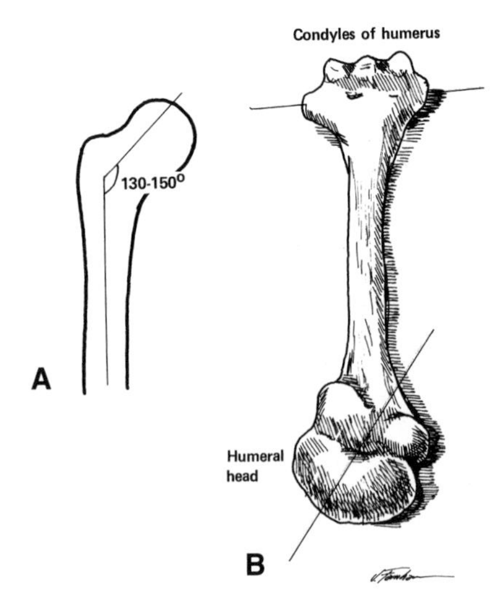

FIGURE 16-7 ■ Angular alignment of the humerus. **(A)** Angle of inclination representing the angle formed by the long axis of the humeral shaft and the axis of the humeral head. **(B)** Angle of torsion representing the relationship between the humeral condyles and the humeral head in the transverse plane. (Courtesy of Norkin, CC, and Levangie, PK: *Joint Structure and Function: A Comprehensive Analysis,* ed 2. Philadelphia, FA Davis, 1992.)

of freedom of motion: ***elevation*** and **depression**, **protraction** and **retraction**, and internal and external rotation. The SC joint axis lies lateral to the joint itself.[3]

The articulation between the manubrium and clavicle is inherently incongruent because the proximal end of the clavicle extends one half of its width above the manubrium (Fig. 16-8). Although the overall stability of the joint is enhanced by the presence of a fibrocartilaginous disk, the SC joint has the poorest bony stability of any of the major joints. Its strong ligamentous structure and protected location, however, makes it one of the least frequently dislocated joints.[4] Surrounded by a synovial membrane, the SC joint is supported by the anterior and posterior SC ligaments, the costoclavicular ligament, and the interclavicular ligament.

The **sternoclavicular disk**, which has qualities similar to the menisci found in the knee, functions as a shock absorber. The upper portion of the disk is attached to the clavicle, and its lower portion is attached to the manubrium and first costal cartilage. This disk divides the joint into two articular cavities, one between the disk and the clavicle and a second between the disk and the manubrium.

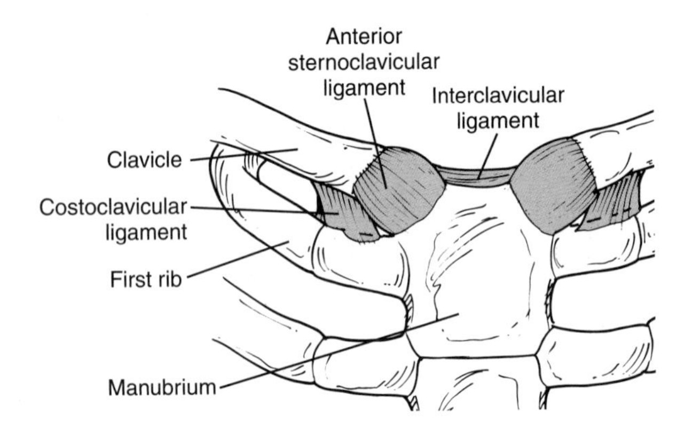

FIGURE 16-8 ■ Ligaments of the SC joint. Although the SC joint does not have inherent bony stability, the ligamentous arrangement provides great strength to the joint.

The synovial membrane is reinforced by the **anterior** and **posterior sternoclavicular ligaments**. Whereas the anterior fibers resist posterior displacement of the clavicle on the manubrium, the posterior fibers resist anterior displacement. The costoclavicular ligament serves as an axis of clavicular elevation and depression and protraction and retraction.

The SC joints are joined to each other by the **interclavicular ligament**. Attaching to the superior proximal ends of the left and right clavicles, the ligament has a common connection on the superior border of the sternum. The interclavicular ligament resists downward movement of the clavicle and assists in dissipating force across the entire upper extremity.

The **costoclavicular ligament** (rhomboid ligament) arises from the superior aspect of the first rib and connects to the inferior aspect of the clavicle. Likewise, the posterior fibers limit elevation and medial movement of the clavicle. The anterior fibers resist clavicular elevation from the superior pull of the sternomastoid and sternohyoid muscles and limits medial translation of the clavicle.[3]

The acromioclavicular joint

The distal end of the clavicle meets the acromion process of the scapula to form the AC joint. A plane synovial joint, the AC joint allows a gliding articulation between the acromion and the clavicle, capable of 3 degrees of freedom of movement, each around an oblique axis: (1) internal and external rotation around a vertical axis, (2) upward and downward rotation around an axis perpendicular to the plane of the scapula, and (3) anterior and posterior **scapular tipping** around a horizontal axis. This articulation allows for the motion necessary to maintain the relationship between the scapula and the clavicle in the early and late stages of the GH joint's ROM.

Surrounded by a synovial membrane, the AC joint is supported by the AC ligament and the **coracoclavicular ligament**, which suspend the scapula from the clavicle (Fig. 16-9). A synovial disk is present between the clavicle and the acromion that disappears by the second decade of life.

Divided into two separate bands, the superior and inferior portions of the AC ligament function to maintain continuity between the articulating surfaces of the acromion and clavicle. With much of its restraint in the horizontal plane, this ligament maintains stability by preventing the clavicle from riding up and over the acromion process.

Most of the AC joint's intrinsic stability arises from the coracoclavicular ligament, a structure extrinsic to the joint. This ligament is divided into two distinct portions: the lateral

Scapular tipping The inferior angle of the scapula moving away from the thorax while its superior border moves toward the thorax.

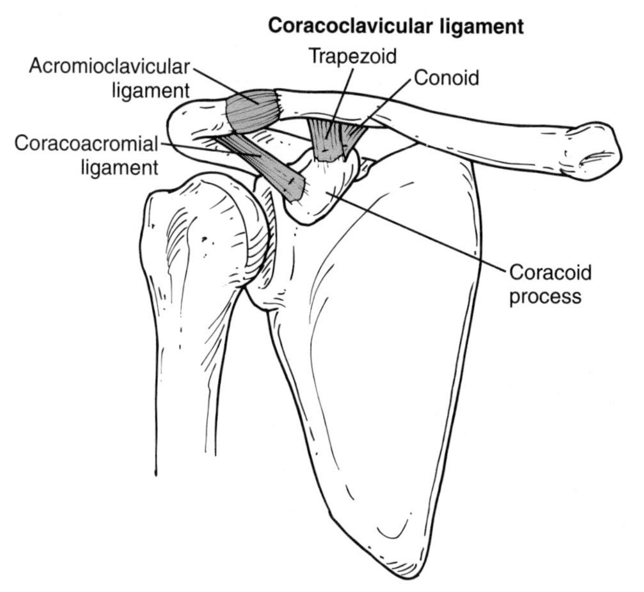

FIGURE 16-9 ■ Ligaments of the acromioclavicular joint. The acromioclavicular ligament provides anterior/posterior stability to the joint. The two portions of the coracoclavicular ligament prevent superior/inferior displacement of the clavicle on the scapula.

quadrilateral-shaped trapezoid ligament and the medial triangular-shaped conoid ligament. Separated by a bursa, the **trapezoid ligament** limits lateral movement of the clavicle over the acromion. The **conoid ligament** restricts superior movement of the clavicle. Acting jointly, these ligaments limit rotation of the scapula and provide some degree of horizontal stability. The conoid portion of the ligament is critical for the passive posterior rotation of the clavicle that occurs during shoulder elevation. However, a horizontal dislocation of the AC joint can occur with the coracoclavicular ligament remaining intact.

The scapulothoracic articulation

The articulation between the scapula and the posterior rib cage is not a true anatomical joint because it lacks the typical synovial joint characteristics of connection by fibrous, cartilaginous, or synovial tissues. The scapulothoracic articulation moves only in response to AC and SC joint movement. For example, when the arm is abducted, the scapulothoracic articulation must upwardly rotate, externally rotate, and posteriorly tip (Fig. 16-10).[3] Changes in mobility at either the AC or SC joints influence the movement of the scapulothoracic articulation.

The glenohumeral joint

Formed by the head of the humerus and the scapula's glenoid fossa, the GH articulation is a ball-and-socket joint capable of

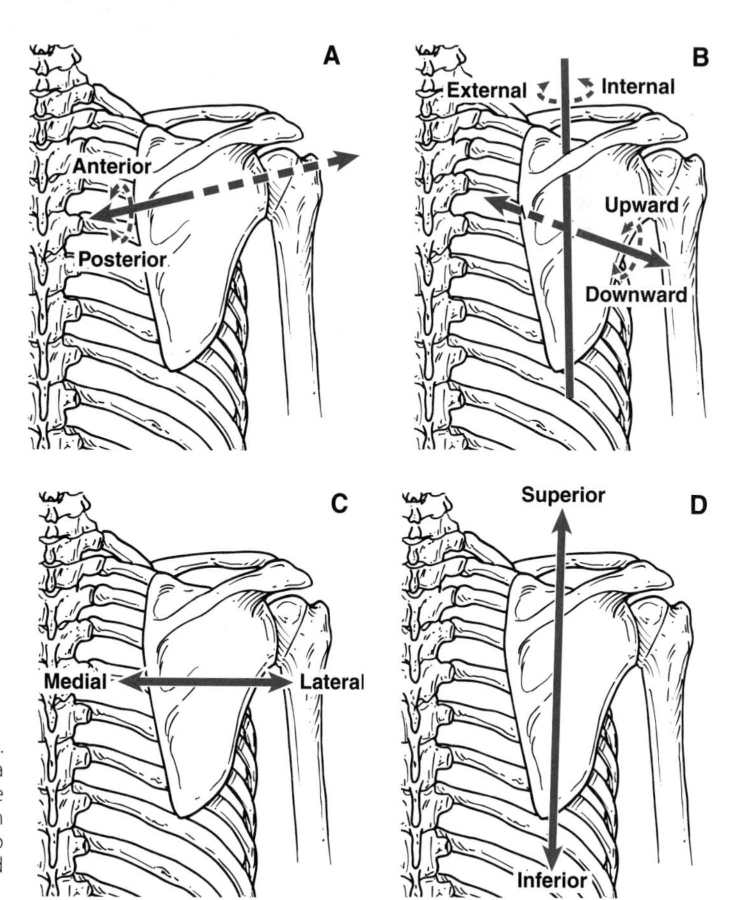

FIGURE 16-10 ■ Motions at the scapulothoracic articulation. **(A)** Anterior and posterior tilt occurs in the sagittal plane around a horizontal axis. **(B)** Upward and downward rotation occurs in the frontal plane about a sagittal axis. Internal and external rotation occurs in the transverse plane about a vertical axis. The scapula also translates medially and laterally (retraction/protraction) **(C)** and superiorly and inferiorly (elevation/depression) **(D)**.

3 degrees of freedom of motion: flexion and extension, abduction and adduction, and internal and external rotation. Although not true anatomical motions, horizontal adduction and abduction (or horizontal flexion and extension) and circumduction also occur at the GH joint. Most upper extremity motions do not occur in a single isolated plane but, rather, are a combination of movements in two or more planes.

The GH joint is inherently unstable because of the relationship in the sizes of the articular surfaces of the glenoid fossa and the humeral head, a loose joint capsule, and relatively weak ligamentous support. The pear-shaped articulating surface of the glenoid fossa is significantly smaller than that of the humeral head and only vaguely resembles the ball-and-socket joint of the hip. The socket is somewhat deepened by the **glenoid labrum**, which also slightly increases the articular surface. Traditionally thought of as a synovium-lined fibrocartilage, recent findings suggest that the glenoid labrum is actually a fold of dense fibrous connective tissue.[8] Disruption of the glenoid labrum is often associated with recurrent shoulder instability.

Possessing a volume twice the size of the humeral head, the joint capsule arises from the glenoid fossa and glenoid labrum to blend with the muscles of the rotator cuff. Studies on cadavers indicate that the laxity of the capsular arrangement allows the humeral head to be distracted 2 cm or more from the glenoid fossa.[9] The capsule is reinforced by the **glenohumeral ligaments** and the **coracohumeral ligament** (Fig. 16-11).

The three GH ligaments—superior, middle, and inferior—are not distinct joint structures but are actually thickenings in the joint capsule. The specific GH ligament that limits motion depends on the position of the humerus (Table 16-1). The inferior GH ligament possesses an anterior and posterior band with a hammock-like structure, the **inferior pouch**, connecting the two. The area between the superior and middle GH ligaments, the **foramen of Weitbrecht**, is a weak site in the capsule often torn during anterior GH dislocations.

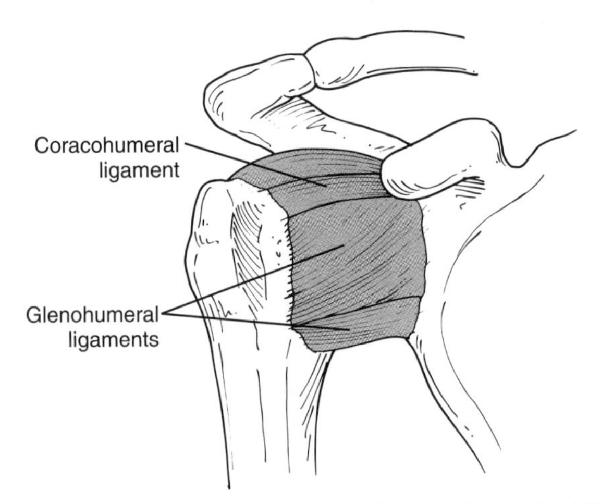

FIGURE 16-11 ■ Ligaments of the GH joint: the coracohumeral and GH ligaments. The GH ligament is divided into superior, middle, and inferior portions. To provide the necessary range of motion to the GH joint, these ligaments must be relatively lax. Much of the stability of this articulation is gained from its muscular arrangement.

Table 16-1 Ligaments Limiting Humeral Motion

Position of the Humerus	Ligamentous Structures Limiting Movement
External rotation in 0° abduction	Superior GH ligament Coracohumeral ligament
External rotation in 45° abduction	Middle GH ligament Anterior band of the inferior GH ligament
External rotation in 90° abduction	Inferior GH ligament
Internal rotation in 90° abduction	Posterior band of the inferior GH ligament
Inferior displacement in 0° abduction	Superior GH ligament Coracohumeral ligament
Inferior displacement in 90° abduction	Inferior GH ligament

GH = glenohumeral.

Emanating from the coracoid process, the **coracohumeral ligament** merges with the superior capsule and the supraspinatus tendon on the greater tuberosity, limiting inferior translation of humeral head when arm is hanging at the side.[3] The anterior fibers of this ligament limit extension while the posterior fibers limit the amount of GH flexion. The coracohumeral ligament and the superior GH ligament limit external rotation of the humerus when the arm is at the side of the body.

When the humerus is hanging at rest in the anatomical position, the articular surfaces of the GH joint have very little contact. Much of the weight of the arm is supported by the superior GH ligament and the inferior portion of the glenoid labrum. When the humerus is abducted to 90 degrees and externally rotated, the entire joint capsule is wound tightly, placing the GH joint in its closed-packed position.

Superior to the humeral head is the **coracoacromial arch**, formed by the **coracoacromial ligament** that traverses from the inferior portion of the acromion process to the posterior portion of the coracoid process (Fig. 16-12). The arch protects the superior portion of the humeral head, the tendons of the rotator cuff muscles, and various bursae from trauma and provides a restraint against superior and anterior GH dislocations. The coracoacromial arch is also involved with shoulder impingement syndrome.

Muscles of the Shoulder Complex

The function of the shoulder complex and arm is controlled by two groups of muscles: those that act primarily on the scapula and those that function primarily on the humerus. Movements of the shoulder complex involve an intricate series of static and dynamic interactions between these two groups of muscles.

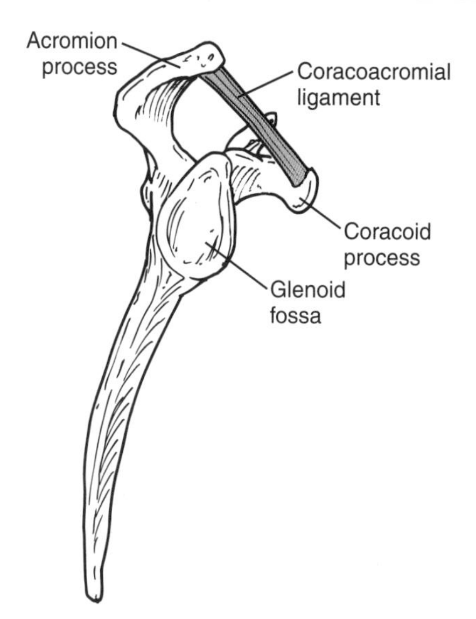

FIGURE 16-12 ■ Coracoacromial arch. The tendons of the rotator cuff, the long head of the biceps brachii tendon, and the subacromial bursa must fit between the space created between the coracoacromial ligament and the humeral head.

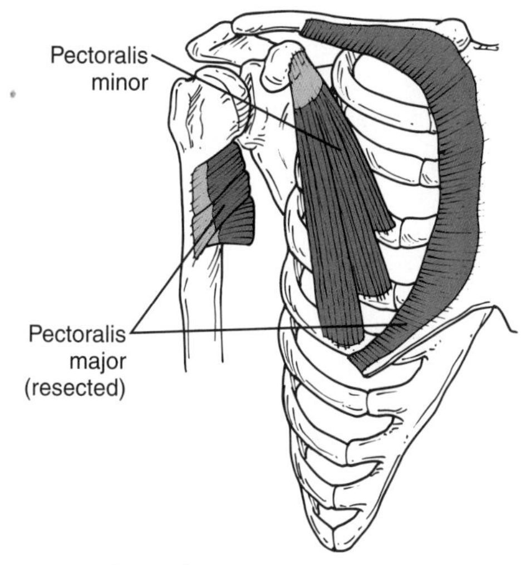

FIGURE 16-13 ■ Pectoralis minor.

Muscles acting on the scapula

The muscles acting on the scapula have two purposes: (1) to control positioning of the scapula's glenoid fossa to allow the shoulder complex increased ROM and (2) to fixate the scapula on the thorax to provide the rotator cuff muscles with a fixed base of support during contractions. The action, origin, insertion, and nerve supply for the muscles acting on the scapula are presented in Table 16-2.

Inserting on the scapula's vertebral border are the **rhomboid minor** and **rhomboid major**. These muscles retract the scapula toward the spine and elevate and downwardly rotate the scapula. The **levator scapulae** acts to elevate and downwardly rotate the scapula. The **serratus anterior**, inserting on the costal surface of the vertebral border, upwardly rotates and protracts the scapula. Working segmentally, the serratus anterior's lower fibers depress the scapula and the upper fibers elevate it. In addition, this muscle plays a primary function in fixating the scapula's vertebral border to the thorax. A weakness of the serratus anterior or injury to the long thoracic nerve innervating it can result in **scapular winging** where the vertebral border lifts away from the thorax. The pectoralis minor tilts the scapula anteriorly so that the inferior angle lifts away from the thorax (Fig. 16-13).

The **trapezius** muscle is divided into upper, middle, and lower segments (Fig. 16-14). Each of these three segments of the trapezius has a unique action on the scapula. The upper fibers elevate and upwardly rotate, the middle fibers retract, and the lower fibers depress and downwardly rotate the scapula.

Two additional muscles have an indirect force on the scapula. The upper fibers from the **latissimus dorsi** depress the shoulder complex. The clavicular portion of the **pectoralis major** depresses the scapula by its attachment to the clavicle at the AC joint.

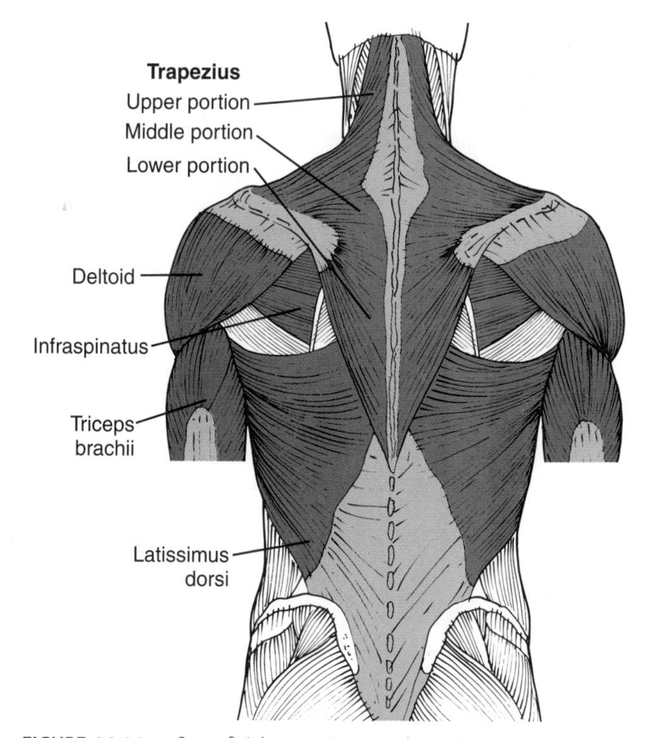

FIGURE 16-14 ■ Superficial posterior muscles acting on the scapula and GH joint. The trapezius (upper, middle, and lower portions), latissimus dorsi, infraspinatus, posterior portion of the deltoid, and the triceps brachii.

Muscles acting on the humerus

Motion at the shoulder complex can occur as GH motion. Generally, however, apparent motion at the shoulder joint is the result of the motion provided by the entire shoulder complex. The action, origin, insertion, and nerve supply for the muscles acting primarily on the humerus are presented in Table 16-3.

Table 16-2 Muscles Acting on the Scapula

Muscle	Action	Origin	Insertion	Innervation	Root
Latissimus Dorsi	Depression of shoulder girdle Internal humeral rotation Humeral extension Humeral adduction	Spinous processes of T6–T12 and the lumbar vertebrae via the lumbodorsal fascia. Posterior iliac crest	Intertubercular groove of the humerus	Thoracodorsal	C6, C7, C8
Levator Scapulae	Elevation Downward rotation Extension of cervical spine Rotation of the cervical spine	Transverse processes of cervical vertebrae C1–C4	Superior medial angle of the scapula	Dorsal scapular	C3, C4, C5
Rhomboid Major	Scapular retraction Scapular elevation Downward rotation of the scapula	Spinous processes of T2, T3, T4, and T5	Vertebral border of scapula (lower two thirds)	Dorsal scapular	C4, C5
Rhomboid Minor	Scapular retraction Scapular elevation	Inferior portion of the ligamentum nuchae Spinous processes C7 and T1	Vertebral border of scapula (near the medial border of the scapular spine)	Dorsal scapular	C4, C5
Serratus Anterior	Upward rotation Protraction Depression (lower fibers) Elevation (upper fibers) Fixation of the scapula to the thorax	Anterior portion of 1st–8th or 9th ribs Aponeuroses of the intercostal muscles	Costal surfaces of the: • Superior angle of scapula • Vertebral border of scapula Inferior angle of scapula	Long thoracic	C5, C6, C7
Trapezius (upper one third)	Elevation of scapula Upward rotation of scapula Rotation of C-spine to the opposite side Extension of C-spine	Occipital protuberance Superior nuchal line of the occipital bone Upper portion of the ligamentum nuchae Spinous process of C7	Distal/lateral one third of clavicle Acromion process Scapular spine	Accessory	CN XI
Trapezius (middle one third)	Retraction of scapula Fixation of thoracic spine	Lower portion of the ligamentum nuchae Spinous processes of the 7th cervical vertebra and T1–T5	Acromion process Spine of the scapula (superior, lateral border)	Accessory	CN XI

Trapezius (lower one third)	Depression of scapula Retraction of scapula Fixation of thoracic spine	Spinous processes and supraspinal ligaments of T8–T12	Spine of the scapula (medial portion)	Accessory	CN XI
Pectoralis Major	Depression of the shoulder girdle (clavicular fibers) Adduction of the humerus Horizontal adduction of the humerus Humeral flexion (clavicular segment) Internal humeral rotation	Medial one-half of the clavicle Anterolateral portion of the sternum	Greater tuberosity of the humerus—lateral lip of the bicipital groove.	Lateral and medial pectoral	C6, C7, C8, T1
Pectoralis Minor	Forward (anterior) tilting	Costal cartilages of ribs 6–7 Anterior portion of 3rd–5th ribs	Coracoid process of scapula	Lateral pectoral	C7, C8, T1

Table 16-3 Muscles Acting on the Humerus

Muscle	Action	Origin	Insertion	Innervation	Root
Biceps Brachii	Flexion Abduction	Long head: Supraglenoid tuberosity of scapula Short head: Coracoid process of scapula	Radial tuberosity and aponeurosis	Musculocutaneous	C5, C6
Coracobrachialis	Flexion Adduction	Coracoid process	Medial shaft of the humerus, adjacent to the deltoid tuberosity	Musculocutaneous	C6, C7
Deltoid (anterior one third)	Flexion Abduction Horizontal adduction Internal rotation	Lateral one third of the clavicle	Deltoid tuberosity	Axillary	C5, C6
Deltoid (middle one third)	Abduction Flexion	Acromion process	Deltoid tuberosity	Axillary	C5, C6
Deltoid (posterior one third)	Extension Horizontal abduction Abduction External rotation	Spine of the scapula	Deltoid tuberosity	Axillary	C5, C6
Infraspinatus	External rotation Horizontal abduction Humeral head stabilization	Infraspinous fossa of the scapula	Lateral portion of the greater tuberosity of the humerus GH joint capsule	Suprascapular	C5, C6
Latissimus Dorsi	Extension Internal rotation Adduction Depression of shoulder girdle	Spinous processes of T6– T12 and the lumbar vertebrae via the lumbodorsal fascia. Posterior iliac crest	Floor of the bicipital groove of the humerus	Thoracodorsal	C6, C7, C8
Pectoralis Major	Adduction of the humerus Horizontal adduction of the humerus Humeral flexion (clavicular segment) Internal humeral rotation Depression of the shoulder girdle (clavicular fibers)	Medial one half of the clavicle Anterolateral portion of the sternum Costal cartilages of ribs 6–7	Greater tuberosity of the humerus	Lateral and medial pectoral	C6, C7, C8, T1

Subscapularis	Internal rotation Humeral head stabilization	Anterior surface (subscapular fossa) and axillary border of the scapula	Lesser tuberosity of the humerus Ventral portion of the GH capsule	Upper and lower subscapular	C5, C6, C7
Supraspinatus	Abduction External rotation Humeral head stabilization	Supraspinous fossa (medial two thirds) of the scapula	Medial aspect of the greater tuberosity GH joint capsule	Suprascapular	C4, C5, C6
Teres Major	Extension Internal rotation Adduction	Inferior angle of scapula Lower one third of the axillary border of the scapula	Medial lip of the bicipital groove	Lower subscapular	C5, C6, C7
Teres Minor	External rotation Horizontal abduction	Lateral upper two thirds of axillary border of the scapula	Lateral aspect of the greater tuberosity	Axillary	C5, C6
Triceps Brachii	Extension (long head) Adduction	Long head: Infraglenoid tuberosity of scapula Lateral head: Lateral and posterior surface of the proximal one half of the humerus Medial head: Distal two thirds of medial and posterior humerus	Olecranon process of ulna	Radial	C6, C7, C8, T1

GH = glenohumeral.

Four muscles arising off the scapula form the **rotator cuff** muscle group (Fig. 16-15). As a group, the rotator cuff internally and externally rotates the humerus and compresses the humeral head in the glenoid fossa, limiting extraneous movement. During the later stages of abduction, the rotator cuff muscle group also provides a downward pull on the humeral head, allowing for its unimpeded passage under the acromion. The **subscapularis muscle** is the only member of the rotator cuff group that internally rotates the humerus. The **supraspinatus** assists in abducting and externally rotating the humerus in addition to compressing the humeral head in the fossa. The remaining two members of the rotator cuff, the **infraspinatus** and **teres minor**, externally rotate the humerus and provide some assistance during horizontal abduction. In addition, the teres minor assists during extension of the GH joint. The eccentric contractions of the infraspinatus and teres minor muscles decelerate the humerus at the end of overhead throwing motions. Closely associated with the muscles of the rotator cuff is the teres major, which assists with internal rotation, adduction, and extension of the humerus.

Although having a common insertion on the deltoid tuberosity of the humerus, each section of the **deltoid muscle group** should be considered independently. As a whole, the deltoid muscle group is the prime mover during abduction. Considered as individual units, the **anterior fibers** flex the GH joint, and horizontally adduct and internally rotate the humerus. The **middle fibers** serve to abduct the humerus. The **posterior fibers** act to extend, horizontally abduct, and externally rotate the humerus. The deltoid group and the upper fibers of the trapezius merge at the AC joint and assume the role of secondary stabilizers of this articulation.

During abduction, a **force couple** is formed between the line of pull between the rotator cuff (specifically the teres minor, infraspinatus, and subscapularis) and the deltoid muscle group. The line of force created by the deltoid's contraction tends to pull the head of the humerus upward against the inferior portion of the acromion process and the coracoacromial ligament. In the early stages of abduction, the rotator cuff's angle of pull must be sufficient to hold the head of the humerus against the glenoid fossa. After the humerus moves past 90 degrees, the rotator cuff's angle of pull changes so that its force slides the humeral head inferiorly on the glenoid fossa, creating clearance to pass under the acromion process and the coracoacromial ligament (Fig. 16-16). A damaged or weak rotator cuff group changes the dynamics of the force couple, resulting in the impingement of the rotator cuff and long head of the biceps brachii tendon between the humeral head, subacromial bursa, and acromion process.

The **pectoralis major** is divided into two portions, the clavicular portion and the sternal portion, each having a common insertion on the greater tuberosity (Fig. 16-17). As a whole, the pectoralis major adducts, horizontally adducts, and internally rotates the humerus. The clavicular portion flexes, internally rotates, and horizontally adducts the humerus. The sternal portion depresses the shoulder girdle and assists in horizontal adduction.

The **latissimus dorsi** has a broad origin on the lumbar spine, thoracodorsal fascia, and iliac crest. Inserting on the intertubercular groove of the humerus, the latissimus dorsi adducts, internally rotates, and extends the humerus. Attaching to the infraglenoid tuberosity of the scapula, the **long head of the triceps brachii** is an adductor and extensor of the humerus, especially when the elbow is flexed.

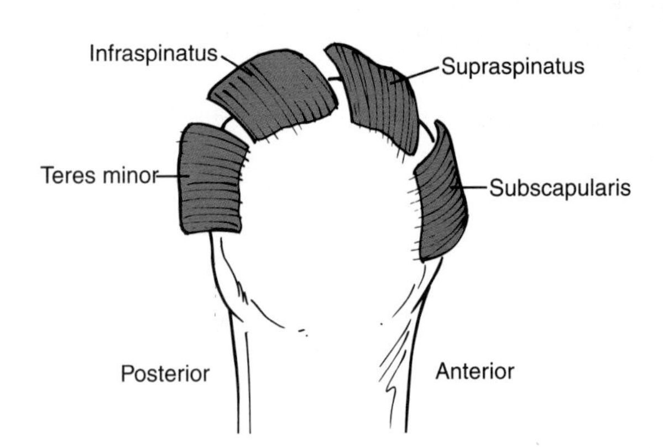

FIGURE 16-15 ■ Muscles of the rotator cuff as they attach to the humeral head.

Force couple Coordination between dynamic and isometric contractions of opposing muscle groups to perform a movement of a joint.

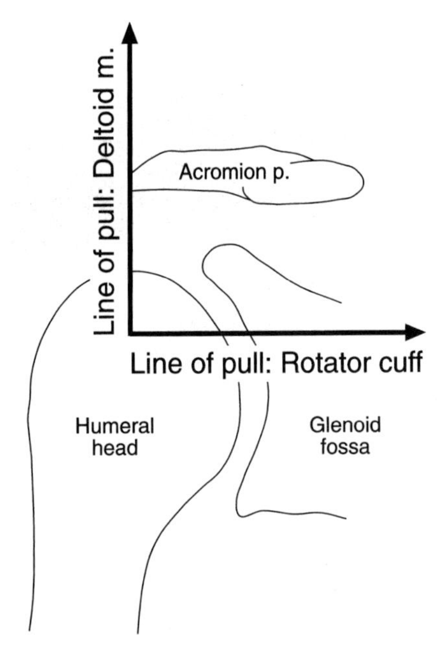

FIGURE 16-16 ■ Scapulohumeral force couple. Contraction of the deltoid muscle pulls the humeral head upward. To prevent contact between the humeral head and the acromion process during abduction, the rotator cuff must hold the humeral head close to the glenoid fossa and, when the humerus approaches 90° of abduction, must serve to glide the humerus inferiorly.

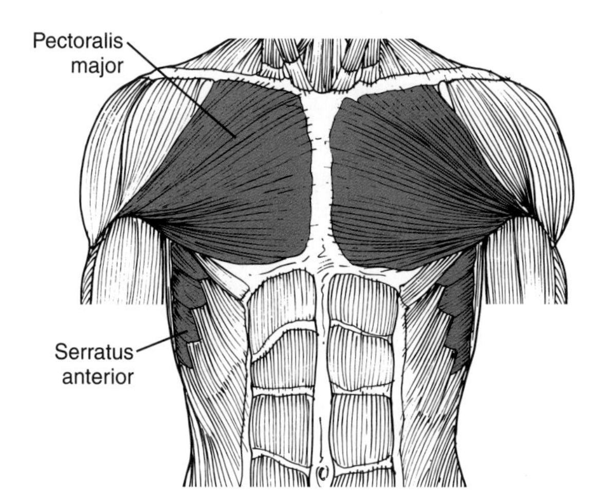

FIGURE 16-17 ■ Pectoralis major and serratus anterior.

The **coracobrachialis** acts on the humerus as a flexor and adductor. Both heads of the **biceps brachii** have an attachment on the scapula (Fig. 16-18). Both heads assist in GH flexion and, when the humerus is externally rotated, the long head assists in GH abduction. The short head attaches to the coracoid process, and the long head passes through the bicipital groove to attach on the supraglenoid tuberosity. Stability within the bicipital groove is maintained by the **transverse humeral ligament**, lined by a capsular sheath emanating from the GH capsule. An inflammatory response or damage to the transverse humeral ligament results in pain and disrupts the normal mechanics of the GH joint.

The long head of the biceps enters the joint capsule between the supraspinatus and subscapularis muscles. Although

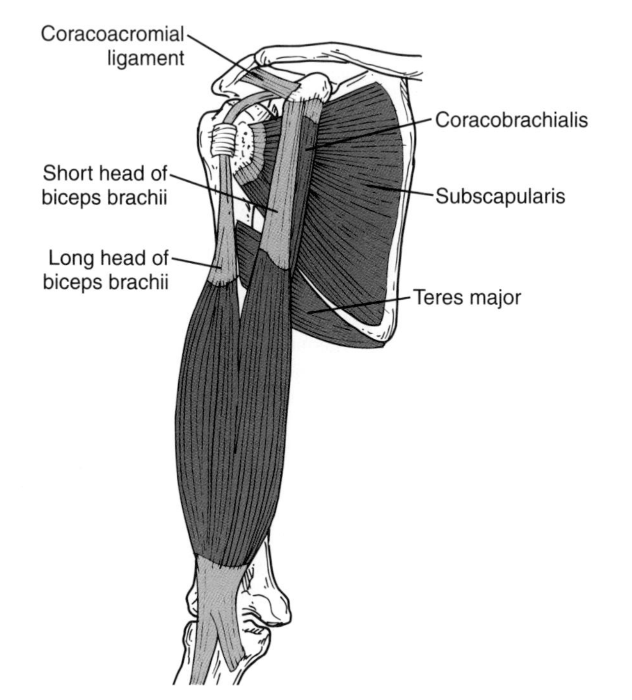

FIGURE 16-18 ■ Coracobrachialis and attachment of the long and short heads of the biceps brachii muscle.

the capsule is penetrated, the tendon does not enter the synovial membrane of the articulation. During the motions of humeral flexion and abduction, the tendon must slide within the bicipital groove. The biceps produces little force during these motions, but the long head tendon may serve to stabilize the humeral head in the anterior and superior directions.

Scapulothoracic Rhythm

For the hand to obtain its maximal arc of motion, the GH and scapulothoracic articulation must combine their available ROMs. If the humeral head were rigidly fixated in the glenoid fossa in a manner eliminating GH movement, the humerus could still be elevated to 60 degrees through movement of the scapula via the AC and SC joints. For the humerus to be elevated to its maximum ROM of 180 degrees, the GH and scapulothoracic articulation must function together. An approximate two-to-one ratio is found between GH elevation and upward scapular rotation, although a wide range of individual variability exists. For 180 degrees of humeral elevation to occur, 120 degrees is from GH movement and 60 degrees is through upward rotation of the scapula.

This ratio is not smooth or consistent. Early in the ROM, elevation occurs primarily at the GH joint, with the scapula fixating to provide stability for the contracting muscles. During the intermediate stages of humeral elevation, the ratio between the GH joint and the scapula is approximately 1:1.[10] At the extremes of these movements, these motions again occur primarily at the GH joint. Maintenance of this rhythm is based on the coordination of the prime movers of the humerus and the synergistic contractions of the scapular stabilizers.

Bursa of the Shoulder Complex

Although commonly fused into a single unit referred to as the subacromial bursa, two bursae are actually located at the GH joint: the **subacromial bursa** and the **subdeltoid bursa**. The subacromial bursa is located above the superior surface of the supraspinatus tendon and lubricates the movement of the overlying fibers of the deltoid muscle, acting as a secondary joint cavity.[11] When the humerus is elevated, the bursa buffers the supraspinatus tendon against its contact with the acromion process and the coracoacromial ligament. When the bursa becomes inflamed, the structures within the subacromial space become compressed, potentially leading to rotator cuff impingement.

Clinical Examination of Shoulder Injuries

Because of the interrelationship of the shoulder complex to the cervical and thoracic spine, torso, abdomen, and elbow, clinicians must be prepared to undertake thorough evaluations of these areas. Likewise, distal pathology, such as elbow pain, may arise from dysfunction at the shoulder. Chapter 14

Examination Map

HISTORY

Past Medical History

History of Present Condition

Mechanism of Injury

Onset of Symptoms

Location of Pain

INSPECTION

Functional Assessment

Inspection of the Anterior Structures

Level of the shoulders
Position of the head
Position of the arm
Contour of the clavicles
Deltoid muscle groups
Humerus

Inspection of the Lateral Structures

Deltoid muscle group
Acromion process
Position of the humerus

Inspection of the Posterior Structures

Vertebral column
Position of the scapula
Muscle development
Position of the humerus

PALPATION

Palpation of the Anterior Structures

Jugular notch
Sternoclavicular joint
Clavicular shaft
Acromion process
Acromioclavicular joint
Coracoid process
Humeral head
Greater tuberosity
Lesser tuberosity
Bicipital groove
Humeral shaft
Pectoralis major
Pectoralis minor
Coracobrachialis
Deltoid muscle group
Biceps brachii
- Long head
- Short head

Palpation of the Posterior Structures

Spine of the scapula
Superior angle
Inferior angle
Rotator cuff
- Infraspinatus
- Teres minor
- Supraspinatus

Teres major
Rhomboids
Levator scapulae
Trapezius
Latissimus dorsi
Posterior deltoid
Triceps brachii

JOINT AND MUSCLE FUNCTION ASSESSMENT

Goniometry

- Flexion
- Extension
- Abduction
- Internal rotation
- External rotation
- Horizontal abduction
- Horizontal adduction

Active Range of Motion

Apley's Scratch Test

Flexion/extension
Abduction/adduction
- Drop arm test

Internal and external rotation
Horizontal adduction/abduction

Manual Muscle Tests

Gerber lift-off test
Flexion/extension
Abduction/adduction
Internal/external rotation
Horizontal abduction/adduction
Scapular muscles
- Retraction and downward rotation
- Retraction
- Protraction and upward rotation
- Depression and retraction
- Elevation

Passive Range of Motion

Flexion
Extension
Abduction
Adduction
Internal rotation
External rotation
Horizontal abduction
Horizontal adduction

JOINT STABILITY TESTS

Joint Play Assessment

Sternoclavicular joint
Acromioclavicular joint
Glenohumeral joint

NEUROLOGIC EXAMINATION

Upper Quarter Screen

PATHOLOGIES AND SPECIAL TESTS

Sternoclavicular Joint

Acromioclavicular Joint

Acromioclavicular traction test
Acromioclavicular compression test

Glenohumeral Joint

Anterior instability
- Apprehension test
- Relocation test
- Anterior release test

Posterior instability
- Posterior apprehension test
- Jerk test

Inferior instability
- Sulcus sign

Multidirectional instability

Rotator Cuff Pathology

Impingement syndrome
- Neer impingement test
- Hawkins impingement test
- Drop arm test

Rotator cuff tendinopathy
- Drop arm test
- Empty can test

Subacromial bursitis

Biceps Tendon Pathology

Bicipital tendinopathy
- Yergason's test
- Speed's test

SLAP lesions
- Active compression test
- Anterior slide test
- Compression–rotation test

discusses pain that originates from the cervical spine, and Chapter 15 describes visceral pain referred into the shoulder and upper arm.

History

Determine the onset and duration of the condition and identify the location of pain. Because the shoulder and upper arm are common sites for referred or radiating pain from orthopedic or visceral origins, a complete examination of the cervical spine, thorax, and abdomen may be indicated, particularly when a patient presents with a vague history of injury to the shoulder complex (see Fig. 15-14). The arm of the dominant hand is subject to more repetitive forces throughout the day and is therefore more susceptible to injury.

The use of standardized self-assessments before and after treatment and rehabilitation aids in determining the patient's outcome and the impact of the subsequent interventions. Standardized and validated self-assessments for the shoulder include the Disabilities of the Arm, Shoulder and Hand (DASH) and the American Shoulder and Elbow Surgeons Shoulder Score Index (ASES).[12,13]

The following information should be obtained during the history-taking process so that the mechanism of injury, influence of prior or current other injuries, structures involved in the injury, and nature of the pain can be determined.

Past Medical History

A history of previous injury to the AC or GH joints can alter the biomechanics of the shoulder complex. Because cervical spine pathology can result in referred or radiating pain to the upper extremity, the previous injury history of the cervical spine must be ascertained. If a history of injury to the cervical spine or thorax has been described, the cervical spine and peripheral nerves are further evaluated so that the possible relationship to the existing condition can be determined.

History of the present condition

- **Location of the pain**: The examination begins by localizing the area of pain, the type of pain, and any dysfunction reported by the patient. Shoulder pathology typically produces pain within the GH joint that may project laterally into the upper arm or medially into the trapezius. Pain that begins in the trapezius and radiates into the upper arm, forearm, or hand implicates cervical nerve root involvement.

*** Practical Evidence**

Patients with rotator cuff pathology or subacromial bursitis typically describe pain in the anterior and lateral shoulder whereas chronic acromioclavicular pathology is commonly associated with pain into the upper trapezius region, especially at night.[14–16]

- **Onset**: The onset of pain often indicates the underlying pathology. Pain with an acute onset may indicate a fracture, GH joint dislocation or subluxation, tendon rupture or an AC sprain. Inflammatory conditions of the shoulder complex, such as tendinopathies, bursitis, or osteoarthritis, usually have an insidious onset. In these cases, pain may first be noticed after activity and then progresses to pain during activity and, eventually, constant pain.
- **Activity and injury mechanism**: An external force applied to the shoulder complex, such as a direct blow or joint force beyond normal limits, results in acute soft tissue or bony injury. A history of repetitive overhead motion activities such as throwing, swimming, or hitting a tennis ball may indicate an overuse injury such as rotator cuff tendon degeneration.
- **Symptoms**: The symptoms to be noted include resting pain, pain with movement, and dysfunction of the shoulder complex. The patient may describe the shoulder as "going out of place," indicating GH instability; decreased velocity or poor accuracy when throwing; or discomfort when performing overhand motions, indicating inflammatory conditions. Question the patient about pain or muscle spasm in the cervical region or radiating pain and altered sensation or numbness possibly indicating nerve pathology. Pain when sleeping on the involved side is often associated with rotator cuff injury.

The preceding list is not all-inclusive for the questions to be asked during the history-taking process. The scope of the questions expands for cases involving an insidious onset. When an acute traumatic injury is being assessed, the history-taking process should become more focused based on the mechanism of injury.

Inspection

The patient should wear clothing that allows full inspection of both shoulders and the cervical, thoracic, and lumbar spine.

Functional assessment

Observe the patient's willingness to move the involved limb throughout the examination. Does the patient raise the involved arm when removing the shirt or jacket or does the arm remain at the side with the clothing dropped down over it? Unwillingness to move the arm may indicate apprehension or a more severe condition.

Observe the patient performing relevant functional activities, such as reaching for an object or throwing, note any pain-provoking motions or adaptations to reduce symptoms. For example, during abduction patients suffering from supraspinatus tendinopathy may laterally flex the trunk to the same side to limit activity of the supraspinatus. Examine the scapular position and motion during elevation, note any scapular winging, excessive elevation, or excessive anterior tilting relative to the contralateral side.

Box 16-1 presents the phases of the pitching motion and relates the structures involved with each. With overhead throwing athletes the arm position that produces pain and throwing deficits yield information regarding the possible underlying pathology[7,16]:

- **Pain on follow-through**: Possible rotator cuff pathology
- **Pain in cocked position**: Instability or impingement
- **Pain in deceleration**: SLAP lesion, biceps tendon pathology
- **Loss of control and/or velocity**: Often proportional to the severity of the condition. Loss of control associated with early ball release is suggestive of internal impingement. Complaints of loss of velocity are associated with a limitation in internal rotation.

Inspection of the anterior structures

- **Level of the shoulders**: Observe the height of the AC joints, the clavicle, and the SC joints. These should align bilaterally, but the dominant shoulder may appear slightly lower than the nondominant one (Fig. 16-19).

  A painful shoulder is often held in its resting position of slight abduction in the plane of the scapula.[4] Unilateral elevation may also indicate upper trapezius hypertrophy on the raised side or atrophy on the depressed side. Another cause of asymmetry is the presence of scoliosis (see the "Inspection of the Posterior Structures" section). Bilaterally raised shoulders may result from well-developed upper trapezius muscles or unwanted spasm in these muscle groups. Shoulders that are abnormally depressed bilaterally may occur as a result of decreased upper trapezius muscle tone. Bilaterally or unilaterally depressed shoulder complexes can place pressure on the arterial, venous, and nervous supply of the arm, predisposing the patient to **thoracic outlet syndrome** (see Chapter 14). Rounded shoulders can indicate tightness of the pectoralis major and minor muscles and result in changes in scapular position.
- **Position of the head**: Observe the position of the head, which normally assumes an upright position. A head that is side bent or rotated may indicate muscle spasm, pressure on a cervical nerve root, or stretching of the cervical nerves. Conditions relating to the cervical spine and its nerve network are discussed in Chapter 14
- **Position of the arm**: Note whether the arm is splinted alongside the body or if it simply hangs limp at the side. Traumatic shoulder injuries are often voluntarily splinted with the humerus along the lateral portion of the rib cage and the forearm supported across the chest. Brachial plexus injuries are characterized by the arm's hanging limply at the side (see Chapter 14). With GH dislocations, the humerus is locked into a fixed position.
- **Contour of the clavicles**: Inspect the clavicle, easily visible in thin patients or those with well-defined upper body musculature. Observe the SC joint, the shaft of the clavicle, and the clavicle's termination at the AC joint for symmetry and compare them bilaterally.

  In adults, acute traumatic conditions involving the clavicle are typically identifiable during the inspection process. SC or AC joint sprains may be marked by a gross deformity at the articulation, with one side having a more predominant protrusion than the other side. Any previous history involving these joints must be established because deformity may be residual from past trauma.

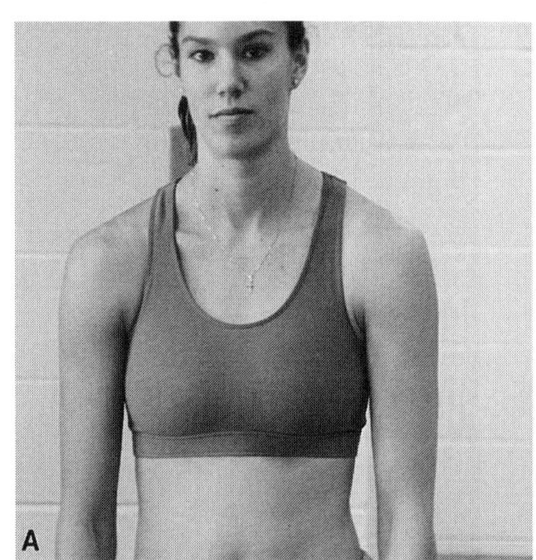

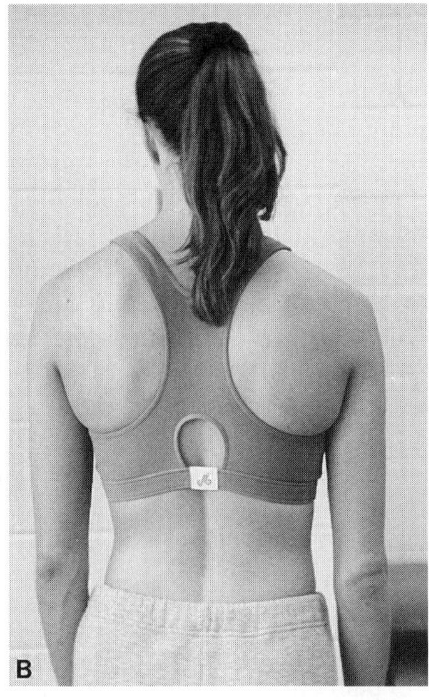

FIGURE 16-19 ■ **(A)** Anterior and **(B)** posterior view of the shoulders. Note that the shoulder of the dominant right arm hangs lower than the shoulder of the nondominant arm.

Box 16-1
Phases of the Pitching Motion

	Wind-up	Cocking	Acceleration	Deceleration	Follow Through
	Wind-up	**Cocking**	**Acceleration**	**Deceleration**	**Follow through**
Glenohumeral Joint Position	Neutral	90° abduction Maximum external rotation	90° abduction Moving to internal rotation	90° abduction Internal rotation	Horizontal abduction Internal rotation Decreasing abduction
Glenohumeral Joint Stresses	Low joint stresses	Anterior joint capsule Inferior joint capsule	Anterior joint capsule	Posterior joint capsule Distraction of GH joint	Posterior joint capsule Distraction of GH joint
Elbow Position	Some degrees of flexion	Approximately 90° flexion Increased valgus forces on the elbow	90° flexion moving into extension	20°–30° flexion moving into extension	Extension
Concentric Muscle Contraction	Muscular forces mostly generated by the lower extremity	External rotators	Internal rotators Serratus anterior Upper trapezius Trunk and lower extremity	Internal rotators Triceps brachii	Internal rotators
Eccentric Muscle Contraction		Internal rotators	External rotators Rhomboids Middle and lower trapezius	External rotators Biceps brachii Brachialis	External rotators
Center of Gravity	Over pivot foot	Over pivot foot	Between pivot foot and plant foot	Over plant foot	Forward of plant foot

GH = glenohumeral.

Complete clavicular fractures are indicated by a clear deformity of the shaft (Fig. 16-20). Although these fractures usually occur at the juncture between the concave and convex bends (the distal third of the shaft), they can occur anywhere along the clavicle. Patients suffering from a fractured clavicle tend to support the involved arm next to the body and rotate the head to the opposite side. If a fractured clavicle is suspected, examine the patient for any other conditions, terminate the evaluation, immobilize the arm with a sling, and refer the patient to a physician.

- **Symmetry of the deltoid muscle groups**: Note the bilateral symmetry of the deltoid muscle tone. Normally, this muscle group has a rounded contour. The deltoid of the dominant arm may be hypertrophied compared with the deltoid of the nondominant side. Atrophy of this muscle group may indicate a lack of use of the involved arm or may reflect pathology to the C5 and C6 nerve roots (axillary nerve involvement).

A dislocated GH joint disrupts the contour of the deltoid group by flattening the area passing over the head of the humerus (Fig. 16-21). With anterior dislocations, the humeral head rests just below the coracoid process. Distal pulses should always be checked with a suspected GH dislocation. The absence of a distal pulse indicates potentially catastrophic impingement of the vascular bundle supplying the arm, wrist, and hand and requires immediate referral for further medical attention.

- **Anterior humerus and biceps brachii muscle group**: Note the shape and contour of the biceps brachii and any unilateral bulges within the muscle. A **long head of the biceps tendon rupture** is characterized by the muscle's shortening away from the involved structure (Fig. 16-22). A careful inspection of the entire muscle is necessary because the distal tendon can rupture from its insertion at the elbow, causing deformity.

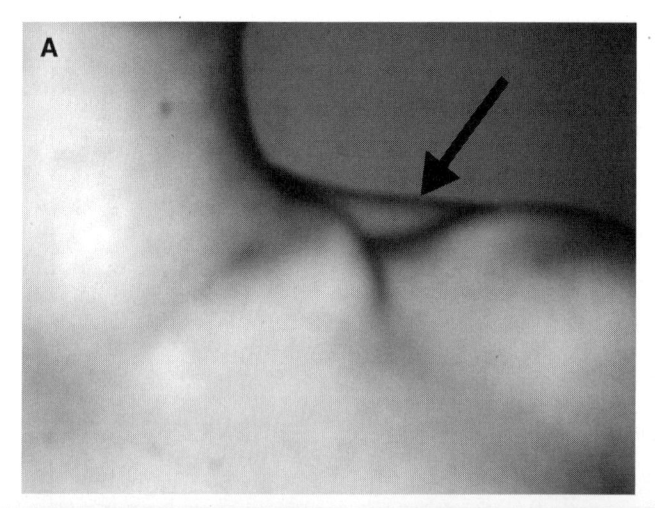

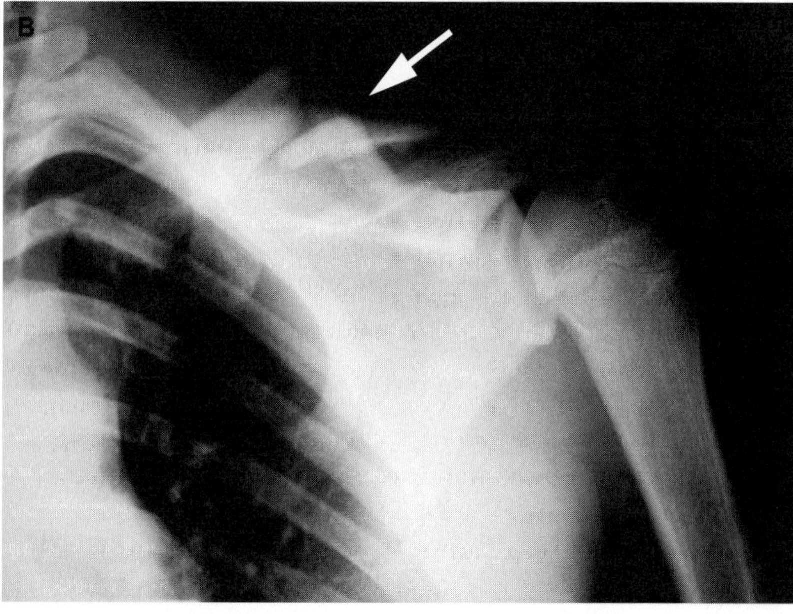

FIGURE 16-20 ■ Fracture of the left clavicle. **(A)** Inspection showing gross deformity. **(B)** Anterior–posterior radiograph demonstrating the fracture lines.

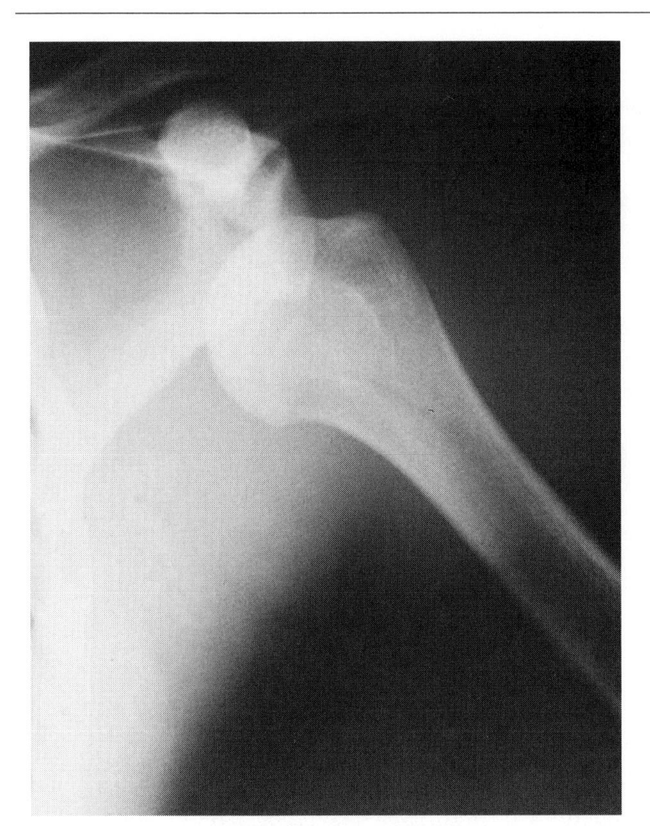

FIGURE 16-21 ■ Radiograph of an anterior GH dislocation.

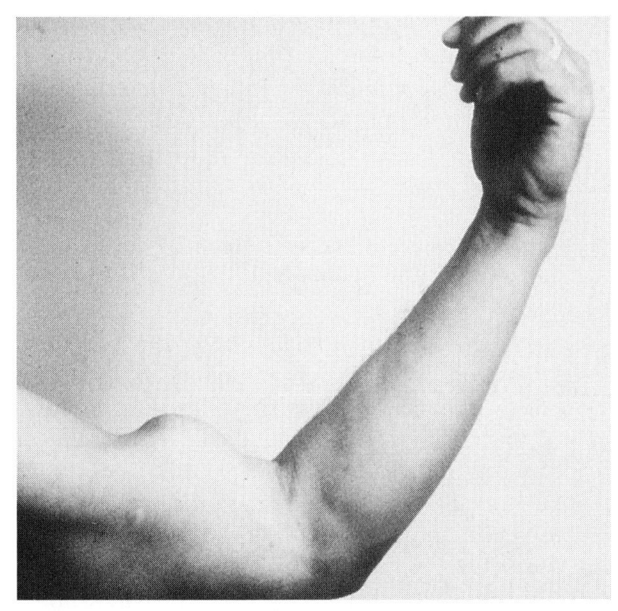

FIGURE 16-22 ■ Rupture of the long head of the biceps brachii tendon.

Inspection of the lateral structures

- **Deltoid muscle group**: This portion of the inspection process is a continuation of the observation of the anterior portion of the deltoid. The contour of this group is noted and compared with the contralateral side, giving special attention to the roundness of the muscle as it passes over the humeral head. Atrophy of the deltoid is associated with C5 or C6 nerve root or axillary nerve involvement.
- **Acromion process**: The junction between the clavicle and the acromion process usually appears smooth and even. Look for the presence of a **step deformity**. This condition involves the clavicle riding above the acromion process, indicating an AC sprain (Fig. 16-23). This finding is confirmed via palpation (**piano key sign**) and during the ligamentous tests portion (**AC traction test**) of the examination.
- **Position of the humerus**: Normally, the humerus hangs in the anatomical position. Adhesions within the GH joint, muscle spasm, or pain associated with bursitis and tendon pathology may cause the patient to splint the arm to the side to guard against motion.

Inspection of the posterior structures

- **Alignment of the vertebral column**: Inspect the alignment of the cervical, thoracic, and lumbar spine to evaluate for scoliosis. This malady can cause altered biomechanics of the shoulder complex.
- **Position of the scapulae**: Observe the vertebral borders of both scapulae, which usually rest an equal distance from the spinous processes of the thoracic vertebrae. The superior angle normally sits at the level of the T2 spinous process and the inferior angle at the T7 spinous process. The most medial aspect of the scapular spine is located at the level of the third thoracic vertebra. In the anatomical position, the scapula is in full contact with the thorax. Note the presence of the inferior angle lifting away from the thorax (winging scapula). Also observe for any unilateral scapular protraction, retraction, or tilting.

  Sprengel's deformity, a congenitally undescended scapula, may occur on one scapula or both. A high-riding scapula may indicate poorly developed or malformed scapular elevators. The clinical ramifications of this condition vary from little or no dysfunction to extreme disability.
- **Muscle development**: Inspect the posterior musculature for symmetry on each side. The superficial muscles of well-developed individuals are usually easily identifiable, as are the prominent bony landmarks. Any spasm, deformity, or discoloration of the musculature or skin should be noted as well.

  Observe the prominence of the scapular spine. Atrophy of the supraspinatus or infraspinatus muscles makes the spine of the scapula more visible and palpable. Chronic rotator cuff tears are classically marked by the wasting of the infraspinatus muscle.[17] The scapular stabilizers should also be observed for symmetry.
- **Position of the humerus**: Check patients with acute shoulder injuries for possible posterior GH dislocation, although it is rare. The head of the humerus, when posteriorly dislocated, usually rests on the infraspinous fossa. This injury is associated with possible

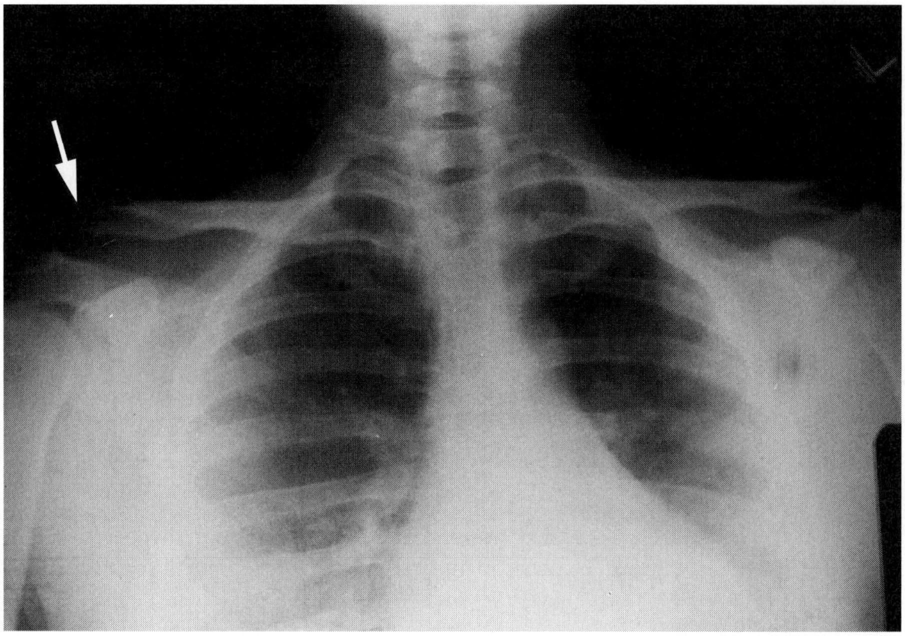

FIGURE 16-23 ■ Radiograph of a third-degree AC sprain. The superior displacement of the clavicle's distal aspect creates a characteristic "step deformity."

bony and articular surface injury and neurovascular damage. This condition may be masked by patients with well-developed shoulder muscles.

PALPATION

The bony structures are palpated prior to the soft tissue structures to rule out fractures, dislocations, and gross joint injury. If palpation reveals any gross deformity, the limb should be examined for neurologic and vascular compromise, the shoulder immobilized, and the patient referred to a physician for a definitive diagnosis.

Palpation of Anterior Shoulder

1 **Jugular notch**: Begin the palpation process by locating the jugular notch on the manubrium. Palpate the common junction provided by the interclavicular ligament between the SC joints.

2 **Sternoclavicular joint**: Proceed laterally to identify the SC joint, checking for point tenderness over the articulation. Dislocations of the SC joint tend to displace the clavicular head medial and superior to the clavicular notch. **Posterior SC dislocations are a medical emergency** because posterior displacement of the clavicle may jeopardize the integrity of the neurovascular structures directly posterior to the joint or may place pressure on the trachea, lung, or both.

3 **Clavicular shaft**: From the SC joint, continue to palpate laterally along the shaft of the clavicle, noting any deformity, crepitus, or pain. The superior surface is easily palpable because of the absence of muscle attachments. Healed clavicular fractures may be marked by palpable bony callus formation over the healed fracture site.

4 **Acromion process and AC joint**: As the clavicle extends laterally, expect that it may become less palpable in patients who have well-developed deltoid muscles. The acromion process may be more easily located by palpating to the lateral end of the scapular spine.

If a step deformity is observed during the observation phase of the examination, note for bobbing of the clavicle when downward pressure is applied, the **piano key sign**, to determine the integrity of the coracoclavicular ligaments.

5 **Coracoid process**: From the most concave portion of the clavicle, move approximately 1 inch inferior to it to locate the coracoid process. Feel for the coracoid process just above and behind the tendon of the pectoralis major. To confirm that the coracoid process has been located, passively move the GH joint through 15 to 30 degrees of flexion and extension and abduction and adduction. No movement of the coracoid process should be felt within this ROM. If movement is felt beneath the fingers, the humeral head is most probably being palpated. In this case, move the fingers medially and attempt this procedure again.

The coracoid process serves as the point of insertion for the pectoralis minor and is the origin of the short head of the biceps brachii tendon and the coracobrachialis muscle. In addition, it provides a source of attachment for several ligaments. Apply pressure carefully when palpating this area because it is easily irritated.

6 **Humeral head**: Moving laterally from the acromion process, palpate the anteromedial portion of the humeral head in the axilla posterior to the tendon of pectoralis major. The relationship of the humeral head to the glenoid fossa must be determined. Direct palpation of the humeral head may not be possible in patients with well-developed

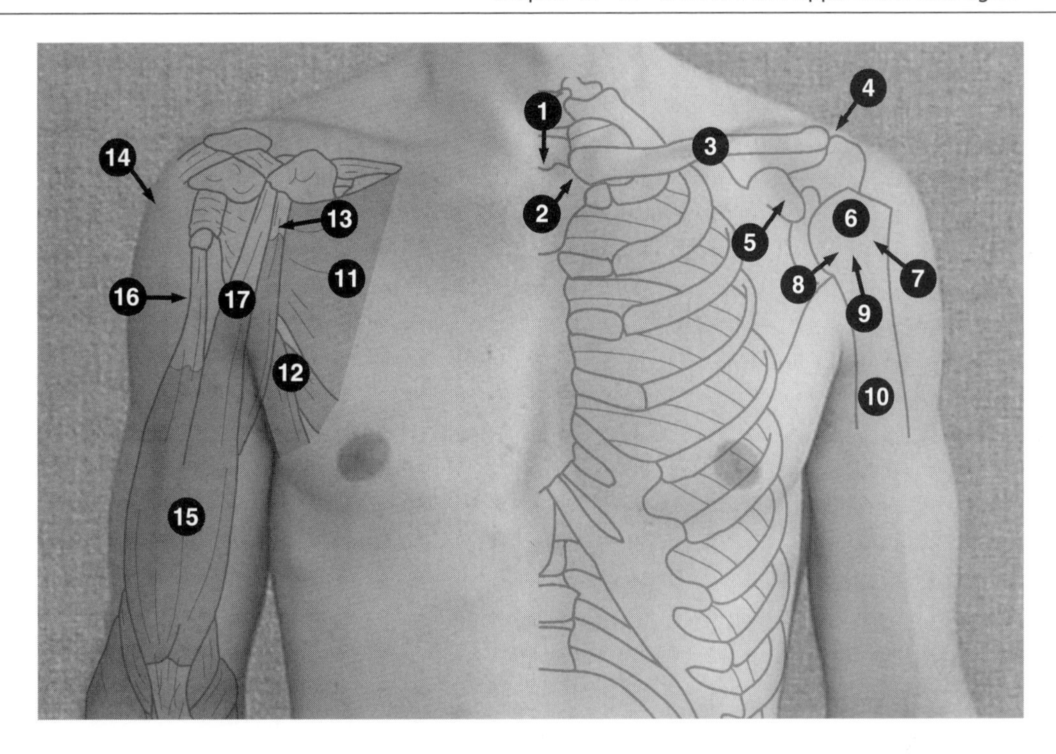

shoulder musculature. However, an anteriorly or inferiorly displaced humeral head is easily palpable.

7 **Greater tuberosity**: Locate the greater tuberosity in the anatomical position approximately one finger breadth inferior to the lateral edge of the anterior portion of the acromion process. This structure is more easily palpated by passively extending the humerus, causing the greater tuberosity to move from beneath the acromion process.

8 **Lesser tuberosity**: With the humerus externally rotated to ease palpation, locate the medial border of the bicipital groove formed by the lesser tuberosity.

9 **Bicipital groove**: Externally rotate the humerus to make the bicipital groove more palpable. The groove is felt as an indentation in the bone just medial to the greater tuberosity. Gently palpate this area along its length to elicit any tenderness caused by pathology of the long head of the biceps tendon or damage to the transverse humeral ligament. Note that this area is typically tender and should be compared with the opposite side to determine a relative difference in pain.

10 **Humeral shaft**: Palpate the shaft of the humerus, more easily palpated along its medial and lateral borders under the belly of the biceps brachii and brachioradialis muscles.

11 **Pectoralis major**: Locate the pectoralis major on the anterior thoracic cavity. Palpate this muscle as it flares into its tendon, noting the integrity and any point tenderness as it crosses the GH capsule and attaches on the greater tuberosity of the humerus.

12 **Pectoralis minor**: Attempt to palpate the tendon insertion on the coracoid process of the pectoralis minor. Located beneath the pectoralis major, the bulk of the pectoralis minor is not palpable.

13 **Coracobrachialis**: Locate the coracobrachialis muscle as it originates off the coracoid process. It may be palpable at this point. Its body and insertion lie deep to the superficial musculature of the humerus and are therefore difficult to palpate. Gentle resistance to forward flexion with the elbow flexed makes this structure more prominent.

14 **Deltoid group**: Palpate each of the three portions of the deltoid from its unique origin to the common insertion on the humerus.

15–17 **Biceps brachii**: From the belly of the biceps brachii, palpate each of the two heads. Feel for the long head of the biceps (**16**) as it travels through its passage in the bicipital groove under the transverse humeral ligament until it passes beneath the anterior deltoid. Palpate the biceps' short head (**17**) along its length as it passes beneath the pectoralis major tendon and attaches on the coracoid process.

Palpation of Posterior Shoulder

1 **Spine of the scapula**: Locate the spine of the scapula by finding the acromion process. Palpate posteriorly along the bony surface of the acromion to meet with the scapular

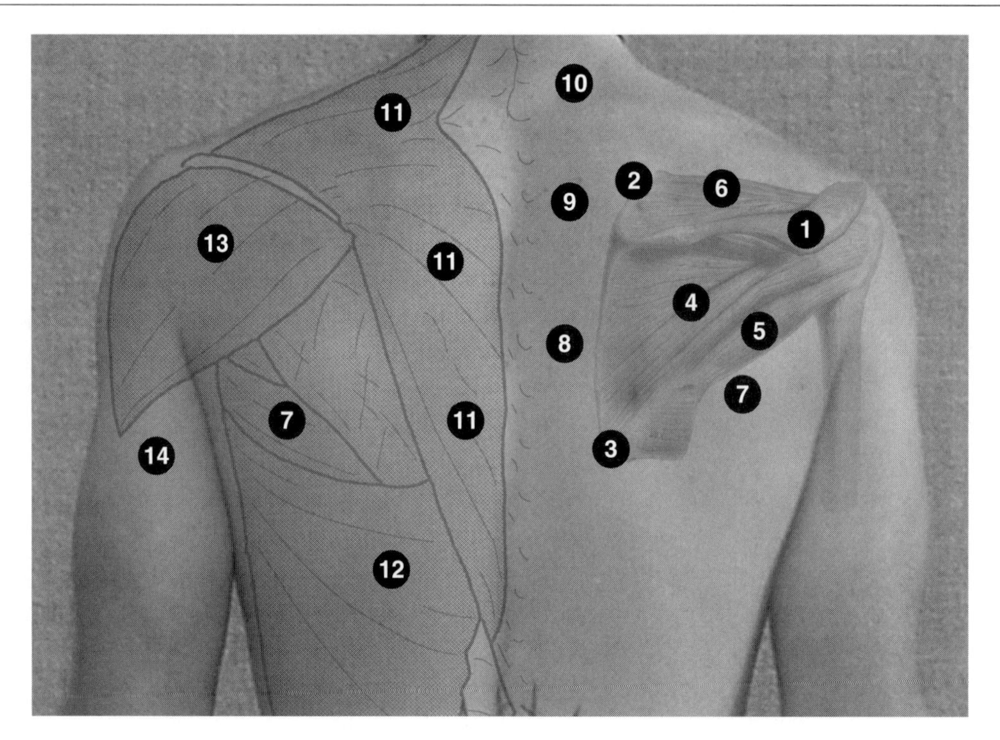

spine. Continue palpation medially along the length of the spine to its termination along the scapula's vertebral border.

2 **Superior angle**: From the vertebral border, palpate upward to find the superior angle of the scapula. This landmark may be obstructed by muscle mass of the upper portion of the trapezius and levator scapulae.

3 **Inferior angle**: Moving inferiorly along the vertebral border, feel for the apex of the inferior angle of the scapula. Ask the patient to touch the inferior angle of the opposite scapula from below, causing the scapula undergoing examination to wing and making the inferior angle and the lower portions of the vertebral and axial borders more easily palpable.

3–6 **Rotator cuff**: Palpate the mass of three of the four rotator cuff muscles on the scapula. Palpate the infraspinatus (**4**), teres minor (**5**), and supraspinatus (partially covered by the trapezius) (**6**) along their lengths until they disappear beneath the mass of the deltoid. By passively extending the GH joint from the anatomical position, the greater tuberosity becomes prominent, allowing for the palpation of these muscles' insertions on the humerus. Although the individual tendons are not distinguishable from each other, any pain or tenderness elicited during palpation should be noted because it may indicate rotator cuff pathology. The origin, mass, and tendinous insertion of the subscapularis muscle are not directly palpable.

7 **Teres major**: Locate the origin and body of the teres major muscle immediately inferior to the teres minor. The insertion of this muscle cannot be directly palpated. This muscle is a common site for trigger points in swimmers and in athletes who participate in sports with overhead movements. Note any hypersensitive areas.

8–9 **Rhomboid**: The rhomboid major (**8**) and rhomboid minor (**9**) cannot be directly palpated and are indistinguishable from each other except for their relative locations.

10 **Levator scapulae**: Although it is largely covered by the upper portion of the trapezius muscle, palpate the origin of the levator scapulae on the transverse processes of the first through the fourth cervical vertebrae to its insertion on the medial border of the scapula, just inferior to the superior angle.

11 **Trapezius**: Palpate the trapezius muscle relative to its upper, middle, and lower portions. This muscle is the most superficial of the muscles acting on the scapula and therefore overlies the levator scapulae and the rhomboid muscle group.

12 **Latissimus dorsi**: Locate the latissimus dorsi tendon inferior to the teres major. Follow this tendon through the axilla to its attachment on the floor of the bicipital groove.

13 **Posterior deltoid**: Palpate the posterior portion of the deltoid muscle group, noting for atrophy, spasm, or localized areas of pain.

14 **Triceps brachii**: Palpate the long head of the triceps brachii tendon superiorly until the insertion disappears under the posterior deltoid.

Joint and Muscle Function Assessment

The motion occurring at the GH, AC, and SC joints, as well as the motion of the scapula, is evaluated during functional assessment, keeping in mind the interrelationship among these articulations. A deficit at one joint affects the motion of the others. These functional tests must not be performed when severe traumatic injuries such as fractures, joint dislocation, or complete muscle tears are suspected.

The amount of motion that the GH joint is capable of producing depends on the position of the greater and the lesser tuberosities relative to the scapula's bony structures. To achieve complete abduction, the humerus must externally rotate to allow the greater tuberosity to clear under the acromion process. The motion of flexion does not depend on relative internal or external rotation of the humerus because the greater tuberosity depresses inferiorly and passes beneath the acromion process.[8]

In healthy individuals, strength is equal in both extremities.[18] This strength relationship may vary among athletes involved in throwing and racquet sports. The dominant shoulder of collegiate tennis players produce a significantly greater amount of torque and power during internal rotation than the nondominant shoulder does.[19] Professional baseball pitchers do not display a significant difference in the amount of peak torque produced during internal rotation when compared bilaterally, but a significant difference does arise at high speeds (greater than or equal to 300° per second) during external rotation, with the dominant arm producing more torque.[20] The strength ratio of internal to external rotators is 3:2 for concentric contractions and 3:4 for eccentric contractions.[21]

Goniometric evaluation of shoulder ROM is presented in Goniometry Boxes 16-1 through 16-4.

Active range of motion

The muscles acting on the scapulothoracic articulation are presented in Table 16-4 and those acting on the glenohumeral joint in Table 16-5. An evaluation of the aggregate

Goniometry Box 16-1
Shoulder Goniometry: Flexion and Extension

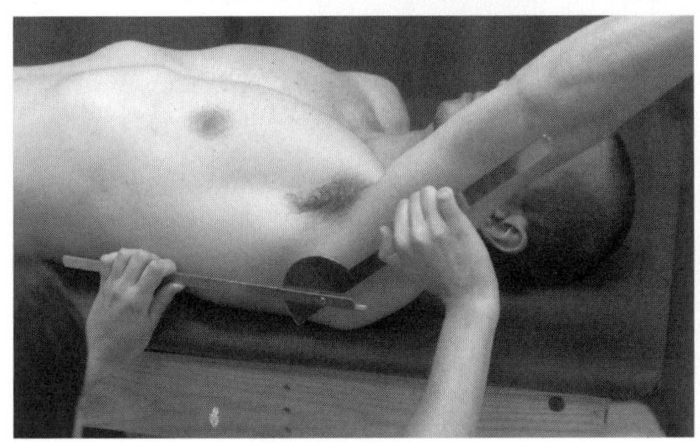

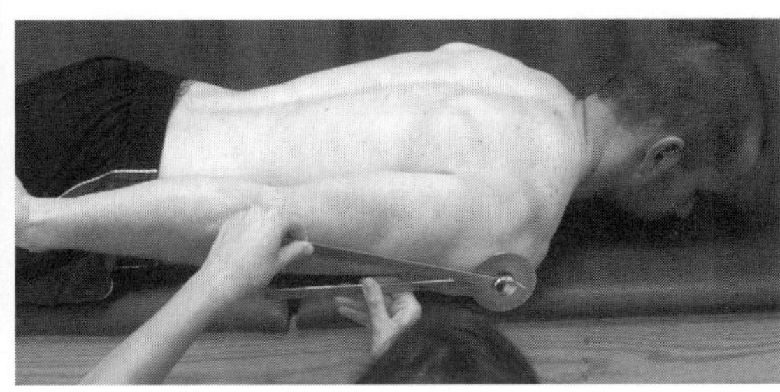

	GH Flexion/0 to 120° Elevation Through Flexion/0 to 180°	GH Extension/0 to 60°
Patient Position	Supine	Prone
Goniometer Alignment		
Fulcrum	Aligned lateral to the acromion process	Aligned lateral to the acromion process
Proximal Arm	The stationary arm is aligned parallel to the thorax.	The stationary arm is aligned parallel to the thorax.
Distal Arm	The movement arm is centered over the midline of the lateral humerus.	The movement arm is centered over the midline of the lateral humerus.
Comments	To isolate GH flexion, stabilize the scapula at its lateral border. Perform the measurement at the point where the scapula begins to move.	Stabilize the scapula on its posterior surface to isolate GH extension.

GH = glenohumeral.

Goniometry Box 16-2
Shoulder Goniometry: Abduction

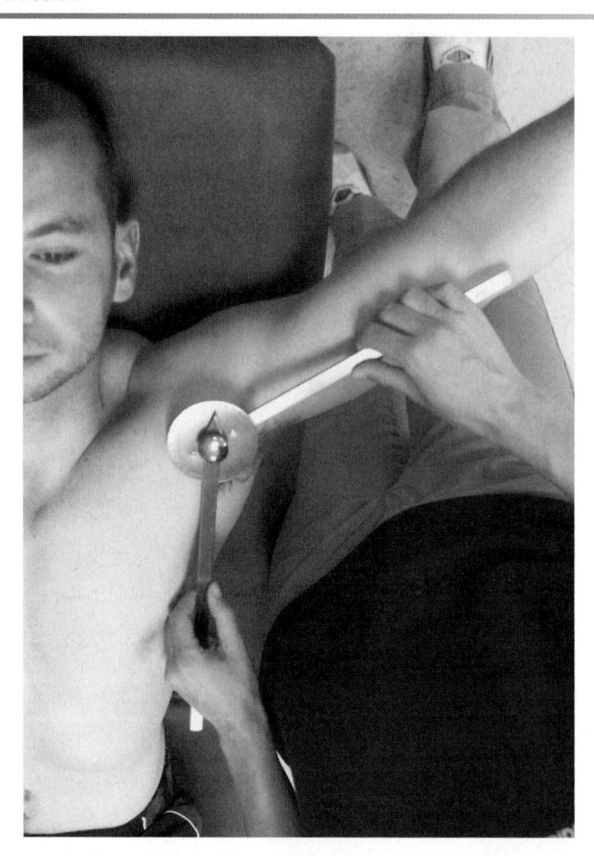

GH Abduction/0 to 120°
Elevation Through Abduction/0 to 180°

Patient Position	Supine or sitting
Goniometer Alignment	
Fulcrum	Anterior to the acromion process
Proximal Arm	The stationary arm is aligned parallel to the long axis of the torso.
Distal Arm	The movement arm is centered over the midline of the anterior humerus.
Comments	To isolate GH abduction, stabilize the scapula at its lateral border. Perform the measurement at the point where the scapula begins to move. Adduction is not normally measured.

GH = glenohumeral.

Goniometry Box 16-3
Shoulder Goniometry: Internal and External Rotation

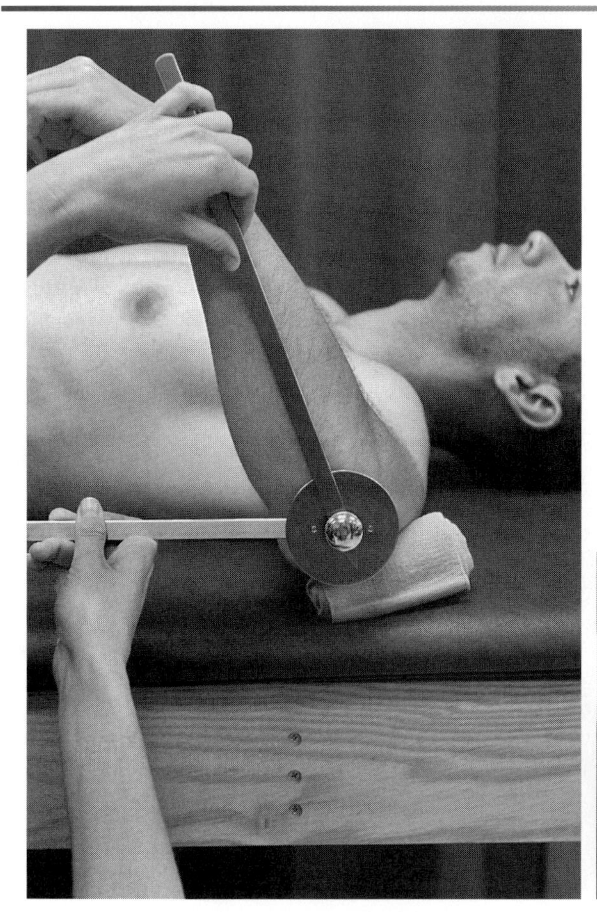

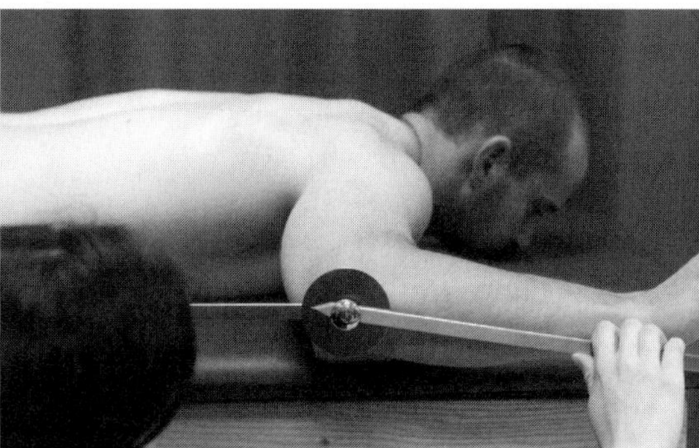

	Internal Rotation 0 to 90°	External Rotation 0 to 100°
Patient Position	Supine with the shoulder abducted to 90° and the elbow flexed to 90°	Prone with the shoulder abducted to 90° and the elbow flexed to 90°
Goniometer Alignment		
Fulcrum	Centered lateral to the olecranon process	
Proximal Arm	The stationary arm is aligned perpendicular to the floor or parallel to the tabletop.	
Distal Arm	The movement arm is centered over the long axis of the ulna.	
Comments	Anterior instability may result in pain and/or apprehension at the end range of external rotation (the apprehension test). To isolate GH motion, stabilize the scapula during external rotation. Perform the measurement at the point where the scapula begins to move. Scapular stabilization is provided by the body weight during internal rotation.	

GH = glenohumeral.

Goniometry 16-4
Shoulder Goniometry: Horizontal Abduction and Adduction

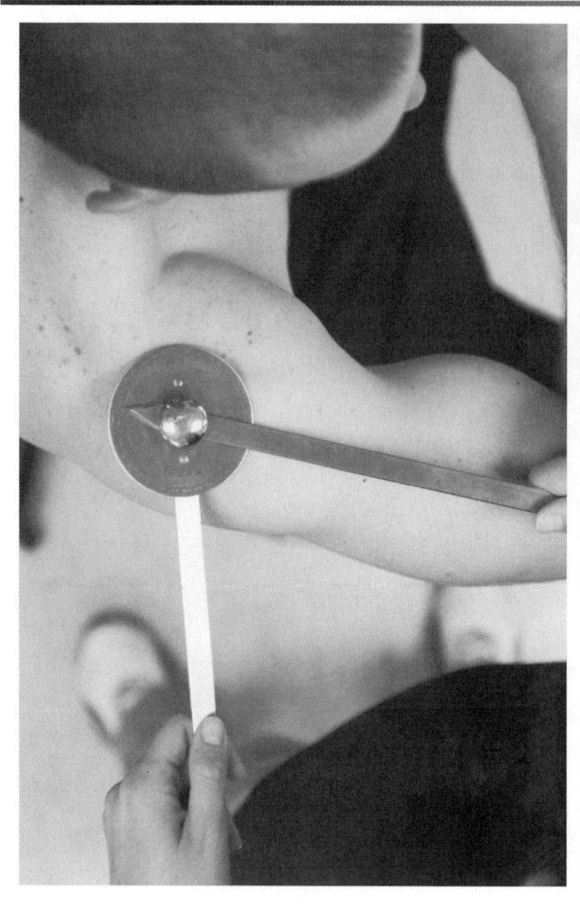

GH Horizontal Abduction 0 to 90°

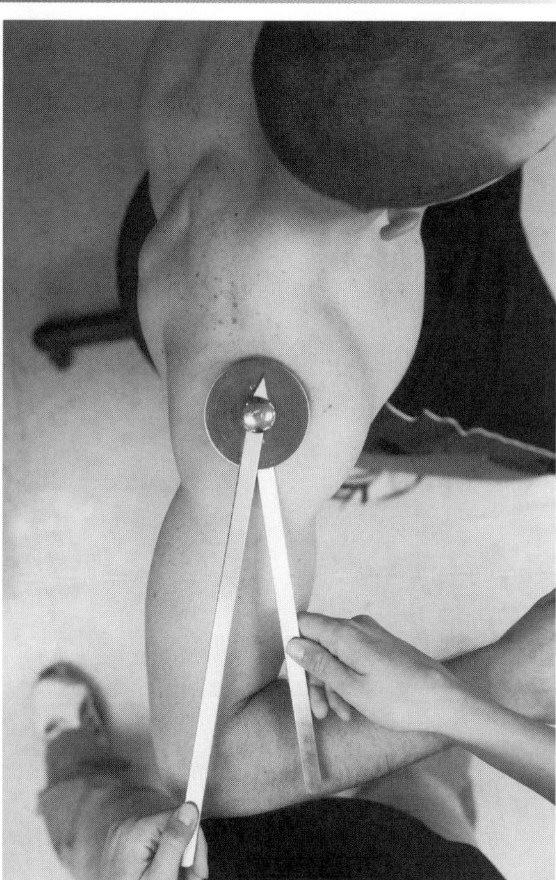

GH Horizontal Adduction 0 to 50°

Patient Position	Seated with the arm abducted to 90º; the elbow is flexed, and the forearm is pronated.
Goniometer Alignment	
Fulcrum	Superior acromioclavicular joint
Proximal Arm	The stationary arm is perpendicular to the trunk.
Distal Arm	The movable arm is parallel to the longitudinal axis of the humerus.
Comment	To isolate glenohumeral motion during horizontal adduction, stabilize the scapula at its lateral border.

motion available to the shoulder complex can be quickly determined through the **Apley's scratch test** (Box 16-2). Each of the three components of this test should be compared bilaterally to determine a decrease in the ROM, pain, and the willingness to move.

- **Flexion and extension**: The shoulder complex is capable of producing 220 to 240 degrees of movement in the sagittal plane (Fig. 16-24). The majority of this ROM, accounting for 170 to 180 degrees of motion from the anatomical position, is provided by flexion. The remaining 50 to 60 degrees occur from the limb's moving from the anatomical position to extension.
- **Abduction and adduction**: Occurring in the frontal plane, the normal ROM for abduction is 170 to 180 degrees (Fig. 16-25). The motion of adduction is blocked in the anatomical position and any further movement requires that the GH joint be flexed or extended so that the humerus can pass in front of or behind the torso. The patient's ability to control adduction should be noticed. An arm that falls uncontrollably from 90 degrees of abduction indicates a positive **drop arm test** for rotator cuff pathology (Special Test 16-1).[23] The

Table 16-4 Muscles Contributing to Scapular Movements

Elevation	**Protraction**	**Upward Rotation**
Levator scapulae	Serratus anterior	Serratus anterior
Rhomboid major		Trapezius (upper and lower portion)
Rhomboid minor		
Serratus anterior (upper portion)		
Trapezius (upper portion)		
Depression	**Retraction**	**Downward Rotation**
Serratus anterior (lower portion)	Rhomboid major	Rhomboid major
Trapezius (lower portion)	Rhomboid minor	Rhomboid minor
Pectoralis major (clavicular portion)	Trapezius (middle fibers)	Levator scapulae
	Trapezius (lower fibers)	Trapezius (lower portion)

Table 16-5 Muscles Contributing to Humeral Movements

Flexion	**Adduction**	**Horizontal Adduction**	**Internal Rotation**
Biceps brachii	Coracobrachialis	Deltoid (anterior one third)	Deltoid (anterior one third)
Coracobrachialis	Latissimus dorsi	Pectoralis major	Latissimus dorsi
Deltoid (anterior one third)	Pectoralis major		Pectoralis major
Deltoid (middle one third)	Teres major		Subscapularis
Pectoralis major (clavicular fibers)	Triceps brachii		Teres major
Extension	**Abduction**	**Horizontal Abduction**	**External Rotation**
Deltoid (posterior one third)	Biceps brachii	Deltoid (posterior one third)	Deltoid (posterior one third)
Latissimus dorsi	Deltoid (anterior one third)	Infraspinatus	Infraspinatus
Teres major	Deltoid (middle one third)	Teres minor	Teres minor
Triceps brachii (long head)	Deltoid (posterior one third)		Supraspinatus
	Supraspinatus		

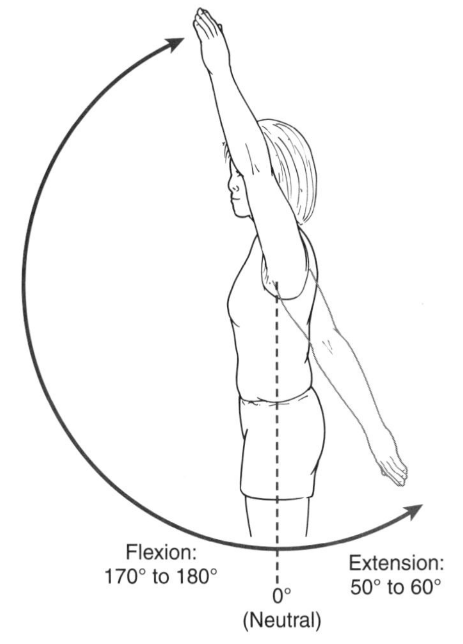

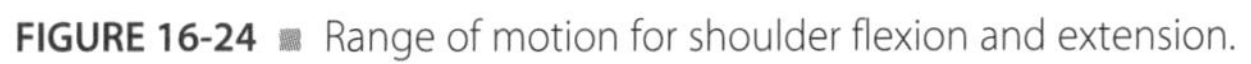
FIGURE 16-24 ■ Range of motion for shoulder flexion and extension.

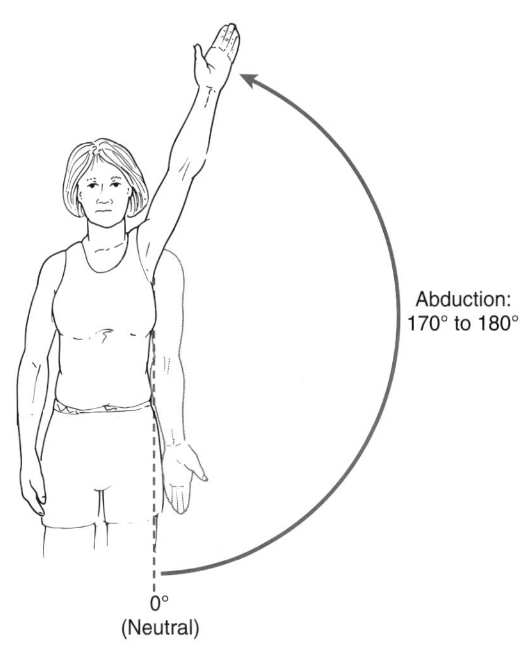

FIGURE 16-25 ■ Range of motion for shoulder abduction and adduction.

Special Test 16-1
Drop Arm Test for Rotator Cuff Tendinopathy

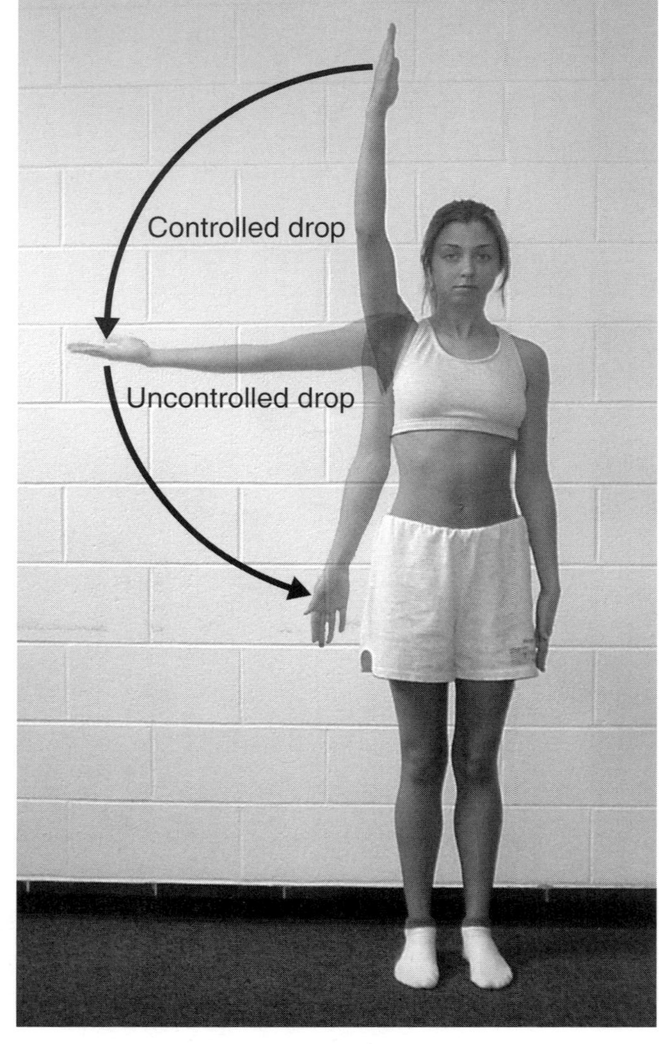

The drop arm test determines the patient's ability to control humeral motion via an eccentric contraction as the arm is slowly lowered from full abduction to adduction.

Patient Position	Standing or sitting The humerus fully abducted and externally rotated and the forearm supinated

Position of Examiner	Standing lateral to, or behind, the involved extremity
Evaluative Procedure	The patient slowly lowers the arm to the side.
Positive Test	The arm falls uncontrollably from a position of approximately 90° abduction to the side. Severe pain may also be described.
Implications	The inability to lower the arm in a controlled manner is indicative of lesions to the rotator cuff, especially the supraspinatus.
Modification	If the patient is able to lower the arm in a controlled manner through the ROM, a derivative of the drop arm test may be implemented: The patient holds the humerus in 90° abduction. The examiner applies gentle pressure on the distal forearm. A positive test result causes the arm to fall against the side of the body, indicating lesions to the rotator cuff.
Evidence	Positive likelihood ratio Not Useful — Useful Very Small — Small — Moderate — Large 0 1 2 3 4 5 6 7 8 9 10 Negative likelihood ratio Not Useful — Useful Very Small — Small — Moderate — Large 1.0 0.9 0.8 0.7 0.6 0.5 0.4 0.3 0.2 0.1 0

ROM = range of motion.

Box 16-2
Apley's Scratch Tests

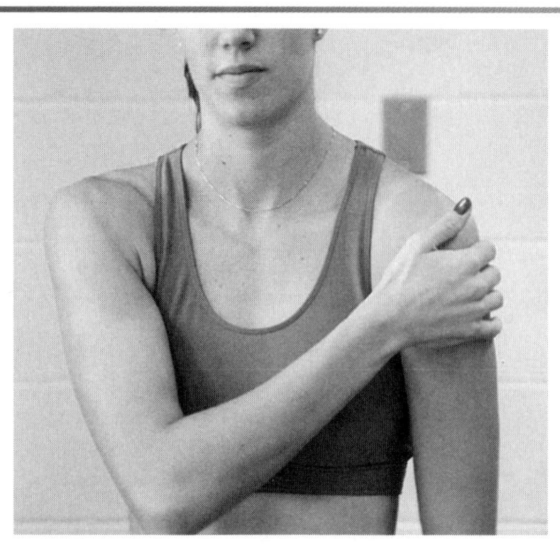

The patient touches the opposite shoulder by crossing the chest.

Motions produced: GH adduction, horizontal adduction, and internal rotation; scapular protraction

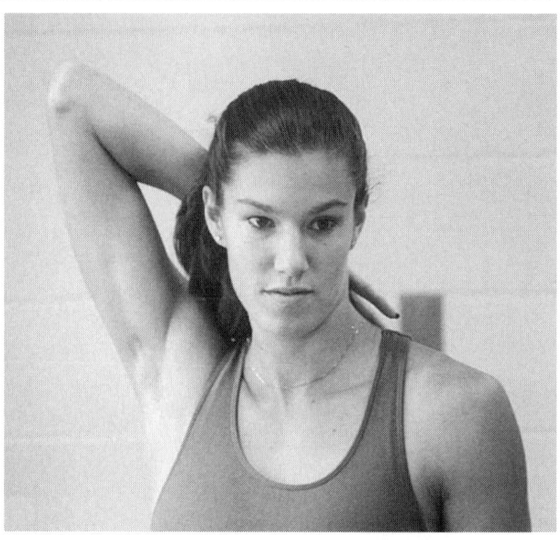

The patient reaches behind the head and touches the opposite shoulder from behind.

Motions produced: GH abduction and external rotation; scapular elevation, and upward rotation

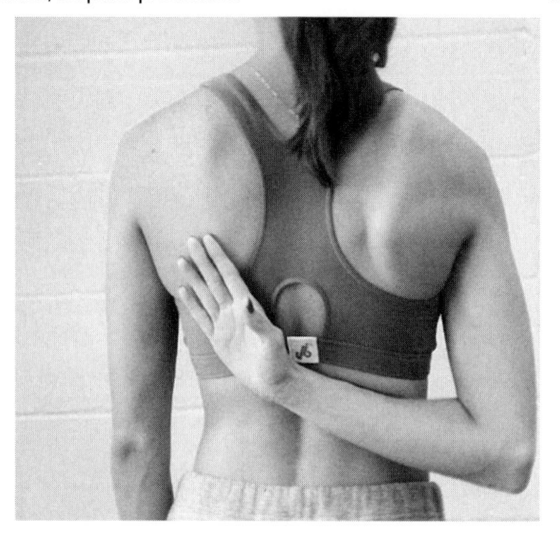

The patient reaches behind the back and touches the opposite scapula.

Motions produced: GH adduction and internal rotation; scapular retraction and downward rotation

GH = glenohumeral.

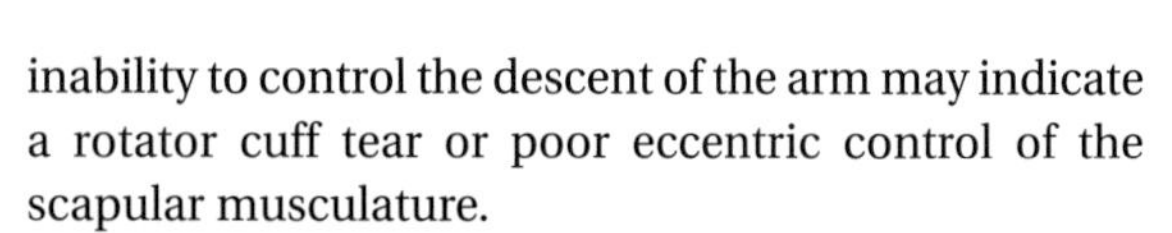

inability to control the descent of the arm may indicate a rotator cuff tear or poor eccentric control of the scapular musculature.

The patient may describe an area within the ROM that elicits pain. This painful arc, usually occurring between 60 and 120 degrees of abduction, is a sensitive indicator identifying impingement of the rotator cuff musculature between the humeral head and the coracoacromial arch.[22]

*** Practical Evidence**

The clinical usefulness of the drop arm test is improved when the results are combined with the findings of other tests. A positive drop arm test with an associated painful arc and a weak infraspinatus manual muscle test increase the probability of a full-thickness rotator cuff tear to 91%.[22]

- **Internal and external rotation**: Internal and external rotation is assessed in both the neutral position and in 90 degrees of abduction. In the neutral position, the humeral head and the greater tuberosity are allowed to rotate beneath the acromion without interference. During internal rotation, the torso blocks the motion. External rotation in this position, usually 40 to 50 degrees, is less than when the humerus is abducted 90 degrees. This motion is limited by the superior GH and coracohumeral ligaments.

When abducted to 90 degrees so that the greater and lesser tuberosities can clear the structures of the scapula, the GH joint can obtain an increased amount of internal and external rotation (Fig. 16-26). With the humerus in 90 degrees of abduction with the elbow flexed to 90 degrees, the normal ROM in this position is 80 to 90 degrees of external rotation and 70 to 80 degrees of internal rotation. These motions are restricted by the inferior GH ligament.

Internal and external rotation can be grossly measured using the Apley's scratch test (see Box 16-2). The amount of available internal rotation can be assessed by having the patient reach behind and up the back (Fig. 16-27). This measurement is more representative of functional motion than standard goniometry. The measurement is taken from the spinal level where the thumb rests at maximal motion. With the dominant hand, the patient should generally be capable of obtaining a spinal level that is equal to or greater than that obtainable on the nondominant side. Pathologic internal impingement is frequently associated with limitations in internal rotation.[24]

- **Horizontal adduction and abduction**: The neutral position for horizontal adduction and abduction is 90 degrees of abduction with the arm flexed at a 30 degree angle from the torso in the plane of the scapula (see Fig. 16-5). Occurring in the horizontal plane, the expected ROM is 120 degrees of horizontal adduction and 45 degrees of horizontal abduction relative to the plane of the scapula. Tightness of the posterior capsule can limit the amount of horizontal adduction.

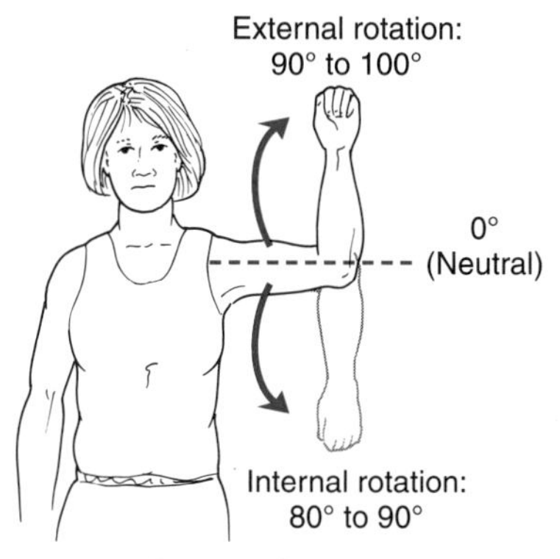

FIGURE 16-26 ■ Range of motion for shoulder internal rotation and external rotation.

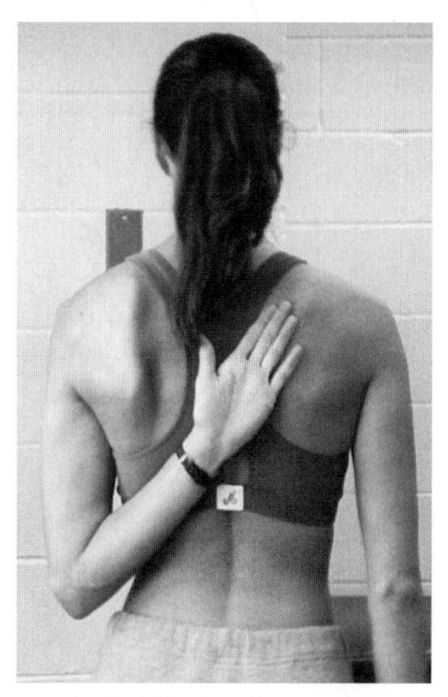

FIGURE 16-27 ■ Method of checking for shoulder internal rotation as recommended by the American Academy of Orthopaedic Surgeons. The amount of internal GH rotation is determined by measuring the distance up the spinal column the patient can reach and comparing this result to that of the opposite shoulder. This method is similar to part of the Apley's scratch test (see Box 16-2).

Manual muscle testing

Following active range of motion (AROM), manual muscle testing is used to detect pain or weakness associated with more specific muscle involvement. While resistance can be applied throughout the range, the results are equivocal because a variety of structures are stressed. The use of an isometric (or break) test in the midrange of motion may minimize other causes of pain and weakness (Manual Muscle Tests 16-1 through 16-4). The **Gerber lift-off test** is a sensitive method of isolating the subscapularis (Special Test 16-2).[25–27,29]

Scapular movements

Observe the motion of the scapula during active humeral movements, noting any winging of the scapula and comparing the scapulothoracic rhythm on one side with that of the opposite side. A greater than normal contribution to humeral elevation is usually observed in patients suffering from GH instability, rotator cuff pathology, or impingement syndromes.[17] Normal elevation includes upward rotation of the scapula coupled with posterior tilting. If the scapula cannot achieve sufficient posterior tilt, which can be caused by tightness of the pectoralis minor, subacromial space is limited increasing the likelihood for impingement.[30]

Winging of the vertebral border may occur during elevation of the humerus and during the eccentric return to the neutral position.[17] Scapular winging (or increased internal rotation) may occur secondary to weakness of the serratus anterior muscle or inhibition of the long thoracic nerve. The most common clinical approach to determining the presence of a winging scapula is to have the patient push

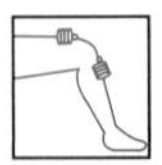

Manual Muscle Test 16-1
Shoulder Flexion and Extension

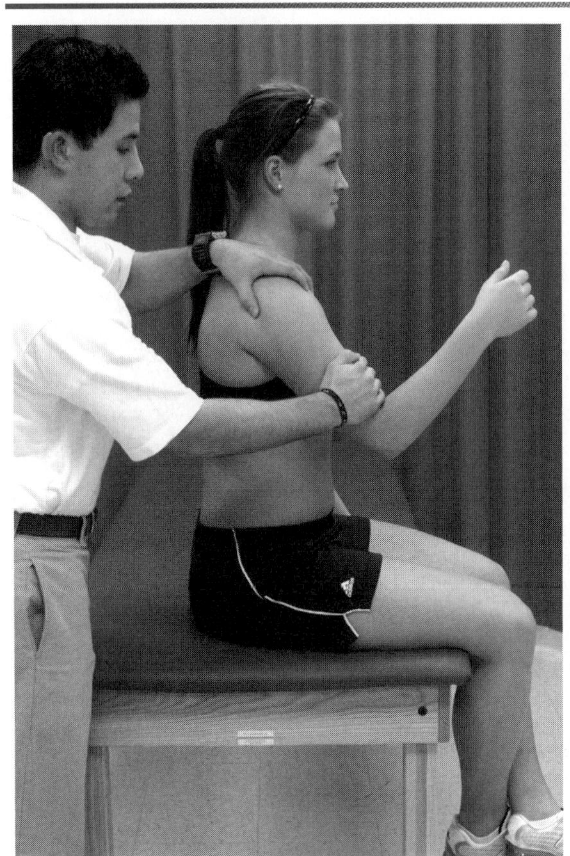

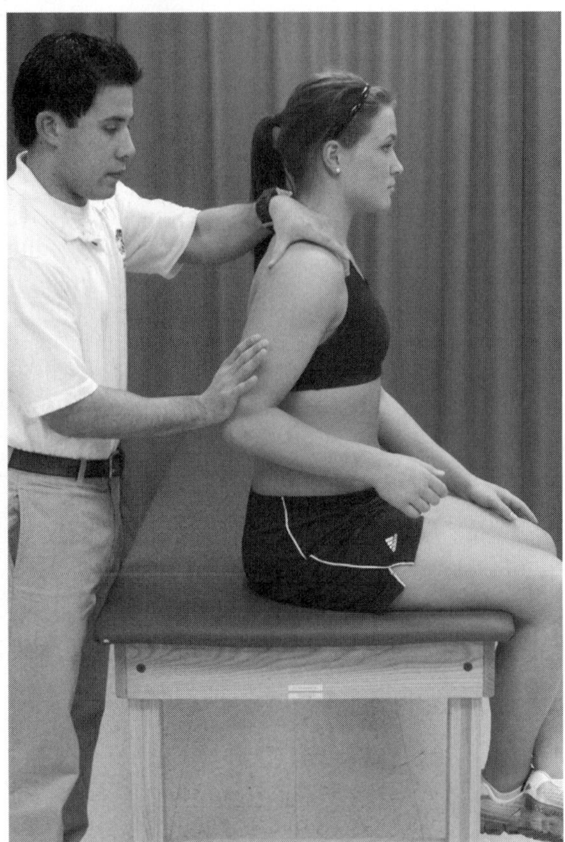

	Flexion	Extension
Patient Position	Seated	
Starting Position	The humerus in the neutral position	
Stabilization	Superior aspect of the shoulder	
Palpation	Anterior shoulder at anterior lateral aspect of clavicle	Latissimus dorsi: Inferior to inferior angle of scapula Teres major: Posterior axilla
Resistance	Distal anterior humerus, just proximal to the cubital fossa	Distal posterior humerus, just proximal to the olecranon
Primary Mover(s) (innervation)	Anterior deltoid (C5, C6)	Latissimus dorsi (C6, C7, C8) Teres major (C5, C6, C7)
Secondary Mover(s) (innervation)	Pectoralis major (clavicular portion) (C6, C7, C8, T1) Coracobrachialis (C6, C7) Middle deltoid (C5, C6) Biceps brachii (C5, C6) Lower trapezius Serratus anterior	Posterior deltoid (C5, C6) Triceps brachii (long head) (C6, C7, C8, T1)
Substitution	Trunk extension, scapular elevation	Scapular protraction (from pectoralis minor)
Comments	Not applicable	Maintain elbow extension to minimize contributions from the triceps.

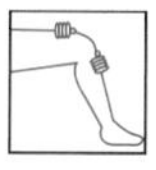

Manual Muscle Test 16-2
Shoulder Abduction and Adduction

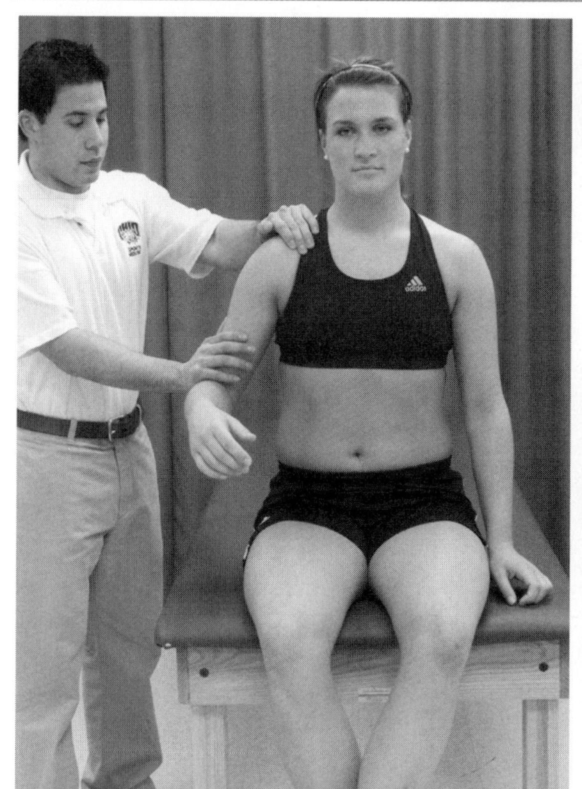

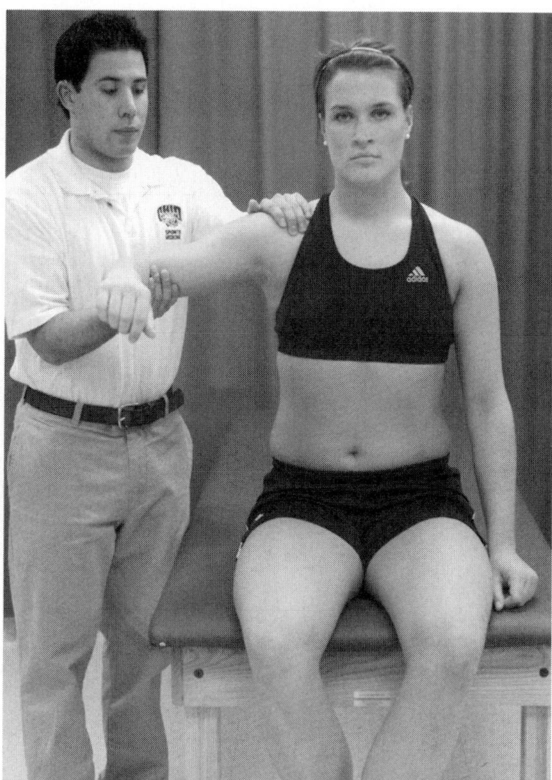

	Abduction	Adduction
Patient Position	Seated	Seated or supine
Starting Position	The humerus abducted to approximately 30°	
Stabilization	Scapula	
Palpation	Deltoid: Just lateral to tip of acromion.	Pectoralis major: Anterior axilla Latissimus dorsi: Inferior to inferior angle of scapula Teres major: Posterior axilla
Resistance	Distal humerus, just proximal to the lateral epicondyle	Distal humerus, just proximal to the medial epicondyle
Primary Mover(s) (Innervation)	Deltoid muscle group (C5, C6) Supraspinatus (C4, C5, C6)	Pectoralis major (C6, C7, C8, T1) Latissimus dorsi (C6, C7, C8) Teres major (C5, C6, C7)
Secondary Mover(s) (Innervation)	Biceps brachii (C5, C6) (greater than 90º abduction)	Coracobrachialis (C6, C7) Triceps brachii (C6, C7, C8, T1)
Substitution	Scapular elevation, external rotation, trunk lateral flexion to same or opposite side	Trunk lateral flexion to same side
Comments		The supine position is used for stabilization. Better isolation of the primary movers is achieved by testing shoulder extension and horizontal adduction.

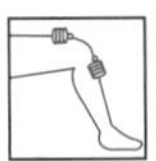

Manual Muscle Test 16-3
Shoulder Internal and External Rotation

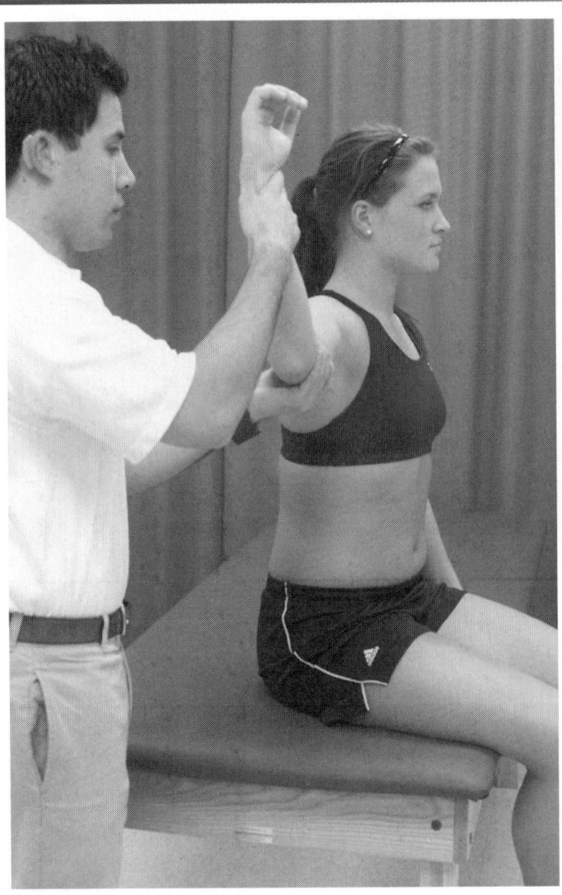

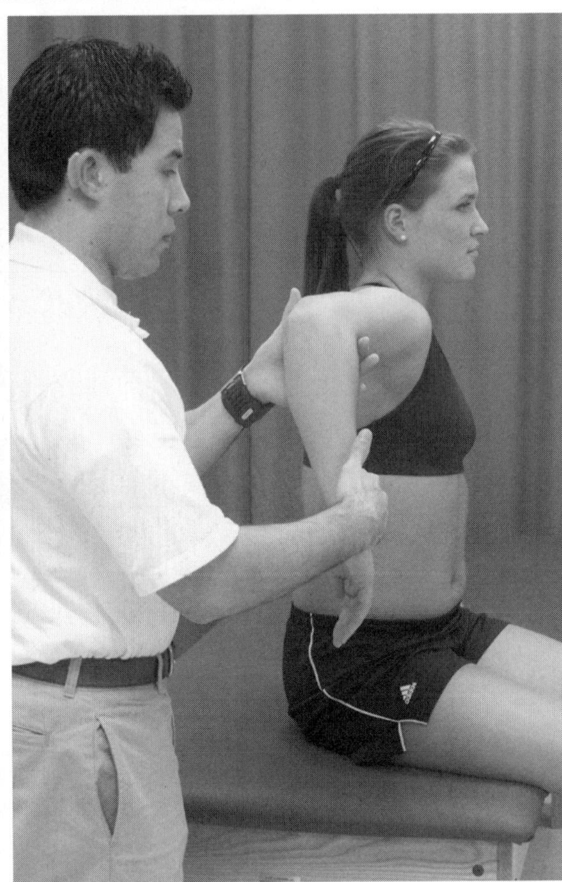

	Internal Rotation	External Rotation
Patient Position	Seated or prone. Stabilization is improved with the patient prone.	
Starting Position	The humerus is in neutral position or abducted to 90°. The elbow is flexed to 90°.	
Stabilization	The distal humerus is stabilized just proximal to the elbow.	
Palpation	Subscapularis: Too deep to palpate	Infraspinatus and teres minor: Inferior to spine of scapula
Resistance	Anterior distal forearm	Posterior distal forearm
Primary Mover(s) (Innervation)	Subscapularis (C5, C6, C7)	Infraspinatus (C5, C6) Teres minor (C5 C6)
Secondary Mover(s) (Innervation)	Teres major (C5, C6, C7) Pectoralis major Latissimus dorsi Anterior deltoid	Posterior deltoid
Substitution	Elbow extension, scapular protraction	Elbow extension, scapular depression
Comments	Optimal isolation of the subscapularis occurs at 45° of internal rotation with the arm at the side.[28] The Gerber lift-off test is also used to assess subscapularis strength.	Optimal isolation of the infraspinatus occurs at 45° of internal rotation with the arm at the side.[28]

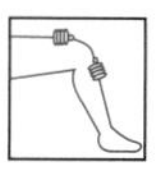

Manual Muscle Test 16-4
Horizontal Adduction and Abduction

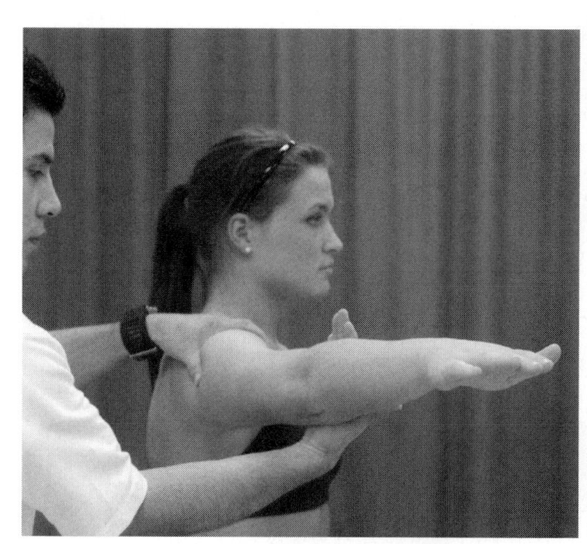

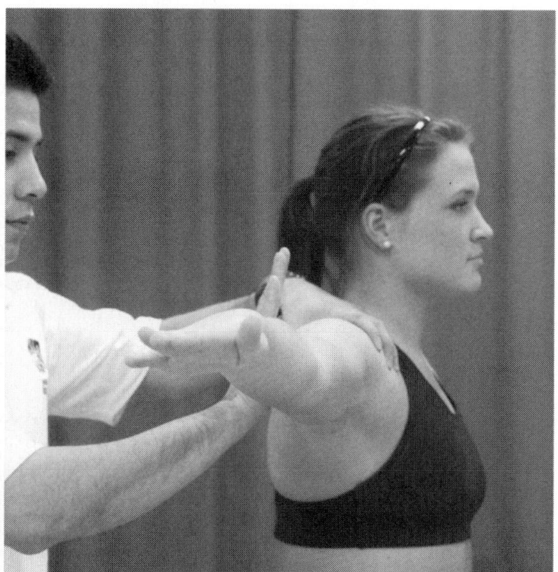

	Horizontal Adduction	Horizontal Abduction
Patient Position	Supine	Prone
Starting Position	The shoulder is abducted to 90°	
Stabilization	Scapula	Scapula
Palpation	Anterior axilla	Inferior to lateral spine of the scapula
Resistance	Anterior portion of the distal humerus	Posterior portion of the distal humerus
Primary Mover(s) (Innervation)	Pectoralis major (C6, C7, C8, T1)	Posterior deltoid (C5, C6)
Secondary Mover(s) (Innervation)	Coracobrachialis (C6, C7) Anterior deltoid (C5, C6)	Infraspinatus (C5, C6) Teres minor (C5, C6)
Substitution	Trunk rotation	Scapular retraction, trunk rotation

Special Test 16-2
Gerber Lift-off Test for Subscapularis Pathology

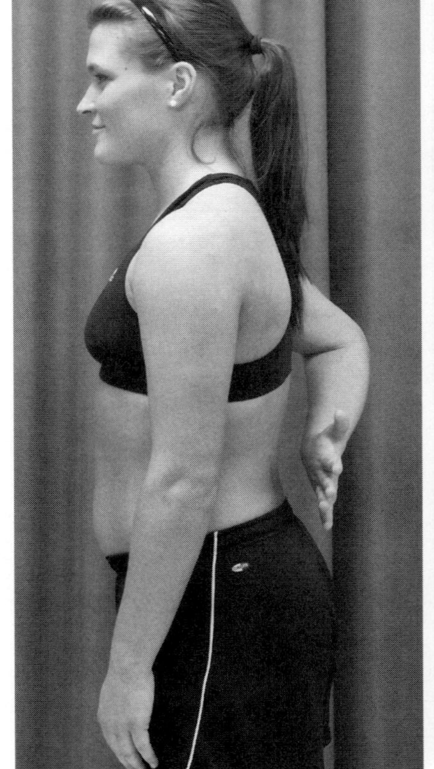
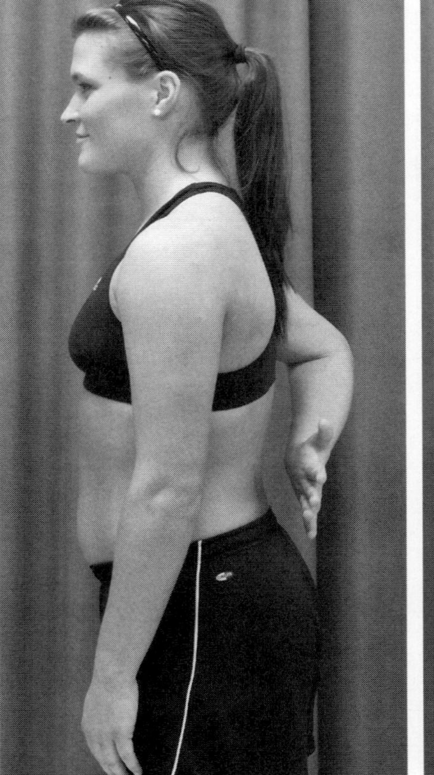
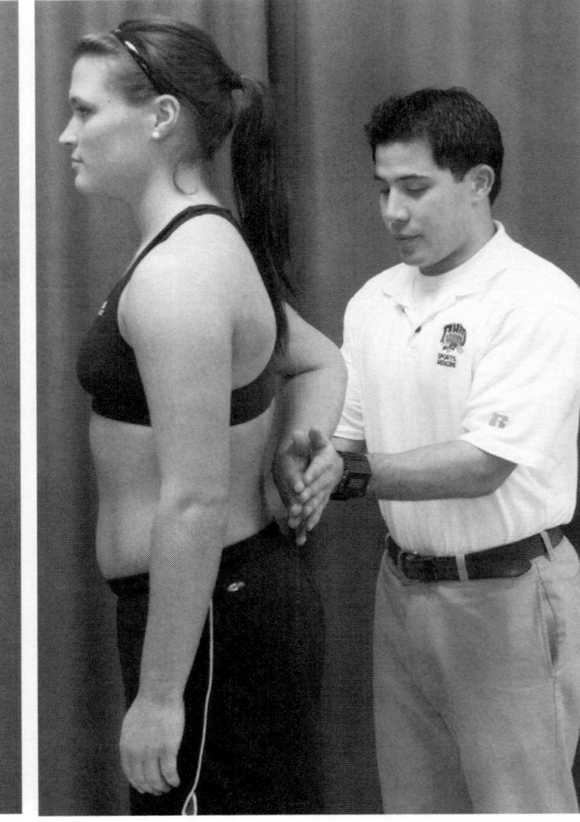

The Gerber lift-off test is a modification of a subscapularis manual muscle test.

Patient Position	Standing with the humerus internally rotated The dorsal surface of the hand placed against the midlumbar spine
Position of Examiner	Standing behind the patient
Evaluative Procedure	The patient attempts to actively lift the hand off the spine while the humerus stays in extension.
Positive Test	Inability to lift the hand off the back
Implications	Positive test findings are associated with tears or weakness of the subscapularis muscle. Possible C5, C6, C7 nerve root pathology

Modification	Resistance can be applied to the patient's palm.
Comments	Test should be performed only if the patient has sufficient internal rotation to reach sacral region or above. Do not allow compensatory motions such as GH extension. With the arm in this position, the subscapularis contributes almost 90% of the force when no resistance is applied. A MMT lower than grade 3 (lift off with no resistance) accurately identifies those with a subscapularis tear 85% of the time.[28]
Evidence	Positive likelihood ratio Not Useful — Useful Very Small · Small · Moderate · Large 0 1 2 3 4 5 6 7 8 9 10 Negative likelihood ratio Not Useful — Useful Very Small · Small · Moderate · Large 1.0 0.9 0.8 0.7 0.6 0.5 0.4 0.3 0.2 0.1 0

GH = glenohumeral; MMT= manual muscle test.

against the wall while observing the relative scapular alignment (Fig. 16-28). Winging of the scapula is immediately apparent when the cause is inhibition of the long thoracic nerve. Winging caused by weakness of the serratus anterior may not become apparent until the muscle is fatigued. For this reason, the patient should perform this standing push-up maneuver a minimum of 10 times. Manual muscle testing of the scapular muscles is presented in Manual Muscle Test Boxes 16-5 through 16-9.

Passive range of motion

Passive range of motion (PROM) assessment helps detect the nature of any joint restriction by detecting the quality and quantity of motion coupled with an assessment of end-feel (Table 16-6). Scapular stabilization is important to differentiate glenohumeral motion from shoulder girdle motion. Glenohumeral capsule involvement results in a characteristic pattern of restriction (see Table 16-6), with external rotation and abduction being limited initially. Patients who present with equal limitations in active and passive motion may have **adhesive capsulitis,** or a frozen shoulder. Usually affecting those older than age of 50, adhesive capsulitis commonly has an idiopathic onset characterized initially by sporadic pain and progressing to constant pain and capsular restriction.

- **Flexion and extension**: PROM may be isolated to the GH joint or may encompass the entire motion allowed by the shoulder complex. To isolate the GH joint, the scapula must be stabilized to prevent its contribution to shoulder motion. When the entire motion provided by the shoulder complex is evaluated, the thorax must be stabilized. Each of these two methods of stabilization is more easily accomplished with the patient sitting or lying supine during flexion and prone during extension (Fig. 16-29).

Table 16-6 Glenohumeral Joint Capsular Patterns and End-Feels

Capsular Pattern: External Rotation, Abduction, Internal Rotation	
Elevation	Firm or hard
Extension	Firm
Flexion	Firm
Abduction	Firm or hard
Horizontal Abduction	Firm
Horizontal Adduction	Firm or soft
Internal Rotation	Firm
External Rotation	Firm

Flexion should have a firm end-feel for both GH and shoulder complex motions. During GH flexion, the terminal motion is checked by the tightening of the GH capsule (especially the coracohumeral ligament and the posterior capsular fibers) and the teres minor, teres major, and infraspinatus muscles. The muscles attaching to the anterior portion of the humerus, especially the pectoralis major and the latissimus dorsi, normally terminate flexion accomplished by the entire shoulder complex.

The two types of passive extension result in a firm end-feel. During isolated GH extension, the coracohumeral ligament and the anterior joint capsule become taut. During extension of the shoulder complex, the pectoralis major (clavicular fibers) and serratus anterior muscles contribute to the end-feel.

Pain occurring at the end range of passive flexion may indicate impingement of the supraspinatus ten-

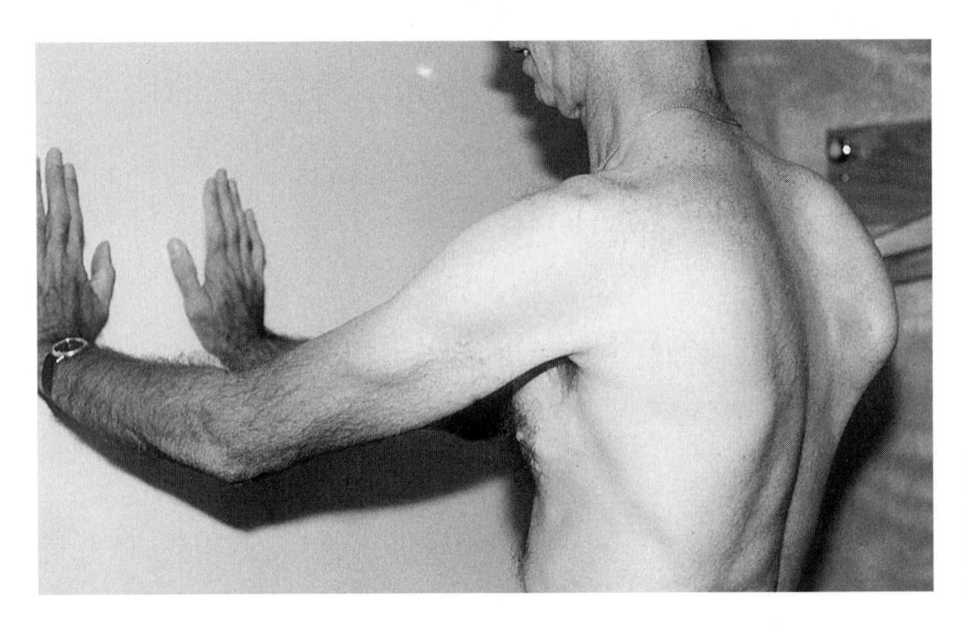

FIGURE 16-28 ■ Test for scapular winging. In the presence of a weakened serratus anterior muscle, or long thoracic nerve injury, performing a "push-up" against a wall causes the vertebral border of the scapula to lift off the thorax.

don, long head of the biceps brachii, or the subacromial bursa between the inferior portion of the acromion process and the humeral head. Pain during passive extension may result from damage to the anterior portion of the GH capsule or the coracohumeral ligament.

- **Abduction and adduction**: As in the case of flexion and extension, abduction is the result of motion's arising from the shoulder complex or isolated to its pure GH movement. When attempting to isolate GH abduction, the scapula is stabilized to prevent its upward rotation and elevation. To restrict motion to the shoulder complex, the thorax is stabilized to eliminate lateral bending of the spine. Passive abduction may be examined with the patient sitting or supine (Fig. 16-30).

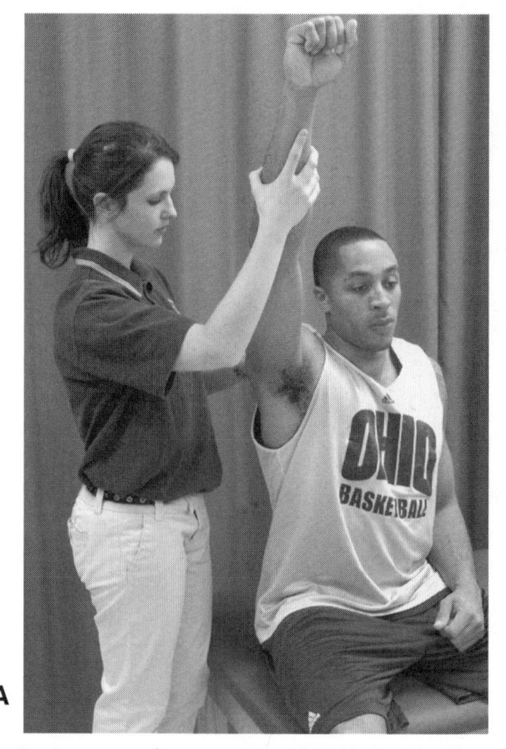

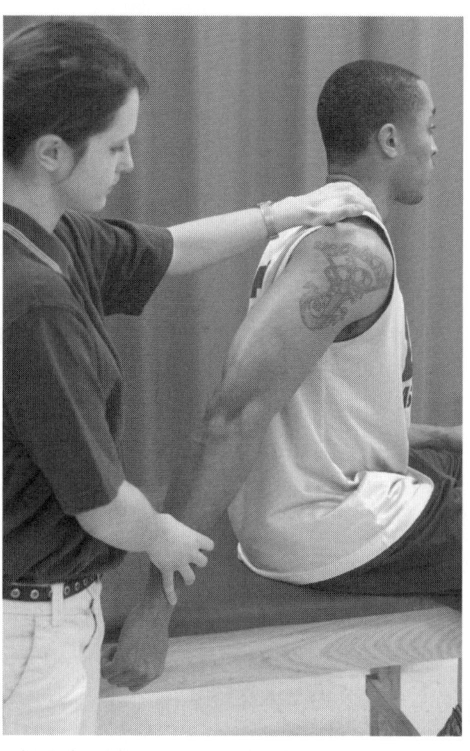

FIGURE 16-29 ■ Passive range of motion testing for **(A)** shoulder flexion and **(B)** shoulder extension. Flex the elbow to reduce biceps brachii tension from restricting the ROM.

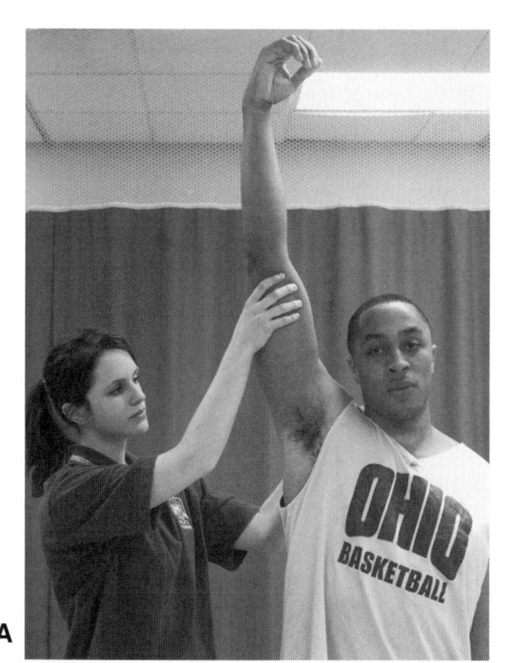

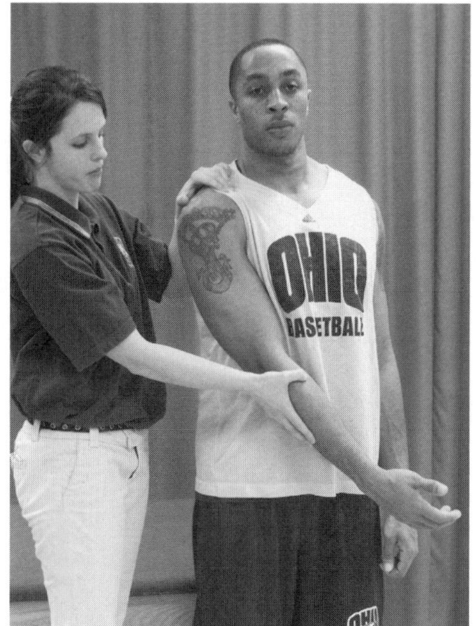

FIGURE 16-30 ■ Passive range of motion testing for shoulder abduction **(A)** and adduction **(B)**.

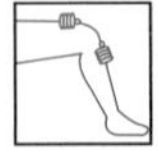

Manual Muscle Test 16-5
Scapular Retraction and Downward Rotation

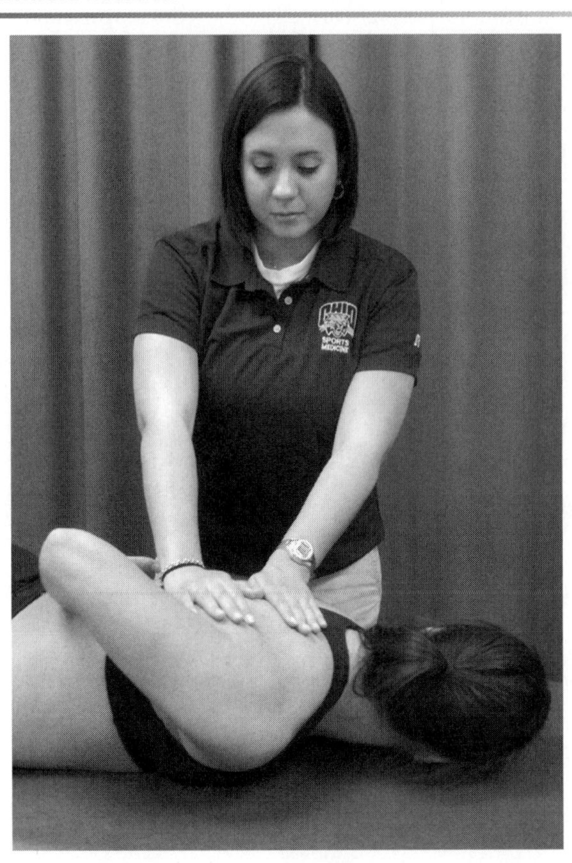

Patient Position	Prone
Starting Position	The arm being tested is behind the patient's back, with the humerus internally rotated.
Stabilization	Trunk
Palpation	Lateral to vertebral border of scapula
Resistance	Lateral scapula as the patient attempts to lift the hand off the back in an upward and lateral direction
Primary Mover(s) (Innervation)	Rhomboid major (C4, C5) Rhomboid minor (C4, C5)
Secondary Mover(s) (Innervation)	Middle trapeziums
Substitution	Trunk rotation, glenohumeral extension, anterior tipping of scapula
Comments	Note the application of resistance on the scapula, which differentiates this from the Gerber lift-off test (see Special Test 16-2).

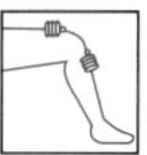

Manual Muscle Test 16-6
Scapular Retraction

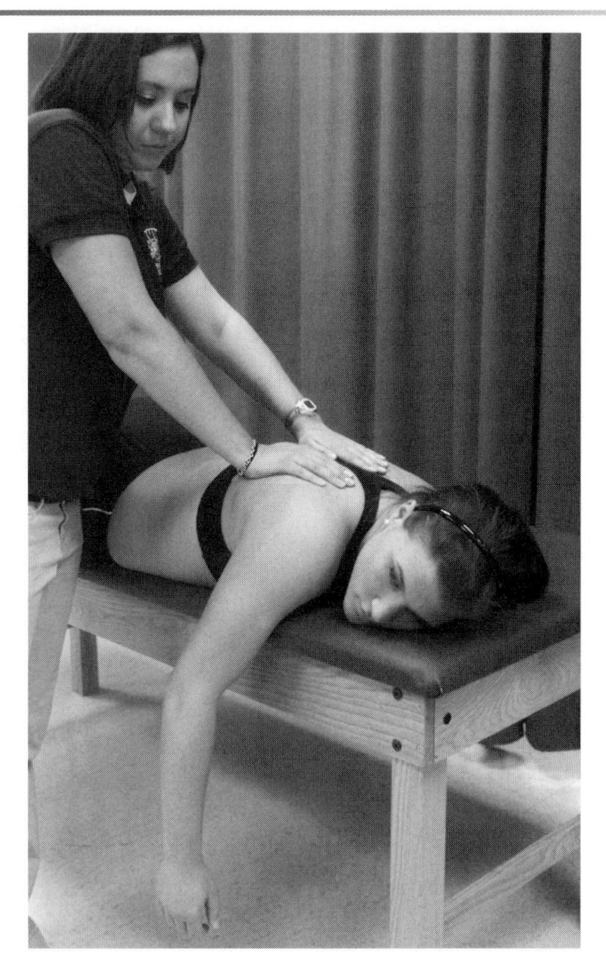

Patient Position	Prone
Starting Position	The elbow is extended and the humerus is flexed to 90°.
Stabilization	Trunk
Palpation	Between spine of scapula and spinous process
Resistance	Scapula
Primary Mover(s) (Innervation)	Middle trapezius (CN XI) Rhomboids
Secondary Mover(s) (Innervation)	Upper and lower trapezius
Substitution	Trunk rotation, glenohumeral horizontal abduction

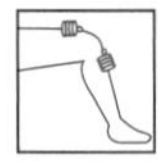

Manual Muscle Test 16-7
Scapular Protraction and Upward Rotation

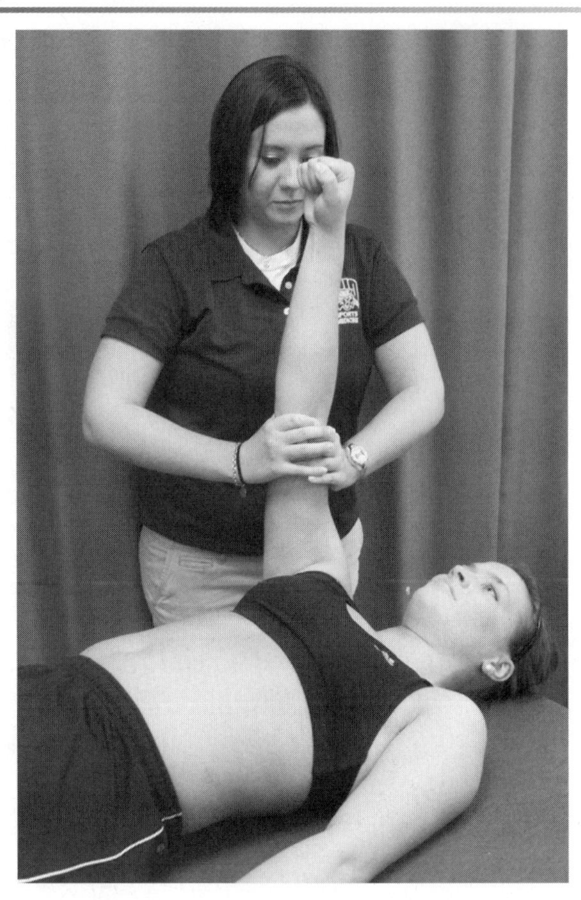

Patient Position	Supine
Starting Position	Test arm is flexed to 90°.
Stabilization	Trunk
Palpation	Lateral trunk
Resistance	Distal humerus, proximal to elbow. Instruct the patient to "punch the ceiling."
Primary Mover(s) (Innervation)	Serratus anterior (C5, C6, C7)
Secondary Mover(s) (Innervation)	Pectoralis minor Trapezius
Substitution	Glenohumeral adduction and horizontal adduction
Comments	Observe the patient performing a wall push-up to functionally assess the serratus anterior.

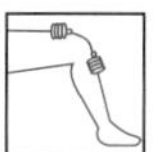

Manual Muscle Test 16-8
Scapular Depression and Retraction

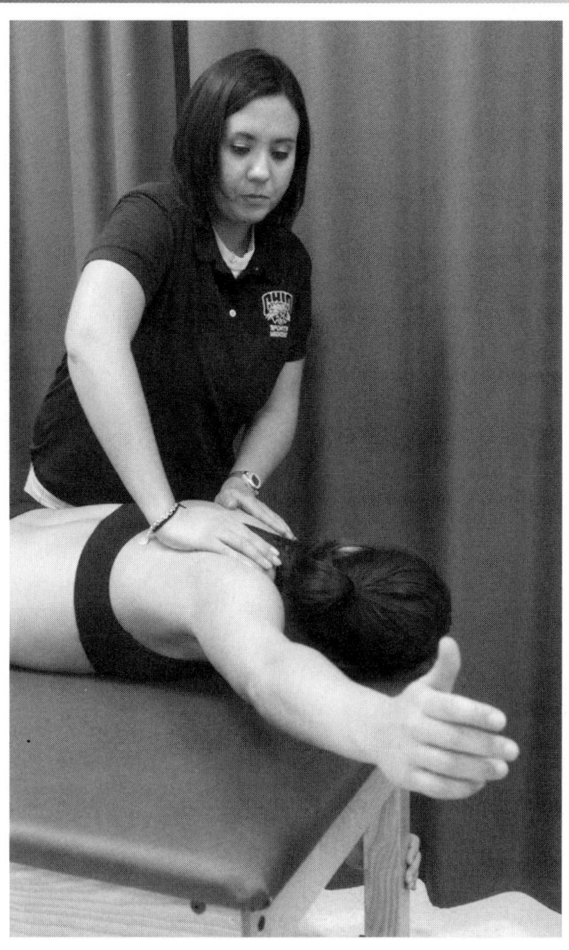

Patient Position	Prone
Starting Position	The arm being tested is abducted to 135° with the forearm supinated and the patient's head rotated to the side opposite that being tested.
Stabilization	Trunk
Palpation	Medial to inferior angle of scapula
Resistance	Scapula. Instruct the patient to "Raise your arm."
Primary Mover(s) (Innervation)	Lower trapezius (CN XI)
Secondary Mover(s) (Innervation)	Middle trapezius
Substitution	Trunk rotation; glenohumeral extension
Comments	Patients suffering from impingement may be unable to achieve this test position. In this case, position the arm at the side and instruct the patient to bring the scapula "down and in."

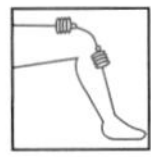

Manual Muscle Test 16-9
Scapular Elevation

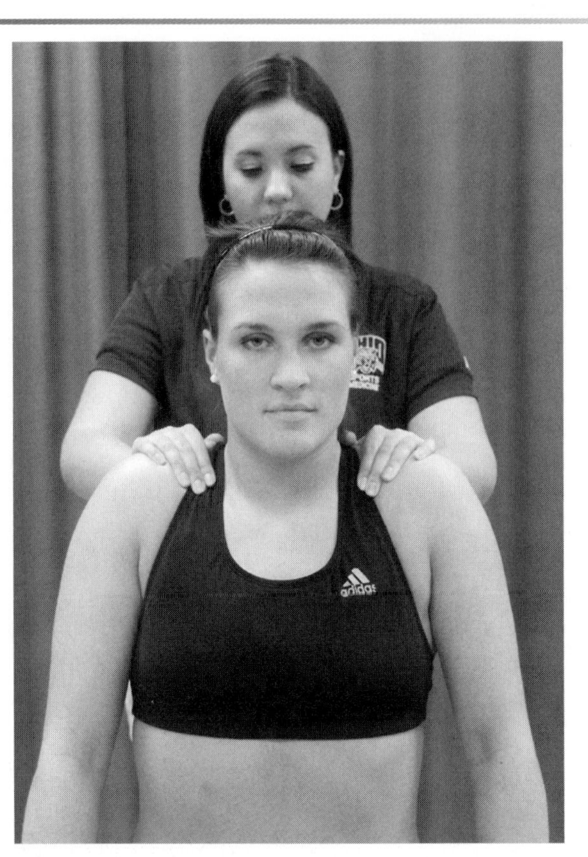

Patient Position	Seated
Starting Position	Seated
Stabilization	Trunk
Palpation	Superomedial to scapula
Resistance	Superior aspect of the shoulder. The patient assumes a shoulder shrug position which the examiner pushes down.
Primary Mover(s) (Innervation)	Upper trapezius (CN XI) Levator scapulae (C3, C4, C5)
Secondary Mover(s) (Innervation)	Not applicable
Substitution	Trunk rotation or side-bending

The normal ROM resulting from purely GH movement has a firm end-feel because of the stress placed on the inferior GH ligament, the inferior capsule, and the pectoralis major and latissimus dorsi muscles. During abduction arising from the entire shoulder complex, the rhomboids and the middle and lower fibers of the trapezius muscle contribute to the end-feel.

PROM measurements and end-feels are not normally taken for adduction because of the humerus striking the body. However, hyperadduction may be measured by moving the arm in front of the torso. Note for the presence of a painful arc, indicating rotator cuff impingement, when passively moving the arm from abduction to adduction. Pain experienced during both passive abduction and passive adduction may indicate inflammation of the subacromial structures.

- **Internal and external rotation**: PROM for rotation of the humerus is measured with the GH joint abducted to 90 degrees and the elbow flexed to 90 degrees. These motions can be tested with the patient in the seated or supine positions although scapular stabilization is more easily accomplished with the patient supine. To isolate rotation at the GH joint, the scapula is stabilized to prevent contributions from the scapulothoracic articulation. When measuring motion produced by the shoulder complex, the thorax is stabilized to prevent flexion or extension of the spine (Fig. 16-31).

The firm end-feel associated with normal internal rotation is caused by tightening of the posterior fibers of the GH capsule and the infraspinatus and teres minor muscles. During internal rotation with the scapula unstabilized, the rhomboid muscle group and the middle and lower fibers of the trapezius contribute to the end-feel.

During external rotation, the GH ligaments, the coracohumeral ligament, and the joint capsule wind tight, resulting in a firm end-feel for both isolated GH movements and the shoulder complex as a whole. Muscular contributions lending to the end-feel for GH external rotation include the subscapularis, pectoralis major, latissimus dorsi, and the teres major muscles.

Athletes who perform overhand motions, such as baseball players, javelin throwers, tennis players, and quarterbacks, often have an increased range of external rotation and decreased internal rotation. Both of these changes alter the mechanics of the shoulder complex. The increased external rotation does not compensate for the limited internal rotation, resulting in a loss of total motion.[7]

Examination of passive external rotation and extension must be delayed until the end of the assessment procedure when a GH dislocation, subluxation, or chronic instability is suspected. In such instances, the examination proceeds with great care. Passive external rotation of the GH joint is the same procedure as the **apprehension test** (see Anterior Glenohumeral Instability).

The GH joint is palpated during passive internal and external rotation to determine the presence of crepitus, which may indicate rotator cuff or bicipital tendinitis and subacromial bursitis, or "clicks," which may indicate a labral tear.

- **Horizontal adduction and abduction**: To isolate GH motion, the scapula must be stabilized to prevent medial and lateral translation. During evaluation of the entire shoulder complex, the torso is stabilized so that spinal motion does not contribute to motion of the shoulder (Fig. 16-32).

Horizontal adduction, also called cross-body adduction, may have a soft end-feel because of soft tissue

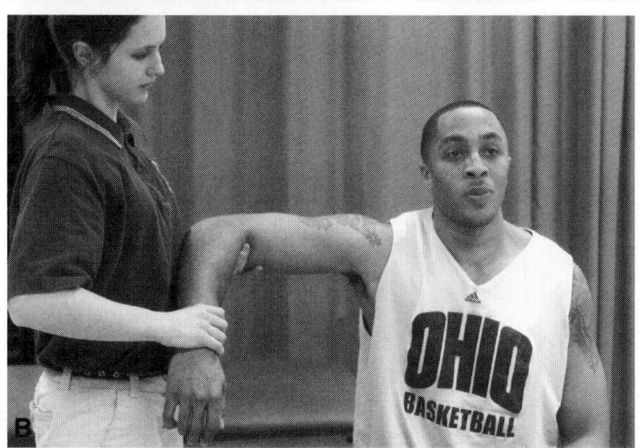

FIGURE 16-31 ■ Passive range of motion assessment of shoulder internal rotation **(A)** and external rotation **(B)**.

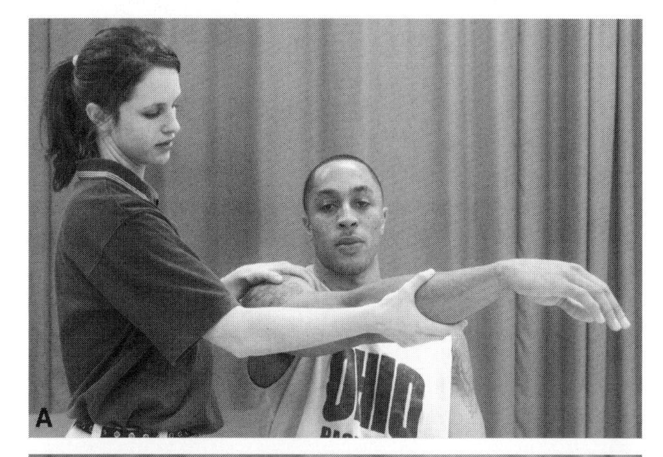
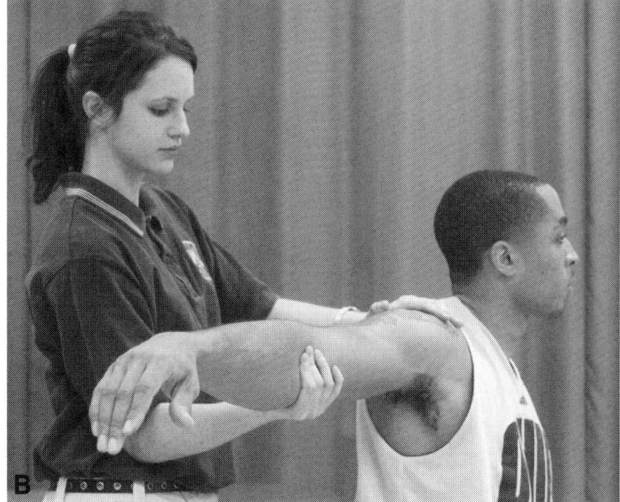

FIGURE 16-32 ■ Passive range of motion assessment of **(A)** shoulder horizontal adduction and **(B)** shoulder horizontal abduction.

approximation when the pectoralis major, biceps, and anterior deltoid muscles are well developed. A soft end-feel also may be found in obese individuals. If this is not the case, a firm end-feel with the scapula stabilized is associated with stretching of the posterior GH capsule and tension developed by the posterior deltoid muscle. Pain at the end-range of horizontal adduction is also associated with AC joint pathology. A restriction may be indicative of glenohumeral impingement.

A firm end-feel is expected during horizontal abduction because of the tightening of the anterior GH capsule and the middle and inferior GH ligaments. Some tension may also be developed by the anterior deltoid and pectoralis major. During horizontal abduction obtained through motions of the entire shoulder complex, additional tension is developed by the pectoralis major.

Joint Stability Tests

The integrity of the ligaments and capsules of the shoulder complex is determined via joint play and stress testing. Because of the relative difficulty in manipulating the clavicle, the findings for tests for SC and AC joint instability are more subtle than the findings for the other joints in the body. Generally, the findings are positive only in the more severe cases. These tests are contraindicated when a fracture or joint dislocation is suspected.

Sternoclavicular joint play

To determine the stability of the SC joint, position the patient supine and while sitting at the head of the patient, grasp the clavicle just distal to the medial clavicular head (Joint Play 16-1).

Pain that is evoked during all movements may result from either damage to the SC joint disk or a complete

Joint Play 16-1
Sternoclavicular Joint Play

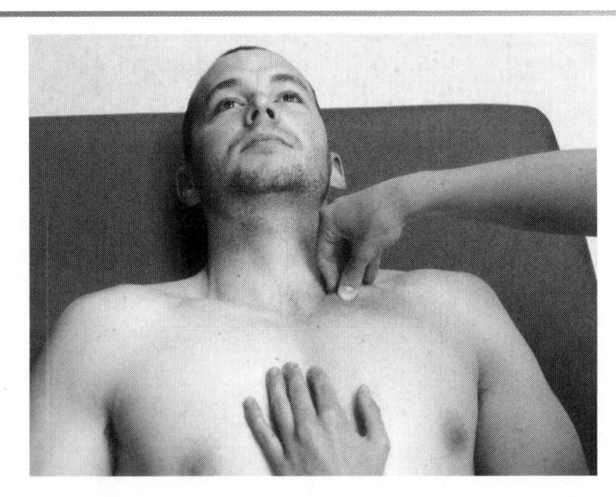

The proximal portion of the clavicle is manipulated to determine the amount of inferior, superior, anterior, and posterior motion available at the joint.

Patient Position	Supine or seated
Position of Examiner	Standing next to the patient, grasping the proximal clavicle
Evaluative Procedure	Apply a gliding pressure that forces the medial clavicle downward, upward, anteriorly, and posteriorly relative to the sternum, noting pain or laxity elicited.

Clavicular Motion	Structures Stressed
Inferior	Interclavicular ligament
Superior	Costoclavicular ligament (anterior and posterior fibers)
Anterior	SC ligament (posterior fibers)
Posterior	SC ligament (anterior fibers)

Positive Test	Pain, hypermobility, or hypomobility
Implications	Hypermobility: Laxity and/or sprain Hypomobility: Joint adhesions

SC = sternoclavicular.

disruption of the joint capsule, indicating a possible dislocation or subluxation of the joint.

Acromioclavicular joint play

With the patient supine, the AC joint is manipulated by grasping the clavicle along its distal one third and gliding the joint in the following directions, noting any pain or laxity (Joint Play 16-2).

Glenohumeral joint play

Assessment of true GH glide involves the sliding of the humeral head relative to the glenoid fossa. The ligaments tested during this procedure are also stressed during many of the special tests used to determine GH laxity. Laxity and instability are not synonymous. A lax shoulder can still be functionally stable. Also, an unstable shoulder may not demonstrate laxity during joint play, especially when the patient is awake (not anesthetized) because of reflexive muscle guarding.

The joint play assessment is performed in three directions—i.e., anterior, posterior, and inferior—with the humerus in the neutral (open pack) position and the scapula stabilized (Joint Play 16-3). Superior glide is not tested because of the bony block formed between the humeral head and the coracoacromial arch.

Joint Play 16-2
Acromioclavicular Joint Play

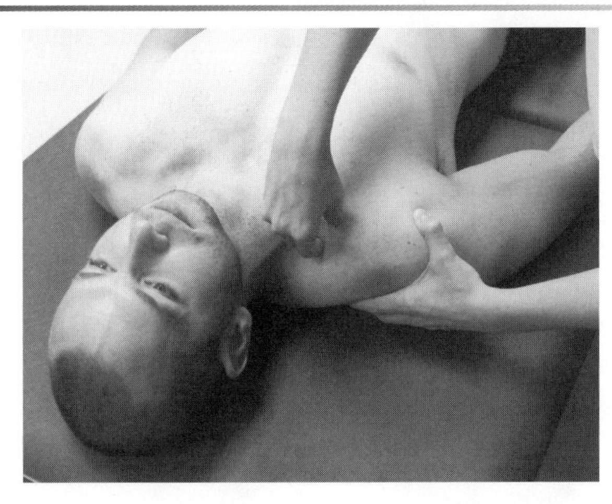

The distal portion of the clavicle is manipulated to determine the amount of inferior, superior, anterior, and posterior motion available at the acromioclavicular joint.

Patient Position	Seated or supine
Position of Examiner	Standing lateral to the patient, grasping the distal portion of the clavicle, just proximal to the AC joint. The opposite hand is stabilizer, the acromian process.
Evaluative Procedure	Apply a gliding pressure that forces the distal clavicle downward, upward, anteriorly, and posteriorly relative to the scapula, noting pain or laxity elicited.

Clavicular Motion	Structures Stressed
Inferior	AC ligament (superior fibers)
Superior	Conoid ligament*
	Trapezoid ligament*
	AC ligament (inferior fibers)
Anterior	AC ligament
	Coracoclavicular ligament (in the absence of the AC ligament)
Posterior	Clavicle contacting acromion (posterior block)
	AC ligament

*Portions of the coracoclavicular ligament.

Positive Test	Pain, hypermobility, or hypomobility
Implications	Hypermobility: Laxity Hypomobility: Joint adhesions

AC = acromioclavicular.

Joint Play 16-3
Glenohumeral Joint Play

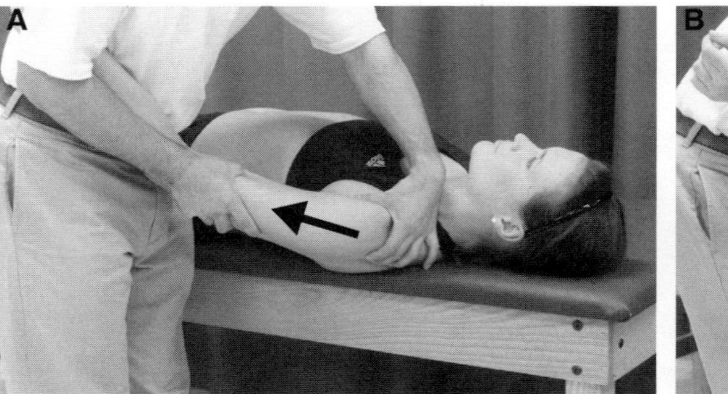

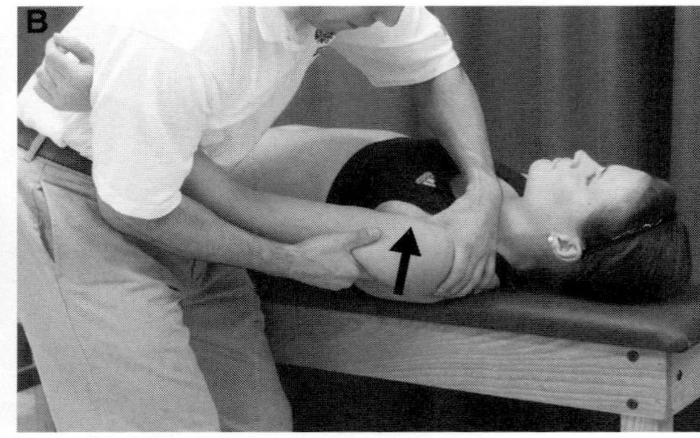

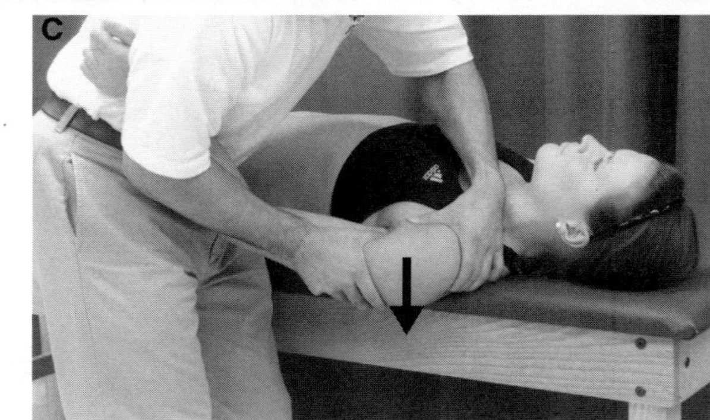

Glenohumeral joint play assesses the amount of mobility allowed by the joint capsule and ligaments.

Patient Position	Seated Place the patient's arm is placed in the resting position (GH joint abducted to approximately 55° and flexed to approximately 30°). The examiner maintains the patient's arm in this position to assure relaxation.
Position of Examiner	**(A) Inferior glide**: One hand supports the arm to maintain the resting position. The opposite hand cups the superior aspect of the humerus. **(B) Anterior glide**: One hand stabilizes the scapula anteriorly by applying pressure to the coracoid process, reaching under the axilla to the scapular body. The opposite hand applies force at the posterior aspect of the humerus. **(C) Posterior glide**: One hand stabilizes the scapula at the acromion process. The opposite hand applies force at the anterior aspect of the humeral head.
Evaluative Procedure	A gentle yet firm force is applied that distracts the joint (to take up the slack) and then moves the humeral head inferiorly, anteriorly or posteriorly.
Positive Test	Pain, increased mobility, or decreased mobility compared with the same direction on the opposite shoulder.

Implications	Hypermobility or hypomobility of the static stabilizers of the GH joint: **(A)** Inferior: Inferior joint capsule, superior GH ligament, coracohumeral ligament (see the description in the "Glenohumeral Instability" section of this chapter) **(B)** Anterior: Coracohumeral ligament, superior and middle GH ligaments, anterior joint capsule, labral tear **(C)** Posterior: Posterior joint capsule, labral tear.
Modification	In the case of large patients, a second examiner can be used to assist in manually stabilizing the scapula or using straps. Load and shift test: Center the humeral head in the fossa by applying an axial load while the patient's humerus is in 20° of abduction and 20° of forward flexion and the scapula stabilized. Joint play is then assessed.
Comment	These results should be interpreted with caution and considered in light of the remaining exam because of the low inter-rater and intra-rater reliability.[32] It is difficult to detect subtle changes (e.g., grade 0 and grade 1). The difference between the inferior glide test and the sulcus sign (see Special Test 16-9) is that the sulcus sign is not performed in the resting position.

GH = glenohumeral.

All motions occur relative to the plane of the scapula. Therefore, anterior glide is not tested by drawing the humerus forward relative to the sagittal plane but, rather, forward relative to the face of the glenoid fossa perpendicular to the plane of the scapula.[31] The degree of laxity is based on the amount of translation relative to the opposite limb. Any situation in which the humeral head can be displaced past the labral rim warrants further examination by a physician. The Pathology and Related Special Tests section of this chapter discusses multidirectional instabilities.

GH joint play can be modified using the **load and shift technique**. During standard GH joint play assessment, the humerus is distracted from the glenoid fossa. During load and shift testing, an axial load is placed on the humerus, compressing the humeral head into the glenoid fossa, centering the joint in its anatomical position. The following scale is used during load and shift testing[33]:

Grade	Amount of Humeral Head Translation
Trace (0)	No translation of the humeral head
Grade I	Translation of the humeral head to the glenoid rim, but not over it
Grade II	Translation of the humeral head over the glenoid rim, but the head spontaneously reduces
Grade III	Dislocation of the humeral head without spontaneous reduction

When a three-point grading scale is used, poor intra- and intertester reliability occurs.[34] If the grading scale is modified to a two-point scale (the humerus does not subluxate or the humerus does subluxate), the reliability of the test greatly improves.[35]

Neurologic Testing

Cervical nerve root trauma, brachial plexus injury, thoracic outlet syndrome, and other nerve pathologies can produce neurologic symptoms in the shoulder and upper extremity (Fig. 16-33). An upper quarter neurologic screen can be used to identify the involved nerve root (or roots) (see Neurological Screening Box 1–2). Chapter 14 describes the brachial plexus and the actual mechanisms and tests for cervical nerve root impingement, and Chapter 15 discusses visceral origins of referred pain into this area.

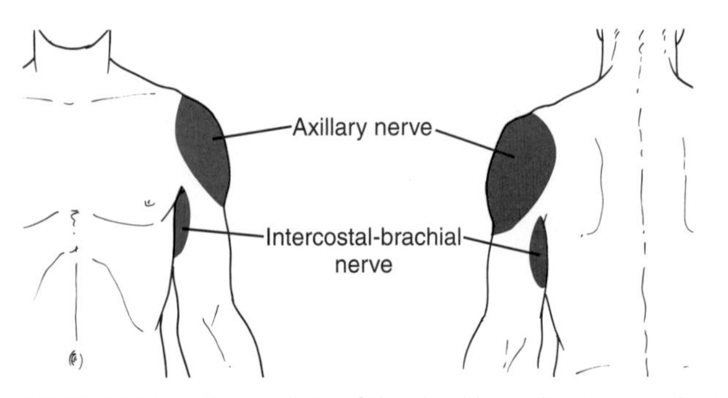

FIGURE 16-33 ■ Neuropathies of the shoulder and upper arm. Pain may also be referred to this area from the thorax (see Fig. 15-14) and the brachial plexus (see Chapter 14 and Neurological Screening Box 1-2).

Pathologies of the Shoulder and Related Special Tests

Because of the number of bones, muscles, articulations, ligaments, and other supporting structures associated with the shoulder complex, this complex is susceptible to a wide range of injuries. This section presents major orthopedic and athletic injuries to each segment and describes the signs, symptoms, and special evaluative procedures used to reach the appropriate conclusions. The clinician should structure the examination approach to include only techniques that are relevant to confirm or reject the suspected pathology.

Sternoclavicular Joint Sprains

Injuries to the SC joint usually occur from a longitudinal force being placed on the clavicle. This mechanism commonly occurs by falling on an outstretched arm or from a force being placed on the lateral portion of the shoulder. Less frequently, traction forces, such as those experienced by gymnasts performing on the rings, high bar, or uneven bars in which the athlete is suspended by the arms, may disrupt the integrity of the joint capsule.

SC sprains are marked by pain during joint play movements. Protraction and retraction of the scapula can reproduce pain associated with ligamentous or disk damage. Dislocations of this joint commonly occur anteriorly, superiorly, or posteriorly relative to the sternum.[36] Anterior dislocations are almost 10 times more common than posterior (retrosternal) dislocations.

Because of the potential threat to the subclavian artery, subclavian vein, trachea, and esophagus, posterior SC dislocations are a medical emergency.[4] Pressure can be placed on the superior mediastinum, blocking the cranial vessels, trachea, and esophagus, producing dizziness, nausea, neurovascular symptoms in the upper extremity, dyspnea, and **dysphagia**. Clinically, patients suffering from SC sprains complain of pain with any shoulder movement that causes motion at the SC joint, particularly when the shoulders are compressed towards each other (Examination Findings 16-1).[4,37]

The clavicle's medial epiphysis does not completely fuse until approximately age 25. The similarities in the signs and symptoms of a SC joint sprain or dislocation and those associated with an epiphyseal injury, a **pseudo-dislocation**, are similar, injuries to the growth plate must be ruled out in patients younger than 25 years old.[4,38] A definitive evaluation of the integrity of the SC joint can be made using magnetic resonance imaging (MRI) or CT. Plain radiographs often result in false-negative readings.

Dysphagia Difficulty with swallowing or the inability to swallow.

Examination Findings 16-1
Sternoclavicular Joint Injury

Examination Segment	Clinical Findings
History	***Onset:*** Acute ***Pain characteristics:*** Limited to the SC joint area Pain is increased with any shoulder motion that causes motion at the SC joint. ***Other symptoms:*** Pressure on the underlying neurovascular network can cause paresthesia in the upper extremity. Pressure on the esophagus and trachea may impede swallowing and breathing. ***Mechanism:*** Force applied longitudinally to the clavicle, such as falling on an outstretched arm, or forceful distraction of the arm and distal shoulder complex Indirect mechanisms include anterior or posterior forces exerted on the anterolateral or posterolateral shoulder.
Inspection	Dislocations are marked by displacement of the clavicular head anteriorly, superiorly, or posteriorly. Sprains may present with localized swelling over the joint; discoloration may or may not be present. The patient's neck may be tilted toward the involved joint.
Palpation	Obvious joint displacement is often felt. Pain may be reported over the SC joint. Crepitus is present over the articulation.
Joint and Muscle Function Assessment	For joint sprains, pain is elicited at any point after 90° of elevation, after which the ligamentous structures are maximally taut. Pain may be elicited during scapular protraction and retraction. ***AROM:*** Increased pain with flexion and abduction ***MMT:*** Isometric testing should not be painful. ***PROM:*** Increased pain with flexion, abduction, and horizontal adduction.
Joint Stability Tests	***Stress tests:*** Ligamentous tests should not be performed on obvious dislocations. ***Joint play:*** Joint play movements elicit pain for 1st-degree sprains; 2nd- and 3rd-degree sprains are marked by hypermobility.
Special Tests	None
Neurologic Screening	Within normal limits
Vascular Screening	Venous congestion of involved arm, neck, and head may occur with posterior dislocation.
Functional Assessment	Increased pain during early phases of elevation
Imaging Techniques	Radiographic, CT, or MR images will reveal joint displacement.
Differential Diagnosis	Proximal clavicle fracture, sternal fracture, 1st rib fracture, medial clavicle epiphyseal injury
Comments	Posterior SC dislocations are considered medical emergencies because of the potential threat to the underlying neurovascular structures, the esophagus, and trachea. Fractures of the medial one third of the clavicle can produce a pseudo-dislocation.

AROM = active range of motion; CT = computed tomography; MMT = manual muscle test; MR = magnetic resonance; PROM = passive range of motion; SC = sternoclavicular.

Examination Findings 16-2
Acromioclavicular Joint Sprains

Examination Segment	Clinical Findings
History	***Onset:*** Acute ***Pain characteristics:*** Localized primarily at the AC joint; also possibly including the upper trapezius, and upper scapula (secondary to trapezius spasm) ***Mechanism:*** Falling on the point of the shoulder, landing on the AC joint Force applied longitudinally to the clavicle, such as falling on an outstretched arm
Inspection	Displacement of the clavicle may be obvious. Step deformities indicate damage to the coracoclavicular ligament.
Palpation	Superior displacement of the clavicle that is reduced with manual pressure (piano key sign).
Joint and Muscle Function Assessment	***AROM:*** Pain with elevation of the humerus and during protraction and retraction of the scapula ***MMT:*** Decreased strength secondary to pain for all muscles having attachment on the acromion or clavicle ***PROM:*** Pain produced during elevation of the humerus owing to movement at the AC joint. Increased pain with horizontal adduction
Joint Stability Tests	***Stress tests:*** Not applicable ***Joint play:*** Joint play movements reveal hypermobility of the AC joint.
Special Tests	AC traction test, AC compression test
Neurologic Screening	Within normal limits
Vascular Screening	Within normal limits
Functional Assessment	Increased pain with overhead motions
Imaging Techniques	AP radiograph to rule out associated clavicular or scapular fracture (primarily the coracoid process) and/or displacement between the acromion and clavicular Stress radiographs are rarely required to identify AC joint dislocations.
Differential Diagnosis	Distal clavicle fracture, scapular fracture (coracoid), rotator cuff pathology, SLAP lesions
Comments	Fractures of the distal clavicle may present with the clinical signs and symptoms of an acromioclavicular joint sprain. Radiographs should be obtained to rule out clavicular fracture and determine the severity of the sprain.

AC = acromioclavicular; AP = anteroposterior; AROM = active range of motion; MMT = manual muscle test; PROM = passive range of motion.

Unstable or irreducible posterior SC dislocations often require surgical repair and internal fixation of the joint.[39] Anterior or superior SC dislocations may be managed through closed reduction and immobilization of the involved arm.

Treatment of a SC joint sprain typically involves palliative measures to decrease the signs and symptoms of inflammation and allow the injury to heal. The use of ice and sling immobilization as necessary to decrease the traction on the joint. ROM for the cervical spine and upper extremity are incorporated initially. As the pain and swelling at the joint decrease, strengthening of the surrounding musculature is initiated with a progressive return to functional activities.

Acromioclavicular Joint Pathology

Horizontal (anterior and posterior) stability of the AC joint is maintained by the AC ligament. Superior stability is maintained by the conoid and trapezoid segments of the coracoclavicular ligament. Commonly referred to as a "separated shoulder," rupture of these ligaments results in instability or dislocation of the joint. Therefore, these ruptures are more

Table 16-7 Classification System for Acromioclavicular Joint Sprains

Grade	Structures Involved	Signs and Symptoms
Type I	Slight to partial damage of the AC ligament and capsule	Point tenderness over the AC joint; no laxity or deformity noted
Type II	Rupture of the AC ligament and partial damage to the coracoclavicular ligament	Slight laxity and deformity of the AC joint Slight step deformity
Type III	Complete tearing of the AC and coracoclavicular ligaments; possible involvement of the deltoid and trapezius fascia	Obvious dislocation of the distal end of the clavicle from the acromion process
Type IV	Complete tearing of the AC and coracoclavicular ligaments and tearing of the deltoid and trapezius fascia	Posterior clavicular displacement into the insertion of the upper fibers of the trapezius.
Type V	Same as type IV	Displacement of the involved clavicle from the acromion one to three times the height of the clavicle as compared with the opposite limb; clavicle posteriorly displaced with stripping away of the deltoid-trapezius aponeurosis
Type VI	Same as type IV	Displacement of the clavicle inferiorly under the coracoid (possible involvement of the brachial plexus)

AC = acromioclavicular.

correctly referred to as sprains. The most common mechanisms for acute injury of the AC joint are characterized by the acromion's being driven away from the clavicle or vice versa. Examples of these mechanisms include:

- Landing on a forward-flexed outstretched arm or the point of the elbow, which drives the scapula posterior to the clavicle
- A blow to the superior acromion process, which drives the scapula inferior to the clavicle
- A force that drives the clavicle away from the scapula when the scapula is fixated

The AC joint may also be injured by overuse, repetitive stress mechanisms. Classification of AC sprains is based on the structures involved, the degree of instability, and the direction in which the clavicle has been displaced relative to the acromion and coracoid process (Table 16-7).

Examination of patients with acute AC injuries reveals a history describing one of the aforementioned mechanisms (Examination Findings 16-2). Pain is located over the distal clavicle, AC joint, anterolateral neck, superior scapula, and the lateral deltoid.[40] On inspection, advanced sprains (type II and above) normally result in noticeable displacement of the clavicle from the acromion process, creating a **step deformity** (see Fig. 16-23). Palpation of the involved area may produce hypermobility of the distal clavicle. The **piano key sign** is a bob of the clavicle vertically, with the distal clavicle depressing and elevating with manual palpation, indicating trauma to the coracoclavicular ligament.

Assessment of AROM and PROM produces pain on most movements, especially those occurring above 90 degrees and during the **Apley's scratch tests** (see Box 16-2). Passive and active horizontal adduction also elicit pain from the AC joint, especially at end range. The **acromioclavicular traction test** (Special Test 16-3) reveals trauma to the coracoclavicular ligament, and the **AC compression test** (Special Test 16-4) reproduces horizontal AC instability.

Patients displaying a hypermobile AC articulation should be referred to a physician for evaluation because, in some instances, fractures of the distal clavicle may clinically mimic a dislocation of the AC joint. Stress radiographs can be used to differentiate between injuries that are isolated to the AC ligament and those that include the coracoclavicular ligament.

Chronic AC joint pain may be the result of a degenerative process within the articulation, previous injury, or aging. Its symptoms may be easily confused with rotator cuff symptoms and may result in, or be caused by, rotator cuff injuries.[42] Pain is produced when the arm is internally rotated or abducted, the AC joint is stressed, or when the GH joint is placed in the classic impingement position of forward flexion and abduction.[43] Pain arising from the AC joint can be differentiated from that arising from the subacromial bursa and rotator cuff by its location. AC joint pain radiates into the scapula and neck. Subacromial joint pathology tends to only radiate pain laterally.[40] During chronic AC joint degeneration, many of the signs and symptoms of an acute AC joint injury are present, but there is no history of trauma to the AC joint.

Special Test 16-3
Acromioclavicular Traction Test

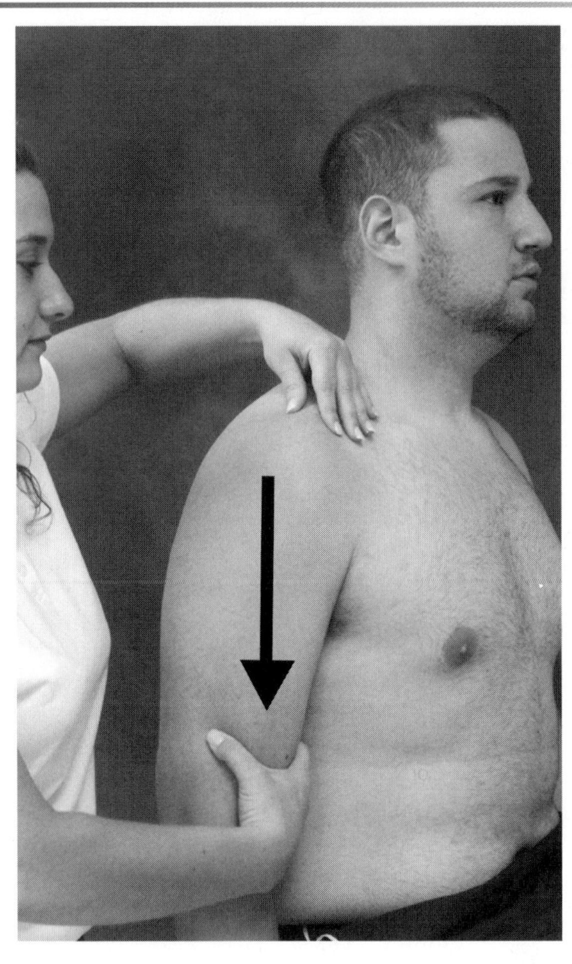

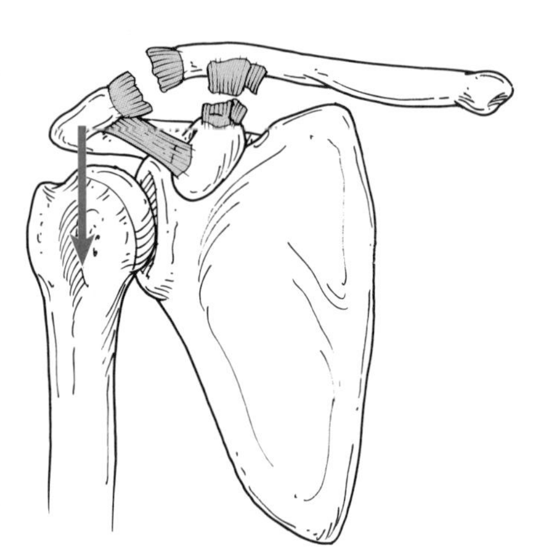

The principle behind the AC traction test is similar to a stress radiograph used to diagnose AC instability.

Patient Position	Sitting or standing The arm hanging naturally from the side
Position of Examiner	Standing lateral to the involved side The clinician grasps the patient's humerus proximal to the elbow. The opposite hand gently palpates the AC joint.
Evaluative Procedure	The examiner applies a downward traction on the humerus.
Positive Test	The humerus and scapula move inferior to the clavicle, causing a step deformity, pain, or both.
Implications	Sprain of the AC or costoclavicular ligaments (see Table 16-7 for grades).
Comments	Patients displaying positive AC traction test results should be referred to a physician for follow-up radiographic stress testing and to rule out a clavicular fracture.
Evidence	Absent or inconclusive in the literature

AC = acromioclavicular.

Special Test 16-4
Acromioclavicular Compression Test

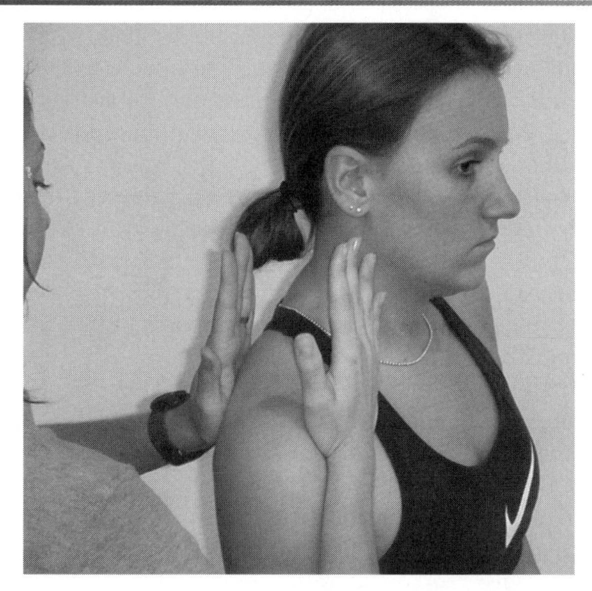

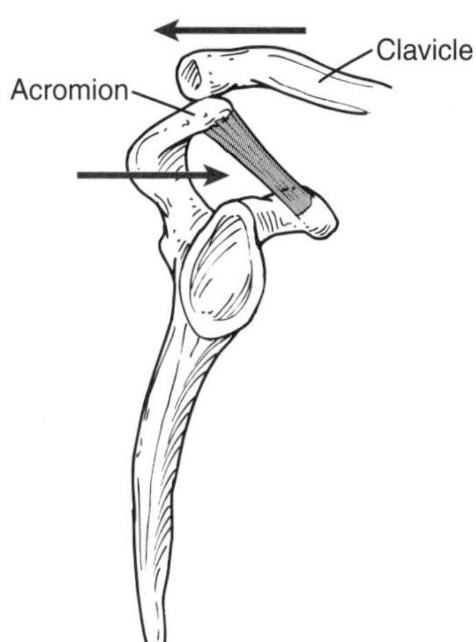

The AC compression test attempts to displace the clavicle over the acromion process, stressing he coracoclavicular ligament.

Patient Position	Sitting or standing with the arm hanging naturally at the side
Position of Examiner	Standing on the involved side with the hands cupped over the anterior and posterior joint structures
Evaluative Procedure	The examiner squeezes the hands together, compressing the AC joint.
Positive Test	Pain at the AC joint or excursion of the clavicle over the acromion process
Implications	Damage to the AC ligament and possibly the coracoclavicular ligament
Modification	Place a thumb on the posterolateral aspect of the acromion process and the index and middle fingers of the same or opposite hand on the midpoint of the clavicle.[41] An anterosuperior force is applied with the thumb and an inferior force on the clavicle. A positive test is marked by pain.
Evidence	Positive likelihood ratio Not Useful — Useful Very Small · Small · Moderate · Large 0 1 2 3 4 5 6 7 8 9 10 Negative likelihood ratio Not Useful — Useful Very Small · Small · Moderate · Large 1.0 0.9 0.8 0.7 0.6 0.5 0.4 0.3 0.2 0.1 0

AC = acromioclavicular.

Although the joint may be painful on palpation, instability is not generally demonstrated. Radiographic examination may show degenerative changes within the joint's articulating space, although bone scans are more sensitive in detecting change.[41]

For patients suffering from grade I AC sprains and those with chronic joint degeneration, conservative management is usually recommended. Local corticosteroid injections can provide short-term relief of symptoms, but they do not alter the long-term progression of the condition.[44]

For patients with AC sprains that are grade II and higher, surgical or conservative management is used. However, there is little difference in the long-term outcome between the two approaches.[45] Conservative management requires a decreased period of immobilization and yields a reduced amount of time lost from activity. Patients being treated conservatively demonstrate strength and ROM that is at least equal to patients who undergo surgery.[45,46] Although the level of function between the two groups is equal, the amount of long-term deformity is higher in patients managed conservatively. For patients being managed surgically, the patient's subjective pain scores commonly are lower after surgery.[45–47]

Conservative management focuses on sling immobilization only for as long as is needed for pain relief. Extended use of a sling or the use of special slings that place pressure on the distal clavicle does not make a difference in long-term results. Local modalities and treatment of subsequent trapezius muscle spasm highlight early treatment. The patient can progress through ROM and shoulder strengthening exercises as tolerated. With grade I AC joint sprains, this may occur within the first week. With more severe injuries, 3 to 4 weeks may be necessary. Because of the increased stress on the AC and GH joints in the terminal ranges of overhead movement, motion and strengthening in these extreme ranges may be limited early on.

Surgical intervention is associated with several potential long-term detriments. Resection of the distal clavicle or disruption of the AC joint capsule can result in dysfunction of both the AC and GH joints.[48]

Glenohumeral Instability

The GH joint may present with instability anteriorly, posteriorly, inferiorly, or in multiple planes. It is the result of ligamentous or labral pathology, capsular instability, or muscular weakness. The severity of the instability is graded based on **joint play movements**, the relative displacement of the humeral head on the glenoid fossa.

The primary passive supports of the GH joint have been described as being the GH ligaments, the joint capsule, and the coracohumeral ligament, which provide stability, limit the extremes of motion, and align the humeral head during movement.[49] These passive restraints are augmented by the rotator cuff and other GH musculature to provide coordinated motion of the shoulder complex. This close relationship between the passive and dynamic stabilizers indicates that pathological changes in the rotator cuff may result in GH instability (Table 16-8).[50]

Anterior instability

Anterior instability is the result of laxity of the anterior stabilizing structures such as the middle GH ligament and, more specifically, the anterior band of the inferior GH ligament.[52] Laxity of the superior and middle GH ligaments,[53] large tears or weakness of the rotator cuff musculature, and dysfunction of the long head of the biceps tendon[54] may also contribute to anterior GH instability.[55] The rotator interval, located in the anterior capsule at the anterior border of the supraspinatus and the superior border of the subscapularis, is a potential area of capsular weakness leading to instability.[56] The inferior GH ligament may be avulsed from the labrum or may be avulsed along with a portion of the labrum, forming a **Bankart lesion**. Bankart lesions are difficult to identify clinically, with the primary complaints being pain and crepitus as the humeral head moves against the anterior labrum during GH joint play assessment, load and shift testing, or external rotation of the humerus. Patients with acutely acquired anterior instability also demonstrate altered activation patterns of the pectoralis major, long head of the biceps, and rotator cuff.[57] These changes in dynamic stabilization capabilities, coupled with damage to static restraints, may contribute to recurrent episodes of instability.

The primary mechanism for anterior dislocations of the humeral head is excessive external rotation and abduction of the humerus. In this position, the anterior capsule is reinforced by the anterior fibers of the deltoid muscle group and the anterior rotator cuff tendons, reducing the anterior shear forces across the glenoid fossa and forcing the humeral head inferiorly.[58] Examination techniques are designed to provoke or alleviate pain and/or the sensation of instability. Passive external rotation of the humerus must be performed with caution, especially when the shoulder is in 90 degrees of flexion as this is replicates the **apprehension test ("crank test") for anterior instability** (Special Test 16-5).[60] Positive apprehension test results are followed up with the **relocation test for anterior instability**, in which posteriorly-directed manual pressure is applied on the anterior humeral head to add artificial stability. The **anterior release (surprise) test** follows the relocation test and is performed by suddenly releasing the posterior pressure applied during the relocation test (Special Test 16-6). Positive findings on any two of the apprehension, relocation and anterior release ("surprise") tests are highly predictive of anterior instability.[59,61,64]

A common MRI finding associated with an anterior GH dislocation is a **Hill–Sachs lesion**, a defect in the posterior humeral head's articular cartilage caused by the impact of the humeral head on the glenoid fossa as the humerus attempts to relocate (Fig. 16-34). The lesion is used as a diagnostic tool in determining the severity of the dislocation. In patients who report that the shoulder dislocated but spontaneously relocated, the lesion may be present on radiographic examination. The lesion itself is rarely symptomatic but may lead to early degeneration of the GH joint.

Posterior instability

Posterior GH instability is relatively rare, accounting for approximately 3 percent of all shoulder instabilities.[65] This type of instability most often occurs when the humerus is flexed and internally rotated while a longitudinal posterior force is placed on the humerus. Although posterior instability may

Table 16-8 Differential Findings of Chronic Glenohumeral Instability

	Anterior Instability	Posterior Instability	Multidirectional Instability
Onset	Chronic	Chronic	Insidious or chronic
Pain	Diffuse ache during ADLs along with the sensation that the shoulder is "loose" when brought into abduction with external rotation	Diffuse ache during ADLs; the patient reports that the shoulder feels unstable when it is brought across the body	Pain in the shoulder that increases with ADLs; the patient reports that theshoulder is "loose" with positions in the extremes of rotation motions Although the instability is multidirectional, the chief complaint is typically pain during external rotation with the shoulder abducted to 90°.
Mechanism	A specific mechanism of injury may be described, but chronic anterior instability is often caused by repetitive microtrauma involving external rotation when the GH joint is abducted to 90°.	Patient may describe a specific mechanism of injury but chronic posterior instability is generally caused by repetitive microtrauma involving longitudinal force on the length of the humerus while internally rotated and the GH joint flexed to 90° and horizontally adducted.	Congenital, acquired from repetitive overhead activity or posttraumatic.[51] A sensation of instability may be described during the midrange of motion.
Predisposition	Joint hypermobility	Joint hypermobility	Joint hypermobility
Inspection	A flattened deltoid is possible as chronic cases can cause atrophy of the deltoid muscle group and the scapular muscles. Possible atrophy of the rotator cuff muscles	Chronic cases can cause atrophy of the deltoid muscle group, rotator cuff muscles, and scapular muscles.	Chronic cases can cause atrophy of the deltoid muscle group and the scapular muscles.
Palpation	Tenderness of the anterior GH joint	Tenderness of the posterior GH joint	Tenderness in the anterior GH joint
Joint and Muscle Function Assessment			
AROM	Decreased external rotation secondary to sensation of instability and/or pain	Decreased internal rotation	Possible limitation at the end ranges of motion secondary to a sensation of instability
MMT	Pain and weakness when assessing external rotation in advanced cases and/or pain	Pain and weakness when assessing internal rotation in advanced cases	Pain and weakness when assessing internal and external rotation
PROM	Decreased external rotation secondary to sensation of instability and/or pain	Decreased internal rotation	Limited end range due to pain and instability
Stress Tests/ Joint Play	Increased anterior glide, although it may not appear increased to the contralateral side due to the bilateral nature of instability in chronic cases	Increased posterior glide, although it may not appear increased to the contralateral side the bilateral nature of instability in due to chronic cases	Increased glide in all directions
Special Tests	Apprehension, relocation, and surprise tests Posterior apprehension test Jerk test	Posterior apprehension test; test for posterior instability in the plane of the scapula	Apprehension test; Relocation test; Posterior apprehension test; Test for posterior instability in the plane of the scapula.
Comments	Chronic cases may have a predisposition to bilateral involvement. Chronic atraumatic instability usually occurs in patients younger than 30 years old.	Chronic cases may have a predisposition to bilateral involvement. Chronic atraumatic instability usually occurs in patients younger than 30 years old.	Chronic cases may have a predisposition to bilateral involvement. Multidirectional instability usually manifests itself in patients younger than 30 years old.

AROM = active range of motion; MMT = manual muscle test; PROM = passive range of motion.

Special Test 16-5
Apprehension Test for Anterior Glenohumeral Laxity

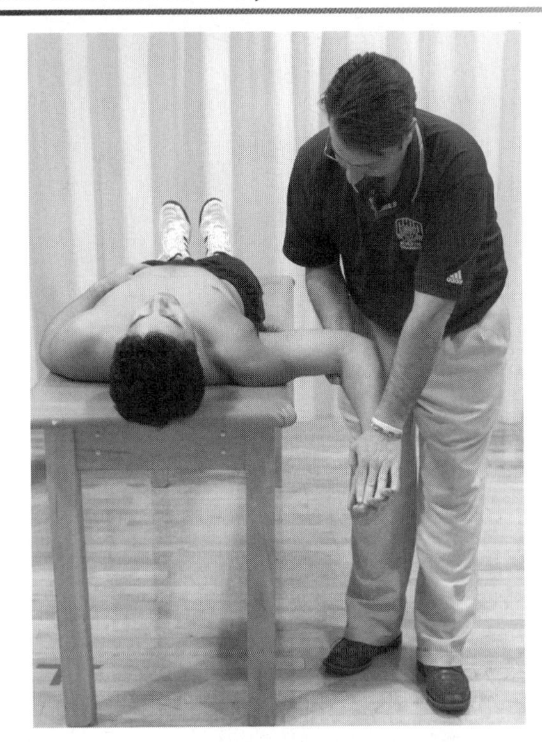

The apprehension test, passive external rotation of the glenohumeral joint, places the joint in the closed-pack position and replicates the mechanism of injury for anterior GH dislocations.

Patient Position	Supine, standing, or sitting The GH joint is abducted to 90° and the elbow is flexed to 90°.
Position of Examiner	Positioned in front of or beside the patient on the involved side The examiner supporting the humerus at midshaft while the forearm is grasped proximal to the wrist
Evaluative Procedure	While supporting the humerus at 90° abduction, the examiner passively externally rotates the GH joint by slowly applying pressure to the anterior forearm.
Positive Test	The patient displays apprehension that the shoulder may dislocate and resists further movement. Pain is centered in the anterior capsule of the GH joint.
Implications	The anterior capsule, inferior GH ligament, or glenoid labrum have been compromised, allowing the humeral head to dislocate or subluxate anteriorly on the glenoid fossa. Apprehension coupled with pain is often associated with instability secondary to rotator cuff pathology.[7] Pain in the deep posterior shoulder may be associated with internal impingement.[7]
Comments	Pressure should be applied gradually and the test terminated at the first sign of apprehension. Do not perform this test when there is obvious dislocation or subluxation of the GH joint. The relocation test is usually performed following a positive apprehension test (see Special Text 16-6).
Evidence	Positive likelihood ratio Not Useful — Useful Very Small / Small / Moderate / Large 18–48.18 0 1 2 3 4 5 6 7 8 9 10 Negative likelihood ratio Not Useful — Useful Very Small / Small / Moderate / Large 1.0 0.9 0.8 0.7 0.6 0.5 0.4 0.3 0.2 0.1 0

GH = glenohumeral.

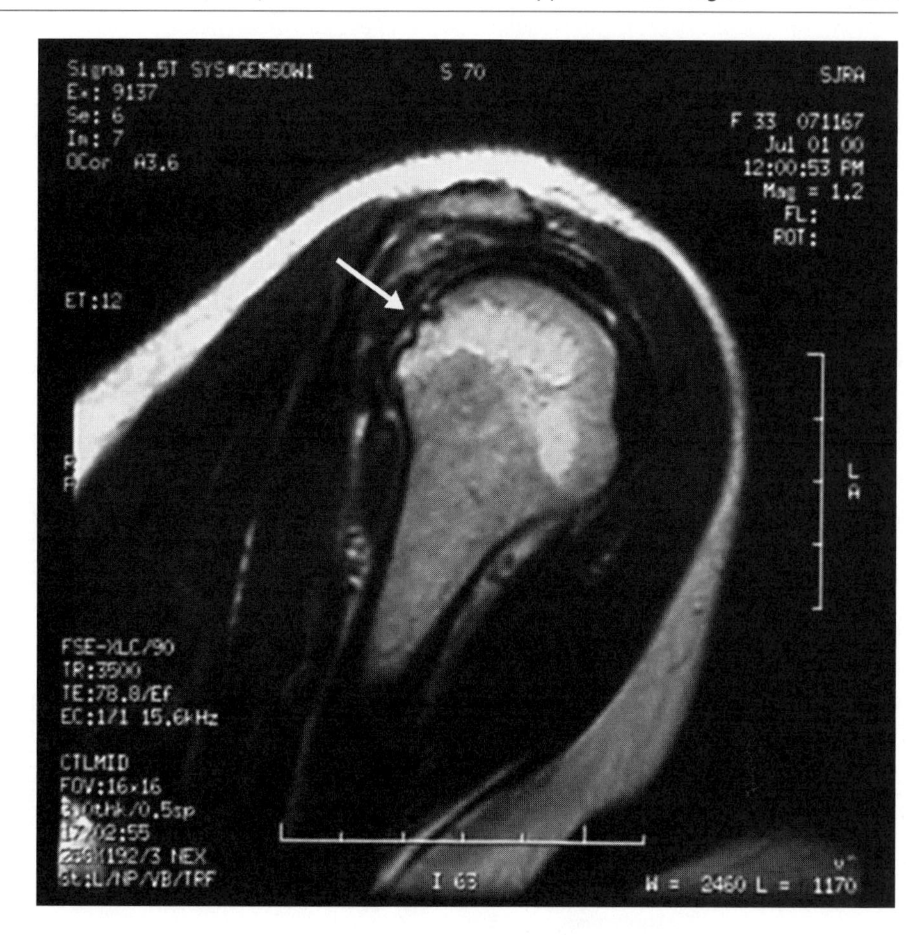

FIGURE 16-34 ■ An MRI of a Hill–Sachs lesion.

be the result of a single traumatic event, it often appears to be the result of accumulated microtrauma secondary to repeated blows on a forward-flexed arm, such as during blocking in football, the follow-through phase of throwing or overhand tennis volleys, or overhead swimming strokes.[65,66]

Posterior instability can result from weakness of the subscapularis muscle, the primary dynamic restraint against posterior humeral displacement. The coracohumeral and posterior band of the inferior GH ligaments also provide restraint when the humerus is in its neutral position or internally rotated, respectively. The long head of the biceps brachii tendon also provides posterior stability.[67] Patients with posterior instability complain of pain with maneuvers that require horizontal adduction, such as the follow-through phase of throwing.[68] The **posterior apprehension test** (Special Test 16-7) and **jerk test** (Special Test 16-8) are used to evaluate posterior GH instability. Lesions found on the anterior portion of the humeral head after a posterior dislocation are termed **reverse Hill–Sachs lesions**.

The jerk test (posterior stress test) is used to detect posteroinferior instability of the glenohumeral joint by applying an axial load to the humerus as it is horizontally adducted. A clunk that is either painful or pain-free will occur as the head of the humerus slides off the fossa. A painless clunk is associated with instability while a painful clunk is associated with a labral tear.[68,69]

Inferior instability

The primary restraint against inferior translation of the GH joint depends on the position of the humerus. In the neutral position, the primary restraint against inferior translation is the superior GH ligament, with little or no assistance provided by the coracohumeral ligament. When the humerus is abducted to 45 degrees in neutral rotation, the anterior portion of the inferior GH ligament is the primary restraint; this position also permits the greatest amount of translation. After further abducting the humerus to 90 degrees, the entire inferior GH ligament is responsible for restricting inferior displacement, but the posterior band is perhaps the most important restraint.[70] The presence of rotator cuff tears or weakness also increases inferior GH laxity.[55] Superior translation of the humeral head is limited by the presence of the coracoacromial arch and the acromion process.

The **sulcus sign** is used to identify the presence of multidirectional instability (Special Test 16-9). If the shoulder demonstrates laxity in the neutral position, it can be assumed to be lax in all positions. A positive sulcus sign with the humerus flexed to 90 degrees may indicate inferior instability.

Multidirectional instability

Multidirectional instabilities (MDIs) are a combination of two or more unidirectional instabilities. The etiology of the MDI is important to determine for the correct intervention.

Special Test 16-6
Relocation and Anterior Release Tests for Anterior Glenohumeral Laxity

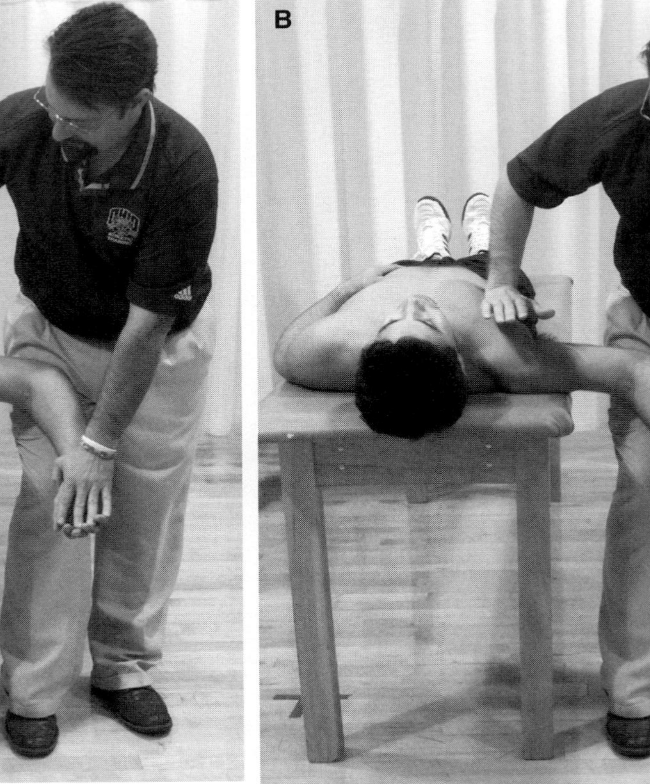

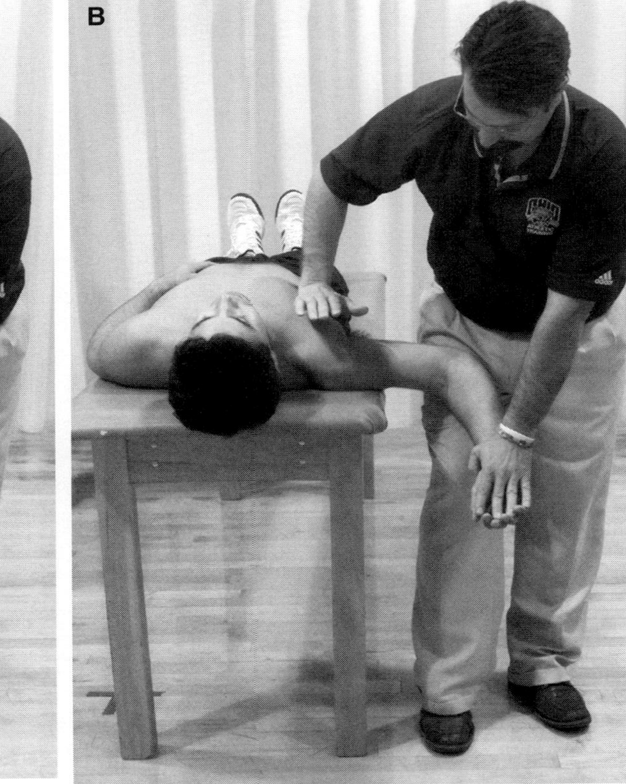

Performed after a positive apprehension test (see Special Test 16-5), the relocation test uses manual pressure to maintain alignment and stability of the GH joint as it moves into external rotation **(A)**. The anterior release test determines apprehension when the pressure applied during the apprehension test is suddenly released ("surprise!") **(B)**. The anterior release test, also known as the surprise test, should be performed with caution.

Patient Position	Supine The GH joint is abducted to 90°. The elbow is flexed to 90°.
Position of Examiner	Standing beside the patient, inferior to the humerus on the involved side The forearm is grasped proximal to the wrist to provide leverage during external rotation of the humerus. The opposite hand is held over the humeral head.
Evaluative Procedure	**(A) Relocation test**: With the patient's arm in the original position, the examiner applies a posterior force to the head of the humerus and maintains that force while externally rotating the humerus. **(B) Anterior release test ("Surprise!" test)**: With the GH in external rotation during the relocation test, the examiner removes the hand applying the posterior pressure.

Positive Test

Relocation test: Decreased pain or increased ROM (or both) compared with the anterior apprehension test

Anterior release test: Apprehension and/or pain when the anterior stabilizing pressure from the relocation test is removed.

Implications

Relocation test: Anterior pain may be the result of increased laxity in the anterior ligamentous and capsular structures or a tear of the labrum. Posterior pain may be from internal impingement of the posterior capsule or labrum.

A positive test result supports the conclusion of increased laxity in the anterior capsule owing to capsular damage or labrum tears. The manual pressure applied by the examiner increases the stability of the anterior portion of the GH capsule, allowing more external rotation to occur.

Anterior release test: Apprehension and/or pain when the anterior stabilizing pressure from the relocation test is removed.

Comments

The relocation test is usually performed after a positive anterior apprehension test. The anterior release test is usually performed after a positive relocation test.

The apprehension test and the relocation test may also be positive in the presence of internal impingement.

Positive findings with the relocation test (e.g., pain reduction) may also be associated with a SLAP lesion, as tension on the disrupted long head of the biceps tendon is reduced.[62,63]

The relocation test adds little predictive value in detecting anterior shoulder instability. It has more predictive when the posterior force reduces the feeling of apprehension rather than pain.

Evidence

Relocation Test

Positive likelihood ratio

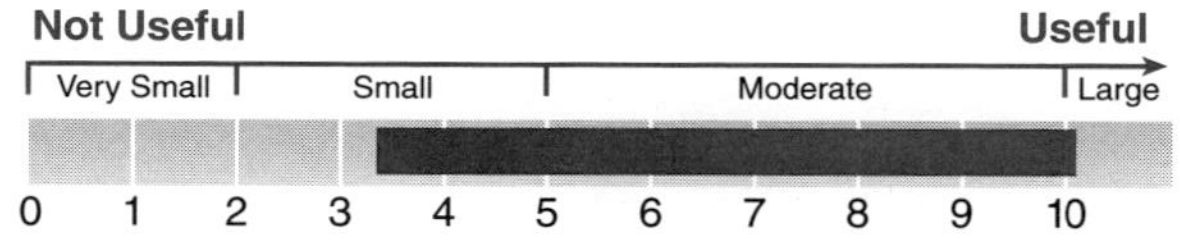

Not Useful Useful
Very Small Small Moderate Large
0 1 2 3 4 5 6 7 8 9 10

Negative likelihood ratio

Not Useful Useful
Very Small Small Moderate Large
1.0 0.9 0.8 0.7 0.6 0.5 0.4 0.3 0.2 0.1 0

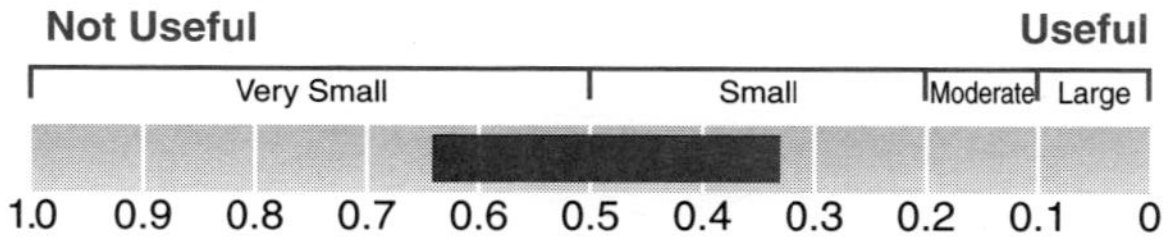

Anterior Release

Positive likelihood ratio

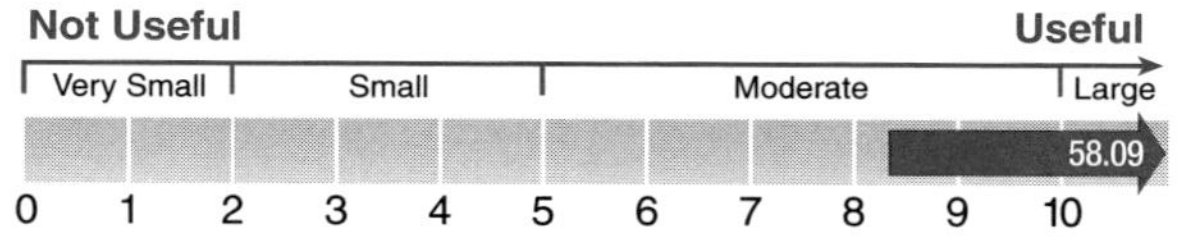

Not Useful Useful
Very Small Small Moderate Large
58.09
0 1 2 3 4 5 6 7 8 9 10

Negative likelihood ratio

Not Useful Useful
Very Small Small Moderate Large
1.0 0.9 0.8 0.7 0.6 0.5 0.4 0.3 0.2 0.1 0

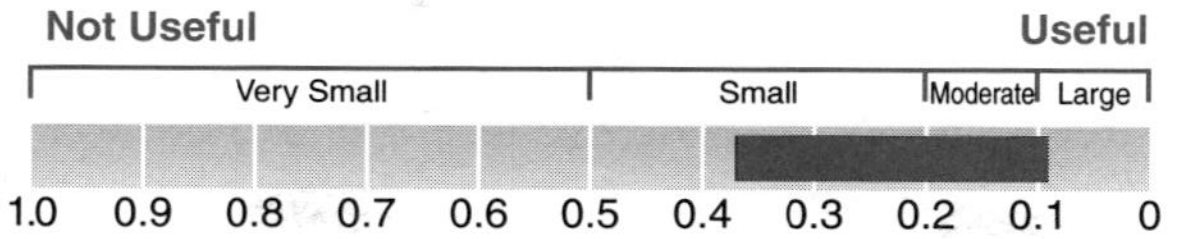

GH = glenohumeral; ROM = range of motion.

Special Test 16-7
Posterior Apprehension Test for Glenohumeral Laxity

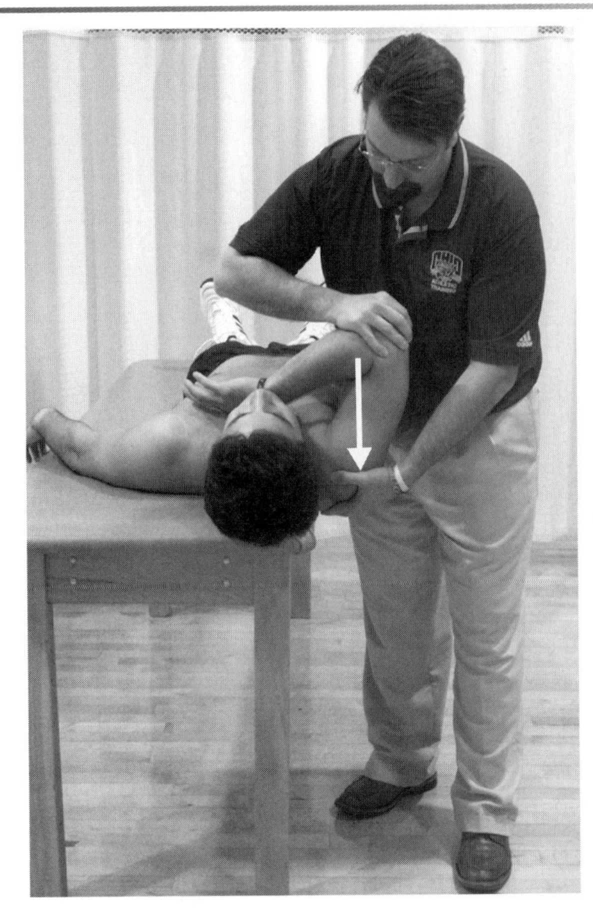

The humeral head is moved posteriorly on the glenoid fossa. In the presence of posterior glenohumeral laxity or instability the patient will abruptly stop the test.

Patient Position	Sitting or supine The shoulder is flexed to 90° and the elbow is flexed to 90°. The GH joint being tested is off to the side of the table.
Position of Examiner	Standing on the involved side One hand grasps the forearm. The opposite hand stabilizes the posterior scapula.
Evaluative Procedure	The examiner applies a longitudinal force to the humeral shaft, encouraging the humeral head to move posteriorly on the glenoid fossa. The examiner may choose to alter the amount of flexion and rotation of the humerus.
Positive Test	The patient displays apprehension and produces muscle guarding to prevent the shoulder from subluxating posteriorly.
Implications	Laxity in the posterior GH capsule, torn posterior labrum
Modification	Horizontally adduct the humerus so that the posterior force is directed perpendicular to the plane of the scapula.
Evidence	Absent or inconclusive in the literature

GH = glenohumeral.

Special Test 16-8
Jerk (Posterior Stress) Test for Labral Tears

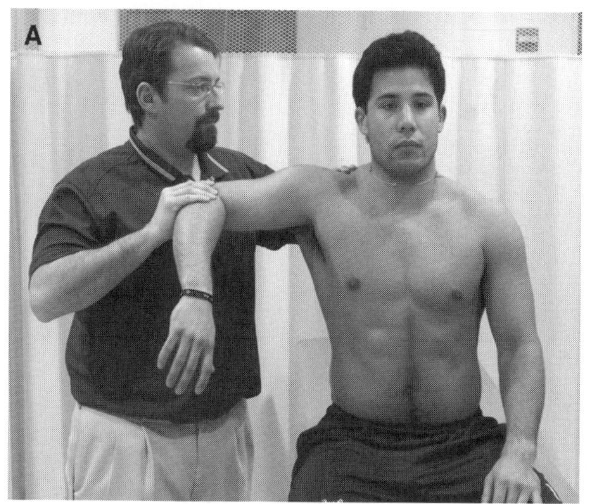

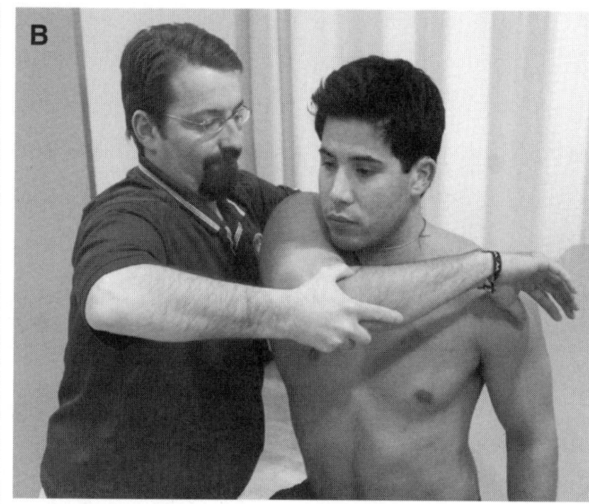

A posterior force is applied to the glenohumeral joint. Pain is associated with posteroinferior instability; a clunk is associated with a tear of the glenoid labrum.

Patient Position	Supine or seated. The supine position provides better scapular stabilization.
Position of Examiner	Behind the patient One hand stabilizes the scapula. The opposite hand holds the affected arm at 90° of flexion and internal rotation **(A)**.
Evaluative Procedure	The affected arm is passively horizontally adducted while the examiner applies a simultaneous axial load to the humerus **(B)**.
Positive Test	Clunk that may or may not be painful
Implications	Posteroinferior instability with or without posteroinferior labral tear
Comments	A painful clunk is frequently associated with a posteroinferior labral tear that must be surgically repaired. Patients with a painless clunk respond well to nonsurgical treatment.[68]
Evidence	Positive likelihood ratio Not Useful — Useful Very Small — Small — Moderate — Large 36.5 0 1 2 3 4 5 6 7 8 9 10 Negative likelihood ratio Not Useful — Useful Very Small — Small — Moderate — Large 1.0 0.9 0.8 0.7 0.6 0.5 0.4 0.3 0.2 0.1 0

The patient with a congenital MDI will present with generalized hyperlaxity of the shoulders and other joints and have no history of trauma. Those with acquired MDI typically participate in overhead activities that impose repetitive microtrauma. These individuals are symptomatic with their activities and present with less laxity than those with congenital MDI. Posttraumatic MDI occurs following a discrete traumatic episode and is usually accompanied by more pain than the other two.[51]

Evaluation of shoulder instability must be performed carefully to differentiate between unidirectional and multidirectional instabilities. Treatment of only one of the unidirectional instabilities in the presence of a multidirectional instability can worsen the condition because only one aspect of the joint is strengthened, potentially increasing the chance of instability in the other involved plane. Those with acquired MDI are most likely to benefit from surgical stabilization.[51]

Special Test 16-9
Sulcus Sign for Inferior Glenohumeral Laxity

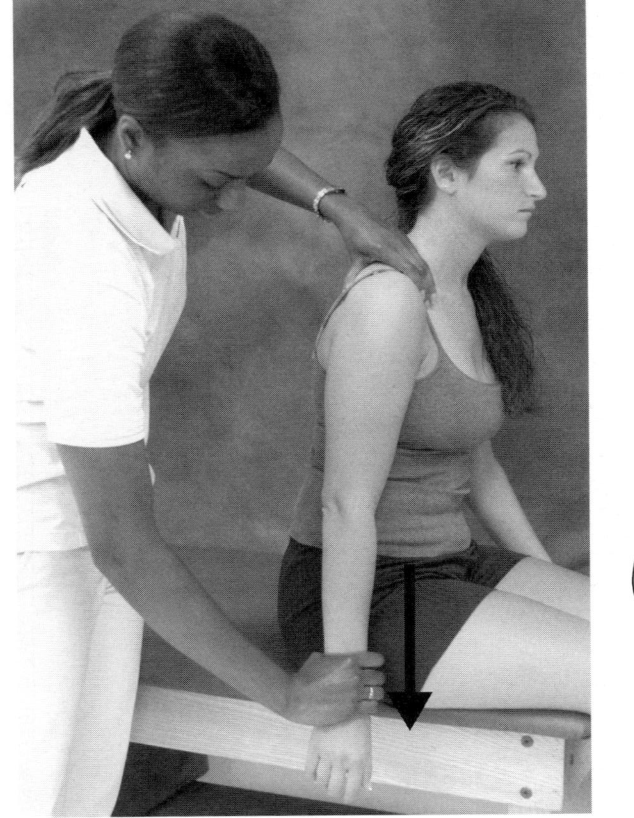

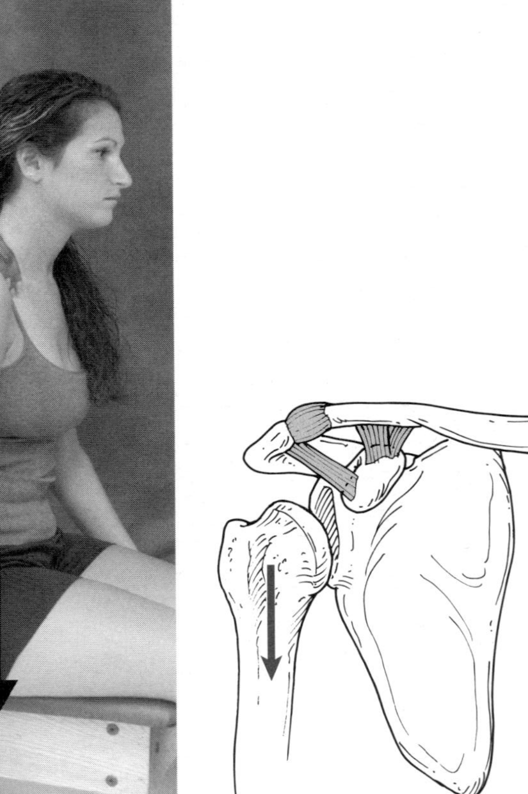

The sulcus sign determines the amount of inferior glide of the humeral head when traction is applied to the humerus.

Patient Position	Sitting Arm hanging at the side
Position of Examiner	Standing lateral to the involved side
Evaluative Procedure	The patient's arm is gripped distal to the elbow. A downward (inferior) traction force is applied to the humerus while the scapula is stabilized.
Positive Test	An indentation (sulcus) appears beneath the acromion process. To differentiate the results of this test from those of the AC traction test for AC joint instability, the movement of the humeral head is away from the scapula and clavicle in this test. In the AC traction test, the humerus and scapula move away from the clavicle.

Implications	The humeral head slides inferiorly on the glenoid fossa, indicating laxity in the superior GH ligament. The grade is based on the widening of the subacromial space:[16] Grade 1: 1 cm or less Grade 2: 1–2 cm Grade 3: Greater than 2 cm
Modification	A positive sulcus sign with the humerus flexed to 90° may indicate inferior instability.
Comments	The results of this test are more meaningful when the patient is anesthetized, indicating the influence of muscle tension on the findings.
Evidence	Positive likelihood ratio Not Useful — Useful Very Small, Small, Moderate, Large 0 1 2 3 4 5 6 7 8 9 10 Negative likelihood ratio Not Useful — Useful Very Small, Small, Moderate, Large 1.0 0.9 0.8 0.7 0.6 0.5 0.4 0.3 0.2 0.1 0

AC = acromioclavicular; GH = glenohumeral.

Rotator Cuff Pathology

The space between the superior glenohumeral joint and the coracoacromial ligament is occupied by the the supraspinatus and infraspinatus tendons, the subacromial bursa, the superior capsule and the long head of the biceps. A cause-and-effect relationship exists between pathology of any or all of these structures and encroachment, or impingement, in the subacromial space.

Impingement

Impingement of the rotator cuff muscles occurs when there is decreased space through which the rotator cuff tendons pass under the coracoacromial arch. In its initial stages, the impingement often results in the inflammation of the rotator cuff tendons. Likewise, inflammation of the rotator cuff tendons results in the enlargement of the tendons, decreasing the subacromial space and increasing the likelihood of impinging the tendons. The source of rotator cuff impingement is classified as being compressive or tensile and further categorized into primary and secondary sources (Table 16-9). Internal impingement results when the posterosuperior aspect of the rotator cuff becomes entrapped between the glenoid labrum and greater tuberosity of the humerus. This impingement occurs at 90 degrees of abduction and 90 degrees of external rotation and is strongly associated with a **glenohumeral internal rotation deficit** (GIRD).[7,71] If untreated, continued internal impingement forces magnified by throwing will result in a SLAP lesion.

This sequence of events creates a closed cycle in which one condition exacerbates the other. When allowed to proceed unchecked, the ultimate outcome is a shoulder with greatly diminished function. To athletes participating in overhead sports or workers who perform repetitive overhead movements, impingement syndrome or rotator cuff pathology can be career threatening.

Table 16-9 Causes of Impingement

Force	Source
Primary Compression	Irregularly shaped acromion
	Coracoacromial ligament
	Enlarged bursa
	Thickened rotator cuff tendons
Secondary Compression	Loss of humeral head depression/ stabilization
	Poor posture
	Repetitive overhead movement
Primary Tensile	Repetitive overload
	Eccentric forces
Secondary Tensile	**Scapular dyskinesis**
	Rotator cuff muscle weakness
	GH instability

Impingement syndrome

Caused by a reduction in the space below the coracoacromial arch, the structures that lie beneath this area, the rotator cuff tendons (primarily the supraspinatus and infraspinatus tendons), the long head of the biceps brachii tendon, the subacromial bursa, the GH joint capsule, and the head of the humerus are compressed between the acromion process and the humeral head (Fig. 16-35). The most common cause of impingement is anatomical variation in the coracoacromial arch that produces a mechanical wear on the rotator cuff, subacromial bursa, and the long head of the biceps tendon.[72] Fatigue from overuse, restricted glenohumeral motion, or decreased strength of the rotator cuff can also contribute to impingement syndrome. Decreased strength or fatigue leads to decreased humeral

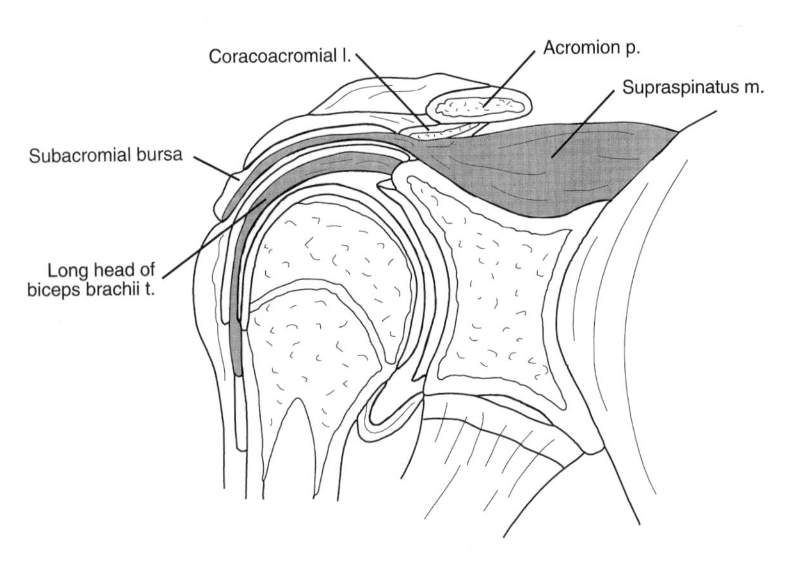

FIGURE 16-35 ■ Structures involved in shoulder impingement syndrome. If the humeral head does not depress during abduction, the long head of the biceps brachii, the subacromial bursa, and the supraspinatus tendon are impinged between the coracoacromial arch and the head of the humerus.

Scapular dyskinesis An improperly moving scapula.

head depression as the humerus is brought into overhead positions, causing impingement of the structures. Tightness of the posterior capsule, as evidenced by restricted posterior joint play, restricted horizontal adduction and restricted internal rotation, causes increased and earlier superior and anterior migration of the humeral head.[73,74] Impingement can occur anywhere along the coracoacromial arch and under the AC joint.

A relationship between poor scapular biomechanics and impingement syndromes has been suggested.[75,76] In this case, the scapula does not upwardly rotate appropriately to allow the tendons of the rotator cuff muscles and the long head of the biceps tendon to pass beneath the coracoacromial arch. In addition, during elevation, activation of the middle and lower trapezius muscles is delayed in those with impingement symptoms. This pattern is consistent with excessive scapular elevation and anterior tilting that further decreases the subacromial space.[77] Tightness of the pectoralis minor may also contribute to these abnormal mechanics.[30]

The chief complaint associated with rotator cuff impingement is pain during overhead movements and an associated painful arc with elevation in the plane of the scapula (Examination Findings 16-3). The patient may describe a relief of symptoms when the GH joint is maintained in slight abduction, or when an inferiorly gliding force is applied to the humeral head during elevation.[78] An injection of anesthetic into the subacromial space with subsequent relief of symptoms is indicative of impingement.[22] In relaxed stance, the patient may present with a forward shoulder posture, where the scapula rests in a protracted and possibly winged position and the humerus is internally rotated. The position further reduces the available subacromial space and influences scapulothoracic mechanics.[74] The physical impingement of the supraspinatus tendon between the acromion process and the greater tuberosity begins when the humerus is abducted to 30 degrees and reaches its peak at 90 degrees of abduction with the humerus internally rotated.[30,79] Common evaluative tests used to evaluate for impingement or its underlying pathologies include the **Neer impingement test** (Special Test 16-10), the **Hawkins (Kennedy–Hawkins) impingement test** (Special Test 16-11), the **drop arm test** (see Special Test 16-1), passive horizontal adduction (which decreases the subacromial space), and manual muscle tests for the infraspinatus and supraspinatus.

*** Practical Evidence**

When examined collectively, positive findings from the Hawkins–Kennedy test coupled with a painful arc and pain and weakness with a manual test of the infraspinatus strongly predict the presence of impingement (positive likelihood ratio = 10.56).[22]

Rotator cuff tendinopathy

Rotator cuff tendinopathy typically presents with a slow onset of the symptoms. Pathology ranges from acute tendinitis after an abrupt change in level of activity to the more common chronic degenerative change in the tissue. Actual tears in the cuff can be partial or complete, with partial tears occurring on the bursal side or articular side of the cuff.

In the early stages of rotator cuff tendinopathy, the chief complaint is pain deep within the shoulder in the subacromial area after activity. The symptoms then progress to pain during activity and, finally, to constant pain with most activities of daily living. Factors contributing to the onset of rotator cuff pathology include a muscle imbalance between the internal and external rotators, capsular laxity, poor scapular control, and impingement syndromes.

The shoulder is predisposed to rotator cuff tendinopathy by the relatively poor vascularization of the tendons, a fact that also hinders the healing process. The supraspinatus tendon is the most susceptible of the rotator cuff group to inflammatory conditions, especially at the convergence zone of the anterior and posterior circumflex arteries, just proximal to the greater tuberosity.[81] In addition to its poor blood supply, pressure is placed on this tendon by the humeral head "wringing" it dry of blood and other vital nutrients.

The shape and location of the acromion process may also precipitate the onset of rotator cuff inflammation. The rate of rotator cuff pathology is markedly increased when the lateral acromion angle is less than 70 degrees, forming an acromial spur.[82] Shoulders that are affected by chronic rotator cuff pathology are also characterized by an increased number of acromial osteophytes (Box 16-3).[83]

The posterior rotator cuff muscles, the infraspinatus and teres minor, play an important role in the throwing motion. In addition to externally rotating the humerus during the cocking phase of the throw, these muscles eccentrically contract to decelerate the arm during the follow-through phase. The eccentric contraction can lead to microtearing or inflammation of these muscles, eventually giving way to larger tears.

The relative severity of rotator cuff pathology is based on the presence of tearing within the tendons (Examination Findings 16-4). Tears to the tendons may result from a single traumatic force or, more commonly and especially in the older population, from the accumulation of microtrauma (overuse injuries). **Partial-thickness tears** are short, longitudinal lesions in the tendon, initially involving the superficial or midsubstance fibers. Tears most commonly occur in the supraspinatus.[84] Partial-thickness tears can occur on the articular side or subacromial side of the rotator cuff. Subacromial tears are more associated with subacromial impingement while articular-side tears are associated with internal impingement.[84] When partial-thickness tears go untreated, a **full-thickness tear** may develop (full-thickness tears may also develop secondary to a single traumatic force). Severe dysfunction of the supraspinatus or infraspinatus muscles may lead to atrophy that is visible during inspection of the scapula.

During the controlled motion from full abduction to adduction, individuals suffering from tears in the rotator cuff tendons are unable to control the rate of fall after the humerus reaches 90 degrees of abduction as demonstrated

Examination Findings 16-3
Impingement Syndrome

Examination Segment	Clinical Findings
History	***Onset:*** Insidious ***Pain characteristics:*** Beneath the acromion process and radiating to the lateral arm Internal impingement: Pain deep in the posterior shoulder ***Other symptoms:*** The patient may complain of popping and clicking, depending on involvement of bursa and rotator cuff musculature. ***Mechanism:*** Repetitive overhead motion impinging the rotator cuff muscles (especially the supraspinatus) and long head of the biceps tendon between the humeral head and coracoacromial arch ***Predisposing conditions:*** Tight posterior capsule and ligamentous tissues, increased anterior laxity, irregularly shaped acromion (curved or hooked), subacromial spurs, scapular dyskinesis, rotator cuff weakness
Inspection	The shoulder may be postured for comfort by holding the arm in slight abduction and avoiding overhead arm motions. A forward shoulder posture where the scapula rests in a protracted position and the humerus is internally rotated is frequently associated with impingement.
Palpation	Tenderness exists beneath the acromion process, over the supraspinatus insertion at the greater tuberosity, and over the bicipital groove. Internal impingement: Pain just inferior to acromion on posterior shoulder
Joint and Muscle Function Assessment	Active, passive, and resisted movements of GH internal and external rotation and flexion result in pain and/or weakness, especially when the arm is abducted above 90°. ***AROM:*** Active abduction in an arc of motion from about 70°–120° results in pain. ***MMT:*** Elevation in plane of scapula (empty can or full can test) External rotation ***PROM:*** Internal impingement: Excessive external rotation; limited internal rotation and horizontal adduction. Pectoralis minor tightness is often associated with impingement.
Joint Stability Tests	***Stress tests:*** A complete ligamentous and capsular screen is necessary to rule out GH and AC laxity. ***Joint play:*** May have hypermobility in all directions. Hypomobile posterior glide is common with impingement.
Special Tests	The Neer and Hawkins impingement tests are usually painful. Internal impingement: Increased pain with apprehension test; reduction of symptoms with relocation test
Neurologic Screening	Within normal limits
Vascular Screening	Within normal limits
Functional Assessment	ADLs and athletic events requiring overhead movement result in pain. Internal impingement: Complain of poor control and loss of velocity with throwing. Increased pain with overhead motions; may be coupled with compensatory scapulothoracic movement, with early and excessive scapular elevation and/or decreased posterior tipping during arm-raising maneuvers.
Imaging Techniques	Radiographs to rule out primary cause of impingement, including a hooked acromion or osteophyte
Differential Diagnosis	Labral tears, SLAP lesions, rotator cuff tendinopathy, subacromial bursitis, long head of the biceps tendinopathy
Comments	Impingement may occur secondary to GH instability in younger patients. The inflammatory response caused by rotator cuff impingement, if untreated, can lead to rotator cuff tears. Temporary relief of symptoms associated with an injection of anesthetic into the subacromial space is indicative of impingement.[22]

AC = acromioclavicular; ADLs = activities of daily living; AROM = active range of motion; GH = glenohumeral; MMT = manual muscle test; PROM = passive range of motion.

by the **drop arm test** (see Special Test 16-1). The **empty can test**, the manual muscle test for the supraspinatus, isolates the supraspinatus tendon for weakness or pain (Special Test 16-12).

Because the supraspinatus contributes so little to general abduction strength, the empty can test may not be able to detect subtle changes in strength resulting from tears in the tendon. The test is most useful in determining the presence of large rotator cuff tears.[14,50] Tears of the subscapularis are associated with weakness with the Gerber lift-off test and weakness with internal rotation.

✱ Practical Evidence

The diagnostic accuracy of the shoulder examination improves when the results are grouped by positive findings. Weakness during the empty can test, weakness in external rotation, and a positive impingement signs is associated with a rotator cuff tear 98% of the time.[23] A positive drop arm test, an associated painful arc, and weakness in external rotation are also highly predictive of a rotator cuff tear.[22]

Subacromial bursitis

Chronic rotator cuff impingement or rotator cuff tears, if untreated, ultimately lead to inflammation of the subacromial bursa and still further encroachment of the subacromial space. Often occurring concurrently, it is difficult to differentiate between rotator cuff pathology and subacromial bursitis. Subacromial bursitis causes positive results from impingement tests and tests for supraspinatus tendinopathy as the three conditions are often related.

Management of rotator cuff pathologies and impingement syndromes

Nonsurgical approaches to managing patients with rotator cuff pathology and impingement syndromes emphasize modification of activity, control of inflammation through the use of medications and therapeutic modalities, and rotator cuff flexibility and strengthening programs.[87] The restoration of capsular flexibility for rotator cuff pathology focuses on decreasing the tightness of the posterior shoulder structures. Tightness of the posterior structures restricts internal rotation (internal rotation deficiency) and increases forces causing elevation of the humeral head under the coracoacromial arch. These structures are isolated during stretching routines by stabilizing the scapula while taking the arm into internal rotation (the sleeper stretch) and during joint mobilization.

Strengthening must focus on the scapular musculature, the rotator cuff, and other shoulder muscles. The strength and use of the legs and trunk also must be analyzed. Much of the forces derived in throwing or swinging originate in the legs, pelvis, and trunk. Decreased contributions from these areas call for increased activity of the rotator cuff muscles, exposing them to potentially injurious force and overuse injuries.

The patient should be able to control the scapula throughout the ROM. Strengthening of the rotator cuff must occur in conjunction with scapular stabilization. Initially, the rotator cuff can be strengthened in the scapular plane with the humerus in slight abduction to prevent overstressing the rotator cuff. As the patient progresses, the humerus can be elevated to overhead positions that place more functional stresses on the tendons. A well-rounded rehabilitation program also includes strengthening of the distal arm musculature.

Surgery may be required to débride the subacromial space, resect the lateral portion of the clavicle (thus increasing the subacromial space), or repair the tear.[87] Based on the pathology, especially the size of any rotator cuff tear, the physician determines if surgery is done arthroscopically, with a mini-open technique (small scar over the superior aspect of the shoulder), or full open repair. Most small to medium sized tears can be repaired with arthroscopy or the mini-open technique.

Postoperatively, rehabilitation is dictated by the type of surgery required. Although débridements of the subacromial space and rotator cuff can progress based on the patient's tolerance, rotator cuff repairs require careful use of active and resisted motions in the repaired tissues for a period of 6 to 8 weeks to allow healing to occur.

Biceps Tendon Pathology

The long head of the biceps tendon provides very little force in moving the GH joint, but pathology of this structure can decrease the strength, ROM, and stability of the GH joint. During overhead movements, the tendon slides within its sheath that is located in the bicipital groove. When the tendon is inflamed, these movements produce pain and decrease the GH joint's functional ability.

Bicipital tendinopathy

Bicipital tendon pathology may result from rotator cuff dysfunction, from overuse of the biceps brachii muscle, or from impingement. The transverse humeral ligament, which holds the tendon in the bicipital groove, may become stretched or torn as the result of sudden forceful extension or external rotation of the shoulder accompanied by elbow flexion. Disruption of the transverse humeral ligament can cause the long head of the biceps tendon to sublux from the bicipital groove, especially when the elbow is flexed and the humerus is externally rotated. Tears of the supraspinatus or infraspinatus tendons are often associated with dislocation or subluxation of the long head of the biceps brachii tendon.[88]

Yergason's test can reproduce subluxation of the long head of the biceps tendon or cause pain in the presence of bicipital tendinopathy or a labral tear (Special Test 16-13). Pain caused by a subluxating tendon can be differentiated by **Speed's test**, which only has positive test results in the presence of bicipital tendinopathy (Special Test 16-14). MRI can also be used to differentiate between the two conditions.[89]

Special Test 16-10
The Neer Shoulder Impingement Test

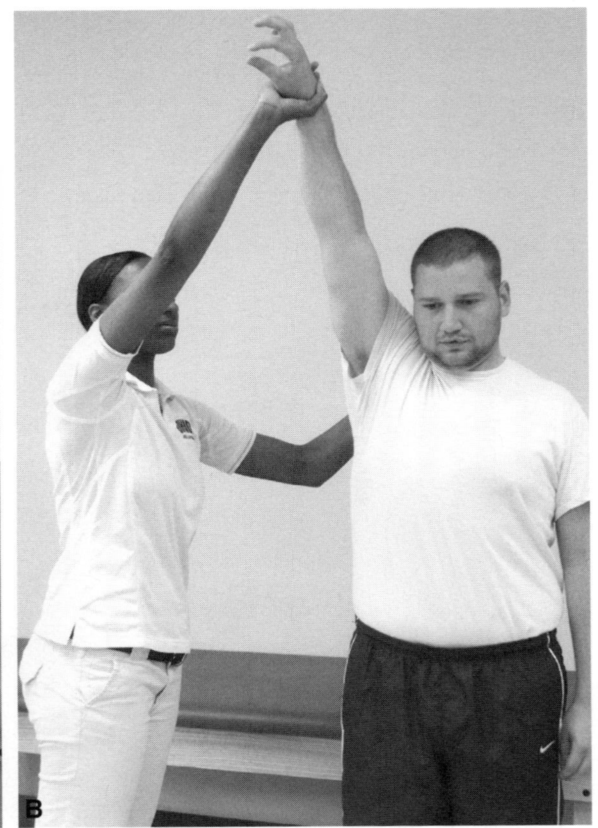

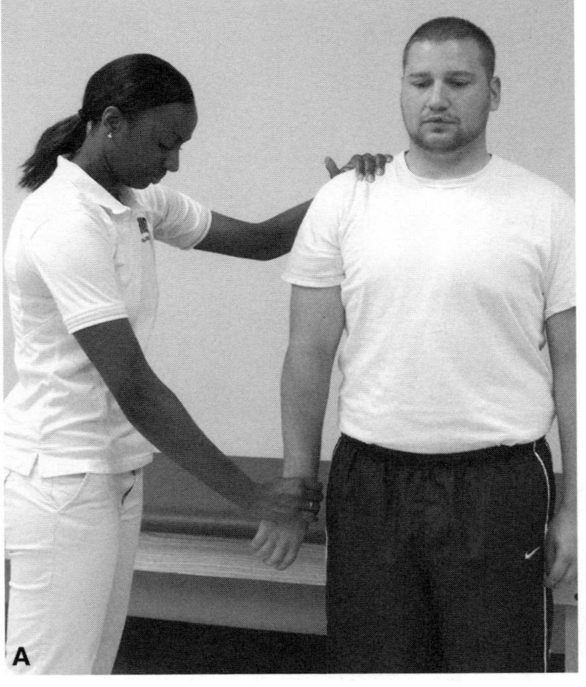

The patient's arm is passively moved through flexion to reproduce the symptoms of rotator cuff impingement, usually between 90° and 180° of flexion.

Patient Position	Standing or sitting The shoulder, elbow, and wrist begin in the anatomical position.
Position of Examiner	Standing lateral or forward of the involved side **(A)** One hand stabilizes the patient's scapula. The opposite hand grasps the patient's arm distal to the elbow joint.
Evaluative Procedure	With the elbow extended, the humerus is placed in internal rotation and the forearm is pronated. The GH joint is then forcefully moved through forward flexion as the scapula is stabilized **(B)**.
Positive Test	Pain in the anterior or lateral shoulder, in range of 90° to full elevation

Implications	Pathology is present in the rotator cuff group (especially the supraspinatus) or the long head of the biceps brachii tendon. The motion of the test impinges these structures between the greater tuberosity and the inferior side of the acromion process and AC joint.
Comments	Bursal involvement only (no rotator cuff damage); the sensitivity improves to 85.7% but the specificity decreases to 49.2% with a positive likelihood ratio of 1.69.[22]
Evidence	Positive likelihood ratio Not Useful — Useful Very Small · Small · Moderate · Large 0 1 2 3 4 5 6 7 8 9 10 Negative likelihood ratio Not Useful — Useful Very Small · Small · Moderate · Large 1.0 0.9 0.8 0.7 0.6 0.5 0.4 0.3 0.2 0.1 0

AC = acromioclavicular; GH = glenohumeral; ROM = range of motion.

Special Test 16-11
The Hawkins Shoulder Impingement Test

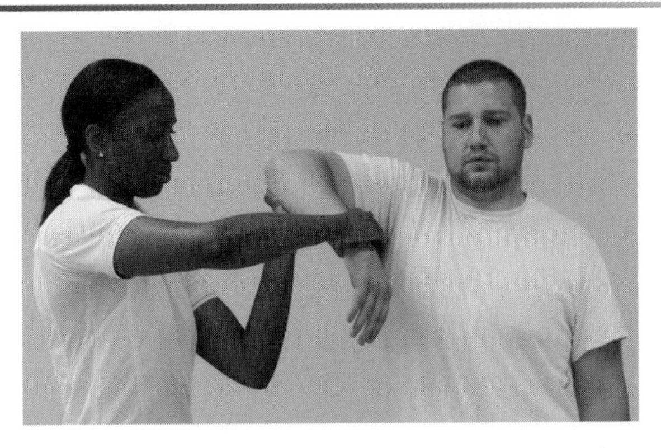

With the glenohumeral joint abducted to 90° in the scapular plane the humerus is internally rotated to reproduce the symptoms of rotator cuff impingement.

Patient Position	Sitting or standing The shoulder, elbow, and wrist are in the anatomical position.
Position of Examiner	Standing lateral or forward of the involved side Grasp the patient's arm at the elbow joint.
Evaluative Procedure	With the elbow flexed, the GH joint is elevated to 90° in the scapular plane. At this point, the humerus is passively internally rotated until painful or scapular rotation is felt or observed.
Positive Test	Pain with motion, especially near the end of the ROM
Implications	Pathology is present in the rotator cuff group (especially the supraspinatus) or the long head of the biceps brachii tendon. The motion of the test impinges these structures between the greater tuberosity and the inferior side of the acromion process.
Comments	If the humerus is brought in toward the sagittal plane, the chance of eliciting a false-positive result secondary to AC joint pathology increases.
Evidence	Positive likelihood ratio Not Useful — Useful Very Small · Small · Moderate · Large 0 1 2 3 4 5 6 7 8 9 10 Negative likelihood ratio Not Useful — Useful Very Small · Small · Moderate · Large 1.0 0.9 0.8 0.7 0.6 0.5 0.4 0.3 0.2 0.1 0

AC = acromioclavicular; GH = glenohumeral; ROM = range of motion.

Bicipital and rotator cuff tendinopathies often occur simultaneously. Conservative rehabilitation includes decreasing inflammation with the use of oral medications, **phonophoresis**, or **iontophoresis**. Stretching and strengthening of the shoulder complex muscles should progress in a manner similar to that used for rotator cuff tendinopathies.

Superior labrum anterior to posterior lesions

Superior labrum anterior to posterior (SLAP) lesions are tears of the superior aspect of the glenoid labrum that extend anteriorly and posteriorly to the biceps insertion.[54] Table 16-10 presents four classifications of SLAP lesions. Type I lesions are most frequently associated with rotator cuff degeneration; GH instability is often the precursor to

Examination Findings 16-4
Rotator Cuff Tendinopathy

Examination Segment	Clinical Findings
History	***Onset:*** Insidious or acute ***Pain characteristics:*** Deep within the shoulder beneath the acromion process. Pain usually radiates into the lateral arm. ***Other symptoms:*** Clicking during certain GH motions ***Mechanism:*** **Insidious**: Chronic impingement or weakening of the rotator cuff tendons over time due to aging; a single traumatic episode may cause the final rupture of a weakened tendon. **Acute**: Dynamic overloading of the tendon ***Predisposing conditions:*** Rotator cuff impingement, chronic rotator cuff tendinopathy, acromion changes, repetitive overhead motion, repetitive eccentric loading
Inspection	In chronic cases, inspection of the scapula possibly revealing atrophy of the infraspinatus and/or supraspinatus.
Palpation	Tenderness in the subacromial space and at the insertion of the supraspinatus tendon into the greater tuberosity
Joint and Muscle Function Assessment	***AROM:*** Painful between 70° and 120° of elevation, especially in abduction ***MMT:*** Pain and/or weakness with abduction, internal rotation, external rotation, and elevation in the plane of the scapula ***PROM:*** Decreased pain compared to AROM, except in positions of impingement
Joint Stability Tests	***Stress tests:*** Tests to rule out GH and AC laxity and impingement ***Joint play:*** Joint play to assess for hyper- or hypomobility
Special Tests	Drop arm test Impingement tests may be positive.
Neurologic Screening	Within normal limits
Vascular Screening	Within normal limits
Functional Assessment	Pain during overhead motions. During elevation, scapula may excessively protract, elevate, or anteriorly tip.
Imaging Techniques	The standard radiographic series consists of scapular plane AP, internal rotation, external rotation, transscapular, and axillary views to rule out rotator cuff tears and bony abnormalities. A subacromial space of less than 7 mm is indicative of a full-thickness cuff tear. MRI has a sensitivity of 0.95 and specificity of 0.95 in identifying rotator cuff tears, degeneration, and partial thickness tears.[80] MR arthrography, ultrasonography
Differential Diagnosis	AC joint degeneration, subacromial impingement, internal impingement, labral tear, long head of the biceps tendinopathy, capsulitis
Comments	Rotator cuff impingement tests are often positive. A history of rotator cuff tendinopathy often precedes a rotator cuff tear.

AC = acromioclavicular; AP = anteroposterior; AROM = active range of motion; GH = glenohumeral; MMT = manual muscle test; MR = magnetic resonance; PROM = passive range of motion.

Phonophoresis The use of therapeutic ultrasound to introduce medication into the body.

Iontophoresis The use of a direct current to introduce medication into the body.

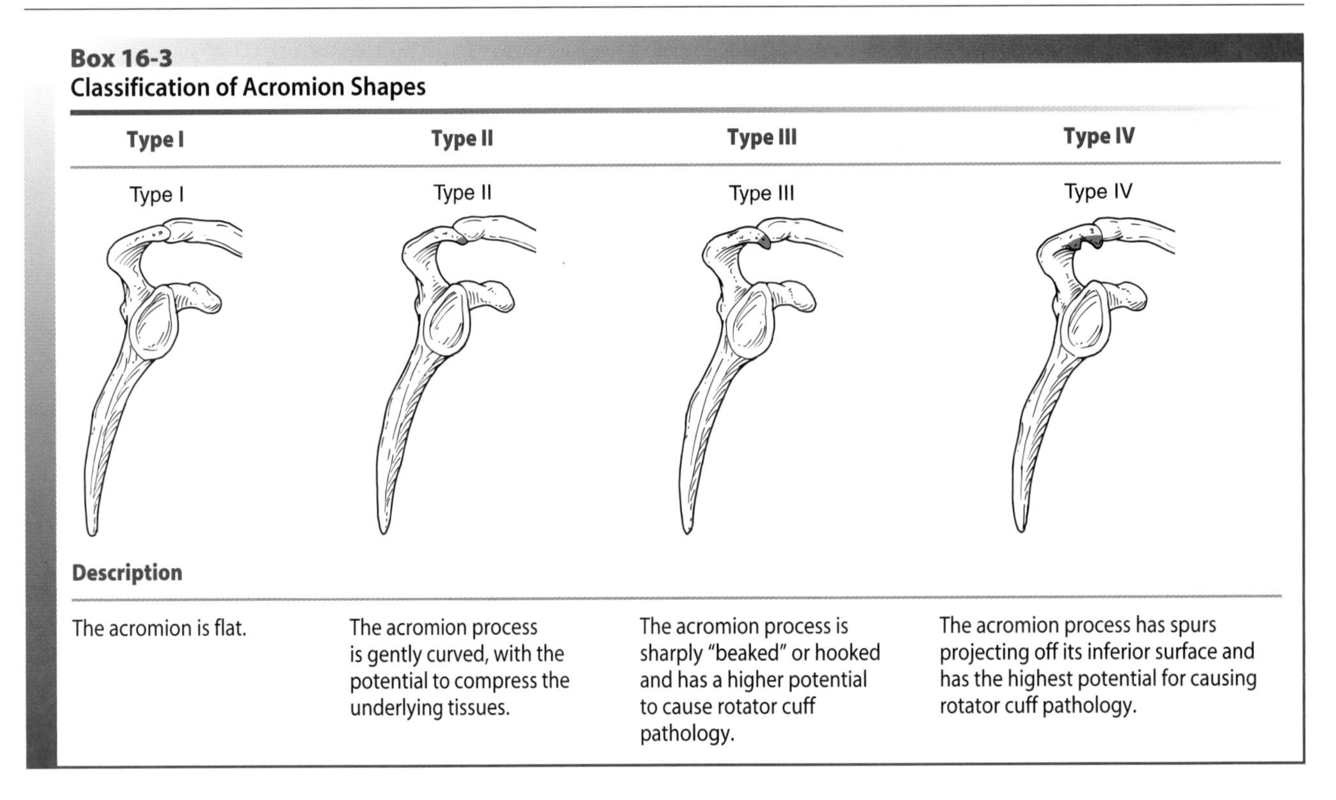

Box 16-3
Classification of Acromion Shapes

	Type I	Type II	Type III	Type IV
Description	The acromion is flat.	The acromion process is gently curved, with the potential to compress the underlying tissues.	The acromion process is sharply "beaked" or hooked and has a higher potential to cause rotator cuff pathology.	The acromion process has spurs projecting off its inferior surface and has the highest potential for causing rotator cuff pathology.

type III and IV lesions. Type II lesions are age-dependent. In younger patients type II lesions tend to clinically resemble those of type III and IV lesions in adults; in older patients, type II lesions more closely resemble type I.[54] SLAP lesions can sometimes be seen on MRI or computed tomography (CT) scans, but are most commonly confirmed during arthroscopy or via MR arthrography.[63,92,95]

Table 16-10 Classification of SLAP Lesions

Type	Pathology
I	Degenerative fraying of the labrum near the insertion of the LHBT
II	Avulsion of the glenoid labrum with an associated tear of the LHBT Type II SLAP lesions have been further classified relative to the detachment of the labrum[54]: • Isolated to the anterior aspect • Isolated to the posterior aspect • Appearing in both aspects
III	A bucket-handle tear of the labrum with displacement of the fragment. No involvement of the LHBT
IV	Bucket-handle tear of the labrum with associated tearing of the LHBT

LHBT = long head of the biceps tendon.

Tension of the long head of the biceps tendon, such as that experienced during the follow-through phase of pitching when the biceps works to decelerate the elbow, pulls the labrum away from the glenoid fossa. Other compression and inferior traction mechanisms can also produce SLAP lesions.[96,97] The LHBT contacting the rotator cuff when the arm is in the cocked position has been associated with posterior-superior tears.[54] Type II lesions can occur by the LHBT being peeled back caused by tendon torsion created as the arm is brought into abduction and external rotation.[54]

With an acute or gradual onset, SLAP lesions present with clinically inconsistent symptoms and are frequently associated with concurrent pathology (Examination Findings 16-5).[92] The chief complaint is of pain between the AC joint and coracoid process during overhead arm movement that is relieved by rest.[71,95] Throwing athletes report "dead arm" symptoms and a loss of throwing control and velocity.

Special tests to evaluate for the presence of SLAP lesions: (1) attempt to reproduce symptoms by recreating tensile forces on the long head of the biceps tendon or (2) apply compressive forces on the labrum. The **active compression test (O'Brien test)** (Special Test 16-15),[98] **anterior-slide test** (Special Test 16-16) and **compression-rotation test (grind test)** (Special Test 16-17) are among the many used clinically. The stated clinical usefulness of these techniques varies widely by investigator.[62–64,94,99–101] Reproduction of symptoms with the Yergason's test, Neer impingement sign, Speed's test, and the relocation test may or may not add predictive value to the diagnosis of SLAP lesions.[63,91,94]

Special Test 16-12
Empty Can Test for Supraspinatus Pathology

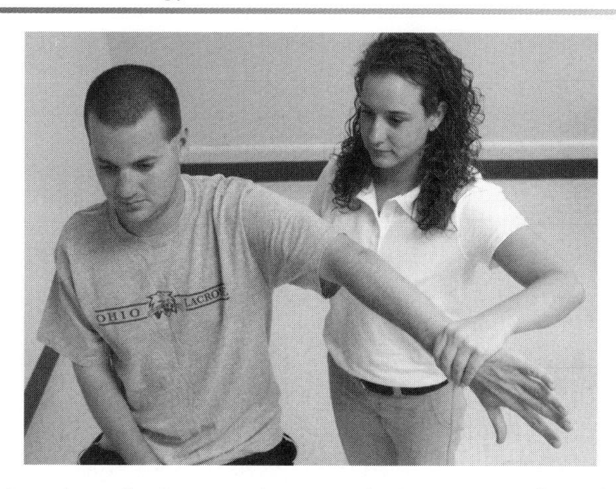

The empty can test is actually a manual muscle test for the supraspinatus muscle. A positive test often indicates subacromial impingement or a lesion to the musculotendinous unit.

Patient Position	Sitting or standing The GH is abducted to 90° in the scapular plane, the elbow extended, and the humerus internally rotated and the forearm pronated so that the thumb points downward.
Position of Examiner	Standing facing the patient One hand is placed on the superior portion of the midforearm to resist the motion of abduction in the scapular plane.
Evaluative Procedure	The evaluator resists abduction (applies a downward pressure).
Positive Test	Weakness or pain accompanying the movement
Implications	The supraspinatus tendon (1) is being impinged between the humeral head and the coracoacromial arch, (2) is inflamed, or (3) contains a lesion.
Modification	This test can be performed with the humerus externally rated and the forearm supinated so that the thumb is facing upward, the full can test.
Comments	The empty can and full can test are about equally accurate in detecting supraspinatus tears. Because the full can test is less pain provoking of impingement symptoms, its use is recommended.[85] Pain alone does not help detect partial-thickness tears or tendinopathy.[86]
Evidence	Positive likelihood ratio Negative likelihood ratio

GH = glenohumeral.

Special Test 16-13
Yergason's Test

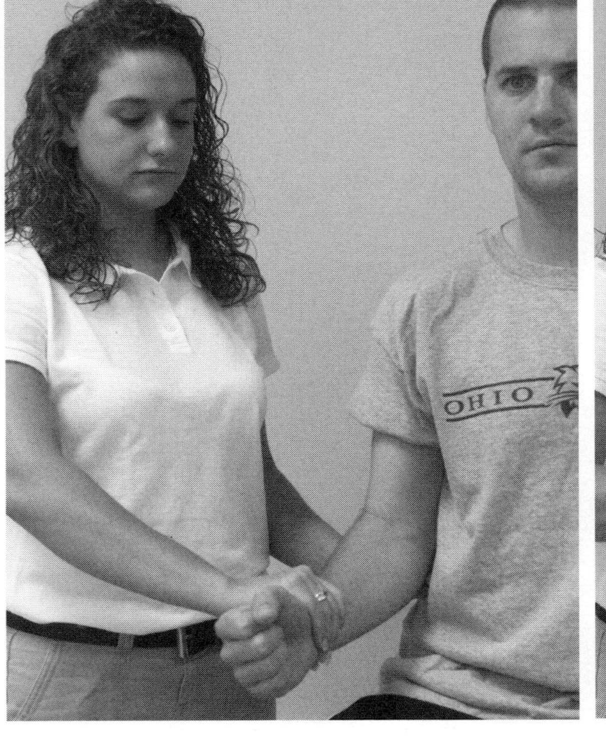

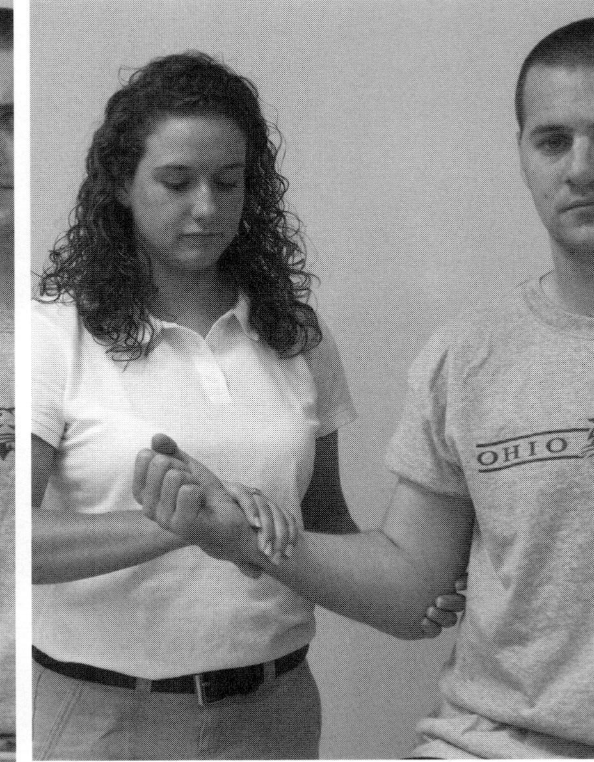

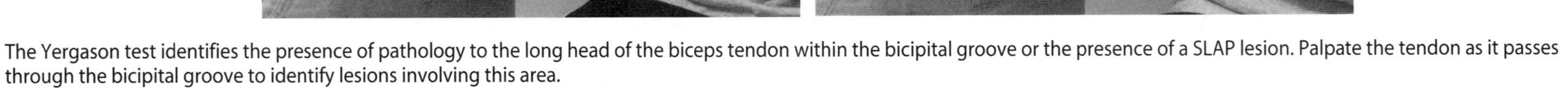

The Yergason test identifies the presence of pathology to the long head of the biceps tendon within the bicipital groove or the presence of a SLAP lesion. Palpate the tendon as it passes through the bicipital groove to identify lesions involving this area.

Patient Position	Sitting or standing GH joint in the anatomical position The elbow is flexed to 90°. The forearm is positioned so that the lateral border of the radius faces upward (neutral position).
Position of Examiner	Lateral to the patient on the involved side, lightly palpating the bicipital groove The olecranon is stabilized inferiorly and maintained close to the thorax. The forearm is stabilized proximal to the wrist.
Evaluative Procedure	The patient provides resistance while the examiner concurrently moves the GH joint into external rotation while resisting supination.

Positive Test	Pain or snapping (or both) in the bicipital groove Pain at the superior glenohumeral joint (SLAP lesion)
Implications	**Primary**: Snapping or popping in the bicipital groove indicates a tear or laxity of the transverse humeral ligament. This pathology prevents the ligament from securing the long head of the tendon in its groove. **Secondary**: Pain with no associated popping in the bicipital groove may indicate bicipital tendinopathy.
Modification	Resist elbow flexion as the humerus moves into external rotation.
Comments	False-positive findings may be the result of rotator cuff impingement.[90] Pain in the superior glenohumeral region are weakly predictive of SLAP lesions.[91]
Evidence	***Slap Lesions*** Positive likelihood ratio Not Useful — Useful Very Small / Small / Moderate / Large 0 1 2 3 4 5 6 7 8 9 10 Negative likelihood ratio Not Useful — Useful Very Small / Small / Moderate / Large 1.0 0.9 0.8 0.7 0.6 0.5 0.4 0.3 0.2 0.1 0 ***Biceps Tendon Pathology*** Positive likelihood ratio Not Useful — Useful Very Small / Small / Moderate / Large 0 1 2 3 4 5 6 7 8 9 10 Negative likelihood ratio Not Useful — Useful Very Small / Small / Moderate / Large 1.0 0.9 0.8 0.7 0.6 0.5 0.4 0.3 0.2 0.1 0

GH = glenohumeral.

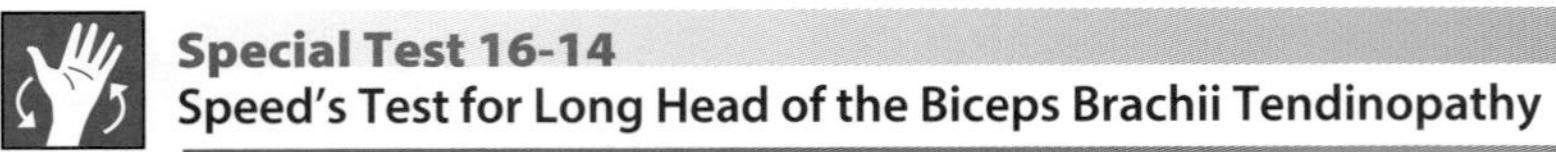

Special Test 16-14
Speed's Test for Long Head of the Biceps Brachii Tendinopathy

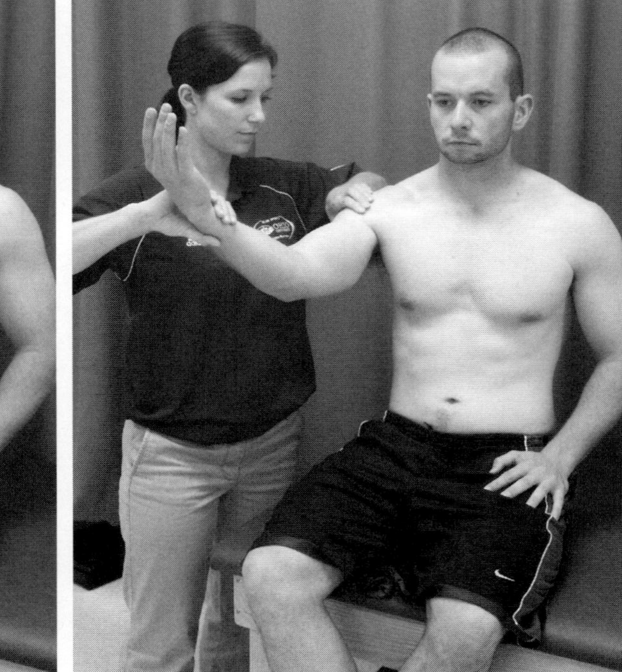

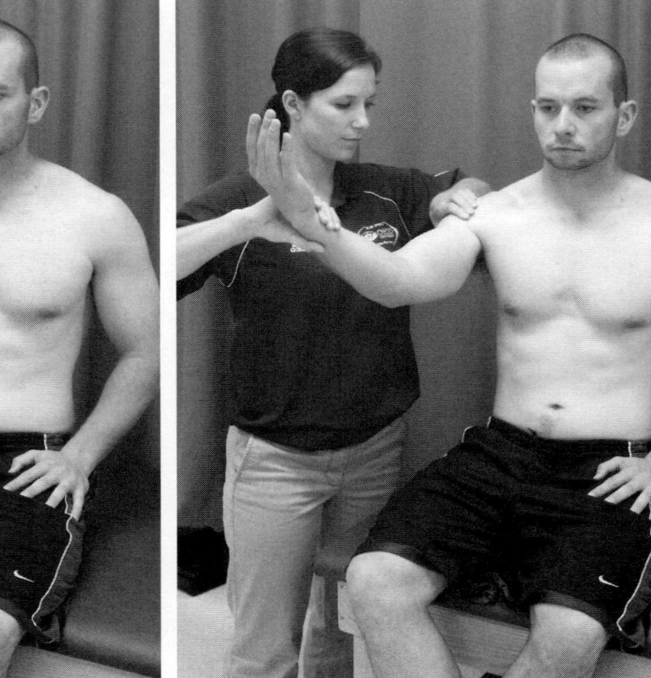

Resisted shoulder flexion with the elbow extended **(A)** or shoulder flexion and elbow flexion **(B)** elicit pain in the bicipital groove in the presence of long head of the biceps tendinopathy, a disruption of the transverse humeral ligament, or a SLAP lesion.

Patient Position	Sitting or standing The elbow is extended. The GH joint is in neutral position or slightly extended to stretch the biceps brachii.
Position of Examiner	Standing lateral to and in front of the involved limb The fingers of one hand are positioned over the bicipital groove while stabilizing the shoulder. The forearm is stabilized proximal to the wrist.
Evaluative Procedure	The clinician resists flexion of the GH joint and elbow while palpating for tenderness over the bicipital groove. Allow the patient to move through flexion range of motion.
Positive Test	Pain along the long head of the biceps brachii tendon, especially in the bicipital groove or at the superior shoulder

Implications	Inflammation of the long head of the biceps tendon as it passes through the bicipital groove Possible tear of the transverse humeral ligament with concurrent instability of the long head of the biceps tendon as it passes through the bicipital groove Pain at the superior shoulder (SLAP lesion)
Modification	The active Speed test where the examiner resists elbow flexion and forward flexion simultaneously may also be helpful in the detection of SLAP lesions.[92]
Comments	Many pathologies can result in positive findings for this test. With the high sensitivity, a negative finding effectively rules out biceps tendon pathology. The small positive likelihood ratio indicates that the test adds little diagnostic value in confirming the presence of biceps tendon pathology.[93]
Evidence	***Slap Lesion*** Positive likelihood ratio Not Useful — Useful Very Small · Small · Moderate · Large 0 1 2 3 4 5 6 7 8 9 10 Negative likelihood ratio Not Useful — Useful Very Small · Small · Moderate · Large 1.0 0.9 0.8 0.7 0.6 0.5 0.4 0.3 0.2 0.1 0 ***Biceps Tendon Pathology*** Positive likelihood ratio Not Useful — Useful Very Small · Small · Moderate · Large 0 1 2 3 4 5 6 7 8 9 10 Negative likelihood ratio Not Useful — Useful Very Small · Small · Moderate · Large 1.0 0.9 0.8 0.7 0.6 0.5 0.4 0.3 0.2 0.1 0

GH = glenohumeral; SLAP = superior labrum anterior to posterior tear.

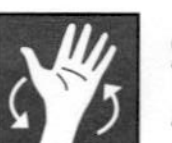

Special Test 16-15
Active Compression Test (O'Brien Test)

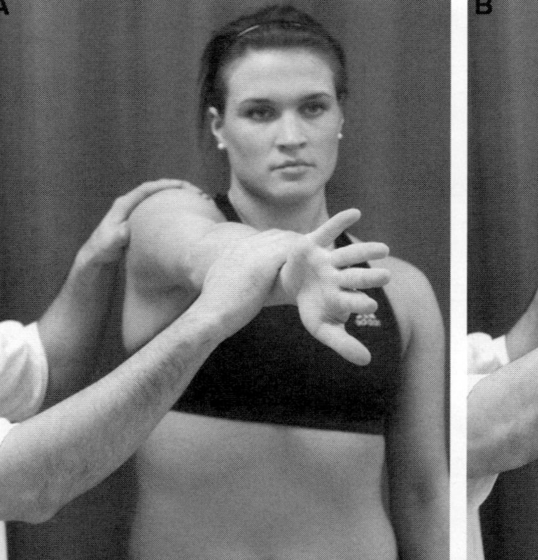
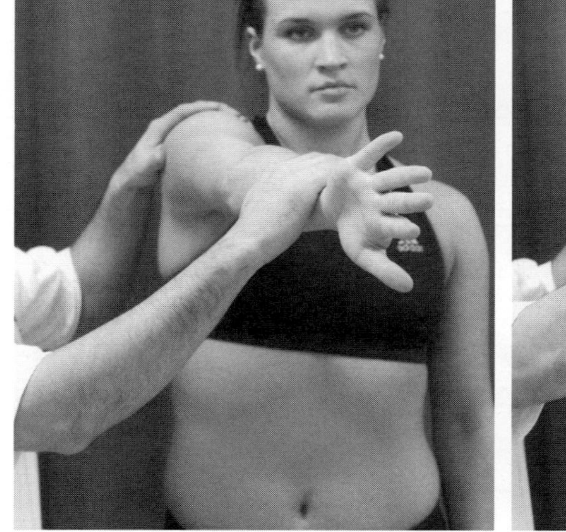

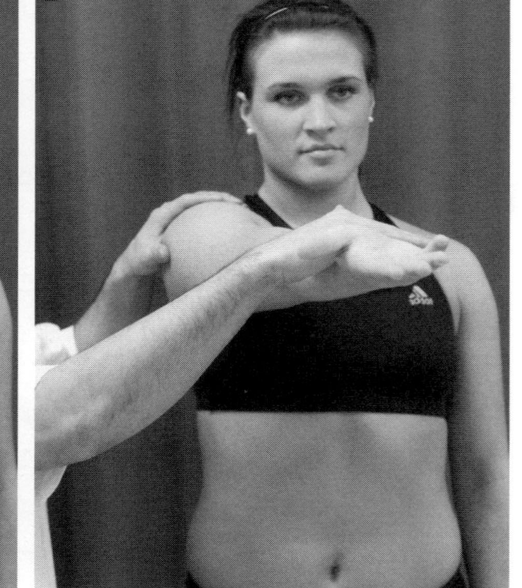

An isometric contraction with the humerus flexed to 90° and horizontally abducted once with the humerus internally rotated **(A)** and then again with the humerus externally rotated **(B)**. Depending on the positions pain is produced, a positive test may indicate a labral tear, AC joint pathology, or a SLAP lesion.

Patient Position	Standing The GH joint is flexed to 90° and horizontally adducted 15° from the sagittal plane. The humerus is in full internal rotation, elbow extended, and the forearm pronated **(A)**.
Position of Examiner	In front of the patient One hand is placed over the superior aspect of the patient's distal forearm.
Evaluative Procedure	The patient isometrically resists the examiner's downward force. The test is repeated with the humerus externally rotated and the forearm supinated **(B)**.
Positive Test	Pain that is experienced with the arm internally rotated but is decreased during external rotation: **1.** Pain or clicking within the GH joint may indicate a labral tear. **2.** Pain at the AC joint may indicate AC joint pathology. Positive SLAP lesion tests are confirmed with pain relief when the hand is supinated; pain with cross-armed horizontal adduction is used to confirm AC pathology.[16]
Implications	SLAP lesion AC joint pathology

Comments The presence of rotator cuff pathology and impingement may produce false-positive results.

Evidence

Inter-rater reliability

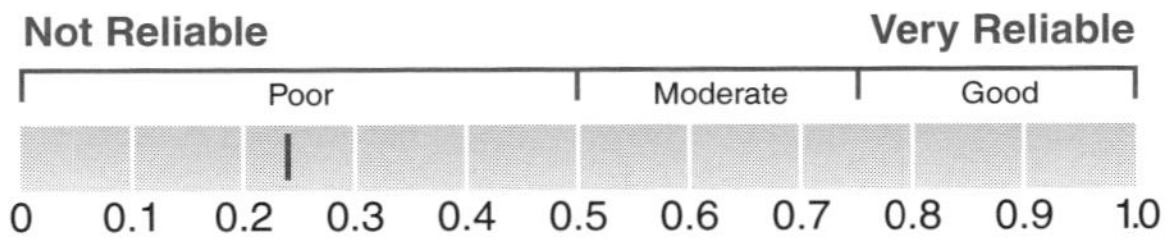

Not Reliable — Very Reliable
Poor | Moderate | Good
0 0.1 0.2 0.3 0.4 0.5 0.6 0.7 0.8 0.9 1.0

AC Joint Pathology

Positive likelihood ratio

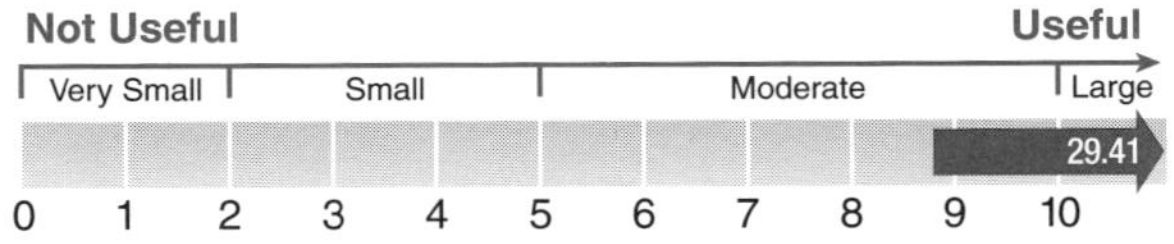

Not Useful — Useful
Very Small | Small | Moderate | Large
29.41
0 1 2 3 4 5 6 7 8 9 10

Negative likelihood ratio

Not Useful — Useful
Very Small | Small | Moderate | Large
1.0 0.9 0.8 0.7 0.6 0.5 0.4 0.3 0.2 0.1 0

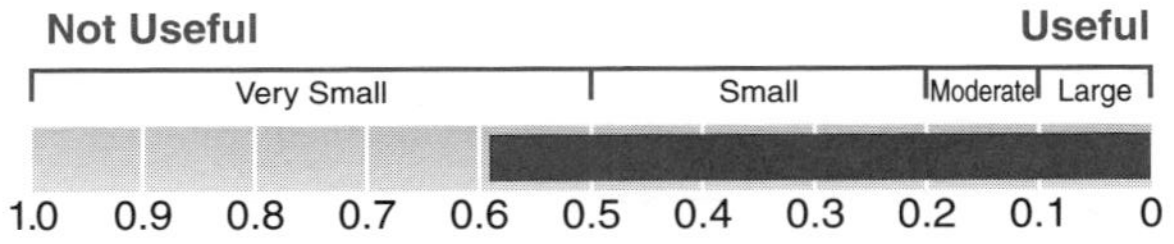

Slap Lesions

Positive likelihood ratio

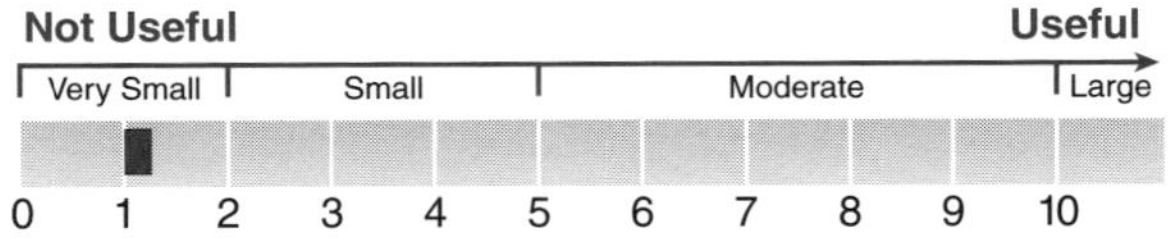

Not Useful — Useful
Very Small | Small | Moderate | Large
0 1 2 3 4 5 6 7 8 9 10

Negative likelihood ratio

Not Useful — Useful
Very Small | Small | Moderate | Large
1.0 0.9 0.8 0.7 0.6 0.5 0.4 0.3 0.2 0.1 0

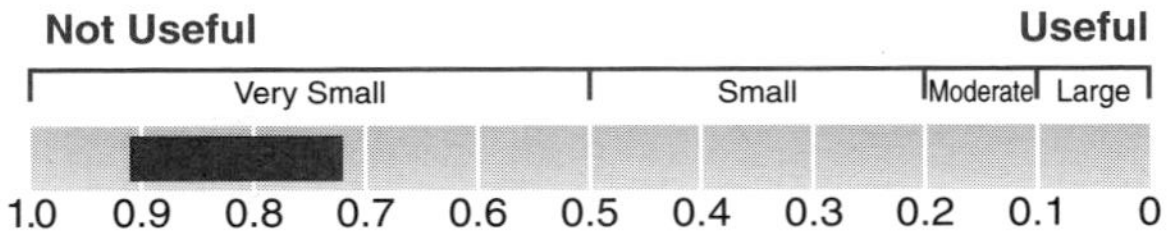

Labral Tears

Positive likelihood ratio

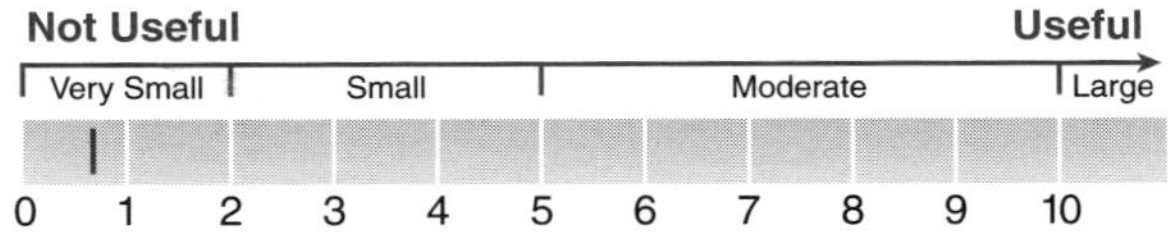

Not Useful — Useful
Very Small | Small | Moderate | Large
0 1 2 3 4 5 6 7 8 9 10

Negative likelihood ratio

Not Useful — Useful
Very Small | Small | Moderate | Large
1.0 0.9 0.8 0.7 0.6 0.5 0.4 0.3 0.2 0.1 0

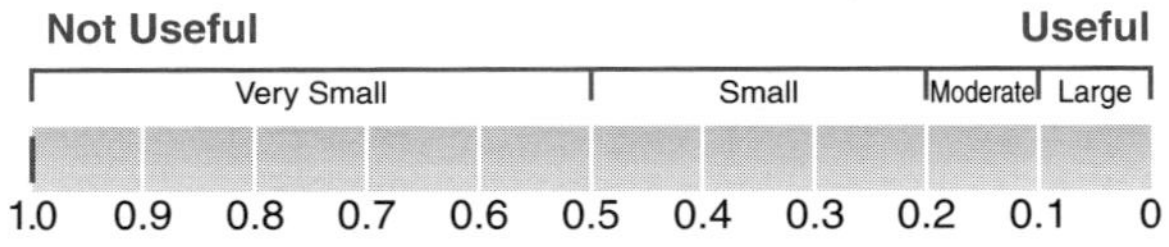

AC = acromioclavicular; GH = glenohumeral; SLAP = superior labrum anterior to posterior tear.

Examination Findings 16-5
SLAP Lesions

Examination Segment	Clinical Findings
History	***Onset:*** Acute or resulting from repetitive microtrauma ***Pain characteristics:*** Pain in the anteroposterior portion of the shoulder Increased pain in position of 90° of abduction and 90° of external rotation Pain is typically not described at rest. ***Other symptoms:*** Patient may complain of clicking or catching. ***Mechanism:*** Landing on a outstretched arm, glenohumeral instability, overhead motions, traction in the LHBT ***Predisposing conditions:*** Glenohumeral instability; hypomobility in posterior capsule
Inspection	Forward shoulder posture The scapula is protracted at rest.
Palpation	Point tender at posterior glenohumeral joint, just inferior to acromion process
Joint and Muscle Function Assessment	***AROM:*** Limited internal rotation and horizontal adduction ***MMT:*** Pain with shoulder and elbow flexion ***PROM:*** Limited horizontal adduction Limited internal rotation
Joint Stability Tests	***Stress tests:*** Not applicable ***Joint play:*** Hypomobile posterior glenohumeral glide consistent with internal impingement
Special Tests	Active compression test Anterior slide test Compression-rotation (grind) test
Neurologic Screening	Within normal limits
Vascular Screening	Within normal limits
Functional Assessment	Complaints of inability to perform (e.g., decreased throwing velocity, decreased accuracy). Increased pain with late cocking phase of throwing
Imaging Techniques	MR arthrography,[92] arthroscopy (anatomical variants make MR less accurate)[63] MR is highly specific for SLAP lesions. If the MR is negative, SLAP lesions can be ruled out.[94]
Differential Diagnosis	Rotator cuff pathology; LHBT tendinopathy; internal impingement, acromioclavicular pathology

AROM = active range of motion; LHBT = long head of the biceps tendon; MMT = manual muscle test; MR = magnetic resonance; PROM = passive range of motion; SLAP = superior labrum anterior to posterior tear.

Special Test 16-16
Anterior Slide Test

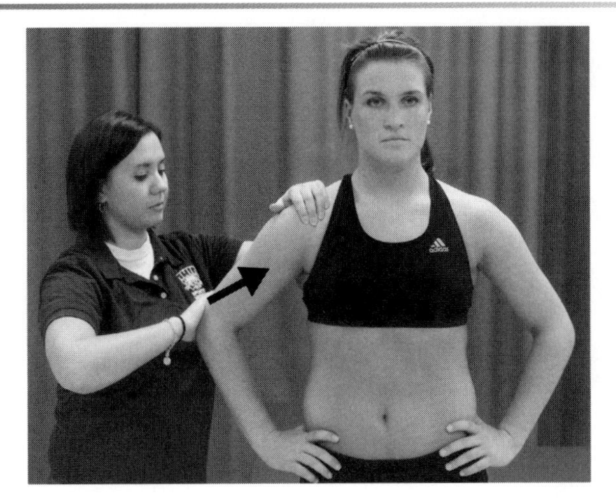

The anterior slide test creates an anteriorly and superiorly directed force that would result in humeral head translation if the superior labrum was torn.

Patient Position	Seated or standing Hands on hips with thumbs pointing posteriorly
Position of Examiner	Behind the patient One hand is placed over the shoulder with the index finger lateral to the acromion and over the glenohumeral joint. The opposite hand is behind the elbow on the test side.
Evaluative Procedure	An anterior and slightly superior force is applied longitudinally through the humerus. The patient resists, or pushes back, against this force.
Positive Test	Shoulder pain or pop or click under the examiner's index finger Patient report of reproduction of symptoms
Implications	SLAP lesion
Comments	A positive anterior slide test partnered with patient complaints of "popping" or "clicking" are strongly associated with a labral tear.[101]
Evidence	***Inter-rater reliability***

Not Reliable — Very Reliable
Poor | Moderate | Good
0 0.1 0.2 0.3 0.4 0.5 0.6 0.7 0.8 0.9 1.0

Positive likelihood ratio

Not Useful — Useful
Very Small | Small | Moderate | Large
0 1 2 3 4 5 6 7 8 9 10

Negative likelihood ratio

Not Useful — Useful
Very Small | Small | Moderate | Large
1.0 0.9 0.8 0.7 0.6 0.5 0.4 0.3 0.2 0.1 0

AC = acromioclavicular; GH = glenohumeral; SLAP = superior labrum anterior to posterior tear.

Special Test 16-17
Compression–Rotation (Grind) Test

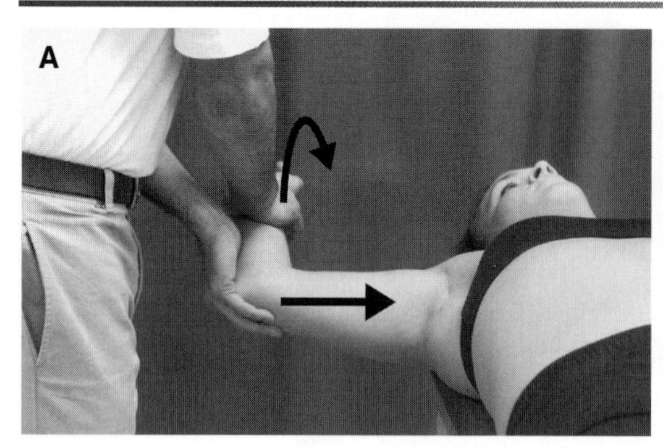

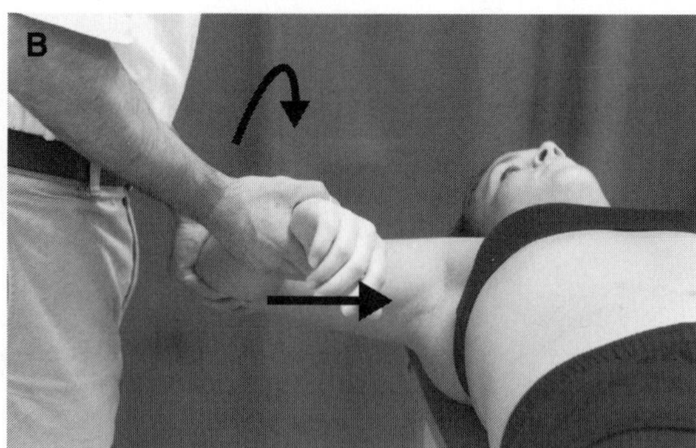

This test is designed to compress the labrum, resulting in reproduction of painful symptoms.

Patient Position	Supine The shoulder is abducted to 90°. The elbow is flexed to 90°.
Position of Examiner	At the test side of the patient
Evaluative Procedure	The examiner maintains an axial load on the humerus while internally and externally rotating it.
Positive Test	Reproduction of symptoms
Implications	SLAP lesion
Modification	The crank test incorporates a similar mechanism with the arm positioned in maximum forward flexion.
Evidence	Positive likelihood ratio Not Useful — Useful Very Small | Small | Moderate | Large 0 1 2 3 4 5 6 7 8 9 10 Negative likelihood ratio Not Useful — Useful Very Small | Small | Moderate | Large 1.0 0.9 0.8 0.7 0.6 0.5 0.4 0.3 0.2 0.1 0

SLAP = superior labrum anterior to posterior tear.

Tests for SLAP tend to yield false-positive results because of the presence of glenohumeral or AC pathologies. In other cases procedures may produce pain caused by a SLAP lesion, but be negative for the pathology being tested. For example, the Neer impingement test may be negative for rotator cuff involvement, but evoke pain caused by a SLAP lesion.[95]

Symptomatic SLAP lesions require surgical repair.[63] Postoperative management of a patient with a SLAP lesion depends on whether the tear was debrided or repaired. Although cases of debridement can usually progress as tolerated, repairs of SLAP lesions progress more slowly. Most importantly after a surgical SLAP repair, contraction of the biceps tendon and other traction forces from the tendon placed on the repair must be controlled for 6 to 8 weeks.

On-Field Examination of Shoulder Injuries

The most important findings to be ruled out during the on-field evaluation of injuries to the shoulder complex are fractures and dislocations, which may often be confirmed through visual inspection or palpation of the area. When a humeral fracture or GH joint dislocation is suspected, the presence of a distal pulse must be determined. The absence of this pulse warrants the athlete's immediate transportation to a hospital.

Pain radiating through the shoulder and into the arms may indicate damage to one or more cervical nerve roots. A complete evaluation of the cervical or thoracic spine must be performed first when the mechanism of injury or description of the symptoms implicates possible cervical spine trauma (see Chapter 21). The athlete is not moved until the possibility of spinal injury has been eliminated. Trauma to the spleen or myocardial dysfunction may also refer pain into the shoulder.

The on-field evaluation of patients with shoulder injuries is complicated by the presence of shoulder pads in sports such as football, ice hockey, and lacrosse. The examiner must become familiar with how to work around these pads and, if necessary, how to remove them without further aggravating the injury.

Equipment Considerations

Palpation under the shoulder pads

Shoulder pads have at least one cantilever that arches over the acromion process and the deltoid muscle group. The space provided by the cantilever provides enough room to reach under the jersey and palpate the humeral head, AC joint, and distal clavicle. By unfastening the strap that passes beneath the axilla and loosening the sternal fasteners, more room may be created. It is also possible to palpate the proximal structures of the shoulder complex by entering the shoulder pads from the neck opening.

Because the clinician is palpating these structures without actually being able to see them, care must be used when applying pressure. The initial palpation must be performed gently, following the contours of the shoulder complex while checking for gross deformity.

Removal of the shoulder pads

Certain injuries such as AC or SC joint sprains, GH dislocations, or clavicular fractures require the removal of the shoulder pads to further evaluate the condition, begin treatment of the area, or transport the athlete. This must be done with as little movement of the injured extremity as possible to prevent further insult to the injured structures.

If the athlete's jersey is loose fitting, the examiner first removes the uninjured arm. After this is completed, the examiner slides the shirt up and over the head, then drops it down over the injured arm. In many cases, it is easier to remove the shirt and shoulder pads as a single unit (Fig. 16-36). If the shirt is extraordinarily tight fitting or is a practice jersey or in the case of a medical emergency, cut it off the athlete.

On-Field History

- **Location of pain**: Trauma to the AC joint is described as pain localized to the upper shoulder, possibly projecting into the deltoid. Pain that involves the upper trapezius and radiates into the shoulder and arm that also is accompanied by weakness may indicate brachial plexus involvement.
- **Mechanism of injury**: A force that internally or externally rotates the GH joint can result in a GH subluxation or dislocation, especially if the humerus was abducted at the time of the injury. Falling on the tip of the shoulder or landing on an outstretched arm can result in a clavicular fracture, AC sprain, or SC sprain.

On-Field Inspection

- **Arm posture**: The position of the shoulder, humerus, and arm can provide useful clues to the possible pathology.
  - **Arm splinted against the torso**: The humerus' being splinted against the ribs with the forearm supported across the body and the athlete's head looking away from the involved side can indicate a clavicular fracture or AC joint pathology.
  - **Arm hanging limply at the side**: The arm's dangling limply to the side often indicates brachial plexus pathology (see Chapter 14).
  - **Arm "locked"**: The humerus' being locked in various positions can indicate a GH dislocation, with the position of the arm providing evidence of the direction of the dislocation. If it is adducted and externally rotated, suspect anterior or inferior GH dislocation; inferior dislocations are marked by a limited amount of abduction. If it is abducted and internally rotated, suspect posterior GH dislocation.

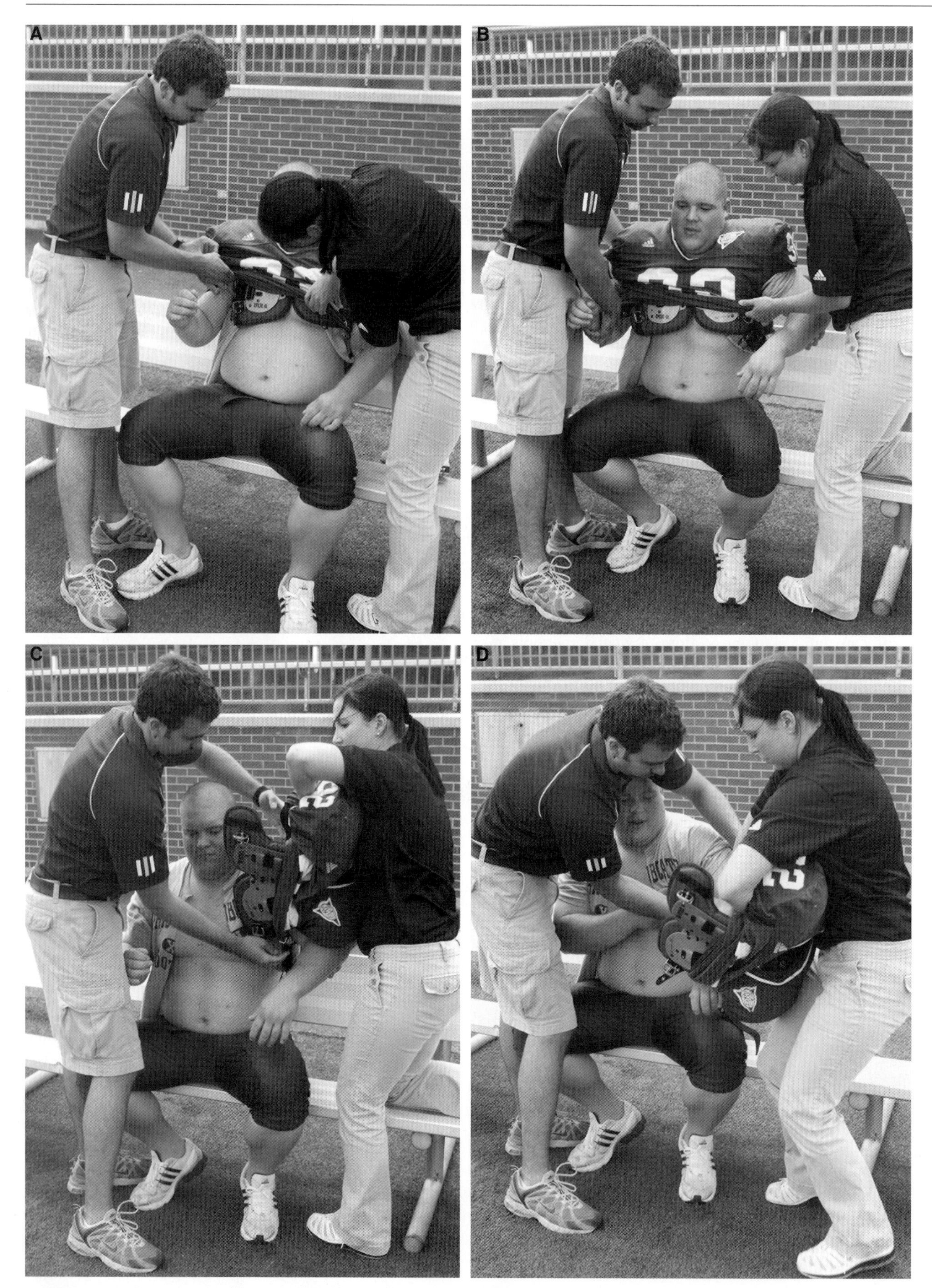

FIGURE 16-36 ■ Removing shoulder pads (the athlete's left arm is injured). **(A)** Unsnap the chest straps. **(B)** Pull the shirt off the uninjured arm. **(C)** Lift the shoulder pads and shirt over the athlete's head. **(D)** Slide the shoulder pads from around the injured arm.

- **Gross deformity**: Initial inspection of the shoulder complex may be hindered by shoulder pads and jerseys. Gross deformity may be identified during palpation or visually after the equipment has been removed.

On-Field Palpation

- **Position of the humeral head**: If the GH joint is dislocated, the humeral head can be palpated sitting anterior, posterior, or inferior relative to the glenoid fossa.
- **AC joint alignment**: The AC joint is palpated for any abnormal motion, including the piano key sign.
- **Clavicle**: Fractures of the clavicle are often readily apparent. If no visible sign of a fracture is present, palpate the length of the clavicle to identify subcutaneous discontinuity or areas of point tenderness.
- **Sternoclavicular joint**: The SC joint is palpated for bilateral symmetry and continuity.
- **Humerus**: The length of the humerus is palpated for signs of a fracture, especially in the area of the surgical neck.

On-Field Neurologic Tests

Brachial plexus injuries cause pain, numbness, and paresthesia in the upper extremity, but the trauma actually involves the cervical nerve roots (see Chapter 14).

Additional On-Field Tests

If the signs of a joint dislocation or bony fracture have been ruled out, the Apley's scratch test (see Box 16-2) can be used as a gross assessment of the athlete's willingness to move the involved extremity and the amount of motion available. The remaining joint and muscle testing can be conducted on the sideline in the manner described in the ROM section of this chapter.

Initial Management of On-Field Shoulder Injuries

The following is suggested protocol for the initial management of major injuries to the shoulder complex and upper arm. In emergencies or when proper splinting materials are not available, the athlete's jersey may be used as a sling or the hand can be tucked into the belt of the pants (Fig. 16-37).

Scapular Fractures

Although rare, reports of scapular fractures in football players have been reported.[102] Incidence of scapular fractures is highest among players who wear relatively small shoulder pads. Fractures may occur to the body of the scapula, but most often in the glenoid fossa, glenoid neck, or coracoid process secondary to a GH dislocation.

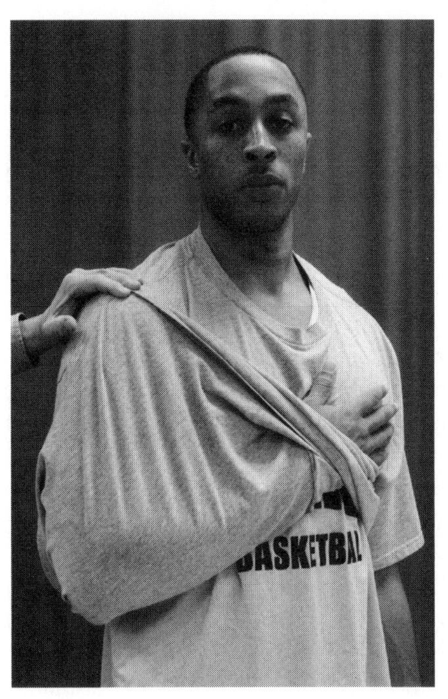

FIGURE 16-37 ■ A temporary sling can be made by pulling the shirt up and over the involved arm.

Patients with fractures of the glenoid fossa may present with many of the signs and symptoms of rotator cuff inflammation through decreased strength during abduction and external rotation. Any athlete suffering from a GH dislocation also needs a radiographic evaluation to rule out a secondary fracture to the glenoid or coracoid process.

To prevent motion, suspected scapular fractures are managed by immobilizing the arm on the affected side in a comfortable position. The athlete then is transported for further medical evaluation.

Clavicular Injuries

Clavicular fractures

When fractures of the clavicle are suspected, the arm must be immobilized to prevent movement of the fractured segments. The athlete also is transported to a physician for a definitive diagnosis. Displaced fractures of the medial one third of the clavicle may require emergency surgery due to neurovascular compromise.[103] Although rare, secondary damage to nerves and blood vessels may result from clavicular fractures.[104]

The shoulder may be immobilized using a sling or triangular bandage. A sling and swath approach may be more comfortable for the athlete by taking the weight of the arm off the involved clavicle. The use of figure-of-eight bandages for stabilization is discouraged as their use is associated with a higher incidence of complications with no difference in functional outcome or appearance.[103]

Sternoclavicular joint injuries

The immediate concern with SC dislocations is the potential compromise to the underlying structures from a posterior dislocation.[4] A neurologic and vascular examination of the extremity and carotid artery on the involved side must be performed immediately. Any absent or diminished findings are considered a medical emergency. The involved arm is immobilized using the procedure described for clavicular fractures and the athlete is immediately transported to an emergency medical facility. To avoid placing pressure on the structures posterior to the SC joint, the athlete must not be transported in the supine position.

Acromioclavicular joint injuries

Athletes displaying the signs and symptoms of an AC joint sprain require immobilization in a position that lessens the displacement between the clavicle and the acromial process. Initially, this may be achieved through the use of a foam pad with a hard shell held in place over the acromial process by a spica wrap and a sling supporting the weight of the arm (Fig. 16-38).

Most commonly, physicians choose to treat all but the most severe AC sprains nonsurgically.[18,105] Comparative follow-up studies of surgical and nonsurgical management of AC dislocations indicate that shoulders treated nonsurgically display little residual decrease in ROM or in strength deficits.[18]

Athletes suffering from AC joint contusions, in addition to the standard modality protocol, need to have the joint protected with additional padding during activity. Such protection may be obtained through the use of a foam doughnut pad with a hard shell held in place by an elastic spica wrap or elastic tape.

Glenohumeral dislocations

Because of the possibility of a dislocated humeral head causing additional trauma to the blood and nerve supply to the arm, it is important to monitor the distal pulses, check for circulation in the fingertips, and perform a sensory screen of the involved arm. Absence of a pulse indicates a medical emergency.

To transport the athlete, the arm is fixed in the position it is found using a moldable splint (metal or vacuum) or towels placed between the humerus and torso. A sling or elastic wrap may be used to support the weight of the arm. It is important to keep the wrist and hand easily accessible so that the pulses may be rechecked.

Because of the threat of causing additional trauma to the GH structures, on-field reductions of GH dislocations should only be performed by those who are trained to do so. Reduction of acute anterior glenohumeral dislocations is obtained by slightly abducting and internally rotating the arm while applying gentle longitudinal traction. Other reduction techniques include elevating the arm while distracting the joint and applying posterior pressure with the thumb and rotating the scapula to align the glenoid while the patient is prone.

Forced reduction of the humeral head may damage the glenoid fossa, the coracoid process, or the neurovascular structures in the area. After reduction, assess distal pulse and active range of motion, avoiding external rotation and abduction. Stabilize the shoulder using a sling and refer the athlete for further examination. The athlete must be immediately transported to a physician as soon as the shoulder has been immobilized.

Humeral fractures

Fractures of the humeral shaft and neck are often marked by extreme pain, dysfunction, and obvious deformity. Most humeral fractures occur as the result of a high-impact force. Spontaneous fractures occurring during pitching also have been reported.[106] Fractures in the region of the surgical neck can threaten the radial nerve. Fractures of the humeral head may occur secondary to GH dislocations

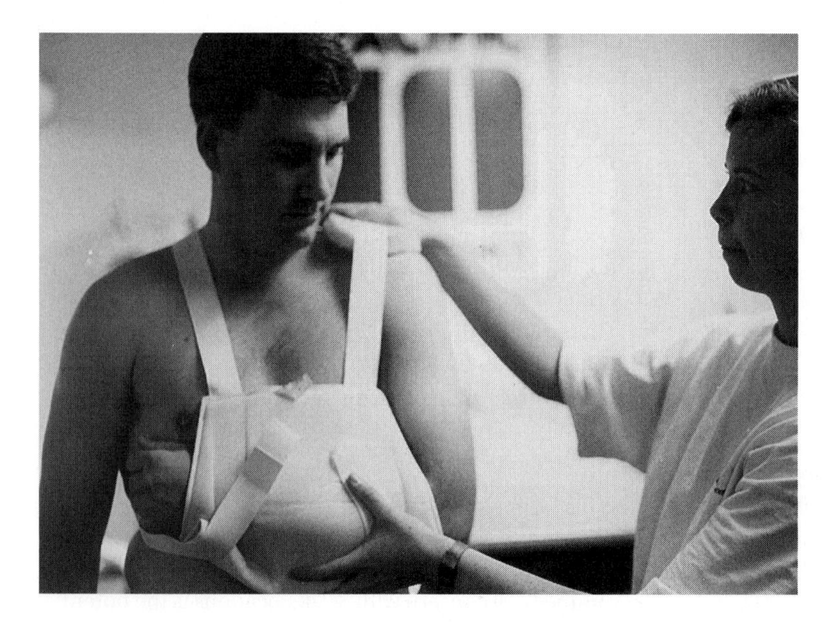

FIGURE 16-38 ■ Management of an acromioclavicular joint sprain. A commercially available device (shown) or a sling and swath can be used to immobilize the shoulder and apply pain-relieving pressure to the AC joint.

and therefore initially go unnoticed because of the attention placed on the joint.

Fractures of the humeral shaft are splinted in the position they are found, using a moldable aluminum splint or a vacuum splint. The wrist and fingers remain exposed so that the radial pulse, circulation to the fingers, and sensation of the fingers can be monitored. The athlete is transported supine or on a stretcher. An immediate physician referral is indicated.

REFERENCES

1. Perry, J: Normal upper extremity kinesiology. *Phys Ther*, 58:265, 1978.
2. Nyland, JA, Caborn, DN, and Johnson, DL: The human glenohumeral joint. A proprioceptive and stability alliance. *Knee Surg Sports Traumatol Arthrosc*, 6:50, 1998.
3. Ludewig, PM, and Borstead, JD: The shoulder complex. In Levangie PK, Norkin CC. *Joint Structure and Function*. Philadelphia, FA Davis, 2005.
4. Wirth, MA, and Rockwood, CA: Acute and chronic traumatic injuries of the sternoclavicular joint. *J Am Acad Orthop Surg*, 4:268, 1996.
5. Culham, E, and Peat, M: Functional anatomy of the shoulder complex. *J Orthop Sports Phys Ther*, 18:342, 1993.
6. Neumann, DA: *Kinesiology of the Musculoskeletal System: Foundations for Physical Rehabilitation*. St. Louis, MO, Mosby, 2002.
7. Meister, K: Injuries to the shoulder in the throwing athlete. Part One: Biomechanics/Pathophysiology/Classification of injury. *Am J Sports Med*, 28:265, 2000.
8. Norkin, CC, and Levangie, PK: The shoulder complex. In Norkin, CC, and Levangie, PK (eds): *Joint Structure and Function: A Comprehensive Analysis* (ed 2). Philadelphia, FA Davis, 1992, p 220.
9. Kessler, RM, and Hertling, D: The shoulder and shoulder girdle. In Hertling, D, and Kessler, RM (eds): *Management of Common Musculoskeletal Disorders. Physical Therapy Principles and Procedures* (ed 2). Philadelphia, JB Lippincott, 1990, p 171.
10. Doody, SG, and Waterland, JC: Shoulder movements during abduction in the scapular plane. *Arch Phys Med Rehabil*, 51:595, 1970.
11. Hollinshead, WH, and Jenkins, DB: The shoulder. In Hollinshead, WH, and Jenkins, DB (eds): *Functional Anatomy of the Limbs and Back* (ed 5). Philadelphia, WB Saunders, 1981.
12. Dowrick, AS, et al: Outcome instruments for the assessment of the upper extremity following trauma: A review. *Injury*, 36:468, 2005.
13. Kirkley, A, Griffin, S, and Dainty, K: Scoring systems for the functional assessment of the shoulder. *Arthroscopy*, 19:1109, 2003.
14. Itoi, E, et al: Are pain location and physical examinations useful in locating a tear site of the rotator cuff? *Am J Sports Med*, 34:256, 2006.
15. Chronopoulos, E, et al: Diagnostic value of physical tests for isolated chronic acromioclavicular lesions. *Am J Sports Med*, 32:655, 2004.
16. Baker, CL, and Merkley, MS: Clinical evaluation of the athlete's shoulder. *J Athl Train*, 35:256, 2000.
17. Boublik, M, and Hawkins, RJ: Clinical examination of the shoulder complex. *J Orthop Sports Phys Ther*, 18:379, 1993.
18. Tibone, J, Sellers, R, and Tonino, P: Strength testing after third degree acromioclavicular dislocations. *Am J Sports Med*, 20:328, 1992.
19. Chandler, TJ, et al: Shoulder strength, power, and endurance in college tennis players. *Am J Sports Med*, 20:445, 1992.
20. Wilk, KE, et al: The strength characteristics of internal and external rotator muscles in professional baseball pitchers. *Am J Sports Med*, 21:61, 1993.
21. Reynolds, RS, and Hirschman, LD: An examination of the concentric and eccentric strength of the shoulder rotators (abstr). *Athl Train: J Natl Athl Train Assoc*, 26:154, 1991.
22. Park, HB, et al: Diagnostic accuracy of clinical tests for the different degrees of subacromial impingement syndrome. *J Bone Joint Surg*, 87-A:1446, 2005.
23. Murrell, GA, and Walton, JR: Diagnosis of rotator cuff tears. *Lancet*, 357:769, 2001.
24. Myers, JB, et al: Glenohumeral range of motion deficits and posterior shoulder tightness in throwers with pathology internal impingement. *Am J Sports Med*, 34:385, 2006.
25. Gerber, C, and Krushell, RJ: Isolated rupture of the tendon of the subscapularis muscle. Clinical features in 16 cases. *J Bone Joint Surg*, 73(B):389, 1991.
26. Kelly, BT, Kadrmas, WR, and Speer, KP: The manual muscle examination for rotator cuff strength. An electromyographic investigation. *Am J Sports Med*, 24:581, 1996.
27. Greis, PE, et al: Validation of the Lift-off test and analysis of subscapularis activity during maximal internal rotation. *Am J Sports Med*, 24:589, 1996.
28. Kelly, BT, Kadrmas, WR, and Speer, KP: The manual muscle examination for rotator cuff strength. An electromyographic investigation. *Am J Sports Med*, 24:581, 1996.
29. Hertel, R, et al: Lag signs in the diagnosis of rotator cuff rupture. *J Shoulder Elbow Surg.*, 5:307, 1996.
30. Borstad, JD, and Ludewig, PM: The effect of long versus short pectoralis minor resting length on scapular kinematics in healthy individuals. *J Orthop Sports Phys Ther*, 35:227, 2005.
31. Speer, KP: Anatomy and pathomechanics of shoulder instability. *Operat Tech Sports Med*, 1:252, 1993.
32. Levy, AS, et al: Intra- and interobserver reproducibility of the shoulder laxity examination. *Am J Sports Med*, 58:272, 1999.
33. Hawkins, RJ, and Bokor, DJ: Clinical evaluation of shoulder problems. In Rockwood, CA, and Masten, FA (eds): *The Shoulder* (vol 1). Philadelphia, WB Saunders, 1990, pp 149–177.
34. Levy, AS, et al: Intra- and interobserver reliability of the shoulder laxity examination. *Am J Sports Med*, 27:460, 1999.
35. McFarland, EG, Campbell, G, and McDowell, J: Posterior shoulder laxity in asymptomatic athletes. *Am J Sports Med*, 24:468, 1996.
36. Prime, HT, Doig, SG, and Hooper, JC: Retrosternal dislocation of the clavicle: A case report. *Am J Sports Med*, 19:92, 1991.
37. Jougon, JB, Lepront, DJ, and Dromer, CE: Posterior dislocation of the sternoclavicular joint leading to mediastinal compression. *Ann Thorac Surg*, 61:711, 1996.
38. Brinker, MR, and Simon, RG: Pseudo-dislocation of the sternoclavicular joint. *J Orthop Trauma*, 13:222, 1999.

39. Brinker, MR, et al: A method for open reduction and internal fixation of the unstable posterior sternoclavicular joint dislocation. *J Orthop Trauma*, 11:378, 1997.
40. Gerber, C, Galantay, RV, and Hersche, O: The pattern of pain produced by irritation of the acromioclavicular joint and the subacromial space. *J Shoulder Elbow Surg*, 7:352, 1998.
41. Walton, J, et al: Diagnostic values of tests for acromioclavicular joint pain. *J Bone Jt Surg*, 86-A:807, 2004.
42. Gartsman, GM: Arthroscopic resection of the acromioclavicular joint. *Am J Sports Med*, 21:71, 1993.
43. Gartsman, GM, et al: Arthroscopic acromioclavicular joint resection: An anatomical study. *Am J Sports Med*, 19:2, 1991.
44. Jacob, AK, and Sallay, PI: Theraputic efficacy of corticosteroid injections in the acromioclavicular joint. *Biomed Sci Instrum*, 34:380, 1997.
45. Phillips, AM, Smart, C, and Groom, AF: Acromioclavicular dislocation. Conservative or surgical therapy. *Clin Orthop*, Aug:10, 1998.
46. Press, J, et al: Treatment of grade III acromioclavicular separations. Operative versus nonoperative management. *Bull Hosp Jt Dis*, 56:77, 1997.
47. Rawes, ML, and Dias, JJ: Long-term results of conservative treatment for acromioclavicular dislocation. J *Bone Joint Surg*, 78(B):410, 1996.
48. Shaffer, BS: Painful conditions of the acromioclavicular joint. *J Am Acad Orthop Surg*, 7:176, 1999.
49. Terry, GC, et al: The stabilizing function of passive shoulder restraints. *Am J Sports Med*, 19:26, 1991.
50. Jobe, FW, et al: Anterior capsulolabral reconstruction of the shoulder in athletes in overhand sports. *Am J Sports Med*, 19:428, 1991.
51. Joseph, TA, Williams, JS, and Brems, JJ: Laser capsulorrhaphy for multidirectional instability of the shoulder. *Am J Sports Med*, 31:26, 2003.
52. Stefko, JM, et al: Strain of the anterior band of the inferior glenohumeral ligament during capsule failure. *J Shoulder Elbow Surg*, 6:473, 1997.
53. Steinbeck, J, Liljenqvist, U, and Jerosch, J: The anatomy of the glenohumeral ligamentous complex and its contribution to anterior shoulder stability. *J Shoulder Elbow Surg*, 7:122, 1998.
54. Kim, TK, et al: Clinical features of the different types of SLAP Lesions. An analysis of one hundred and thirty cases. *J Bone Joint Surg*, 85(A):66, 2003.
55. Hsu, HC, et al: Influence of rotator cuff tearing on glenohumeral stability. *J Shoulder Elbow Surg*, 6:413, 1997.
56. Levine, WM, and Flatow, EL: The pathophysiology of shoulder instability. *Am J Sports Med*, 28:910, 2000.
57. Myers, JB, et al: Reflexive muscle activation alterations in shoulders with anterior glenohumeral instability. *Am J Sports Med*, 32:1013, 2004.
58. Tsia, L, et al: Shoulder function in patients with unoperated anterior shoulder instability. *Am J Sports Med*, 19:469, 1991.
59. Lo, IK, et al: An evaluation of the apprehension, relocation and surprise tests for anterior shoulder instability. *Am J Sports Med*, 32:301, 2004.
60. Luime, JJ, et al: Does this patient have an instability of the shoulder or a labrum lesion? *JAMA*, 292:1989, 2004.
61. Farber, AJ, et al: Clinical assessment of three common tests for traumatic anterior shoulder instability. *J Bone Joint Surg*, 88(A): 1467, 2006.
62. Tripp, BL, et al: Functional multijoint position reproduction acuity in overhed throwing athletes. *J Athl Train*, 41:146, 2006.
63. Parentis, MA, et al: An evaluation of the provocative tests for superior labral anterior posterior lesions. *Am J Sports Med*, 34:265, 2006.
64. Guanche, CA, and Jones, DC: Clinical testing for tears of the glenoid labrum. *Arthroscopy*, 19:517, 2003.
65. Hurley, JA, et al: Posterior shoulder instability: Surgical versus conservative results with evaluation of glenoid version. *Am J Sports Med*, 20:396, 1992.
66. Greenan, TJ, et al: Posttraumatic changes in the posterior glenoid and labrum in a handball player. *Am J Sports Med*, 21:153, 1993.
67. Blasier, RB, et al: Posterior glenohumeral subluxation: active and passive stabilization in a biomechanical model. *J Bone Joint Surg*, 79(A):433, 1997.
68. Kim, SH, et al: Painful jerk test: A predictor of success in nonoperative treatment of posteroinferior instability of the shoulder. *Am J Sports Med*. 32:1849, 2004.
69. Kim S-H, et al: The Kim Test: A novel test for posteroinferior labral lesion of the shoulder—a comparison to the jerk test. *Am J Sports Med*, 33:1188, 2005.
70. Warner, JJP, et al: Static capsuloligamentous restraints to superior-inferior translation of the glenohumeral joint. *Am J Sports Med*, 20:675, 1992.
71. Burkhart, SS, Morgan, CD, and Kibler, WB: The disabled throwing shoulder: Spectrum of pathology. Part I: Pathoanatomy and biomechanics. *Arthroscopy*, 19:404, 2003.
72. Burns, TP, and Turba, JE: Arthroscopic treatment of shoulder impingement in athletes. *Am J Sports Med*, 20:13, 1992.
73. Harryman, DT, et al: Translation of the humeral head on the glenoid with passive glenohumeral motion. *J Bone Joint Surg*, 72-A:1334, 1990.
74. Michener, LA, McClure, PW, and Karduna, AR: Anatomical and biomechanical mechanisms of subacromial impingement syndrome. *Clin Biomech*, 18:369, 2003.
75. Kamkar, A, Irrgang, JJ, and Whitney, SL: Nonoperative management of secondary shoulder impingement syndrome. *Am J Sports Med*, 17:212, 1993.
76. Shankwiler, JA, and Burkhead, WZ: Diagnosis, evaluation, and conservative treatment of impingement syndrome. *Operative Techniques in Sports Medicine*, 1:89, 1994.
77. Cools, AM, et al: Scapular muscle recruitment patterns: Trapezius muscle latency with and without impingement symptoms. *Am J Sports Med*, 31:542, 2003.
78. Corso, G: Impingement relief test: An adjunctive procedure to traditional assessment of shoulder impingement syndrome. *J Orthop Sports Phys Ther*, 22:183, 1995.
79. Brossmann, J, et al: Shoulder impingement syndrome: Influence of shoulder position on rotator cuff impingement: An anatomic study. *Am J Roetgenol*, 167:1511, 1996.
80. Wilson, JJ, and Best, TM: Common overuse tendon problems: A review and recommendations for treatment. *Am Fam Phys*, 72:811, 2005.
81. Determe, D, et al: Anatomic study of the tendinous rotator cuff of the shoulder. *Surg Radiol Anat*, 18:195, 1996.
82. Banas, MP, Miller, RJ, and Totterman, S: Relationship between the lateral acromion angle and rotator cuff disease. *J Shoulder Elbow Surg*, 4:454, 1995.
83. Cuomo, F, et al: The influence of acromioclavicular joint morphology on rotator cuff tears. *J Shoulder Elbow Surg*, 7:555, 1998.

84. Matava, MJ, Purcell, DB, and Ridzki, JR: Partial-thickness rotator cuff tears. *Am J Sports Med*, 33:1405, 2005.
85. Itoi, E, et al: Which is more useful, the "full can test" or the "empty can test" in detecting the torn supraspinatus tendon? *Am J Sports Med*, 27:65, 1999.
86. Holtby, R, and Razmjou, H: Validity of the supraspinatus test as a single clinical test in diagnosing patients with rotator cuff pathology. *J Orthop Sports Phys Ther*, 34:194, 2004.
87. McConville, OR, and Iannotti, JP: Partial-thickness tears of the rotator cuff: Evaluation and management. *J Am Acad Orthop Surg*, 7:32, 1999.
88. Walch, G, et al: Subluxations and dislocations of the tendon of the long head of the biceps. *J Shoulder Elbow Surg*, 7:100, 1998.
89. Zanetti, M, et al: Tendinopathy and rupture of the tendon of the long head of the biceps brachii muscle: Evaluation with MR arthography. *Am J Rotentgenol*, 170:1557, 1998.
90. Çaliş, M, et al: Diagnostic values of clinical diagnostic tests in subacromial impingement syndrome. *Ann Rheum Dis*, 59:44, 2000.
91. Holtby, R, and Razmjou, H: Accuracy of the Speed's and Yergason's tests in detecting biceps pathology and SLAP lesions: comparison with arthroscopic findings. *Arthroscopy*, 20:231, 2004.
92. Wilk, KE, et al: Current concepts in the recognition and treatment of superior labral (SLAP) lesions. *J Orthop Sports Phys Ther*, 35:273, 2005.
93. Bennett, WF: Specificity of the Speed's test: arthroscopic technique for evaluating the biceps tendon at the level of the bicipital groove. *Arthroscopy*, 14:789, 1998.
94. Stetson, WB, and Templin, K: The crank test, the O'Brien test, and routine magnetic imaging scans in the diagnosis of labral tears. *Am J Sports Med*, 30:806, 2002.
95. Alessandro, DF, Fleischli, JE, and Connor, PM: Superior labral lesions: Diagnosis and management. *J Athl Train*, 35:286, 2000.
96. Handelberg, F, et al: SLAP Lesions: A retrospective multicenter study. *Arthroscopy*, 14:856, 1998.
97. Morgan, CD, et al: Type II SLAP lesions: Three subtypes and their relationships to superior instability and rotator cuff tears. *Arthroscopy*, 14:553, 1998.
98. O'Brien, SJ, et al: The active compression test: A new and effective test for diagnosing labral tears and acromioclavicular joint abnormalities. *Am J Sports Med*, 26:610, 1998.
99. McFarland, EG, Kim, TK, and Savino, RM: Clinical assessment of three common tests for superior labral anterior-posterior lesions. *Am J Sports Med*, 30:810, 2002.
100. Kibler, WB: Specificity and sensitivity of the anterior slide test in throwing athletes with superior glenoid labral tears. *Arthroscopy*, 11:296, 1995.
101. Walsworth, MK, et al: Reliability and diagnostic accuracy of history and physical examination for diagnosing glenoid labral tears. *Am J Sports Med*, e-pub, 2007.
102. Cain, TE, and Hamilton, WP: Scapular fractures in professional football players. *Am J Sports Med*, 20:363, 1992.
103. Quillen, DM, Wuchner, M, and Hatch RL: Acute shoulder injuries. *Am Fam Phys*, 70:1947, 2004.
104. Bartosh, RA, Dugdale, TW, and Nelson, R: Isolated musculocutaneous nerve injury complicating closed fracture of the clavicle: A case report. *Am J Sports Med*, 20:356, 1992.
105. Martel, JR: Clavicular nonunion: Complications with the use of mersilene tape. *Am J Sports Med*, 20:360, 1992.
106. Branch, T, et al: Spontaneous fractures of the humerus during pitching: A series of 12 cases. *Am J Sports Med*, 20:468, 1992.

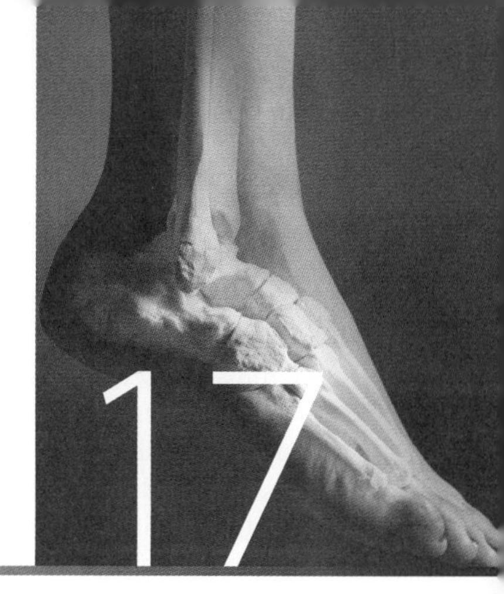

CHAPTER 17

Elbow and Forearm Pathologies

Serving as the link between the powerful movements of the shoulder and the **fine motor control** of the hand, the elbow is often overlooked as an area of potentially disabling injury. Even minor injuries to the elbow can severely hamper the ability to perform the most rudimentary movements. Fractures or other trauma involving the elbow or forearm can result in impairment of the neurovascular structures supplying the wrist, hand, and fingers. Therefore, examination of the elbow and forearm is often expanded to include the hand and shoulder.

Clinical Anatomy

The humerus, radius, and ulna form the elbow joint. The radius and ulna continue on to form the proximal and distal radioulnar joints of the forearm. The distal end of the humerus flares to form the medial and lateral epicondyles. The larger of these epicondyles, the **medial epicondyle**, is demarcated on its distal anteromedial border by the **trochlea**. Covered by articular cartilage, this epicondyle serves as the axis for rotation of the ulna on the humerus. Separated from the trochlea by the trochlear groove, the **capitellum** forms the lateral humeral articulating surface on the distal border of the **lateral epicondyle**. Unlike the trochlea, the dome-shaped capitellum does not extend to the posterior aspect of the humerus. Located immediately above the capitellum, the **radial fossa** is an indentation in the lateral epicondyle that accepts the radial head during elbow flexion (Fig. 17-1). The distal end of the humerus is anteriorly rotated 30 degrees relative to the humeral shaft.[1]

The **ulna** forms the medial border of the forearm. Proximally, the ulna articulates with the humerus and radius. The **semilunar notch**, an indentation lined with articular cartilage, fits snugly around the humeral trochlea. The proximal border of the ulna is formed by the **olecranon**

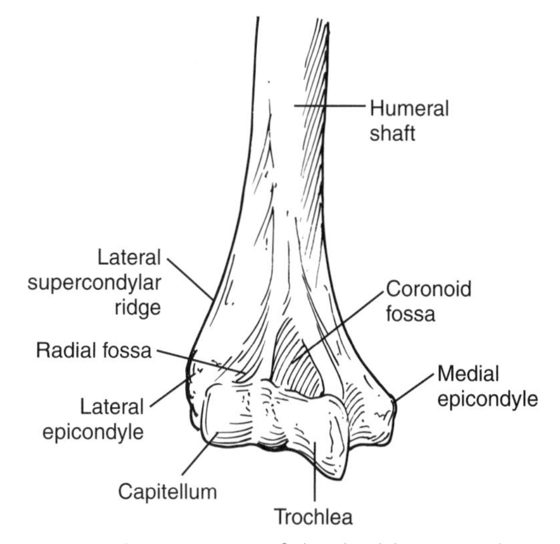

FIGURE 17-1 ■ Bony anatomy of the distal humerus. The trochlea articulates with the ulna; the capitellum, with the radial head.

Fine motor control Specific control of the muscles allowing for completion of small, delicate tasks.

process, a projection that fits into the humeral **olecranon fossa** during complete extension of the elbow. The distal border of the semilunar notch is formed by the **coronoid process**. The ulnar coronoid process is received by the **coronoid fossa** of the humerus during elbow flexion. Lateral and slightly distal to the coronoid process, the **radial notch** is an indentation that accepts the radial head to form the **proximal radioulnar joint** (Fig. 17-2).

Located on the thumb-side of the forearm, the **radius** is lateral to the ulna when the body is in its anatomical position. The proximal articulating surface, the **radial head**, is disk shaped and concave to allow gliding and rotation on the capitellum, significantly enhancing the elbow's stability.[2] The border of the proximal radius is also covered with articular cartilage to allow it to rotate on the ulna. Distal to the radial head is the **bicipital tuberosity** (radial tuberosity), the insertion site for the biceps brachii. The **radial shaft** is triangular in shape and broadens medially and laterally at its distal end. The **radial styloid process** projects off the lateral border of the distal radius. **Lister's tubercle** projects off the dorsal surface of the distal radius.

Articulations and Ligamentous Anatomy

To function properly, the elbow relies on the integrity of four individual articulations: the humeroulnar joint, humeroradial joint, proximal radioulnar joint, and distal radioulnar joint. The elbow relies almost equally on its bony configuration and ligamentous structure for support.[3] The three proximal joints share a common joint capsule, such that injury at one joint impacts function at the others. This complex, interrelated architecture often results in injury at one of the elbow articulations influencing the remaining ones. This interrelationship is particularly problematic when the elbow is immobilized.

The motion of elbow flexion and extension occurs at the humeroulnar and humeroradial joint. The motion of forearm **supination** and **pronation** occurs at the humeroradial, superior radioulnar, and inferior radioulnar joints.

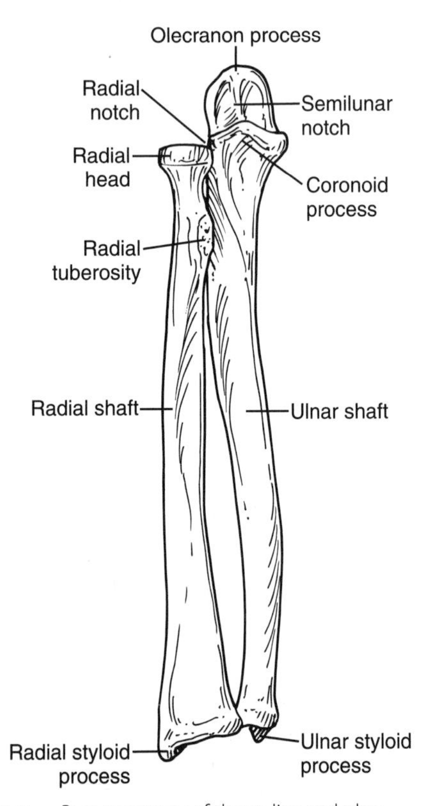

FIGURE 17-2 ■ Bony anatomy of the radius and ulna.

Humeroulnar and humeroradial joints

A modified hinge joint, the **humeroulnar articulation**, allows for 1 degree of freedom of movement: flexion and extension. The design of this joint may allow up to 5 degrees of internal rotation of the ulna on the humerus, but this motion is an accessory one.

Also a modified hinge joint, the **humeroradial joint** permits 2 degrees of freedom of movement: (1) flexion and extension as the radial head glides around the capitellum and (2) rotation of the radius on the capitellum during the movements of pronation and supination.

Proximal and distal radioulnar joints

The **proximal radioulnar joint** is formed by the convex radial head and the concave radial notch of the ulna. The **distal radioulnar joint** is formed by an articular disk between the radius and ulna where the concave ulnar notch of the radius articulates with the convex region of the ulna. The radioulnar joints have 1 degree of freedom of movement, pronation and supination. Their alignment is maintained by an interosseous membrane spanning the median (facing) borders of the bones, classifying it as a syndesmotic joint. During pronation, proximal joint motion occurs as the radius rotates within the radial notch of the ulna, causing the radius to cross over the ulna. At the distal joint, the disk and ulnar notch of the radius sweep across the ulna. The reverse occurs during supination.

Ligamentous support

Valgus support of the medial elbow is obtained from the **ulnar collateral ligament** (UCL), also referred to as the medial collateral ligament, which is divided into three unique sections: the anterior, transverse, and posterior bundles (Fig. 17-3). The **anterior bundle** originates from the inferior surface of the medial epicondyle and passes anterior to the axis of rotation to insert on the medial aspect of the coronoid process. Unlike the other elbow ligaments, the anterior bundle is easily distinguishable from the joint capsule. Taut throughout the elbow's range of

Supination (forearm) Movement at the radioulnar joints allowing for the palm to turn upward, as if holding a bowl of soup.

Pronation (forearm) Movement at the radioulnar joints allowing for the palm to be turned downward.

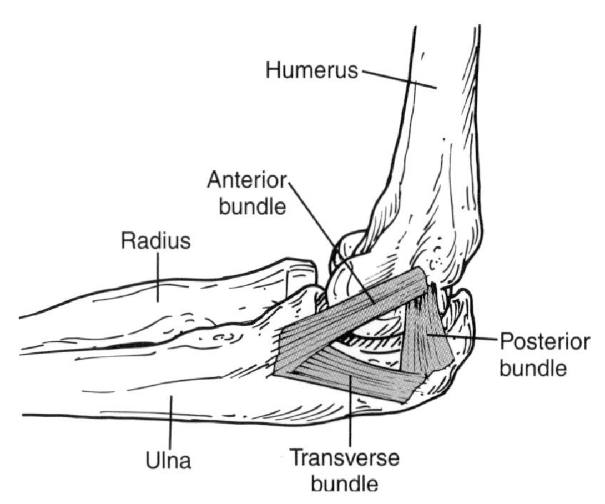

FIGURE 17-3 ■ Ulnar collateral ligament complex. This ligament is formed by the anterior oblique ligament, the posterior oblique ligament, and the transverse oblique ligament.

motion (ROM), this band is the primary restraint against valgus force. The anterior bundle is further divided into anterior and posterior bands. The anterior band resists valgus stress until about 90 degrees of flexion; the posterior band is the primary restraint when the elbow is flexed beyond 60 degrees and is primarily stressed in overhead throwing athletes.[3] The **transverse bundle**, originating from the medial epicondyle and inserting on the coronoid process, does not cross the axis of the elbow and therefore provides little, if any, medial support.[1] Inserting on the olecranon process, the **posterior bundle** is taut in flexion beyond 90 degrees and is subject to stress only if the anterior bundle is completely disrupted.[3]

Lateral support of the elbow is derived from the radial collateral, annular, lateral ulnar collateral, and the accessory lateral collateral ligaments (Fig. 17-4). The **lateral ulnar collateral ligament** (LUCL) is the most important lateral stabilizing structure. Arising from the middle of the lateral epicondyle and inserting on the tubercle of the ulna, the LUCL provides lateral support of the ulna that is independent of the other lateral ligaments. Disruption of this ligament results in rotatory instability of the elbow joint.

The **radial collateral ligament** (RCL) is a thickened area in the lateral joint capsule between the lateral epicondyle and the annular ligament. In addition to resisting varus stresses, the RCL assists in maintaining the close relationship between the humeral and radial articulating surfaces.

Encircling the radial head, the **annular ligament** is a fibro-osseous structure that permits internal and external rotation of the radial head on the capitellum of the humerus. Both ends of the annular ligament attach to the coronoid process and form four fifths of a circle. The remaining one fifth of the circle is formed by the radial notch. This articulation receives additional support from the attachment of the RCL and the fibrous attachment of the supinator muscle. The distal end of the annular ligament narrows to conform to the shape of the radial head, preventing the radius from sliding distally.

During excessive supination, the anterior fibers of the annular ligament become taut; at the end of pronation, the posterior fibers are taut. When a varus stress is applied to the elbow, the **accessory lateral collateral ligament** (ALCL) assists the annular ligament and the RCL in preventing the radius from separating from the ulna.

Interosseous membrane

A dense band of fibrous connective tissue, the fibers of the interosseous membrane run obliquely from the radius to the ulna and span the distance between the proximal and distal radioulnar joints (Fig. 17-5). This fibrous arrangement

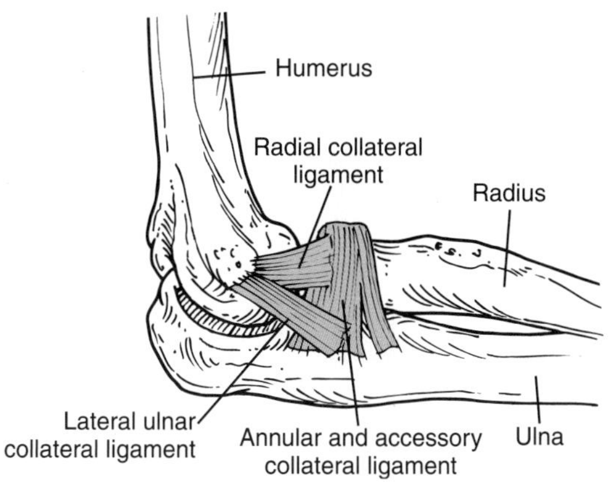

FIGURE 17-4 ■ Lateral ligaments of the elbow. This group is formed by the radial collateral ligament, the lateral ulnar collateral ligament, and the annular ligament. The annular ligament is responsible for maintaining the relationship between the proximal radius and ulna.

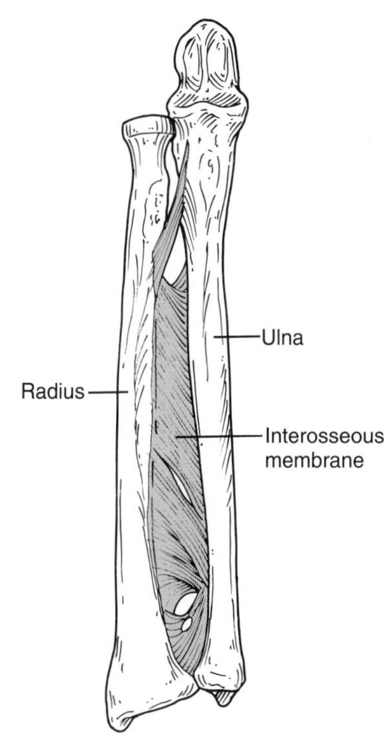

FIGURE 17-5 ■ Interosseous membrane. The fibrous arrangement of this structure transmits force absorbed by the radius at the wrist to the ulna.

serves as a stabilizer against axial forces applied to the wrist, transmitting force from the radius to the ulna. This force is then transmitted to the humerus. The interosseous membrane also serves as the origin for many of the muscles acting on the wrist and hand. Dislocation of the proximal or distal radioulnar joint may also injure the interosseous membrane.[2]

Muscular Anatomy

The muscles inserting on the proximal radius and ulna act to flex or extend the elbow and pronate or supinate the forearm. Many of the prime movers of the wrist and hand originate from the humeral epicondyles and the proximal radius and ulna. The actions, origins, insertions, and innervation of the muscles producing elbow and forearm motion are presented in Table 17-1. Chapter 18 discusses the forearm muscles acting on the wrist and hand.

Elbow flexor and supinator group

The **biceps brachii**, **brachialis**, and **brachioradialis** are the primary elbow flexors. The relative position (pronated, supinated, or neutral) of the forearm determines which of the muscles provides the primary contribution to the movement. The biceps brachii is the prime elbow flexor when the forearm is supinated; when the forearm is pronated, the brachialis is the prime flexor.[4] The contribution of the biceps brachii to forearm supination increases with the amount of elbow flexion until approximately 90 degrees where the maximum length–tension relationship is reached.[4] When the forearm is in its neutral position (radial side upward), the brachioradialis is the primary elbow flexor. The **supinator** is assisted by the biceps brachii during forceful supination. The brachioradialis contributes to both pronation and supination when the forearm is at the end of the opposite motion (i.e., the brachioradialis contributes to pronation when the forearm is fully supinated). The lateral bulk of the forearm muscles is formed by the extensor carpi radialis longus, extensor carpi radialis brevis, extensor carpi ulnaris, and extensor digitorum communis muscles (Fig. 17-6).

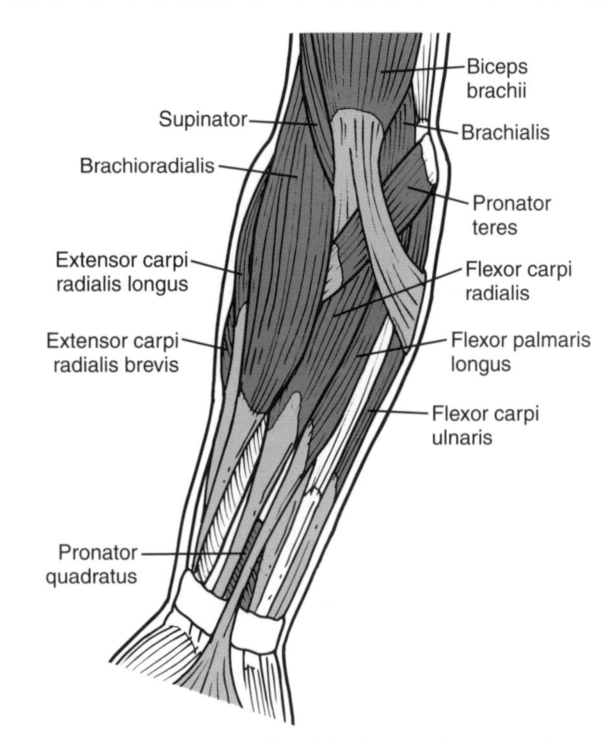

FIGURE 17-6 ■ Anterior muscles of the forearm. These muscles serve primarily to flex the wrist and fingers and rotate the forearm.

Elbow extensor and pronator group

The muscles acting to extend the elbow, the **triceps brachii** and **anconeus**, do not influence pronation or supination of the forearm. However, the anconeus does stabilize the ulna during these movements (Fig. 17-7). The primary pronators of the forearm are the **pronator teres**, arising from just above the medial epicondyle of the humerus and inserting on the anterolateral aspect of the radius, and the **pronator quadratus**, located on the distal forearm running obliquely from the medial aspect of the ulna to the radius. The remaining medial bulk of the proximal forearm is formed by the flexor carpi radialis, palmaris longus, flexor digitorum superficialis, and

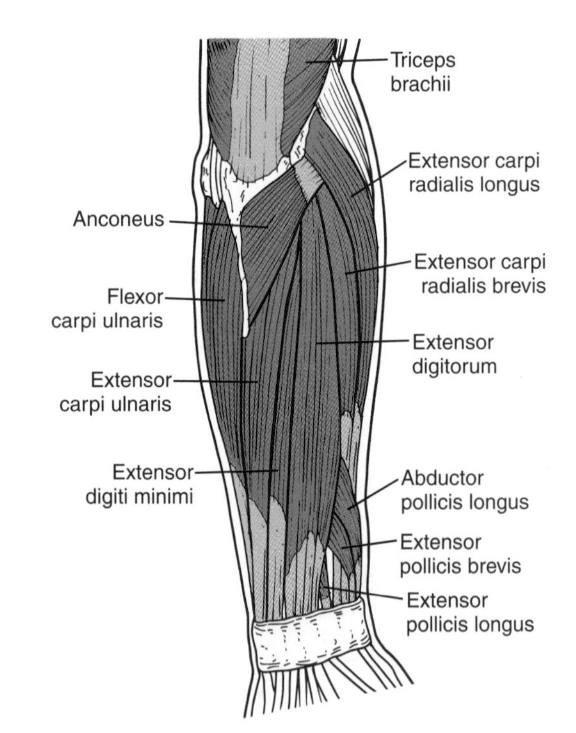

FIGURE 17-7 ■ Posterior muscles of the forearm. These muscles serve to extend the wrist and fingers.

flexor carpi ulnaris muscles, which are discussed in Chapter 18.

Nerves

Three primary nerves cross the elbow: the median nerve, ulnar nerve, and radial nerve. Their relatively superficial course across the elbow and in the distal portion of the forearm predisposes them to acute traumatic injury; their anatomical locations predispose them to entrapment-type conditions (Fig. 17-8).

Median nerve

Crossing the anterior elbow in the same path as the brachial artery, the median nerve travels deep within the forearm muscles to follow the flexor digitorum superficialis down the middle of the anterior forearm. As it approaches the wrist, the median nerve becomes superficial once again as it passes between the flexor digitorum superficialis and flexor carpi radialis tendons (beneath the palmaris longus) to pass through the carpal tunnel and enter the hand. With the exception of the flexor carpi ulnaris and the medial portion of the flexor digitorum profundus, the median nerve supplies all of the wrist flexor muscles and the pronator teres and pronator quadratus. Shortly after crossing the elbow joint, the **anterior interosseous nerve** projects off the median nerve to pass under the two heads of the pronator teres.

Ulnar nerve

The ulnar nerve enters the elbow via the **arcade of Struthers**, located approximately 8 cm proximal to the medial epicondyle, and then passes between the olecranon process and the medial epicondyle. After superficially crossing the joint line, it courses deep to follow the ulnar artery to the middle of the forearm. At this point, it moves medial to the flexor carpi ulnaris tendon and crosses the wrist joint superficial to the flexor retinaculum, traveling between the pisiform and the hook of the hamate (**tunnel of Guyon**) to provide sensory and motor innervation to the hand. The ulnar nerve innervates the flexor carpi ulnaris muscle and the medial portion of the flexor digitorum profundus in the forearm.

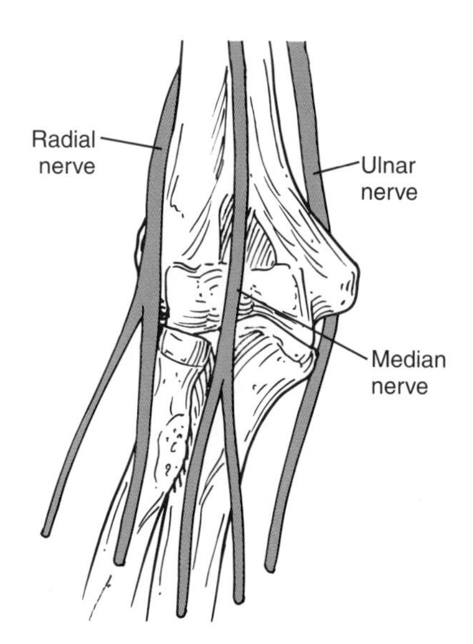

FIGURE 17-8 ■ Primary nerves of the elbow.

Radial nerve

The radial nerve courses distally on the posterior aspect of the humerus and then crosses the lateral aspect of the elbow's joint line between the brachioradialis and brachialis muscles. Then it diverges into two branches, the superficial and deep branches approximately 1.3 cm proximal to the radiohumeral joint. The **superficial branch**, the direct continuation of the radial nerve, provides sensation to the dorsum of the wrist, hand, and thumb. The **deep branch** (deep radial nerve) passes through the radial tunnel and the extensor carpi radialis brevis muscle to provide motor innervation exclusively to the extensor carpi radialis longus and brevis, supinator, brachioradialis, extensor pollicis longus, abductor pollicis longus, extensor pollicis brevis, and extensor digitorum muscles. Therefore, it is possible to injure the deep branch of the radial nerve without experiencing any sensory loss. However, critical motor loss does occur.

Bursae

Several bursae are found in the elbow region, but few have clinical significance. The **subcutaneous olecranon bursa**, located between the olecranon process and the skin, is susceptible to trauma and infection. This bursa is usually injured after a direct blow to the olecranon process. The other significant bursa is the **subtendinous olecranon bursa**. This structure is located between the tendon of triceps brachii and the olecranon process. This bursa may become inflamed secondary to repetitive stresses applied to the joint.

Clinical Examination of the Elbow and Forearm

The elbow may be traumatized by valgus or varus forces, forced hyperextension, direct blows to the olecranon process or the epicondyles, or most commonly, secondary to overuse from the inherently unnatural motion of throwing. The stresses placed on the elbow are increased when improper technique is used or when an individual compensates for shoulder pain or decreased ROM by altering elbow motion.

Table 17-1 Muscles Acting on the Elbow and Forearm

Muscle	Action	Origin	Insertion	Innervation	Root
Anconeus	Elbow extension Stabilization of ulna during pronation and supination	Posterior surface of the lateral epicondyle	Lateral border of the olecranon process	Radial	C7, C8
Biceps Brachii	Elbow flexion Forearm supination Shoulder flexion	Long head: Supraglenoid tuberosity of scapula Short head: Coracoid process of scapula	Radial tuberosity	Musculocutaneous	C5, C6
Brachialis	Elbow flexion	Distal one half of anterior humerus	Coronoid process of ulna Ulnar tuberosity	Musculocutaneous	C5, C6
Brachioradialis	Elbow flexion Forearm pronation May assist with forearm supination	Lateral supracondylar ridge of humerus	Styloid process of radius	Radial	C5, C6
Extensor Carpi Radialis Brevis	Wrist extension Radial deviation	Lateral epicondyle via the common extensor tendon Radial collateral ligament	Base of the 3rd metacarpal	Radial	C6, C7
Extensor Carpi Radialis Longus	Wrist extension Radial deviation	Supracondylar ridge of humerus	Radial side of the 2nd metacarpal	Radial	C6, C7
Extensor Carpi Ulnaris	Wrist extension Ulnar deviation	Lateral epicondyle via the common extensor tendon	Ulnar side of the base of the 5th metacarpal	Deep radial	C6, C7, C8
Extensor Digitorum Communis	Wrist extension MCP extension PIP extension	Lateral epicondyle via the common extensor tendon	Into the dorsal surface of the base of the middle and distal phalanges of each of the four fingers	Deep radial	C6, C7, C8
Flexor Carpi Radialis	Forearm pronation Wrist flexion Radial deviation Elbow flexion	Medial epicondyle via the common flexor tendon	Palmar aspect of the bases of the 2nd and 3rd metacarpal bones	Median	C6, C7
Flexor Carpi Ulnaris	Wrist flexion Ulnar deviation Elbow flexion	Humeral head: Medial epicondyle via the common flexor tendon • Ulnar head: Medial border of the olecranon; proximal two-thirds of the posterior ulna	Pisiform Hamate Palmar aspect of the base of the 5th metacarpal	Ulnar	C8, T1

Flexor Digitorum Profundus	DIP flexion PIP flexion Wrist flexion	Anteromedial proximal three fourths of the ulna and associated interosseous membrane	Bases of the distal phalanges of the second through fifth digits	Lateral: Median nerve Medial: Ulnar nerve	C8, T1
Flexor Digitorum Superficialis	PIP flexion MCP flexion Wrist flexion	Humeral head: Medial epicondyle via the common flexor tendon; ulnar collateral ligament Ulnar head: Coronoid process Radial head: Oblique line of radius	Middle phalanges of the second through fifth digits	Median	C7, C8, T1
Palmaris Longus	Wrist flexion	Medial epicondyle via the common flexor tendon	Flexor retinaculum Palmar aponeurosis	Median	C6, C7
Pronator Quadratus	Forearm pronation	Anterior surface of the distal one fourth of ulna	Lateral portion of the distal one fourth of the radius	Anterior interosseous nerve	C8, T1
Pronator Teres	Forearm pronation Elbow flexion	Humeral head: Proximal to the medial epicondyle of humerus Ulnar head: Coronoid process	Middle one third of the lateral radius	Median	C6, C7
Supinator	Forearm supination	Lateral epicondyle Radial collateral ligament Annular ligament Supinator crest of ulna	Proximal one third of radius	Deep radial	C6, C7, C8
Triceps Brachii	Elbow extension Shoulder extension	Long head: Infraglenoid tuberosity of scapula Lateral head: Posterolateral surface of the proximal one-half of the humeral shaft Medial head: Posteromedial surface of the humerus	Olecranon process of the ulna	Radial	C7, C8

DIP = distal interphalangeal; MCP = metacarpophalangeal; PIP = proximal interphalangeal.

Examination Map

HISTORY

Past Medical History

General medical health

History of the Present Condition

Location and onset of symptoms

Mechanism of injury

INSPECTION

Functional Assessment

Inspection of the Anterior Structures

Carrying angle

Cubital fossa

Inspection of the Medial Structures

Medial epicondyle

Flexor muscle mass

Inspection of the Lateral Structures

Alignment of the wrist and forearm

Cubital recurvatum

Extensor muscle mass

Inspection of the Posterior Structures

Bony alignment

Olecranon process and bursa

PALPATION

Palpation of the Anterior Structures

Biceps brachii

Cubital fossa

Brachioradialis

Wrist flexor group
- Pronator teres
- Flexor carpi radialis
- Palmaris longus
- Flexor carpi ulnaris

Palpation of the Medial Structures

Medial epicondyle

Ulna

Ulnar collateral ligament

Palpation of the Lateral Structures

Lateral epicondyle

Radial head

Radial collateral ligament

Capitellum

Annular ligament

Lateral ulnar collateral ligament

Palpation of the Posterior Structures

Olecranon process

Olecranon fossa

Triceps brachii

Anconeus

Ulnar nerve

Wrist extensors
- Extensor carpi ulnaris
- Extensor carpi radialis brevis
- Extensor carpi radialis longus

Finger extensors
- Extensor digitorum
- Extensor digiti minimi

Thumb musculature
- Extensor pollicis brevis
- Abductor pollicis longus

Radial tunnel

JOINT AND MUSCLE FUNCTION ASSESSMENT

Goniometry

Flexion

Extension

Pronation

Supination

Active Range of Motion

Flexion

Extension

Pronation

Supination

Manual Muscle Tests

Flexion

Extension

Pronation

Supination

Passive Range of Motion

Flexion

Extension

Pronation

Supination

JOINT STABILITY TESTS

Stress Testing

Valgus stress test

Varus stress test

Joint Play Assessment

Humeroulnar distraction

Radioulnar

Humeroulnar radiohumeral

NEUROLOGIC EXAMINATION

Upper Quarter Screen

PATHOLOGIES AND SPECIAL TESTS

Elbow Dislocations

Elbow Fractures

Elbow Sprains

Ulnar collateral ligament
- Valgus extension overload
- Posterolateral rotatory instability

Radial collateral ligament

Epicondylalgia

Lateral epicondylalgia
- Tennis elbow test

Medial epicondylalgia

Distal Biceps Tendon Rupture

Osteochondritis Dissecans of the Capitulum

Nerve Pathology

Ulnar nerve pathology

Radial nerve pathology

Median nerve pathology

Forearm compartment syndrome

History

A thorough history includes questioning regarding any pain or functional limitations in the cervical, shoulder and wrist and hand regions, as impairments in these regions can impact function at the elbow. For example, weakness of the scapular stabilizers of the shoulder may result in increased forces at the elbow. Question the patient regarding any changes in sensation or temperature, which may signal vascular or nerve compromise.

Past medical history

- **Previous history:** Pain that is associated with seasonal athletic activity may be related to poor conditioning. Because of the possibility of referred pain, patients with nontraumatic origin of pain or suspected of having referred pain from the cervical spine require investigation about a history of previous trauma, paresthesia, strength loss, or other dysfunction in this area.
- **General medical health:** A history of other medical conditions needs to be ascertained. Certain vascular problems, neurologic involvement, or systemic diseases may predispose the elbow to inflammatory or degenerative injuries or illnesses. Osteoporosis is associated with an increased risk of forearm and wrist fractures.[5]

History of the present condition

The onset and location of the symptoms are among the most important history findings surrounding elbow trauma. Determining the cause-and-effect relationship between the mechanism and the onset of the symptoms is helpful in developing a successful treatment plan. In addition, because the elbow may be the site of radicular symptoms from the cervical nerve roots, all other possible sources of pain must be ruled out.

- **Location of the symptoms:** Begin the examination by localizing the area of pain, the type of pain, and any dysfunction that is reported, remembering the possibility of these symptoms being referred by pathology that is proximal or distal to the elbow (Table 17-2). Referred pain usually presents with symptoms localized within the distribution of a peripheral nerve or nerve root. Nerve entrapment around the elbow may manifest itself with symptoms in the hand and forearm.
- **Onset of the symptoms:** Elbow pain may have an acute or chronic onset. Traumatic injury is traced to a specific onset of pain and symptoms. Chronic conditions of the elbow may initially produce minor symptoms related to activity but can rapidly progress to constant pain during all activities of daily living (ADLs).
- **Mechanism of injury:** The elbow is well protected at the side of the body and is not subjected to an overburden of harmful stress. The elbow can be acutely injured by the high amount of stress generated while throwing or during weight lifting. Acute injury can occur if the hand is planted on the ground so that it is away from the side of the body and forces are transmitted across the joint.

Table 17-2 Possible Pathology Based on the Location of Pain

	Location of Pain			
	Lateral	**Anterior**	**Medial**	**Posterior**
Soft Tissue Injury	Annular ligament sprain Radial collateral ligament sprain Radiocapitellar chondromalacia Lateral epicondylalgia (tennis elbow) Radial head dislocation Radial nerve pathology	Biceps brachii tendinopathy Rupture of the biceps brachii tendon Median nerve trauma Anterior capsule sprain	Ulnar collateral ligament sprain Medial epicondylalgia Ulnar nerve pathology	Olecranon bursitis Triceps brachii tendinopathy Triceps tendon rupture
Bony Injury	Avulsion of the common extensor tendon Lateral epicondyle fracture Radius fracture Radial head fracture Radial head dislocation	Osteochondral fracture Avulsion of the biceps brachii tendon	Avulsion of the common flexor tendon Medial epicondyle fracture Ulna fracture Osteophyte formation	Fracture of the olecranon process Osteophyte formation

Most elbow injuries tend to be caused by repetitive low-load stresses. Throwing a ball or using a racquet can cause stresses capable of resulting in tendinopathy or neuritis in the elbow. Adolescents are vulnerable to repetitive stress injuries at open growth plates as stresses are transmitted across these areas. Question athletes who are involved in throwing activities about the level of activity, including the number of throws, time span in which the throws occurred, and any changes in the throwing technique. The use of computers, musical instruments, or machinery that requires repetitive wrist and finger motions may also produce symptoms or exacerbate the current symptoms.

*** Practical Evidence**

Adolescent pitchers who throw high-velocity pitches and participate in showcase events are more likely to sustain serious injuries.[6]

- **Technique:** Overuse injuries commonly lead to suspicion of improper technique or poor elbow biomechanics or weak muscles. Ask the patient about changes in technique or equipment or increases in the intensity or duration of play. Although frequently cited as a causative factor in elbow problems for tennis players, inappropriate grip size in tennis does not alter muscle activation strength.[7] However, a further biomechanical analysis of elbow function during the pain-causing activity may be needed.
- **Associated sound and sensations:** An elbow that chronically locks, clicks, or pops during movement may indicate osteochondritis dissecans or an unstable joint. These conditions are confirmed through diagnostic imaging.

Inspection

The upper arm, elbow, and forearm are inspected for the evidence of contusions, ecchymosis, scars, and swelling. These conditions can place pressure on the radial, median, and ulnar nerves, causing symptoms to radiate to the forearm and hand.

Functional observation

Patients with the acutely injured elbow will frequently assume the resting position of approximately 70 degrees of flexion to minimize stresses on the joint.

Observe the patient performing common daily tasks and those tasks that provoke symptoms. Limitations in elbow motion results in characteristic adaptations at the shoulder and wrist and hand. For example, a limitation in elbow extension may result in increased scapular protraction during elevation. Patients with limited pronation or supination may compensate with increased internal and external glenohumeral motion, respectively.

Throwing athletes with medial elbow instability frequently complain of pain during the late cocking and acceleration phases of throwing, as these periods invoke the most stresses on the ulnar collateral ligament (see Box 16-1).[8]

Inspection of the anterior structures

- **Carrying angle:** The angle formed by the long axis of the humerus and ulna, the carrying angle, ranges from 10 to 15 degrees of valgus in women and 5 to 10 degrees in men. Normally this angle is reduced or entirely eliminated during flexion.[1] With the elbow fully extended and the forearm supinated, note the presence of an increased carrying angle, **cubitus valgus**, or a decreased angle, **cubitus varus** (Fig. 17-9).

  Baseball pitchers may exhibit cubitus valgus in the throwing arm, an adaptation to repeated valgus loading during the throwing motion.[9] Other deviations of this angle may reflect a fracture of one or more bones or their epiphyseal plates. Cubitus varus may be associated with ulnar neuropathy, avascular necrosis, osteoarthritis, posterolateral rotatory instability, and other conditions.[10]
- **Cubital fossa:** Swelling within the cubital fossa can place pressure on the local neurovascular structures, raising the suspicion of injury to the nearby soft tissues, including the distal biceps tendon (Fig. 17-10).

Inspection of the medial structures

- **Medial epicondyle:** The medial epicondyle is the most prominent structure on the medial aspect of the

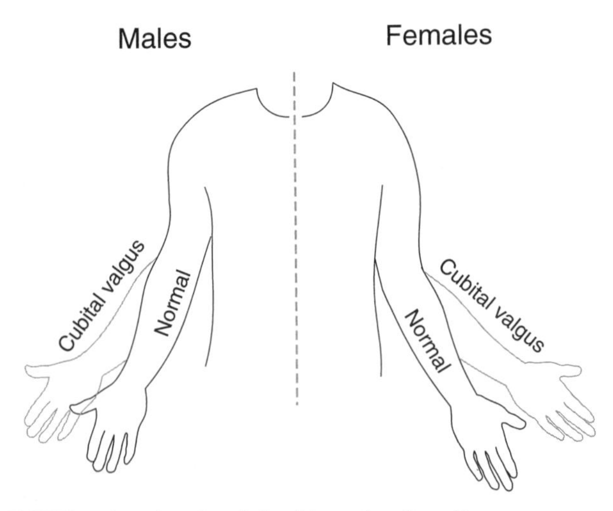

FIGURE 17-9 ■ Angular relationships at the elbow. On average, women have an increased angle between the midline of the forearm and the humerus (the "carrying angle") relative to men. Long term participation in overhand throwing sports increases this angle in the dominant arm.[9]

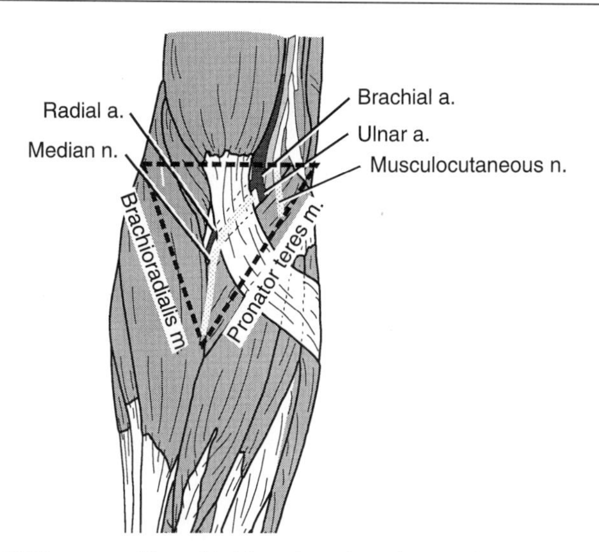

FIGURE 17-10 ■ The cubital fossa is a triangular area demarcated by the brachioradialis muscle laterally and the pronator teres medially. The brachial artery and its two subdivisions (the radial and ulnar arteries), the median nerve, and the musculocutaneous nerve pass through this fossa.

elbow, but it may become masked by excessive swelling.

- **Flexor muscle mass:** The wrist flexor muscle mass is observable along the medial aspect of the elbow and forearm. The mass widens approximately 2 to 3 inches below the elbow. Loss of girth along the medial forearm may occur secondary to prolonged immobilization or disuse associated with long-term tendinopathy.

Inspection of the lateral structures

- **Alignment of the wrist and forearm:** The wrist should be centered on the forearm. Compression of the radial nerve as it crosses the elbow joint can inhibit the wrist extensors, resulting in drop wrist syndrome (see Chapter 18).[1]
- **Cubital recurvatum:** The alignment of the forearm and humerus when the elbow is fully extended is noted. Although normally a straight line, extension beyond 0 degrees (cubital recurvatum) is common, especially in women (Fig. 17-11).

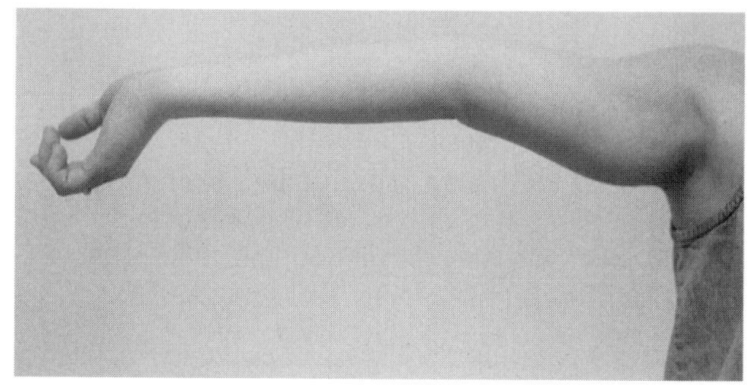

FIGURE 17-11 ■ Cubital recurvatum. A normal hyperextension of the elbow.

- **Extensor muscle mass:** The wrist extensor muscle mass is observable along the lateral aspect of the elbow and forearm. The mass widens approximately 1 to 2 inches below the elbow. Loss of girth along the lateral forearm can occur secondary to prolonged immobilization or disuse after long-term tendinopathy or radial nerve involvement.

Inspection of the posterior structures

- **Bony alignment:** When the elbow is flexed to 90 degrees, the medial epicondyle, lateral epicondyle, and olecranon process form an isosceles triangle. When the elbow is extended, these structures typically lie within a straight line. Deviation from this alignment may reflect bony pathology.
- **Olecranon process and bursa:** Flexion of the elbow makes the bony contour of the olecranon process visible. Acute injury or overuse conditions may cause the olecranon bursa to rupture or swell masking the outline of the olecranon (Fig. 17-12).

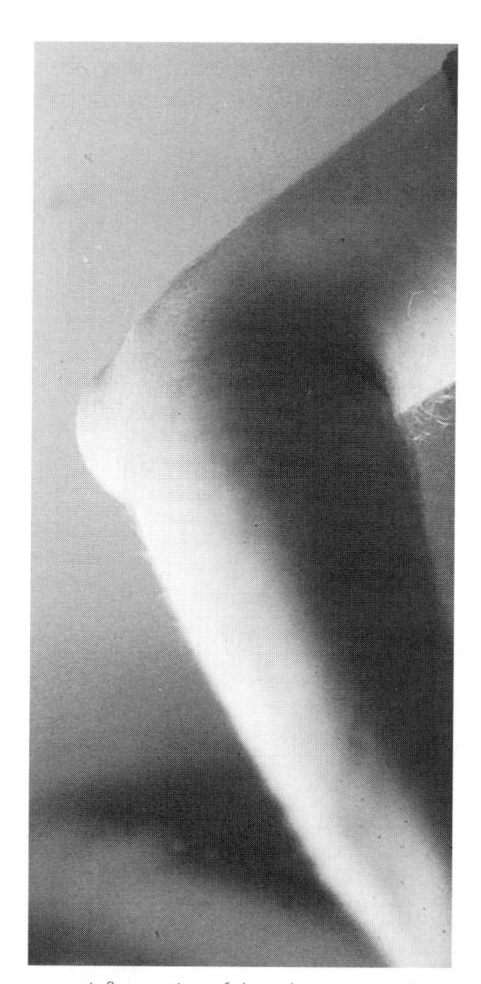

FIGURE 17-12 ■ Inflammation of the subcutaneous olecranon bursa. This structure is often traumatized by a direct blow to the olecranon process.

PALPATION

Many of the structures of the upper extremity insert or originate at the elbow, making careful, precise palpation a must for the examiner. Tenderness elicited with palpation must be correlated with other subjective and physical objective findings. Some areas, such as the humeral condyles, may be tender in the uninjured elbow.

Palpation of the Anterior Structures

1 Biceps brachii: Palpate the muscle belly of the biceps brachii along the anterior aspect of the humerus until its tendon inserts onto the radius. The tendon is more easily recognized if the elbow is held in 90 degrees of flexion. The distal biceps brachii tendon can be ruptured with a forceful eccentric contraction, resulting in deformity of the muscle.

2 Cubital fossa: Passing within the cubital fossa, palpate the brachial artery medial to the biceps brachii tendon. In some individuals, the median nerve can be palpated within the fossa. The musculocutaneous nerve also passes through this area but cannot be palpated because it runs underneath the pronator teres muscle (see Fig. 17-10).

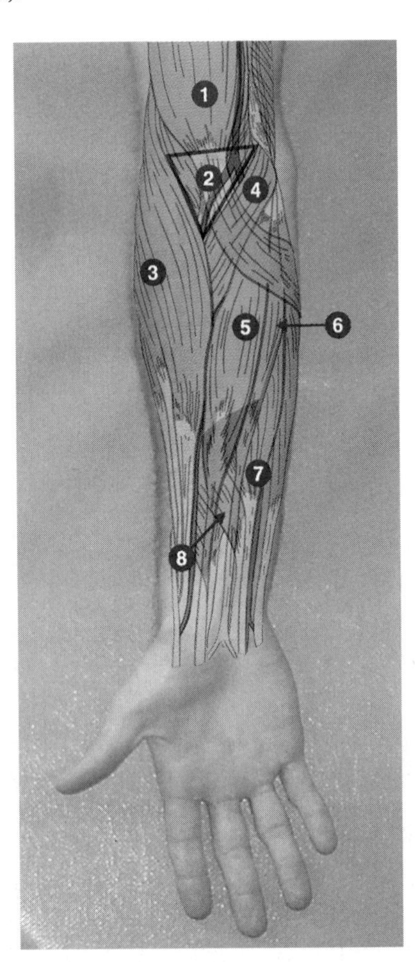

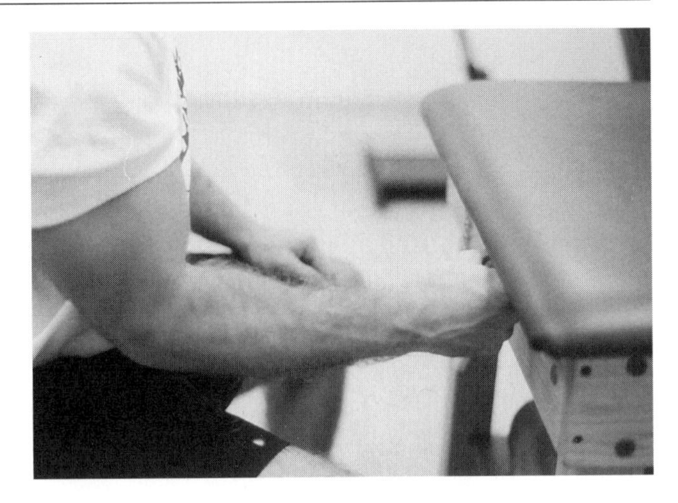

FIGURE 17-13 ■ Making the brachioradialis more prominent. An isometric contraction with the forearm in the neutral position and the elbow flexed to 90° causes the brachioradialis to become prominent.

3 Brachioradialis: To palpate the brachioradialis, place the forearm in the neutral position. The most lateral of the elbow flexor muscles, the brachioradialis is made prominent by resisting elbow flexion while the forearm is held in this position (Fig. 17-13). Palpate the length of the brachioradialis muscle from its attachment on the lateral supracondylar ridge to the distal attachment on the radial styloid process. The distal tendon of the brachioradialis is also the site to assess the deep tendon reflex of the C6 nerve root.

4–7 Wrist flexor group: Near their origin on the medial epicondyle, the bellies of the wrist flexors cannot be distinguished from one another. As they progress distally, the individual tendons of the pronator teres **(4)**, flexor carpi radialis **(5)**, palmaris longus (absent in some individuals) **(6)**, and the flexor carpi ulnaris **(7)** become identifiable as they near the wrist. Figure 17-14 presents a memory aid to assist in identifying these muscles.

8 Pronator quadratus: Laying deep to the wrist and finger flexors, palpate the area over the pronator quadratus muscle on the distal aspect of the anterior forearm.

Palpation of the Medial Structures

1 Medial epicondyle: Locate the medial epicondyle, prominent along the distal aspect of the humerus as it flares away from the shaft of the bone. The common wrist flexor tendon attaches at the epicondyle; palpation of the epicondyle elicits exquisite tenderness in the presence of medial epicondylalgia.

2 Ulna: Identify the base of the ulna, located distal to the elbow's medial joint space. The shaft is prominent throughout its length, especially along its medial and posterior (dorsal) surfaces. The anterior aspect of the shaft

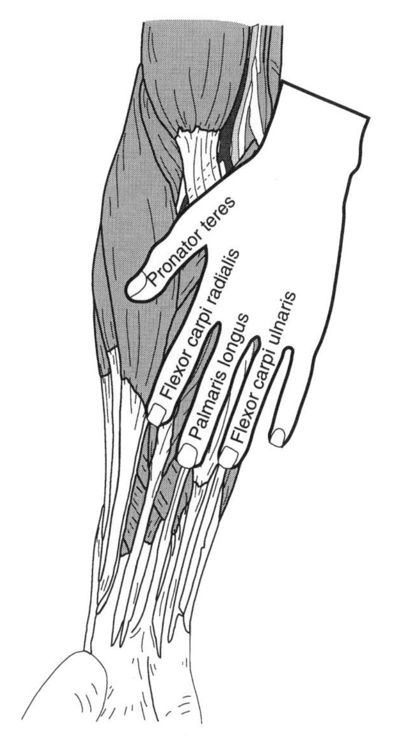

FIGURE 17-14 ■ Method of approximating the superficial muscles of the flexor forearm.

can be palpated along the distal two thirds of its length as it arises from beneath the mass of the wrist flexors to its point of articulation with the wrist.

3–5 Ulnar collateral ligament: To uncover the UCL from the more superficial flexor-pronator muscles, have the patient flex the elbow to between 50 and 70 degrees.[8] The anterior band **(3)** of this ligament can be directly palpated as it crosses the angle formed by the humerus and ulna. Continue around the medial aspect of the elbow to palpate the area over the posterior **(4)** and transverse bundles **(5)** of the UCL, although these are usually not distinguishable.

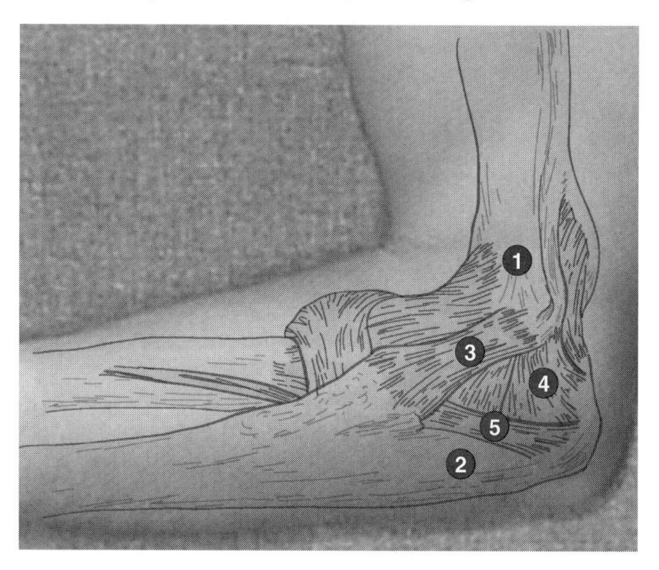

Palpation of the Lateral Structures

1 Lateral epicondyle: Smaller than the medial epicondyle, identify the lateral epicondyle, prominent as it projects from the distal end of the humerus. Palpate this structure for tenderness caused by pathology of the common origin of the wrist extensors.

2 Radial head: Moving slightly distal from the lateral joint line, locate and palpate the head of the radius underneath the posterior aspect of the wrist extensor muscles. It becomes more identifiable as it rolls beneath the examiner's finger as the forearm is pronated and supinated. During flexion and extension of the elbow, the radial head moves with the forearm.

3 Radial collateral ligament: Locate the RCL between the radial head and the lateral epicondyle. Although the RCL is not normally identifiable, its length is palpated for tenderness.

4 Capitellum: Moving proximally from the radial head across the joint line, find the rounded capitellum. While passively pronating and supinating the forearm with the elbow flexed to various degrees, palpate the capitellum and radial head for the presence of crepitus, which indicates radiocapitular chondromalacia.[12]

5 Annular ligament: Although this structure cannot be identified directly during palpation, palpate the area overlying the radial head for evidence of tenderness, crepitus, or swelling.

6 Lateral ulnar collateral ligament: Move superiorly and anteriorly from the radial head to locate the LUCL as it crosses the lateral joint line. Passively extending the forearm may make this structure more palpable.

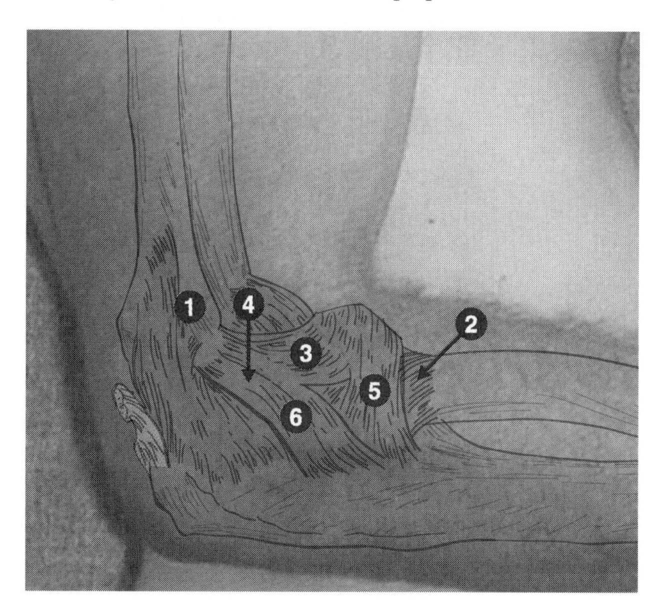

Palpation of the Posterior Structures

1 Olecranon process: Locate the ulna's olecranon process, the prominent rounded bone on the posterior aspect of the elbow. Palpate this structure for tenderness and mobility. A forced hyperextension of the elbow or a direct backward fall on the elbow may cause a fracture. The olecranon bursa is not palpable unless it is inflamed, in which case it can potentially result in a large amount of swelling and tenderness and mask the underlying bone.

2 Olecranon fossa: With the elbow partially flexed and the triceps muscle relaxed, palpate the olecranon fossa on the posterior humerus, located just superior to the olecranon process. Posteromedial tenderness resulting from impingement is associated with valgus extension overload.

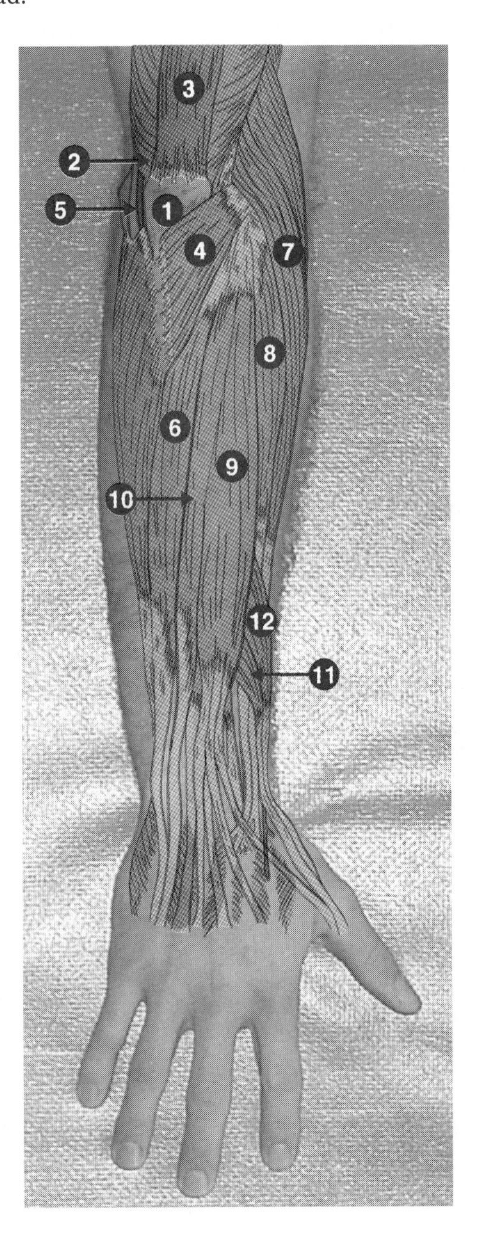

3 Triceps brachii: Slightly flex the elbow to make the fibers of the triceps brachii tendon stand out from its attachment on the olecranon. The posterolateral portion of this muscle is formed by the lateral head of the triceps and the posteromedial portion by the long head. The medial head runs deep to the long head but becomes palpable over the medial aspect of the distal humerus. The length of the triceps brachii is palpated for tenderness or deformity.

4 Anconeus: Palpate the anconeus between the lateral epicondyle and the olecranon process.

5 Ulnar nerve: With the elbow in full extension, palpate the sulcus formed by the medial epicondyle and the medial border of the olecranon process for the ulnar nerve, identifiable as a thin, cordlike structure. Determine if the ulnar nerve can be displaced from the sulcus by gently moving it medially and laterally. Inflammation of the nerve may result in a positive Tinel's sign, burning, pain, or paresthesia along the medial border of the forearm and little finger during palpation. Also palpate the ulnar nerve as the elbow is flexed and extended to determine if the nerve subluxates out of its groove.

6–8 Wrist extensors: Resist wrist extension with the fingers relaxed to make the extensor carpi ulnaris **(6)**, extensor carpi radialis brevis **(7)**, and extensor carpi radialis longus **(8)**, muscles become prominent. With the forearm pronated, the wrist extensors can be palpated distal to the lateral epicondyle. The superficial muscle is the extensor carpi radialis longus; the inferior, the extensor carpi radialis brevis.

9–10 Finger extensors: Resist finger extension to make the extensor digitorum **(9)** and extensor digiti minimi muscles **(10)** prominent.

11–12 Thumb musculature: Ask the patient to extend and abduct the thumb to more easily identify the extensor pollicis brevis **(11)** and abductor pollicis longus muscles **(12)**.

13 Radial tunnel: Place the patient's forearm in neutral. Approximately as long as 4 fingertips, the radial tunnel can be located on the posterior aspect of the forearm on a line anterior to the radiohumeral joint to the forearm's midpoint. Patients who demonstrate the clinical signs of lateral epicondylalgia but are more sensitive to palpation over the radial tunnel should also be examined to rule out radial tunnel syndrome.[13]

Joint and Muscle Function Assessment

The motions at the elbow joints are limited to flexion and extension and pronation and supination. Testing of strength and length of the wrist and long finger flexors and extensors is routinely included in an examination of the elbow, as these structures are closely associated with elbow function. Entrapment of the median, radial or ulnar nerve around the elbow may manifest itself with distal symptoms. Refer to Chapter 18 for a description of muscle function at the wrist and hand.

Goniometry Boxes 17-1 and 17-2 provide goniometric measurement of elbow flexion and extension and pronation and supination. Baseball pitchers typically demonstrate reduced flexion and extension on the dominant side, although this change is not associated with a change in function.[14]

Active Range of Motion

- **Flexion and extension:** Most of the elbow's ROM is composed of flexion, ranging between 145 and 155 degrees from the neutral position and occurs in the sagittal plane around a coronal axis (Fig. 17-15). Extension is usually limited at 0 degrees by the olecranon process, but hyperextension is common (see Fig. 17-11).
- **Pronation and supination:** The neutral position for forearm pronation and supination is the thumb and radius pointing upward. The total ROM is 170 to 180 degrees, with approximately 90 degrees of motion in each direction. This movement occurs in the transverse plane around the longitudinal axis relative to the anatomical position.

Manual Muscle Testing

Manual muscle testing procedures are presented in Manual Muscle Tests 17-1 and 17-2. Because of the interrelated functioning of the elbow and wrist and hand musculature, assuring relaxation of the wrist and hand during testing of the elbow muscles is important to the validity of the MMT.

Even injured patients are capable of overpowering the clinician during pronation and supination testing. An alternative method of resisting pronation and supination is through the use of a 1-inch diameter dowel. The patient grasps the middle of the dowel as if holding a hammer. The examiner then applies resistance to both ends of the dowel as the patient pronates and supinates the forearm (Fig. 17-16). This test for pronation and supination is more functionally oriented than the clinical test, but the patient is more likely to compensate using humeral movements.

Goniometry Box 17-1
Elbow Goniometry: Flexion and Extension

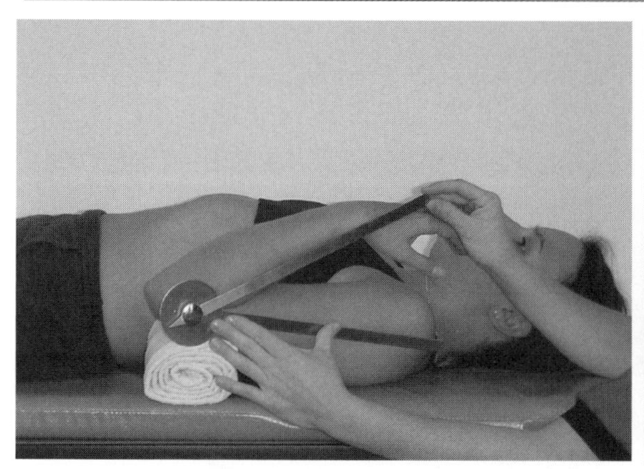

Flexion 0° to 145°–155°

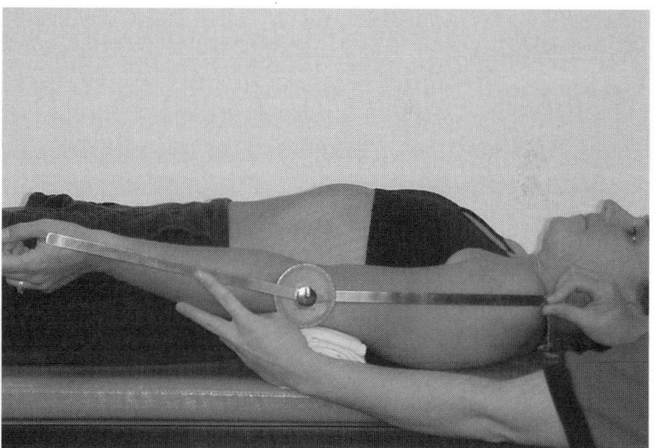

Extension 0°

Patient Position	Supine with the humerus close to the body, the shoulder in the neutral position, and the forearm supinated A bolster is placed under the distal humerus.
Goniometer Alignment	
Fulcrum	Centered over the lateral epicondyle
Proximal Arm	The stationary arm is aligned with the long axis of the humerus, using the acromion process as the proximal landmark.
Distal Arm	The movement arm is aligned with the long axis of the radius, using the styloid process as the distal landmark.

Goniometry Box 17-2
Elbow Goniometry: Pronation and Supination

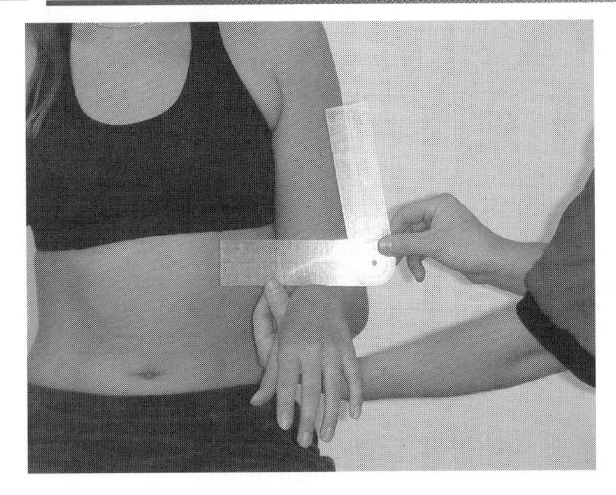

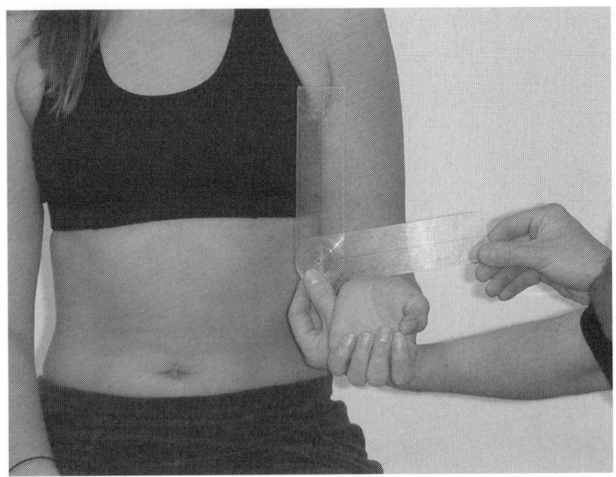

	Pronation 0°–90°	Supination 0°–90°
Patient Position	Sitting with the humerus held against the torso The elbow is flexed to 90°.	
Goniometer Alignment		
Fulcrum	Centered lateral to the ulnar styloid process	
Proximal Arm	Align the stationary arm parallel to the midline of the humerus.	
Distal Arm	The movement arm is positioned across the dorsal portion of the forearm, proximal to the radiocarpal joint.	The movement arm is positioned across the ventral portion of the forearm, proximal to the radiocarpal joint.
Modifications	The motion arm is aligned parallel to a pencil held in the hand, using the 3rd metacarpal as the axis.[15] This method captures a more functional range by incorporating movement at the wrist. Both measurement strategies demonstrate high inter- and intrarater reliability.[16]	

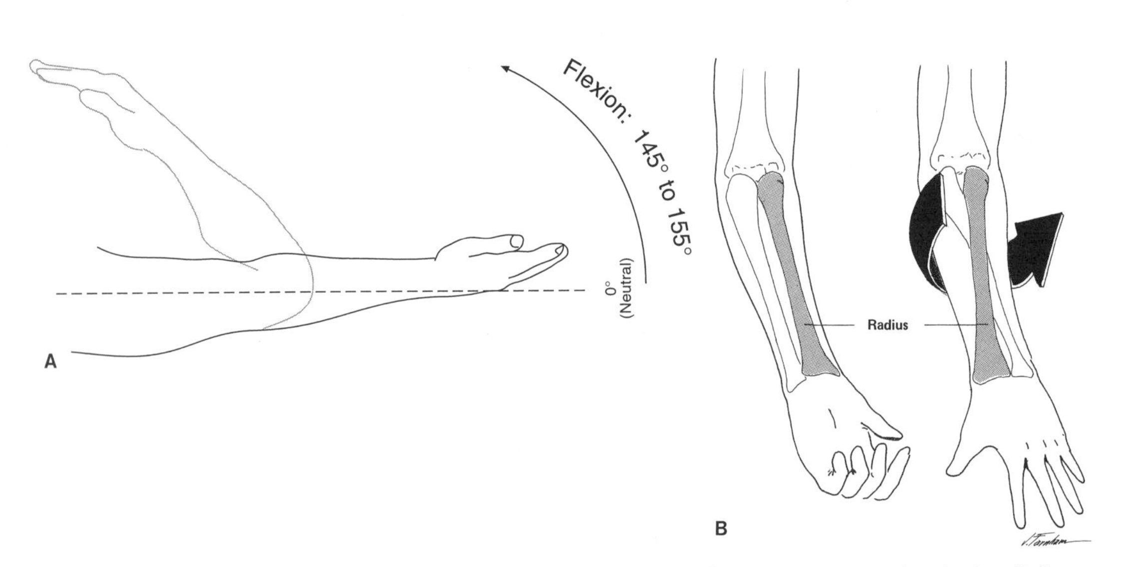

FIGURE 17-15 ■ Active range of motion at the elbow. **(A)** Elbow flexion and extension; **(B)** forearm pronation and supination. (**B**, Courtesy of Norkin, CC, and Levangie, PK: *Joint Structure and Function: A Comprehensive Analysis*, ed 2. Philadelphia, FA Davis, 1992.)

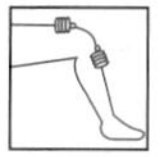

Manual Muscle Test 17-1
Elbow Flexion and Extension

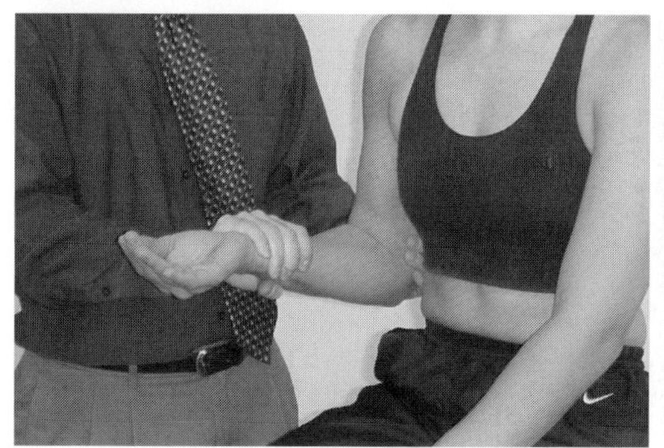

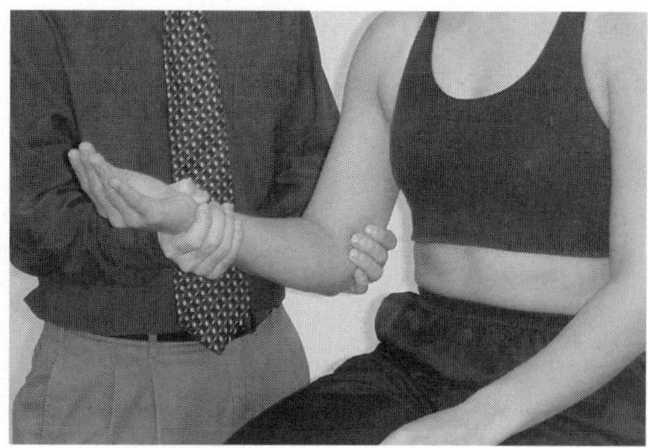

	Flexion	Extension
Patient Position	Sitting, standing, or supine.	Prone or sitting
Starting Position	The shoulder in the neutral position To isolate a specific muscle during the test: Forearm supinated Forearm pronated Forearm in midposition	The shoulder is abducted to 90°. The elbow is flexed and the forearm pronated.
Stabilization	Anterior humerus, being careful not to compress the involved muscles	Posterior humerus, being careful not to compress the involved muscles
Palpation	Over the corresponding muscle belly on the humerus	Posterior upper arm
Resistance	Over the distal forearm	Over the posterior aspect of the distal forearm
Primary Mover(s) (Innervation)	Forearm supinated: Biceps brachii (C5, C6) Forearm pronated: Brachialis (C5, C6) Forearm neutral: Brachioradialis (C5, C6)	Triceps brachii (C7, C8)
Secondary Mover(s) (Innervation)	Flexor carpi ulnaris (C8, T1)	Anconeus (C7, C8)
Substitution	Wrist and finger flexion, shoulder elevation	Wrist and finger extension, glenohumeral horizontal abduction, scapular retraction.
Comments	The patient should keep the fingers relaxed.	An alternative test position is supine, with the shoulder flexed to 90° and the elbow flexed.

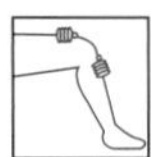

Manual Muscle Test 17-2
Pronation and Supination

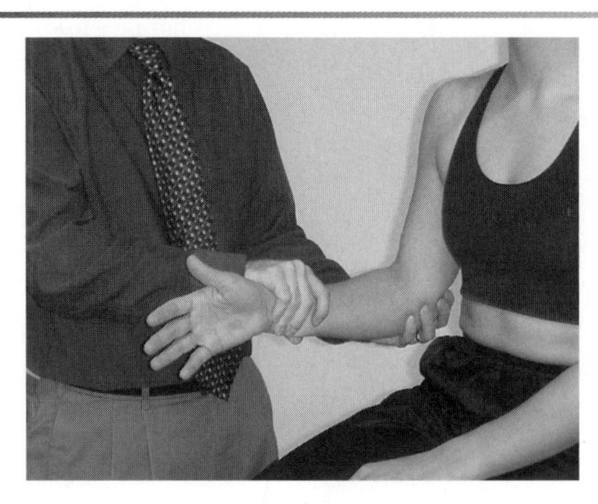

Pronation and Supination

Patient Position	Seated	
Starting Position	The shoulder in the neutral position and the elbow flexed to 90°. The thumb is facing upward.	
Stabilization	Proximal to the elbow to prevent abduction or adduction of the glenohumeral joint	
Palpation	Proximal anterior forearm	Anterior upper arm
Resistance	Resistance is applied to the ventral aspect of the forearm.	Resistance is applied to the dorsal surface of the forearm.
Primary Mover(s) (Innervation)	Pronator quadratus (C8, T1) Pronator teres (C6, C7)	Biceps brachii (C5, C6)
Secondary Mover(s) (Innervation)	Brachioradialis (C5, C6) Flexor carpi radialis (C6, C7)	Brachioradialis (C5, C6) Supinator (C6, C7, C8)
Substitution	Finger flexion, glenohumeral internal rotation	Wrist extension, glenohumeral external rotation
Comments	A more functional assessment of pronation and supination strength is performed by having the patient grip the examiner's hand and rotating. The brachioradialis assists in returning the forearm to neutral from a pronated or supinated position. Pronator weakness is commonly associated with C6 radiculopathy.[17]	

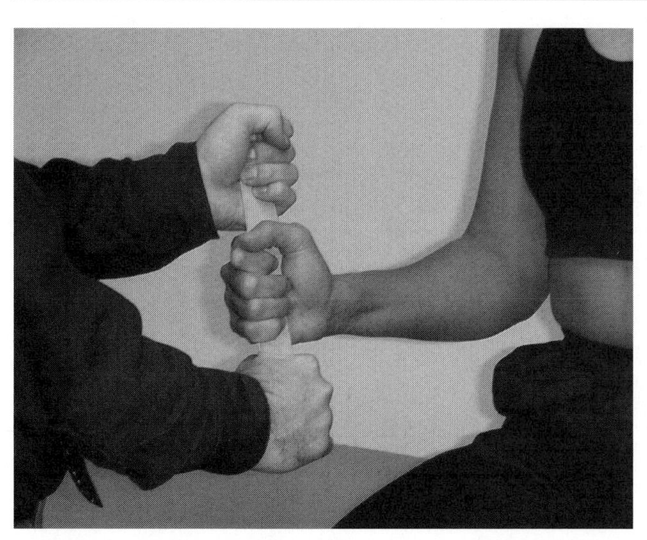

FIGURE 17-16 ■ Alternate method for resisted range of motion testing during pronation and supination.

Passive Range of Motion

Elbow: Ulnohumeral and Radiohumeral Joint Capsular Patterns and End-feels	
Capsular Pattern: Flexion, Extension	
Extension	Hard
Flexion	Soft
Elbow: Superior Radioulnar Joints	
Capsular Pattern: Supination and Pronation Equally	
Radioulnar supination	Firm
Radioulnar pronation	Hard or firm
Forearm: Distal Radioulnar Joint	
Capsular Pattern: Supination and Pronation Equally	
Radioulnar supination	Firm
Radioulnar pronation	Firm

- **Flexion and extension:** Position the elbow in extension with the forearm supinated and the shoulder joint stabilized to prevent compensatory motion (Fig. 17-17). Flex the elbow until soft tissue approximation between the bulk of the biceps brachii muscle and the muscles of the anterior forearm limits the motion, creating a soft end-feel. A hard end-feel during passive flexion is indicative of osteophyte formation or a loose body in the joint.[8] Extension produces a hard end feel by the bony contact between the olecranon process and the olecranon fossa.
- **Pronation and supination:** Position the shoulder in the neutral position and flex the elbow to 90 degrees. Support the forearm so that the radius and thumb are pointing upward and the elbow is stabilized against the torso to prevent shoulder motion. During pronation, the end-feel may be hard as the radius and ulna contact each other or firm secondary to stretching of the proximal and distal radioulnar ligaments and the interosseous membrane. Supination normally meets with a firm end-feel caused by the stretching of the proximal and distal radioulnar ligaments and the interosseous membrane.

Joint Stability Tests

Stress testing

Single-plane instability of the elbow joint can be tested only in the frontal plane when the joint is not fully extended. Valgus and varus stress ligamentous testing of the fully extended elbow is meaningless in detecting ligamentous instability because the olecranon process is locked securely within its humeral fossa. However, laxity demonstrated in this position may indicate an epiphyseal or olecranon fracture.

Stress tests for medial ligament laxity. The anterior oblique portion of the UCL is the primary restraint of the medial elbow against valgus stress. Trauma to this structure is assessed using the **valgus stress test** (Stress Test 17-1), although detecting subtle laxity is clinically difficult. Injury to the other medial ligaments is unlikely without first damaging the anterior oblique portion of the UCL.

Stress tests for lateral ligament laxity. Less common than medial ligament laxity, straight-plane varus laxity of the elbow occurs when the RCL is damaged. Involvement of the annular ligament, ALCL, or LUCL increases the laxity by allowing the radial head to separate from the ulna. The integrity of these structures is determined through **varus stress tests** (Stress Test 17-2).

Joint play

If passive flexion and extension at the elbow or pronation and supination at the forearm is restricted, examination of the accessory motions is warranted. The common joint capsule of all three elbow articulations means that restriction at all three joints is possible in the event of elbow injury (Joint Play 17-1).

Neurologic Testing

The muscles innervated by the brachial plexus range from the shoulder into the elbow, forearm, and hand. Nerve impingement occurring in the cervical or shoulder region can result in disruption of the sensory or motor function (or both) in the elbow, forearm, and hand. Likewise, nerve trauma in the elbow refers its symptoms into the wrist, hand, and fingers (Fig. 17-18). Neurologic testing may also require that an upper quarter screen be performed (see Neurologic Screening Box 1-2).

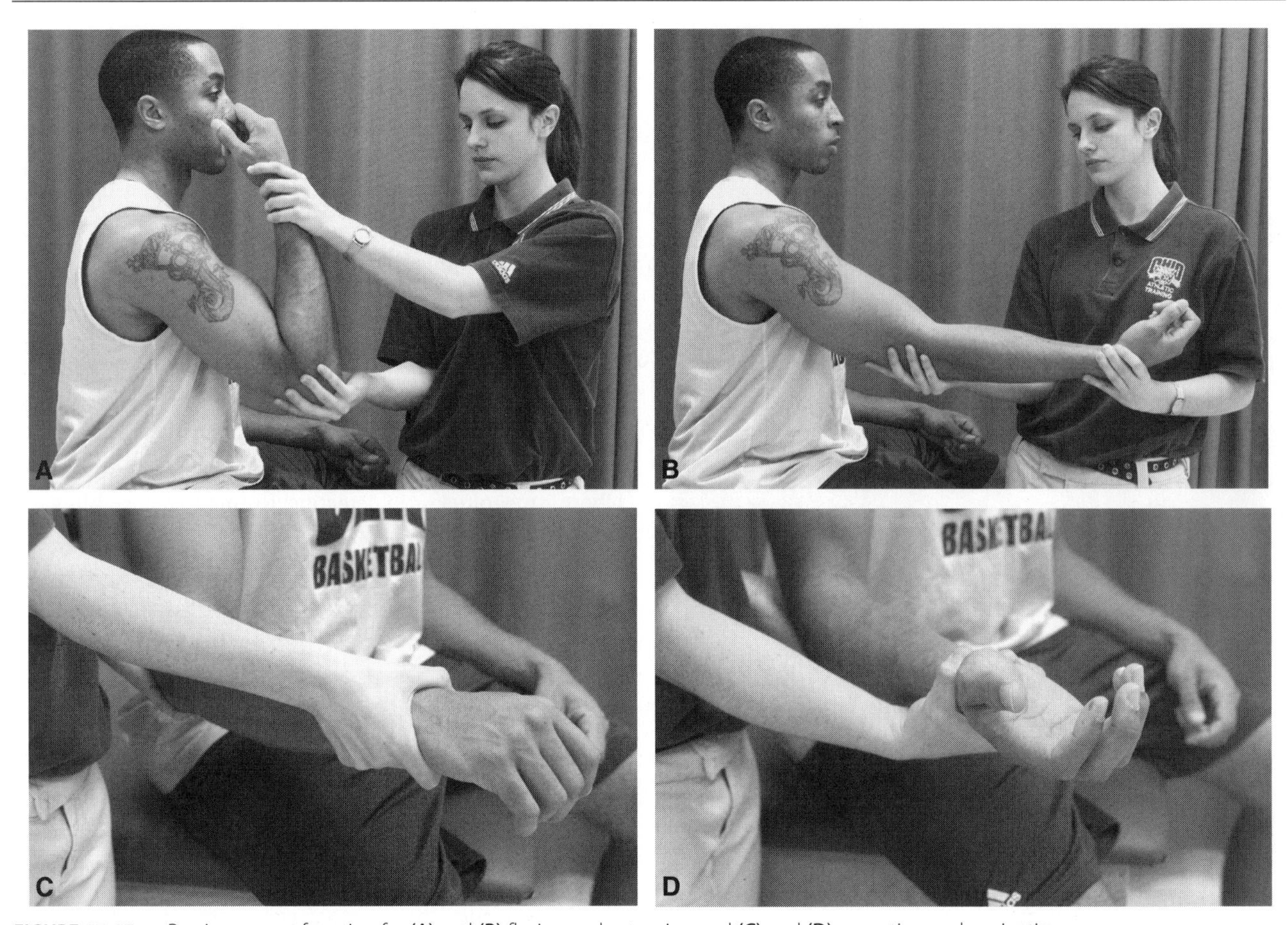

FIGURE 17-17 ■ Passive range of motion for (A) and (B) flexion and extension and (C) and (D) pronation and supination.

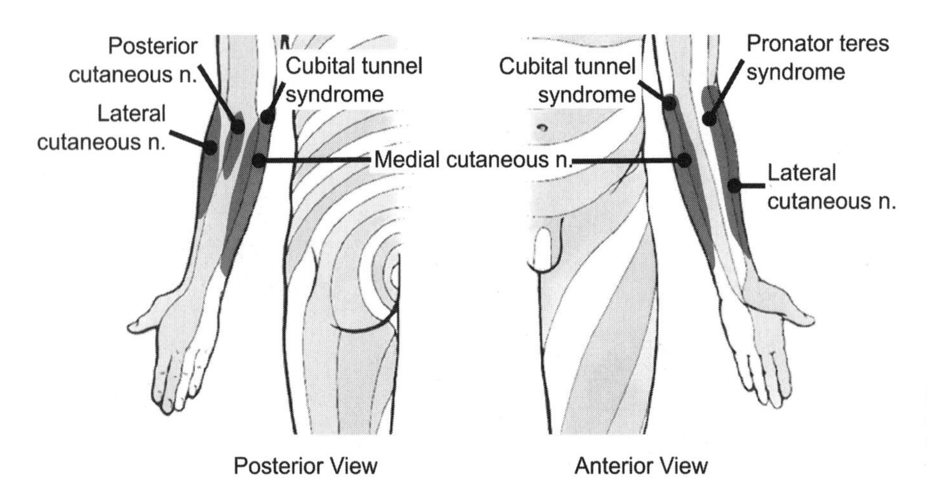

FIGURE 17-18 ■ Local neuropathies of the elbow, forearm, and hand. Correlate these findings with those of an upper quarter neurologic screen (see Box 1-6).

Pathologies and Related Special Tests

This section discusses the evaluation of patients with acute and chronic elbow injuries. The number of special tests for the elbow is relatively limited compared with those associated with the other joints described in this text. The conclusion of specific injuries is largely based on the correlation between the history of injury and examination findings.

Elbow Dislocations

Large forces are required to cause an elbow dislocation, typically requiring an axial force through the forearm while the elbow is slightly flexed. Injuries of this magnitude cause extreme pain and perhaps hysteria. The involved elbow is obviously deformed and the ability to actively move the elbow is lost. The forearm is displaced posteriorly or posterolaterally relative to the humerus in approximately 90% of the cases (Fig. 17-19).[18]

A dislocation where the coronoid process is displaced posterior to the ulna involves more ligamentous disruption than dislocations where the coronoid process remains anterior to or even with the trochlea.[19] Rarely the elbow will dislocate in an anterior or lateral direction.[18] The possibility of fracture must be ruled out, specifically the "**terrible triad of the elbow**": posterior dislocation, fracture of the radial head, and fracture of the coronoid.[20] Chronic posterolateral instability may also result. Complete dislocations result in articular surface damage in up to 50% of cases.[19]

The onset of swelling can be rapid, possibly masking the underlying deformity if there is a delay in evaluating the condition (Examination Findings 17-1). Because of the potential compromise of the blood vessels and nerves crossing the joint, the patient's distal neurovascular function must be assessed. Closed reduction by trained personnel as quickly as possible is the preferred intervention. Capillary refill and distal pulses should be assessed before and after reduction. Following reduction, early active motion that avoids extremes of the range is initiated as soon as initial pain has been reduced.

Fracture About the Elbow

Supracondylar fractures are almost exclusively found in adolescent athletes, resulting from a fall directly onto a flexed elbow or a hyperextension mechanism. Pain occurs over the supracondylar region. Angular deformity of the humerus may be noted, except in the case of nondisplaced fractures.

Fractures of the olecranon process are more common in skeletally mature patients (Fig. 17-20).[6] Being relatively unprotected by overlying muscle, the olecranon is most predisposed to direct blows such as falling on a flexed elbow. Pain, crepitus, and deformity are noted on palpation. Acute swelling may arise directly from the trauma to the

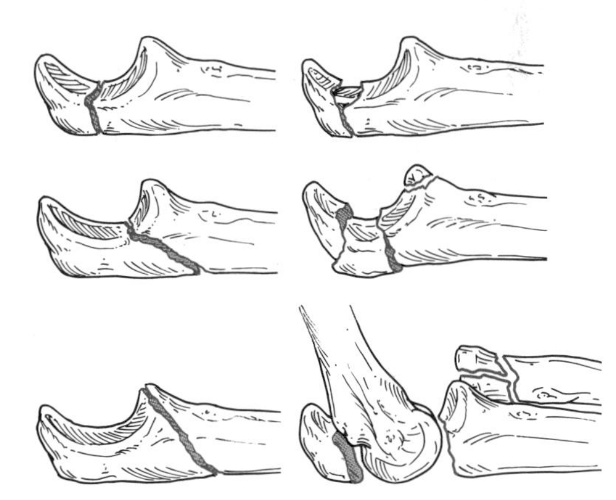

FIGURE 17-20 ■ Fracture of the olecranon process.

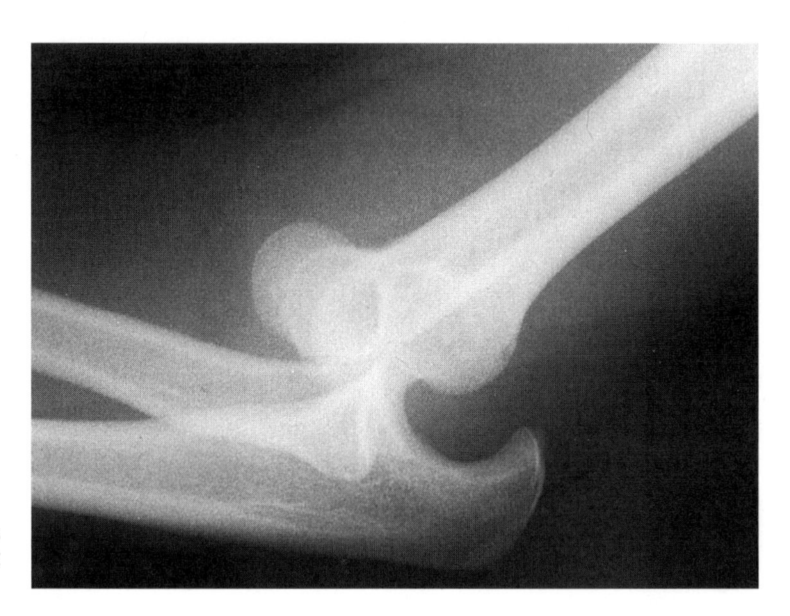

FIGURE 17-19 ■ Posterior dislocation of the elbow. This condition results in obvious deformity of the joint. Note that the humeroulnar and humeroradial joints are involved.

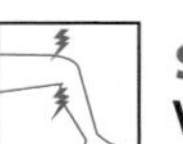

Stress Test 17-1
Valgus Stress Test

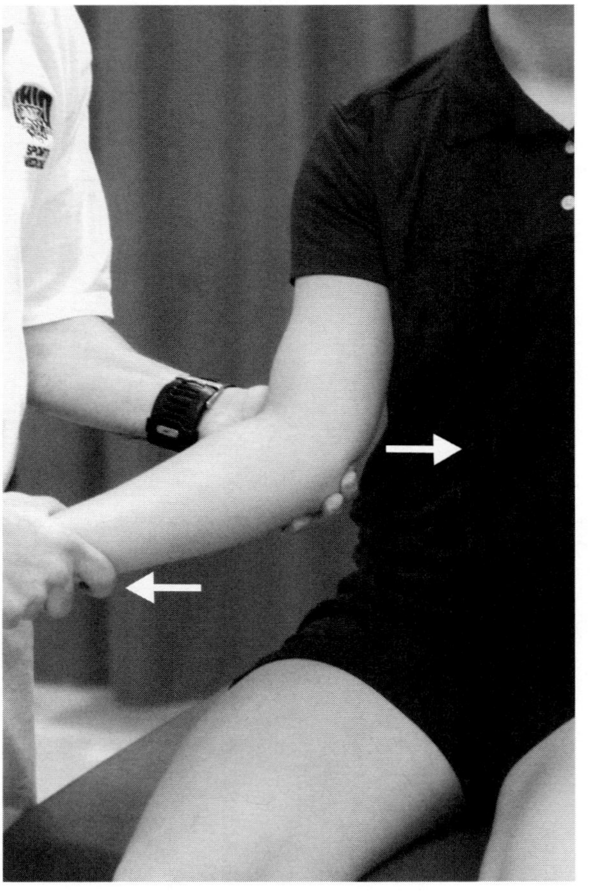

The valgus stress test determines the integrity of the ulnar collateral ligament. Also see the Moving Valgus Stress Test (see Special Test 17-1).

Patient Position	Standing, sitting, or supine The humerus is internally rotated. The elbow is flexed to 10°–25°.
Position of Examiner	Standing lateral to the joint being tested One hand supports the lateral elbow with the fingers reaching behind the joint to palpate he medial joint. The opposite hand grasps the distal forearm.

Evaluative Procedure	A valgus force is applied to the joint. The procedure is repeated with the elbow in various degrees of flexion.
Positive Test	Increased laxity compared with the opposite side, or pain, or both
Implications	Sprain of the ulnar collateral ligament, especially the anterior oblique portion Laxity beyond 60° of flexion also implicates involvement of the posterior oblique fibers.
Modification	The patient can be positioned with the humerus in external rotation for better stabilization. This position should be avoided in patients with anterior glenohumeral instability.
Comments	Laxity may also indicate epiphyseal injury. Laxity in full extension is indicative of an olecranon or humeral fracture.
Evidence	***For laxity:*** Positive likelihood ratio (see scale below); Negative likelihood ratio (see scale below) ***For pain:*** Positive likelihood ratio (see scale below); Negative likelihood ratio (see scale below)

For laxity:

Positive likelihood ratio

Not Useful — Useful
Very Small | Small | Moderate | Large
0 1 2 3 4 5 6 7 8 9 10
19.0

Negative likelihood ratio

Not Useful — Useful
Very Small | Small | Moderate | Large
1.0 0.9 0.8 0.7 0.6 0.5 0.4 0.3 0.2 0.1 0

For pain:

Positive likelihood ratio

Not Useful — Useful
Very Small | Small | Moderate | Large
0 1 2 3 4 5 6 7 8 9 10

Negative likelihood ratio

Not Useful — Useful
Very Small | Small | Moderate | Large
1.0 0.9 0.8 0.7 0.6 0.5 0.4 0.3 0.2 0.1 0

Stress Test 17-2
Varus Stress Test

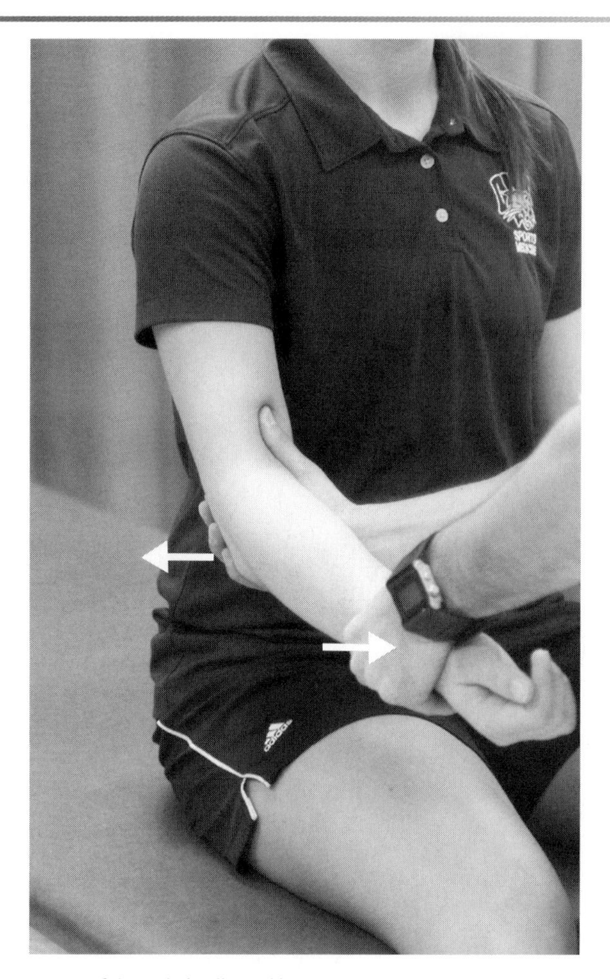

The varus stress test determines the integrity of the radial collateral ligament.

Patient Position	Standing or sitting The elbow is flexed to 25°. The humerus is in neutral.
Position of Examiner	Standing medial to the joint being tested One hand supports the medial elbow with the fingers reaching behind the joint to palpate the lateral joint line. The opposite hand grasps the distal forearm.
Evaluative Procedure	A varus force is applied to the elbow. This process is repeated with the joint in various degrees of flexion.
Positive Test	Increased laxity compared with the opposite side, and/or pain is produced.
Implications	Moderate laxity reflects trauma to the radial collateral ligament. Gross laxity may also indicate damage to the annular or accessory lateral collateral ligament, causing the radius to displace from the ulna.
Comments	Laxity may also indicate epiphyseal injury.
Evidence	Absent or inconclusive in the literature

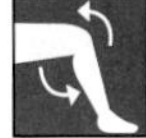

Joint Play 17-1
Elbow Joint Play

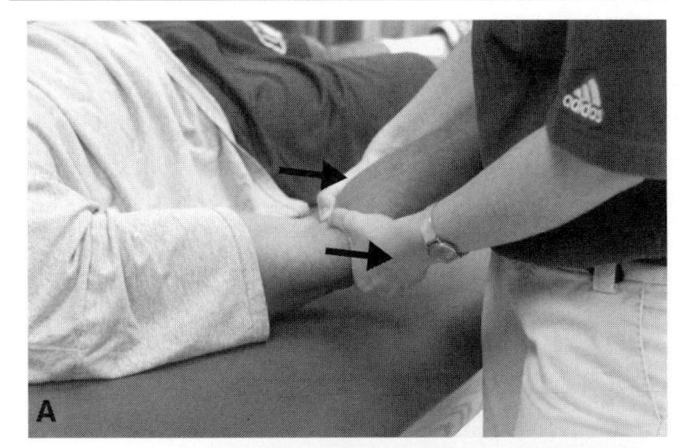

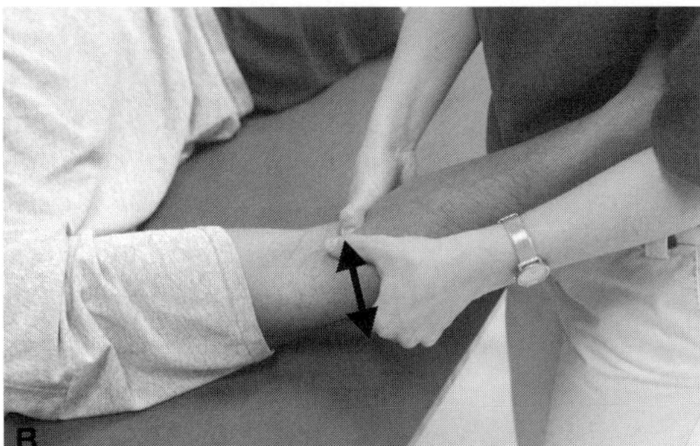

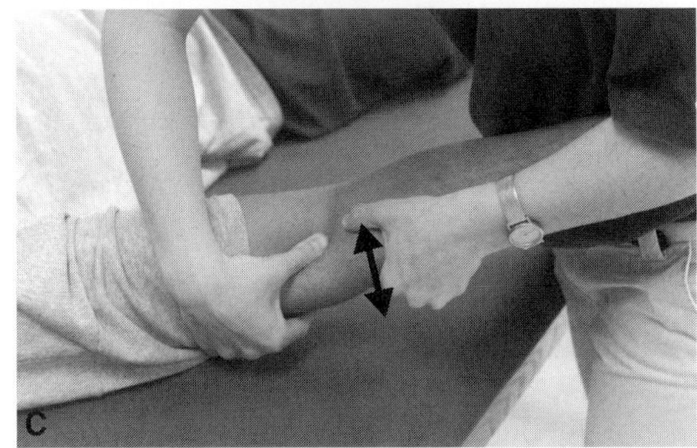

Joint play at the elbow assesses the amount of mobility allowed by the joint capsule and ligaments.

Patient Position	Humeroulnar: Supine; elbow in about 70° of flexion Radioulnar: Sitting or supine; elbow in 70° of flexion and 35° of supination Radiohumeral: Sitting or supine; elbow extended and forearm supinated
Position of Examiner	At the side of the patient
Evaluative Procedure	Humeroulnar: The examiner places thumbs on the proximal ulna while stabilizing distal forearm between his forearm and body. Applies a distracting force to the elbow Radioulnar: The examiner stabilizes the proximal ulna and applies an anterior and then posterior force at the humeral head. Radiohumeral: The examiner stabilizes the proximal ulna and applies an anterior and then posterior force at the humeral head.
Positive Test	Hypomobility or hypermobility
Implications	Restrictions in all articulations may accompany loss of physiologic elbow motion. Hypomobility at the radioulnar joint is associated with restricted supination and pronation.
Comment	Note that only the patient's position differs when assessing the radioulnar and radiohumeral articulations. The pressure needed to grasp the patient's radial head may be painful in noninjured patients. Joint movement is easier to detect in the posterior direction. Joint play of radial and ulnar deviation is performed as in valgus and varus stress testing of the elbow.

Examination Findings 17-1
Elbow Dislocations

Examination Segment	Clinical Findings
History	***Onset:*** Acute ***Pain characteristics:*** Localized to the elbow; radicular symptoms may be described in the forearm, wrist, and hand if there is associated nerve involvement. ***Mechanism:*** An axial load placed on the forearm when the arm is weight-bearing (e.g., falling on an outstretched arm). ***Predisposing conditions:*** History of elbow instability Shallow olecranon fossa with a prominent olecranon tip may be a predisposition to anterior and lateral dislocations.[18] The rate of elbow dislocations is notably higher in children.
Inspection	Obvious bony deformity and edema
Palpation	The disarticulation may be readily palpable; the area is tender.
Joint and Muscle Function Assessment	***AROM:*** Limited or absent due to bony displacement ***MMT:*** Not performed ***PROM:*** Not performed
Joint Stability Tests	***Stress tests:*** Not performed ***Joint play:*** Not performed
Special Tests	Not performed
Neurologic Screening	Assess the radial, ulnar, and median nerve distribution for sensory and motor function.
Vascular Screening	Assess the radial pulse and capillary refill Note any blood pooling distally that may indicate insufficient venous return.
Functional Assessment	The ability to use the elbow, and possibly the wrist and hand, is limited by the joint disarticulation and pain.
Imaging Techniques	AP and lateral radiographs are used to identify the magnitude and direction of the dislocation. MRI may be ordered to identify associated soft tissue injury.
Differential Diagnosis	Epiphysis fracture in children; humeral shaft fracture
Comments	Elbow dislocations may result in fractures of the coronoid process, radial head, and/or olecranon process. Associated nerve and/or vascular damage must be ruled out.

AP = anteroposterior; AROM = active range of motion; MMT = manual muscle test; MRI = magnetic resonance imaging; PROM = passive range of motion.

olecranon or arise secondary to injury of the olecranon bursa (Examination Findings 17-2). Pain is also described during active extension of the elbow and with passive overpressure during extension. By their nature, olecranon fractures are intra-articular and require anatomical alignment to restore the articular surfaces.[6]

Radial head fractures can occur following a longitudinal compression, such as when falling on an outstretched arm and often occur concurrently with an elbow dislocation. Because this fracture affects both the radiohumeral and radioulnar articulations, the patient will experience pain with flexion/extension and pronation and supination. If the fracture is displaced, restoration of normal alignment through open reduction and internal fixation is critical to avoid chronic instability and subsequent loss of function.[21]

Forearm fractures are classified by three descriptors: open or closed, simple or compound, and the degree of angulation, rotation or displacement.[22] The management decision is based on restoring anatomical congruency so that long-term function is not compromised. Fractures of the radius and ulna may compromise the neurovascular supply to the wrist and hand. Because of this, distal pulses must be monitored constantly after the injury. At that time, the elbow, forearm, and wrist must be immobilized to minimize movement of the fractured bones. After the area has been stabilized, the athlete must be immediately transported and treated for shock.

*** Practical Evidence**

Forearm fractures in children are often treated with closed reduction and casting because of young bone's ability to remodel. In adults, the same fracture frequently requires open reduction and fixation to achieve good alignment and ultimate function.[22]

Elbow Sprains

Because the elbow is stabilized by the locking of the olecranon process in its fossa when the joint is extended, strain is placed on the ligaments when the elbow is flexed. A valgus or varus stress from a blow or forceful motion delivered to a flexed elbow is dissipated by the collateral ligaments. The elbow's collateral ligament structure and bony arrangement create a mechanism whereby tensile forces on one side of the joint result in compressive forces on the opposite side.[23]

Trauma becomes more complex when a rotational component is added to the elbow. When a valgus or varus force is placed on an extended elbow, the olecranon process, in addition to the collateral ligament, must be evaluated for injury. A hyperextension mechanism can stress the elbow's anterior capsule or compress the posterior structures.

Ulnar collateral ligament

The UCL is stressed secondary to a valgus loading of the humeroulnar joint. Acutely, this stress results from a force delivered to the lateral elbow. Valgus loading of the UCL occurs during normal athletic movements and is significantly increased during the overhand pitching motion. The force generated during this motion is so great that the UCL cannot tolerate the tension on its own. As a result, the UCL must rely on the triceps brachii, the wrist flexor–pronator muscles, and the anconeus to provide dynamic stabilization to counteract the valgus force placed on this joint.[26] The LUCL can also be injured if the force is sufficient. When the forces generated during the cocking and acceleration phases of throwing are greater than the tensile strength of the UCL, insidious tearing of the ligament begins.[3]

The chief complaint is pain on the medial aspect of the elbow that intensifies with motion. Compression of the radial nerve may produce radicular pain in the forearm and fingers. Tensile forces placed on the ulnar nerve can cause paresthesia in the distal ulnar nerve distribution. Swelling may be present on the anterior, medial, and posterior borders of the joint. In most medial sprains, the anterior oblique section of the UCL is traumatized. Tenderness is noted along its length from the medial epicondyle to the coronoid process. If the elbow is flexed past 60 degrees, the posterior oblique band may also be painful. ROM testing may reveal pain secondary to stretching of the ligaments or from joint instability. Valgus stress testing demonstrates pain and laxity at various degrees of flexion (Examination Findings 17-3). The **moving valgus stress test** identifies UCL instability within the range of maximal dynamic pressure, normally between 120 and 70 degrees, closely approximating the late cocking and early acceleration phases of throwing (Special Test 17-1).[25,27] Because of the relationship of the ulnar nerve to the medial elbow, a neurologic examination of the forearm, wrist, hand, and fingers may also be required.

Valgus extension overload: Attenuation of the anterior bundle of the UCL leads to **valgus extension overload**, a collection of tensile, shear, and compressive forces that result from mild UCL laxity.[25] In addition to tensile stresses on the ulnar nerve and ulnar collateral ligament, compressive and shear forces are created at the radial head and posterior medial olecranon process. Consequences of this compression and shear include osteophyte formation and loose bodies on the posterior medial olecranon process and fossa and loose bodies at the radiohumeral articulation. This collection of forces begins with medial laxity. Potential symptoms of valgus extension overload include posteromedial and lateral elbow pain, along with ulnar nerve paresthesia as the nerve is stretched.

Elbow posterolateral rotatory instability: Tears of the LUCL permit a transient rotational subluxation of the radius

Examination Findings 17-2
Elbow Fractures

Examination Segment	Clinical Findings
History	***Onset:*** Acute ***Pain characteristics:*** Localized to the elbow ***Mechanism:*** Fall onto the elbow Hyperextension ***Predisposing conditions:*** Skeletal immaturity
Inspection	Although fractures around the elbow may result in obvious deformity, distal humeral fractures, coronoid process fractures, olecranon process fractures, and radial head fractures may not have evident bony displacement. Swelling and ecchymosis may be noted.
Palpation	Point tender over the fracture site (excluding intra-articular fractures)
Joint and Muscle Function Assessment	***AROM:*** Limited by pain and possible instability. ***MMT:*** Painful and weak with muscle attachment on involved bone Do not perform in the presence of obvious fracture. Not performed if a fracture is suspected. ***PROM:*** Pain with movement; olecranon process fractures elicit pain with passive overpressure. Radial head fracture elicits pain with pronation and supination. Do not perform in the presence of obvious fracture.
Joint Stability Tests	***Stress tests:*** Apparent ligamentous laxity may be caused by bony instability. Do not perform in the presence of obvious fracture. ***Joint play:*** Apparent increased joint mobility may be caused by bony instability. Do not perform in the presence of obvious fracture.
Special Tests	Not applicable
Neurologic Screening	Assess of the radial, ulnar, and median nerve distribution for sensory and motor function.
Vascular Screening	Assess the radial pulse and capillary refill. Note any blood pooling distally that may indicate insufficient venous return.
Functional Assessment	The ability to use the elbow, and possibly the wrist and hand, is limited by the fracture and pain.
Imaging Techniques	AP and lateral radiographs are used to identify the magnitude and direction of the fracture. The fat pad sign, representing bleeding into the joint, may be noted on radiographs.
Differential Diagnosis	Elbow dislocation; biceps tendon rupture; collateral ligament sprain
Comments	Distal humeral fractures are often intra-articular. The fracture may be open. Concurrent dislocation of the elbow may occur.

AP = anteroposterior; AROM = active range of motion; MMT = manual muscle test; MRI = magnetic resonance imaging; PROM = passive range of motion.

Examination Findings 17-3
Ulnar Collateral Ligament Sprain

Examination Segment	Clinical Findings
History	***Onset:*** Acute or insidious ***Pain characteristics:*** Medial aspect of elbow ***Mechanism:*** Acute: Valgus stress placed on the ulnar collateral ligament Insidious: Repeated valgus loading of the elbow ***Predisposing conditions:*** Repeated activities that exert tensile stresses on the medial aspect of the elbow (e.g., throwing); internal rotation deficits in the throwing athlete Cubitus varus may predispose posterolateral rotatory instability.[10]
Inspection	Effusion may be present in the anterior medial, and posterior aspects of the elbow. Edema may extravasate distally if the capsule is torn. Ecchymosis may be present over the medial aspect of the elbow.
Palpation	Palpation of the medial elbow from the medial epicondyle to the coronoid process may elicit tenderness and crepitus.
Joint and Muscle Function Assessment	***AROM:*** Elbow motion is limited secondary to pain because of stretching of the ligaments or joint instability, especially moving into extension. Wrist flexion is painful. ***MMT:*** Decreased strength and pain in wrist flexors ***PROM:*** Pain elicited at end range of supination and extension Extension may be limited by a flexion contracture in chronic cases Wrist extension is painful at the end range.
Joint Stability Tests	***Stress tests:*** Valgus testing at 10°–25° of flexion demonstrates increased laxity and pain at the medial elbow and may elicit paresthesia in the ulnar nerve distribution. Testing at other degrees of flexion (e.g., 45°, 60°, and 90°) may elicit symptoms. ***Joint play:*** Humeroulnar, radiohumeral, radioulnar
Special Tests	Posterolateral rotatory instability test of the elbow Moving valgus stress test
Neurologic Screening	Sensory and motor testing of the ulnar nerve distribution may be affected. Tinel sign at the ulnar nerve may be positive if the nerve has been traumatized.
Vascular Screening	Within normal limits
Functional Assessment	Overhand throwing athletes will describe a significant decrease in velocity.
Imaging Techniques	Valgus stress radiographs may be obtained. An opening of the medial joint line greater than 2–3 mm is consistent with instability.[3,24] Ligament disruption and surrounding soft tissue involvement is visualized via MRI. Asymptomatic overhead throwing athletes may demonstrate increased medial opening on stress radiographs.[25]
Differential Diagnosis	Pronator muscle strain, supinator muscle sprain, arthritis, ulnar neuropathy, flexor carpi radialis strain, flexor carpi ulnaris strain
Comments	Not applicable

AROM = active range of motion; MRI = magnetic resonance imaging; MMT = manual muscle test; PROM = passive range of motion.

Special Test 17-1
Moving Valgus Stress Test

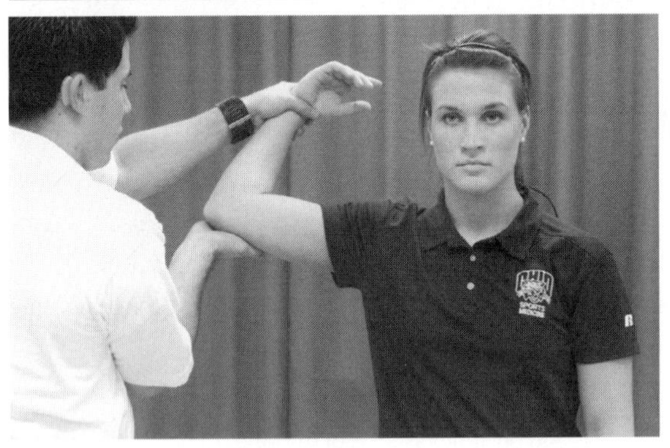

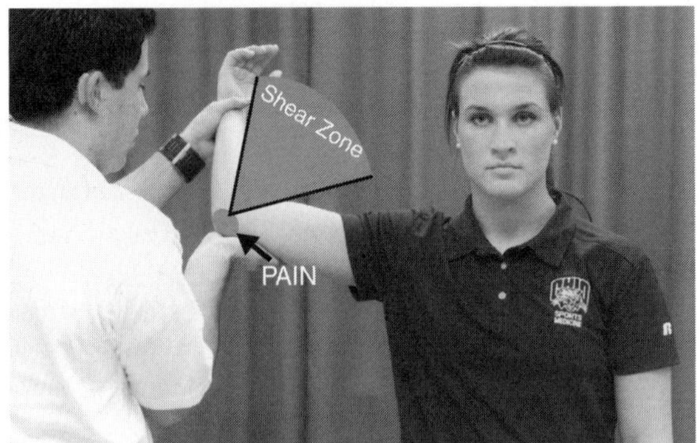

The moving valgus stress test places tensile forces on the ulnar collateral ligament through elbow flexion and extension to identify dynamic elbow instability.

Patient Position	Sitting The shoulder is abducted to 90°. The elbow is flexed to the end of the ROM.
Position of Examiner	Standing next to the patient One hand stabilizes the distal humerus. The opposite hand grasps the ulnar side of the distal forearm.
Evaluative Procedure	While applying a valgus force on the elbow, the examiner externally rotates the humerus. The examiner extends the elbow to approximately 30° while maintaining a valgus force on the joint, noting the position(s) that pain is evoked. The examiner then moves the elbow from extension into flexion while maintaining a valgus stress on the joint.
Positive Test	(1) Pain at the medial elbow that reproduces functional pain, often producing an apprehension response AND (2) Pain that occurs between 120° and 70° (representing the position of the late cocking and early acceleration throwing phases) A positive test is marked by the reproduction of pain at the same point in the ROM during both the flexion and extension segments of the examination.
Implications	Partial tear or attenuation of the UCL
Comments	Shoulder pathology may elicit pain during this procedure. Do not perform in the presence of known GH instability.
Evidence	Positive likelihood ratio Not Useful — Useful Very Small (0–2) | Small (2–5) | Moderate (5–10) | Large (10+) Scale: 0 1 2 3 4 5 6 7 8 9 10; marker at 4 Negative likelihood ratio Not Useful — Useful Very Small (1.0–0.5) | Small (0.5–0.2) | Moderate (0.2–0.1) | Large (0.1–0) Scale: 1.0 0.9 0.8 0.7 0.6 0.5 0.4 0.3 0.2 0.1 0; marker at 0

GH = glenohumeral; ROM = range of motion; UCL = ulnar collateral ligament.

and ulna relative to the humerus, **posterolateral rotatory instability**, causing external rotation of the radius and ulna, and valgus opening of the elbow (Fig. 17-21).[10,28,29] This results in the radius and ulna acting as a single unit as they rock away from the articulating surfaces of the humerus. A classic complaint of patients with an insufficiency of the LUCL is an ability or reluctance to push out of a chair and fully extend the elbow with the forearms supinated and the arms abducted greater than shoulder width (chair sign). In addition, patients will be unable to fully extend or apprehensive in performing a push-up from the floor with the forearms supinated and the arms abducted greater than shoulder width (pushup sign).[30] Clinically, patients with this condition may be evaluated through the **posterolateral rotatory instability test** (Special Test 17-2).

*** Practical Evidence**

A patient's inability to perform a pushup or push out of a chair (with the forearms supinated and greater than shoulder width apart) is a better indicator of posterolateral rotatory instability than the posterolateral rotatory instability (pivot shift) test in an unanesthetized patient.[30]

In cases of chronic overload to the medial side of the elbow, the initial treatment is to alleviate any repetitive forces on the elbow. Local modalities are helpful to decrease pain and inflammation. ROM is progressed in a pain-free manner. Strengthening of the muscles surrounding the joint is performed to assist in stabilizing the elbow against valgus forces. In athletes who perform throwing motions, the ROM at the shoulder also requires assessment. Over time, throwers lose shoulder internal rotation and gain excessive amounts of external rotation. A tremendous amount of valgus force is placed on the medial elbow during the cocking and acceleration phases of overhead pitching. ROM exercises for increasing internal rotation of the shoulder are often needed to balance the stresses at the medial elbow.

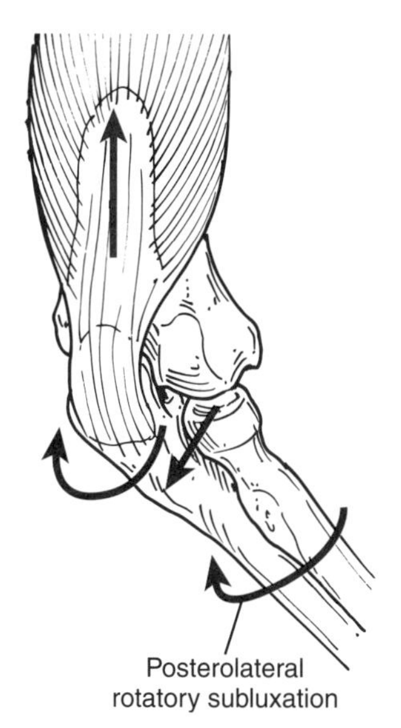

FIGURE 17-21 ■ Posterolateral rotational subluxation of the radius. Contraction of the triceps brachii against resistance result in a varus stress and external rotation of the ulna. This causes the radius to externally rotate. The subluxation occurs when the radial head rotates off the capitellum.

Radial collateral ligament

Injury to the RCL complex is rare because in most positions, the body shields the elbow from varus forces. In addition, the stresses placed on the elbow joint during throwing and racquet sports are absorbed by the UCL and the wrist extensor muscles.

Varus forces placed on the lateral elbow ligaments can result in trauma to the RCL and, possibly, the annular ligament. Trauma to the RCL or its component parts (see Fig. 17-4) not only results in varus laxity but also may disrupt the articulation between the radial head and the capitellum. The signs and symptoms of RCL sprains are similar to those of UCL trauma but may be compounded by pain, laxity, or weakness during pronation and supination.

The treatment for patients with radial collateral ligament sprains is similar to that for those with medial elbow sprains. With radial collateral sprains, strengthening focuses on the wrist extensors, supinators, brachioradialis, and the surrounding elbow muscles to provide dynamic stabilization against varus stresses.

Epicondylalgia

Both the lateral and medial epicondyles serve as the origin for many of the muscles acting on the wrist and fingers. Although commonly used, the term epicondylitis does not accurately capture most conditions at these origins; chronic pathology is more likely a degenerative tendinosis than an actual inflammatory tendinitis condition. The term epicondylalgia is a better description of the changes at the medial or lateral epicondyle.

Lateral epicondylalgia

Inflammation or repetitive stresses at the lateral epicondyle irritates the common attachment of the wrist extensor group (extensor carpi ulnaris, extensor carpi radialis longus, extensor carpi radialis brevis, extensor digitorum communis, and supinator). Although any or all of these muscles may be involved, the extensor carpi radialis brevis is the muscle most commonly affected. Underlying the extensor carpi radialis longus, the brevis has a broad origin from the common extensor tendon on the lateral epicondyle, lateral collateral ligament, annular ligament, and associated muscular fascia.[34] Repeated, forceful eccentric contractions of the wrist extensor muscles result in the accumulation of degenerative forces at their attachment site, creating microtears.[34,35] The relatively small area of attachment for these muscles causes a great force load to be applied to the bone as these muscles contract.

Special Test 17-2
Posterolateral Rotatory Instability Test (Pivot Shift)

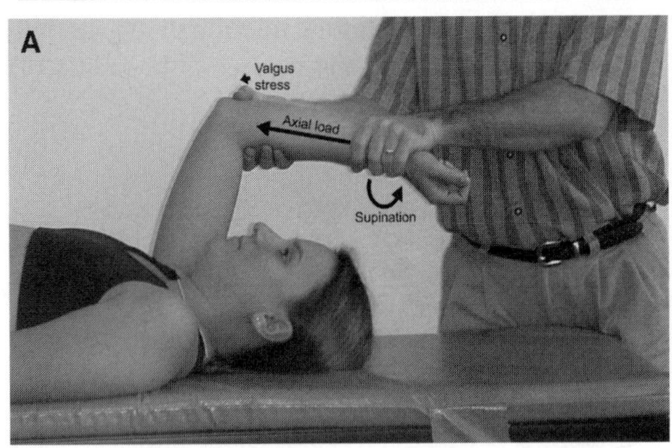

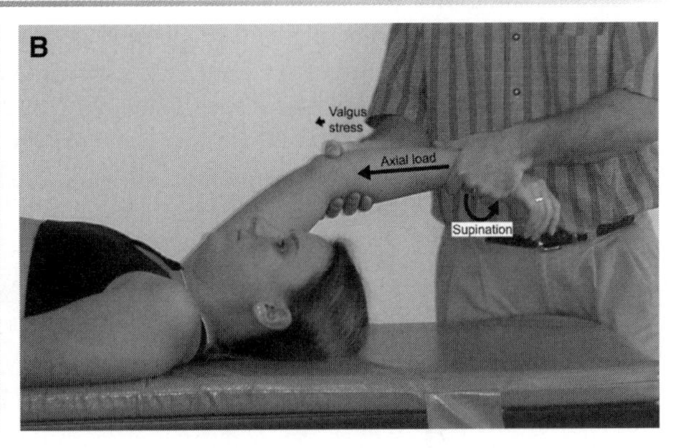

Test for posterolateral rotatory instability of the elbow consists of extending the elbow with a axial load, valgus stress, and forearm supination. The elbow subluxates as it nears full extension. A palpable reduction may be felt as the elbow is moved back into flexion.

Patient Position	Supine The shoulder and elbow are flexed to 90° and the forearm is fully supinated.
Position of Examiner	Standing at the head of the patient One hand grasps the proximal forearm and the other hand grasps the distal forearm at the wrist **(A).**
Evaluative Procedure	While applying a valgus stress and axial compression, the elbow is extended and the forearm is maintained in full supination **(B)**. The elbow then can be taken back into flexion (not shown).
Positive Test	The elbow subluxates as it is extended and can be felt to relocate as it is flexed.
Implications	Chronic instability of the elbow
Comments	When performed with the patient under anesthesia, the posterolateral rotatory instability test was positive only when the entire lateral collateral ligament was sectioned.[29]
Evidence	Absent or inconclusive in the literature

Lateral epicondylalgia is prevalent in racquet sports, affecting more than half of all regular tennis players, leading to its colloquial name, "tennis elbow." Most common in individuals older than 40 years of age, the chief complaint and most significant clinical finding is pain over the lateral epicondyle, decreased grip strength, and pain with gripping.[36] In patients who play racquet sports, the symptoms are increased during backhand strokes.

Inspection of the painful area may reveal swelling, and palpation of the area may produce pain. Active wrist extension results in pain that worsens with resisted motion. Pain elicited during passive stretching of the extensor muscles and resisted finger extension has also been demonstrated to be a reliable indicator of this condition.[37] Active and passive wrist flexion, elbow extension, and forearm pronation, all of which stretch the common extensor tendon, are routinely limited for the patient with lateral epicondylalgia.[30] The **tennis elbow test** is sensitive to even mild cases of lateral epicondylalgia (Special Test 17-3). Entrapment of the radial nerve may produce symptoms that are similar to lateral epicondylalgia (Examination Findings 17-4).

Treatment of lateral epicondylalgia involves avoiding the activities that aggravate the condition. Oral anti-inflammatory medications and local anti-inflammatory modalities may reduce pain but do not otherwise affect the condition. Local corticosteroid injections may be beneficial for short-term gains in pain reduction, although structured rehabilitation or simply waiting produces better long-term outcomes.[27,30] Patients who have occupations that require extensive computer use have worse outcomes than those in other occupations.[31] Therapeutic exercises involve stretching and strengthening around the elbow with the main focus on the wrist extensor group. Although many advocate the use of "tennis elbow" straps, the true benefit of these devices is inconclusive.[1]

As the patient recovers, a return to the initial activities creating the condition may require an assessment of the equipment being used (i.e., racquet size and stiffness,

Special Test 17-3
Test for Lateral Epicondylalgia ("Tennis Elbow" Test)

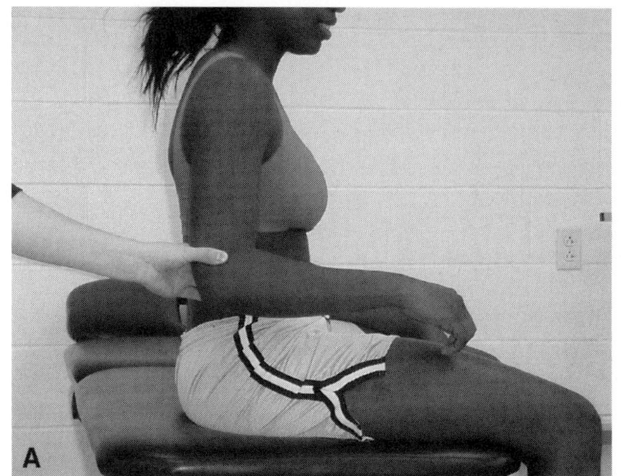

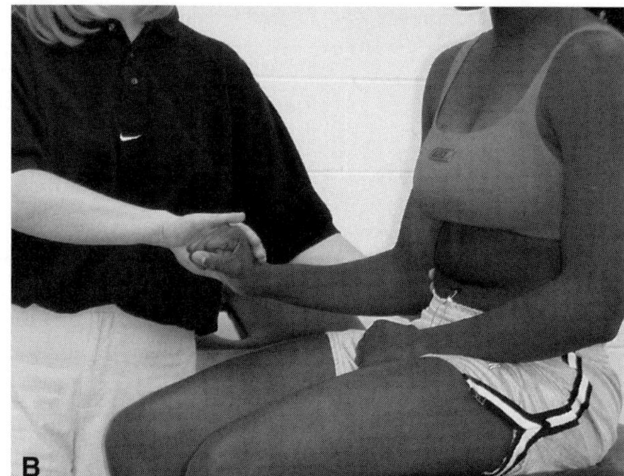

(A) The location of the thumb on the lateral epicondyle. **(B)** Resisted wrist extension.

Patient Position	Seated with the tested elbow flexed to 90°, the forearm pronated, and the fingers flexed
Position of Examiner	Standing lateral to the patient with one hand positioned over the dorsal aspect of the wrist and hand
Evaluative Procedure	The examiner resists wrist extension while palpating the lateral epicondyle and common attachment of the wrist extensors.
Positive Test	Pain in the lateral epicondyle
Implications	Lateral epicondylalgia ("tennis elbow")
Modification	This test may also be performed with the elbow in extension.
Comments	This is the manual muscle test for wrist extension performed through a full range of motion instead of midrange.
Evidence	Absent or inconclusive in the literature

ergonomic assessment of computer work station) and the technique being used. Many patients who develop this condition from athletic participation may benefit from an expert's lesson to improve their techniques. Activity modifications that reduce or eliminate repetitive contraction of the wrist extensors may be beneficial.

Medial epicondylalgia

Activities involving the swift, powerful snapping of the wrist and pronation of the forearm load the medial epicondyle. As with its lateral counterpart, medial epicondylalgia involves point tenderness at the origin of the pronators teres, flexor carpi radialis, palmaris longus, and flexor carpi ulnaris tendon on the medial epicondyle. The length of the pronator teres muscle also may be tender and the patient's grip strength may be markedly decreased (Examination Findings 17-5).[21] In young baseball pitchers, the tension build-up in the medial epicondyle may result in avulsion of the common tendon from its attachment site, "Little Leaguer's elbow" (Fig. 17-22). Radiographic changes involving separation or fragmentation of the medial epicondyle are commonly detected in Little League pitchers and catchers, although the individuals may or may not complain of pain.[38] Medial epicondylalgia may cause neuropathy of the ulnar nerve, causing symptoms to radiate into the medial forearm and fingers.[39]

The treatment of patients with medial epicondylalgia follows the interventions described for those with lateral epicondylalgia.

Distal Biceps Tendon Rupture

Biceps tendon ruptures are most common in males older than the age of 40.[4,40] The incident of rupture is 7.5 times greater in patient who smoke than those with no history of smoking.[40] The tendon and its aponeurosis degrades with time, ultimately resulting in a spontaneous rupture of the tendon often occurring in the hypovascular zone between

Examination Findings 17-4
Lateral Epicondylalgia

Examination Segment	Clinical Findings
History	***Onset:*** Insidious ***Pain characteristics:*** Lateral epicondyle and proximal portion of the common tendons of the wrist extensors; radicular pain into the wrist extensor muscles is possible with advanced cases. ***Mechanism:*** Overuse syndrome involving repeated, forceful wrist extension; radial deviation, supination, or grasping in an overhand position ***Predisposing conditions:*** Repeated eccentric loading of the wrist extensor muscles Occupation requiring prolonged computer use[31] Inexperience or newness in playing racquet sports[23]
Inspection	Swelling possibly present over the lateral epicondyle
Palpation	Pain and possible crepitus over the lateral epicondyle and proximal portion of the common wrist extensor tendon
Joint and Muscle Function Assessment	Wrist flexion, elbow extension, and pronation are all limited passively and actively. ***AROM:*** Pain with combined wrist extension and elbow flexion; radial deviation also possibly painful. Pronation and supination may be limited in patients with chronic lateral epicondylalgia.[23] ***MMT:*** Pain with wrist extension and MCP joint extension when elbow extended. ***PROM:*** Pain at the end range of passive wrist flexion, especially with elbow extended Limitation in wrist flexion with the elbow extended.
Joint Stability Tests	***Stress tests:*** Unremarkable ***Joint play:*** Restricted radioulnar and radiohumeral glide.
Special Tests	Test for lateral epicondylalgia ("tennis elbow" test)
Neurologic Screening	Rule out radial nerve entrapment
Vascular Screening	Within normal limits
Functional Assessment	Pain and weakness with gripping activities Decreased grip strength as measured on a dynamometer[32] Pain and weakness in combined elbow flexion and wrist extension motions
Imaging Techniques	Plain radiography is used to image (or rule out) osteophyte formation, arthritis, osteochondritis dissecans, or fracture.[33] Diagnostic ultrasound may demonstrate thickening in the tendon.[33] MRI can image tendon degeneration.[33]
Differential Diagnosis	Radial tunnel syndrome or other neuropathy, arthritis, acute epicondylar fracture, stress fracture
Comments	Lateral epicondylalgia, LCL, and/or radial nerve trauma may occur in any combination.[23] In racquet sports, pain is worsened with the backhand stroke and may be related to improper size of the racquet handle grip or a racquet that is too tightly strung.

AROM = active range of motion; LCL = lateral collateral ligament; MCP = metacarpophalangeal; MMT = manual muscle test; MRI = magnetic resonance imaging; PROM = passive range of motion.

Examination Findings 17-5
Medial Epicondylalgia

Examination Segment	Clinical Findings
History	***Onset:*** Insidious ***Pain characteristics:*** Medial epicondyle and the proximal portion of the adjacent wrist flexor and pronator muscles ***Mechanism:*** Repeated, forceful flexion or pronation of the wrist (or both) ***Predisposing conditions:*** Repeated activities that eccentrically load the medial elbow muscles (e.g., throwing, golfing)
Inspection	Swelling in the area over the medial epicondyle
Palpation	Point tenderness and crepitus over the medial epicondyle; tenderness in the proximal portion of the wrist flexor group, especially the pronator teres
Joint and Muscle Function Assessment	***AROM:*** Pain during wrist flexion; wrist extension possibly resulting in pain secondary to stretching the involved muscles ***MMT:*** Decreased strength and pain during testing of the wrist flexors and forearm pronators ***PROM:*** Pain at the end range of wrist extension, especially with the elbow extended
Joint Stability Tests	***Stress tests:*** Unremarkable ***Joint play:*** Unremarkable
Special Tests	Not applicable
Neurologic Screening	Sensory and motor tests to identify potential ulnar nerve neuropathy
Vascular Screening	Within normal limits
Functional Assessment	Patient may demonstrate decreased grip strength.
Imaging Techniques	Plain radiography is used to image (or rule out) osteophyte formation, arthritis, osteochondritis dissecans, or fracture.[33] Diagnostic ultrasound may demonstrate thickening in the tendon.[33] MRI can image tendon degeneration.[33]
Differential Diagnosis	Ulnar neuropathy, medial epicondylalgia, arthritis, acute epicondylar fracture, stress fracture
Comments	Medial epicondylalgia, UCL, and/or ulnar nerve trauma may occur in any combination.[23]

AROM = active range of motion; MMT = manual muscle test; MRI = magnetic resonance imaging; PROM = passive range of motion; UCL = ulnar collateral ligament.

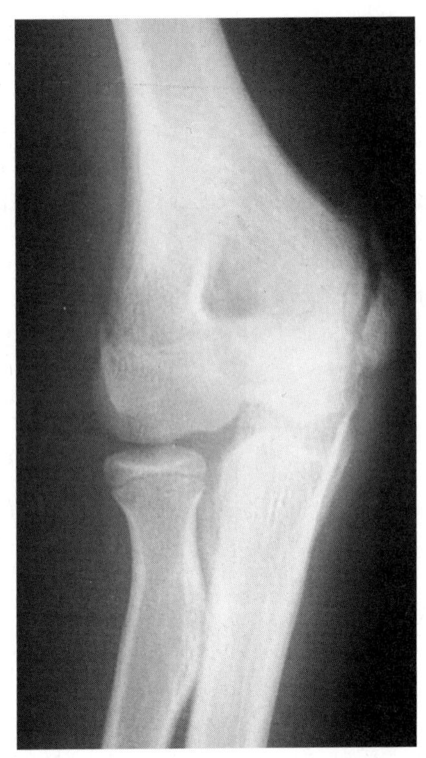

FIGURE 17-22 ■ Avulsion of the origin of the wrist flexor muscles, "Little Leaguer's elbow." This condition can mimic medial epicondylalgia .

the proximal and distal blood supply.[4] The mechanism of injury involves the eccentric loading of the biceps brachii when the elbow is flexed to 90 degrees.[4,41–43] Ruptures are classified as being complete or partial. Clinically, the distal tendon is still palpable along its length when it is partially ruptured.

Rupture of the distal biceps tendon is debilitating because of the loss of strength during elbow flexion and supination. The patient reports immediate pain and the sensation of a "pop" within the elbow. A loss of arm strength during elbow flexion and forearm supination is also apparent. Inspection of the cubital fossa reveals swelling and ecchymosis. A palpable defect in the distal biceps tendon may also be noted. Active ROM (AROM) and passive ROM (PROM) may remain within normal limits, but a definitive decrease in strength during manual muscle testing for elbow flexion and supination is present (Examination Findings 17-6). Most biceps tendon ruptures involve the avulsion of the bicipital (radial) tuberosity, a diagnosis made using radiographs, MR, or CT scans.

✱ Practical Evidence

When the patient actively supinates, by approaching from the lateral side the examiner will be able to hook a finger under an intact distal biceps tendon (hook test). Initial evaluation of this test reveals that it is both sensitive and specific.[44]

Although biceps tendon ruptures may be managed conservatively, surgical repair is the preferred method of treatment for both complete and partial ruptures.[4,45–47] Postsurgical rehabilitation consists of a progressive return of ROM after a 1-week period of total immobilization. Submaximal strengthening is begun at 4 weeks and progressed as tendon healing in the bone solidifies by week 8.[43]

Osteochondritis Dissecans of the Capitellum

Osteochondritis dissecans of the capitellum develops gradually because of increased valgus loading compressing the radial head and capitellum with overhead throwing. The resulting valgus load on the elbow places compressive and shear forces on the capitellum.[48] Osteochondritis dissecans develops secondary to disrupted blood flow to the area creating an osteochondral defect over time. Osteochondritis dissecans is frequently associated with other orthopedic conditions such as osteochondral fracture, avascular necrosis, and detached bony fragments.[48]

The patient complains of lateral elbow pain that increases with activity. A flexion contracture is usually present. Radiographic examination reveals either a nondisplaced fragmented defect or a loose body within the joint (Examination Findings 17-7). If the fragment has not separated, rest along with a progressive program of ROM and strengthening is used. A loose body warrants surgical intervention to remove the fragment and curettage the defect. In either case, the return to previous athletic endeavors is guarded, especially in the throwing athlete.

Nerve Pathology

The peripheral nerves emanating from the brachial plexus can be compromised by chronic entrapment, repetitive tension or trauma. Anatomical structures including the **arcade of Struthers**, intramuscular fascia, tunnels beneath ligaments, and bony tracts through which the nerve passes are common sites are entrapment.[49] Postinjury fibrosis or postsurgical scarring can also compress the nerve. Abnormal tension resulting from instability, such as when the ulnar nerve is stretched secondary to medial elbow laxity, can result in nerve symptoms. Acute trauma can directly damage the nerves. With humeral fractures, the radial nerve is damaged around 12 percent of the time.[50]

The anatomic tunnels through which the ulnar, radial, and median nerves pass can result in entrapment symptoms. Inhibition of these nerves in the area of the elbow causes the symptoms to radiate distally, resulting in dysfunction in the wrist, hand, and fingers. This dysfunction is characterized by paresthesia, decreased grip strength, and the inability to actively extend the wrist depending on the nerve involved (Examination Findings 17-8). Figure 17-23 presents the sensory distribution of these nerves in the hand.

Examination of a patient with unexplained neurologic symptoms in the elbow, forearm, wrist, and/or hand should include a thorough examination of the cervical region (see Chapter 18).

Examination Findings 17-6
Distal Biceps Tendon Rupture

Examination Segment	Clinical Findings
History	***Onset:*** Acute ***Pain characteristics:*** Pain in the cubital fossa that decreases over time ***Mechanism:*** Eccentric loading of the biceps brachii while the elbow is flexed ***Predisposing conditions:*** More commonly seen after the third decade of life as the tensile strength of the tendon decreases A history of cigarette smoking Anabolic steroid use
Inspection	Swelling and ecchymosis in the cubital fossa
Palpation	Palpable defect in the distal biceps tendon; the lesion may be more easily recognized if the patient attempts to hold the elbow in 90° of flexion. The defect is more difficult to detect when the aponeurosis is intact than when it is ruptured along with the tendon.
Joint and Muscle Function Assessment	***AROM:*** Possibly within normal limits or slightly decreased during elbow flexion and extension and forearm pronation and supination secondary to pain ***MMT:*** Decreased strength for elbow flexors and forearm supinators ***PROM:*** Within normal limits; a partial tearing of the tendon may produce pain at the end range of elbow extension and pronation as the remaining fibers are stretched.
Joint Stability Tests	***Stress tests:*** Unremarkable ***Joint play:*** Unremarkable
Special Tests	Hook test
Neurologic Screening	Radial neuropathy may arise secondary to the trauma or the surgical technique.
Vascular Screening	Within normal limits
Functional Assessment	Patient will describe or demonstrate weakness in activities that require lifting.
Imaging Techniques	Radiographs, MRI, or CT scans are obtained to determine if an avulsion of the radial tuberosity has occurred and to rule out concomitant fractures.
Differential Diagnosis	Biceps tendon strain; avulsion fraction of the radial tuberosity
Comments	The long head of the biceps tendon may rupture in the shoulder.

AROM = active range of motion; CT = computed tomography; MMT = manual muscle test; PROM = passive range of motion.

Examination Findings 17-7
Osteochondritis Dissecans of the Capitellum

Examination Segment	Clinical Findings
History	***Onset:*** Insidious ***Pain characteristics:*** Dull, lateral elbow pain that is increased with activity ***Mechanism:*** Repetitive valgus loading of the elbow joint; compressive loading of the humeroulnar joint ***Predisposing conditions:*** Improper biomechanics Valgus instability
Inspection	Arm possibly postured with the elbow in flexion
Palpation	Tenderness over the capitellum, lateral epicondyle, and lateral joint line
Joint and Muscle Function Assessment	***AROM:*** Decreased extension; flexion contracture possible ***MMT:*** Pain secondary to compression placed through the joint ***PROM:*** Decreased extension; flexion contracture possible
Joint Stability Tests	***Stress tests:*** Valgus stress test ***Joint play:*** Unremarkable
Special Tests	Unremarkable
Neurologic Screening	Within normal limits
Vascular Screening	Within normal limits
Functional Assessment	Throwing: Increased lateral pain during late cocking and acceleration phase of cocking
Imaging Techniques	Abnormalities of the capitellum may be observed on MRI or on ultrasonic images
Differential Diagnosis	Radial nerve entrapment, epiphyseal fracture, posterolateral rotatory instability
Comments	Typically seen in adolescents participating in throwing athletics. The prognosis for a full return to activity is guarded.

AROM = active range of motion; MMT = manual muscle test; MRI = magnetic resonance imaging; PROM = passive range of motion.

Ulnar nerve pathology

As the ulnar nerve crosses the medial aspect of the elbow's joint line, it is relatively superficial, predisposing it to concussive forces. If the nerve's supporting structures are unstable, the nerve may chronically subluxate as the forearm is flexed, resulting in a progressive inflammation. The ulnar nerve is subject to additional traction forces during throwing, especially in the presence of medial elbow instability. The increased size of the inflamed structures causes a decrease in the cross-sectional size of the cubital tunnel leading to compression of the ulnar nerve.[51] The pressure within the ulnar nerve is elevated to more than three times the resting level when the elbow is flexed and the wrist is extended.[3]

Impairment of the ulnar nerve manifests its symptoms through decreased sensory and motor function in the hand and fingers. Patients will complain of increased symptoms when the elbow is flexed for prolonged periods. Increased night pain is common if the patient sleeps in with the elbow flexed. Acute trauma of the ulnar nerve causes a burning sensation in the medial forearm, little finger, and ring finger and decreased strength of the finger flexor muscles, lumbricals, interossei, thumb abductors, and flexor carpi ulnaris.

Examination Findings 17-8
Nerve Pathology at the Elbow

Examination Segment	Clinical Findings
History	***Onset:*** Insidious ***Pain characteristics:*** **Ulnar nerve:** Medial aspect of the elbow and forearm **Radial nerve**: Proximal forearm, wrist extensor region **Median nerve**: Anterior (volar) forearm ***Other symptoms:*** Numbness or paresthesia radiating into the nerve patterns (see Fig. 17–23): **Ulnar nerve**: Medial forearm, little finger and medial one half of ring finger **Radial nerve**: Lateral first metacarpal, dorsal lateral ventral hand, distal forearm. **Median nerve**: Ventral lateral hand (thumb to lateral one half of ring finger, anterior lateral forearm Pain may radiate from the elbow into the shoulder and cervical spine. ***Mechanism:*** Compression, traction, or inflammation of the nerve ***Predisposing conditions:*** Arthritis of the epicondylar groove or osteophytes can result in insidious nerve irritation. Diabetes Circulatory impairments Fractures
Inspection	Swelling may be noted.
Palpation	Pain may be elicited around the course of the nerve.
Joint and Muscle Function Assessment	***AROM:*** May be limited due to neurologic impairment. ***MMT:*** Weakness in the muscles serviced by the involved nerve ***PROM:*** Increased symptoms when nerve is maximally tensioned
Joint Stability Tests	***Stress tests:*** As needed to rule out underlying instability placing additional tension on nerve ***Joint play:*** As needed to rule out underlying instability placing additional tension on nerve
Special Tests	Tinel sign
Neurologic Screening	Assess the nerve distribution of the forearm, wrist, and hand. Electrodiagnostic studies may be required to definitively diagnose the condition.
Vascular Screening	Within normal limits
Functional Assessment	The function of the elbow, wrist, and hand may deteriorate with time.
Imaging Techniques	AP, oblique, and lateral views are used to identify neuropathy caused by bony defects.
Differential Diagnosis	Cervical nerve root compression, wrist compression, lateral epicondylalgia, carpal tunnel syndrome
Comments	A nerve can be compressed at multiple points along its path.

AP = anteroposterior; AROM = active range of motion; MMT = manual muscle test; PROM = passive range of motion.

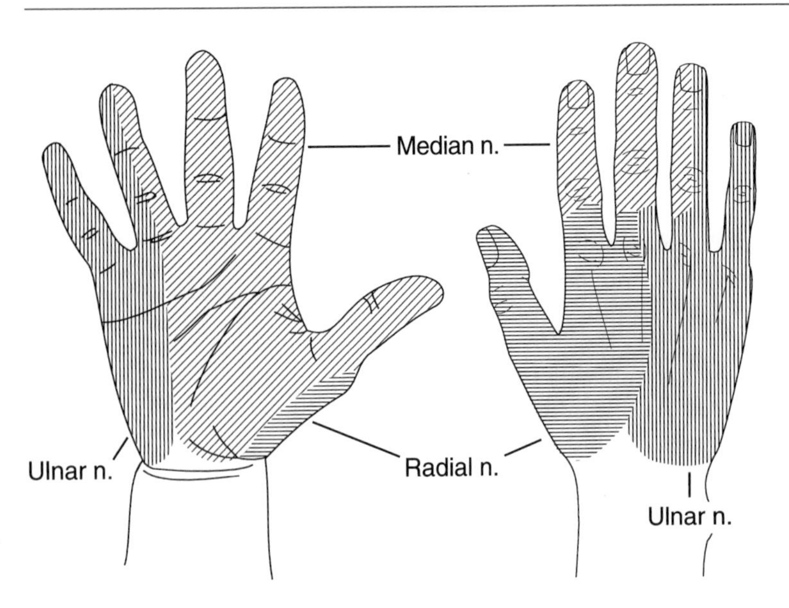

FIGURE 17-23 ■ The median, ulnar, and radial nerve sensory distribution in the hand. Note that texts differ on the exact delineation between the cutaneous distribution of the individual nerves.

Numbness on the dorsal aspect of the hand is indicative of ulnar neuropathy in the area of the elbow. Numbness on only the palmar side of the ulnar nerve distribution is indicative of ulnar nerve compression distal to the tunnel of Guyon where the nerve diverges into palmar and dorsal branches.[49]

Chronic neurologic deficit to these muscles causes the hand to deviate radially during flexion and results in the inability to maintain adduction of the little finger leaving it resting in an abducted position (**Wartenberg sign**).[40] This deficit also inhibits the individual's ability to make a fist because of a lack of flexion in the fourth and fifth distal interphalangeal (DIP) joints, characterized by a **clawhand** position (see Chapter 18).

Radial nerve pathology

The radial nerve is most often injured by deep lacerations of the elbow or secondary to fractures of the humerus or radius. The posterior interosseous nerve, the deep branch of the radial nerve, is dedicated to motor function of the thumb's extensors, wrist extensors, finger extensors, and supinators. Thus, there is no sensory loss associated with trauma to this nerve segment. If the superficial branch is lacerated or entrapped, sensory loss or paresthesia results on the posterior forearm and hand. Inflammation or irritation of the ulnar and radial nerves as they cross the elbow joint can be detected through Tinel's sign (Fig. 17-24).

Entrapment of the radial nerve, **radial tunnel syndrome** (RTS), clinically resembles lateral epicondylalgia.[13] Radial tunnel syndrome differs from epicondylalgia in that the symptoms of RTS are located more distally on the forearm. RTS can persist for more than 6 months with tenderness over the radial tunnel. Also, the symptoms may reproduced with resisted supination and during resisted extension of the middle finger, possibly resembling the findings of lateral epicondylalgia.[52]

Median nerve pathology

The median nerve is typically injured or compressed on the distal portion of the forearm. However, pressure in the cubital fossa may compress the nerve as it crosses the joint line. The most common clinical manifestation of median nerve trauma, **carpal tunnel syndrome**, is discussed in Chapter 18. A branch of the median nerve, the anterior interosseous nerve, can become compressed by the pronator teres, causing **pronator teres syndrome**. This syndrome is characterized by the patient's inability to pinch the tips of the thumb and index fingers together.

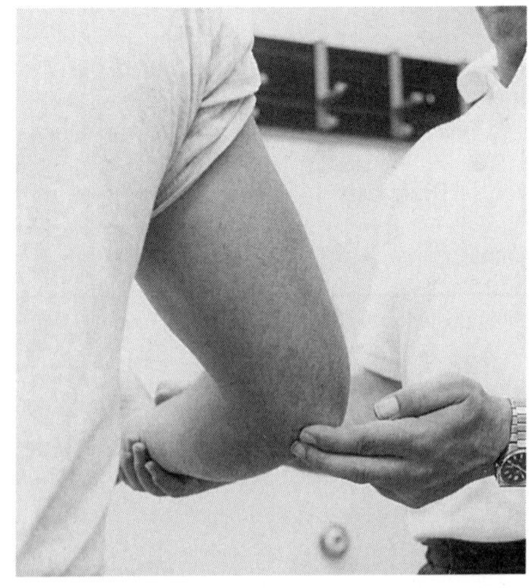

FIGURE 17-24 ■ Tinel's sign for neuropathy. In the presence of neuropathy, tapping on the ulnar (shown) or radial nerve results in a burning sensation in the hand.

Clawhand Positioning characterized by hyperextension of the metacarpophalangeal joints and flexion of the middle and distal phalanges resulting from trauma to the median and ulnar nerves.

Forearm compartment syndrome

The forearm contains three identifiable compartments: the volar, dorsal, and mobile wads.[53] Increased pressures within these compartments, possibly the result of hypertrophic muscles, hemorrhage, or fractures of the mid forearm, distal radius, or supracondylar area, increases the risk for compromising circulation and neurologic function of the hand.[53,54] As in the lower leg, forearm compartment syndromes can be exertional, subsiding with cessation of the offending activity, or acute.

In its early stages, forearm compartment syndrome is marked by complaints of pressure in the forearm, sensory disruption in the hand and fingers, decreased muscular strength, and pain during passive elongation of the involved muscles. Because of their deep location, the flexor digitorum profundus and the flexor pollicis longus are the most commonly affected muscles.[53] As the condition becomes more chronic or increases in severity, a decrease or absence of the radial or ulnar pulses are noted and **Volkmann's ischemic contracture** may develop (see Chapter 18). Surgery is often required to relieve the increased intracompartmental pressure. An acute forearm compartment syndrome can develop following fracture of the radius or ulna.

On-Field Evaluation of Elbow and Forearm Injuries

In most instances, acute injuries of the elbow do not require an on-field evaluation and subsequent management of the condition. The exceptions to this are elbow dislocations and fractures of the forearm or humerus. In these cases, the athlete remains down on the playing surface.

On-Field History

After the possibility of a fracture or dislocation has been ruled out, the circumstances surrounding the injury must be established:

- **Position of the arm:** When the hand is supporting the body weight, the arm is in a closed kinetic chain. Blows to the forearm, elbow, or humerus must be absorbed by the elbow's supportive structures, increasing the suspicion of acute ligamentous injuries.
- **Type of force involved:** The nature of the force delivered to the elbow must be determined. Landing on the palm of the hand delivers a longitudinal force up the radius that is transferred to the ulna by the interosseous membrane. A force to the lateral side of the elbow places stress on the UCL, and a medial force stresses the RCL. A force from the posterior aspect of the elbow results in hyperextension of the joint and places shear forces on the olecranon process. A blunt force places compressive forces on the tissues beneath the location of the impact.

On-Field Inspection

The primary tool in the evaluation of these conditions is inspection of the injured area. Elbow dislocation and forearm or humeral fractures tend to result in gross deformity, but radial and ulnar fractures are inherently more noticeable.

- **Alignment of forearm and wrist:** Observe the length of the radius and ulna for gross deformity and note the relationship between the forearm and wrist. A complete fracture of either of the long bones may alter the wrist's position relative to the forearm.
- **Posterior triangle of the elbow:** Note the alignment of the medial epicondyle, lateral epicondyle, and the olecranon process. These structures should form an isosceles triangle when the elbow is flexed to 90 degrees. Any deviation of this relationship may indicate a dislocation. In the event of a posterior dislocation, the olecranon process becomes overly prominent. If either condition exists, the evaluation must be terminated immediately and the athlete must be referred to a physician after appropriate immobilization.

On-Field Palpation

Palpation is performed to confirm the suspicion of injury established during the history-taking process while also ruling out any other gross trauma.

- **Alignment of the elbow:** Palpate the medial epicondyle, lateral epicondyle, and olecranon for tenderness, crepitus, and improper alignment.
- **Collateral ligaments:** Palpate the RCL and UCL along their lengths to identify any pain or crepitus along these structures. Crepitus at the ligament's origin or insertion may indicate an avulsion.
- **Radius and ulna:** Palpate the length of the radius and ulna for tenderness, deformity, or false joints indicative of a fracture.

On-Field Joint and Muscle Function Tests

Before deciding whether to splint the arm, the athlete's willingness and ability to move the elbow must be established:

- **Active range of motion:** Ask the athlete to wiggle the fingers, move the wrist through flexion and extension and radial and ulnar deviation, and then through forearm pronation and supination and elbow flexion and extension. The inability to perform any one of these steps or significant pain with these motions warrants the immobilization of the elbow, forearm, and wrist before the athlete is removed from the field. If the patient can fully extend the elbow it is unlikely that an elbow fracture is present.[55]
- **Manual muscle tests:** Although this portion of the examination can be delayed until the athlete is removed to the sideline, establish a baseline of strength

for future comparison. Nerve root compression may result in a short-term loss of strength that rapidly returns to normal.

- **Passive range of motion:** After the athlete has displayed the ability to actively and willingly move the elbow, passively move the joint through its ROMs. Osteochondral fractures cause a premature end-point in the ROM. Fractures of the olecranon process cause pain at the terminal range of extension.

On-Field Neurologic Tests

The immediate evaluation of elbow injuries may necessitate the neurologic assessment of the forearm and hand. Refer to the section of this chapter on neurologic testing and see Figure 17-23.

On-Field Management of Elbow and Forearm Injuries

The most significant injuries facing athletic trainers during the on-field evaluation are dislocations of the elbow joint and fractures of the forearm. These conditions require careful management to prevent further trauma to the involved structures and protect the neurovascular network supplying the hand. Fractures of the forearm or dislocations of the elbow may lead to the onset of Volkmann's ischemic contracture (see Chapter 15).

Elbow Dislocations

The elbow is immobilized in the position in which it is found, while still allowing the distal pulse to be monitored. Concomitant injury to the glenohumeral joint, proximal humerus, and wrist must be ruled out. The athlete must be immediately transported for further medical treatment by a physician.

Fracture About the Elbow

Fractures of the radius and ulna may compromise the neurovascular supply to the wrist and hand. Because of this, distal pulses must be monitored constantly after the injury. At that time, the elbow, forearm, and wrist must be immobilized to minimize movement of the fractured bones. After the area has been stabilized, the athlete must be immediately transported and monitored for shock.

REFERENCES

1. Stroyan, M, and Wilk, KE: The functional anatomy of the elbow complex. *J Orthop Sports Phys Ther,* 17:279, 1993.
2. Smith, AM, et al: Radius pull test: Predictor of longitudinal forearm instability. *J Bone Joint Surg,* 84(A):1970, 2002.
3. Chen, FS, Rokito, AS, and Jobe, FW: Medial elbow problems in the overhead-throwing athlete. *J Am Acad Orthop Surg,* 9:99, 2001.
4. Ramsey, ML: Distal biceps tendon injuries: Diagnosis and management. *J Am Acad Orthop Surg,* 7:199, 1999.
5. McClung, MR: Do current management strategies and guidelines adequately address fracture risk? *Bone,* 38:S13, 2006.
6. Hak, DJ, and Golladay, GJ: Olecranon fractures: Treatment options. *J Am Acad Orthop Surg,* 8:266, 2000.
7. Hatch, GF, et al: The effect of tennis racket grip size on forearm muscle firing patterns. *Am J Sports Med,* 34:1997, 2006.
8. Cain, EL, et al: Elbow injuries in throwing athletes: A current concepts review. *Am J Sports Med,* 31:621, 2003.
9. King, JW, Brelsford, HJ, and Tullos, HS: Analysis of the pitching arm of the professional baseball pitcher. *Clin Orthop,* 67:116, 1969.
10. O'Driscoll, SW, et al: Tardy posterolateral rotatory instability of the elbow due to cubitus varus. *J Bone Joint Surg,* 83:1358, 2001.
11. Doughty, MP: Drop wrist: Complications following a comminuted fracture of the radius. Orthotic glove designed to permit participation. *Athl Train: J Natl Athl Train Assoc,* 22:221, 1987.
12. Andrews, JR, et al: Physical examination of the thrower's elbow. *J Orthop Sports Phys Ther,* 17:269, 1993.
13. Ekstrom, RA, and Holden, R: Examination of and intervention for a patient with chronic lateral elbow pain with signs of nerve entrapment. *Phys Ther,* 82:1077, 2002.
14. Wright, RW, et al: Elbow range of motion in professional baseball pitchers. *Am J Sports Med,* 34:190-193, 2006.
15. Gajdosik, RL: Comparison and reliability of three goniometric methods for measuring forearm supination and pronation. *Percept Mot Skills,* 93:353, 2001.
16. Karagiannopoulos, C, Sitler, M, and Michlovitz, S: Reliability of 2 functional goniometric methods for measuring forearm pronation and supination active range of motion. *J Orthop Sports Phys Ther,* 33:523, 2003.
17. Rainville, J, et al: Assessment of forearm pronation strength in C6 and C7 radiculopathies. *Spine,* 32:72, 2007.
18. Cohen, MS, and Hastings, H: Acute elbow dislocation: Evaluation and management. *J Am Acad Orthop Surg,* 6:15, 1998.
19. Morrey, BF: Acute and chronic instability of the elbow. *J Am Acad Orthop Surg,* 4:117, 1996.
20. Ring, D, Jupiter, JB, and Zilberfarb, J: Posterior dislocation of the elbow with fractures of the radial head and coronoid. *J Bone Joint Surg,* 84(A):547, 2002.
21. Rosenberg, N, Soudry, M, and Stahl, S: Comparison of two methods for the evaluation of treatment in medial epicondylitis: Pain estimation vs grip strength measurements. *Arch Orthop Trauma Surg,* 124:363, 2004.
22. Arnander, MWT, and Newman, KJH: Forearm fractures. *Surgery (Oxford),* 24:426, 2006.
23. Hume, PA, Reid, D, and Edwards, T: Epicondylar injury in sport. Epidemiology, type, mechanisms, assessment, management, and prevention. *Sports Med,* 36:151, 2006.
24. Chen, AL, et al: Imaging of the elbow in the overhead throwing athlete. *Am J Sports Med,* 31:466, 2003.
25. O'Driscoll, SWM, Lawton, RL, and Smith, AM: The "Moving valgus stress test" for medial collateral ligament tears of the elbow. *Am J Sports Med,* 33:231, 2005.
26. Werner, SL, et al: Biomechanics of the elbow during baseball pitching. *J Orthop Sports Phys Ther,* 17:274, 1993.
27. Smidt, N, et al: Corticosteroid injections, physiotherapy, or a wait-and-see policy for lateral epicondylitis: A randomised controlled trial. *Lancet,* 359:657, 2002.

28. Nestor, BJ, O'Driscoll, SW, and Morrey, BF: Ligamentous reconstruction for posterolateral rotatory instability of the elbow. *J Bone Joint Surg Am,* 74:1235, 1992.
29. Dunning, CE, et al: Ligamentous stabilizers against posterolateral rotatory instability of the elbow. *J Bone Joint Surg,* 83(A):1823, 2001.
30. Bisset, L, et al: Mobilisation with movement and exercise, corticosteroid injection, or wait and see for tennis elbow: Randomized trial. *BMJ,* doi:10.1136/bmj.38961.584653.AE (published 29 September 2006).
31. Waugh, EJ, Jaglal, SB, and Davis, AM: Computer use associated with poor long-term prognosis of conservatively managed lateral epicondylalgia. *J Orthop Sports Phys Ther,* 34:770, 2004.
32. Pienimä, TT, Siira, PT, and Vanharanta, H: Chronic medial and lateral epicondylitis: A comparison of pain, disability, and function. *Arch Phys Med Rehabil,* 83:317, 2002.
33. Wilson, JJ, and Best, TM: Common overuse tendon problems: A review and recommendations for treatment. *Am Fam Phys,* 72:811, 2005.
34. Jobe, FW, and Ciccotti, MG: Lateral and medial epicondylitis of the elbow. *J Am Acad Orthop Surg,* 2:1, 1994.
35. Lieber, RL, Ljung, BO, and Friden, J: Sarcomere length in wrist extensor muscles. Changes may provide insights into the etiology of chronic lateral epicondylitis. *Acta Orthop Scand,* 68:249, 1997.
36. Smidt, N, et al: Interobserver reproducibility of the assessment of severity of complaints, grip strength, and pressure pain thresholds in patients with lateral epicondylitis. *Arch Phys Med Rehabil,* 83:1145, 2002.
37. Haker, E: Lateral epicondylalgia: Diagnosis, treatment, and evaluation. *Crit Rev Phys Rehabil Med,* 5:129, 1993.
38. Hang, DW, Chao, CM, and Hang, Y-S: A clinical and roentgenographic study of Little League elbow. *Am J Sports Med,* 32:79, 2004.
39. Gabel, GT, and Morrey, BF: Operative treatment of medial epicondylitis. Influence of concomitant ulnar neuropathy at the elbow. *J Bone Joint Surg,* 77(A):1065, 1995.
40. Safran, MR, and Graham, SM: Distal biceps tendon ruptures: Incidence, demographics, and the effect of smoking. *Clin Orthop Relat Res,* 404:275, 2002.
41. Agins, HJ, et al: Rupture of the distal insertion of the biceps tendon. *Clin Orthop,* 234:34, 1988.
42. D'Allesandro, DF, et al: Repair of distal biceps tendon ruptures in athletes. *Am J Sports Med,* 21:114, 1993.
43. D'Arco, P, et al: Clinical, functional, and radiographic assessments of the conventional and modified Boyd-Anderson surgical procedures for repair of distal biceps tendon ruptures. *Am J Sports Med,* 26:254, 1998.
44. O'Driscoll, SW, Goncalves, LBJ, and Dietz, P: The hook test for distal biceps tendon avulsion. *Am J Sports Med,* 35:1865, 2007.
45. Baker, BE, and Bierwagen, D: Rupture of the distal tendon of the biceps brachii: Operative versus non-operative treatment. *J Bone Joint Surg,* 67(A):414, 1985.
46. Friedmann, E: Rupture of the distal biceps brachii tendon: Report on 13 cases. *J Am Med Assoc,* 184:60, 1963.
47. Morrey, BF, et al: Rupture of the distal tendon of the biceps brachii: A biomechanical study. *J Bone Joint Surg,* 67(A):418, 1985.
48. Takahara, M, et al: Early detection of osteochondritis dissecans of the capitellum in young baseball players. Report of three cases. *J Bone Joint Surg,* 80(A):892, 1998.
49. Posner, MA: Compressive ulnar neuropathies at the elbow: I. Etiology and diagnosis. *J Am Acad Orthop Surg,* 6:282, 1998.
50. Shao, YC, et al: Radial nerve palsy associated with fractures of the shaft of the humerus. *J Bone Jt Surg (Br.),* 87-B:1647, 2005.
51. Barker, C: Evaluation, treatment, and rehabilitation involving a submuscular transposition of the ulnar nerve at the elbow. *Athl Train: J Natl Athl Train Assoc,* 23:10, 1988.
52. Lutz, FR: Radial tunnel syndrome: An etiology of chronic lateral elbow pain. *J Orthop Sports Phys Ther,* 14:14, 1991.
53. Botte, MJ, and Gelberman, RH: Acute compartment syndrome of the forearm. *Hand Clin,* 14:391, 1998.
54. Peters, CL, and Scott, SM: Compartment syndrome in the forearm following fractures of the radial head or neck in children. *J Bone Joint Surg,* 77(A):1070, 1995.
55. Docherty, MA, Schwab, RA, and Ma, OJ: Can elbow extension be used as a test of clinically significant injury? *South Med J,* 95:539, 2002.

CHAPTER 18

Wrist, Hand, and Finger Pathologies

The shoulder is equipped for mobility and gross placement of the arm in space. The elbow is equipped for stability. The wrist, hand, and fingers, the final links in the chain, are perfectly equipped for strength and precision. Injury to this area includes impairment of gross and fine motor movements. The extent of an individual's disability after injury to these areas depends on the nature of necessary tasks and whether or not the dominant extremity is involved. In football, a hand injury that has little consequence to a lineman could be disabling to a quarterback or wide receiver. In a sport such as basketball, injuries to the nonshooting hand impact the athlete's ability less than those involving the shooting hand.

Clinical Anatomy

The distal portions of the radius and ulna, eight carpal bones, five metacarpals, and 14 phalanges, form the skeleton of the wrist, hand, and fingers (Fig. 18-1). The **distal radius** broadens to form a small **ulnar notch** on its medial surface to accept the ulnar head, and the **radial styloid process** projects off its anterolateral border. The **ulnar head** is more circular, with the **ulnar styloid process** arising from its medial surface.

Having unusual shapes and irregular surfaces, the **carpal bones** are aligned in two rows (Fig. 18-2). From the radial to ulnar sides, the proximal row consists of the scaphoid, lunate, triquetrum, and the pisiform bones. The distal row is formed by the trapezium, trapezoid, capitate, and hamate bones. In the distal carpal row, the trapezium aligns with the first **metacarpal**, the trapezoid with the second metacarpal, the capitate with the third metacarpal, and the fourth and fifth metacarpals with the hamate. The pisiform "floats" on the triquetrum, acting as a sesamoid bone to improve the mechanical efficiency of the flexor carpi ulnaris muscle. The scaphoid is the most commonly fractured of the carpals, and the lunate is the most commonly dislocated.

Much of the length of the hand is formed by the metacarpals, numbered from I (thumb) to V (little finger). Shaped similarly to long bones, the proximal articulating surfaces are concave to accept the convex surface of the

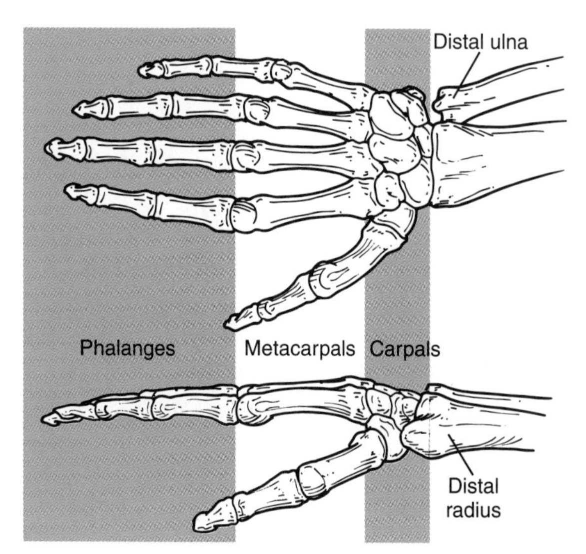

FIGURE 18-1 ■ Bones of the wrist and hand, formed by the radius and ulna, 8 carpals, 5 metacarpals, and 14 phalanges.

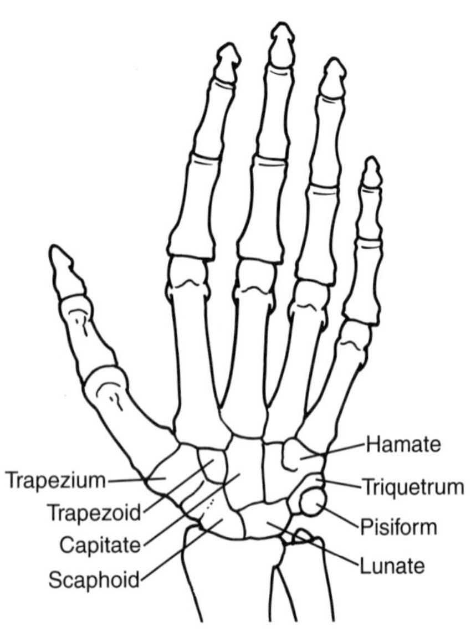

FIGURE 18-2 ■ Carpal bones of the hand.

carpals. The distal surfaces are convex to accept the concave surface of the proximal phalanx of each of the fingers. Each finger (except the thumb, which has only a proximal and distal phalanx) has a **proximal**, **middle**, and **distal** phalanx. The proximal aspect of these bones is referred to as the base, and the distal aspect is referred to as the head.

Two small sesamoid bones are located over the palmar aspect of the distal end of the first metacarpal (see Fig. 18-2). These mobile bones improve the mechanical line of pull of the flexor pollicis brevis, abductor pollicis brevis, and adductor pollicis muscles.

Articulations and Ligamentous Support

The motion produced by the wrist, hand, and fingers occurs through the interaction of several joints. Several force couples among each joint's associated muscles facilitate the precise coordination needed at the wrist and hand. An overview of the interactions involving specific joints is described in this section.

Distal radioulnar joint

The distal radioulnar articulation, formed by the ulnar head and the ulnar notch of the radius, allows 1 degree of freedom of movement: pronation and supination. The distal and proximal radioulnar joints work together to produce those motions. Restriction of motion at either of these joints limits pronation and supination of the entire forearm. At the distal radioulnar joint, pronation and supination is produced by the radius' gliding around the ulna. However, the ulna moves slightly palmarly and medially during supination and posteriorly and laterally during pronation.

Radiocarpal joint

The radiocarpal articulation is an ellipsoid joint that provides 2 degrees of freedom of movement: flexion and extension and radial and **ulnar deviation**. The joint is formed by the distal end of the radius' articulation with the scaphoid and lunate. Through its connection to the distal radius, the triangular fibrocartilage functionally extends this joint to incorporate the triquetrum.

The joint is covered by a fibrous capsule reinforced by ligamentous thickenings (Fig. 18-3). The **radial collateral ligament** (RCL), originating off the styloid process and inserting on the scaphoid and trapezium, limits ulnar deviation and becomes taut when the wrist is at the extreme ranges of flexion and extension.

The most important ligament for controlling motion and wrist stability is the **palmar radiocarpal ligament**.[1] This structure originates from the anterior surface of the distal radius and courses obliquely and medially to split into three individual segments, each named for the bone to which it attaches: the **radiocapitate ligament**, **radiotriquetral ligament**, and **radioscaphoid ligament**. As a unit, these

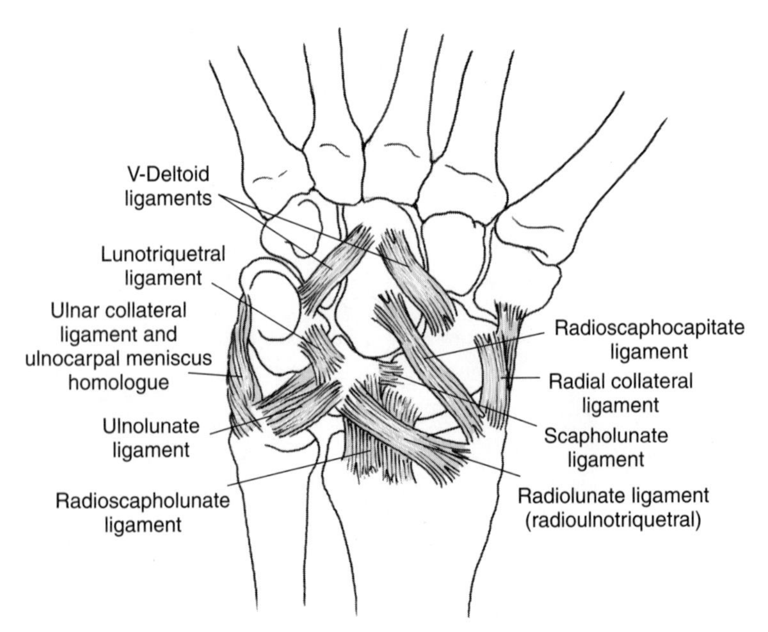

FIGURE 18-3 ■ Palmar (volar) ligaments of the left wrist and hand. Note the three bands of the palmar radiocarpal ligament: radioscaphocapitate, radiolunate, and radioscapholunate ligaments. (Courtesy of Norkin, CC, and Levangie, PK: *Joint Structure and Function: A Comprehensive Analysis*, ed 4. Philadelphia: FA Davis, 2005.)

ligaments maintain the alignment of the associated joint structures and limit hyperextension of the wrist.

The **dorsal radiocarpal ligament** is the only major ligament on the **dorsal** surface of the wrist (Fig. 18-4). Arising from the posterior surface of the distal radius and styloid process, this ligament attaches to the lunate and triquetrum to limit wrist flexion.

The ulna is buffered from the proximal row of carpals by the **triangular fibrocartilaginous complex** (TFCC). The TFCC is composed of the articular disk (or fibrocartilage), the dorsal and palmar radioulnar ligaments, the ulnar collateral ligament, and the meniscus homolog (meaning like a meniscus), which attaches the fibrocartilage to the triquetrum (Fig. 18-5).[2] The TFCC dissipates stresses imposed on the forearm during loading, stabilizes the distal radioulnar joint, and extends the radiocarpal articulation by stabilizing the ulnar side carpals.[3]

The **ulnar collateral ligament** (UCL) arises from the ulna's styloid process and attaches on the medial aspect of the triquetrum dorsally and the pisiform palmarly. This ligament checks **radial deviation** and becomes taut at the end-ranges of flexion and extension. Medially, the small palmar ulnocarpal ligament originates from the distal ulna, blends in with the UCL, and attaches to the lunate and triquetrum.

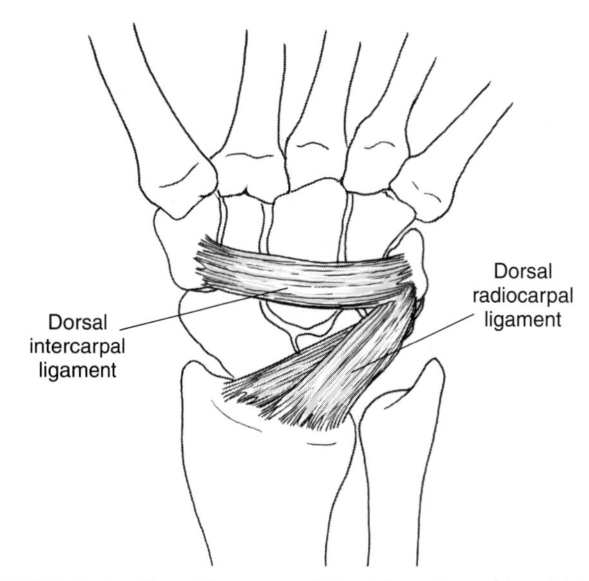

FIGURE 18-4 ■ Dorsal ligaments of the right wrist and hand. Note the horizontal "V" configuration of these ligaments that adds to radiocarpal stability. (Courtesy of Norkin, CC, and Levangie, PK: *Joint Structure and Function: A Comprehensive Analysis*, ed 4. Philadelphia: FA Davis, 2005.)

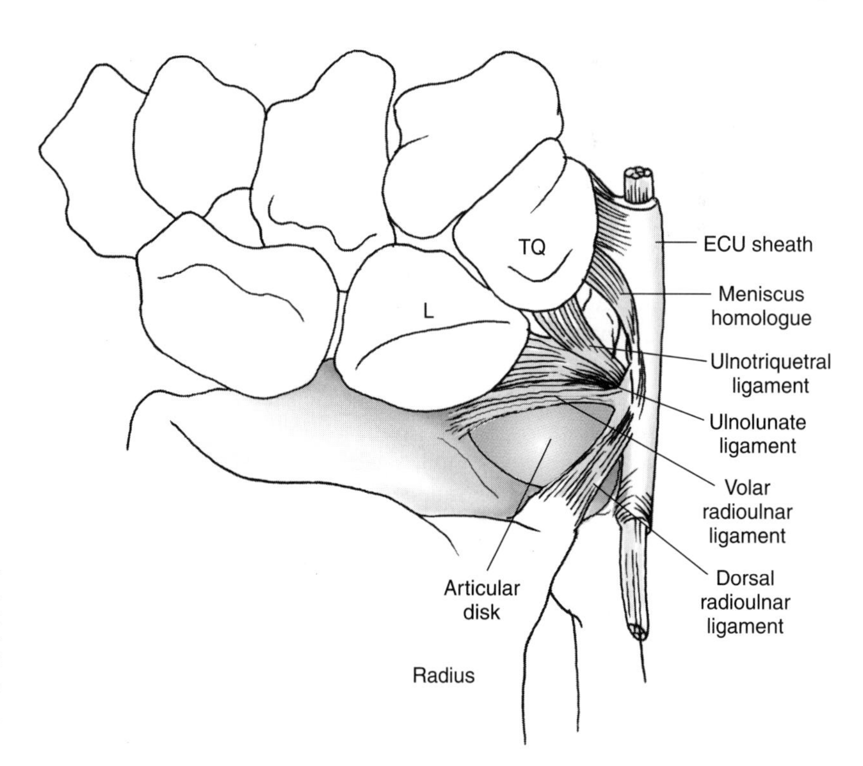

FIGURE 18-5 ■ The triangular fibrocartilage complex (TFCC). Several ligaments and other fibrous structures attach to the fibrocartilage. As a unit the TFCC provides support to the distal radioulnar joint. L = lunate; TQ = triquetrum. (Courtesy of Norkin, CC, and Levangie, PK: *Joint Structure and Function: A Comprehensive Analysis*, ed 4. Philadelphia: FA Davis, 2005.)

Ulnar deviation Movement of the hand toward the ulnar side of the forearm.

Dorsal (upper extremity) The posterior aspect of the hand and forearm relative to the anatomical position.

Radial deviation Movement of the hand toward the radial (thumb) side.

Intercarpal joints

Capsular and interosseous ligaments bind the carpal bones tightly together. Each carpal bone is fixated to its contiguous carpal in the same row by small palmar, dorsal, and **interosseous ligaments**. The capsular ligaments arise from the radius and insert on the individual carpals.[4] This ligamentous arrangement allows for very little gliding movement between the bones adjacent to one another within a row.

The interosseous C-shaped **scapholunate** and **lunotriquetral** ligaments span the dorsal and palmar aspects of the palmar edges of the scaphoid, lunate, and triquetrum. The palmar segments of these ligaments are stronger than the dorsal. Balancing the lunate between the scaphoid and the triquetrum leads to the lunate exerting a flexion force through the scapholunate ligament and an extension force through the lunotriquetral ligament.[5] Disruption of one of these carpals and/or its associated ligament can result in profound dysfunction of the carpal group's biomechanics.

Midcarpal joints

The proximal and distal carpal rows are separated by a single joint cavity with small fibrous projections connecting the rows. This structure allows limited gliding movements of flexion and extension and radial and ulnar deviation that are needed to obtain the normal amount of wrist flexion and extension.

Carpometacarpal joints

Each of the first three metacarpals articulates primarily with a single carpal: metacarpal I with the trapezium and metacarpal III with the capitate. The broad base of the second metacarpal articulates primarily with the trapezoid, but also has an articulation with the trapezium and capitate. The fourth and fifth metacarpals articulate with the hamate to form one of the **carpometacarpal (CMC) joints** (see Fig. 18-2).

The first CMC joint, that of the thumb, has a synovial cavity separate from the lateral four joints. Classified as a saddle joint, the first CMC joint is capable of 2 degrees of freedom of movement: flexion and extension and abduction and adduction. An accessory rotational component occurs concurrently with these motions, allowing for **opposition**, a combined movement that allows the thumb to touch each of the four fingers (the return motion from opposition is **reposition**).

The CMC joints II through IV are **plane synovial joints** that have 1 degree of freedom of movement: flexion and extension. The fifth CMC joint has 2 degrees of movement: flexion and extension and abduction and adduction. Several small ligaments support these joints and allow progressively more motion with each medial joint. The second and third CMC joints are practically immobile, but the fourth and fifth have greater mobility, allowing the hand to strongly grip small objects.

Plane synovial joint A synovial joint formed by the gliding between two or more bones.

Metacarpophalangeal and interphalangeal joints

The condyloid metacarpophalangeal joints are capable of 2 degrees of freedom of movement: flexion and extension, and abduction and adduction. The five metacarpophalangeal (MCP) articulations represent the union between the concave articular surface of the proximal phalanx of each finger and the convex articular surface of the associated metacarpal. Although the thumb is capable of abducting and adducting at any point in the range of motion (ROM), the maximum amount of this abduction and adduction in the lateral four fingers is possible only when they are fully extended.

Support against valgus and varus forces is provided by pairs of collateral ligaments running obliquely from the dorsal aspect of the side of the metacarpal to the palmar aspect of the phalanx. As the fingers are flexed, these ligaments tighten, limiting the amount of abduction and adduction available to the joint in this position. This feature makes gripping less dependent on dynamic stability.

The palmar aspect of the MCP joints is reinforced by a thick fibrocartilaginous **palmar ligament**. The dorsal aspects of the lateral four MCP joints are reinforced by the expansion of the extensor hood. Reinforcement is also provided by the deep transverse metacarpal ligament. These strong bands limit abduction and adduction and reinforce the palmar ligaments. MCP hyperextension is primarily limited by the intrinsic musculature.[6]

With one on the thumb and two on the remaining fingers, the interphalangeal (IP) joints have 1 degree of freedom: flexion and extension. Like the MCP joints, the IP joints have a thick palmar ligament (Volar plate) that restricts extension and radial and ulnar collateral ligaments that restrict abduction and adduction. The shallow bony configuration of the IP joints results in a reliance on soft tissue structures for stability.

Muscular Anatomy

The muscles of the wrist and hand function under a broad spectrum of circumstances and demands. The same muscles that are used to grip strongly are also called on to perform the most delicate of fine motor skills. The extrinsic muscles acting on the wrist, including the long muscles of the fingers, are described in Table 18-1. The intrinsic muscles of the hand are presented in Table 18-2.

The natural, relaxed position of the hand and fingers is one of slight flexion. This positioning is caused by the relative shortness of the finger flexors. This concept is demonstrated by noting how the fingers flex as the wrist is passively extended.

Extensor muscles

Located on the posterolateral portion of the forearm, the wrist and finger extensor muscles form six compartments in the dorsal aspect of the wrist and are primarily innervated by the radial nerve (Fig. 18-6). The wrist extensor muscles stabilize the wrist in extension so that the refined finger flexors are optimally positioned to function. Figures 17–6 and 17–7 show the locations of these muscles relative to the forearm, and Figures 18-7 and 18-8 show the locations of their insertions on the wrist and hand.

The superficial muscles originating on the posterior humerus and forearm, the **extensor carpi radialis longus and brevis** and **extensor carpi ulnaris**, are the primary wrist extensors. The **extensor digitorum communis**, the primary extensor of the interphalangeal (IP) joints of the lateral four fingers, assists in wrist extension. The brachioradialis is also located in the superficial compartment, but it does not directly influence wrist movement.

The deep compartment contains the thumb's extensors, the **extensor pollicis longus** and the **extensor pollicis brevis**, and its primary abductor, the **abductor pollicis longus**. The long extensor of the second finger, the **extensor indicus**, is also located in this compartment. The remaining deep muscle, the **supinator**, is capable of supinating the forearm at all angles of elbow flexion but has no action on the hand or fingers.

The extensor muscles are secured to the posterior portion of the distal radius and ulna by the **extensor retinaculum.** This strong, transverse band increases the efficiency of the muscles' pull and prevents "bow stringing" when the wrist is extended.

Flexor muscles

The anteromedial forearm is also divided into two compartments, superficial and deep. The superficial compartment houses the wrist's flexor muscles, the **flexor carpi radialis**, **palmaris longus** (absent in approximately 12% to 15% of the population), and **flexor carpi ulnaris.** The **flexor digitorum superficialis**, responsible for flexion of the four proximal interphalangeal (PIP) joints, and the **pronator**

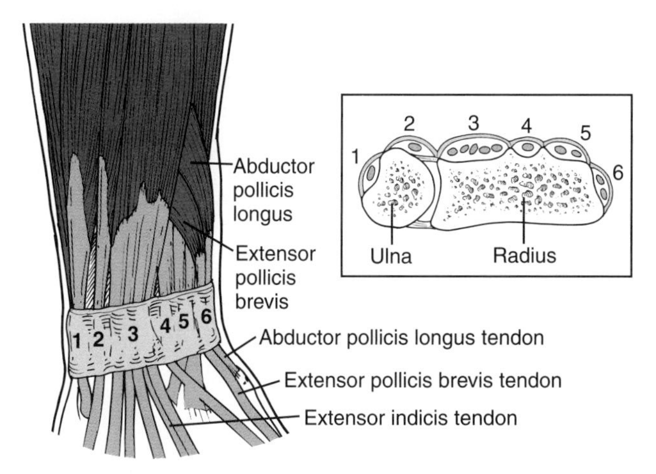

FIGURE 18-6 ■ Extensor compartment. Each group passes beneath the extensor retinaculum and contained within a compartment. From ulnar to radial: *1*, extensor digiti minimi; *2*, extensor carpi ulnaris; *3*, extensor digitorum communis and extensor indicus; *4*, extensor pollicis longus; *5*, extensor carpi radialis longus and extensor carpi radialis brevis; *6*, abductor pollicis longus and extensor pollicis brevis.

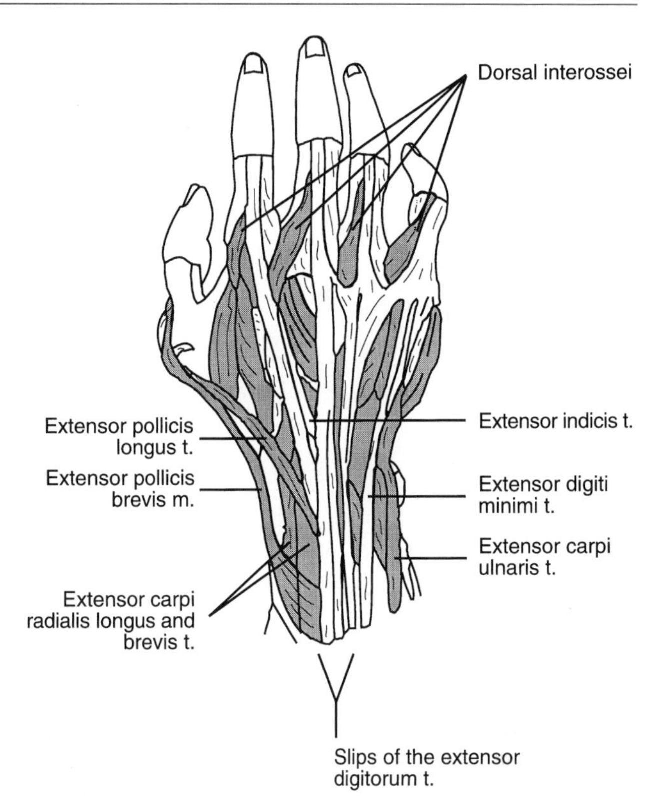

FIGURE 18-7 ■ Intrinsic muscles of the dorsal hand and attachments of the long finger extensors.

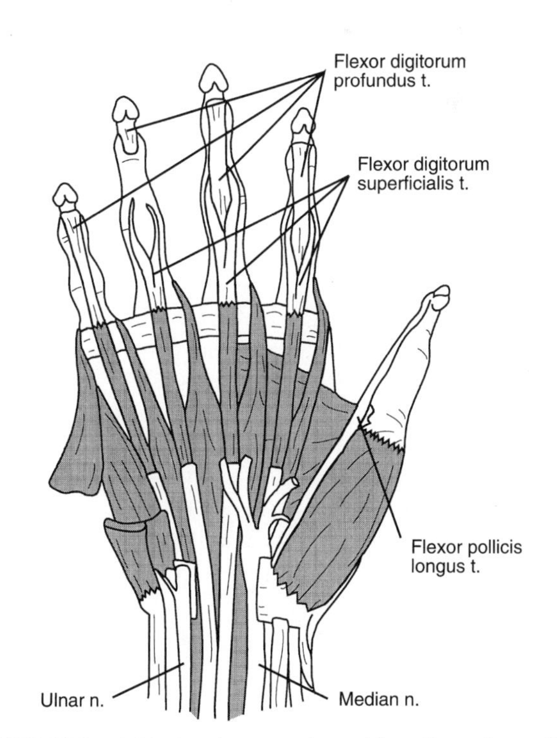

FIGURE 18-8 ■ Intrinsic palmar muscles and long finger flexors. Note the location of the ulnar and median nerves.

Table 18-1 Extrinsic Muscles Acting on the Wrist and Hand

Muscle	Action	Origin	Insertion	Innervation	Root
Abductor Pollicis Longus	1st CMC joint abduction 1st CMC joint extension Assists in radial deviation of the wrist	Posterior surface of the distal ulna Posterior surface of the distal radius Adjoining interosseous membrane	Radial side of the base of the 1st metacarpal	Median	C6, C7
Extensor Carpi Radialis Brevis	Wrist extension Radial deviation	Lateral epicondyle via the common extensor tendon Radial collateral ligament	Base of the 3rd metacarpal	Radial	C6, C7
Extensor Carpi Radialis Longus	Wrist extension Radial deviation	Supracondylar ridge of humerus	Radial side of the base of the 2nd metacarpal	Radial	C6, C7
Extensor Carpi Ulnaris	Wrist extension Ulnar deviation	Lateral epicondyle via the common extensor tendon	Ulnar side of the base of the 5th metacarpal	Deep radial	C6, C7, C8
Extensor Digiti Minimi	5th MCP joint extension 5th DIP and PIP extension, working with the lumbricalis and interossei	Lateral epicondyle via the common extensor tendon Deep antebrachial fascia	To the middle and distal phalanx of the 5th finger via the extensor digitorum longus tendon	Radial	C6, C7, C8
Extensor Digitorum Communis	Wrist extension MCP extension IP extension Radial deviation of the wrist	Lateral epicondyle via the common extensor tendon	Dorsal surface of the proximal base of the middle and distal phalanges of each of the four fingers	Deep radial	C6, C7, C8
Extensor Indicis	2nd MCP extension (index finger) 2nd DIP and PIP extension, working with the lumbricalis and interossei	Posterior surface of the ulna, distal to the extensor pollicis longus Interosseous membrane	To the middle and distal phalanx of the index finger via the extensor digitorum longus tendon	Radial	C6, C7, C8
Extensor Pollicis Brevis	1st MCP joint extension 1st CMC joint extension 1st CMC joint abduction Assists in wrist radial deviation	Posterior surface of the distal radius Adjoining interosseous membrane	Dorsal surface of the base of the proximal phalanx of the thumb	Deep radial	C6, C7
Extensor Pollicis Longus	1st IP joint extension 1st MCP joint extension 1st CMC joint extension Assists in wrist extension Assists in wrist radial deviation	Posterior surface of the middle one third of the ulna Adjoining interosseous membrane	Dorsal surface of the base of the distal phalanx of the thumb	Deep radial	C6, C7, C8

Flexor Carpi Radialis	Wrist flexion Forearm pronation Radial deviation	Medial epicondyle via the common flexor tendon	Bases of the 2nd and 3rd metacarpals	Median	C6, C7
Flexor Carpi Ulnaris	Wrist flexion Ulnar deviation	Humeral head • Medial epicondyle via the common flexor tendon Ulnar head • Medial border of the olecranon • Proximal two thirds of the posterior ulna	Pisiform Hamate 5th metacarpal	Ulnar	C8, T1
Flexor Digitorum Profundus	DIP flexion PIP flexion Wrist flexion	Anteromedial proximal three fourths of ulna and associated interosseous membrane	Bases of the medial phalanges of digits II–V	Palmar interosseous	C8, T1
Flexor Digitorum Superficialis	PIP flexion MCP flexion Wrist flexion	Humeral head • Medial epicondyle via the common flexor tendon • Ulnar collateral ligament Ulnar head • Coronoid process Radial head • Oblique line of radius	Sides of the middle phalanges of digits II–V	Median	C7, C8, T1
Flexor Pollicis Longus	1st IP joint flexion 1st MCP joint flexion Assists in wrist flexion	Anterior surface of the radius Adjoining interosseous membrane Coronoid process of ulna	Palmar surface of the base of the distal phalanx of the thumb	Palmar interosseous	C8, T1
Palmaris Longus	Wrist flexion	Medial epicondyle via the common flexor tendon	Flexor retinaculum Palmar aponeurosis	Median	C6, C7

CMC = carpometacarpal; DIP = distal interphalangeal; IP = interphalangeal; MCP = metacarpophalangeal; PIP = proximal interphalangeal.

Table 18-2 Intrinsic Muscles Acting on the Hand

Muscle	Action	Origin	Insertion	Innervation	Root
Abductor Digiti Minimi	Abduction of the 5th finger Assists in opposition	Tendon of flexor carpi ulnaris Pisiform	By two slips into the 5th finger • Ulnar side of the base of the proximal phalanx • Ulnar border of the extensor expansion	Ulnar	C8, T1
Abductor Pollicis Brevis	1st CMC joint abduction 1st MCP joint abduction Assists in opposition	Flexor retinaculum Trapezium Scaphoid	Radial surface of the base of the proximal phalanx of the thumb Via a slip into the extensor expansion	Median	C6, C7
Adductor Pollicis	1st CMC joint adduction 1st MCP joint adduction 1st MCP joint flexion Assists in opposition	Capitate bone Bases of 2nd and 3rd metacarpals Palmar surface of 3rd metacarpal	Ulnar surface of the base of the proximal phalanx of the thumb Via a slip into the extensor expansion	Deep palmar branch	C8, T1
Dorsal Interossei	Abduction of the 3rd, 4th and 5th fingers Assists in MCP flexion Assists in extension of the IP joints	Thumb • Ulnar border of 1st metacarpal • Radial border of 2nd metacarpal 2nd, 3rd, and 4th fingers • Adjacent sides of metacarpals	Thumb • Radial border of the 2nd finger 2nd • Radial side of the 3rd finger 3rd • Ulnar side of 3rd finger 4th • Ulnar side of 4th finger	Deep palmar branch	C8, T1
Flexor Digiti Minimi	5th MCP joint flexion Assists in opposition	Hook of the hamate bone Flexor retinaculum	Ulnar border of the proximal phalanx of the 5th finger	Ulnar	C8, T1
Flexor Pollicis Brevis	1st MCP joint flexion 1st CMC joint flexion Assists in opposition	Flexor retinaculum Trapezoid Capitate	Radial surface of the base of the proximal phalanx Via a slip into the extensor expansion	Median Deep palmar branch	C6, C7 C8, T1

Lumbricales	Flexion of the 2nd through 5th MCP joints Extension of the PIP and DIP joints	1st and 2nd • Radial surface of flexor profundus tendons 3rd • Adjacent sides of flexor profundus tendons of 3rd and 4th fingers 4th • Adjacent sides of flexor profundus tendons of the 4th and 5th fingers	Radial border of the extensor tendons of the respective digits	1st and 2nd: Median 3rd and 4th: Deep palmar branch	C6, C7 C8, T1
Opponens Digiti Minimi	Opposition of the 5th finger	Hook of the hamate bone Flexor retinaculum	Ulnar border of the length of the 5th metacarpal	Ulnar	C8, T1
Opponens Pollicis	Thumb opposition	Flexor retinaculum Trapezium	Length of the 1st metacarpal	Median	C6, C7
Palmar Interossei	Adducts 1st, 2nd, 4th, and 5th fingers Assists in flexion of the MCP joints	Thumb • Ulnar border of the 1st metacarpal 2nd • Ulnar border of the 2nd metacarpal 3rd • Radial border of the 4th metacarpal 4th • Radial border of the 5th metacarpal	Thumb • Ulnar border of thumb 2nd • Ulnar side of 2nd finger 3rd • Radial side of ring finger • Radial side of little finger	Deep palmar branch	C8, T1

CMC = carpometacarpal; DIP = distal interphalangeal; IP = interphalangeal; MCP = metacarpophalangeal; PIP = proximal interphalangeal.

teres are also located in this compartment. The location of these muscles is presented in Figure 17-6, and their insertion on the wrist and hand is given in Figure 18-8. The deep compartment is formed by the **flexor digitorum profundus**, flexing both the PIP and distal interphalangeal (DIP) joints; the **flexor pollicis longus**; and the **pronator quadratus**.

The flexor muscles are innervated by the **median nerve**. The exception is the flexor carpi ulnaris and the fourth and fifth portions of the flexor digitorum profundus. These are supplied by the **ulnar nerve**.

Palmar muscles

The hand's intrinsic muscles are grouped into the thenar, central, hypothenar, and adductor interosseous compartments. The **thenar eminence**, the mass found over the thumb's palmar surface, is formed by the **abductor pollicis brevis**, **flexor pollicis brevis**, and **opponens pollicis** muscles and the tendon of the **flexor pollicis longus muscle** (Fig. 18-9). On the ulnar aspect, the fleshy mound at the base of the little finger, the **hypothenar eminence**, contains the **abductor digiti minimi**, **flexor digiti minimi brevis**, and the **opponens digiti minimi muscles**.

The tendons of **flexor digitorum superficialis** (FDS) and **flexor digitorum profundus** (FDP) pass through the central compartment. Proximally, the FDP lies directly underneath the FDS tendon. Near the distal phalanx the FDS splits into two sections, allowing the profundus tendon to become superficial while the FDS tendons pass posteriorly and laterally to insert on the distal phalanx. This divergence results in the FDP's ability to flex the MCP, PIP, and DIP joints. The FDS only acts on the MCP and PIP joints.

To prevent bowstringing, a series of pulleys restrain and guide the tendons as they travel across the length of the fingers (Fig. 18-10). During flexion and extension of the fingers, the flexor tendons require almost four times the amount of excursion than the extensor tendons.[7] The **annular pulleys** arise from the palmar aspects of the MCP, PIP, and DIP joints. Numbered from proximal to distal, the annual pulleys act as tunnels through which the tendons pass to maintain their alignment with the finger. The **cruciate pulleys**, also numbered from proximal to distal, are more pliable and collapse to allow the annular pulleys to move towards each other during finger flexion. The **palmar aponeurosis pulley**, located on the distal aspect of the metacarpal, is the most proximal member of the pulley system.[7]

Four **lumbrical** muscles originate off the radial side of each slip of the flexor digitorum profundus tendon. Crossing the MCP joint on the palmar side, the lumbrical muscle continues around the phalanx to insert into the extensor hood. Because of their attachment on the extensor hood, the lumbrical muscles serve to flex the MCP joints and extend the PIP and DIP joints. The entire central compartment is covered by the **palmar aponeurosis** (volar plate).

The palmar adductor interosseous compartment fills the void between metacarpals. The webspace between the thumb and index finger is filled by the **adductor pollicis muscle**. Three spaces between the remaining metacarpals are filled by three palmar and four dorsal interosseous

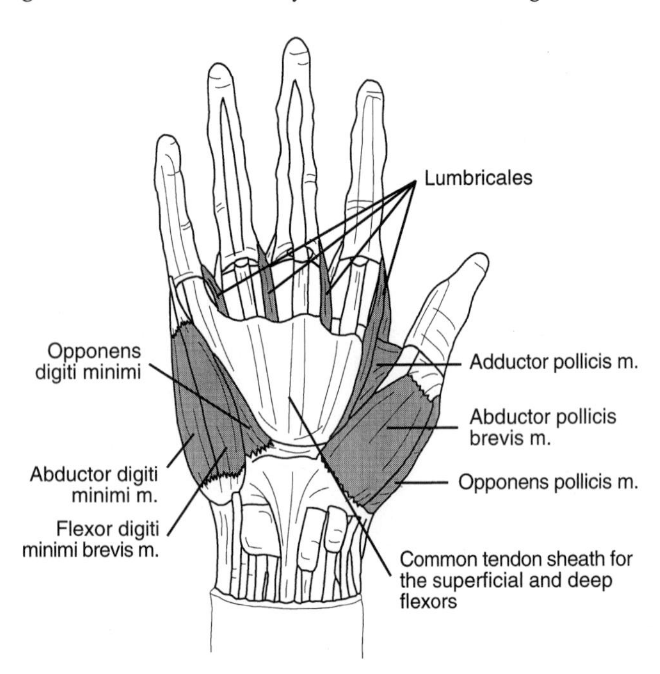

FIGURE 18-9 ■ Intrinsic muscles of the thumb and little finger.

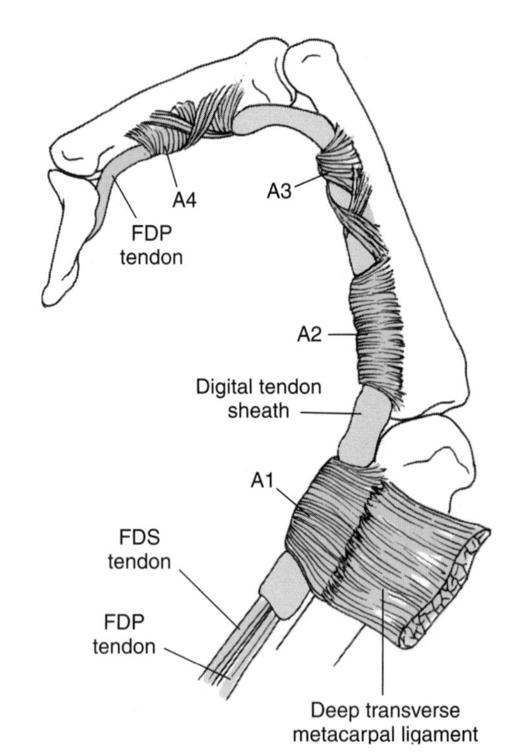

FIGURE 18-10 ■ The flexor pulley system. The annular pulleys (A's) hold the tendons close to the bone. The cruciate pulleys (C's) are pliable to allow full flexion of the finger. The palmar aponeurosis pulley (PA) improve the efficiency of the pulley system. (Courtesy of Norkin, CC, and Levangie, PK: *Joint Structure and Function: A Comprehensive Analysis*, ed 4. Philadelphia: FA Davis, 2005.)

muscles. Using the third metacarpal as the midline reference, the palmar interossei adduct the fingers, and the dorsal interossei abduct them. The palmar interossei have no attachment on the third finger.

Nerves

Three peripheral nerves provide motor and sensory input to the wrist and hand. Proximal entrapment of these nerves can manifest itself with symptoms in the wrist and hand.

Ulnar nerve

The ulnar nerve travels superficially through the palmar aspect of the wrist just medial to the carpal tunnel then passes through the Tunnel of Guyon formed by the hamate and pisiform. At its end, the ulnar nerve divides into superficial and deep branches. The superficial branch provides sensory input to the palmar surface of the little finger and medial one-half of the ring finger. The deep branch innervates the muscles of the hypothenar eminence, the medial two lumbricales, the interossei, and the adductor pollicis.[8]

Median nerve

Following its course with the flexor digitorum superficialis through the forearm, the median nerve travels through the carpal tunnel lateral and divides into a motor and palmar digital branches.[9] The motor branches supply the muscles of the thenar eminence. The palmar digital branch provides sensation to the palmar surface of the thumb, index finger, middle finger and lateral one half of the index finger in addition to innervating the lateral two lumbricals.[9]

Radial nerve

The radial nerve divides into motor (posterior interosseous nerve) and sensory branches (superficial radial nerve) in the proximal forearm. The posterior interosseous nerve innervates the wrist and finger extensors. The superficial radial nerve travels down the dorsal forearm and supplies sensation to the dorsal hand.[10]

The Carpal Tunnel

Many of the anterior muscles acting on the wrist and fingers cross the radiocarpal joint through the carpal tunnel (Fig. 18-11). A fibro-osseous structure, the tunnel's floor is formed by the proximal carpal bones. Its roof is formed by the transverse carpal ligament. Ten structures pass through the tunnel: the median nerve, the flexor pollicis longus tendon, the four tendons of the flexor digitorum superficialis, and the four flexor digitorum profundus tendons. Inflammation of these structures compresses the median nerve, resulting in paresthesia in the median nerve distribution in the palmar aspect of the second, third, and fourth fingers. Grip strength is decreased because of pain and inhibition of the motor nerves supplying the thumb's flexors and opposition muscles.

Clinical Examination of Injuries to the Wrist, Hand, and Fingers

An evaluation of the elbow, shoulder, and cervical spine may also be indicated when a patient's history, mechanism, or symptoms suggest involvement of these structures. Impairment of the nerves in these proximal areas may manifest their symptoms through decreased sensation and strength in the hand. The level of disability must be ascertained by determining the impact of limitations imposed by the problem.

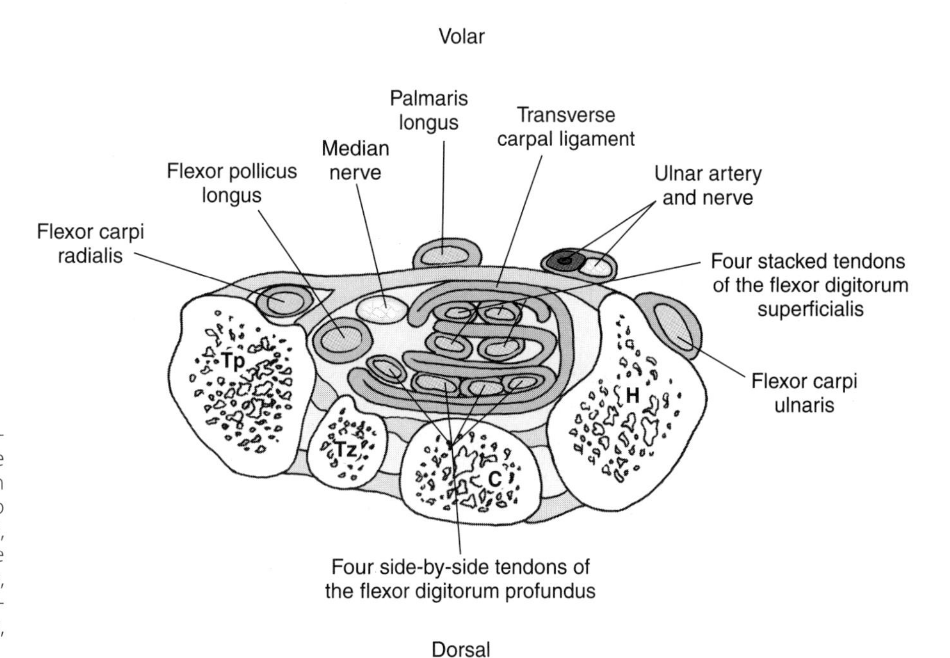

FIGURE 18-11 ■ The carpal tunnel. Inflammation of the tendons passing through the carpal tunnel increases the volume within this fixed space. If the volume continues to increase, the median nerve is compressed, resulting in neurologic symptoms in the hand. (Courtesy of Norkin, CC, and Levangie, PK: *Joint Structure and Function: A Comprehensive Analysis*, ed 4. Philadelphia: FA Davis, 2005.)

Examination Map

HISTORY

Past Medical History

Previous injury history

General medical health

History of the Present Condition

Location of pain

Mechanism of injury

Onset and severity of symptoms

Changes in activity

INSPECTION

Functional Assessment

General Inspection

Wrist and hand posture

Gross deformity

Palmar creases

Lacerations or scars

- Russell's sign

Inspection of the Wrist and Hand

Continuity of the radius and ulna

Continuity of the carpals and metacarpals

Alignment of the MCP IP joints

Ganglion cyst

Inspection of the Thumb and Fingers

Skin and fingernails

Subungual hematoma

Felon

Paronychia

Alignment of fingernails

Muscle contour

Finger posture

PALPATION

Palpation of the Wrist and Finger Flexor Muscle Group

Medial epicondyle

Flexor carpi ulnaris

Flexor digitorum profundus

Flexor digitorum radialis

Flexor carpi radialis

Palmaris longus

Carpal tunnel

Palpation of the Wrist and Finger Flexor Muscle Group

Lateral epicondyle

Extensor digitorum communis

Extensor pollicis longus

Abductor pollicis longus

Extensor pollicis brevis

Abductor pollicis longus

Palpation of the Hand

Metacarpals

MCP joint collateral ligaments

Phalanges

IP joint collateral ligaments

Thenar compartment

- Opponens pollicis
- Abductor pollicis brevis
- Flexor pollicis brevis

Thenar webspace

- Adductor pollicis

Central compartment

Hypothenar compartment

Palpation of the Wrist

Ulna

Ulnar styloid process

IP joint ulnar collateral ligament

IP joint radial collateral ligament

Radius

Radial styloid process

Lister's tubercle

Palpation of the Carpals

Scaphoid

- Anatomic snuffbox

Lunate

Triquetrum

Pisiform

Trapezium

Trapezoid

Capitate

Hamate

JOINT AND MUSCLE FUNCTION ASSESSMENT

Goniometry

Wrist

- Flexion
- Extension
- Radial deviation
- Ulnar deviation

Finger

- Flexion
- Extension
- MCP abduction

Thumb

- CMC flexion
- CMC extension
- CMC abduction

Active Range of Motion

Wrist

- Flexion
- Extension
- Radial deviation
- Ulnar deviation

Finger

- Flexion
- Extension
- Abduction
- Adduction

Thumb

- CMC flexion
- CMC extension
- CMC abduction
- CMC adduction
- Opposition
- Reposition

Manual Muscle Tests

Wrist

- Flexion and radial deviation
- Flexion and ulnar deviation
- Extension and radial deviation
- Flexion and ulnar deviation

Thumb

- MCP flexion
- MCP extension
- IP flexion
- IP extension
- CMC abduction
- CMC adduction
- Opposition

Finger (MCP, PIP, and DIP)

- Flexion
- Extension
- MCP abduction
- MCP adduction

Grip dynamometry

Passive Range of Motion

Wrist

- Flexion
- Extension
- Radial deviation
- Ulnar deviation

Finger (MCP, PIP, and DIP)

- Flexion
- Extension
- MCP abduction
- MCP adduction

Thumb

- CMC flexion
- CMC extension
- CMC abduction
- CMC adduction
- Opposition
- Reposition

JOINT STABILITY TESTS

Stress Testing

Wrist

- Radial collateral ligament
- Ulnar collateral ligament

Examination Map—cont'd

Finger (PIP and DIP)
- Radial collateral ligament
- Ulnar collateral ligament

Joint Play Assessment

Wrist
- Radial glide
- Ulnar glide
- Dorsal glide
- Palmar glide

Hand
- Intercarpal glide

NEUROLOGIC EXAMINATION

Upper Quarter Screen

Tinel Sign

PATHOLOGIES AND SPECIAL TESTS

Wrist Pathologies

Distal forearm fracture
- Colles' fracture
- Smith's fracture

Scaphoid fracture
- Scaphoid compression test

Preiser's disease

Hamate fracture

Perilunate/lunate dislocation
- Dissociative carpal instability
- Kienböck's disease

Wrist sprains
- Watson test

Triangular fibrocartilage complex Injury

Carpal tunnel syndrome

Hand Pathologies

Metacarpal fractures

Finger Pathologies

Collateral ligament injuries

Boutonniere deformity
- Pseudo-boutonniere deformity

Finger fractures

Tendon ruptures and avulsion fractures

Thumb Pathologies

De Quervain's syndrome

Thumb sprains

MCP joint dislocations

Thumb fractures

History

Past history

- **Previous history:** Determine the previous history of injury and any resulting loss of function. Wrist instabilities may result from a seemingly resolved prior trauma.
- **General medical health:** Question the patient about a history of other disorders. Systemic diseases such as gout or rheumatoid arthritis often affect the wrist and fingers before the other joints in the body.[11] This area is often the first to be affected by **peripheral vascular disease** (PVD) or **Raynaud's phenomenon**. Vascular insufficiencies may result in a sensation of coolness and thickness in the hand. Chronic wrist pain is a common complaint among people with diabetes and associated neuropathies.[12] Pregnancy increases the risk of acquiring carpal tunnel syndrome.[13]

History of the present condition

- **Location of pain:** Because the structures of the wrist and hand are so close to one another, enough details should be gained during the history-taking process to localize the symptoms as specifically as possible. Trauma to the cervical spine, shoulder, elbow, and forearm can radiate symptoms into the wrist and hand. Injury to the median, ulnar, and radial nerves can radiate symptoms into their specific sensory or motor distributions in the hand (Fig. 18-12).

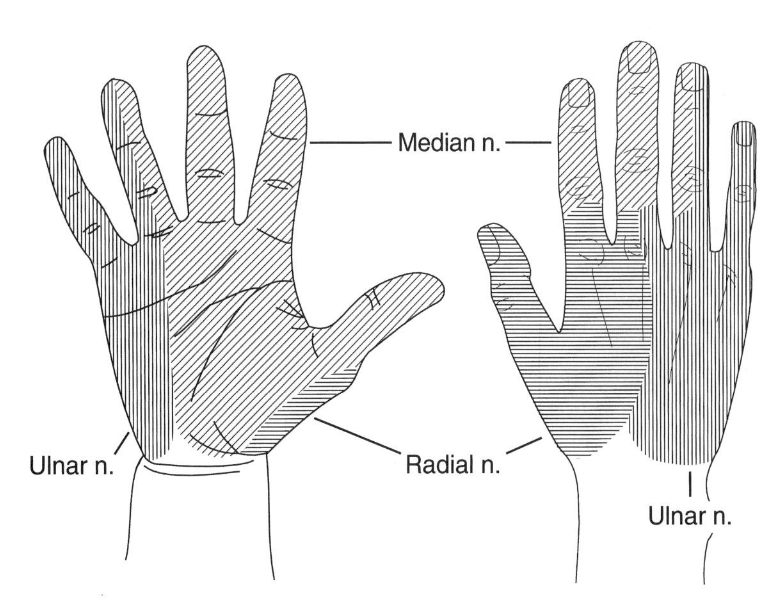

FIGURE 18-12 ■ Nerve distribution in the hand.

Peripheral vascular disease (PVD) A syndrome involving an insufficiency of arteries or veins in maintaining proper circulation.

- **Mechanism of injury:** In the case of acute trauma, identify the mechanism of injury to localize the injured structure or structures. Ask patients describing an injury of insidious onset about activities that increase or decrease the symptoms. When evaluating patients with hand injuries that have an insidious onset, pay particular attention to specific postures that may be assumed for long periods of time, such as when working at a computer.
- **Relevant sounds or sensations:** Question the patient about any sounds or sensations experienced. Fractures, dislocations, and tendon pathology such as a **trigger finger** may have an associated popping sound that is accompanied by a sensation of snapping (Box 18-1). "Clicking" on the ulnar side of the wrist is often associated with **triangular fibrocartilaginous complex** (TFCC) tears.
- **Duration of symptoms:** Correlate the injury mechanism with the duration of symptoms. Nagging wrist pain that does not decrease in severity may indicate a **scaphoid fracture**, a tear of the TFCC or carpal instability.
- **Description of symptoms:** Ask the patient to describe the symptoms. Pain that is described as "aching" or "throbbing" is often associated with trauma to the involved bony or soft tissues. "Burning" or "tingling" sensations suggest neurologic or vascular involvement.
- **Changes in activity:** Question the patient regarding any changes in positioning associated with activities of daily living (ADLs) or sport activities. Sustained postures, such as those associated with working at a computer, may predispose an individual to tendinopathies of the wrist flexors or extensors. Technique changes or adopting new activities such as rowing may overstress tissues, leading to acute or chronic pathologies.

Inspection

Inspection of the wrist, hand, and fingers should be performed with the arm exposed and, when applicable, include inspection of the elbow and shoulder. Injuries to the wrist, hand, or fingers often result in observable functional limitations and/or deformities.

Functional observation

When observing the patient's replication of activities that produce pain or during specific functional testing, compensation for a lack of mobility in the distal arm is demonstrated by using extra motion at the elbow and shoulder. Several pathologies such as a fracture, scapholunate instability, carpal dislocation, or carpal tunnel syndrome limit grip strength and cause the patient to describe an increase in symptoms with ADLs such as opening a door, brushing teeth or shaking hands. The patient may be able to voluntarily reproduce subluxation at the distal radioulnar joint or at the scapholunate joint.[11]

Box 18-1
Trigger Finger

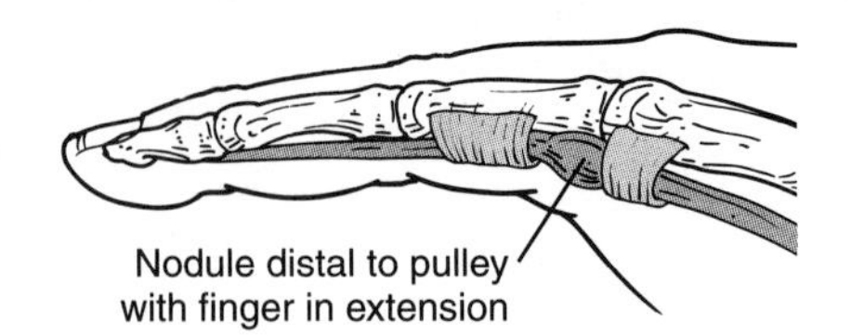

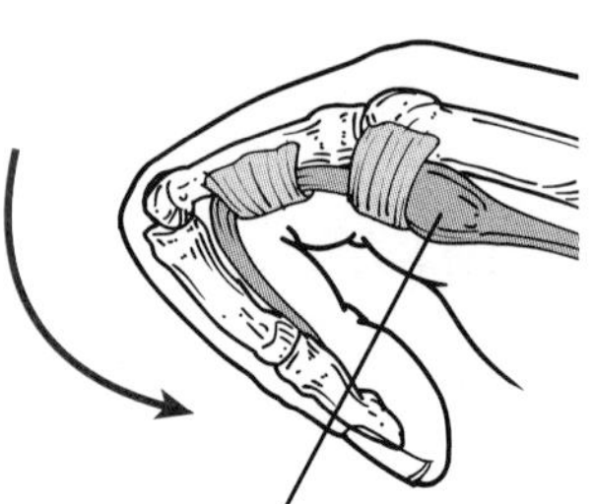

Trigger finger is the result of stenosing tenosynovitis that leads to the formation of a nodule in a flexor tendon, most frequently affecting the flexor digitorum profundus or flexor pollicis longus.[14] Normal flexion and extension of the MCP joint is affected as the nodule passes proximal to the A1 pulley (see Fig. 18-10) during flexion and distal to this pulley during extension. The finger will hesitate and then "snap" as the nodule is wedged beneath the pulley, often resulting in an audible pop as it passes through the opening.

More prevalent in females than males, trigger finger may affect multiple digits and occur bilaterally. The patient may be reluctant or hesitant to make a fist. Initially the nodule and joint motion are painless, but discomfort increases with time. Although the restriction to motion is occurring at the MCP joint, the patient may describe the PIP joint being involved. As the nodule enlarges the nodule will become palpable and painful to the touch. In advanced cases the patient will be unable to fully flex or extend the finger.[14]

If the diagnosis is made early, trigger finger can be successfully treated using oral or injected anti-inflammatory medication. Significantly enlarged nodules, thickening of the A1 pulley, and/or the formation of adhesions within sheath may require surgical correction.

General inspection

- **Posturing of the wrist and hand:** The natural, relaxed posture of the wrist and hand is that of mild extension of the wrist and slight flexion of the hand, with a subtle arch in the palm. The absence of this arch may indicate an avulsion of one or more finger flexors or atrophy of the hand's intrinsic muscles in the case of chronic injuries or prolonged nerve compression (Inspection Findings 18-1).
- **Gross deformity:** Note areas of swelling, discoloration, or gross deformity. Dislocation of the MCP or IP joints results in obvious deformity of the joint's articulating surfaces (Fig. 18-13). A fracture of the metacarpal shows as a protrusion or depression along the usually flat dorsal surface of the hand.

Inspection Findings 18-1
Pathological Hand and Finger Postures

	Ape Hand	Bishop's Deformity	Claw Hand
	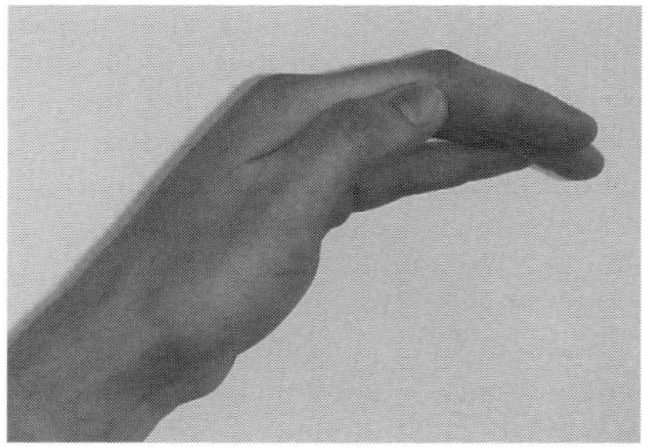	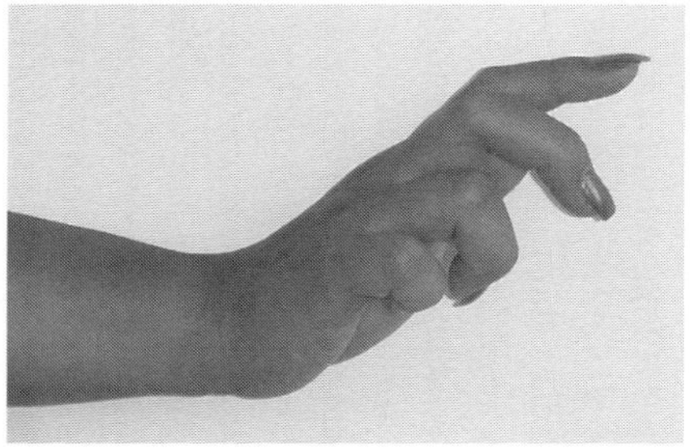	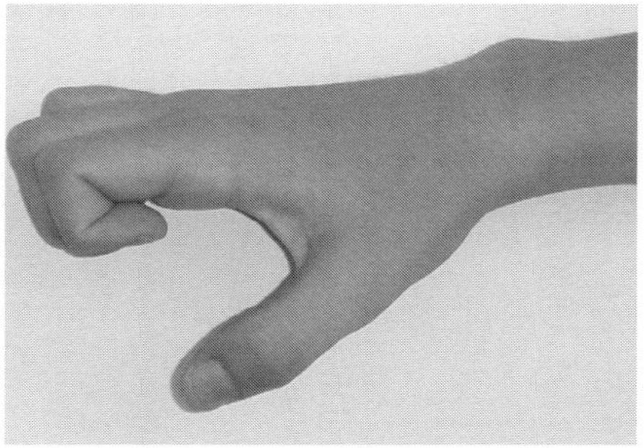
Impairments	Weakness and atrophy of the muscles of the thenar eminence results in overemphasis of the extensor muscles, which pull the thumb parallel with the fingers. Opposition and flexion of the MCP and IP are weakened.	Weakness and atrophy of the hypothenar, interossei, and medial two lumbricals causes the medial fingers to assume a resting posture of flexion in the PIP and DIP joints. Extension of these joints is limited.	Weakness and atrophy of the hand intrinsic muscles results in extension of the MCP joint and flexion of the PIP and DIP joints.
Pathology	Median nerve neuropathy	Inhibition of the ulnar nerve; also known as "Benediction deformity"	Ulnar and median nerve involvement

	Dupuytren's Contracture	Swan-Neck Deformity	Volkmann's Ischemic Contracture
	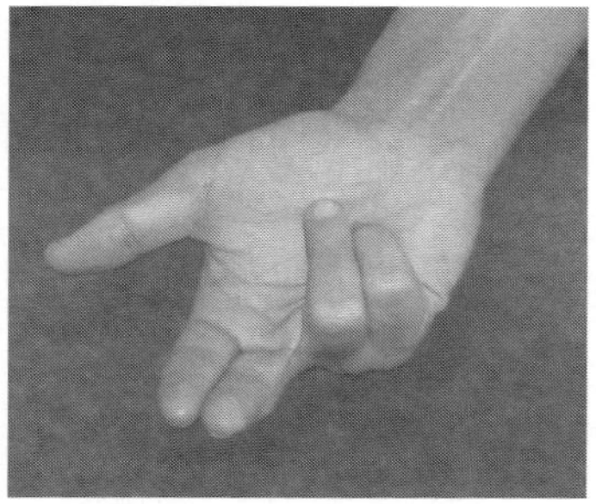	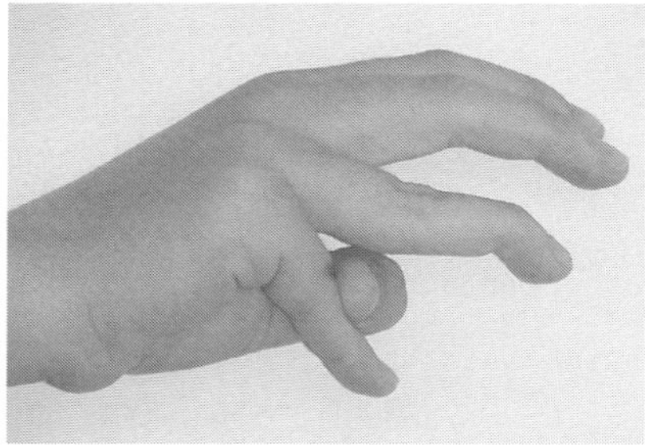	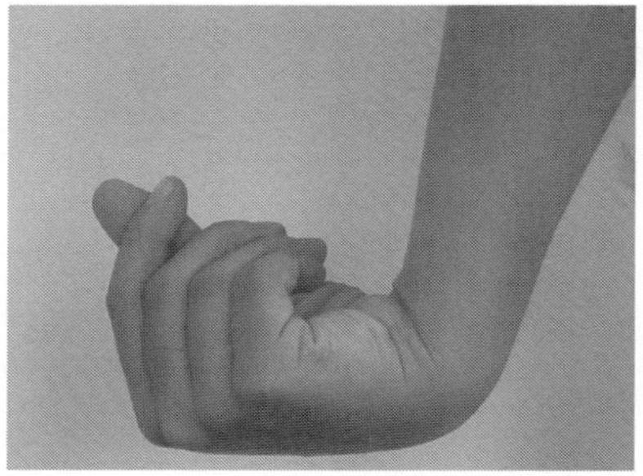
Impairments	Involved finger(s) assume excessively flexed resting position. Inability to passively or actively extend the MCP and PIP joints of the involved finger	Characterized by flexion of the MCP and DIP joints and hyperextension of the PIP joint	Flexion contraction of the wrist and fingers (claw fingers) resulting in limited extension at these joints
Pathology	Flexion contracture of the MCP and PIP joints is caused by a shortening or adhesion (or both) of the palmar fascia. This hereditary condition most commonly affects the 4th and 5th fingers.	Can be caused by a wide range of pathologies, including volar plate injuries, malunion fractures of the middle phalanx, trauma to the finger flexor or extensor muscles, or rheumatoid arthritis.	A decrease in the blood supply to the forearm muscles; Volkmann's contracture can occur after a forearm fracture, fracture or dislocation of the elbow, or forearm compartment syndrome.

DIP = distal interphalangeal; MCP = metacarpophalangeal; PIP = proximal interphalangeal.

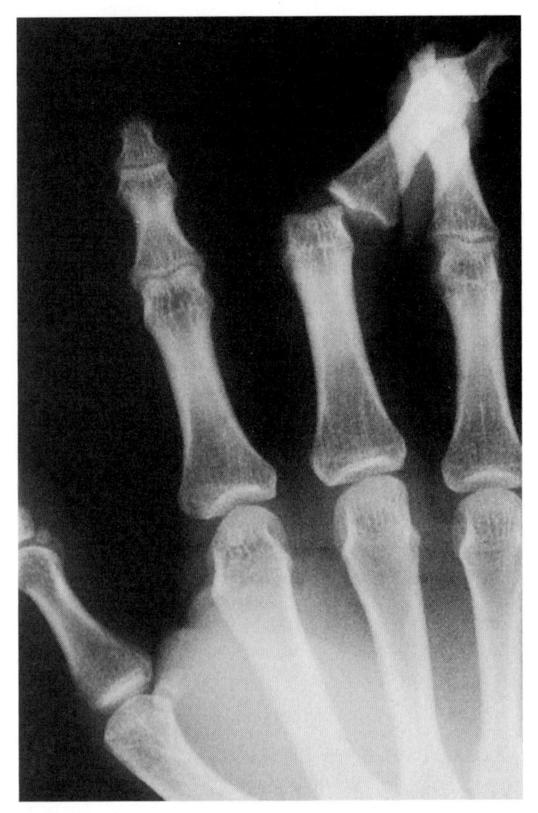

FIGURE 18-13 ■ Dislocation of the proximal interphalangeal joint of the third finger. This type of injury results in obvious visible deformity.

- **Palmar creases:** Swelling in one or more of the hand compartments can obliterate the normal palmar creases.
- **Lacerations or scars:** The superficial nature of the wrist and hand tendons and nerves makes them vulnerable to even minor cuts. Prior lacerations or surgery may have permanently injured the underlying structures, resulting in paresthesia or the loss of function in one or more fingers. Skin laceration over a joint, especially those caused by a bite, should be referred to a physician for prophylactic antibiotic treatment.

Abrasions, small cuts, or callosities over the dorsal surface of the MCP or IP joints, **Russell's sign**, can be one of the few outward signs of bulimia. These lesions are caused by repeated contact with the teeth during self-induced vomiting.[15]

Inspection of the wrist and hand

- **Continuity of the distal radius and ulna:** Observe the symmetry of the distal radius and ulna. A loss of continuity in one bone relative to the other may indicate a fracture.
- **Continuity of the carpals and metacarpals:** Although the carpal bones are normally indistinguishable from one another during inspection of the hand, observe the metacarpal shafts for gross discontinuity. Also observe the dorsal area overlying the lunate for an abnormal contour that may indicate a dislocation (palmar-side dislocations are less easily observed).
- **Alignment of the MCP joints:** Look for the MCP joints to be normally aligned relative to the noninvolved side. A depressed or shortened metatarsal head may indicate a metacarpal fracture.
- **Posture of the wrist and hand:** Note the posture of the wrist and hand. Trauma to the structures that lie between the cervical spine and wrist may cause the wrist and hand to assume an abnormal posture such as **Volkmann's ischemic contracture** (see Box 15-1). Inhibition of the radial nerve may result in paralysis of the wrist and finger extensors and cause **drop-wrist deformity**, indicating the inability to extend the wrist.
- **Ganglion cyst:** Note any collection of fluid or the formation of a mass. A benign collection of thick fluid within a tendinous sheath or joint capsule, ganglion cysts are commonly found in the wrist and hand complex (Fig. 18-14). When the cyst becomes symptomatic, pain is caused by motion and the ganglion is tender to the touch and hardens with time. Patients with symptomatic cysts should be referred to a physician for further evaluation and treatment.

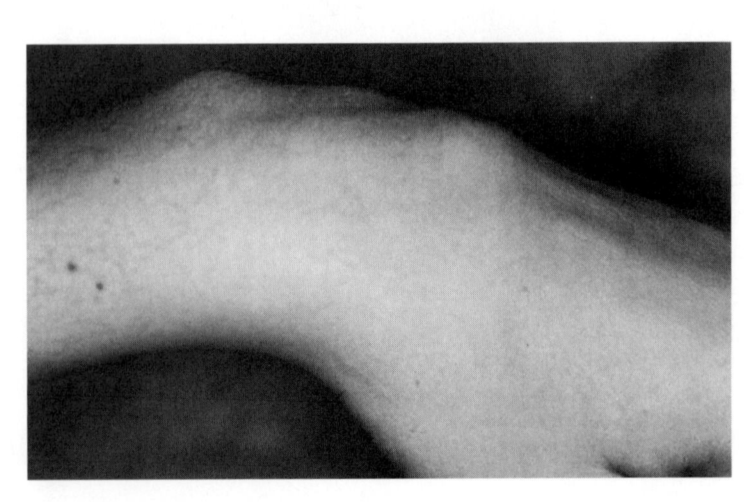

FIGURE 18-14 ■ Ganglion cyst of the wrist extensor tendon. These deformities, caused by a build-up of fluid within the tendon's sheath or joint capsule, are often asymptomatic.

Inspection of the thumb and fingers

- **Inspection of the skin and fingernails:** Trophic changes such as discoloration and changes in hair patterns or skin and nail texture may indicate peripheral vascular disease, complex regional pain syndrome, or Raynaud's phenomenon. Clubbing or cyanosis of the nail sometimes indicates pulmonary disease, Marfan syndrome, cardiovascular disorder, or other disease states.
- **Subungual hematoma:** The formation of a hematoma is characterized by discoloration beneath the fingernail. Observe for the presence of the crescent-shaped **lumina**. If the lumina is absent, the fingernail will eventually fall off.
- **Felon:** An infection or abscess at or distal to the DIP joints, felons arise secondary to contusions or lacerations. The distal end of the finger is red, enlarged, tender to the touch, and warm. Felons must be treated with antibiotics to prevent them from spreading proximally in the finger and hand.
- **Paronychia:** An infection around the periphery of the fingernail, a paronychia results in redness, swelling, and possible drainage around the nailbed (Fig. 18-15). A paronychia should be treated with warm soaks. A physician may prescribe oral antibiotics or drain the affected area.
- **Alignment of fingernails:** During finger flexion, the lateral four fingernails usually assume approximately the same alignment. A finger that deviates from the rest may indicate a spiral fracture of a phalanx or metacarpal.
- **Muscle contour:** Atrophy of the muscles of the thenar eminence is associated with prolonged compression of the median nerve, frequently associated with carpal tunnel syndrome. Entrapment of the ulnar nerve proximal or at the level of the pisiform (before the Tunnel of Guyon) may result in atrophy of the hypothenar eminence.
- **Individual finger deformities:** Irregular posture of one finger may indicate an acute injury or previous trauma (Inspection Findings 18-2). Deformities along the shaft of the bone may indicate a fracture; deformities at the joint indicate a dislocation.

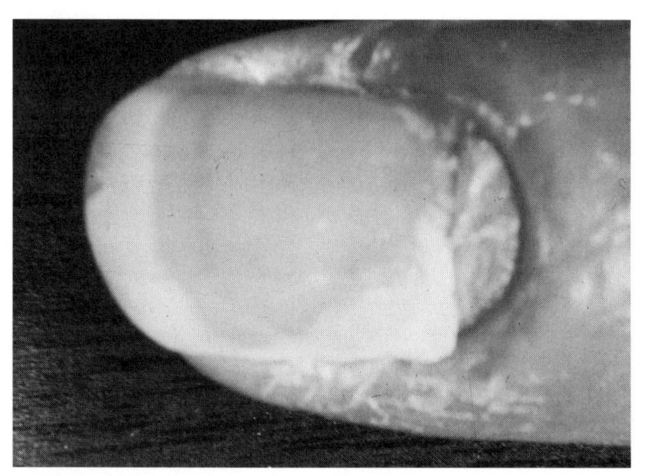

FIGURE 18-15 ■ A paronychia, infection of the fingernail bed. (Courtesy of Goldsmith LA, Lazarus GS, and Tharp MD: *Adult and Pediatric Dermatology. A Color Guide to Diagnosis and Treatment.* Philadelphia: FA Davis, 1997.)

Lumina The growth plate of a fingernail or toenail.

PALPATION

Detailed palpation of the muscles that originate on the elbow and act on the wrist and hand is described in Chapter 17.

Palpation of Wrist and Finger Flexor Muscle Group

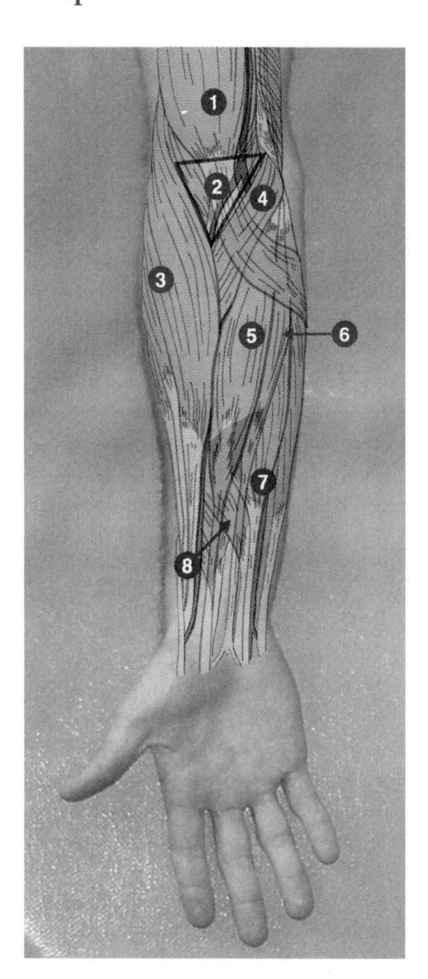

1. Starting at their origin on the medial humeral epicondyle, palpate the wrist flexor group **3–7** through its mass to the point where the individual tendons become distinguishable.

2. Although the tendons may not be individually identifiable, palpate the area over the **7** flexor carpi ulnaris, and flexor carpi radialis **5** from their origin on the anterior arm to their respective attachment on the hand and wrist.

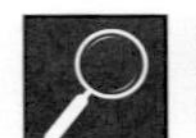

Inspection Findings 18-2
Finger Deformities

	Jersey Finger	Mallet Finger*	Boutonnière Deformity*
Observation	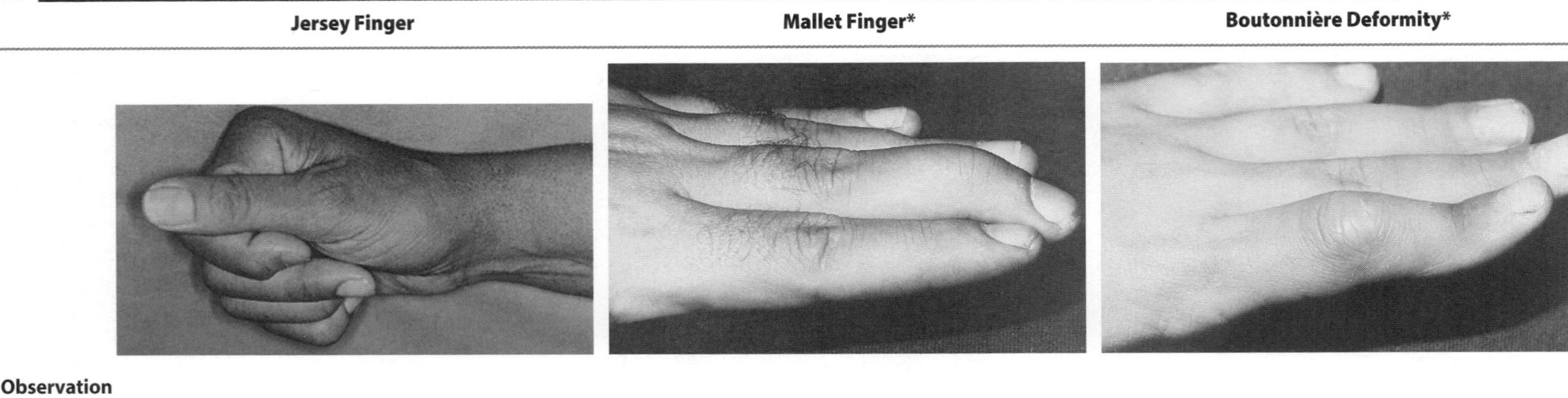		
Illustration	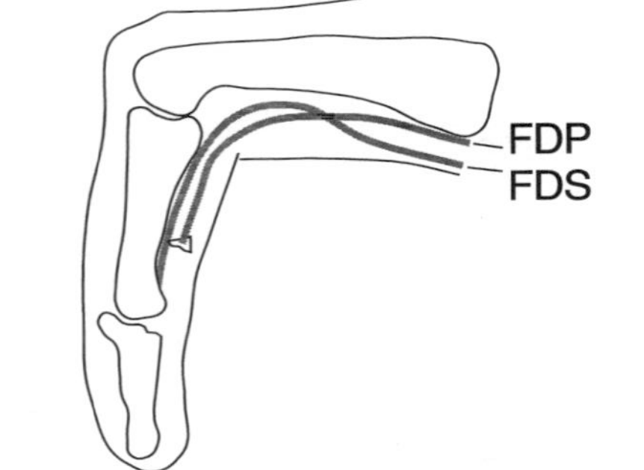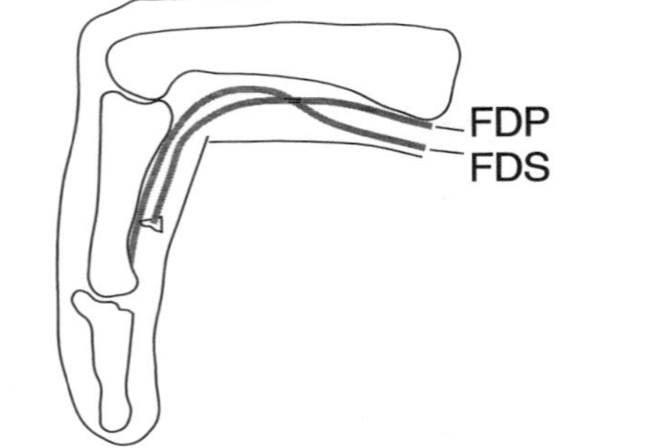	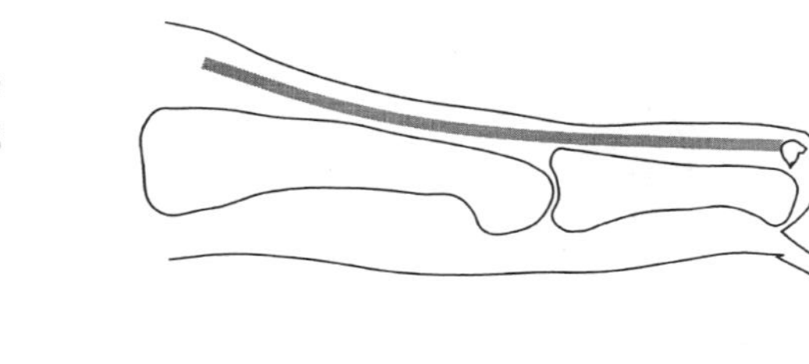	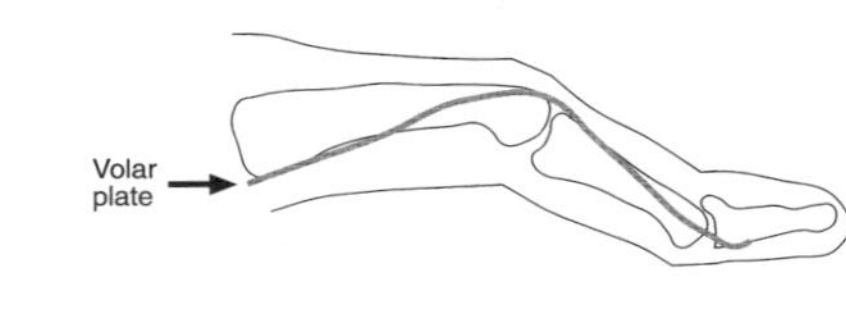
Pathology	Avulsion of the flexor digitorum profundus tendon	Avulsion of the extensor digitorum longus tendon 	Boutonnière deformity: A rupture of the central extensor tendon Pseudo-boutonnière deformity: A rupture of the volar plate
Impairment	Inability to actively flex the DIP joint	Inability to actively extend the distal phalanx, which assumes the posture of 25°–35° of flexion	Extension of the MCP and DIP joints and flexion of the PIP joint; acutely, the PIP joint can be passively extended in those with boutonnière deformities but active PIP extension is absent. In pseudo-boutonnière deformities, passive and active PIP extension are limited.

DIP = distal interphalangeal; MCP = metacarpophalangeal; PIP = proximal interphalangeal.
*Courtesy of Stanley BG and Tribuzi SM: Concepts in Hand Rehabilitation. Philadelphia: FA Davis, 1992.

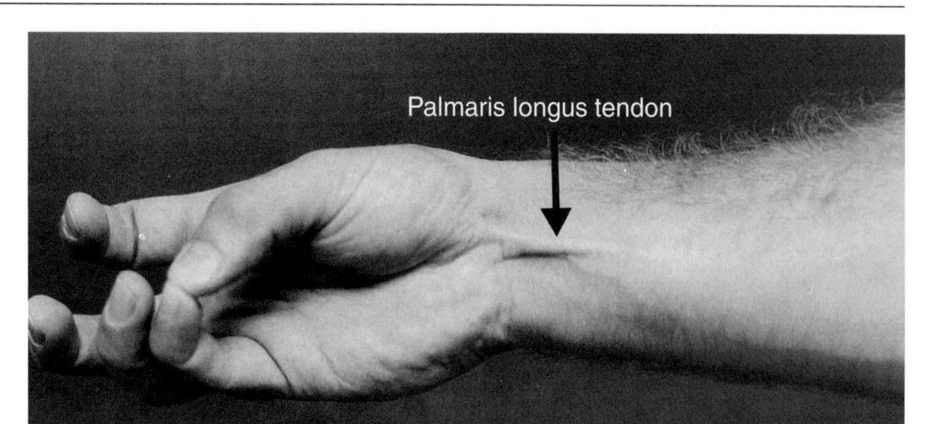

FIGURE 18-16 ■ The palmaris longus tendon becomes prominent during wrist flexion and opposition of the thumb and little finger.

3. Locate the **3** palmaris longus as it travels up the middle of the forearm by moving medially from the flexor carpi radialis. Absent in 12% to 15% of the population, the palmaris longus is more easily identified when the thumb and fifth finger are opposed and the wrist is flexed (Fig. 18-16).

4. On the anterior portion of the wrist, palpate the area of the carpal tunnel for edema or tenderness that may radiate distally into the hand (see Fig. 18-11).

Palpation of the Wrist and Finger Extensor Muscle Group

1. Starting at their common origin on the lateral epicondyle of the humerus **6–10**, palpate the wrist and finger extensor group.

2. The **9** extensor digitorum is palpated along its distal length, where it becomes tendinous and splits into the four tendons leading to the fingers.

3. The thumb extensors, extensor **12** pollicis longus, and **11** extensor pollicis brevis (radial side) are identifiable by their location around the anatomical snuffbox. The extensor pollicis longus tendon forms the medial (ulnar) border; the abductor pollicis longus and extensor pollicis brevis tendons form the lateral (radial) border. Palpate the length of these tendons to their insertion on the thumb.

4. A portion of the abductor pollicis longus may also be palpable.

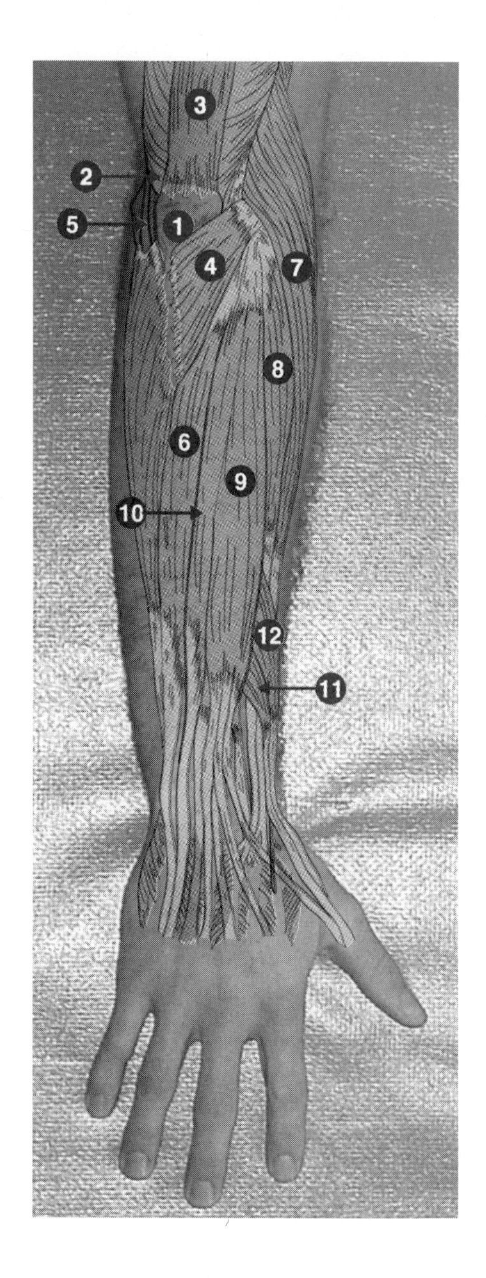

Palpation of the Hand

The intrinsic muscles of the hand cannot be individually identified during palpation. The palpation of these structures is broken down into compartmental zones: thenar eminence, central compartment, and hypothenar eminence (Fig. 18-17).

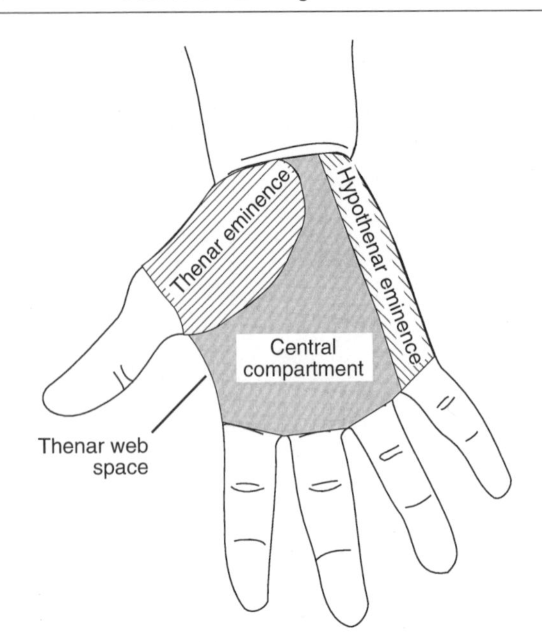

FIGURE 18-17 ■ Zones of the hand.

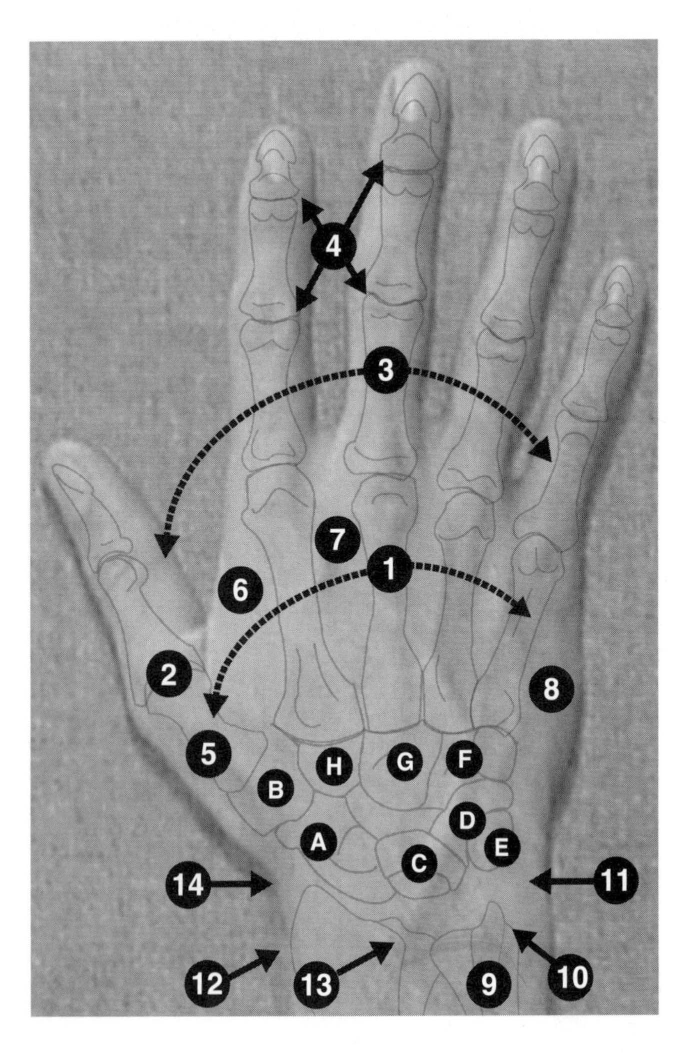

1 Metacarpals: All five metacarpals are palpable along their entire length. Begin the palpation of each metacarpal at the MCP joint and proceed proximally to the CMC joint, noting for areas of pain, deformity, or crepitation.

2 Collateral ligaments of the metacarpophalangeal joints: The UCL and RCL of the thumb are relatively subcutaneous as they cross the first MCP joint. The RCL of the second MCP joint and the UCL of the fifth MCP joint are the only other collateral ligaments directly palpable.

3 Phalanges: Each phalanx of the fingers is palpated for the presence of pain, crepitus, or deformity. The flares adjoining the bases and heads with the shafts are frequent sites of avulsion fractures. Abduction, adduction, or other injury to the IP joints may result in a fracture through these areas.

4 Collateral ligaments of the IP joints: The collateral ligaments of each of the nine IP joints are easily palpated as they cross the joint line. Palpate these ligaments from their origin on the proximal bone to their insertion on the distal bone.

5 Thenar compartment: The small but prominent thenar muscle mass is palpated on the palmar surface of the hand near the base of the thumb. The opponens pollicis sits deep within the compartment, covered by the abductor pollicis brevis and the flexor pollicis brevis muscles and the tendon of the flexor pollicis longus tendon.

6 Thenar webspace: The adductor pollicis is palpated within the webspace between the thumb and index finger and is more easily identified if the thumb is actively extended.

7 Central compartment: Lying between the thenar and hypothenar compartments, the palmar aponeurosis is the most superficial structure within the central compartment. Palpation along the metacarpals may reveal the fingers' flexor tendons.

8 Hypothenar compartment: The hypothenar mass is palpated along the ulnar border of the palm. The muscles within this area (i.e., the abductor digiti minimi, flexor digiti minimi brevis, and opponens digiti minimi muscles) cannot be identified specifically.

9 Ulna: The distal two thirds of the ulna is palpated starting at the point where it emerges from the bulk of the wrist flexors on the dorsal aspect of the forearm. As the ulna approaches the wrist articulation, its head becomes prominent and palpable on its anterior, medial, and posterior borders.

10 **Ulnar styloid process:** The ulnar styloid process is palpated on the distal posteromedial border for tenderness or crepitus.

11 **Ulnar collateral ligament:** The wrist's UCL is palpated as it arises from the styloid process and crosses the joint space to attach to the triquetrum dorsally and the pisiform palmarly.

12 **Distal radius and styloid process:** The distal radius is palpated on the anterior, lateral, and posterior sides of the forearm. The small styloid process can be located on the most distal aspect of the lateral radius.

13 Lister's tubercle is palpable on the dorsal surface of the distal radius.

14 **Radial collateral ligament:** After locating the RCL from its attachment on the radial styloid process, this structure is palpated as it crosses the joint line to its attachment on the scaphoid.

Palpation of the Carpals

The individual carpals are not easily identifiable from one another, but the area overlying these bones can be palpated on the dorsal side of the hand.

A **Scaphoid:** Locate the scaphoid bone, which serves as the floor of the **anatomical snuffbox**, making it easily identifiable and a good starting point for palpating the carpals. Actively extending the thumb and first metacarpal makes the abductor pollicis longus, extensor pollicis brevis, and extensor pollicis longus more distinct. The scaphoid is located within these two boundaries (Fig. 18-18). To differentiate between the scaphoid and trapezium bones, palpate the wrist just distal from the radius while the wrist is ulnarly deviated. The scaphoid bone will be felt to "pop" into position under the finger. The distal tuberosity of the scaphoid can be palpated on the palmar side of the hand.

B **Trapezium:** Locate and palpate the trapezium between the scaphoid bone and the thumb's metacarpal.

C **Lunate:** Return to the scaphoid bone and then move toward the ulna. The lunate is prominent across the joint line from the medial radial head, approximately in line with the third metacarpal. Locate the lunate by first finding Lister's tubercle on the dorsal aspect of the distal radius. From there palpate distally and slightly medially to locate a depression in the joint line. The lunate will fill this void as the patient's wrist is passively flexed. The space between the scaphoid and lunate, the scapholunate interval is a frequent site of sprains and is palpable 1.5 cm distal to Lister's tubercle.[13]

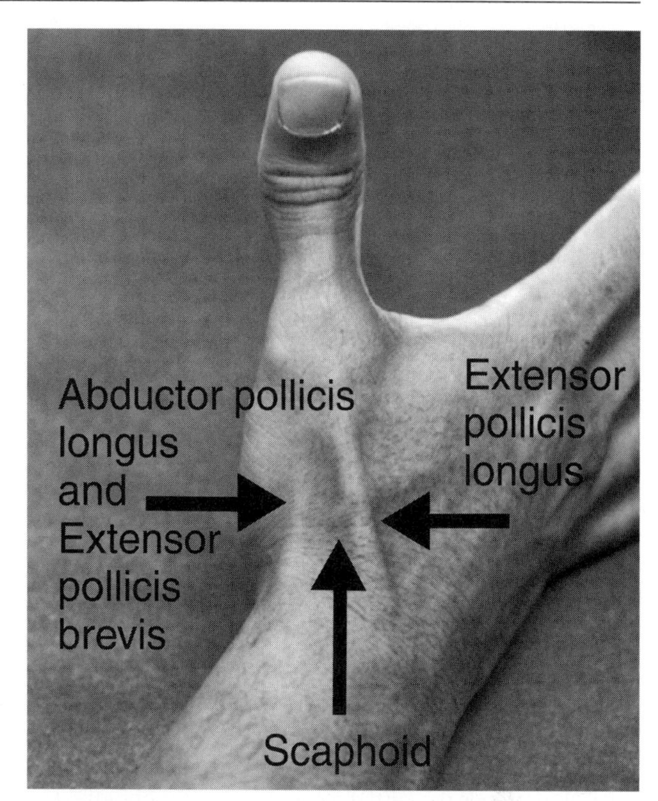

FIGURE 18-18 ■ Borders of the anatomical snuffbox.

D **Triquetrum:** Palpate the triquetrum along the most proximal aspect of the hand approximately one finger's breadth distal to the ulnar styloid process.

E **Pisiform:** Palpate directly anterior to the triquetrum for the pisiform, prominent as a small, rounded protuberance on the palmar side of the most proximal aspect of the hypothenar group. This bone is mobile when the wrist is passively flexed as it lies in the tendon of the flexor carpi ulnaris muscle.

F **Hamate:** Identify the hamate by its palmarly projecting hook. Locate the center of the ulna and palpate immediately across the joint line, distal to the pisiform. The hook of the hamate feels like a hard palmar projection that moves with the hand as the wrist is flexed and is palpated on the palmar side.

G **Capitate:** From the hamate, move toward the thumb side of the hand to locate the capitate, just proximal to the base of the third metacarpal on the palmar aspect of the hand.

H **Trapezoid:** Locate the trapezoid lying at the base of the second metacarpal. This structure is more easily palpated from the dorsal aspect of the hand.

Joint and Muscle Function Assessment

A summary of the end-feels obtained from passive ROM (PROM) assessment of the wrist, hand, fingers, and thumb is presented in Table 18-3. Refer to Tables 18-1 and 18-2 for the innervations of these muscles. Goniometric evaluation of the wrist is presented in Goniometry Box 18-1, the fingers in Goniometry Box 18-2, and the thumb in Goniometry Box 18-3.

Wrist joint and muscle function assessment

The motions of pronation and supination of the forearm are described in Chapter 14.

Active range of motion:

- **Flexion and extension:** A total of 155 to 175 degrees of motion occurs in the sagittal plane around a coronal (medial–lateral) axis. Flexion accounts for 80 to 90 degrees and extension ranges from 75 to 85 degrees. The fingers should be relaxed to assess the maximum amount of motion (Fig. 18-19A). Holding the fingers extended while extending the wrist and flexed while flexing the wrist helps determine the length of the FDP/FDS and EDC, respectively.
- **Radial and ulnar deviation:** Approximately 55 degrees of motion is permitted through the range of radial and ulnar deviation. This motion occurs in the frontal plane around an anteroposterior axis. From the neutral position, 35 degrees of ulnar deviation and 20 degrees of radial deviation are permitted by the joint structure (Fig. 18-19B). Normally, the proximal carpal

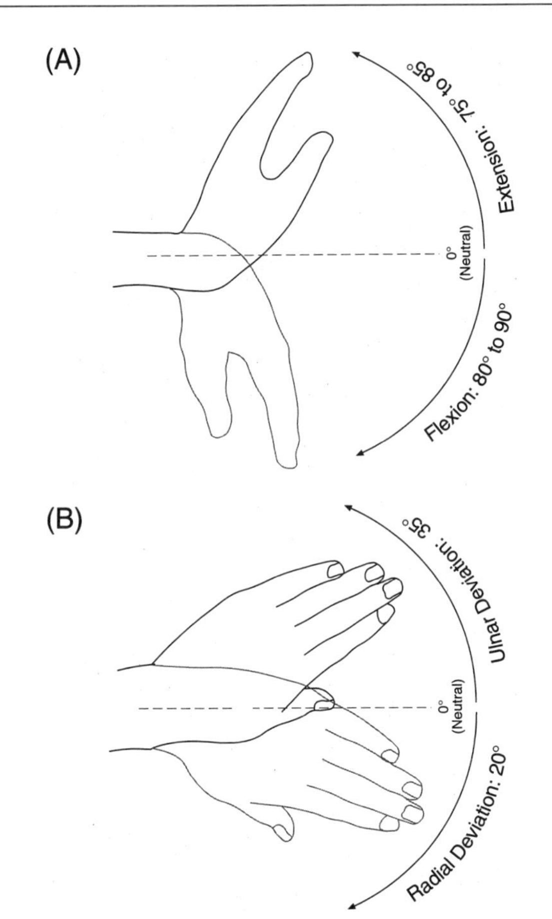

FIGURE 18-19 ■ (A) Active range of motion for wrist flexion and extension. (B) Active range of motion for radial and ulnar deviation of the wrist.

Table 18-3 Normal End-Feels Obtained During Passive Range-of-Motion Testing

Area	Motion	End-Feel	Tissues
Wrist	Flexion	Firm	Dorsal radiocarpal ligament and joint capsule
	Extension	Firm	Palmar radiocarpal ligament and joint capsule
	Radial deviation	Hard	Scaphoid striking styloid process of radius
	Ulnar deviation	Firm	Radiocarpal ligaments and tendons
Thumb (CMC)	Flexion	Soft	Approximation of thenar eminence and the palm
	Extension	Firm	Palmar joint capsule, flexor pollicis brevis, opponens pollicis, first interossei
	Abduction	Firm	Stretching of the webspace
	Adduction	Soft	Approximation of thenar eminence and palm
Fingers and Thumb (MCP)	Flexion	Hard	Proximal phalanx contacts the metacarpal
	Extension	Firm	Tension in the volar plate
	Abduction	Firm	Stretching of the collateral ligaments and webspace
	Adduction	Firm	Stretching of the collateral ligaments and webspace
Fingers (PIP)	Flexion	Hard	Proximal and middle phalanges contact
	Extension	Firm	Stretching of the volar plate
Fingers (DIP) and Thumb (IP)	Flexion	Firm	Tension in dorsal joint capsule and collateral ligaments
	Extension	Firm	Stretching of palmar joint capsule and volar plate

CMC = carpometacarpal; DIP = distal interphalangeal; IP = interphalangeal; MCP = metacarpophalangeal; PIP = proximal interphalangeal.

Goniometry Box 18-1
Wrist

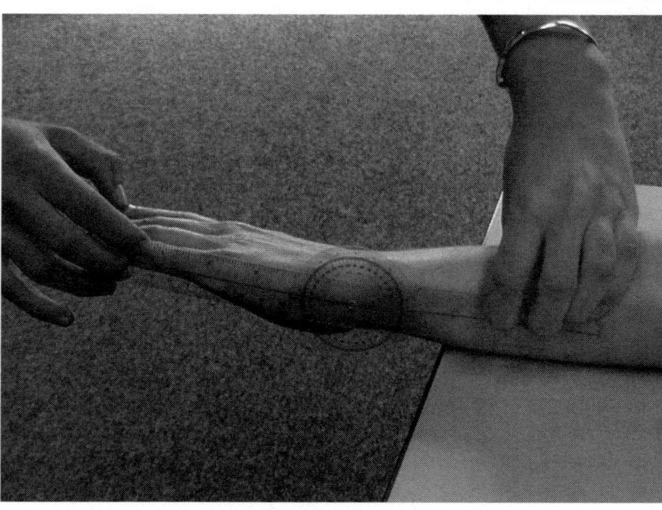

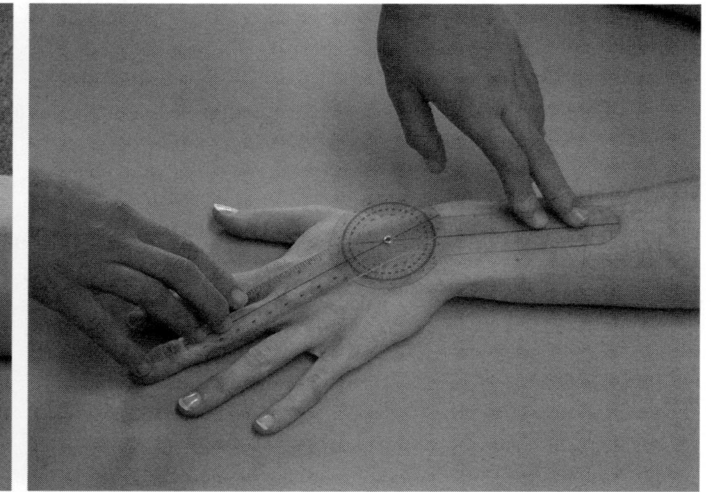

	Flexion and Extension 0° to 90°; 0° to 85°	Radial and Ulnar Deviation 0° to 20°; 0° to 35°
Patient Position	Forearm is pronated with the hand off the edge of the table. Elbow is flexed to 90°. During wrist flexion, the fingers are allowed to extend. During wrist extension, the fingers are allowed to flex.	Forearm is pronated with the hand resting on the table. Elbow is flexed to 90°.
Goniometer Alignment		
Fulcrum	Aligned with the ulnar styloid process	Aligned with the capitate on the dorsal aspect of the wrist
Proximal Arm	The stationary arm is centered on the midline of the ulnar shaft.	The stationary arm is centered over the midline of the forearm.
Distal Arm	The movement arm is parallel to the longitudinal axis of the fifth metacarpal.	The movement arm is centered over the third metacarpal.
Comments	During measurement of PROM, apply the overpressure evenly at the dorsum of the metacarpals to avoid rotation at the wrist.	Avoid wrist extension during the measurement. Popping during ulnar deviation may be indicative of tear of the triangular fibrocartilage complex.

PROM = passive range of motion.

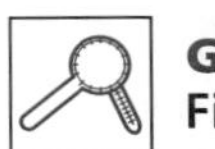

Goniometry Box 18-2
Finger

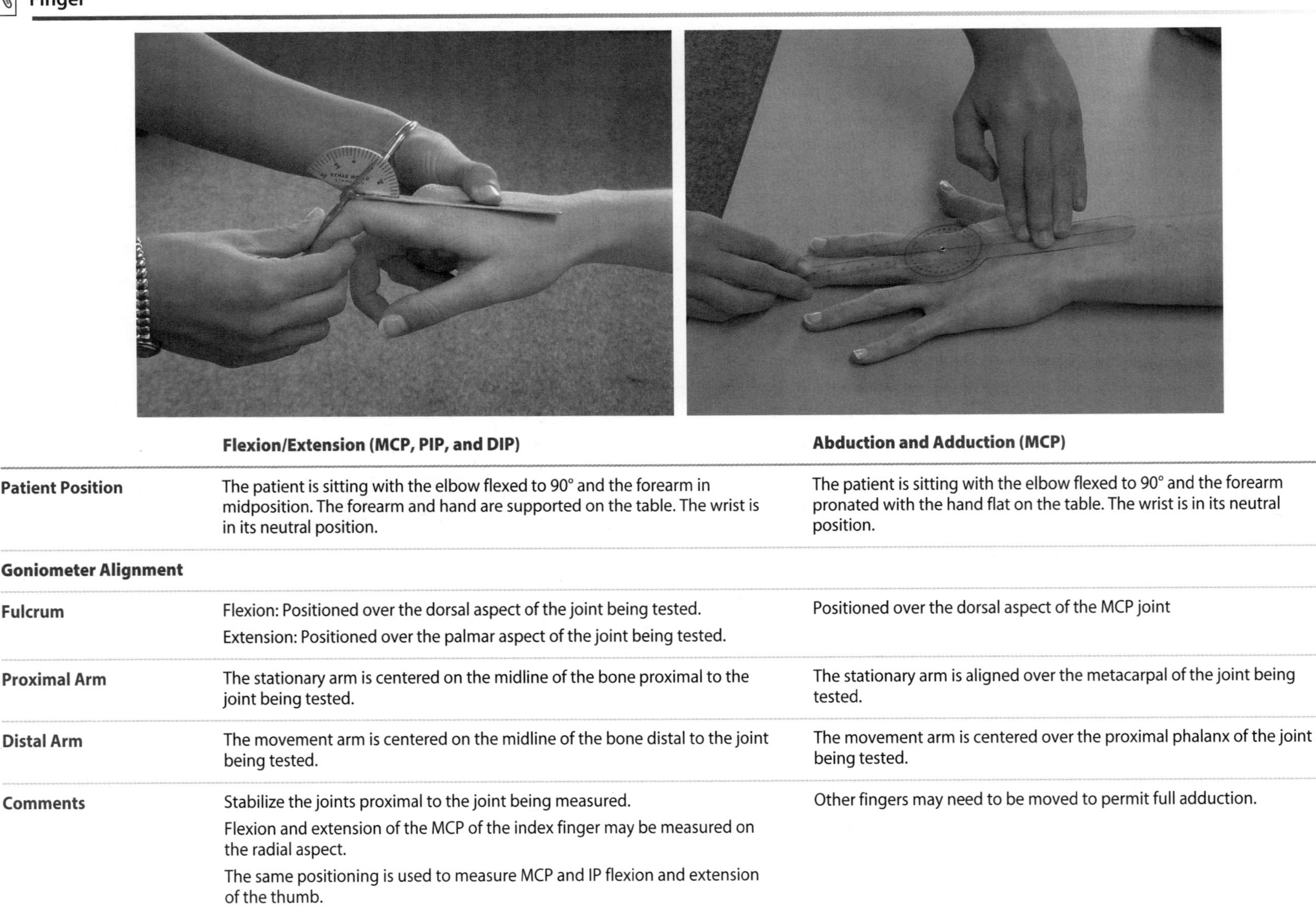

	Flexion/Extension (MCP, PIP, and DIP)	Abduction and Adduction (MCP)
Patient Position	The patient is sitting with the elbow flexed to 90° and the forearm in midposition. The forearm and hand are supported on the table. The wrist is in its neutral position.	The patient is sitting with the elbow flexed to 90° and the forearm pronated with the hand flat on the table. The wrist is in its neutral position.
Goniometer Alignment		
Fulcrum	Flexion: Positioned over the dorsal aspect of the joint being tested. Extension: Positioned over the palmar aspect of the joint being tested.	Positioned over the dorsal aspect of the MCP joint
Proximal Arm	The stationary arm is centered on the midline of the bone proximal to the joint being tested.	The stationary arm is aligned over the metacarpal of the joint being tested.
Distal Arm	The movement arm is centered on the midline of the bone distal to the joint being tested.	The movement arm is centered over the proximal phalanx of the joint being tested.
Comments	Stabilize the joints proximal to the joint being measured. Flexion and extension of the MCP of the index finger may be measured on the radial aspect. The same positioning is used to measure MCP and IP flexion and extension of the thumb.	Other fingers may need to be moved to permit full adduction.

DIP = distal interphalangeal; IP = interphalangeal; MCP = metacarpophalangeal; PIP = proximal interphalangeal.

Goniometry Box 18-3
Thumb

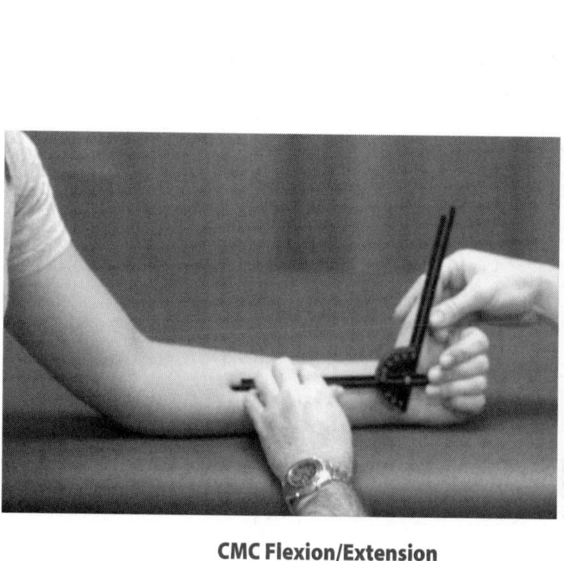

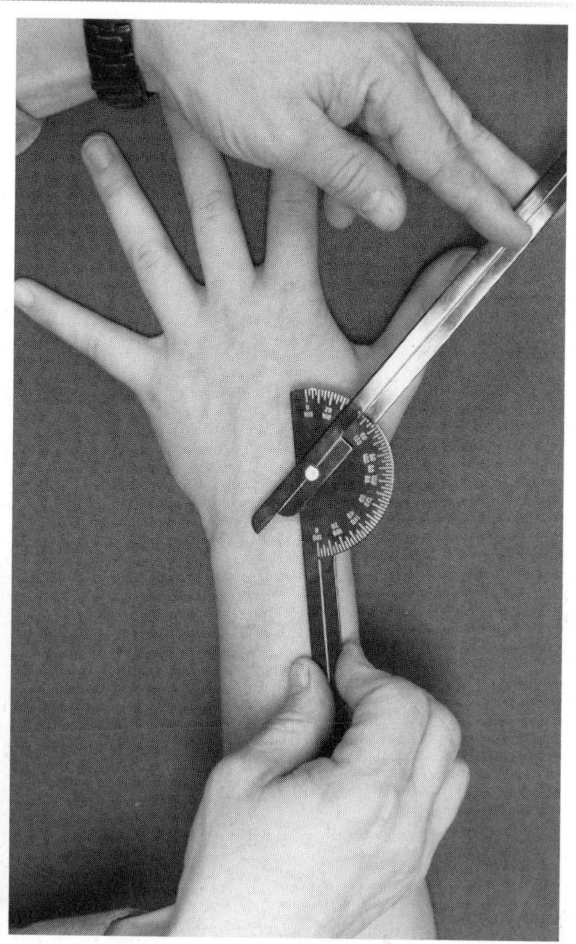

	CMC Flexion/Extension	CMC Abduction
Patient Position	The patient is sitting with the elbow flexed to 90° and the forearm in midposition. The forearm and hand are supported on the table. The wrist is in its neutral position.	Patient is seated with the forearm pronated. The palm is flat on the table.
Goniometer Alignment		
Fulcrum	The axis is centered at the palmar aspect of the CMC.	The axis is centered at the dorsal aspect of the CMC, where the bases of the first and second metacarpals meet.
Proximal Arm	The stationary arm is aligned parallel to the shaft of the radius.	The stationary arm is aligned parallel to the shaft of the second metacarpal.
Distal Arm	The movement arm is aligned parallel to the shaft of the first metacarpal.	The movement arm is aligned parallel to the shaft of the first metacarpal.
Comments	Flexion and extension occur in the frontal plane. When measuring PROM, apply overpressure at the distal metacarpal instead of the proximal phalanx. The initial position of the goniometer is considered the start or zero position.	When measuring PROM, apply overpressure at the distal metacarpal instead of the proximal phalanx. Stabilize the 2nd metacarpal. The initial position of the goniometer is considered the start or zero position.

CMC = carpometacarpal; PROM = passive range of motion.

row smoothly moves from a flexed position to an extended position as the wrist moves from radial to ulnar deviation. In individuals with a midcarpal instability, this transition may be abrupt, resulting in a clunk as the wrist moves from radial to ulnar deviation.[16] "Popping" during ulnar deviation can indicate a tear of the triangular fibrocartilage complex (see p. 801).

Manual muscle tests: Single-plane motions such as wrist extension and wrist flexion are less capable of differentiating between specific muscles; therefore, the components of ulnar and radial deviation should be evaluated (Manual Muscle Test 18-1). Because resisting range of motion throughout the range can provoke symptoms from tissues other than the muscle, an isometric test in the midrange of a movement is recommended to detect muscle weakness or pain. Innervation for wrist flexion and radial deviation is primarily supplied by the median nerve, flexion and ulnar deviation from the ulnar nerve. Extension and radial deviation of the wrist is derived from the radial nerve, extension and ulnar deviation from the deep radial nerve.

Passive range of motion:

- **Flexion and extension:** Position the wrist over the edge of the table with the elbow flexed to 90 degrees, the forearm pronated and the hand facing downward. Stabilize the forearm to prevent pronation and supination. The fingers should be relaxed (Fig. 18-20A and B). **Radial and ulnar deviation:** Position the wrist and forearm in the same manner as for passive flexion and extension (Fig. 18-20C and D).

Thumb joint and muscle function assessment: Carpometacarpal joint

The degrees of freedom of motion and the ROM allowed by the first CMC joint are markedly different from the other CMC joints. Although abduction and adduction of the fingers occur in the frontal plane, abduction and adduction of the CMC joint (palmar abduction and adduction) occurs in the sagittal plane. Likewise, flexion and extension of the fingers occur in the sagittal plane. At the CMC joint, these motions occur in the frontal plane. CMC motions are confusing. Extension occurs when the thumb is put in a "hitch hiker position"; the CMC joint is placed in abduction when gripping a can.

Active range of motion:

- **Flexion and extension:** Thumb CMC flexion and extension occur in the frontal plane around an anteroposterior axis. The majority of this motion, 60 to 70 degrees, is flexion (Fig. 18-21A). Only a trace amount of true CMC extension occurs from the anatomical position.
- **Abduction and adduction:** In the anatomical position, this motion occurs in the sagittal plane around a coronal axis at the CMC. Abduction accounts for the

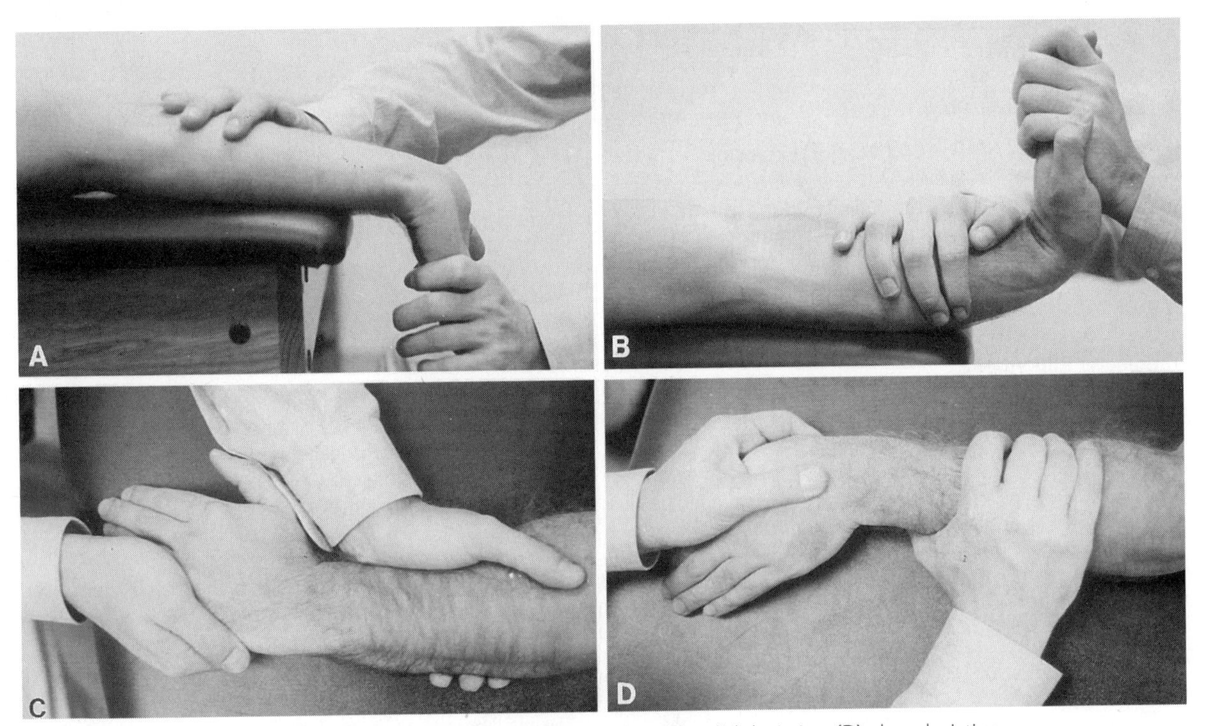

FIGURE 18-20 ■ Passive range of motion of the wrist: (A) flexion; (B) extension; (C) radial deviation; (D) ulnar deviation.

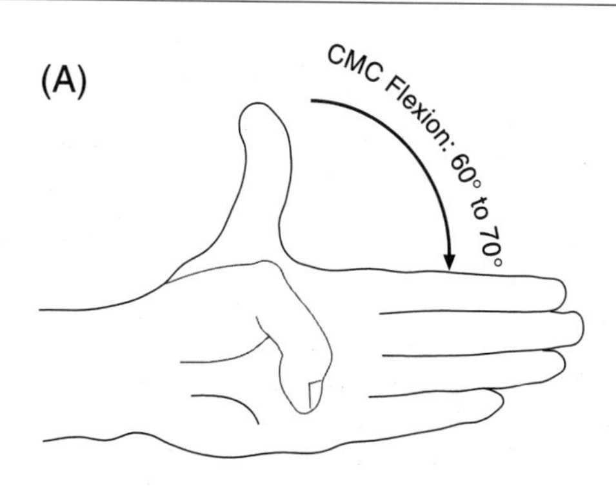

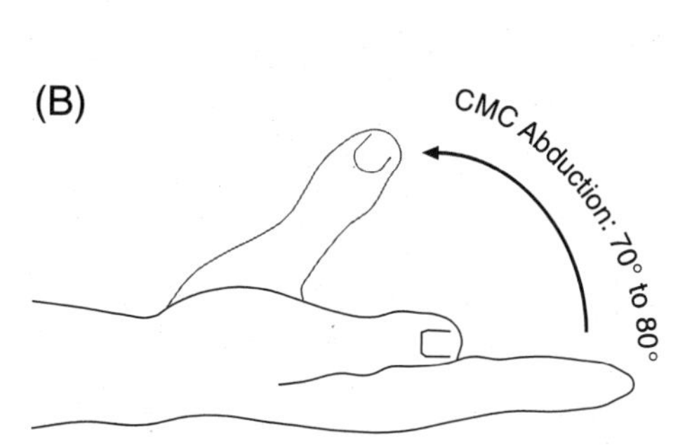

FIGURE 18-21 ■ Active range of motion of the first carpometacarpal joint: (A) flexion/extension (extension is placing the hand in the hitch-hikers position); (B) abduction/adduction (abduction is holding a can).

total motion of 70 to 80 degrees (Fig. 18-21B). True adduction is limited by the phalanx striking the second metacarpal.

- **Opposition:** Opposition is the combined motion of flexion, abduction, and rotation of the thumb and is demonstrated by touching the thumb to the little finger (see Fig. 18-16).

  Manual muscle tests. MMTs for the muscles controlling the thumb are presented in Manual Muscle Tests 18-2, 18-3, and 18-4.

Passive range of motion:

- **Flexion and extension:** Flexion and extension are measured with the forearm supinated and resting on a table with the wrist and IP joint in the neutral position. The carpal bones are stabilized to prevent wrist motion (Fig. 18-22A and B).
- **Abduction and adduction:** The medial forearm is rested on the table in the neutral position. The wrist, CMC, MCP, and IP joints are placed in 0 degrees of extension. Stabilization is provided to the carpal bones and second metacarpal (Fig. 18-22C and D).
- **Opposition:** The forearm is fully supinated and the wrist is placed in its neutral position. The examiner brings the thumb and fifth finger toward each other. Normally, the two fingers should touch each other.

Finger joint and muscle function assessment

Active range of motion:

- **Flexion and extension of the MCP joints:** Flexion and extension of the MCP joints occur in the sagittal plane around a coronal axis. A maximum of 105 to 135 degrees of motion is allowed at the MCP joint, with 20 to 30 degrees occurring during extension and the remaining 85 to 105 degrees accounted for during flexion (Fig. 18-23A).

  Locking that occurs during finger flexion can indicate "**trigger finger**," adhesions in the flexor tendon sheath (see Box 18-1). During active flexion, the sheath adheres to the surrounding tissues and requires additional effort to gain flexion. As the tendon releases, an audible snap is heard and the finger snaps into flexion. During the latter stages of this condition, full flexion may be restricted.
- **Abduction and adduction of the MCP joints:** Twenty to 25 degrees of motion are allowed during abduction and the return motion of adduction. The movement occurs in the frontal plane around an anteroposterior axis with the third metacarpal serving as the reference point (Fig. 18-23B).
- **Flexion and extension of the IP joints:** Flexion and extension of the IP joints range from 80 to 90 degrees at the thumb, 110 to 120 degrees at the PIP, and 80 to 90 degrees at the DIP joints of the fingers (Fig. 18-23C and D).

  Manual muscle tests. MMTs for the finger are presented in Manual Muscle Tests 18-5, 18-6, and 18-7. A manual dynamometer can be used to quantitatively measure grip strength (Special Test 18-1).[18]

Passive range of motion:

- **Flexion and extension of the MCP joints:** While stabilizing the metacarpal, grasp the proximal phalanx of the finger being tested (Fig. 18-24A and B).
- **Abduction and adduction of the MCP joints:** Grasp the finger over the PIP joint. The patient's arm is positioned so that the palm is resting flat against the table with the metacarpals stabilized to prevent wrist motion.
- **Flexion and extension of the interphalangeal joints:** Stabilize the phalanx proximal to the joint being tested while applying force to the phalanx of the distal bone. The normal end-feel for the PIP joint is hard during flexion as the two phalanges contact each other, but a soft end-feel can occur by soft tissue approximation (Fig. 18-24C and D).

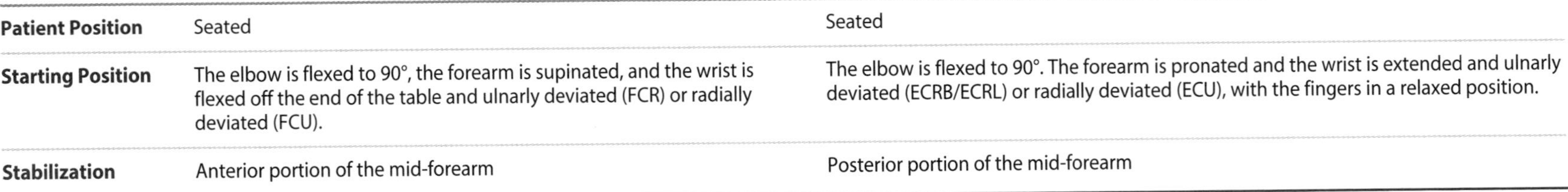

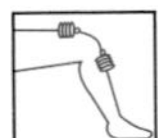

Manual Muscle Test 18-1
Wrist Flexion and Extension

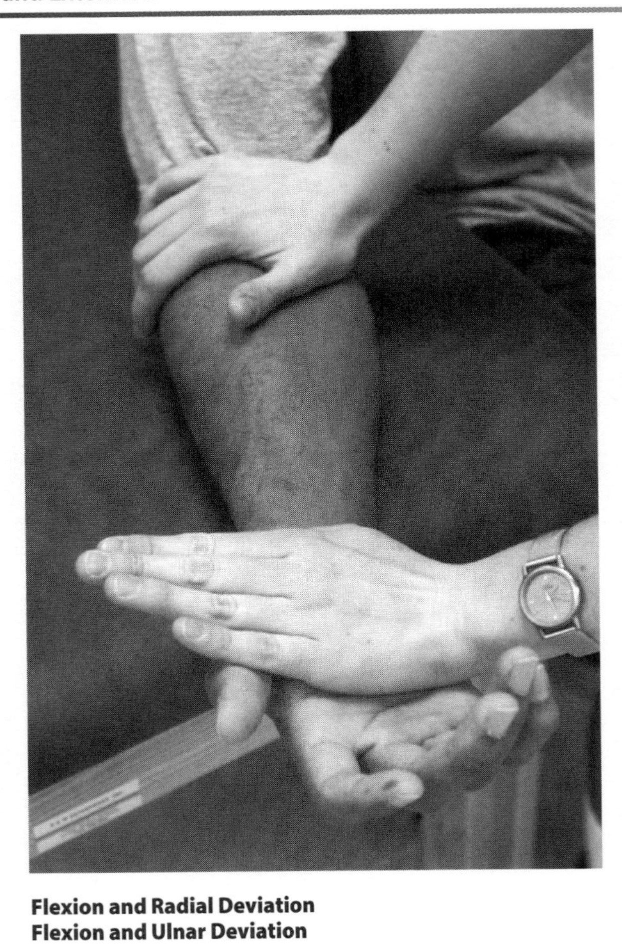

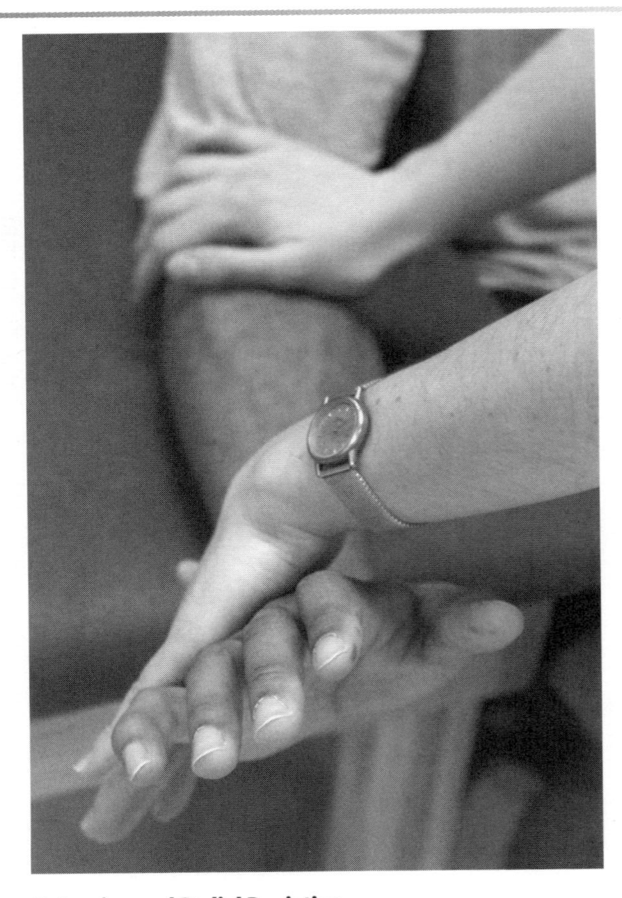

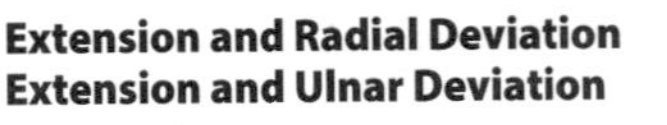

	Flexion and Radial Deviation Flexion and Ulnar Deviation	Extension and Radial Deviation Extension and Ulnar Deviation
Patient Position	Seated	Seated
Starting Position	The elbow is flexed to 90°, the forearm is supinated, and the wrist is flexed off the end of the table and ulnarly deviated (FCR) or radially deviated (FCU).	The elbow is flexed to 90°. The forearm is pronated and the wrist is extended and ulnarly deviated (ECRB/ECRL) or radially deviated (ECU), with the fingers in a relaxed position.
Stabilization	Anterior portion of the mid-forearm	Posterior portion of the mid-forearm

Palpation	FCR: Anterior lateral wrist in line with second web space[17] FCU: Anterior medial wrist just proximal to pisiform.	ECRL/ECRB: ECRL—dorsal base of 2nd metacarpal; ECRB—dorsal base of 3rd metacarpal. ECU: dorsal wrist between base of 5th metacarpal and distal ulna.
Resistance	FCR: Thenar eminence FCU: Hypothenar eminence	Dorsal surface of the hand
Primary Mover(s) (Innervation)	***Flexion and radial deviation:*** Flexor carpi radialis (median: C6, C7) ***Flexion and ulnar deviation:*** Flexor carpi ulnaris (ulnar: C8, T1)	***Extension and radial deviation:*** Extensor carpi radialis longus (radial: C6, C7) Extensor carpi radialis brevis (radial: C6, C7) ***Extension and ulnar deviation:*** Extensor carpi ulnaris (DR: C6, C7, C8)
Secondary Mover(s) (Innervation)	***Flexion and radial deviation:*** Flexor carpi ulnaris (ulnar: C8, T1) Palmaris longus (median: C6, C7) Flexor digitorum profundus (PI: C8, T1) Flexor digitorum superficialis (median: C7, C8, T1) Flexor pollicis longus (PI C8, T1) ***Flexion and ulnar deviation:*** Flexor carpi radialis (median: C6, C7) Palmaris longus (median: C6, C7) Flexor digitorum profundus (ulnar: C8, T1) Flexor digitorum superficialis (Median: C7, C8, T1) Flexor pollicis longus (PI: C8, T1)	***Extension and radial deviation:*** Extensor carpi ulnaris (DR: C6, C7, C8) Extensor digitorum communis (DR: C6, C7, C8) Extensor pollicis longus (DR: C6, C7, C8) ***Extension and ulnar deviation:*** Extensor carpi radialis longus (radial: C6, C7) Extensor carpi radialis brevis (radial: C6, C7) Extensor digitorum communis (DR: C6, C7, C8) Extensor pollicis longus (DR: C6, C7, C8)
Substitution	***Flexion and radial deviation:*** Ulnar deviation, finger flexion ***Flexion and ulnar deviation:*** Radial deviation, finger flexion	***Extension and radial deviation:*** Ulnar deviation, finger extension ***Extension and ulnar deviation:*** Radial deviation, finger extension
Comments	To minimize contributions from the FDS and FDP, the fingers should not flex during the test.	To minimize contributions from the extensor pollicis longus and extensor digitorum communis, instruct the patient to keep the fingers relaxed during the test.

DR = deep radial nerve; PI = palmar interosseous nerve.

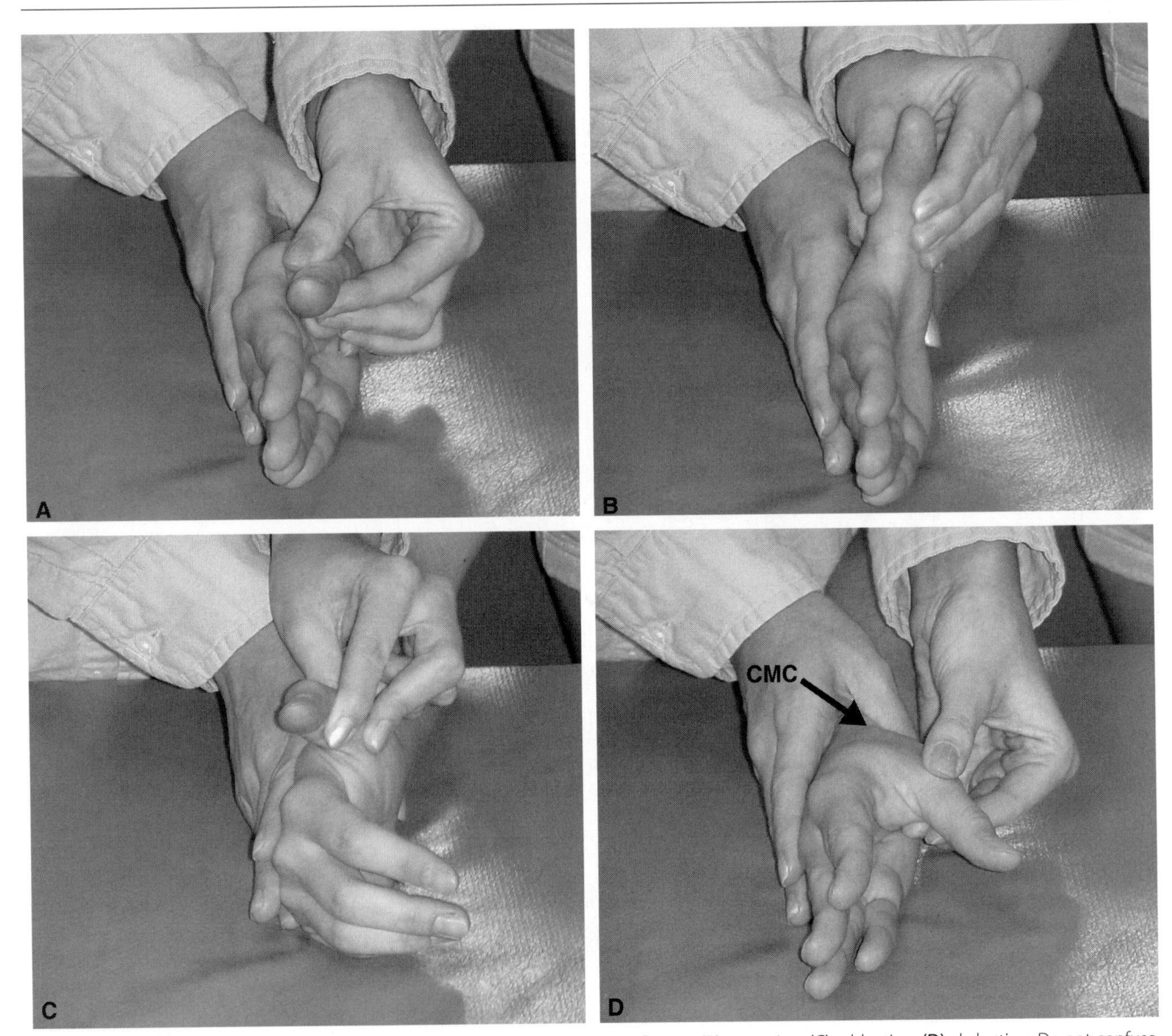

FIGURE 18-22 ■ Passive range of motion of the first carpometacarpal joint: **(A)** flexion, **(B)** extension, **(C)** adduction, **(D)** abduction. Do not confuse CMC motion with motion produced by the MP joint (refer to Fig. 18-21D for the location of the CMC joint).

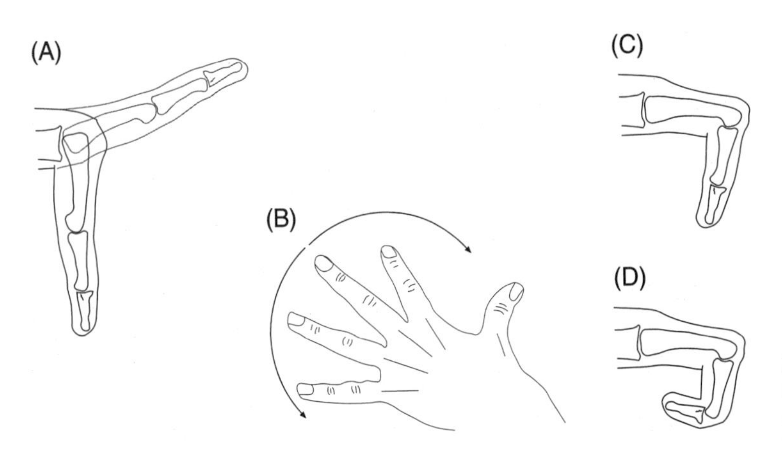

FIGURE 18-23 ■ Finger range of motion: **(A)** metacarpophalangeal flexion and extension; **(B)** metacarpophalangeal abduction; **(C)** flexion of the proximal interphalangeal joint; **(D)** flexion of the proximal and distal interphalangeal joints.

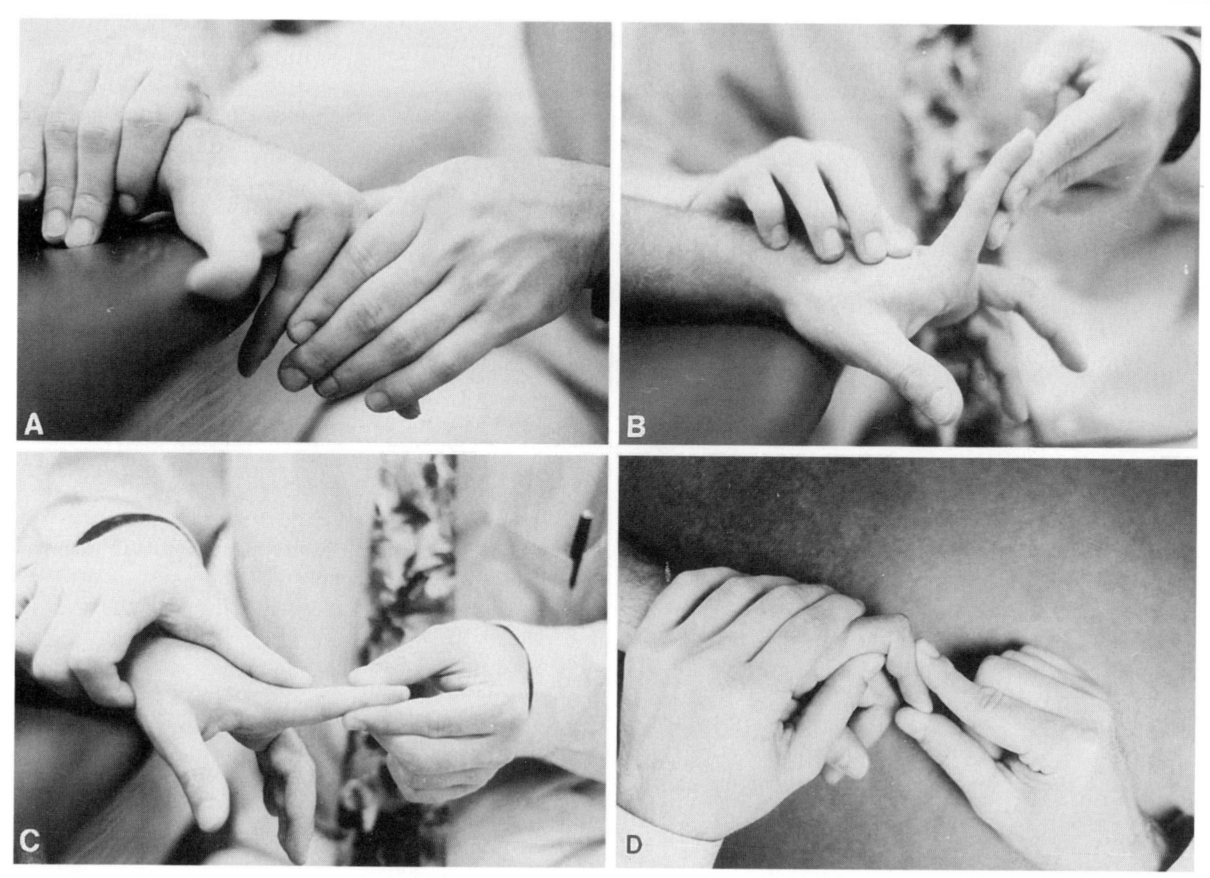

FIGURE 18-24 ■ Passive finger range of motion: (A) flexion and (B) extension of the metacarpophalangeal joint; (C) extension of the proximal interphalangeal joint; (D) flexion of the proximal interphalangeal joint.

Joint Stability Tests

The ligaments of the wrist are stressed with overpressure during the evaluation of PROM (Table 18-4). Avulsion fractures of a ligament's attachment may produce positive results during stress testing. Because the fracture can involve the joint's articular surface, radiographs should be taken to rule out bony pathology.

Table 18-4 Ligaments Stressed During Wrist Passive Range of Motion

	Ligaments Stressed	
Passive Movement	Primary	Secondary
Extension	Palmar ulnocarpal Palmar radiocarpal	Radial collateral Ulnar collateral
Flexion	Dorsal radiocarpal	Radial collateral Ulnar collateral
Radial Deviation	Ulnar collateral	Palmar ulnocarpal
Ulnar Deviation	Radial collateral	Palmar radiocarpal

Stress testing

Tests for collateral support of the wrist ligaments. The UCL provides lateral support against valgus forces (radial deviation), and the RCL checks varus forces (ulnar deviation). These two ligaments also function cooperatively to limit wrist flexion and extension. Although rarely injured in isolation, their integrity can be established through valgus and varus stress testing (Stress Test 18-1) and by assessing glide between the proximal carpal row and the radius (see joint play assessment). These tests check the integrity of the collateral ligaments and may elicit signs of trauma to the triangular fibrocartilage.

Tests for collateral support of the interphalangeal joints. The integrity of the IP joints' collateral ligaments can be determined through stress testing the radial and ulnar ligaments. Although these tests demonstrate laxity in cases of a complete rupture of the ligament or avulsion fracture, pain may also be used as a measure of the relative severity of the injury (Stress Test 18-2).

Test for support of the ulnar collateral ligament. The only MCP joint that is routinely stress tested is the thumb's UCL (Stress Test 18-3). Because of the alignment of the fingers, the only other MCP collateral ligaments commonly injured are the UCL of the MCP joint of the index finger and the RCL of the little finger.

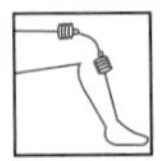

Manual Muscle Test 18-2
Thumb: MCP and IP Flexion and Extension

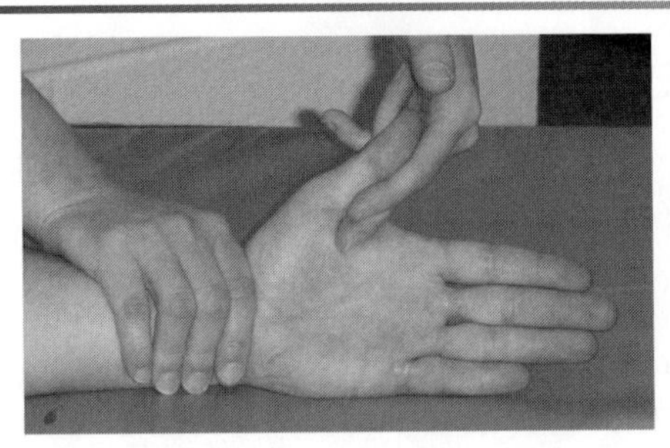

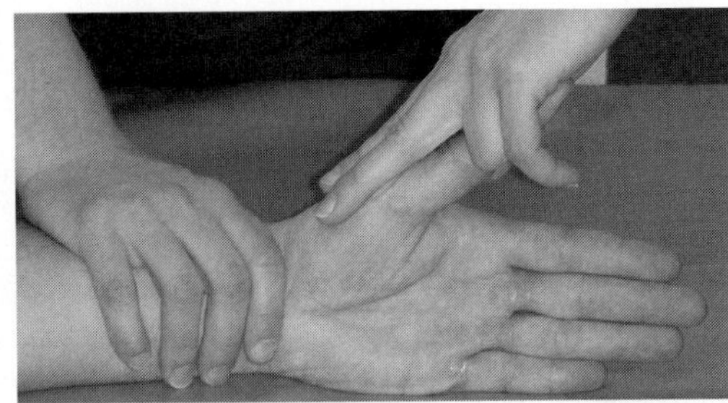

	Flexion	Extension
Patient Position	Seated; elbow flexed 90°; forearm supinated and test hand resting on the table top	Seated; elbow flexed 90°; forearm in midposition and test hand resting on the table top
Starting Position	Wrist in neutral with thumb extended	Wrist in neutral with MCP and IP joints flexed (MCP extension) or IP joint flexed (IP extension)
Stabilization	MCP flexion: First metacarpal IP flexion: Proximal phalanx	MCP extension: First metacarpal IP extension: Proximal phalanx
Palpation	MCP flexion: Thenar eminence, medial to abductor pollicis brevis IP flexion: Palmar aspect, proximal phalanx	MCP extension: Radial border of anatomic snuffbox; medial to tendon of abductor pollicis longus IP extension: Ulnar border of anatomic snuffbox
Resistance	MCP flexion: Palmar aspect, proximal phalanx IP flexion: Palmar aspect, distal phalanx	MCP extension: Dorsal aspect, proximal phalanx IP extension: Dorsal aspect: distal phalanx
Primary Mover(s) (Innervation)	***MCP flexion:*** Flexor pollicis brevis (DPB: C6, C7, C8, T1) ***IP flexion:*** Flexor pollicis longus (PI: C8, T1)	***MCP extension:*** Extensor pollicis brevis (DR: C6, C7) ***IP extension:*** Extensor pollicis longus (DR: C6, C7, C8)
Secondary Mover(s) (Innervation)	***MCP flexion:*** Flexor pollicis longus (PI: C8, T1) IP flexion: None	***MCP extension:*** Extensor pollicis longus (DR: C6, C7, C8) IP extension: None
Substitution	MCP flexion: Do not allow IP joint flexion.	MCP extension: Do not allow IP joint extension.

DR = deep radial nerve; DPB = deep palmar branch (median nerve); IP = interphalangeal; MCP = metacarpophalangeal; PI = palmar interosseous nerve.

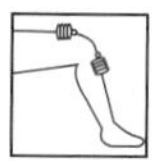

Manual Muscle Test 18-3
First Carpometacarpal Joint Abduction and Adduction

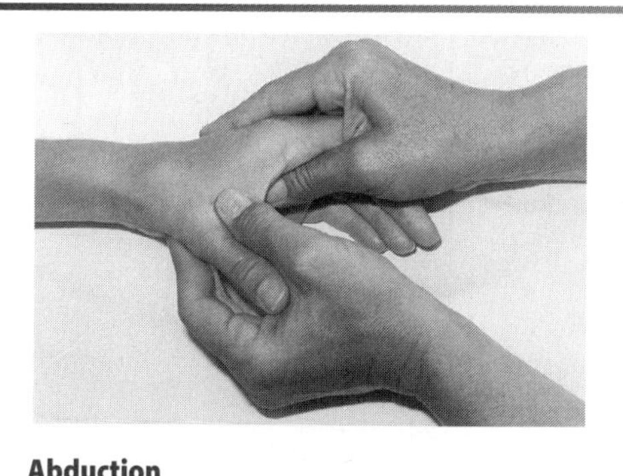

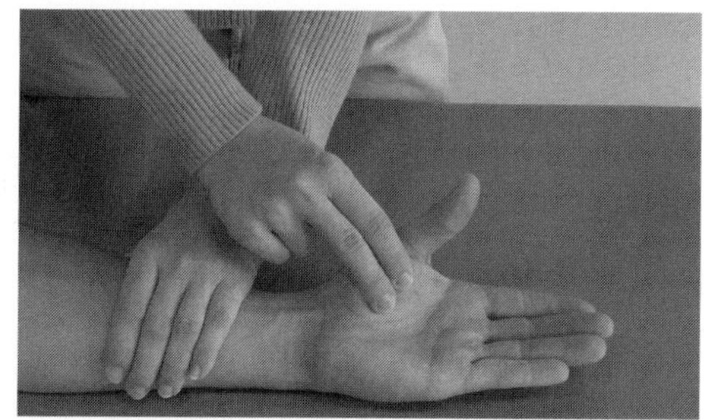

	Abduction	Adduction
Patient Position	Seated; elbow flexed to 90°; forearm supinated with hand resting on table top	Seated; the elbow flexed to 90°; forearm supinated with hand resting on table top
Starting Position	Neutral hand position	Thumb in palmar abduction with MCP and IP joints flexed
Stabilization	Wrist and lateral four metacarpals	Wrist and lateral four metacarpals
Palpation	Lateral aspect of first metacarpal	Palmar surface at thenar eminence between 1st and 2nd metacarpal
Resistance	Lateral aspect of proximal phalanx	Medial border of the proximal phalanx
Primary Mover(s) (Innervation)	Abductor pollicis brevis (median: C6, C7)	Adductor pollicis (DPB: C8, T1)
Secondary Mover(s) (Innervation)	Abductor pollicis longus (median: C6, C7) Extensor pollicis brevis (DR: C6, C7)	Flexor pollicis brevis (DPB: C6, C7, C8, T1)
Substitution	Radial abduction	Not applicable
Comments	Provide resistance to abduction with the thumb at a 45° angle from the sagittal plane to better isolate the abductor pollicis longus. This is sometimes called radial abduction.	Maintain IP and MCP flexion during the test.

DR = deep radial nerve, DPB = deep palmar branch (median nerve); IP = interphalangeal; MCP = metacarpophalangeal.

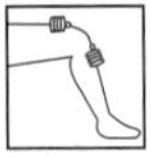

Manual Muscle Test 18-4
Opposition (First and Fifth Carpometacarpal Joint Flexion)

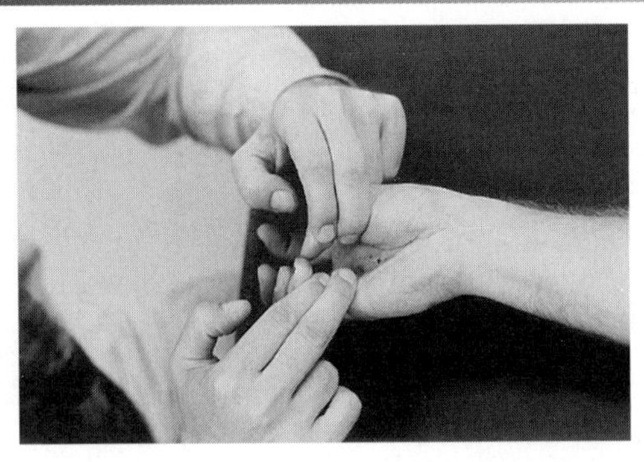

Patient Position	Seated; elbow flexed to 90°; forearm supinated with hand resting on table top
Starting Position	The thumb and 5th fingers opposed
Stabilization	Not applicable
Palpation	Thenar and hypothenar eminences
Resistance	The examiner attempts to separate the fingers, applying resistance at the distal 1st and 5th metacarpals.
Primary Mover(s) (Innervation)	Opponens pollicis (median: C6, C7) Opponens digiti minimi (ulnar: C8, T1)
Secondary Mover(s) (Innervation)	Abductor pollicis brevis (median: C6, C7) Flexor pollicis brevis (DPB: C6, C7, C8, T1)
Substitution	IP joint and wrist flexion

DPB = deep palmar branch (median nerve); IP = interphalangeal.

Wrist and hand joint play assessment

Joint play of the many articulations of the wrist is performed using standard principles: stabilize one bone and glide the adjacent bone, noting any changes in mobility relative to the uninvolved side. Hypermobility may be associated with sprains and is common at the scapholunate articulation. Hypomobility frequently follows periods of immobilization. Radiocarpal and midcarpal joint play is presented in Joint Play 18-1; intercarpal joint play is presented in Joint Play 18-2.

Neurologic Testing

Most commonly, nerves of the hand, wrist, and fingers are affected by pathology proximal to the forearm, but trauma in this region can lead to localized symptoms. **Carpal tunnel syndrome** (CTS), discussed later in this chapter, causes dysfunction in the distal median nerve distribution (Fig. 18-25). The ulnar nerve can become compressed as it passes through the Tunnel of Guyon, located between the hook of the hamate and the pisiform. Radial nerve pathology in the elbow can result in **drop wrist syndrome**, which is the inability to actively extend the wrist and fingers. A complete upper quarter screen may be indicated (see Neurologic Screening Box 1-2). Paresthesia relating to a specific nerve root or peripheral nerve follows defined patterns.

Numbness on the dorsal aspect of the hand is indicative of ulnar nerve neuropathy in the area of the elbow. Numbness on only the palmar side of the ulnar nerve distribution is indicative of ulnar nerve compression distal to the Tunnel of Guyon where the nerve diverges into palmar and dorsal branches.[19]

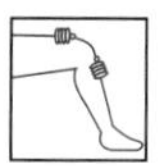

Manual Muscle Test 18-5
PIP and DIP Flexion

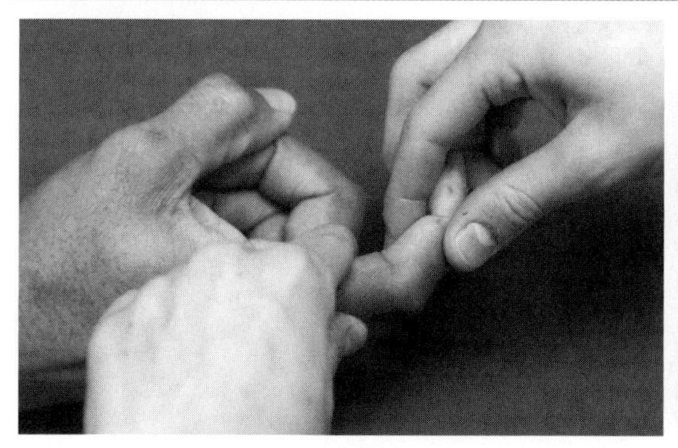

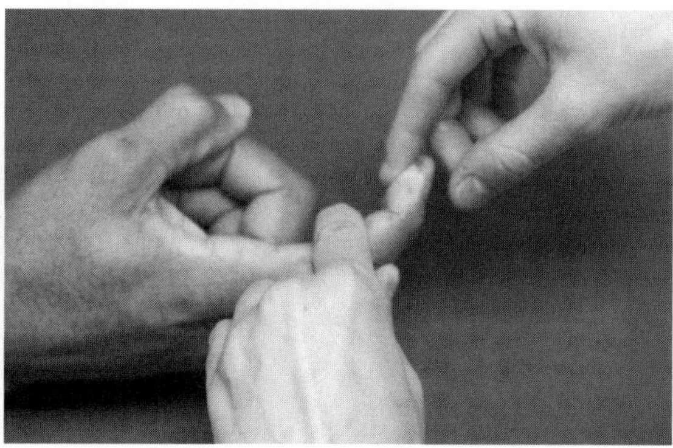

	PIP Flexion	DIP Flexion
Patient Position	Seated; forearm in supination and resting on table	Seated; forearm in supination and resting on table
Starting Position	Test finger in extension	Test finger in extension
Stabilization	Proximal phalanx	Middle phalanx
Palpation	Palmar surface, proximal phalanx	Palmar surface
Resistance	Palmar surface, middle phalanx	Palmar surface, distal phalanx
Primary Mover(s) (Innervation)	Flexor digitorum superficialis (C7, C8, T1)	Flexor digitorum profundus (C8, T1)
Secondary Mover(s) (Innervation)	Flexor digitorum profundus (C8, T1)	None
Substitution	DIP flexion (FDP)	None
Comments	Maintain nontest fingers in extension to limit contribution from the FDP.[17]	

DIP = distal interphalangeal; PIP = proximal interphalangeal.

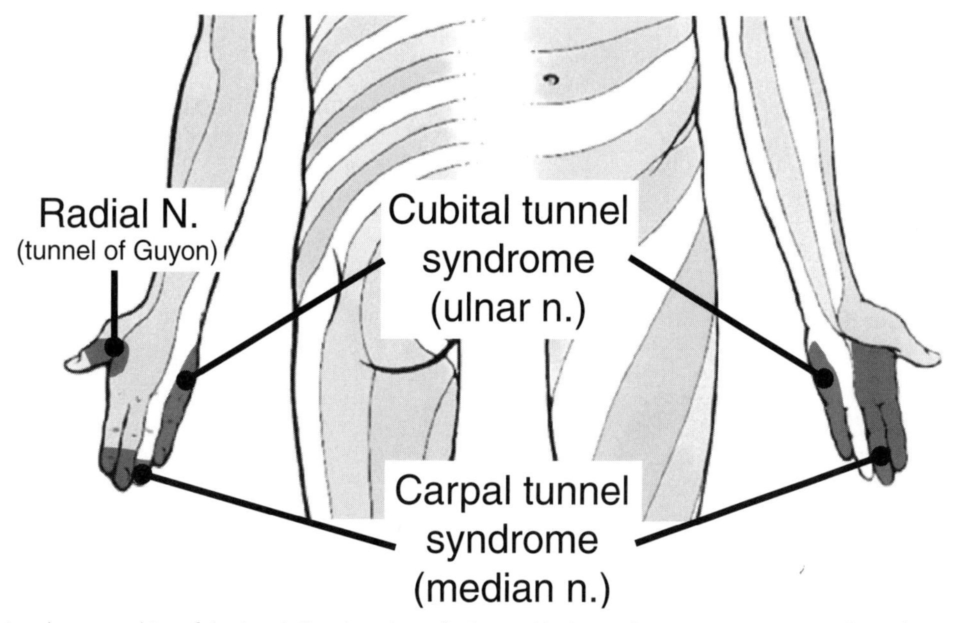

FIGURE 18-25 ■ Local neuropathies of the hand. Correlate these findings with those of an upper quarter neurological screen (see Neurological Testing Box 1–2).

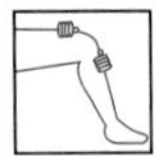

Manual Muscle Test 18-6
MCP Abduction and Adduction

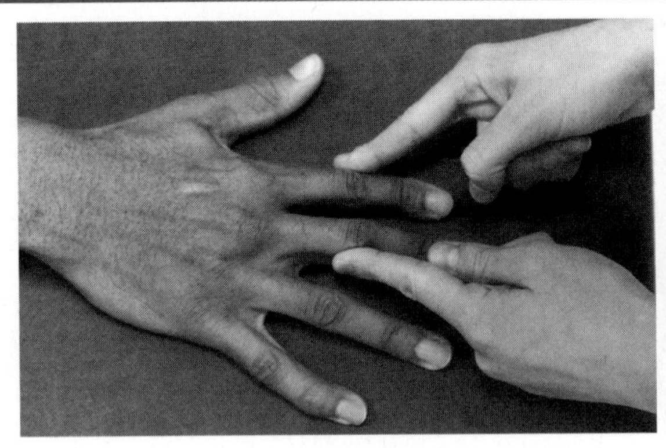

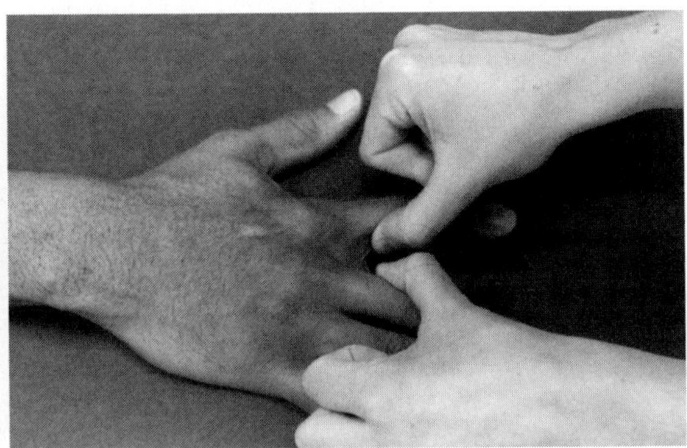

	Abduction	Adduction
Patient Position	Seated; elbow flexed to 90°; forearm pronated and hand resting on table	Seated; elbow flexed to 90°; forearm supinated and hand resting on table
Starting Position	The joint being tested is placed in the neutral position	The fingers are abducted.
Stabilization	Dorsum of hand	Dorsum of hand
Palpation	1st DI: radial aspect, 2nd metacarpal Abductor digiti minimi: ulnar aspect, 5th metacarpal	Cannot be palpated.
Resistance	Proximal phalanx of test finger	Proximal phalanx of test finger
Primary Mover(s) (Innervation)	Dorsal interossei (C8, T1) Abductor digiti minimi (5th finger) (C8, T1)	Palmar interossei (C8, T1)
Secondary Mover(s) (Innervation)	None	None
Substitution	MCP flexion	None
Comments	To test all four dorsal interossei, apply resistance to abduction at the ulnar aspect of the ring finger, at the radial and ulnar aspect of the middle finger and at the radial aspect of the index finger.	To test the three palmar interossei, apply resistance to adduction at the radial aspect of the little finger, the radial aspect of the ring finger, and the radial aspect of the index finger.

MCP = metacarpophalangeal.

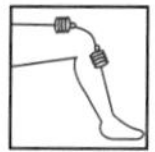

Manual Muscle Test 18-7
Finger MCP Extension and Flexion with IP Extension

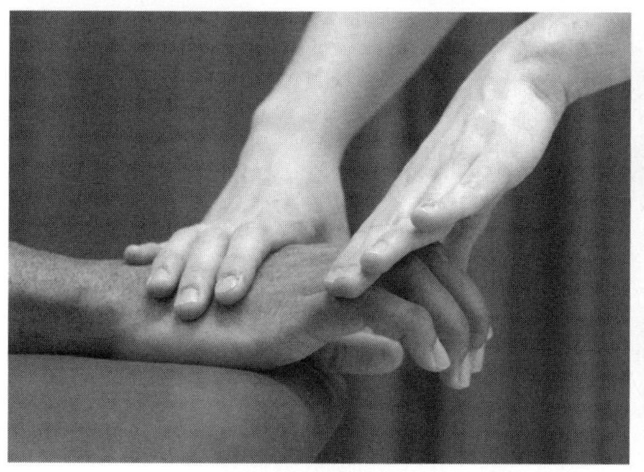

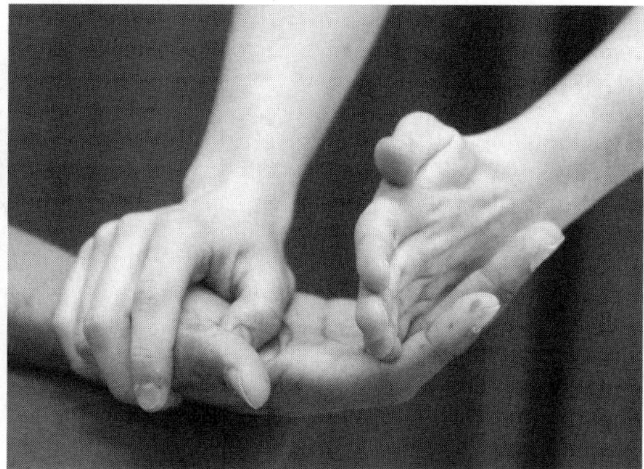

	MCP Extension	Flexion with IP Extension
Patient Position	Seated; elbow in 90° of flexion; forearm pronated; wrist in neutral	Seated; elbow in 90° of flexion; forearm supinated and resting on the table
Starting Position	MCP and IP joints flexed over the end of the table	MCP joints extended and adducted; IP joints flexed
Stabilization	Metacarpals	Metacarpals
Palpation	The tendon to each finger is palpated on the dorsum of the hand. The extensor indicis is medial to the extensor digitorum communis tendon to the index finger. The extensor digiti minimi is lateral to the extensor digitorum communis tendon of the little finger.	Cannot be palpated.
Resistance	Dorsal aspect, proximal phalanx of the test finger	Palmar aspect, proximal phalanx (to resist MCP flexion); dorsal aspect, middle phalanx (to resist PIP extension)
Primary Mover(s) (Innervation)	Extensor digitorum communis (C6, C7, C8) Extensor indicis (radial: C6, C7, C8) Extensor digiti minimi (radial: C6, C7, C8)	Lumbricales (C6, C7, C8, T1)
Secondary Mover(s) (Innervation)	None	Flexor digiti minimi (Ulnar: C8, T1) Dorsal interossei (C8, T1) Palmar interossei (C8, T1)
Substitution	Wrist extension	Wrist flexion
Comments	Test MCP extension of all fingers at the same time. IP joint flexion should be maintained during the test. To assess for extensor digitorum communis tendon rupture, have the patient attempt to actively extend the involved joint while stabilizing the proximal segment.	Resist PIP extension and MCP flexion simultaneously. MCP flexion also occurs via the interossei. The flexor digiti minimi can be tested by resisting MCP flexion of the little finger.

IP = interphalangeal; MCP = metacarpophalangeal; PIP = proximal interphalangeal.

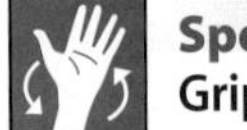

Special Test 18-1
Grip Dynamometry

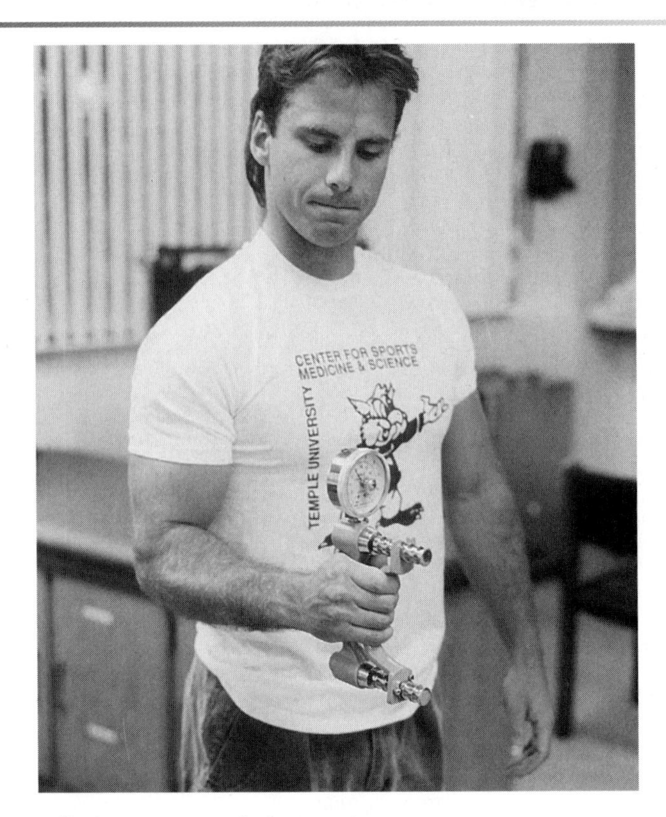

Use of a grip dynamometer provides a qualitative assessment of grip strength.

Patient Position	Holding the grip dynamometer with the elbow flexed to 90° and the radioulnar joint in its neutral position
Position of Examiner	Standing in front of the patient, viewing the dynamometer's gauge
Evaluative Procedure	The dynamometer is set at one of five specified settings (1, 1.5, 2, 2.5, and 3 inches). The patient squeezes the dynamometer's handle with maximum force at every setting, with adequate recovery time allowed between bouts. The values are recorded and the test is repeated on the opposite hand.
Positive Test	***Injured nondominant hand:*** More than 10% bilateral strength deficit compared with the dominant hand ***Injured dominant hand:*** More than 5% bilateral strength deficit compared with the nondominant hand
Implications	Pathology that inhibits grip strength; the underlying cause of the weakness must be determined.
Comments	Because of the wide range of variation in grip strength, the outcome of each of these tests is most meaningful when compared with a baseline measure. This test can be repeated three times at any one setting and the results averaged.
Evidence	***Inter-rater reliability:***

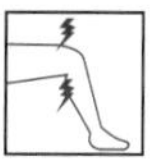

Stress Test 18-1
Radial Collateral and Ulnar Collateral Ligament Stress Tests of the Wrist

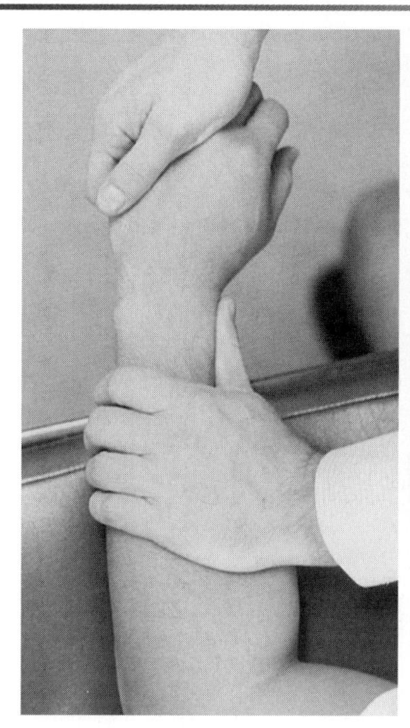

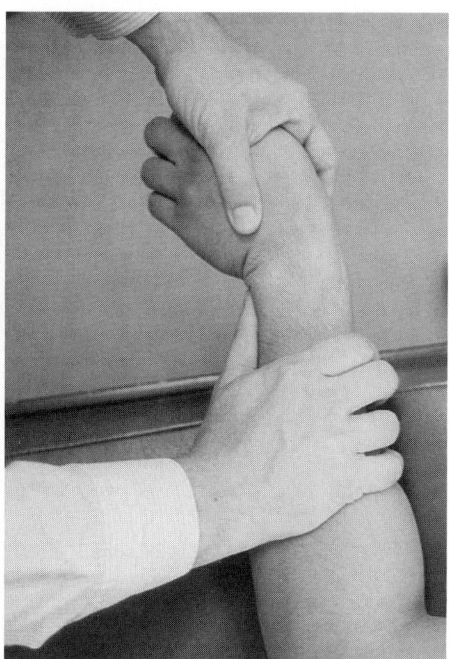

Although of limited clinical use, a valgus stress assesses the ulnar collateral ligament. A varus test stresses the radial collateral ligament of the wrist.

Patient Position	Sitting The elbow flexed to 90°, the forearm pronated, and the fingers assuming the relaxed position of flexion
Position of Examiner	Sitting or standing lateral to the wrist being tested One hand grips the distal forearm and the other grasps the hand across the metacarpals.
Evaluative Procedure	UCL: A valgus stress is applied, radially deviating the wrist. RCL: A varus stress is applied, ulnarly deviating the wrist.
Positive Test	Pain or laxity (or both) compared with the same ligament on the opposite wrist
Implications	Sprain of the UCL or RCL
Comments	Pain may be elicited in the presence of trauma to the triangular fibrocartilage, scaphoid fractures, or the palmar or dorsal radiocarpal or ulnocarpal ligaments. These tests are rarely positive for hypermobility.
Evidence	Absent or inconclusive in the literature

RCL = radial collateral ligament; UCL = ulnar collateral ligament.

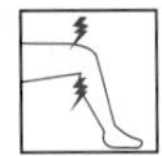

Stress Test 18-2
Valgus and Varus Testing of the Interphalangeal Joints

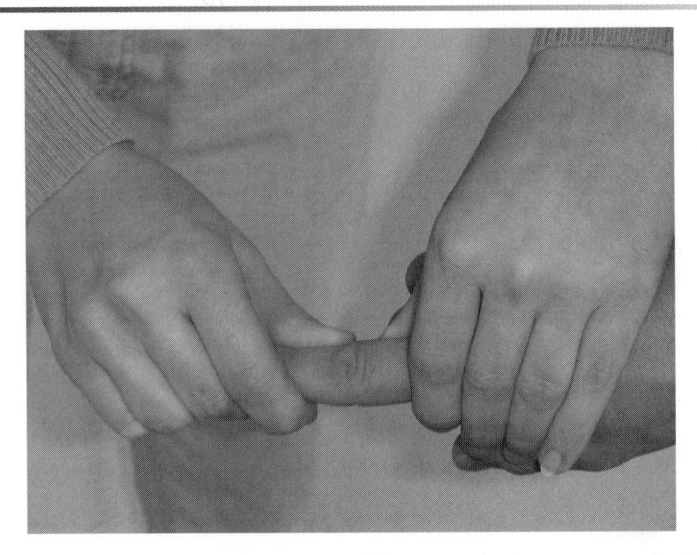

Stress testing the ulnar collateral ligament of the PIP joint. This test should be repeated using varus stress for the radial collateral ligament.

Patient Position	Sitting or standing The joint being tested is in extension.
Position of Examiner	Standing if front of the patient, stabilizing the phalanx proximal to the joint being tested
Evaluative Procedure	The examiner grasps the phalanx distal to the joint being tested and applies a valgus stress to the joint. A varus stress is then applied to the joint.
Positive Test	Increased gapping, compared with the same motion on the same finger of the opposite hand Pain
Implications	Collateral ligament sprain Avulsion fracture
Comments	Except in the case of a complete disruption of the ligament, the degree of injury to the ligament cannot be established. Avoid placing the stabilizing finger over the ligament.
Evidence	Absent or inconclusive in the literature

PIP = proximal interphalangeal.

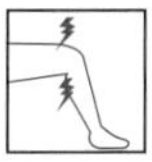

Stress Test 18-3
Test for Laxity of the Thumb MCP Collateral Ligaments

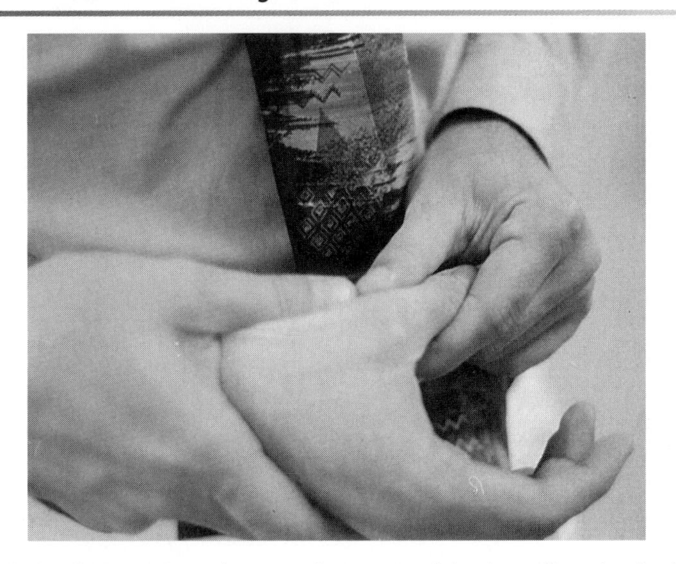

A valgus and varus stress is applied to the MCP joint to determine the integrity of the ulnar collateral and radial collateral ligaments.

Patient Position	Sitting or standing
Position of Examiner	Standing in front of the patient
Evaluative Procedure	The examiner stabilizes the first metacarpal with one hand and its proximal phalanx with the other. While stabilizing the first metacarpal with the thumb slightly abducted and extended, the examiner applies a valgus stress to the ulnar collateral ligament. In extension, the test stresses the accessory collateral ligament. In full flexion, the collateral ligament proper is stressed.
Positive Test	The ulnar side of the first MCP joint gaps farther than the uninjured side or the patient describes pain (or both).
Implications	Sprain of the ulnar collateral ligament Avulsion fracture
Comments	Avoid stabilizing over the MCP ligament stressed.
Evidence	Absent or inconclusive in the literature

MCP = metacarpophalangeal.

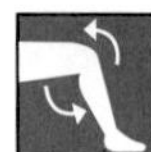

Joint Play 18-1
Radiocarpal and Midcarpal Joint Play

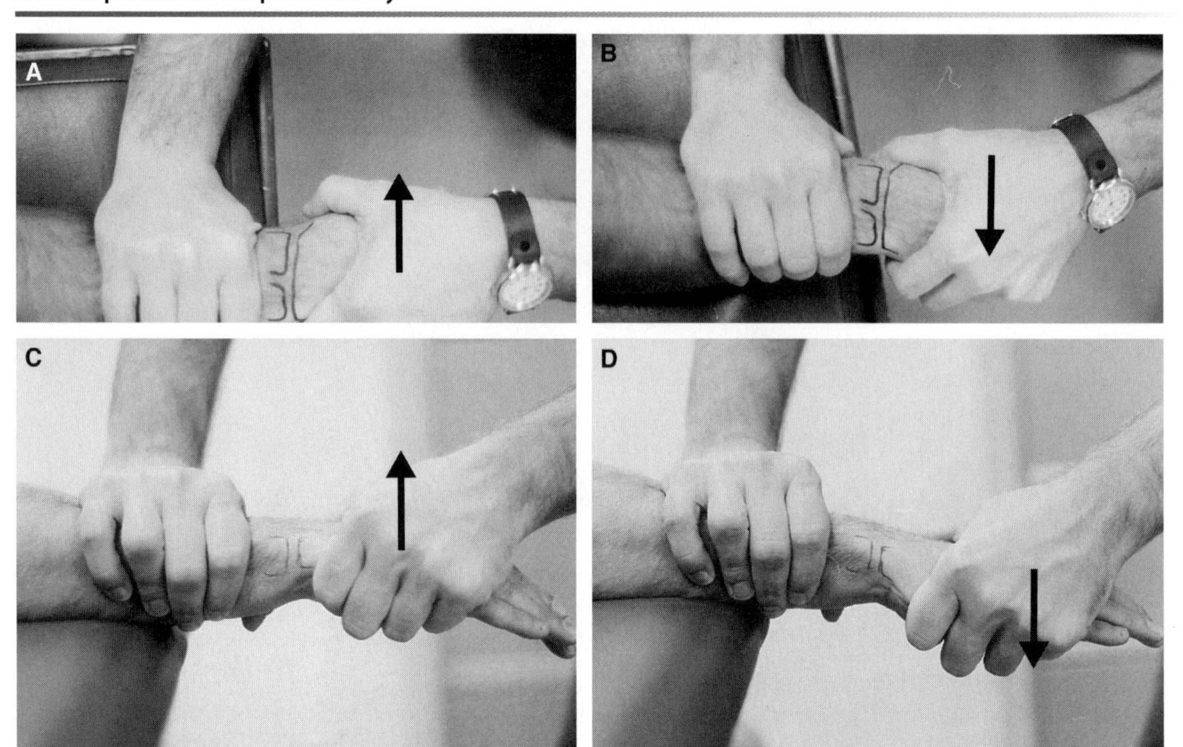

Joint play of the radiocarpal joint: radial glide **(A)**; ulnar glide **(B)**; dorsal glide **(C)**; and palmar glide **(D)**. Note that the hands are spread to allow visualization of the bones in the photographs. When performed clinically the hands should almost be touching.

Patient Position	Sitting The elbow is flexed to 90°, the forearm pronated, and the fingers in a relaxed position.
Position of Examiner	Sitting or standing lateral to the wrist being tested Radiocarpal joint: One hand grips the distal radius and the other hand grasps the proximal carpal row. Midcarpal joint: The proximal hand stabilizes the proximal carpal row, immediately distal to the radius. The other hand is immediately distal to the proximal row.
Evaluative Procedure	A shear force is applied to the wrist by gliding the distal segment in a radial and ulnar direction and then in a dorsal and palmar direction.
Positive Test	Pain or significant change in glide compared with the opposite side
Implications	Sprain of the collateral or intercarpal ligaments or trauma to the triangular fibrocartilage. Decreased glide may indicate adhesions and capsular stiffness after injury or surgery.
Comment	Radial and ulnar glide stresses both collateral ligaments; the determination of which ligament is involved is based on the location of pain.
Evidence	Absent or inconclusive in the literature

Joint Play 18-2
Intercarpal Joint Play

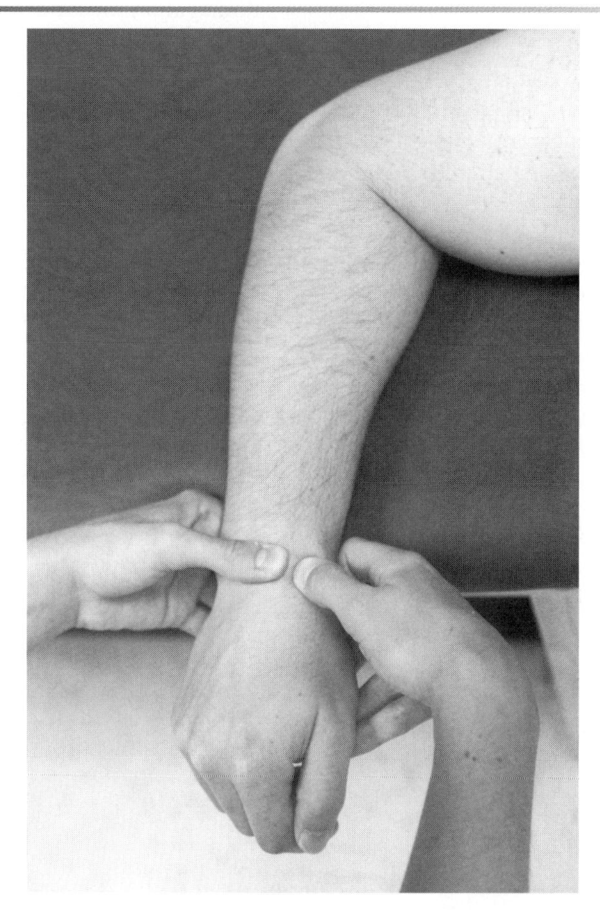

Joint play of the intercarpal articulations. Joint play of the scapholunate articulation is shown above.

Patient Position	Sitting The elbow is flexed to 90°, the forearm pronated, and the fingers in a relaxed position.
Position of Examiner	Sitting or standing lateral to the wrist being tested The thumb and index finger of one hand stabilize one carpal, with the thumb and index finger of the other hand stabilizing the other (or the radius).
Evaluative Procedure	A dorsal or palmar shear force is applied to one carpal while stabilizing the other.
Positive Test	Pain or significant change in glide compared with the opposite side
Implications	Tear or stretching of the intercarpal ligaments. Decreased glide may indicate adhesions and capsular stiffness after injury or surgery.
Modification	Apply slight traction to the wrist during the test.
Comment	A systematic approach to testing each intercarpal articulation is required.
Evidence	Absent or inconclusive in the literature

Pathologies of the Wrist, Hand, and Fingers and Related Special Tests

Any injury to this area involves the possible ramification of significant disability in both athletic competition and ADLs. Although similar in nature, trauma to the thumb and trauma to the fingers are discussed in separate sections because of the potential differences in the functional outcomes.

Wrist Pathology

Trauma to the wrist can affect the distal portion of the radius and ulna; the collateral, palmar, and dorsal ligaments; the triangular fibrocartilage; or the neurovascular structures. Resulting hyper- or hypomobility at these small articulations changes the demands on proximal and distal structures. The mechanisms of injury for most of these conditions are similar, calling for careful inspection, palpation, and functional testing of the involved structures.

Distal forearm fractures

Fractures of the distal radius or ulna frequently occur secondary to landing on an outstretched arm. This region and its epiphyses are particularly vulnerable in the child and adolescent. The term "**Colles' fracture**" is often used to describe any fracture of the distal radius. However, a true Colles' fracture is a nonarticular fracture of the radius approximately 1.5 inches proximal to the radiocarpal joint, where the distal radius is displaced dorsally.[20] On a lateral radiographic view, the wrist appears as an upside-down fork (Fig. 18-26). The terms "**Smith's fracture**" and "**reverse Colles' fracture**" are used to describe a fracture in which the distal radius is displaced palmarly (Examination Findings 18-1).[21]

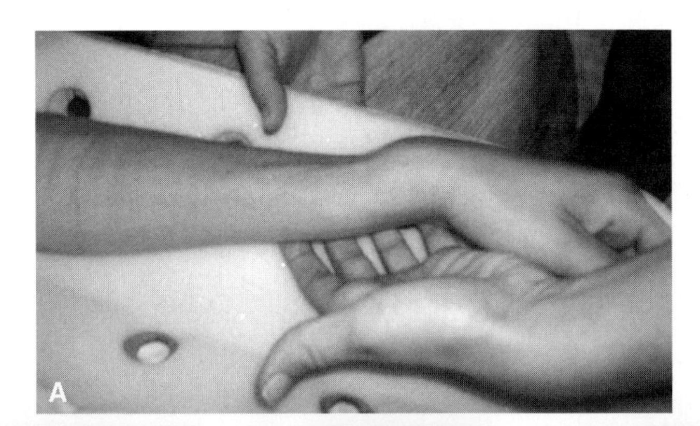

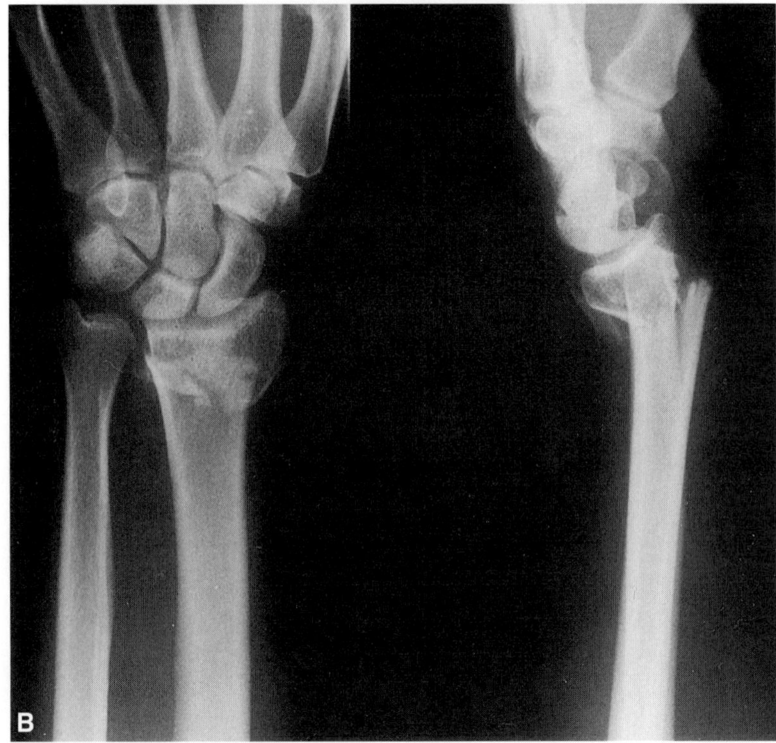

FIGURE 18-26 ■ Colles' fracture. **(A)** Inspection of obvious deformity. **(B)** Radiographic view.

Examination Findings 18-1
Distal Forearm Fractures

Examination Segment	Clinical Findings
History	***Onset:*** Acute ***Pain characteristics:*** Sharp at distal forearm, proximal wrist ***Other symptoms:*** The patient may describe hearing and feeling a cracking sensation. ***Mechanism:*** A hyperextension mechanism, possibly combined with a rotatory component, placing tensile, compressive, or shear forces on the radius, ulna, or both (e.g., landing on an outstretched arm) ***Predisposing conditions:*** Osteoporosis
Inspection	Gross deformity of the radius and/or ulna possible; rapid onset of swelling Open fractures are readily apparent.
Palpation	Bony palpation may be omitted if gross deformity is present. Discontinuity of the long bones may be felt and the area is tender to the touch.
Joint and Muscle Function Assessment	In the event of obvious gross deformity of the long bones, ROM testing is not conducted. ***AROM:*** Not applicable ***MMT:*** Not applicable ***PROM:*** Not applicable
Joint Stability Tests	***Stress tests:*** Should not be conducted if fracture is suspected. ***Joint play:*** Should not be performed if fracture is suspected.
Special Tests	Not applicable
Neurologic Screening	Determine distal neurologic function in the radial, median, and ulnar nerve distributions.
Vascular Screening	The examiner must locate the radial and ulnar pulses and check capillary refill to ensure an adequate blood supply to the hand and fingers.
Functional Assessment	None indicated
Imaging Techniques	Radiographs
Differential Diagnosis	Distal radioulnar dislocation, radiocarpal dislocation, epiphyseal fracture
Comments	Suspected fractures should be appropriately splinted and the patient immediately referred to a physician. The patient should be monitored for shock.

AROM = active range of motion; MMT = manual muscle test; PROM = passive range of motion.

Scaphoid fractures

The majority (70%) of all carpal fractures involve the scaphoid bone because of its function as a bony block limiting wrist extension.[23,24] Scaphoid fractures are most prevalent in the 15 to 30 year old population. In the very young and elderly populations, the scaphoid is spared at the expense of the weaker distal radius.[25] Receiving its blood supply from the radial artery at the distal end, a fracture compromises nutrition to the proximal portion, causing a high incidence of nonunion fractures and malunion fractures secondary to avascular necrosis (Fig. 18-27).[26] Unresolved fractures or chronically impaired circulation to the scaphoid may result in the development of **Preiser's disease**.

*** Practical Evidence**

Scaphoid fractures are rare in patients older than the age of 50. The older the person, the more likely it is that the wrist will fracture at the distal radial metaphysis than at the scaphoid.[22]

A fractured scaphoid can lead to instability of the proximal carpal row. When the scaphoid becomes bipartite, the lunate rotates dorsally around the triquetrum while the proximal pole of the scaphoid rotates with the lunate.

Preiser's disease Osteoporosis of the scaphoid, resulting from a fracture or repeated trauma.

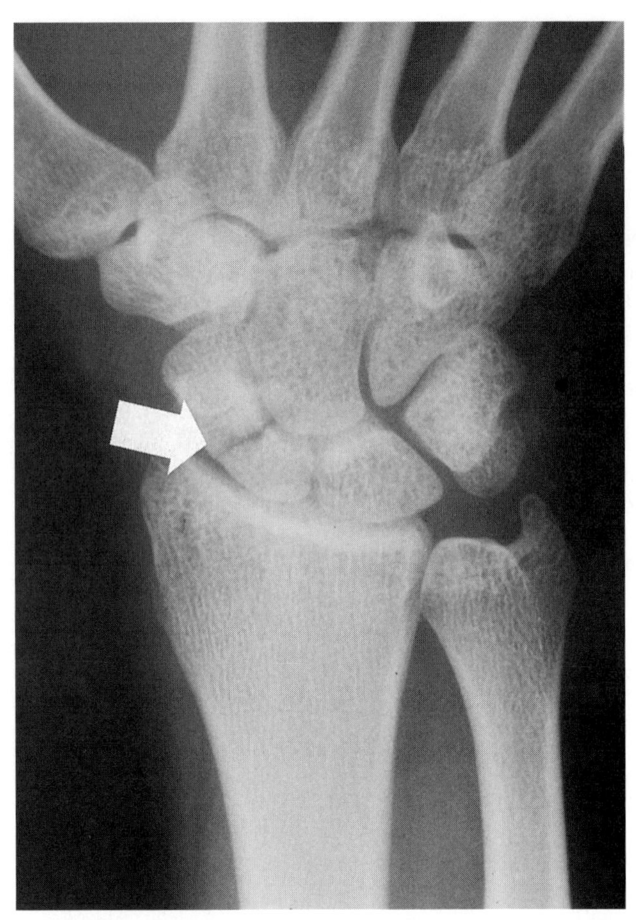

FIGURE 18-27 ■ Radiograph of a scaphoid fracture.

A **humpback** deformity results from the dorsal and radial angulation of the scaphoid fragments.[22]

The chief complaint is of an ache in the area of the anatomical snuffbox that is worsened with palpation at the snuffbox and scaphoid tubercle (see Fig. 18-18). Pain at the scaphoid tubercle is an even stronger indicator of a scaphoid fracture. To locate the scaphoid tubercle, palpate at the intersection of the distal wrist crease and tendon of the flexor carpi radialis and ulnarly deviate the wrist.[27] The scaphoid is the prominent bump. Pain occurs with active and resisted wrist extension near the end of the ROM, where the scaphoid contacts the radius. Severe pain is produced with overpressure during passive flexion, extension, and radial deviation. Grip strength may be decreased on the involved side. The **scaphoid compression test,** an axial load placed on the first metacarpal toward the scaphoid, may also produce pain.[22] Swelling may or may not be present, depending on the timing from the original injury (Examination Findings 18-2).

✱ Practical Evidence

Absence of pain in the anatomical snuffbox pain is highly sensitive to the absence of a scaphoid fracture; however, point tenderness in the snuffbox demonstrates a low specificity, indicating that many false-positive results are associated with the test.[25,27]

Patients with an injury that produces pain in the area of the anatomical snuffbox after a hyperextension mechanism, such as falling on an outstretched arm, must be treated as having a fracture of the scaphoid. The wrist and thumb require immobilization and the patient is referred to a physician. Fracture lines are not always visible on the initial radiographic examination, and follow-up radiographs may be ordered as indicated.[28] Bone scans, computed tomography (CT) scans, and magnetic resonance imaging (MRI) scans can identify the presence of a scaphoid fracture earlier than can standard radiographs.

No one course of treatment for patients with scaphoid fractures is universally accepted. Some physicians choose to treat these fractures in a short arm cast. Others elect to use a long arm thumb spica cast for 6 weeks followed by a short arm thumb spica cast for 6 weeks. The long arm cast eliminates movement at the fracture site caused by forearm pronation and supination. This treatment course may decrease the number of non- and malunions with these fractures. After adequate healing has taken place and the cast has been removed, the initial treatment focuses on restoration of ROM followed by strengthening. Any amount of displacement warrants operative treatment, typically open reduction and internal fixation.[22,25] For some athletes, the treatment of choice may also be to immediately surgically fixate the fracture. This allows for an increased chance of healing as well as earlier motion with less chance of motion loss.

Nonunion or malunion scaphoid fractures can lead to significant long-term disability. Most commonly associated with displaced fractures, fractures of the proximal pole, and in unrecognized fractures, decreased grip strength, reduced ROM, radiocarpal arthrosis, and pain significantly limit function.[22]

Hamate fractures

The hook of the hamate functions as a muscular attachment site for the flexor digiti minimi and the opponens digiti minimi and the point of attachment for the transverse carpal ligament and the pisohamate ligament. Hook of the hamate fractures occur following falls on an outstretched arm or, more commonly, as a result of trauma to the palm when using a golf club or swinging a baseball bat.[13] The body of the hamate is fractured through an axial load applied to the fourth or fifth metacarpal and frequently occurs concurrently with a metacarpal fracture. The body may also be fractured secondary to a direct blow.

Although acute injuries may be initially unremarkable during inspection, with time swelling in the hypothenar eminence and/or a noticeable protrusion over the hamate may be noted (Examination Findings 18-3). The patient may be tender during firm palpation of the hamate. The multiple attachments to the hook of the hamate result in pain when the fifth finger is actively abducted or adducted, or flexion and abduction are resisted. Pain occurs during passive extension of the fifth finger.

Examination Findings 18-2
Scaphoid Fractures

Examination Segment	Clinical Findings
History	***Onset:*** Acute, although the patient may delay seeking assistance because of the initial "minor" nature of the injury ***Pain characteristics:*** Proximal portion of the lateral wrist in the anatomic snuffbox and at the scaphoid tubercle ***Mechanism:*** Forceful hyperextension of the wrist that compresses the scaphoid ***Predisposing conditions:*** Younger than 50 years old
Inspection	Swelling possible in the anatomic snuffbox
Palpation	Palpation of the scaphoid as it sits in the anatomical snuffbox elicits pain and tenderness; crepitus may be present. Pain may also be produced during palpation of the distal tuberosity of the scaphoid on the palmar aspect of the hand. Compression of the first metacarpal toward the scaphoid may elicit pain.
Joint and Muscle Function Assessment	***AROM:*** Pain is produced at the terminal wrist ROM, especially during extension. Radial deviation increases pain as the scaphoid is impinged between the radius, lunate, and trapezium. ***MMT:*** Weakness secondary to pain with CMC extension and abduction and wrist extension with radial deviation ***PROM:*** Overpressure produces exquisite pain during extension and radial deviation. Pressure during flexion may also produce pain.
Joint Stability Tests	***Stress tests:*** Stress of UCL increases lateral wrist pain due to compression. ***Joint play:*** May have increased pain with radiocarpal joint play.
Special Tests	Scaphoid compression test
Neurologic Screening	Within normal limits
Vascular Screening	Within normal limits
Functional Assessment	Reduced grip strength May complain of pain and weakness with gripping actions and those that require radial deviation.
Imaging Techniques	PA radiographs with the wrist in neutral and ulnarly deviated, lateral view, and 45° pronation and supination views are obtained. The sensitivity and specificity of plain film radiographs are low in the days immediately after the trauma.[22] MRI are sensitive for identifying scaphoid fractures within 48 hours after trauma.[22] Up to 20% of scaphoid fractures are not detected using radiographs.[12]
Differential Diagnosis	Scapholunate sprain, fracture at the base of the first metacarpal (Bennett's fracture), trapezium fracture
Comments	Patients describing pain in the anatomical snuffbox after a mechanism involving forced hyperextension of the wrist should be managed as if they have a scaphoid fracture until it is ruled out by a physician. Scaphoid fractures may not appear on standard radiographs until several weeks after the injury but may be recognized on a bone scan within 72 hours after injury.

AROM = active range of motion; CMC = carpometacarpal; MRI = magnetic resonance images; MMT = manual muscle test; PROM = passive range of motion.

Examination Findings 18-3
Hamate Fractures

Examination Segment	Clinical Findings
History	***Onset:*** Acute ***Pain characteristics:*** Pain on the ulnar side of the hand, proximal to the 5th MC Diffuse pain in the wrist and hand ***Mechanism:*** The hook of the hamate may be fractured secondary to a fall on the hand. The probability of a fracture is increased if the patient is gripping an object such as a bat, racquet, golf club, or hammer. An axial load applied to the 4th or 5th MC Direct blow to the hamate
Inspection	Often unremarkable Swelling may develop in the hypothenar eminence. A callus-like projection may develop over the hamate.
Palpation	Pain during palpation of the hamate Hook of the hamate fractures will elicit pain during palpation of the palmar aspect of the hand.
Joint and Muscle Function Assessment	***AROM:*** Pain occurs during abduction and adduction of the 5th finger. ***MMT:*** Pain during resisted flexion of the 5th finger MCP, DIP, or IP Pain during resisted abduction of the 5th MCP ***PROM:*** Pain during passive extension of the wrist, 5th and possibly 4th, MCP
Joint Stability Tests	***Stress tests:*** Within normal limits ***Joint play:*** Within normal limits
Special Tests	None
Neurologic Screening	Paresthesia may be present in the 4th and 5th fingers secondary to ulnar nerve trauma.
Vascular Screening	Within normal limits
Functional Assessment	Reduced grip strength, complaints of pain and secondary weakness when gripping objects
Imaging Techniques	Radiographs are obtained using the carpal tunnel view and with the wrist supinated. CT scans are more specific for fractures of the hamate.[29]
Differential Diagnosis	CMC dislocation, fracture of the 4th or 5th MC, intercarpal sprain, ulnar nerve palsy
Comments	Misdiagnosed or untreated hamate fractures may lead to a nonunion or malunion.

AROM = active range of motion; CT = computed tomography; CMC = carpometacarpal; DIP = distal interphalangeal; IP = interphalangeal; MC = metacarpal; MCP = metacarpophalangeal; MMT = manual muscle test; PROM = passive range of motion.

An unstable hamate can compress the ulnar nerve as it passes through the Tunnel of Guyon, leading to paresthesia of the fourth and fifth fingers. Decreased innervation of the fifth slip of the flexor digitorum profundus can lead to its rupture.[29]

Perilunate and lunate dislocation

The biomechanics of the carpals causes the lunate to act as the keystone of the carpal group.[4] Perilunate and lunate dislocations fall on the same spectrum of injury and also involve the scaphoid and capitate.[30] Lunate dislocations occur when the lunate is disassociated from its contiguous carpals; perilunate dislocations involve the proximal carpal row being stripped from around the lunate.

High-energy forced hyperextension of the wrist and hand may disassociate the lunate from the rest of the carpals, resulting in its displacement either dorsally or palmarly. As the limits of the wrist and hand extension are exceeded, the scaphoid bone strikes the radius, rupturing the palmar interosseous ligaments connecting the scaphoid to the lunate. As the force continues, the distal carpal row is stripped away from the lunate, resulting in the lunate's resting dorsally relative to the other carpals, a perilunate dislocation. Further extension leads to rupture of the dorsal ligaments, relocating the carpals and rotating the lunate. Each of these types of dislocations may spontaneously reduce. Laxity of the interosseous ligaments alters the synchronous motion of the lunate, scaphoid, and triquetrum, **dissociative carpal instability**.[4] As the scaphoid is bound to both the proximal and distal carpal rows, an associated scaphoid fracture and/or instability of the associated carpals must be considered.[4]

The chief complaint is pain along the radial side of the palmar or dorsal aspect of the wrist that limits ROM. A bulge may be visible on the palmar or dorsal aspect of the hand proximal to the third metacarpal (Examination Findings 18-4). The displacement of the lunate or swelling can cause paresthesia in the middle finger. With a lunate dislocation, the third knuckle is level with the other knuckles (it normally appears to be more distal).[31] A fracture of the scaphoid bone should be suspected with any lunate dislocation because of the similarity in their mechanisms of injury. However, patients with these injuries may present with no significant physical findings other than pain, so a definitive diagnosis of a lunate dislocation is made via radiographs or MRI.

Mobilization of the carpal joints can reproduce the patient's symptoms. A compressive force placed on the ulnar side of the triquetrum, compressing the proximal carpal row radially and a palmar to dorsal force applied over the lunotriquetral joint stress the lunotriquetral ligament (Fig. 18-28).

Repeated trauma to the lunate may compromise its vascular supply, resulting in **Kienböck's disease**. Untreated, Kienböck's disease may result in a loss of ulnar deviation; tenderness, pain, and swelling over the lunate; decreased grip strength; and weakness during wrist extension. A characteristic finding of Kienböck's disease is pain during passive extension of the third finger.

Lunate dislocations that are seen early after the injury may be amenable to closed reduction. If reduction is successful, the wrist is then immobilized in flexion for 6 to 8 weeks. Frequent follow-up evaluations with radiographic examination are needed to make sure that the reduction is maintained. If the reduction is lost, percutaneous pinning of the lunate in the reduced position or open reduction may be needed.

If the patient is seen within 3 weeks of the initial injury, perilunate dislocations may be treated with closed reduction. If good anatomic reduction is demonstrated on radiographic

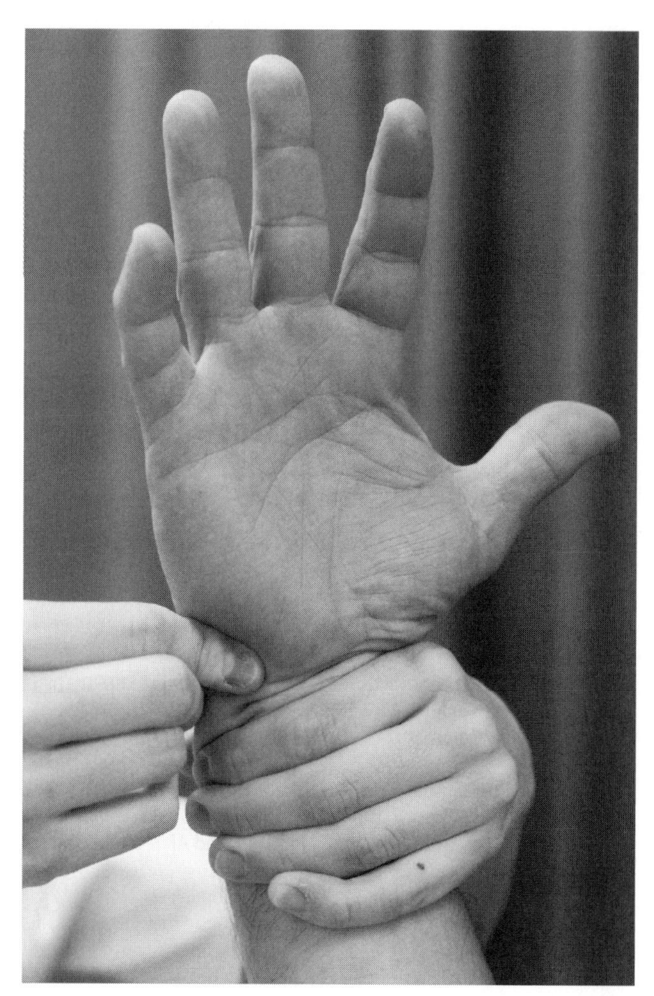

FIGURE 18-28 ■ A compressive force placed on the ulnar side of the triquetrum, compressing the proximal carpal row radially and a palmar to dorsal force applied over the lunotriquetral joint stress the lunotriquetral ligament.

Kienböck's disease Osteochondritis or slow degeneration of the lunate bone.

Examination Findings 18-4
Perilunate or Lunate Dislocation

Examination Segment	Clinical Findings
History	***Onset:*** Acute ***Pain characteristics:*** Lateral (ulnar) wrist and hand ***Other symptoms:*** Paresthesia along the ulnar nerve distribution Descriptions of the wrist and hand giving way ***Mechanism:*** Forced hyperextension of the wrist and hand. A ulnar deviation component may result in a perilunate dislocation. ***Predisposing conditions:*** Participation in activities that require repetitive resisted wrist extension, such as weight lifting and football (offensive linemen)
Inspection	A bulge caused by the displacement of the lunate may be seen on the palmar or dorsal aspect of the hand. If the dislocation spontaneously reduces, this may not be present. The fingers may be postured in a semiflexed position.[4]
Palpation	The lunate can be prominent during palpation, especially if it is dorsally displaced. Ballottement of the triquetrum is indicative of lunotriquetral ligament tears.[5] Malalignment of the carpals may be noted. Point tenderness and crepitus are present over the lunate.
Joint and Muscle Function Assessment	ROM in all planes is limited secondary to pain. ***AROM:*** Limited wrist extension. Finger flexion may be painful. ***MMT:*** Pain and weakness with PIP and DIP flexion; possibly WNL with isometric testing in neutral position ***PROM:*** Limited wrist extension; patient will be apprehensive at end-range. Passive extension of the fingers may produce pain.
Joint Stability Tests	***Stress tests:*** Not applicable in the event of an obvious dislocation ***Joint play:*** Not applicable in the event of an obvious dislocation Radial translation of the proximal carpal row relative to the radius and ulna will produce pain.
Special Tests	None
Neurologic Screening	Median nerve may be impinged, resulting in paresthesia in its distribution.
Vascular Screening	Within normal limits
Functional Assessment	Pain and decreased strength with gripping activities
Imaging Techniques	Lateral, PA, and AP radiographs are required for diagnosis.[4]
Differential Diagnosis	Distal radioulnar joint subluxation, triangular fibrocartilage pathology, distal radius fracture, scaphoid fracture, hamate fracture, carpal instability, carpal tunnel syndrome, or other neuropathy
Comments	An associated scaphoid fracture must be suspected with both perilunate and lunate dislocations.

AP = anteroposterior; AROM = active range of motion; DIP = distal interphalangeal; MMT = manual muscle test; PA = posteroanterior; PIP = proximal interphalangeal; PROM = passive range of motion.

examination, the wrist is then immobilized with slight flexion for 6 to 8 weeks. Loss of the reduction, even with casting, is common. Percutaneous pinning or open reduction is generally needed to maintain stable reduction.

Wrist sprains

Because wrist ligament sprains are caused by many of the same mechanisms as for other pathologies of the wrist and hand, the conclusion of a wrist sprain is often based on the exclusion of other injuries.[32] The possibilities of carpal fractures (especially the scaphoid), triangular fibrocartilage tears, and CTS must first be eliminated before making the determination of a wrist sprain. Sprains of the distal radioulnar ligaments can lead to a dislocation of the distal ends of these two bones, especially in the presence of an associated fracture.[33]

*** Practical Evidence**

Because standard imaging techniques such as radiographs and MRI do not capture the dynamic instability associated with scapholunate dissociation. Arthroscopy is considered the gold standard for diagnosis.[34]

Sprains of the scapholunate ligaments are the most common and outnumber sprains to the lunotriquetral joint by six to one.[16] Either can result in disabling instability if undetected and lead to static or dynamic instability.[5] Some scapholunate ligament sprains result in the scaphoid assuming a static flexed position while the lunate and triquetrum are relatively extended, a dorsal intercalated segmental instability (DISI). In other cases, the flexed position is assumed only during motion, a dynamic instability.[34,35] Patients with acute scapholunate injury will present with pain and swelling at the dorsal scapholunate articulation, coupled with decreased range of motion (Examination Findings 18-5). The **Watson test** may be positive and is particularly meaningful if a clunk is accompanied by pain (Special Test 18-2).[36] Radiographs, especially using a clenched-fist view, may show a gap between the scaphoid and lunate.[16] Arthroscopy is the gold standard for diagnosing ligamentous injuries to the wrist. MR and CT imaging are also used but these are most helpful in detecting complete tears and are less effective in detecting partial disruption. Diagnostic ultrasound lacks the sensitivity (46.2%) to detect all of those with the pathology.[34] Often misdiagnosed as a sprain, nontreatment of scapholunate instability will create a chronic condition, with the patient describing pain and weakness with wrist motion during functional tasks.

Triangular fibrocartilage complex injury

Trauma or repeated insult to the TFCC and the UCL can result in permanent disability of the wrist if left unrecognized and untreated.[2] Athletes who compete in sports that place the upper extremity in a closed kinetic chain are at an increased risk of TFCC injury. A positive ulnar variance, where the ulna is unusually long compared to the radius, increases compressive forces on the TFCC and predisposes this structure to injury (Fig. 18-29).[16]

When the TFCC is injured traumatically, forced hyperextension results in pain along the ulnar side of the wrist and is accompanied by decreased wrist motion secondary to pain. Acute injury can also occur by a force that distracts the ulnar aspect of the wrist.[3] Repeated weight-bearing,

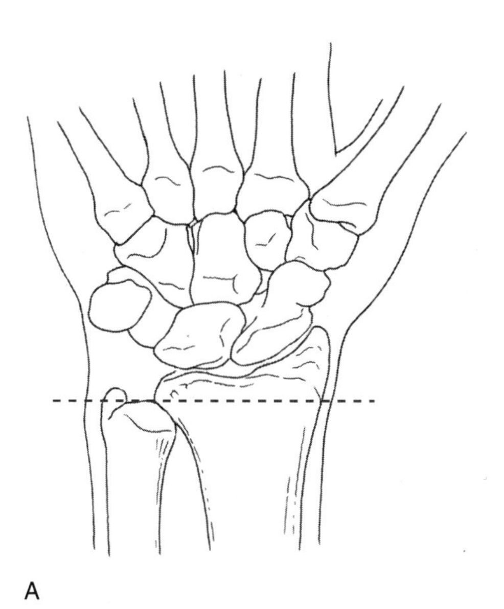

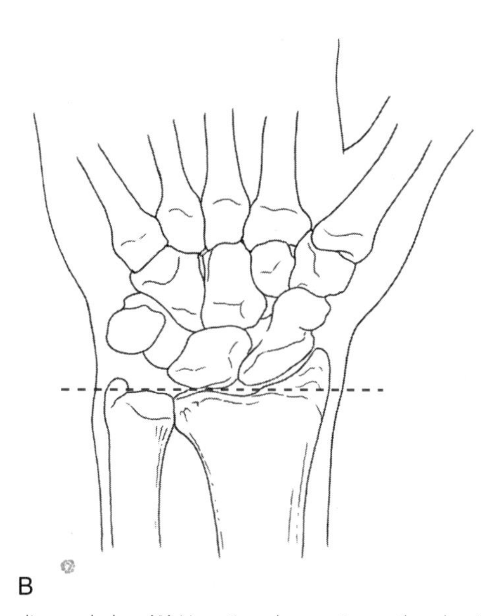

FIGURE 18-29 ■ Ulnar variance. The length relationship between the distal radius and ulna. **(A)** Negative ulnar variance: the ulna is shorter than the radius. **(B)** Positive ulnar variance: the ulna is longer than the radius. (Courtesy of Norkin, CC, and Levangie, PK: *Joint Structure and Function: A Comprehensive Analysis*, ed 4. Philadelphia: FA Davis, 2005.)

Examination Findings 18-5
Scapholunate Dissociation

Examination Segment	Clinical Findings
History	***Onset:*** Acute; diagnosis may be made much later. ***Pain characteristics:*** Pain emanating from the palmar and dorsal aspects of the wrist near the joint line ***Mechanism:*** Tensile forces placed on the ligaments as the joint is forced past its normal ROM ***Predisposing conditions:*** Not applicable
Inspection	Acutely, significant swelling at the proximal wrist
Palpation	Tenderness at scapholunate joint. usually more diffuse over the wrist region than with other wrist injuries such as scaphoid fractures or tears of the triangular fibrocartilage
Joint and Muscle Function Assessment	***AROM:*** Decreased wrist flexion and extension ***MMT:*** Pain possibly absent with isometric testing in a neutral position ***PROM:*** Limited wrist flexion and extension as the sprained tissues are placed on stretch
Joint Stability Tests	***Stress tests:*** Associated hypermobility of radiocarpal joint ***Joint play:*** Hypermobility at the scapholunate articulation
Special Tests	Watson test
Neurologic Screening	Within normal limits
Vascular Screening	Within normal limits
Functional Assessment	Pain and weakness in gripping activities. Restricted range may further limit function.
Imaging Techniques	MRI is more specific than CT. A clenched fist AP view may reveal increased space between the scaphoid and lunate.
Differential Diagnosis	Scaphoid fracture, lunotriquetral sprain, midcarpal joint sprain, TFCC tear radioulnar instability, lunate subluxation
Comments	The diagnosis of a wrist sprain is made after the possibility of carpal fractures, triangular fibrocartilage tears, and other traumatic injury has been ruled out.

AP = anteroposterior; AROM = active range of motion; CT = computed tomography; MRI = magnetic resonance image; MMT = manual muscle test; PROM = passive range of motion; ROM = range of motion.

such as during gymnastic maneuvers, may cause degeneration of the TFCC, especially at its ulnar insertion.

Functionally the patient will describe pain when weight-bearing on the arms, such as pushing up from a chair.[11] During palpation, close attention must be devoted to the ulnar styloid process because it can be avulsed by the UCL concurrently with injury to the TFCC (Examination Findings 18-6). Any suspicion of injury to the TFCC warrants referral to a physician for further evaluation.

Symptomatic TFCC tears are usually managed operatively. Tears to the avascular central articular disk, common in traumatic cases, respond well to debridement. Tears in the well-vascularized periphery can be repaired using open or arthroscopic procedures.[3] When a positive ulnar variance is the cause of degenerative changes, a procedure to shorten the ulna is required to prevent further damage.[16]

Carpal tunnel syndrome

Carpal tunnel syndrome refers to the signs and symptoms caused by the compression of the median nerve as it passes through the carpal tunnel (see Fig. 18-11). The most frequently cited cause of CTS is fibrosis of the synovium of the flexor tendons secondary to tenosynovitis.[38,39] CTS may occur with repetitive microtrauma, with acute trauma to the carpal tunnel, or as the result of progressive degeneration of the carpal tunnel's structures. The resulting symptoms of CTS can have detrimental effects on both athletic ability and ADLs.

Paresthesia and pain are described along the median nerve distribution (thumb, index, middle, and lateral half of the ring finger), with the symptoms often occurring at night and relieved with shaking.[37,40] Inspection of the hand may reveal atrophy of the thenar muscles, and grip strength is often

Special Test 18-2
Watson Test for Scapholunate Instability

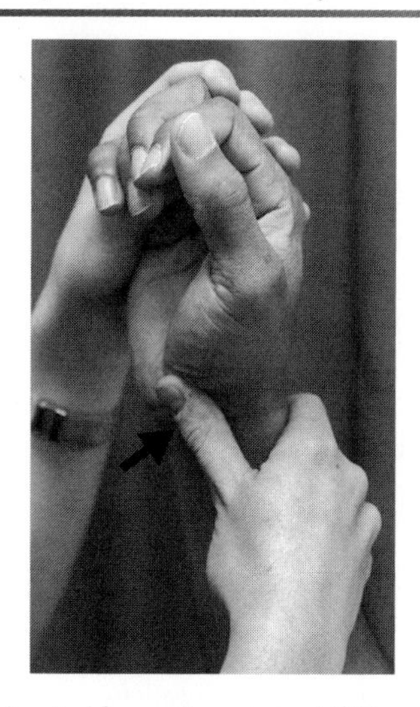
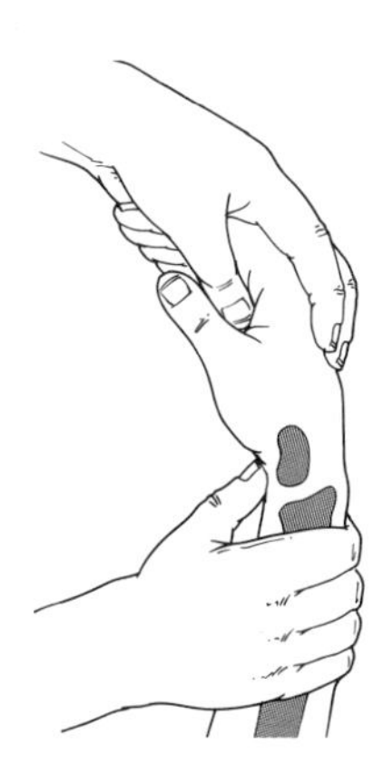
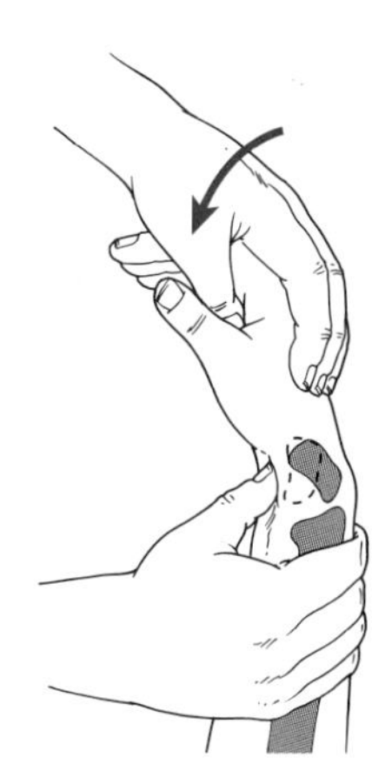

Application of a dorsally directed force attempts to shift the scaphoid from the lunate.

Patient Position	Seated with the elbow flexed and supported on the table and the forearm and hand pointing up, resembling the starting position for arm wrestling The wrist is ulnarly deviated.
Position of Examiner	In front of the patient
Evaluative Procedure	The examiner's thumb applies dorsal pressure to the distal pole of the scaphoid and then moves the patient's wrist from ulnar to radial deviation.
Positive Test	Reproduction of pain and notable pop at the scapholunate articulation
Implications	Scapholunate dissociation
Comments	This test may be difficult to perform on the acutely injured patient. Bilateral comparison is important because many patients have nonpathologic but positive findings.[16]
Evidence	Positive likelihood ratio Not Useful — Useful Very Small, Small, Moderate, Large 0 1 2 3 4 5 6 7 8 9 10 Negative likelihood ratio Not Useful — Useful Very Small, Small, Moderate, Large 1.0 0.9 0.8 0.7 0.6 0.5 0.4 0.3 0.2 0.1 0

Examination Findings 18-6
Triangular Fibrocartilage Complex Injury

Examination Segment	Clinical Findings
History	***Onset:*** Traumatic or degenerative Acute: The patient may not report the injury for some time after its onset. ***Pain characteristics:*** Distal to the ulna along the medial one half of the wrist; the UCL of the wrist may also be tender. ***Other symptoms:*** May complain of clicking on the ulnar side of the wrist with active motion. Click may be audible. ***Mechanism:*** Forced or repeated hyperextension of the wrist, compressing the triangular fibrocartilage ***Predisposing conditions:*** Positive ulnar variance
Inspection	Diffuse swelling around the wrist is possible, although acutely, no swelling may be visible.
Palpation	Point tenderness distal to the ulna along the medial one half of the wrist's joint line; the UCL may also display tenderness.
Joint and Muscle Function Assessment	***AROM:*** Motion is limited, especially into extension and ulnar deviation. ***MMT:*** Isometric testing may be normal; resistance through the ROM is limited, especially as the wrist is brought into extension and ulnar deviation. ***PROM:*** Motion is limited, especially into extension and ulnar deviation. Reproduction of clicking symptoms with ulnar deviation
Joint Stability Tests	***Stress tests:*** Stressing the UCL elicits pain, although laxity may not be present Ulnar deviation produces pain. ***Joint play:*** Pain during lateral and/or medial radiocarpal glide
Special Tests	None
Neurologic Screening	Within normal limits
Vascular Screening	Within normal limits
Functional Assessment	Increased symptoms with weight bearing activities on the arm (e.g., pushing off from table or chair, handstands) or activities that require repeated ulnar deviation and extension (e.g., hammering).
Imaging Techniques	MRI, MRI arthrogram
Differential Diagnosis	Lunotriquetral instability, extensor/flexor tendinopathy or subluxation, degeneration of distal radioulnar joint
Comments	Triangular fibrocartilage complex tears may be easily confused or occur in conjunction with a sprain of the wrist's UCL; persistence of symptoms should alert the examiner to injury beyond a simple wrist sprain. Patients suspected of suffering from triangular fibrocartilage complex tears should be referred to a physician for further evaluation.

AROM = active range of motion; MRI = magnetic resonance imaging; MMT = manual muscle test; PROM = passive range of motion; ROM = range of motion; UCL = ulnar collateral ligament.

decreased.[41] Manual muscle testing of the abductor pollicis brevis and the opponens pollicis reveals weakness on the involved side (Examination Findings 18-7).[42] A positive **Tinel's sign** is elicited over the carpal tunnel and **Phalen's test** is positive (Special Test 18-3). Sustained pressure applied with both thumbs directly over the carpal tunnel (carpal tunnel test) will reproduce neurological symptoms.[40] An achy pain may be described in the palmar aspect of the forearm. The results of two-point discrimination testing at less than 5mm will be diminished.[43]

Replication of the functional demands that induce symptoms is important to determine the underlying cause of CTS. Repetitive motions, such as those associated with typing with the wrist in an extended position may be cause the problem. The postural examination may also reveal contributing factors, such as forward head and shoulders, that cause an increased demand and less than optimal biomechanics on the smaller distal joints and muscles.

The signs and symptoms of CTS closely resemble the peripheral symptoms associated with impingement of the C7 nerve root and proximal neuropathy of the median nerve. A careful differential evaluation must be made to identify the cause of the symptoms. An examination of the cervical spine and/or elbow is warranted if the patient reports a history of injury in these regions.

Initially, patients with CTS are managed conservatively. The basic treatment plan focuses on rest from aggravating activities, postural training, activity modification and ergonomic changes in work stations and computer usage. Initial treatments also include the use of nonsteroidal anti-inflammatory drugs (NSAIDs) to decrease inflammation and splinting to remove harmful physical stresses.[45] Initially splinting may be used only at night. Severe or nonresponsive cases may require splint use throughout the day. Attempts at stretching and strengthening the surrounding wrist musculature usually do not affect the course of the treatment.

Surgery may be required to relieve the compression on the median nerve. After an initial period of taking NSAIDs and immobilization to allow for healing, AROM and strengthening exercises are begun.

Hand Pathology

The majority of injuries to the hand have an acute onset. Injury to the metacarpals and phalanges typically follows axial loading of the bone. Both groups of bones are also susceptible to crushing forces. Tendon ruptures or bony avulsions occur with eccentric stresses to the muscle–tendon unit.

Metacarpal fractures

The metacarpals are typically fractured secondary to a compressive force along the bone's shaft, such as improperly punching with a fist. In football players, the incidence of fractures involving metacarpals is evenly divided among the five digits. In basketball players, most fractures involve the fourth and fifth metacarpals.[16] It is common for the patient to hear the bone snapping as it fractures and describe immediate pain along one or more metacarpals. Gross deformity at the fracture site may be observed as one end of the bone rides over the other end, or the fracture site may be obscured by localized swelling along the dorsum of the hand (Fig. 18-30). Palpation reveals local tenderness over the fracture site. The actual bony fragments or crepitus may be palpated and the presence of a false joint established. The presence of a nondisplaced fracture may be confirmed through a variation of the long bone compression test (Fig. 18-31). The AROM of the involved finger, and possibly the hand, is limited by pain. The patient is unable to make a fist (Examination Findings 18-8). As the patient attempts to flex the hand, the fingers should remain parallel to one another. With metacarpal fractures, the involved segment may rotate so that the finger flexes under or on top of the finger next to it.

Fractures of the fifth metacarpal are termed "**boxer's fractures**" because of their common incidence after an improperly thrown punch. This type of fracture is characterized by a depressed fifth MCP joint that, on radiographic examination, reveals an overlapping of the bone fragments.

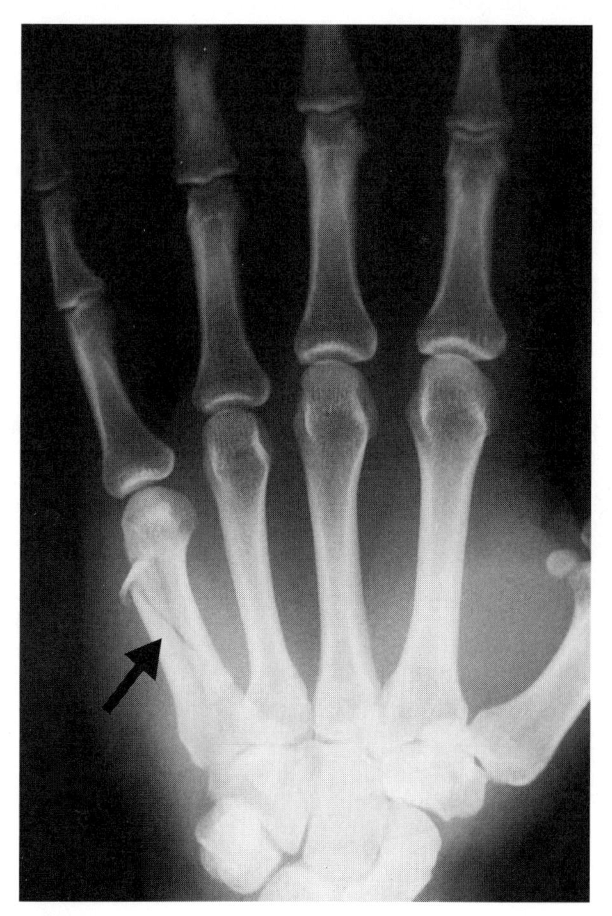

FIGURE 18-30 ■ Radiograph of a fractured 5th metacarpal, the so-called "boxer's fracture."

Examination Findings 18-7
Carpal Tunnel Syndrome

Examination Segment	Clinical Findings
History	***Onset:*** Insidious ***Pain characteristics:*** Pain in the hand, wrist, and fingers, possibly radiating up the length of the arm and worsening during sleep secondary to a flexed posture of the elbow, wrist, and fingers ***Other symptoms:*** Paresthesia in the forearm, wrist, or hand (median nerve distribution) ***Mechanism:*** Repetitive wrist movement involving flexion and extension or finger flexion and extension ***Predisposing conditions:*** Poor posture or biomechanics; Pregnancy[13]; Hypothyroidism[13]; Diabetes[13]; Carpal instability; Age older than 45 years[37]
Inspection	Palmar aspect of the wrist possibly appearing thickened; atrophy of the thenar eminence after long duration of symptoms
Palpation	Possible tenderness on palpation or sustained pressure (carpal compression test) directly over the palmar aspect of the wrist
Joint and Muscle Function Assessment	***AROM:*** The wrist motion may be slightly limited owing to stiffness, although AROM may be normal. ***MMT:*** In chronic cases, the strength of the abductor pollicis brevis, flexor pollicis brevis, or opponens pollicis may be decreased. ***PROM:*** Median nerve symptoms may increase as the wrist is fully extended or fully flexed.
Joint Stability Tests	***Stress tests:*** Not applicable ***Joint play:*** Hypermobility of intercarpal or radiocarpal articulations may be an underlying pathology.
Special Tests	Tinel's sign; Phalen's test
Neurologic Screening	Possible decreased sensation along the median nerve distribution of the hand (palmar aspect of the thumb, fingers II and III, and the lateral aspect of IV) Decreased 2-point discrimination tests within the median nerve distribution
Vascular Screening	Capillary refill and venous return are usually normal.
Functional Assessment	Forward head, neck, and/or shoulder posture may be observed with activities of daily living. Shaking hands relieves symptoms.[37]
Imaging Techniques	Radiographs to rule out bony impingement within the tunnel MRI can be used to assist in identifying soft tissue compression of the tunnel.
Differential Diagnosis	Thoracic outlet syndrome, nerve root compression, proximal median nerve compressions (pronator syndrome, anterior interosseous nerve syndrome)
Comments	This condition is typically found in individuals who perform repetitive wrist and hand movements such as typing and may become more pronounced in a student-athlete population with the increase in computer use in academic work. Nerve conduction studies may reveal latency of the median nerve.

AROM = active range of motion; MMT = manual muscle test; MRI = magnetic resonance imaging; PROM = passive range of motion.

Special Test 18-3
Phalen's Test for Carpal Tunnel Syndrome

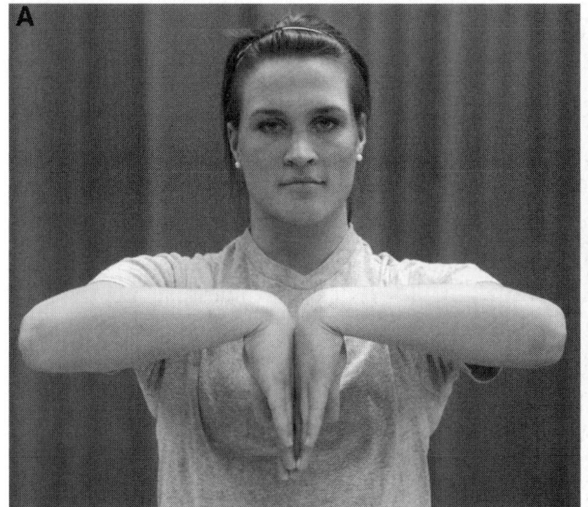

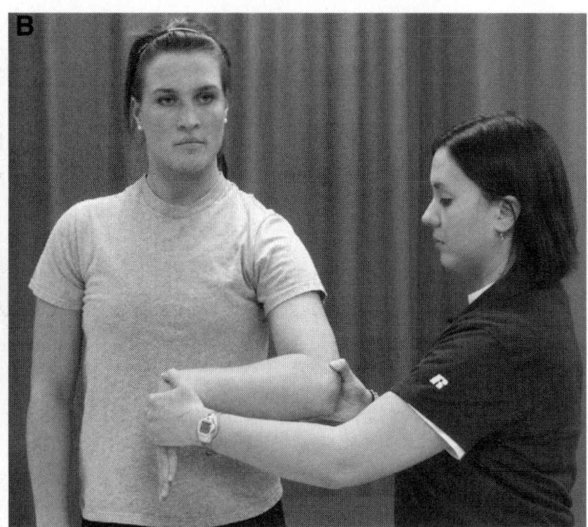

(A) Original test as described by Phalen. **(B)** Modification of Phalen's test (described below).

Patient Position	Standing
Position of Examiner	Standing in front of the patient
Evaluative Procedure	The examiner applies overpressure during passive wrist flexion and holds the position for 1 minute. Repeat this procedure for the opposite extremity.
Positive Test	Tingling develops or increases in the distribution of the median nerve distal to the carpal tunnel.
Implications	Median nerve compression
Modification	The traditional version of this test, in which the patient maximally flexes the wrists by pushing the dorsal aspects of the hands together, is not recommended because the patient may shrug the shoulders, causing compression of the median branch of the brachial plexus as it passes through the thoracic outlet. Reverse Phalen's, with the wrist positioned in maximum extension, is an alternate position to stress the median nerve, with approximately the same diagnostic value **(B)**.[43,44]
Comments	Patients with numbness may not have an exacerbation of symptoms with this test, leading to a false-negative result.[43]
Evidence	***Inter-rater reliability:***

Not Reliable — Very Reliable
Poor | Moderate | Good
0 0.1 0.2 0.3 0.4 0.5 0.6 0.7 0.8 0.9 1.0

Positive likelihood ratio

Not Useful — Useful
Very Small | Small | Moderate | Large
0 1 2 3 4 5 6 7 8 9 10

Negative likelihood ratio

Not Useful — Useful
Very Small | Small | Moderate | Large
1.0 0.9 0.8 0.7 0.6 0.5 0.4 0.3 0.2 0.1 0

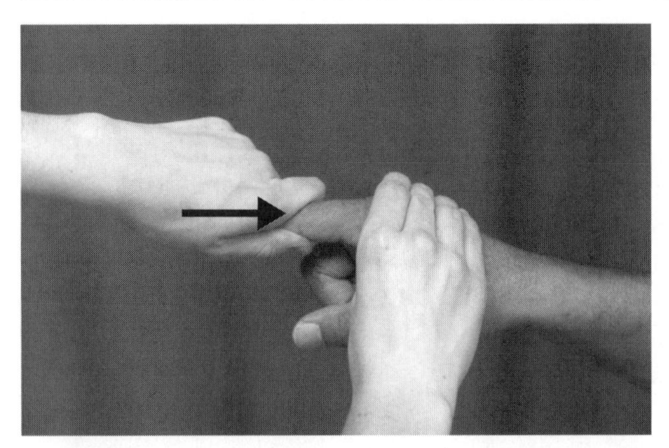

FIGURE 18-31 ■ Long bone compression test for phalanx fracture. For the middle and proximal phalanx and the metacarpals an axial load is applied to the ray. For the distal phalanx, the examiner flicks the tip of the finger.

Treatment for metacarpal fractures depends on the presence of rotation and extent of angulation at the fracture site. In the absence of rotation, a conservative approach of casting may be used. The presence of rotation at the fracture site that cannot be resolved with closed reduction necessitates open reduction with internal fixation to ensure favorable functional outcomes.[46] The amount of angulation deformity that can be tolerated while maintaining function differs among the metacarpals. At the fifth metacarpal, with its extensive mobility at its CMC, angulation of up to 70 degrees may be acceptable.[47] After adequate healing has taken place, AROM can be started and progressed to PROM, if needed, at about 8 weeks after the fracture. Strengthening of the wrist and hand is incorporated to counteract the effects of immobilization on the surrounding soft tissue.

Finger Pathology

Frequently finger injuries go unreported or there is a significant lapse between the onset of the injury and its report. Often gross deformity is associated with these conditions, especially with joint dislocations. However, the patient may self-reduce a dislocation before seeking medical attention.

Collateral ligament injuries

Trauma to the collateral ligaments can range from simple sprains to complete dislocations caused from a unilateral stress being applied to an extended finger. Pain is experienced at the affected joint. Active motion and passive motion are limited secondary to pain and swelling. With the exception of a complete disruption of the ligament, valgus and varus stress testing does not accurately distinguish the severity of the injury.

Boutonnière deformity

A rupture of the central extensor tendon causes the lateral bands to slip palmarly on each side of the PIP joint, changing its line of pull on this joint from that of an extensor to one of a flexor. The resulting position of the finger is extension of the DIP and MCP joints and flexion of the PIP joint, a boutonnière deformity (see Inspection Findings 18-2). The patient describes a longitudinal force on the finger, such as being struck with a ball. Pain occurs on the dorsal aspect of the PIP joint, and the boutonnière deformity is visible. In acute cases, the PIP joint cannot be actively extended, but the examiner can passively return the joint to its normal position. The signs and symptoms of a tendon rupture may not be recognized for some time after the injury.[48] In chronic cases, the remaining tendon becomes fibrotic, forming a mechanical block against even passive extension of the joint.

An injury to the volar plate can cause a flexion deformity of the PIP joint that resembles a boutonnière deformity, a **pseudo-boutonnière deformity** (see Inspection Findings 18-2). Hyperextension of the finger causes the volar plate to split along the finger's long axis and slide dorsally past the joint's axis. The PIP joint cannot be extended either actively or passively.

Finger fractures

Fractures of the **distal phalanx**, the most common fractures of the hand, occur most frequently in the thumb and middle finger. One reason for this high incidence of injury is the attachments of the flexor and extensor tendons. Avulsions of these tendons result in the inability to completely flex or extend the distal phalanx. The distal phalanx is also vulnerable to crushing mechanism (e.g., being stepped on) and longitudinal compression and rotation (e.g., a blow to the tip of the finger). The **middle phalanx** is the least frequently fractured phalanx and tends to fracture at the distal portion of the shaft. Injuries to the **proximal phalanx** usually have concurrent tendon and skin trauma. A direct blow to the finger often results in a transverse or comminuted fracture; a twisting or rotational force causes a spiral fracture (Fig. 18-32).

The signs and symptoms of phalanx fractures are similar to those of metacarpal fractures (see Examination Findings 18-8). An audible "snap" at the time of injury may be reported, especially when the proximal or middle phalanx is injured. Pain is centered over the fracture site, and gross deformity may be present in the finger's alignment. Soft tissue swelling and hematoma formation increase the amount of pain associated with the fracture and impair the ability to palpate the injured area. AROM is limited by pain or bony derangement. During finger flexion, a spiral or oblique fracture causes the portion of the finger distal to the fracture site to rotate so that the fingernails are not in line with each other (Fig. 18-33). Fractures that extended into the joint's articular surface can result in the long-term loss of ROM if not surgically realigned.

Finger fractures are managed similarly to metacarpal fractures.

Tendon ruptures and avulsion fractures. Mallet finger occurs when an avulsion or rupture of an extensor tendon results in the inability to fully extend the distal phalanx (see Inspection Findings 18-2). This occurs when the DIP is forced into flexion, such as when the fingertip is struck with

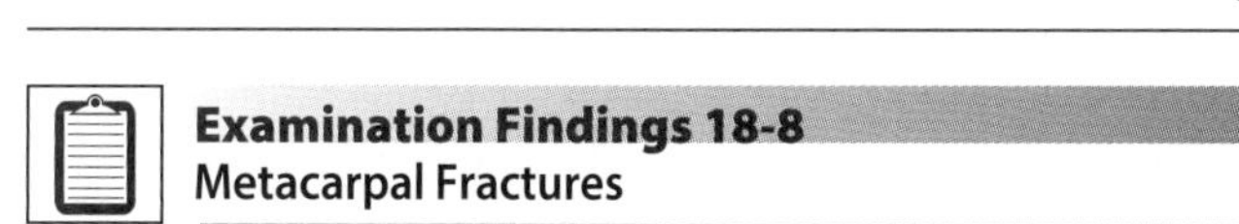

Examination Findings 18-8
Metacarpal Fractures

Examination Segment	Clinical Findings
History	***Onset:*** Acute ***Pain characteristics:*** Along the shaft of one or more metacarpals ***Mechanism:*** Longitudinal compression of the bone (direct contact), a crushing force (being stepped on), or a shear force (hyperextension of the finger)
Inspection	Gross deformity of the bone may be visible. There is localized swelling over the involved metacarpal(s), and MCP joint(s), which may spread to the entire dorsum of the hand. Fractures of the 5th, and possibly 4th, metacarpals may result in a depression or shortening of the knuckles. The fingernail may be abnormally rotated when a fist is made.
Palpation	Palpation should not be performed if a fracture is evident. Severe tenderness is present over the fracture site. Bony fragments or crepitus may be present. A false joint may be displayed.
Joint and Muscle Function Assessment	ROM testing should not be performed if a fracture is evident. ***AROM:*** Limited secondary to pain; in some instances, the patient is unable to make a fist. ***MMT:*** Do not assess in presence of suspected fracture. ***PROM:*** Do not assess in presence of suspected fracture.
Joint Stability Tests	***Stress tests:*** Not applicable ***Joint play:*** Not applicable
Special Tests	Long bone compression test
Neurologic Screening	Within normal limits
Vascular Screening	Within normal limits
Functional Assessment	Difficulty and pain when grasping objects
Imaging Techniques	Radiographs
Differential Diagnosis	MCP or CMC dislocation
Comments	If a fracture is evident during inspection, the evaluation should be immediately terminated, the hand appropriately splinted, and the patient immediately referred to a physician.

AROM = active range of motion; CMC = carpometacarpal; MCP = metacarpophalangeal; MMT = manual muscle test; PROM = passive range of motion; ROM = range of motion.

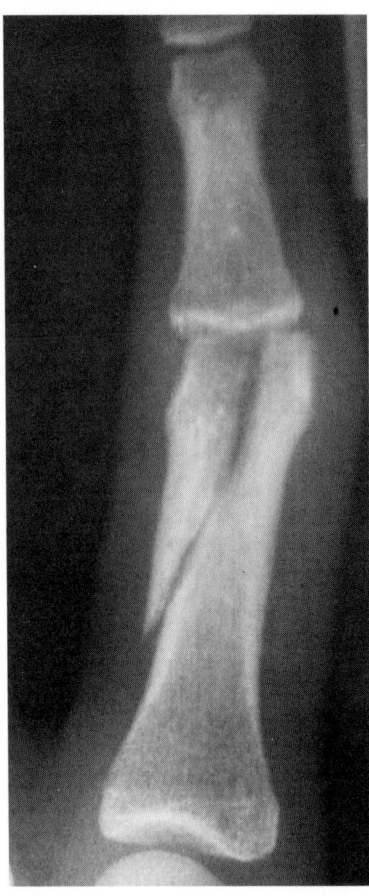

FIGURE 18-32 ■ Radiograph of a phalanx fracture. Note that this is a spiral fracture involving the articular surface.

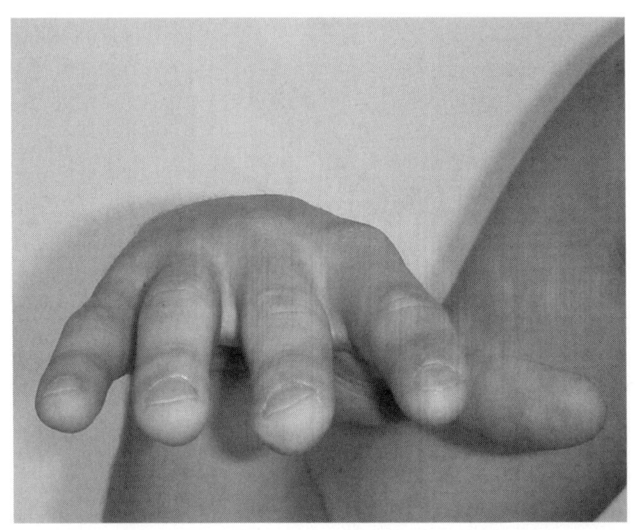

FIGURE 18-33 ■ Rotational malalignment associated with a spiral fracture of the phalanx or metacarpal. Note the rotational displacement of the third fingernail.

a ball. In addition to being unable to actively extend the finger, the patient will report pain at the distal phalanx, which rests at approximately 25 to 35 degrees of flexion. Active flexion is still present and the phalanx can be passively moved into extension.

An avulsion of the flexor digitorum profundus tendon off the palmar aspect of the DIP joint, **jersey finger**, results in the inability to flex the distal phalanx (see Inspection Findings 18-2). This commonly occurs when an athlete grasps another athlete's jersey, forcing the finger into extension as the finger is attempting to flex and hold onto the opponent. The jersey finger injury is described as being one of three types.[49]

- **First degree:** The bony attachment is left intact and the ruptured tendon retracts to the PIP joint.
- **Second degree:** A portion of the bony attachment is avulsed and the tendon retracts to the palm.
- **Third degree:** A fragment of bone is avulsed with the tendon's insertion and retracts to the PIP joint.

On casual inspection and functional testing, the involved finger appears to be normal. The finger is painful, but little swelling or disfiguration is noted. The fingers appear to flex and extend normally, with an increase in pain noted during flexion. The telltale sign occurs when the examiner stabilizes the PIP joint in extension and requests that the patient flex the DIP joint but the patient is unable to do so.

Thumb Pathology

The thumb is involved in most aspects of ADLs and athletics and the position it assumes when gripping, catching, or in the "ready position" exposes it to potentially injurious forces in all planes. Unlike the other digits, the thumb is also susceptible to overuse conditions.

De Quervain's syndrome

De Quervain's syndrome is a tenosynovitis of the extensor pollicis brevis and abductor pollicis longus tendons, which are encased by a fibrous sheath having a common synovial lining. De Quervain's syndrome is most common in women between the ages of 20 and 40.[50] Repetitive stress results in the compartment's becoming inflamed. Consequently, prolonged inflammation causes a thickening and narrowing of the tendon's sheath. A history of this condition reveals a mechanism of repetitive motions usually involving radial deviation.[51] Pain is located at the radial styloid process and dorsum of the thumb and radiates proximally into the forearm. Swelling may be located over the styloid process and thenar eminence. Radial and ulnar deviation of the wrist results in pain, as do flexion, extension, and abduction of the thumb (Examination Findings 18-9). Although not conclusive, **Finkelstein's test** may be used to support or refute the presence of de Quervain's syndrome (Special Test 18-4).

Patients with de Quervain's syndrome are best treated corticosteroid injections.[52] Rest, ice, NSAIDs, and splinting to limit ulnar deviation may also be used. The use of iontophoresis may be helpful to decrease the inflammation in the tissues. Activity modification and long-term splinting may be needed to eliminate excessive stress on the tendons with repetitive ulnar deviation.

Examination Findings 18-9
De Quervain's Syndrome

Examination Segment	Clinical Findings
History	***Onset:*** Insidious ***Pain characteristics:*** Over the length of the extensor pollicis brevis and abductor pollicis longus, the radial styloid process and thenar eminence, possibly extending into the distal forearm; complaints of pain increased during radial and ulnar deviation ***Mechanism:*** Repetitive stress often involving radial deviation ***Predisposing conditions:*** Repetitive motion accompanied by poor biomechanics
Inspection	Swelling over the styloid process and in the involved tendons
Palpation	Pain felt over the styloid process, thenar eminence, and the length of the extensor pollicis brevis and abductor pollicis longus muscles
Joint and Muscle Function Assessment	***AROM:*** Wrist: Pain with radial and ulnar deviation Thumb: Pain with flexion and adduction and extension and abduction ***MMT:*** Wrist: Pain with radial deviation Thumb: Pain with extension and abduction of CMC ***PROM:*** Wrist: Pain at the end range of ulnar deviation Thumb: Pain with flexion and adduction CMC
Joint Stability Tests	***Stress tests:*** Not applicable ***Joint play:*** Not applicable
Special Tests	Finkelstein's test
Neurologic Screening	Within normal limits
Vascular Screening	Within normal limits
Functional Assessment	Increased symptoms with activities requiring radial and ulnar deviation
Imaging Techniques	Generally none used
Differential Diagnosis	Extensor carpi radialis brevis (ECRB), extensor carpi radialis longus (ECRL) tendinopathy, ganglion, cervical radiculopathy, scaphoid fracture
Comments	Not applicable

AROM = active range of motion; CMC = carpometacarpal; MMT = manual muscle test; PROM = passive range of motion.

Thumb sprains

The UCL of the thumb's MCP joint is injured 10 times more often than its radial counterpart is.[53] This structure may be acutely sprained by hyperabduction or hyperextension of the MCP joint or it may be traumatized secondary to a repetitive stress. In the case of acute trauma, an associated avulsion fracture may occur around the MCP joint. The term "gamekeeper's thumb" was coined to describe the stretching of this ligament suffered by individuals whose duty it was to snap the neck of small game that had just been captured during hunting. This injury is commonly seen in skiers, football players, and basketball players. UCL sprains limit opposition of the thumb and decrease grip strength.

The chief complaint is pain along the ulnar aspect of the MCP joint that hinders the ability to forcefully pinch or grasp smaller objects. Swelling, which can be extensive, is usually localized in the adductor compartment and thenar eminence. Ecchymosis may also be present. During palpation, tenderness is elicited over the UCL, with special attention paid to its proximal and distal attachments, noting for signs of an avulsion. Pain is produced and a strength deficit is noted during opposition of the thumb and index finger (Examination Findings 18-10). Valgus stress testing

Special Test 18-4
Finkelstein's Test for De Quervain's Syndrome

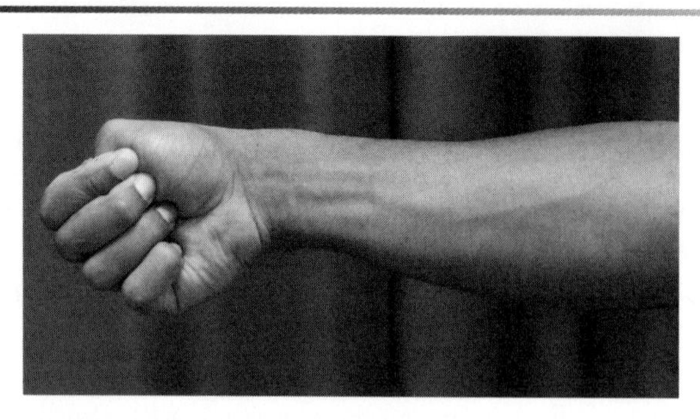

The patient ulnarly deviates the wrist while the thumb is clasped by the fingers.

Patient Position	Seated or standing
Position of Examiner	Standing in front of the patient
Evaluative Procedure	The patient tucks the thumb under the fingers by making a fist. The patient then ulnarly deviates the wrist.
Positive Test	Increased pain in the area of the radial styloid process and along the length of the extensor pollicis brevis and abductor pollicis longus tendons
Implications	De Quervain's syndrome (tenosynovitis of the extensor pollicis brevis and abductor pollicis longus tendons)
Comments	This test often produces false-positive results, so the results must be correlated with other findings of the evaluation.
Evidence	Absent or inconclusive in the literature

of the UCL demonstrates an increase in the amount of gapping present as compared with the uninjured hand. Stress testing should be carried out with the first MCP joint extended and then again with the joint flexed to account for the geometry of the joint and to test the various bands of the UCL.[54]

The treatment of patients with sprains of the UCL of the first MCP joint is determined by the severity of the sprain. Instability of this joint will adversely affect ADLs as simple as gripping a soda can as well as more vigorous sports activities. Patients with incomplete tears with a firm endpoint and less than 30 degrees of opening compared with the opposite side during stress testing may be treated with a thumb spica splint for 4 to 6 weeks. Complete ruptures require early surgical repair to avoid long-term complications, but surgery can usually be attempted up to 3 weeks after the injury.[55] Periods longer than 3 weeks after the injury may require a reconstruction of the ligament with a graft versus a primary repair of the tissue. **Stener lesions**, in which the proximal end of the UCL dislocates from under the adductor aponeurosis, must be treated with surgery.[47]

Metacarpophalangeal joint dislocation

Dislocation of the MCP joint is most common in the thumb and occurs when the volar plate is avulsed from the head of the first metacarpal. The mechanism of injury is extension and abduction. A fracture of the proximal phalanx or first metacarpal joint may occur concurrently. The involved joint has obvious deformity and is unable to demonstrate AROM because of pain.

Thumb fractures

Fractures of the first metacarpal are similar to the description given for metacarpal fractures of the hand. Fractures of the base of the first metacarpal that extend into the articular surface are termed **Bennett's fractures** (Fig. 18-34). Because of the thumb's potential loss of function secondary to instability at the CMC joint, patients with this type of fracture often require internal fixation of the bony fracture.

Examination Findings 18-10
Ulnar Collateral Ligament Sprains

Examination Segment	Clinical Findings
History	***Onset:*** Acute or chronic ***Pain characteristics:*** Along the ulnar aspect of the first MCP joint ***Mechanism:*** Acute: Hyperextension or hyperabduction (or both) of the first MCP joint Chronic: Repetitive flexion or adduction (or both) of the joint ***Predisposing conditions:*** Repetitive motion that applies a valgus force to the MCP joint
Inspection	Localized swelling in the adductor compartment and thenar eminence Possible ecchymosis
Palpation	Pain is felt along the ulnar border of the MCP joint. The examiner should note for the presence of bony fragments indicating an avulsion of the ligament.
Joint and Muscle Function Assessment	***AROM:*** Pain during extension, abduction, and opposition of the thumb ***MMT:*** Weakness experienced during MCP flexion and CMC adduction; pinch strength decreased ***PROM:*** Pain during thumb extension and abduction
Joint Stability Tests	***Stress tests:*** Test for ulnar collateral ligament instability Valgus stress test for the MCP joint ***Joint play:*** Increased ulnar glide of MCP joint
Special Tests	None
Neurologic Screening	Within normal limits
Vascular Screening	Within normal limits
Functional Assessment	Increased pain or weakness with any tasks requiring gripping
Imaging Techniques	Radiographs to rule out avulsion fracture
Differential Diagnosis	Metacarpal or proximal phalanx fracture, volar plate injury
Comments	UCL sprains should be referred to a physician for further evaluation to rule out an avulsion fracture.

AROM = active range of motion; CMC = carpometacarpal; MCP = metacarpophalangeal; MMT = manual muscle test; PROM = passive range of motion; UCL = ulnar collateral ligament.

On-Field Evaluation and Management of Wrist, Hand, and Finger Injuries

Most often, athletes with a wrist, hand, or finger injury leave the field on their own, cradling and protecting the injured extremity. The examiner must carry out a complete inspection of the injured area, a task that is somewhat eased by the relatively superficial nature of the structures. With the exception of trauma to the carpal bones, deformity is usually obvious and may involve open or closed fractures or dislocation of the fingers.

Typically the injured hand and wrist are not covered by equipment. In certain sports such as football, ice hockey, and lacrosse, the athlete may wear a glove. In these cases, the glove is removed most easily, and with the least amount of pain, by the athlete.

Wrist Fractures and Dislocations

Fractures of the radius or ulna as well as dislocations of the radiocarpal joint must be immobilized in the position in which they are found, using a vacuum-type splint (Fig. 18-35). Before splinting the area, the radial and ulnar

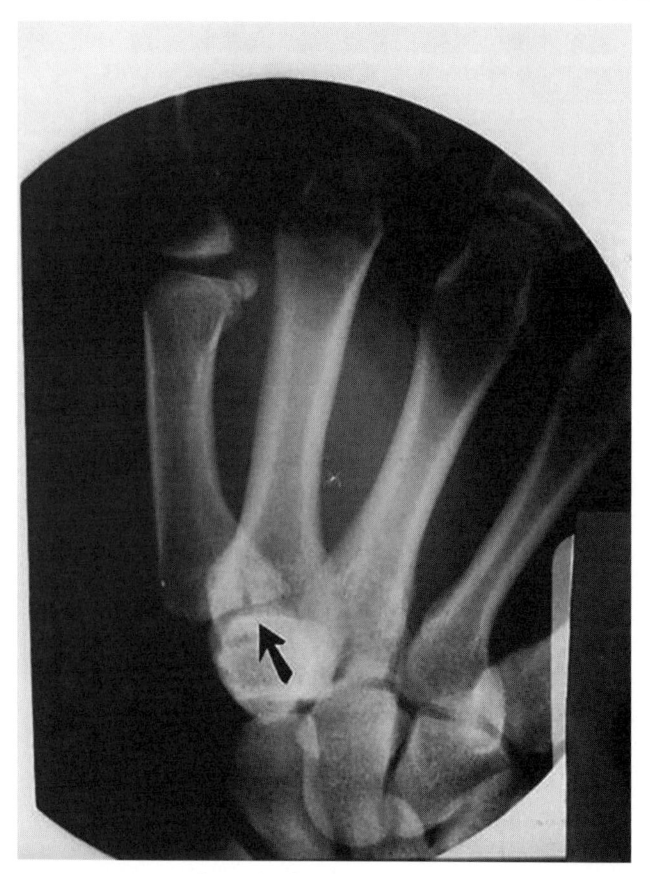

FIGURE 18-34 ■ Radiograph of a Bennett's fracture.

Interphalangeal Joint Dislocations

Dislocation of an IP joint results in obvious deformity. In some instances, the athlete instinctively reduces the dislocation by applying traction to the finger. The on-field reduction of IP joint dislocations should be performed by trained personnel and followed by splinting, referral, and appropriate imaging.

For unreduced dislocations the palmar aspect of the injured finger must be splinted in the position in which it was found. An ice pack is applied to the dorsal side, and the athlete is referred to a physician.

Hand and Finger Fractures

When fractures of the hand are suspected, the hand is splinted so that the wrist and fingers are also immobilized. However, the fingernails must remain uncovered so that distal blood flow can be checked. Finger fractures are splinted in the position in which they are found using an aluminum splint that also immobilizes the MCP joint. Often a standard tongue depressor can be used to sufficiently splint the area. Table 18-5 describes the splinting position for other common finger injuries. Correct immediate management and arterial pulses must be evaluated. As with any fracture, the joint itself or the joint above and below the fracture site needs to be immobilized. Open fractures should be managed using universal precautions and with the fracture site bandaged.

Suspected fractures or dislocations of the carpal bones can be carefully supported and the athlete moved off the field for further evaluation. If a fracture is suspected, the wrist is immobilized as previously described.

Table 18-5 Splinting of Common Finger Injuries

Deformity	Splinting Position
Jersey finger	DIP joint in flexion
Mallet finger	DIP joint in extension
Boutonnière deformity	PIP and DIP joints in extension
Phalanx fracture	Position found
Metacarpal fracture	Palmar surface of wrist and hand
Unreduced dislocations	Position found

DIP = distal interphalangeal; PIP = proximal interphalangeal.

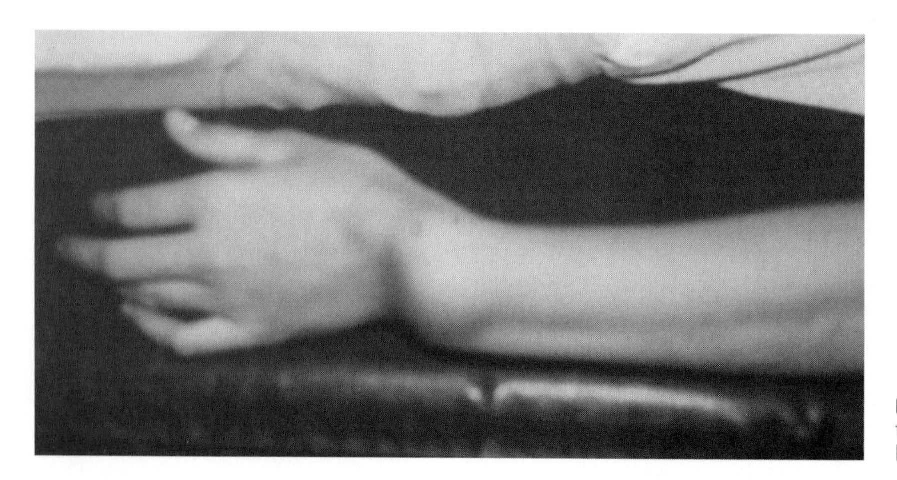

FIGURE 18-35 ■ Wrist dislocation. Note that the radius and ulna are displaced dorsally to the hand.

proper immobilization techniques reduce the chance that the injury will require surgical correction.

Lacerations

Because of the relatively superficial location of the tendons and nerves in the wrist, hand, and fingers, they are vulnerable to damage from even shallow lacerations. As with any cut, the possibility of infection exists, especially when the laceration involves the joints. Any laceration involving the fascia below the cutaneous level requires referral to a physician to rule out the possibility of trauma to the underlying tendons and nerves and determine the possible need for suturing.

REFERENCES

1. Austin, NM: The wrist and hand complex. In Levangie, PK, and Norkin, CC (eds): *Joint Structure and Function: A Comprehensive Analysis* (ed 4). Philadelphia, FA Davis, 2005, p 305.
2. Nishikawa, S, and Satoshi, T: Anatomical study of the carpal attachment of the triangular fibrocartilage complex. *J Bone Joint Surg [Br]*, 84-B:1062, 2002.
3. Shih, J-T, Lee, H-M, and Tan, C-M: Early isolated triangular fibrocartilage complex tears: Management by arthroscopic repair. *J Trauma*, 53:922, 2002.
4. Kozin, SH: Perilunate injuries: Diagnosis and treatment. *J Am Acad Orthop Surg*, 6:114, 1998.
5. Shin, AY, Battaglia, MJ, and Bishop, AT: Lunotriquestral instability: Diagnosis and treatment *J Am Acad Orthop Surg*, 8:170, 2000.
6. Newport, ML: Extensor tendon injuries in the hand. *J Am Acad Orthop Surg*, 5:59, 1997.
7. Strickland JW. Flexor tendon injuries: I. Foundations of treatment. *J Am Acad Orthop Surg*, 3:44, 1995.
8. McNamara, B: Clinical anatomy of the ulnar nerve. *ACNR*, 3:25, 2003.
9. McNamara, B: Clinical anatomy of the median nerve. *ACNR*, 2:18, 2003.
10. McNamara, B: Clinical anatomy of the radial nerve. *ACNR*, 3:28, 2003.
11. Nagle, DJ: Evaluation of chronic wrist pain. *J Am Acad Orthop Surg*, 8:45, 2000.
12. van Vugt, RM, Bijlsma, JWJ, and van Fugt, AC: Chronic wrist pain: Diagnosis and management. Development and use of a new algorithm. *Ann Rheum Dis*, 58:665, 1999.
13. Forman, TA, Forman, SK, and Rose, NE: A clinical approach to diagnosing wrist pain. *Am Fam Phys*, 72:1753, 2005.
14. Saldana, MJ: Trigger digits: Diagnosis and treatment. *J Am Acad Orthop Surg*, 9:246, 2001.
15. Daluiski, A, Rahbar, B, and Meals, RA: Russell's sign. Subtle hand changes in patients with bulimia nervosa. *Clin Orthop*, 343:107, 1997.
16. Rettig, AC: Athletic injuries of the wrist and hand. Part I: Traumatic injuries of the wrist. *Am J Sports Med*, 31:1038, 2003.
17. Clarkson, HM: *Musculoskeletal Assessment. Joint Range of Motion and Manual Muscle Strength.* (ed 2). Philadelphia: Lippincott Williams & Wilkins, 2000.
18. Schreuders, TAR, et al: Measurement error in grip and pinch force measurements in patients with hand injuries. *Phys Ther*, 83:806, 2003.
19. Posner, MA: Compressive ulnar neuropathies at the elbow: I. Etiology and diagnosis. *J Am Acad Orthop Surg*, 6:282, 1998.
20. Colles, A: On the fracture of the carpal extremity of the radius. *Edinb Med Surg J*, 10:182, 1814.
21. Thoms, FB: Reduction of Smith's fractures. *J Bone Joint Surg Br*, 39:463, 1959.
22. Ring, B, Jupiter, JB, and Herndon, JH: Acute fractures of the scaphoid. *J Am Acad Orthop Surg*, 8:225, 2000.
23. Cave, EF: The carpus with reference to the fractured navicular bone. *Arch Surg*, 40:54, 1940.
24. Rettig, AC, and Patel, DV: Epidemiology of elbow, forearm and wrist injuries in the athlete. *Clin Sports Med*, 14:289, 1995.
25. Phillips, TG, Reibach, AM, and Slomiany, WP: Diagnosis and management of scaphoid fractures. *Am Fam Phys*, 70:879, 2004.
26. Taleisnick, J, and Kelly, PJ: The extraosseous and intraosseous blood supply to the scaphoid bone. *J Bone Joint Surg Am*, 48:1126, 1966.
27. Schubert, HE: Scaphoid fracture. Review of diagnostic tests and treatment. *Can Fam Physician*, 46:1825, 2000.
28. Dobyns, JH, and Linsheid, RL: Fractures and dislocations in the wrist. In Rockwood, CA, and Green, DP (eds): *Fractures in Adults* (ed 2). Philadelphia, JB Lippincott, 1984, p 411.
29. David, TS, Zemel, NP, and Mathews, PV: Symptomatic, partial union of the hook of the hamate fracture in athletes. *Am J Sports Med*, 31:106, 2003.
30. Green, DP, and O'Brien, ET: Classification and management of carpal dislocations. *Clin Orthop Relat Res*, 149:55, 1980.
31. Campbell, RD, Lance, EM, and Yeoh, CB: Lunate and perilunate dislocations. *J Bone Joint Surg Br*, 46:55, 1964.
32. Frykman, GK, and Nelson, EF: Fractures and traumatic conditions of the wrist. In Hunter, J, et al (eds): *Rehabilitation of the Hand: Surgery and Therapy* (ed 3). St Louis, CV Mosby, 1990, p 267.
33. Trousdale, RT, et al: Radio-ulnar dissociation. A review of twenty cases. *J Bone Joint Surg Am*, 74:1486, 1992.
34. Dao, KD, et al: The efficacy of ultrasound in the evaluation of dynamic scapholunate ligamentous instability. *J Bone Joint Surg [Am]*, 86-A:1473, 2004.
35. Seradge, H, et al: Treatment of dynamic scaphoid instability. *J Trauma*, 56:1253, 2004.
36. Park, MJ: Radiographic observation of the scaphoid shift test. *J Bone Jt Surg [Br]*, 85-B: 358, 2003.
37. Salerno, DF, et al: Reliability of physical examination of the upper extremity among keyboard operators. *Am J Ind Med*, 37:423, 2000.
38. Phalen, GS: The carpal tunnel syndrome: Seventeen years' experience in diagnosis and treatment of 654 hands. *J Bone Joint Surg Am*, 48:211, 1966.
39. Phalen, GS: The carpal tunnel syndrome: Clinical evaluation of 598 hands. *Clin Orthop*, 83:29, 1972.
40. Szabo, RM, et al: The value of diagnostic testing in carpal tunnel syndrome. *J Hand Surg*, 24A:704, 1999.
41. Bechtol, C: Grip test: The use of a dynamometer with adjustable handle spacings. *J Bone Joint Surg Am*, 36:L820, 1954.
42. Zimmerman, GR: Carpal tunnel syndrome. *J Athl Train*, 29:22, 1994.

43. MacDermid, JC, and Wessel, J: Clinical diagnosis of carpal tunnel syndrome. A systematic review. *J Hand Ther,* 17:309, 2004.
44. Aird, J, et al: The impact of wrist extension provocation on current perception thresholds in patients with carpal tunnel syndrome: A pilot study. *J Hand Ther,* 19:299, 2006.
45. Brininger, TL, et al: Efficacy of a fabricated customized splint and tendon and nerve gliding exercises for the treatment of carpal tunnel syndrome: a randomized controlled trial. *Arch Phys Med Rehabil,* 88:1429, 2007.
46. Capo, JT, and Hastings, H: Metacarpal and phalangeal fractures in athletes. *Clin Sports Med,* 17:491, 1998.
47. Leggit, JC, and Meko, CJ: Acute finger injuries: Part II. Fractures, dislocations, and thumb injuries. *Am Fam Phys,* 73:827, 2006.
48. Dawson, WJ: The spectrum of sports-related interphalangeal joint injuries. *Hand Clin,* 10:315, 1994.
49. Leddy, JP, and Packer, JW: Avulsion of the profundus tendon insertion in athletes. *J Hand Surg Am,* 2:66, 1977.
50. Rossi, C, et al: De Quervain disease in volleyball players. *Am J Sports Med,* 33:424, 2005.
51. Lipscomb, PR: Stenosing tenosynovitis at the radial styloid process. *Ann Surg,* 134:110, 1951.
52. Richie, CA 3rd, and Briner, WW, Jr: Corticosteroid injection for treatment of de Quervain's tenosynovitis: A pooled quantitative literature evaluation. *J Am Board Fam Pract,* 16:102, 2003.
53. Lane, LB: Acute grade III ulnar collateral ligament ruptures: A new surgical and rehabilitation protocol. *Am J Sports Med,* 19:234, 1991.
54. McCue, FC, Mayer, V, and Moran, DJ: Gamekeeper's thumb: Ulnar collateral ligament rupture. *J Musculoskel Med,* 5:53, 1988.
55. Langford, SA, Whitaker, JH, and Toby, EB: Thumb injuries in the athlete. *Clin Sports Med,* 17:553, 1998.

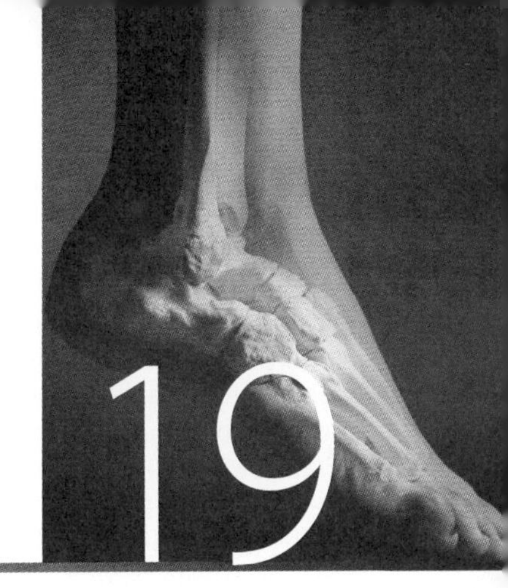

CHAPTER 19

Eye Pathologies

Resulting from a direct blow, impalement, or chemical invasion, trauma to the eye requires an accurate assessment so that proper management and further evaluation by an **ophthalmologist** can be initiated. Failure to recognize and properly manage eye trauma can result in permanent dysfunction, including blindness.

Racquet sports (in which the ball can reach speeds up to 140 mph), boxing, and golf are most often associated with catastrophic injury to the eye. However, traumatic injury to the eye can occur in all sports, with basketball being the most common.[1,2] An estimated 90% of all eye injuries can be prevented through the use of approved protective eye wear.

Clinical Anatomy

The eye, except for its anterior aspect, sits encased within the conical bony **orbit** (Fig. 19-1). In addition to protecting and stabilizing the eye, the orbit also serves as an attachment site for some of the extrinsic muscles acting on the eye. The **orbital margin** (periorbital region) is composed of the **frontal bone**, forming the supraorbital margin; the **zygomatic bone** and a portion of the frontal bone, forming the lateral margin; and the zygomatic bone and **maxillary bone**, forming the infraorbital margin.

The anterior portion of the orbit's roof is formed by the frontal bone. A portion of the **sphenoid bone** forms its posterior aspect. Medially, the orbit is formed by the thin **lacrimal**, **ethmoid**, **maxillary**, and **sphenoid bones**. The floor is formed by the maxillary, zygomatic, and **palatine bones**. Laterally, the orbit is composed of the zygomatic bone and the sphenoid bone. Here the orbit is the thickest. The **superior orbital fissure**, an opening between the lesser and greater wings of the sphenoid bone, is located between the lateral wall and the roof. This fissure allows the cranial nerves, arteries, and veins to communicate with the eye. The orbit's posterior aspect is marked by the **optic canal**, the foramen through which the optic nerve passes to reach the brain.

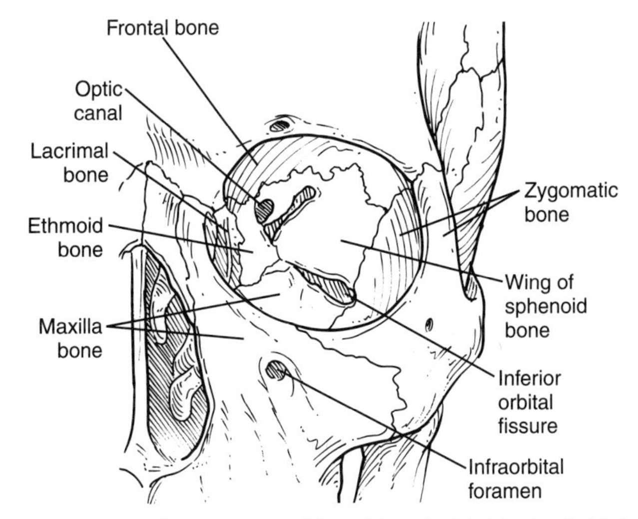

FIGURE 19-1 ■ Bony anatomy of the orbit and orbital rim (periorbital region).

Ophthalmologist A medical doctor specializing in injury, diseases, and abnormalities of the eye.

Eye Structures

The mass of the eye is a fibrous, fluid-filled structure collectively referred to as the **globe**. Its white layering, the **sclera**, encompasses the posterior five sixths of the globe and becomes continuous with the sheath of the optic nerve as the nerve continues posteriorly and merges with the brain's fibrous lining. The dark central aperture of the eye, the **pupil**, is surrounded by pigmented contractile tissue, the **iris** (Fig. 19-2). The **conjunctiva**, a thin mucous membrane, covers the sclera and lines the inside of the eyelids. Anteriorly, the conjunctiva is continuous with the transparent **cornea**. The cornea is the main structure involved in focusing light rays entering the eye.

Suspended by ligaments arising from the **ciliary body**, the **lens** is a clear elastic structure located behind the iris that serves to sharpen and focus visual rays on the globe's posterior surface, the **retina**. The area of the retina facing the center of the globe contains nervous tissues. The outer layer is composed of darkly pigmented vascular tissue, the **choroid**. Light rays strike the nervous tissues, stimulating the **rods** and **cones**, which are photoreceptors located on the globe's posterior surface. Each receptor passes its stimulus through a complex network of nerves until the impulses are collected and transmitted to the brain via the optic nerve. Rods and cones are absent at the **optic nerve**, thus causing a blind spot in the field of vision (Fig. 19-3).

Eyelids act as shutters to protect the eye from accidental direct contact by reflexively closing when an object comes close to the exposed globe and by preventing airborne dust and dirt from entering the eye. The conjunctiva of the globe is continuous with the inner surfaces of the eyelids. The **blink reflex** aids in lubricating the eye's ocular surface.

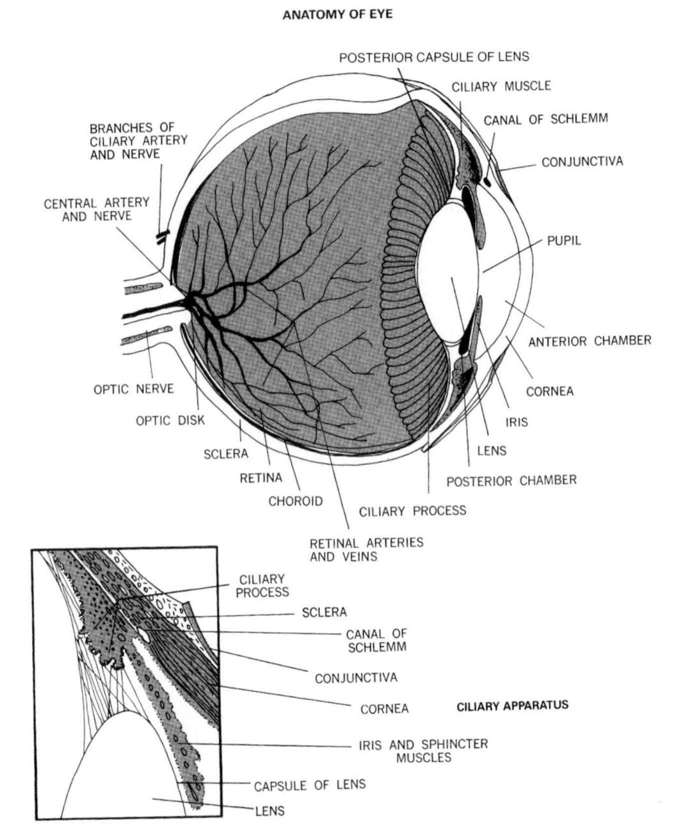

FIGURE 19-2 ■ Cross-sectional view of the anatomy of the eye with an enlargement of the ciliary apparatus. (From Venes D [ed]: *Taber's cyclopedic medical dictionary*, ed 21, Beth Anne Willert, MS, medical illustrator. Philadelphia: FA Davis, 2009.)

Muscular Anatomy

Six muscles control the movement of the globe (Fig. 19-4). The inferior, medial, lateral, and superior **rectus muscles** rotate the globe toward the contracting muscle (e.g., the inferior rectus rotates the eye downward). The **inferior** and **superior oblique muscles** function to provide a torsion (circular) motion to the globe (Table 19-1).

Visual Acuity

Proper anatomy and correct geometry of the lens are required for perfect vision. The quality of vision, visual acuity, can be assessed using a **Snellen chart** (Fig. 19-5). This method determines the person's ability to clearly see letters based on a normalized scale. **Emmetropia**, 20/20 vision, is the ability to read the letters on the 20-foot line of an eye chart when standing 20 feet from the chart, indicating that the light rays are focused precisely on the retina. **Myopia**, or nearsightedness, occurs when the light rays are focused in front of the retina, making only objects very close to the eyes distinguishable. **Hypermetropia** (hyperopia), or farsightedness, results when the light rays are focused at a point behind the retina. Diminished visual acuity may require further assessment to enhance performance and ensure safe participation in sports through corrective methods such as eyeglasses or contact lenses.

Clinical Examination of Eye Injuries

Blunt trauma to the eye can result in injury to the globe and its related structures, laceration of the periorbital skin, or a fracture of the bony orbit. Infections, diseases, allergies, and brain trauma can also lead to dysfunction of the eye. Because of the eye's delicate nature, all maladies involving

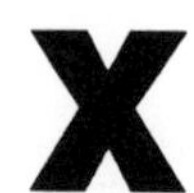

FIGURE 19-3 ■ Determining the blind spot in the field of vision. Close one eye and focus on the "X." Move the page toward or away from you until the round spot disappears, indicating the blind area in your field of vision.

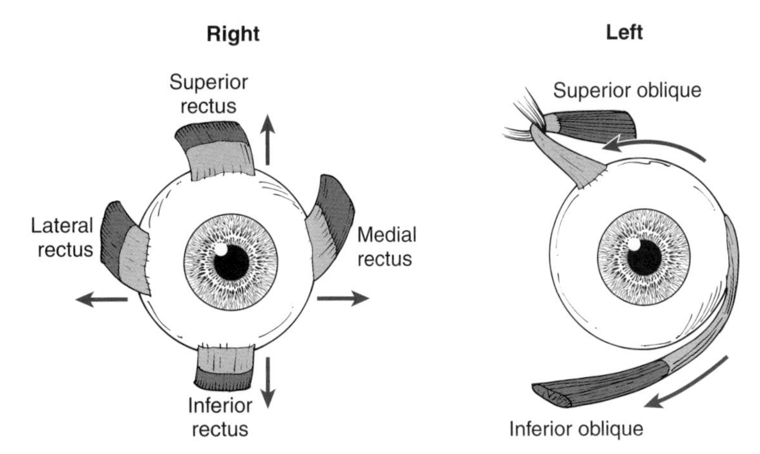

FIGURE 19-4 ■ Extrinsic muscles of the eye. The right eye is used to present the rectus muscles, which move the globe in the cardinal planes. The left eye describes the oblique muscles, which abduct and adduct the globe.

the eye must be managed with the utmost care and urgency. The supplies necessary for the evaluation and management of eye injuries are presented in Table 19-2.

History

Past medical history

- **Prior visual assessment:** Ask the patient about prior visual acuity, the need for corrective lenses (glasses or contact lenses), congenital pupillary changes, **nystagmus** (involuntary shaking of the eyes), other prior existing conditions, and any relevant history of previous eye injuries. This information should be noted in the medical file and be available for comparison with any subsequent examination findings.
- **General health:** Question the patient about any chronic illness. Certain conditions, such as diabetes, are associated with increased **retinopathy**.

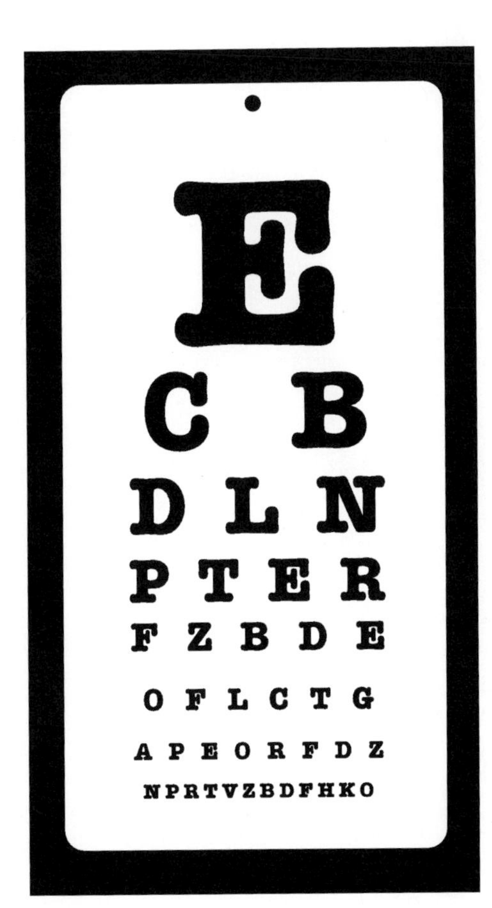

FIGURE 19-5 ■ Snellen-type chart. This device is commonly used to determine an individual's visual acuity.

History of the present condition

With the exception of dysfunction occurring secondary to infection, disease, or allergy, all eye injuries have an acute onset.

- **Location and description of the symptoms:** The patient may complain of **photophobia**. Complaints of scratchiness or "something in the eye" may be caused by a foreign body, a displaced contact lens, or a **corneal abrasion**. Itching of the eye is usually associated with edema of the conjunctiva (**chemosis**) caused by an allergy or infection, such as conjunctivitis. Disruption of the normal visual field may also be described. These findings are discussed in the "Functional Assessment" section of this chapter.
- **Injury mechanism:** The size and elastic properties of the object striking the eye are key indicators of the subsequent injury (Table 19-3). Hard objects that are larger than the orbital rim transmit forces directly to the eye's bony margin. Elastic objects or objects smaller than the orbital margin may deliver forces directly to the eye. Elastic objects are of particular concern because the expansive force may be of a magnitude sufficient to rupture the globe.

Injury may also be caused by chemicals or other foreign substances entering the eye. In addition to dirt and sand, athletes commonly encounter substances such as lime (or other field marking agents), chlorine, and fertilizers and pesticides used for maintaining grass fields. If a foreign substance enters the eye, transport a sample of the substance to the hospital with the patient.

Retinopathy A degenerative disease of the blood vessels supplying the retina, often associated with diabetes.

Photophobia The eye's intolerance to light.

Table 19-1 Extrinsic Muscles Acting on the Eye

Muscle	Action	Origin	Insertion	Innervation	Root
Inferior Rectus	Downward rotation of the globe	From a tendinous ring on the posterior aspect of the orbit	Middle of the inferior aspect of the anterior globe	Oculomotor	CN III
Superior Rectus	Upward rotation of the globe	From a tendinous ring on the posterior aspect of the orbit	Middle of the superior aspect of the anterior globe	Oculomotor	CN III
Medial Rectus	Medial rotation of the globe	From a tendinous ring on the posterior aspect of the orbit	Middle of the medial aspect of the anterior globe	Oculomotor	CN III
Lateral Rectus	Lateral rotation of the globe	From a tendinous ring on the posterior aspect of the orbit	Middle of the lateral aspect of the anterior globe	Abducens	CN VI
Inferior Oblique	Adduction of the globe Elevation of the globe Rotation of the globe when abducted	From the periosteum of the maxilla	Inferolateral quadrant of the globe	Oculomotor	CN III
Superior Oblique	Abduction of the globe Depression of the globe Rotation of the globe when adducted	Greater wing of the sphenoid	Superolateral quadrant of the globe	Trochlear	CN IV

CN = cranial nerve.

Examination Map

HISTORY

Past Medical History
Prior vision assessment
Mental health status

History of the Present Condition
General health status
Location of pain
Radicular symptoms
Mechanism of injury
Onset of condition

INSPECTION

Periorbital Area
Discoloration
Gross deformity

Inspection of the Globe
General appearance
- Eyelids
- Cornea
- Conjunctiva
- Sclera
- Iris
- Pupil shape and size

PALPATION

Orbital Margin

Frontal Bone

Nasal Bone

Zygomatic Bone

Soft Tissue

FUNCTIONAL ASSESSMENT

Vision Assessment

Pupillary Reaction to Light

NEUROLOGIC EXAMINATION

CN III, IV, VI

PATHOLOGIES AND SPECIAL TESTS

Orbital Fractures
Blowout fractures

Corneal Abrasion

Corneal Laceration

Iritis

Hyphema

Retinal Detachment

Ruptured Globe

Conjunctivitis

Foreign Bodies

Table 19-2 Supplies Needed for the Evaluation and Management of Eye Injuries

Evaluation Supplies	Management Supplies
Snellen chart or similar	Eye shield
Occluder to cover the eye not being tested	Eye patch
	Tape
Penlight	Plunger for removing hard contact lenses
Cobalt blue light	Sterile irrigation solution
Small mirror	Sterile cotton swabs
Fluorescein strips	Sterile gauze
	Antibiotic eyedrops
	Contact lens case
	Steri-Strips or butterfly bandages
	Telephone number of consulting ophthalmologist
	Telephone number of hospital or poison control center

Inspection

Because all but the most anterior portion of the eye is hidden from view, trauma to its external structures, the eyelid and the eyebrow, may mask underlying pathology. A relatively normal outward appearance of the eye does not correlate well with possible internal damage. The presence of the findings listed in Table 19-4 indicates the need for immediate referral for further assessment by an ophthalmologist.

Inspection of the periorbital area

- **Discoloration:** A simple periorbital hematoma (or black eye) is common with blunt injuries and may have no consequence other than its abnormal appearance. However, external trauma to the eyelid, orbit, or conjunctiva may alter function and indicate trauma to the eye itself.
- **Gross deformity:** Gross bony deformity of the orbit, although rare, indicates a significant condition requiring immediate medical intervention. The loose skin surrounding the eye and eyelid is easily swollen after an injury, and the swelling is often less significant than it appears. Lacerations are common secondary to direct trauma and require management using the appropriate standard precautions.

Inspection of the globe

- **General appearance:** The appearance of the globe is evaluated as it sits within the orbit relative to the uninvolved eye. Orbital fractures may cause the globe to be displaced medially, inferiorly, or posteriorly (**enophthalmos**) or to bulge anteriorly (**exophthalmos**) within the orbit.
- **Eyelids:** The eyelids are inspected for signs of acute injury, such as swelling, ecchymosis, or lacerations, which may obscure serious underlying pathology of the globe (Fig. 19-6). A **stye**, an infection of a **ciliary gland** or **sebaceous gland**, is caused by bacteria.

Ciliary gland A form of sweat gland on the eyelid.
Sebaceous gland Oil-secreting gland of the skin.

Table 19-3 Blunt Eye Trauma and the Resulting Eye Pathology*

Size Relative to the Orbit	Elastic Property	Resulting Pathology
Larger	Hard	Orbital fracture, periorbital contusion
Larger	Elastic	Blow-out fracture, ruptured globe, corneal abrasion, traumatic iritis, periorbital contusion
Smaller	Hard	Ruptured globe, corneal abrasion, corneal laceration, traumatic iritis
Smaller	Elastic	Ruptured globe, blow-out fracture, corneal abrasion, traumatic iritis

*All of these mechanisms of injury can result in subconjunctival hemorrhage and retinal pathology.

Table 19-4 Findings that warrant for an Immediate Referral to an Ophthalmologist

History	Inspection	Palpation	Functional Tests	Neurological Tests
Loss of all or part of the visual field Persistent blurred vision Diplopia Photophobia Throbbing or penetrating pain around or within the eye Description of mechanism for a ruptured globe Air escaping from the eyelid or pain when blowing the nose	Foreign body protruding into the eye Laceration involving the margin of the eyelid Deep laceration of the lid Inability to open the eyelid because of swelling Protrusion of the globe (or other obvious displacement) **Injected** conjunctiva with a small pupil Loss of corneal clarity Hyphema Pupillary distortion Unilateral pupillary dilation or constriction	Crepitus of the orbital rim	Restricted eye movement Double vision occurring with eye movement	Numbness or paresthesia over the lateral nose and cheek Pupillary reaction abnormality

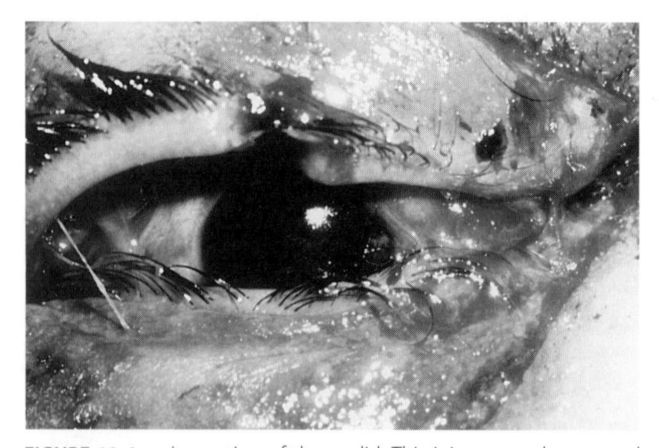

FIGURE 19-6 ■ Laceration of the eyelid. This injury may also conceal underlying eye trauma.

General eyelid edema, focal tenderness, and redness of the involved lid usually are noted.

- **Cornea:** Normally crystal clear, any discoloration of the cornea indicates trauma warranting the immediate termination of the evaluation and subsequent referral to an ophthalmologist. Increased intraocular pressure may result in corneal cloudiness. **Hyphema**, the collection of blood within the anterior chamber of the eye, is caused by the rupture of a blood vessel supplying the iris (Fig. 19-7). See page 828 for further description of hyphema.

Injected (injection) Congested with blood or other fluids forced into an area.

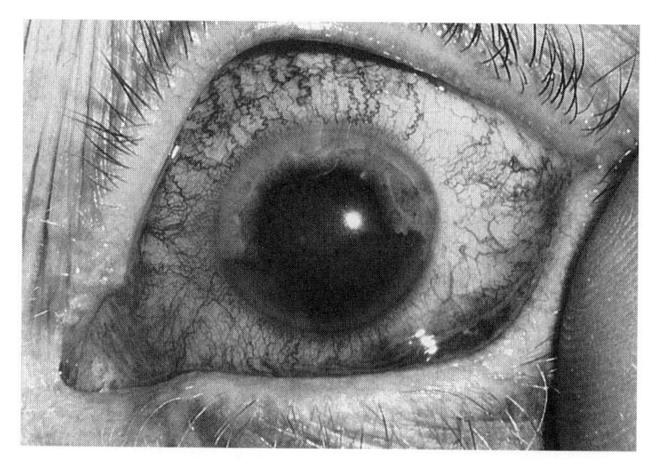

FIGURE 19-7 ■ Hyphema, a collection of blood within the anterior chamber of the eye.

- **Conjunctiva:** Normally, the conjunctiva appears transparent as it covers the white sclera anteriorly. To view the inferior portion of the conjunctiva, gently pull down on the eyelid as the patient looks upward. To view the upper conjunctiva, gently lift the upper eyelid while the patient looks downward. If a foreign body is suspected, the upper conjunctiva is viewed by gently inverting the upper eyelid using a cotton-tipped applicator. In some situations, the patient may be more comfortable doing this on his or her own (Fig. 19-8). Leakage of the superficial blood vessels, **subconjunctival hematoma**, is a common benign condition but is of concern because of its potential to conceal underlying pathology (Fig. 19-9).[3]
- **Sclera:** The appearance of a black object on the sclera must be viewed with concern because it may actually be the inner tissue of the eye that is bulging outward through a wound.
- **Iris:** Marked conjunctival injection adjacent to the cornea indicates the presence of inflammation, **iritis**.
- **Pupil shape and size:** The pupils are normally equal in size and shape, but **anisocoria** may be congenital or associated with brain trauma. Any irregularity in the pupil's shape is an ominous sign of a serious injury. An elliptical or **"teardrop" pupil** is of serious concern because of the possibility of a **corneal laceration** or **ruptured globe** (Fig. 19-10).

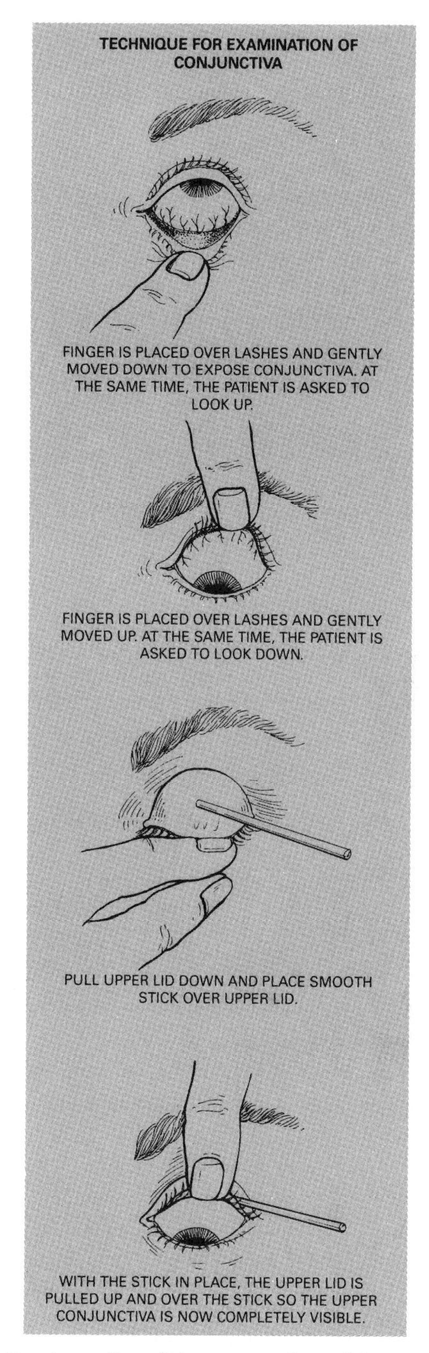

FIGURE 19-8 ■ Inspection of the upper surface of the eye. The upper eyelid is inverted around a cotton-tipped applicator to expose the upper portion of the sclera and conjunctiva. (From Venes D (ed): Taber's *cyclopedic medical dictionary*, ed 21, Beth Anne Willert, MS, medical illustrator. Philadelphia: FA Davis, 2009.)

Anisocoria Unequal pupil sizes; possibly a benign congenital condition or secondary to brain trauma.

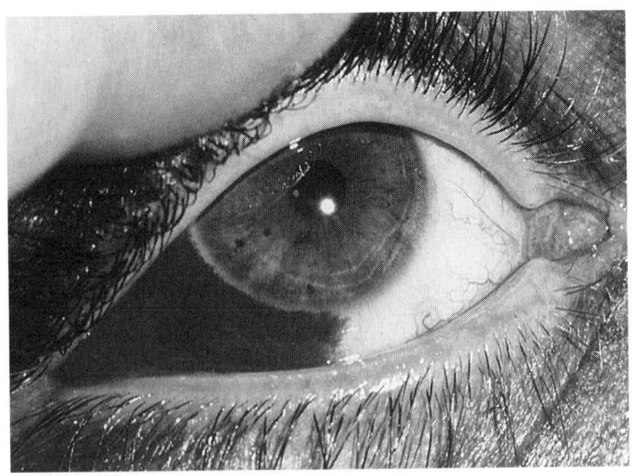

FIGURE 19-9 ■ Subconjunctival hemorrhage. This condition by itself is usually benign but may conceal underlying pathology.

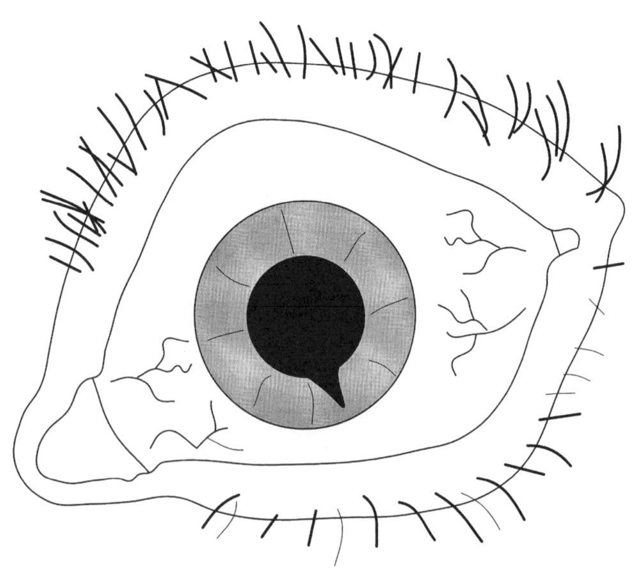

FIGURE 19-10 ■ Teardrop pupil. This condition, or any other deviation in the normally round shape of the pupil, indicates serious underlying pathology such as a corneal laceration or ruptured globe.

PALPATION

Assessment of eye injuries should not include palpation or probing of the globe itself. However, the superficial bony structures and the soft tissue surrounding the eye may be safely palpated for signs of an injury.

1 **Orbital margin:** Palpate the circumference of the orbital rim for signs of tenderness or crepitus indicating the presence of an orbital fracture. The bony prominence of the orbit may become obscured secondary to swelling.

2–4 **Related areas:** Include a general palpation of the frontal **(2)**, nasal **(3)**, and zygomatic **(4)** bones to rule out concurrent injuries caused by blunt trauma.

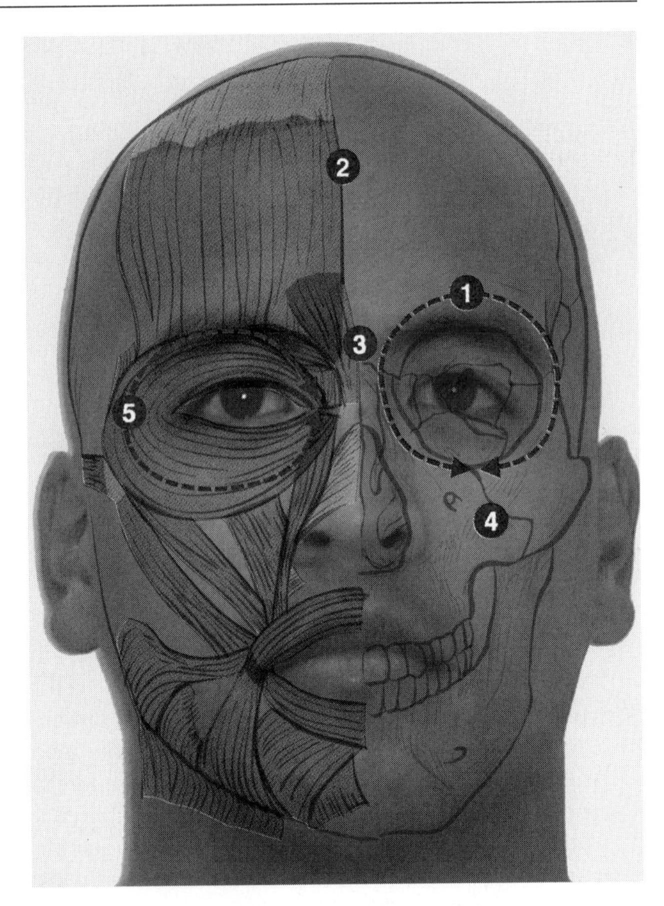

5 **Soft tissue:** Palpate the eyelid and skin surrounding the eye, if appropriate. Keep in mind that injury to these areas is usually apparent during inspection.

Functional Assessment

Vision assessment

Vision can be assessed using the Snellen chart (see Fig. 19-5), a near-vision card, a newspaper, or a game program. Vision assessment is performed monocularly (one eye) and binocularly (both eyes). Individuals who require the use of glasses or contact lenses should be wearing these at the time of the vision assessment. A person younger than age 40 years who has 20/20 vision should be able to read standard newspaper print held 16 inches from the eye. Individuals older than age 40 years may have 20/20 distance vision but may have **presbyopia** and require the use of reading glasses.

If the patient is unable to read the chart, fingers may be used. When testing, the fingers are held at different distances and vision is evaluated. The lack of normal visual acuity or the onset of **diplopia** after an injury to the eye requires a referral to an ophthalmologist for further

Presbyopia Loss of near vision as the result of aging.
Diplopia Double vision.

evaluation. If these symptoms develop following a head injury the patient should be examined for a concussion.

Blurred vision that clears on blinking the eye indicates the formation of mucus or other debris floating in the surface of the eye. This is not a significant finding. Blinking that clears the vision momentarily can indicate a corneal abrasion. Loss of portions of the visual field, typically described as resembling a shade or curtain's being pulled over the eye, may indicate a detached retina. Diplopia may indicate an orbital fracture, brain trauma, damage to the optic or cranial nerves, or injury to the eye's extrinsic muscles.

Pupillary reaction to light

Pupillary dysfunction is also associated with significant head trauma and may include dilatation, diminished reactivity to light, or asymmetry (Special Test 19-1).

Eye motility

The eyes' ability to perform a complete sweep of the range of motion (ROM) in a smooth, symmetrical manner through the eye's field of gaze is a key examination finding (Special Test 19-2). Asymmetrical motion or movement that results in diplopia is considered significant.

Neurologic Testing

The muscles of the eye are controlled sympathetically or parasympathetically by cranial nerves III, IV, and VI. A discussion of these nerves and their direct influence on the eyes is provided in Chapter 21. Numbness in the cheek and lateral nose corresponds to the distribution of the infraorbital nerve and may indicate an orbital floor fracture.

Eye Pathologies and Related Special Tests

Injury to the globe usually results in some degree of visual impairment, with or without outward signs of trauma. Periorbital injuries usually have no associated visual change. Following a recent history of head injury, associated brain pathology must be considered for those who complain of visual disturbances.

Orbital Fractures

A blow to the periorbital area from an object that is larger than the orbit itself may result in a fracture of the frontal, zygomatic, or maxillary bones of the orbital rim. A deformable or irregularly shaped object, such as a ball or an elbow, may also deliver force to the globe with a magnitude sufficient to cause the orbit to rupture at its weakest point, usually in the medial wall or the floor of the orbit (Fig. 19-11).[4] Fractures of the medial wall or floor are termed **blowout fractures**, and fractures of the orbital roof are termed **blow-up fractures.**[5]

After an orbital fracture, the globe may be sunken, medially displaced, or retracted (enophthalmos) in relation to

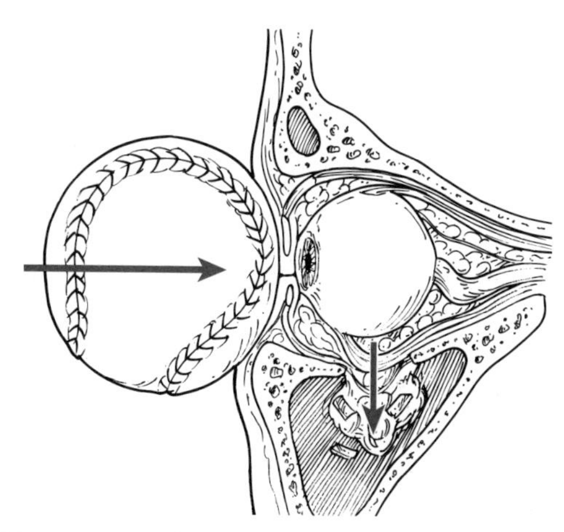

FIGURE 19-11 ■ Mechanism for an orbital floor "blow-out" fracture. The object striking the eye causes the globe to expand downward, rupturing the relatively thin floor.

the location and magnitude of the fracture (i.e., a fracture of the orbital floor would cause the globe to sit low within the orbit). Numbness may also be present in the infraorbital area. However, none of these symptoms may be present.[6,7] Pieces of the maxillary portion of the orbital floor may entrap the inferior rectus muscle, mechanically limiting the ability to look upward (Fig. 19-12).

✱ Practical Evidence

Plain radiographs are often inconclusive in diagnosing orbital floor fractures. CT imaging is the imaging gold standard.[8]

Initially, fractures of the medial wall of the orbit may be asymptomatic, remaining undiagnosed until the person attempts to blow his or her nose, at which time air escapes the nasal passage, enters the orbit, and exits from under the eyelids. A floor fracture or its subsequent swelling may cause infraorbital nerve entrapment, resulting in numbness in the lateral nose and cheek. Fracture of the lateral wall of the orbit can result in pain when the mouth is opened.[2]

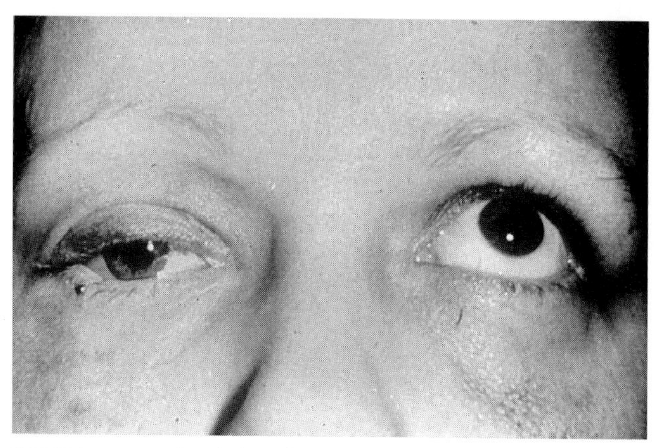

FIGURE 19-12 ■ Restriction of eye motion following a blow-out fracture of the orbital floor. The person's right eye is unable to gaze upward, indicating an entrapment of the inferior rectus muscle.

Special Test 19-1
Pupillary Reaction Assessment

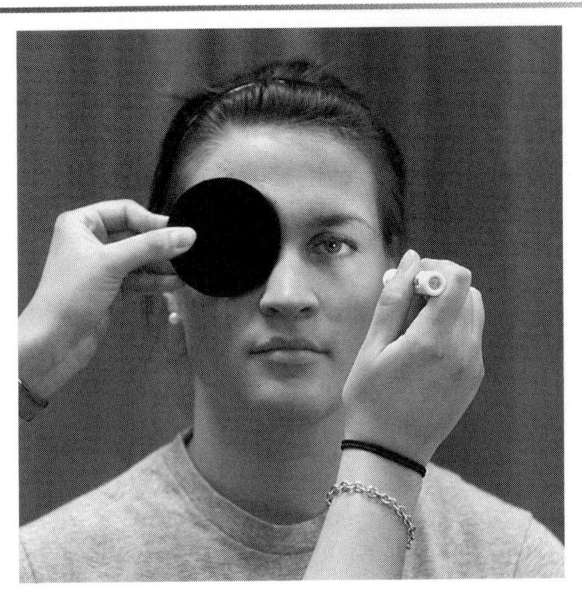

Checking for normal pupil reaction to light. If a penlight is not available, the eye tested can be covered and the pupil observed for constriction when the eye is exposed to light.

Patient Position	Sitting or standing
Position of Examiner	Standing in front of the patient
Evaluative Procedure	A card, an occluder, or the patient's hand is held in front of the eye not being tested. A penlight is used to shine light into the pupil for 1 s and then removed. The examiner observes for the pupil constricting when the light is applied and dilating when the light is removed. This process is repeated for the opposite eye.
Positive Test	A pupil that is unresponsive to light, reacts sluggishly compared with the opposite eye, or paradoxically dilates or constricts.
Implications	***Afferent lesion (retina or optic nerve):*** The involved pupil enlarges as the light is moved from the unaffected side to the affected side (paradoxical dilation). ***Efferent lesion (CN III or pupillary muscle lesion):*** The involved pupil does not react to light.[2]
Evidence	Absent or inconclusive in the literature

CN = cranial nerve.

Special Test 19-2
Assessment of Eye Motility

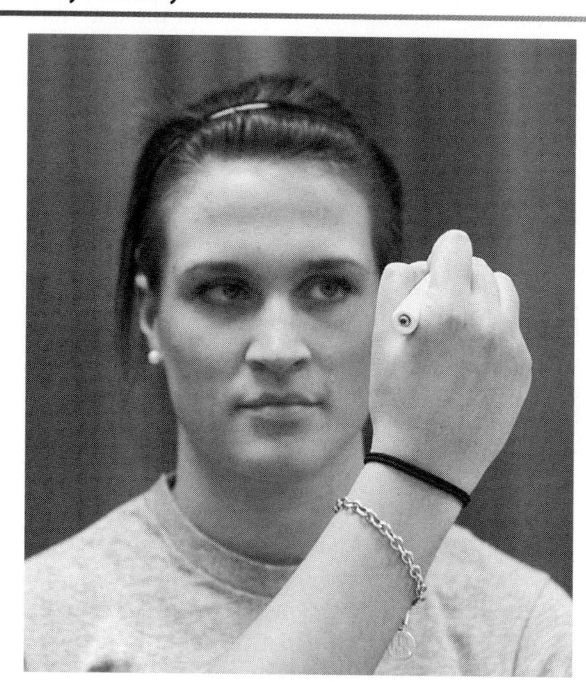

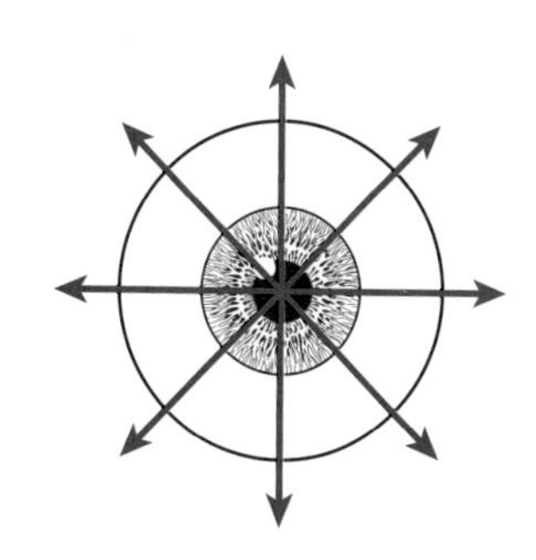

Checking the range of motion, motility, of the eye. The eyes should track smoothly and travel an equal distance.

Patient Position	Sitting or standing
Position of Examiner	Standing in front of the patient, holding a finger approximately 2 ft. from the patient's nose
Evaluative Procedure	The patient focuses on the examiner's finger and instructed to report any double vision experienced during test. The examiner moves the finger upward, downward, left, and right relative to the starting point. The patient follows this motion using only the eyes and is allowed to fix the gaze at the terminal end of each movement. The finger is then moved through the diagonal fields of gaze.
Positive Test	Asymmetrical tracking of the eyes or double vision produced at the end of the ROM.
Implications	Decreased motility of the eyes as the result of neurologic or muscular trauma or decreased vision.
Evidence	Absent or inconclusive in the literature

ROM = range of motion.

Any deformity of the orbit, caused by bony fractures, entrapment of a muscle, or edema can disrupt the eye's alignment and result in diplopia. Although not always associated with a blow-out fracture, fractures of the orbital rim may produce focal tenderness and crepitus during palpation (Examination Findings 19-1). The definitive diagnosis of orbital fractures may require radiographic examination, computed tomography (CT) scanning, or magnetic resonance imaging (MRI).

Corneal Abrasions

Scratching of the cornea may be caused by an external force directly striking the eye or by a foreign object such as sand or dirt being caught between the cornea and the eyelid. Contact lenses may also create a corneal abrasion. Subsequent blinking of the eyelids results in pain and the sensation of a foreign body on the eye, which may or may not still be present.

The eye sympathetically tears in an attempt to wash any invading particles from the eye. Subsequent exposure of the corneal nerves may result in a sharp, stabbing pain. If the abrasion involves the central visual axis, the vision may be blurred (Examination Findings 19-2). Under normal conditions, the abrasion is not visible to the unaided eye. Definitive diagnosis is made using fluorescein strips and a cobalt blue light. The fluorescein strips serve as a dye absorbed only by the cells exposed after a corneal laceration (Special Test 19-3). When a cobalt blue light is shined on the area, the abrasion becomes obvious.

An ophthalmologist will prescribe antibiotic and anesthetic eye drops. A patch may or may not be used to cover the eye.[11]

Corneal Lacerations

Direct trauma to the eye from a sharp object can result in partial- or full-thickness tears of the cornea.[3] Partial-thickness tears are similar in their signs and symptoms to corneal abrasions (see Examination Findings 19-2). However, with these lacerations, the actual trauma to the cornea may be visible. Full-thickness tears are readily apparent by the disruption in the normal translucent appearance of the cornea, a shallow anterior chamber, or the obvious opening of the laceration and subsequent spilling of its contents. An irregularly shaped (elliptical or teardrop) pupil is suggestive of a corneal laceration.

Iritis

Minor blunt trauma to the eye can activate an inflammatory reaction within the anterior chamber, resulting in the "red eye" appearance associated with iritis. Inflammation of the iris itself may occur without pain, but the sensation of pressure within the globe may be described along with marked sensitivity to light. On inspection, the involved pupil is constricted relative to the opposite side. In certain cases, however, the pupil appears dilated or normal. The inflammatory cells within the anterior chamber may cause blurred vision. Assessment of pupillary reaction, determined with a penlight, reveals that the pupil reacts sluggishly when compared with the pupil of the uninjured eye (Examination Findings 19-3).

Hyphema

A hyphema, blood in the anterior chamber of the eye, can result from blunt eye trauma. Less frequently, hyphemas occur spontaneously with no evidence of trauma. An increase in intraocular pressure is associated with hyphema approximately one third of the time.[10] An individual presenting with a traumatic hyphema should be examined for other ocular injuries.

The management of a hyphema includes patching and shielding the eye with immediate referral to an emergency room. The patient should be placed in a semi-reclined position to encourage blood pooling in the inferior anterior chamber. Conservative treatment including relative rest, medications for pain and to reduce the incidence of secondary hemorrhage or decrease intraocular pressure, are generally effective; however, permanent visual impairment can result, particularly in the case of a total hyphema. Close monitoring is essential to insure that the hyphema is resolving and that ocular pressure is decreasing. Hyphemas typically resolve in 5 to 7 days.

Retinal Detachment

A jarring force to the head can result in an interruption in the communication of the retina and the choroid. Although this mechanism can be delivered to the head, the jarring motion associated with sneezing may also be sufficient. The actual detachment of the retina involves the interruption of the nerve pulses being relayed to the optic nerve, often occurring when the vitreous humor seeps between the retina and the choroid.

The patient may complain of flashes of light, halos, or blind spots within the normal field of vision. The patient may also describe a "curtain" or shape being pulled over the field of vision. Retinal detachment, only able to be diagnosed by an ophthalmologist, often requires surgical correction. Spontaneous retinal detachment may be indicative of Marfan syndrome (see Chapter 15).

Ruptured Globe

The most catastrophic injury to the eye is a ruptured globe. Severe blunt trauma delivered to the globe itself (i.e., little or no force being dissipated by the orbital rim) can result in a rupture of the cornea or sclera, subsequently causing it to spill its contents. Commonly, these tears occur behind the insertion of the eye's extrinsic muscles (where the sclera is

Examination Findings 19-1
Orbital Fracture

Examination Segment	Clinical Findings
History	***Onset:*** Acute ***Pain characteristics:*** Orbital margin and possibly within the eye and orbit ***Other symptoms:*** Asymptomatic or possible complaints of air escaping from beneath the eyelid ***Mechanism:*** A direct blow to the periorbital area or the globe itself. A blow-out fracture occurs when a blow increases the amount of pressure within the orbit, causing the orbital floor or medial wall to fracture.
Inspection	Ecchymosis and swelling may be present in the periorbital area. The eye may appear sunken inferiorly or posteriorly into the socket (enophthalmos), may bulge outward (exophthalmos), or may be medially displaced. A laceration of the periorbital area or eyelid may be associated with trauma.
Palpation	Possible tenderness in the periorbital area, but no tenderness may be elicited with a blow-out fracture
Joint and Muscle Function Assessment	***AROM:*** Although not a prerequisite symptom, blow-out fractures may result in the affected eye's inability to look upward or outward.
Joint Stability Tests	***Stress tests:*** Not applicable ***Joint play:*** Not applicable
Special Tests	Not applicable
Neurologic Screening	Sensory testing of the cheek and lateral nose for infraorbital nerve involvement
Vascular Screening	Not applicable
Functional Assessment	***Vision:*** Diplopia, especially on end-gaze, is caused by an alteration in the shape of the orbit or possibly secondary to the bony impingement of the eye's intrinsic musculature or to edema; blurred vision may also be described. ***Jaw function:*** Fracture of the lateral orbital wall will produce pain when opening the mouth (trismus).[2]
Imaging Techniques	Radiography, CT scan, or MRI is used to view the orbit.
Differential Diagnosis	Hyphema, corneal or scleral abrasion, detached retina, infraorbital nerve entrapment
Comments	Individuals who are suspected of suffering from an orbital fracture should be referred to an ophthalmologist for further evaluation. Patients suspected of suffering a blow-out fracture should be instructed to refrain from blowing their nose.

AROM = active range of motion; CT = computed tomography; MRI = magnetic resonance imaging.

Examination Findings 19-2
Corneal Abrasion

Examination Segment	Clinical Findings
History	***Onset:*** Acute ***Pain characteristics:*** Over the cornea and the surrounding conjunctiva, normally reported as "something in my eye;" pain possibly intense ***Other symptoms:*** Blurred vision, photophobia ***Mechanism:*** Direct contact to the cornea or a foreign object (e.g., sand) between the cornea and the eyelid, causing an abrasion ***Predisposing conditions:*** Not applicable
Inspection	The patient's eyes may water. Conjunctival redness is present. A small foreign object may be present. The actual abrasion is not visible under normal conditions.
Special Tests	A corneal abrasion is definitively diagnosed through fluorescein strips and a cobalt blue light.
Neurologic Screening	Not applicable
Vascular Screening	Not applicable
Functional Assessment	Vision possibly blurred secondary to increased watering of the eye or to scratching of the central cornea
Imaging Techniques	Ocular CT scan; nonmetallic MRI studies
Differential Diagnosis	Laceration, orbital fracture, hyphema, retinal detachment
Comments	The visual symptoms of a corneal abrasion may momentarily clear when the surface is lubricated during blinking; however, the blurring of vision soon returns. Patients suspected of having a corneal abrasion should be immediately referred to an ophthalmologist, with the eye closed and patched.

CT = computed tomography; MRI = magnetic resonance imaging.

Special Test 19-3
Fluorescent Dye Test for Corneal Abrasions

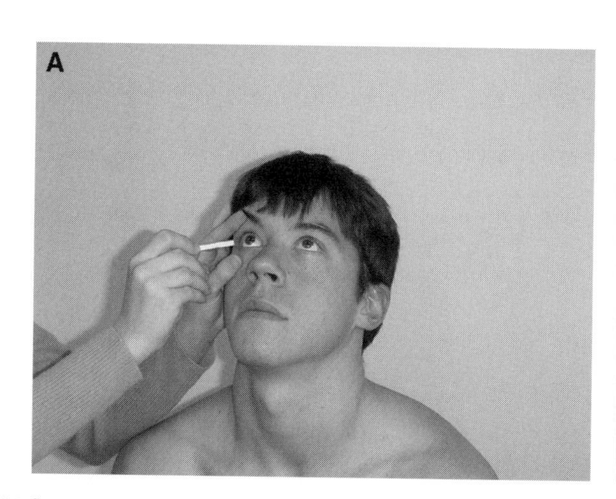

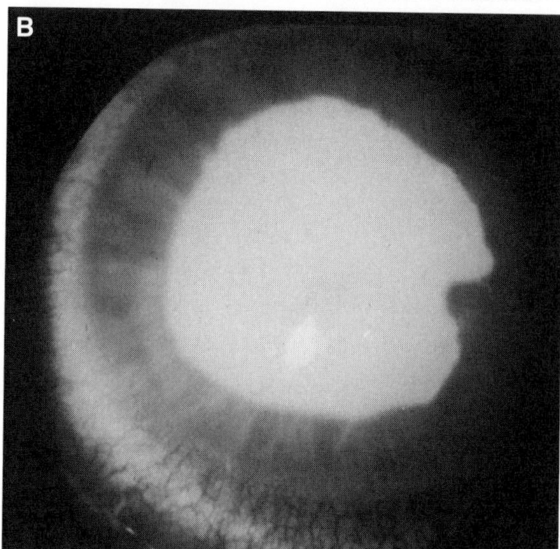

(A) A fluorescein strip is lightly touched to the conjunctiva. **(B)** A cobalt-blue light is shined into the eye to highlight the abraded area.

Patient Position	Seated or supine
Position of Examiner	Standing in front of or beside the patient
Evaluative Procedure	Soak the fluorescein strip with sterile saline solution. Lightly touch the wet fluorescein strip to the conjunctiva of the lower eyelid for a few seconds. Avoid placing the strip directly on the cornea. Ask the patient to blink the eye a few times to spread the solution. Darken the room and use a cobalt blue light to illuminate the eye.
Positive Test	When viewed with the cobalt blue light, corneal abrasions appear as a bright yellow-green pattern on the eye.
Implications	A corneal abrasion
Evidence	Absent or inconclusive in the literature

Examination Findings 19-3
Traumatic Iritis

Examination Segment	Clinical Findings
History	***Onset:*** Acute ***Pain characteristics:*** Pain and burning in the eye ***Other symptoms:*** Photophobia ***Mechanism:*** A traumatic force to the eye that elicits an inflammatory response
Inspection	The conjunctiva adjacent to the cornea may be injected (profused with blood). The involved pupil may be constricted. On occasion, the pupil may be dilated or normal.
Special Tests	Not applicable
Neurologic Screening	Pupillary reaction (CN III)
Vascular Screening	Not applicable
Functional Assessment	The pupil is sluggishly reactive to light. Photophobia is usually described.
Imaging Techniques	Not applicable
Differential Diagnosis	Scleral or corneal abrasion
Comments	Blunt trauma can result in a tearing of the iris sphincter, leading to permanent pupillary deformity.

CN = cranial nerve.

the thinnest) and therefore may not be visible. However, black specks on the sclera are indicative of the contents of the eye's spilling outward.

The primary complaints after a ruptured globe are pain and total or partial loss of vision. On inspection, the globe may appear disoriented in the orbit and the anterior chamber may seem unusually deep. The conjunctiva has marked edema (**chemosis**), and the pupil may be elliptical or teardrop shaped. Hyphema or a dark, coffee ground–like substance also may be viewed within the anterior chamber (Examination Findings 19-4). However, many ruptured globes are often outwardly asymptomatic.

Placement of an eye shield over the eye and immediate transport to the hospital are necessary for individuals suspected of suffering from a ruptured globe. Do not administer any type of eye drops or touch the globe. Because of the possibility of the need for immediate surgery, advise the person not to eat or drink.

Conjunctivitis

Conjunctivitis is the result of a viral or bacterial infection of the conjunctiva. The first symptoms of conjunctivitis are usually experienced upon waking in the morning when the eyelids may stick together and the eye burns and itches. The involved eye typically is red and swollen. The nature of the discharge usually dictates the etiology. A watery discharge accompanied by redness of the conjunctiva indicates a viral infection (pink eye), while a yellow or green discharge indicates a bacterial infection. The affected eye may also be sensitive to light (Examination Findings 19-5). This condition may develop secondary to improper cleaning and care of contact lenses.

Patients with conjunctivitis, a highly contagious condition, must be instructed not to touch the affected eye to avoid spreading the contamination to the uninvolved eye. Likewise, athletes diagnosed with this condition must be barred from contact sports or from entering a swimming pool to prevent transmission of the disease to other athletes. Bacterial conjunctivitis is easily treated with antibacterial eyedrops. Therefore, individuals suspected of suffering from conjunctivitis should be referred to a physician immediately.

Foreign Bodies

A foreign body in the eye is a troublesome but usually benign condition that clears after the object has been removed from the eye. On occasion, a foreign object can lead to corneal abrasions. Do not confuse foreign bodies with impalement of the eye by an object.

An attempt to locate the material causing the discomfort, as described in the section of this chapter on inspection, is necessary. After the particle has been located, it may

Examination Findings 19-4
Ruptured Globe

Examination Segment	Clinical Findings
History	***Onset:*** Acute ***Pain characteristics:*** Throughout the eye; asymptomatic cases have also been reported. ***Mechanism:*** Severe blunt trauma to the globe
Inspection	The globe may be obviously deformed. The anterior chamber may appear deepened. Hyphema or a black, grainy substance may be visible within the anterior chamber. Elliptical or teardrop-shaped pupil may be observed. The contents of the globe may bulge outward through the sclera, appearing as a black "foreign object" on the eye.
Joint and Muscle Function Assessment	***AROM:*** Eye tracking may be absent.
Special Tests	Not applicable
Neurologic Screening	Not applicable
Vascular Screening	Not applicable
Functional Assessment	Vision is lost or markedly decreased in the affected eye.
Imaging Techniques	Not applicable
Differential Diagnosis	Orbital fracture, hyphema, retinal detachment, laceration
Comments	Patients suspected of having a ruptured globe should immediately be transported to the hospital, with a shield covering the eye. Patches should not be used because direct pressure on the globe is to be avoided. No food or fluids should be permitted because immediate surgery may be required.

AROM = active range of motion.

Examination Findings 19-5
Conjunctivitis

Examination Segment	Clinical Findings
History	***Onset:*** Acute; symptoms normally appearing on awakening ***Pain characteristics:*** Itchy, burning sensation in the affected eye Photophobia also possible ***Other symptoms:*** Patient complaints of the eyelids sticking together upon awakening. ***Mechanism:*** Viral or bacterial infection ***Predisposing conditions:*** Improper cleaning and care of contact lenses
Inspection	Reddening of the involved eye Eyelid swelling possibly present Discharge commonly seen; if a discharge is present, the color should be noted: • Clear or watery discharge: Viral infection • Yellow or green discharge: Bacterial infection
Palpation	Palpation is performed wearing gloves to prevent the infection from spreading to the examiner. The eyelids feel fluid filled and boggy.
Special Tests	None
Neurologic Screening	Not applicable
Vascular Screening	Not applicable
Functional Assessment	Vision possibly hindered in the affected eye secondary to the inability to open the eye, swelling, and discharge.
Imaging Techniques	Not applicable
Differential Diagnosis	Iritis, acute glaucoma, subconjunctival hemorrhage, allergic reaction
Comments	Viral conjunctivitis is highly contagious and will likely spread to the other eye. Individuals suffering from viral conjunctivitis should refrain from physical contact with other people or from entering a swimming pool. People suspected of suffering from conjunctivitis should be referred to a physician for further evaluation. The individual must refrain from wearing contact lenses. Patients with viral conjunctivitis should be advised to not share wash clothes or make-up with others and to wash their hands frequently.

be flushed out of the eye using a saline solution or water. A moistened cotton applicator or the corner of a gauze pad may also be used to blot the contaminant from the eye. Dry cotton should not be used on the eye because the fibers will stick to it, possibly inducing a corneal abrasion. Instruct the person to not rub the eye because this may worsen the problem. Discomfort may be reduced by having the person hold the upper eyelid outward, allowing the eye to tear, possibly washing the particle from the eye.

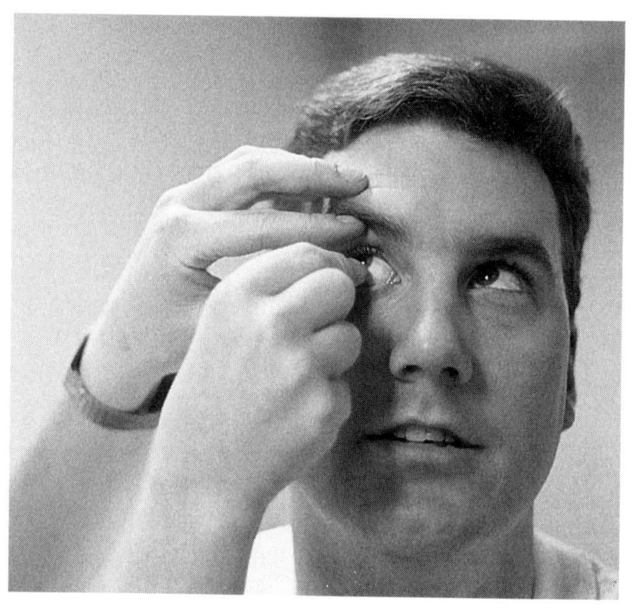

FIGURE 19-13 ■ Removing a soft contact lens. Care must be taken not to insult the cornea or conjunctiva during this procedure.

On-Field Evaluation and Management of Eye Injuries

The correct initial management of eye injuries greatly increases the chances of the long-term viability of the eye. Likewise, improper management can worsen the severity of the injury and increase the likelihood of permanent disability.

Contact Lens Removal

Trauma to the eye when swelling is imminent, such as with a periorbital contusion, requires that contact lenses be removed as soon as possible after the injury. Ideally, this is best performed by the athlete. However, in certain circumstances, the person may require assistance, because either the athlete is unable to do so or he or she cannot find the contact lens on the eye.

Hard contact lenses may be removed through the use of a plungerlike device or may be manually manipulated from the eye in the following manner:

1. The patient opens the eyes as wide as possible.
2. The examiner laterally pulls the outer margin of the eyelids.
3. While holding a hand under the eye to catch the lens, the patient blinks, forcing the lens out of the eye.

Never pluck soft contact lenses directly from the eye, especially when they are resting on the cornea. Doing so may result in serious trauma to the eye. The following procedure is recommended for the removal of soft contact lenses (Fig. 19-13):

1. The patient is asked to look upward.
2. A clean finger is placed on the inferior edge of the contact lens.
3. The lens is manipulated inferiorly and laterally, to where it can be pinched between the fingers and safely removed from the eye.
4. If the contact lens is torn, it is important to remove all pieces from the eye.

Do not attempt to remove the contact lens if a ruptured globe is suspected because of the risk of further damaging the cornea or other structures.

Orbital Fractures

Fractures to the orbital rim that are asymptomatic (other than pain) may require no extraordinary treatment other than ice packs loosely applied to the periorbital area, avoiding direct pressure on the globe.[10] Fractures that cause pain during eye movement need to be shielded with a plastic or metal guard, again avoiding direct pressure on the globe (Fig. 19-14). Because the eyes move in unison, the athlete is instructed to gaze straight ahead with the uninvolved eye, thus limiting voluntary eye movement.

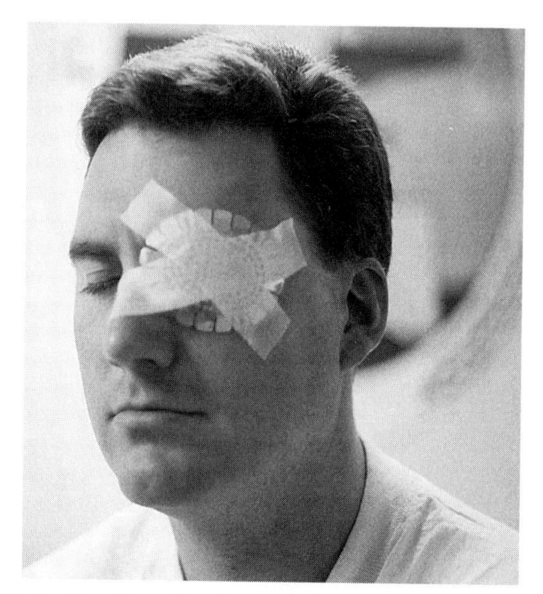

FIGURE 19-14 ■ Protecting the eye with a metal shield. Because the eyes move in unison, it is recommended that the person close the uninvolved eye or stare straight ahead.

Penetrating Eye Injuries

Eye shields, as described previously, are used to manage corneal lacerations and ruptured globes. Do not attempt to remove an object that is impaling the eye, and avoid applying direct pressure on the globe. If the object is protruding some distance outside of the eye, a foam, plastic, or paper cup may be used to cover and protect the eye. In this case, both eyes are covered to minimize movement. The patient must then be immediately transported to the hospital.

Chemical Burns

After a chemical burn, thoroughly irrigate the eye with large amounts of saline solution or water. Then patch the eye. The athlete, along with a sample of the invading substance, is immediately transported to a hospital.

REFERENCES

1. McGwin, G, et al: Consumer product-related eye injury in the United States, 1998–2002. *J Safety Res,* 37:501, 2006.
2. Rodriguez, JO, Lavina, AM, and Agarwal, A: Prevention and treatment of common eye injuries in sports. *Am Fam Physician,* 67:1481, 2003.
3. Boyd-Monk, H: Bringing common eye emergencies. *Nursing,* 35:46, 2005.
4. Burm, JS, Chung, S, and Oh, SJ: Pure orbital blowout fracture: New concepts and importance of medial orbital blowout fracture. *Plast Reconstr Surg,* 103:1839, 1999.
5. Rothman, MI, et al: Superior blowout fracture of the orbit: The blowup fracture. *AJNR Am J Neuroradiol,* 19:1448, 1998.
6. Yab, K, Tajima, S, and Ohba, S: Displacements of eyeball in orbital blowout fractures. *Plast Reconstr Surg,* 100:1409, 1997.
7. Forrest, LA, Schuller, DE, and Strauss, RH: Management of orbital blow-out fractures. Case reports and discussion. *Am J Sports Med,* 17:217, 1989.
8. Ceallaigh, PÓ, et al: Diagnosis and management of common maxillofacial injuries in the emergency department. Part 4: Orbital floor and midface fractures. *Emerg Med J,* 24:292, 2007.
9. Flynn, CA, D'Amico, F, and Smith, G: Should we patch corneal abrasions? A meta-analysis. *J Fam Pract,* 47:264, 1998.
10. Walton, W, et al: Management of traumatic hyphema. *Surv Opthalmol,* 47:297, 2002.
11. Seiff, SR, and Good, WV: Hypertropia and the posterior blowout fracture: Mechanism and management. *Ophthalmology,* 103:152, 1996.

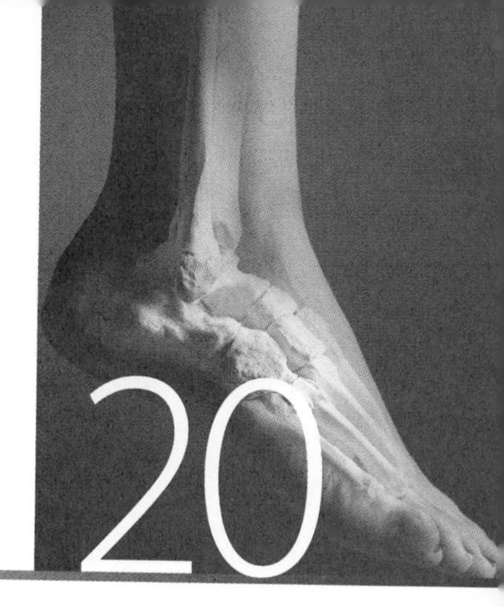

CHAPTER 20

Face and Related Structure Pathologies

Even when appropriate equipment is used, the face, nose, mouth, and ears are vulnerable to injury. However, rules requiring the use of facemasks and mouthguards have reduced the number and severity of injuries to the maxillofacial area. For maximum protection, these devices must be properly fitted. The use of mouthguards during practices and games should be encouraged, even in low-risk sports in which their use is not mandated.

Injuries to the facial structures are significant because of their relationship to neurologic function, the potential of permanent physical deformity and disability, and, in the case of throat injuries, the threat of a compromised airway. An accurate evaluation of injury to these areas is necessary to determine severity and initiate appropriate treatment and management immediately, lessening the probability of any long-term consequences.

Clinical Anatomy

The face is formed by the **frontal**, **maxillary**, **nasal**, and **zygomatic bones** (Fig. 20-1). Comprising a large portion of the anterior face, the maxilla forms a portion of the inferior orbit of the eye, nasal cavity, and oral cavity. The superior row of teeth is fixed within the **alveolar process** along the inferior border of the maxilla. The **zygoma** is fused to the maxilla anteriorly and the **temporal bones** posteriorly, forming the prominent **zygomatic arch** beneath the eyes. Providing the cheek with its surface structure, disruption of the zygomatic arch can drastically affect the face's physical appearance. The zygoma also serves an important role in ocular function by forming a portion of the lateral and inferior rim of the eye's orbit.

Anteriorly, the body of the **mandible** forms the chin. Diverging laterally from the point of the chin, the **ramus** of the mandible begins at the angle of the jaw and continues its course posteriorly and superiorly. The convex **mandibular condylar processes** are located at the end of the ramus, forming the inferior aspect of the **temporomandibular joint**

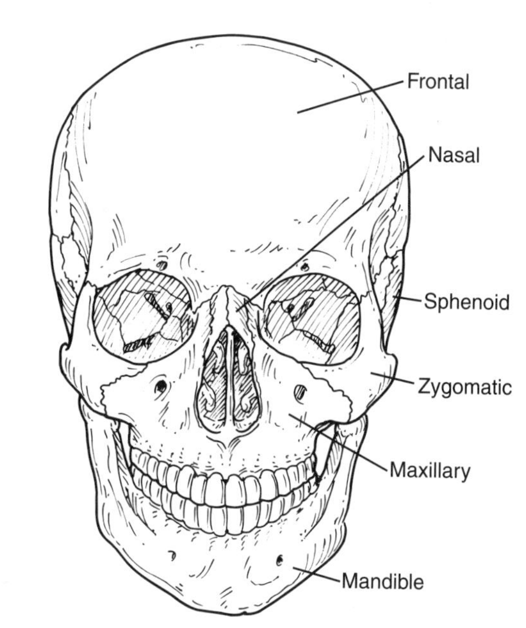

FIGURE 20-1 ■ Bony anatomy of the face.

(TMJ). Anterior to the mandibular condylar process is the site of attachment of the temporalis muscle, the **coronoid process**. Injury to the mandible can potentially involve the alveolar process and thus affect the **occlusion** of the teeth.

Temporomandibular Joint Anatomy

The TMJ joint is a synovial articulation located between the mandibular condylar process and the temporal bone. Pathology to the TMJ can result in **malocclusion** of the teeth, and is often cited as the cause of headaches, cervical muscle strain, and overall muscle weakness.[1,2] Correction of the malocclusion with specially formed mouthpieces has been suggested to solve these problems.

Movement at the TMJ is necessary for communication and the **mastication** of food. The superior temporal articulation, from anterior to posterior, consists of the **articular tubercle**, **articular eminence**, **glenoid fossa**, and **posterior glenoid spine** (Fig. 20-2). The actual articulating area for the mandibular condylar process is the convex articular eminence. The anterosuperior portion of the mandibular condylar process and the articular eminence are covered with the thickest area of fibrocartilaginous tissue, enabling these surfaces to withstand the stresses associated with joint movement.

The entire TMJ joint is encased by a synovial joint capsule. An **articular disk** is located between the two bones, dividing the joint into two separate cavities. The disk is concave on both its superior and inferior surfaces, allowing for a smooth articulation between two convex bones. The disk has sturdy attachments to the mandible, attaching anteriorly and posteriorly to the capsule and surrounding tissues and divides the joint space into upper and lower compartments. Medially and laterally, there are no attachments to the joint capsule so that the disk has freedom of movement in the anteroposterior direction as the mouth opens and closes.

To allow the mouth to open the TMJ's mandibular condyles must roll and translate.[3] As the muscles of mastication (masseter, temporalis, medial pterygoid, and lateral pterygoid) relax, gravity causes the mandibular condyles to roll anterior on the articular disk as the disk rotates posteriorly until the midpoint of motion. At approximately the midpoint of the ROM the lateral pterygoid muscle contracts, translating the disk and condyle forward. Closing the mouth reverses this sequence of events. TMJ biomechanics tend to degrade with age as the articular disk begins to degenerate.[4]

The Ear

The ear is composed of three sections: the external ear, middle ear, and inner ear (Fig. 20-3). The design of the ear permits it to focus acoustical energy and convert it into an electrical signal that can be interpreted by the brain. The inner ear components also function to maintain balance.

The external ear

The shape of the external ear is maintained by an accumulation of cartilaginous tissue, the **auricle (pinna)**. The shape of the external ear functions as a funnel, collecting and focusing sound waves into the **external auditory meatus** to be passed on to the middle ear. Although the auricle is sturdy enough to maintain the shape of the ear, the cartilage

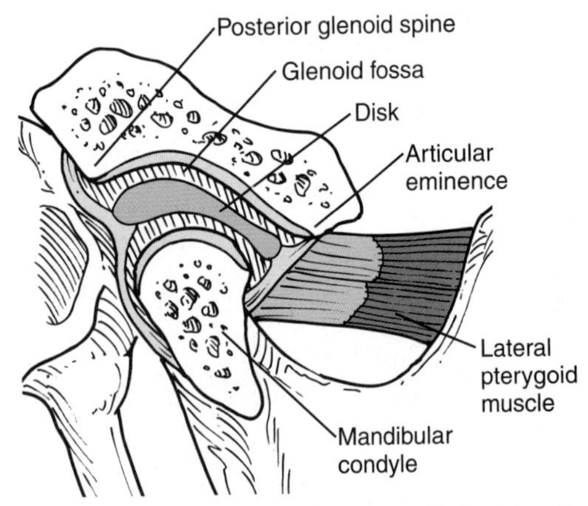

FIGURE 20-2 ■ Anatomy of the temporomandibular joint. The joint structure allows the mandibular condyle to glide forward as the mouth is opened. Trauma to the disk results in a locking or catching as the mouth is opened and closed.

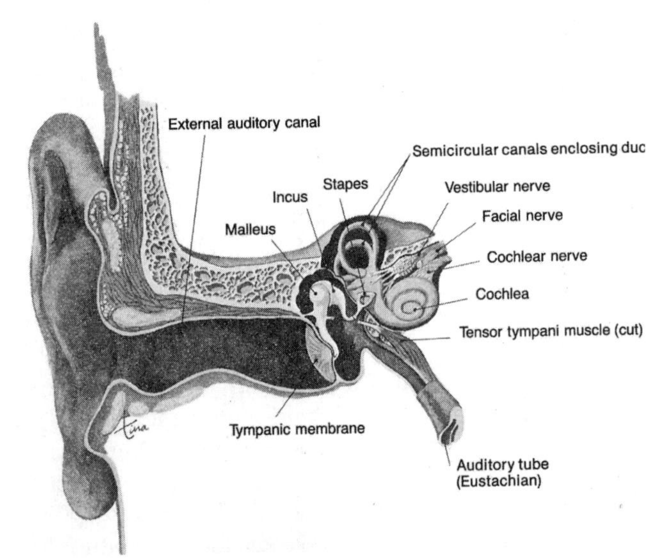

FIGURE 20-3 ■ Anatomy of the ear. The external and middle ear are separated by the tympanic membrane. The middle and inner ear are divided by the oval window. (Courtesy of Rothstein, JM, Roy, SH, and Wolf, SL: *The Rehabilitation Specialist's Handbook*. Philadelphia: FA Davis, 1991.)

Occlusion The process of closing or being closed.

Malocclusion A deviation in the normal alignment of two opposable tissues (e.g., the mandible and maxilla).

Mastication The chewing of food.

is capable of being deformed and quickly returning to its original shape, a mechanism that efficiently disperses many of the forces to which the external ear is exposed.

The middle ear

The **tympanic membrane**, or eardrum, is the outer barrier of the middle ear. Functioning similarly to a microphone that is picking up sound, sound waves strike the tympanic membrane, causing it to oscillate. Three small bones, the **auditory ossicles,** consisting of the **malleus**, **incus**, and **stapes**, are aligned in a chain. These bones transmit the vibrations of the tympanic membrane to the oval window of the inner ear.

The middle ear is connected to the nasal passages by the **eustachian tube**, which regulates the amount of pressure within the middle ear.

The inner ear

Within the inner ear, the mechanical vibrations caused by sound waves are encoded into electrical impulses to be interpreted by the brain. The structures of the inner ear, the **cochlea** and the **semicircular canals**, sit within a bony, fluid-filled labyrinth formed within the temporal bone (Fig. 20-4). Acoustic signals are passed along the cochlea, a bony structure that moves up and down in response to these signals. This movement is detected by fine hair cells and subsequently translated into electrical impulses by the **vestibulocochlear nerve**.

The semicircular canals are filled with fluid. As the head moves, the fluid in the canals shifts. The feedback from this movement is provided to the brain, assisting in maintaining balance and an upright posture of the head and body.

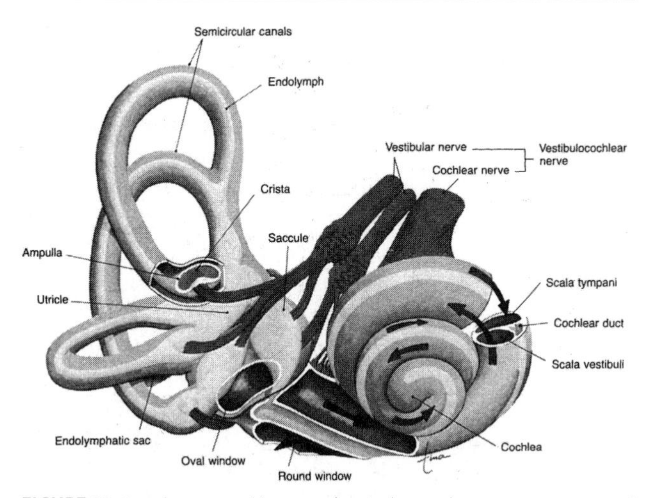

FIGURE 20-4 ■ Inner ear. Here mechanical sound waves are converted into nervous impulses that are sent along to the brain for processing. (Courtesy of Rothstein, JM, Roy, SH, and Wolf, SL: *The Rehabilitation Specialist's Handbook*. Philadelphia: FA Davis, 1991.)

The Nose

The paired, wafer-thin **nasal bones** arise off the facial bones to meet with extensions of the **frontal bones** and **maxillary bones**, forming the **nasal bridge**. The **nasal septum**, formed on its posterior half by the vomer bone and the perpendicular plate of the **ethmoid bone**, meets with the **nasal cartilage** anteriorly to separate the nasal passage into two halves.[5] The floor of the nasal cavity is formed by the **hard palate** anteriorly and the **soft palate** posteriorly (Fig. 20-5).

The external nasal openings, the nostrils, allow air to flow into the nasal passages, through the inferior, middle, and superior **conchae**, and into the **pharynx** to be transmitted to the lungs via the trachea. The nasal passages are lined with **mucosal cells** that warm and humidify cool, dry air before inspiration into the lungs. These cells also produce mucus that acts in conjunction with the nasal hairs to trap foreign particles, preventing them from being passed along to the lungs.

Blood supply to the nasal passage is provided by the highly vascular **Kiesselbach's plexus**, a common source of epistaxis. Bleeding as the result of nasal fracture usually results from the **anterior ethmoid artery** (anterior bleeding) or the **sphenopalatine artery** (posterior bleeding).[5]

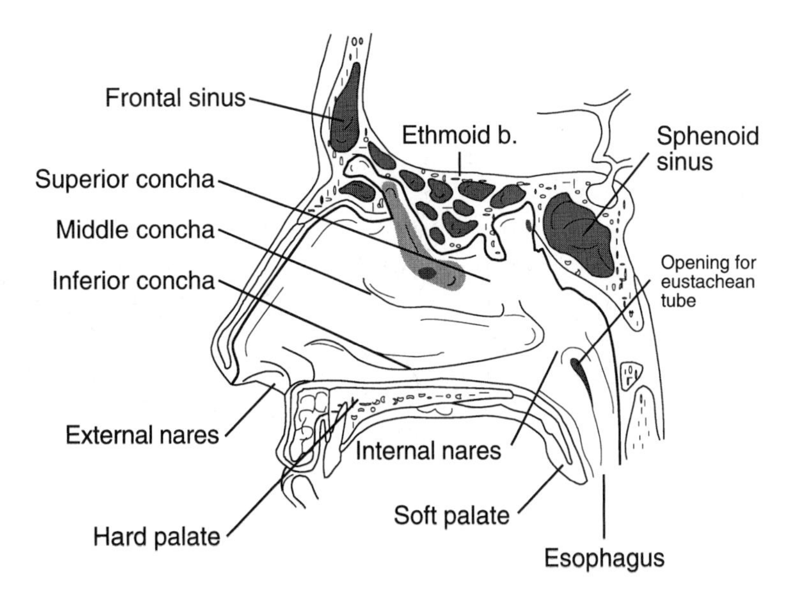

FIGURE 20-5 ■ Cross section of the nasal passage.

The Throat

Because the **larynx** is the most superficial and prominent structure of the throat, it is the area most susceptible to traumatic injury. Covered superiorly by the prominent **thyroid cartilage** (Adam's apple) and inferiorly by the **cricoid cartilage**, the larynx is well protected from all but the most severe blows. Inferior to the cricoid cartilage, the trachea's semicircular cartilage serves as its protective covering until it descends behind the sternum (Fig. 20-6).

The **hyoid bone**, located in the anterior neck between the mandible and the larynx, functions as the tongue's attachment site. This U-shaped bone is suspended by ligaments arising from the temporal bones. The hyoid bone, the only bone in the body that does not articulate with another bone, consists of a central body with two pairs of laterally and posteriorly projecting structures, the greater and lesser **cornua**.

The Mouth

Formed by connective tissue and a thin covering of skin, the lips contain a small layer of transparent cells over a network of vascular capillaries. The lips meet the skin of the face at the **vermillion border**. The rest of the oral cavity is covered by a membrane that produces protective mucus throughout the digestive system (see Chapter 15). The mouth is divided into the **oral vestibule**, delineated as the area from the lips to the teeth, and the **oral cavity**, including everything past the teeth, leading to the trachea.

Lymphatic structures are located at the juncture between the oral cavity and throat. The **tonsils** and **adenoids** prevent bacteria and other germs from entering the respiratory and/or digestive system. Their function is more pronounced in the early years of life and decrease with time.

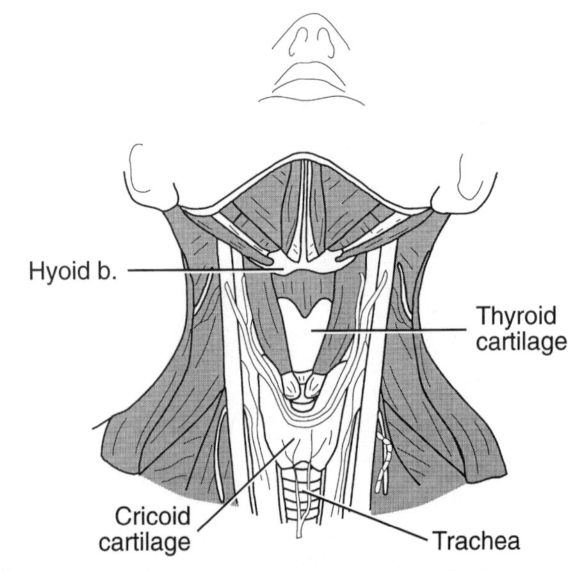

FIGURE 20-6 ■ Anatomy of the upper trachea. The larynx lies behind the thyroid and cricoid cartilages.

The tongue is a skeletal muscle covered by mucous membrane (Fig. 20-7). Its surface is covered with **papillae** and **taste buds**. The papillae are small, rough projections on the surface of the tongue that assist in the movement of food during chewing. The taste buds allow us to appreciate the flavor of whatever we are eating. The tongue is connected on its underside to the floor of the oral cavity by the **lingual frenulum**. This small piece of mucous membrane can be injured during trauma to the tongue or mouth.

The Teeth

A total of 32 permanent teeth, divided equally into upper and lower rows, are normally present. Each row is formed by four different types of teeth, each serving a different function (see Fig. 20-7; Table 20-1). Individually, each tooth has three major anatomical areas: the **root**, the **neck**, and the **crown**. The roots are anchored to the alveolar process by **cementum** and small **periodontal ligaments**. The **gums** cover the alveolar process and root to the base of the tooth's neck.

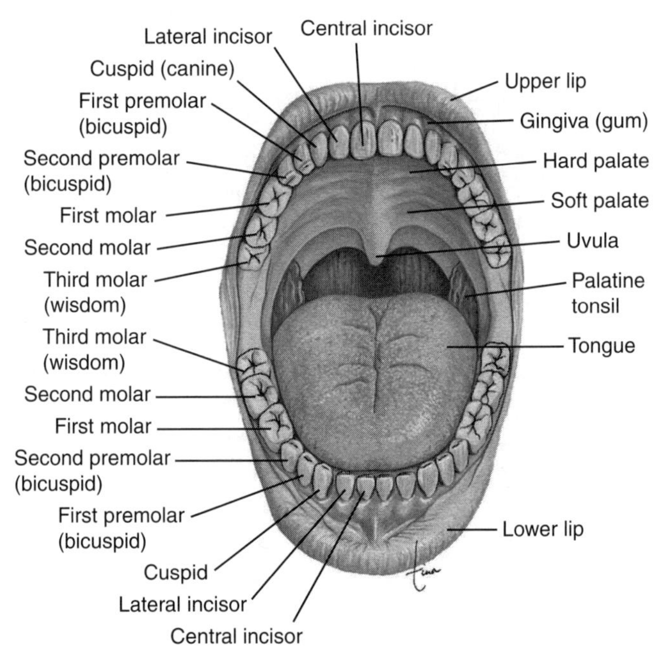

FIGURE 20-7 ■ Oral cavity.

Table 20-1 Classification and Function of the Teeth per Row

Type	Number	Function
Incisors	4	Cutting
Cuspids (Canines)	2	Tearing
Bicuspids (Premolars)	4	Crushing and grinding
Molars	6	Crushing and grinding

Each tooth is formed by **dentin**, a hard, calcified substance covered by an even harder substance, **enamel**. The tooth's core is formed by the **pulp chamber**, housing a strong connective tissue **(pulp)**, nerves, and blood vessels (Fig. 20-8). The nerves and blood vessels enter from the underlying bone through the apical foramen and course through the root canal up into the pulp cavity.

Muscular Anatomy

For the purposes of this chapter, the maxillofacial muscles are classified as being either the muscles of mastication or muscles of expression. Dysfunction of these muscles occurs secondary to lacerations, dislocations, fractures, or cranial nerve involvement. Additional facial muscles acting on the eye and eyelids are discussed in Chapter 19.

Muscles of mastication

The primary muscle for flexing the jaw (closing the mouth) is the masseter, which spans the distance between the mandibular angle and the inferior portion of the zygomatic arch. The mouth is opened by the contraction of the **digastric**, **mylohyoid**, **medial pterygoid**, and **lateral pterygoid** muscles.

Muscles of expression

The muscles of expression—those that move the lips, cheeks, nose, eyebrows, and forehead—are presented in Table 20-2 and Figure 20-9. The lack of symmetrical movement or hypertonicity of the facial muscles indicates that there is trauma or disease to one or more cranial nerves, **Bell's palsy**, which may be caused by infection, disease, or stroke.

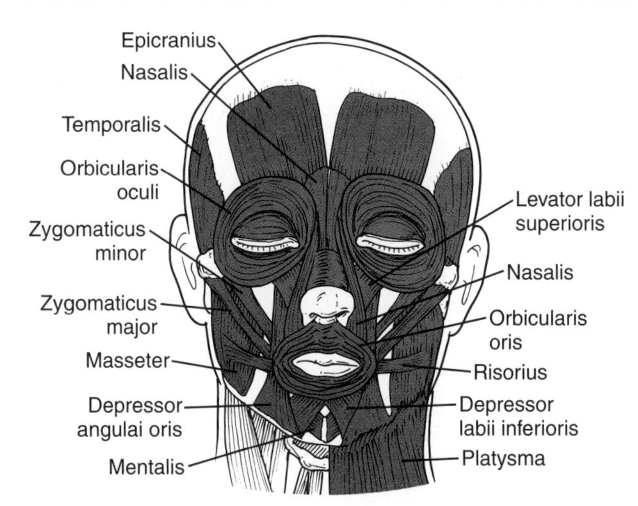

FIGURE 20-9 ■ The muscles of expression.

Clinical Examination of Facial Injuries

The evaluation of a specific segment of the face need not encompass all aspects of otherwise unrelated structures. However, a secondary screen of these areas should be conducted to rule out concurrent injury. For example, a direct

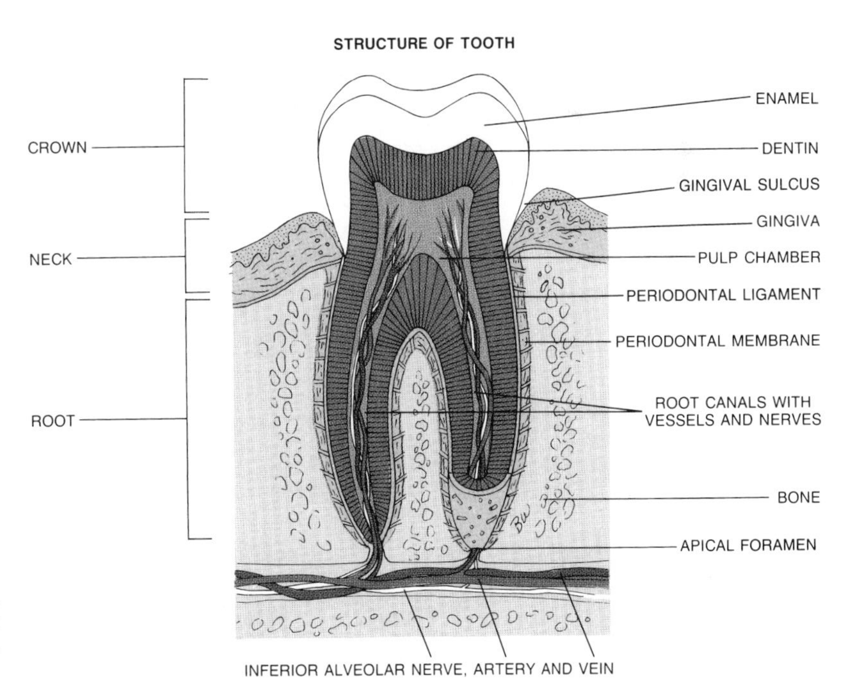

FIGURE 20-8 ■ Cross-sectional anatomy of a tooth. (Courtesy of Venes D (ed): *Taber's cyclopedic medical dictionary*, ed 21, Beth Anne Willert, MS, medical illustrator. Philadelphia: FA Davis, 2009.)

Bell's palsy Inhibition of the facial nerve secondary to trauma or disease, resulting in flaccidity of the facial muscles. In individuals suffering from Bell's palsy, the face on the involved side appears elongated.

Table 20-2 Muscles of Expression (Partial List)

Muscle	Action	Origin	Insertion	Innervation	Root
Buccinator	Depresses the cheeks	Alveolar process of the maxilla and mandible.	Angle of the mouth	Facial	CN VII
Depressor Anguli Oris	Draws the angle of the mouth downward (frowning)	Oblique line of the mandible	Angle of the mouth	Facial	CN VII
Depressor Labii Inferioris	Lowers the mouth	Oblique line of the mandible	Lower lip	Facial	CN VII
Digastric	Opens mouth	Inferior border of the mandible	Superior aspect of the hyoid bone	Trigeminal	CN V
Geniohyoid	Opens mouth	Median ridge of the mandible	Body of the hyoid bone	Ansa cervicalis	CN I, CNII
Levator Anguli Oris	Raises each side of the mouth (a bilateral muscle)	Just superior to the canine teeth	Angle of the mouth	Facial	CN VII
Masseter	Aids in biting	Superficial portion: Zygomatic process of maxilla; anterior two-thirds of zygomatic arch Profundus portion: Posterior one-third of the zygomatic arch	Superficial portion: Inferior one-half of the lateral ramus of the mandible Profundus portion: Superior one-half of the ramus and coronoid process of the mandible	Trigeminal	CN V
Mentalis	Elevates the skin of the chin.	Incisive fossa of the mandible	Point of the mandible	Facial	CN VII
Mylohyoid	Opens mouth	Inferior border of the mandible	Superior aspect of the hyoid bone	Trigeminal	CN V
Orbicularis Oris	"Puckers" lips	Originates off of the muscles surrounding the mouth	Skin surrounding the lips	Facial	CN VII
Procerus	Wrinkles the nose	Lower portion of the nasal bone Lateral nasal cartilage	Lower portion of the forehead between the eyebrow	Facial	CN VII
Temporalis	Aids in biting	Temporal fossa	Coronoid process and ramus of themandible	Trigeminal	CN V
Zygomaticus Major	Used for smiling	Zygomatic bone	Angle of the mouth	Facial	CN VII

CN = cranial nerve.

Examination Map

HISTORY

Location of Pain

Onset

Activity and Injury Mechanism

Symptoms

INSPECTION

Inspection of the Ear
Auricle
Tympanic membrane
Periauricular area

Inspection of the Nose
Alignment
Epistaxis
Septum and mucosa
Eyes and face

Inspection of the Nose
Respiration
Thyroid and cricoid cartilage

Inspection of the Face and Jaw
Bleeding
Ecchymosis
Symmetry
Muscle tone

Inspection of the Oral Cavity
Lips
Teeth
Tongue
Lingual frenulum
Gums

PALPATION

Palpation of the Anterior Structures
Nasal bone
Nasal cartilage
Zygoma
Maxilla
Temporomandibular joint
Periaricular area
External ear
Teeth
Mandible
Hyoid bone
Cartilages

Palpation of the Lateral Structures
Temporalis
Masseter
Buccinator

FUNCTIONAL ASSESSMENT

Ear
Hearing
Balance

Nose
Smell

Temporomandibular Joint
Range of motion
Tracking

NEUROLOGIC EXAMINATION

Cranial Nerve Assessment

PATHOLOGIES AND SPECIAL TESTS

Ear Pathologies
Auricular hematoma
Tympanic membrane rupture
Ostitis externa
Ostitis media

Nasal Pathologies

Throat Pathologies

Facial Pathologies
Mandibular fracture
Zygoma fracture
Maxillary fracture
LeFort fracture

Dental Conditions
Tooth fracture
Tooth luxation
Dental caries

Temporomandibular Joint Dysfunction

blow to the face may fracture bones and damage teeth. In the event of direct blows to the head, brain and cervical spine injury must also be ruled out (see Chapter 21).

History

Despite the presence of an obvious injury to a particular structure, trauma to adjacent areas must also be ruled out. Injuries to the larynx may impede the ability to breathe and/or speak.

History involving the ear

- **Location of the pain:** Direct blows to the external ear result in pain in the affected area. Complaints of pressure within the middle or inner ear indicate an infection or a tympanic membrane rupture. Otitis externa, the infection of the external auditory meatus, causes intense, unremitting pain and itching.
- **Activity and injury mechanism:** Most ear injuries stem from a blunt trauma to the auricle, especially prevalent in sports in which headgear is not mandated. A tympanic membrane rupture can be caused by a slapping blow to the ear that produces pressure on the middle ear, thereby causing the membrane to rupture, an injury that is predisposed by infection of the middle ear. A physical puncture of the tympanic membrane may occur from an object entering the external auditory meatus. Infections to the middle ear are usually preceded by **upper respiratory infections**, resulting in inflamed mucous membranes that block the eustachian tubes. The tympanic membrane can also be injured secondary to external pressures during diving and airplane travel.
- **Other symptoms:** An infection of the inner ear, or **labyrinth**, can occasionally result from an upper respiratory infection. In the acute stages patients with labyrinthitis may complain of **vertigo**, nausea, and vomiting.[6] With infection, pressure changes within the middle or inner ear cause the ear to feel congested.

Upper respiratory infection (URI) A categorical term encompassing a wide range of viral or bacterial infections of the nasal pathway, pharynx, and/or bronchi. The common cold is a form of URI.

Vertigo Dizziness.

This condition may be aggravated by pressure changes associated with airplane travel.

History involving the nose

- **Location of the pain:** Pain may be located over the nose but may also radiate throughout the eyes, face, and forehead.
- **Onset:** The onset of injury is often, if not always, acute. The insidious onset of nasal symptoms is suggestive of diseases such as **sinusitis** or upper respiratory infection.
- **Activity and injury mechanism:** The mechanism of injury is a direct blow to the nasal bone or nasal cartilage. Spontaneous **epistaxis** may occur as the result of a hot, dry environment's drying out the highly vascularized nasal membrane.
- **Symptoms:** Pain and bleeding may be present. The patient requires evaluation for a possible concussion and orbital damage because the forces needed to fracture a nose may be sufficient to cause eye injury or closed head trauma (see Chapter 21).
- **Medical history:** Questioning the patient about a history of past nasal trauma is important. A prior nasal fracture may result in deformity that can be mistaken for an acute injury.

History involving the throat

- **Location of the pain:** Acute throat trauma causes pain in the anterior portion of the neck. Pain arising from illness (e.g., sore throat) is described as being deep within the neck.
- **Onset:** Throat injuries typically have acute onsets.
- **Activity and injury mechanism:** The throat is usually injured when it is struck with an object such as a bat, ball, or an opponent's elbow.
- **Symptoms:** A blow that crushes the larynx may result in the inability to speak. Respiratory distress may occur secondary to an obstruction of the airway and may result in the patient's speaking in a hoarse, raspy voice. This constitutes a medical emergency.

History involving maxillofacial injuries

- **Location of the pain:** Normally, the exact site of pain can be located. Dental injuries usually can be pinpointed to one or more teeth. Oral pain may also be the result of neuralgia, temporomandibular joint (TMJ) conditions, sinusitis, migraine headaches, and myofascial inflammation.[7]
- **Onset:** Maxillofacial injuries are usually acute and the direct result of trauma. The exceptions are nonathletic dental problems (e.g., **dental caries**) and nerve conditions (e.g., Bell's palsy, **trigeminal neuralgia**).
- **Activity and injury mechanism:** The typical mechanism of injury is blunt trauma from an object or competitor. Balls, various forms of sticks and bats, and opponents all pose potential risks for inflicting maxillofacial injuries. Lacerating trauma to the lips or tongue can be accidentally self-inflicted by the patient's teeth.
- **Bruxing:** Bruxism (clenching or grinding of the teeth) may occur subconsciously or during sleep, can be habitual, the result of stress, or caused by TMJ dysfunction.[8] With time, bruxing can result in degeneration of the teeth's enamel and TMJ structures.
- **Other symptoms:** The facial bones are a large component of the eye orbit. The patient may report visual impairment and difficulty with eye movements. Initially, TMJ injuries may not be reported, but the patient may begin to notice pain or clicking in the TMJ while chewing. Difficulty chewing may indicate malocclusion of the teeth. Patients in the early stages of oral cancer may complain of gingivitis-like symptoms, and the tongue may feel thick and swollen (angioedema).

Inspection

Close inspection of the facial structures is vital for the accurate evaluation and management of injuries to this area. The primary inspection includes a check for obvious lacerations to the face and mouth because these injuries are usually found concurrently with other trauma. Because trauma to the face and mouth involves the respiratory system, the patency of the airway must also be immediately assessed. In cases of injury to the mouth, the oral cavity requires inspection for blockage by a mouthguard, piece of tooth, or other object that could become lodged in the airway.

Inspection of the ear

- **The auricle:** Observe the outer ear for signs of a contusion or laceration. High-velocity impact of the auricle, as occurs when hit with a baseball, may cause a piece of the outer ear to be avulsed (Fig. 20-10). Formation of a hematoma within the auricle can result in the characteristic **pinna** or **auricular hematoma** (cauliflower ear) (Fig. 20-11). **Otitis externa** is evident as the external ear, including the external auditory meatus, is inflamed.
- **The tympanic membrane:** Inspect the eardrum using an otoscope (Inspection Findings 20-1). The membrane normally appears shiny, convex, translucent, and smooth without any perforations. Suspected disruption of the tympanic membrane or fluid within the auditory canal requires immediate referral for

Sinusitis Inflammation of the nasal sinus.

Epistaxis A nosebleed.

Dental caries A destructive disease of the teeth; cavities.

Trigeminal neuralgia A painful condition involving cranial nerve V, with possible motor involvement to one side of the mouth and paresthesia in the cheek.

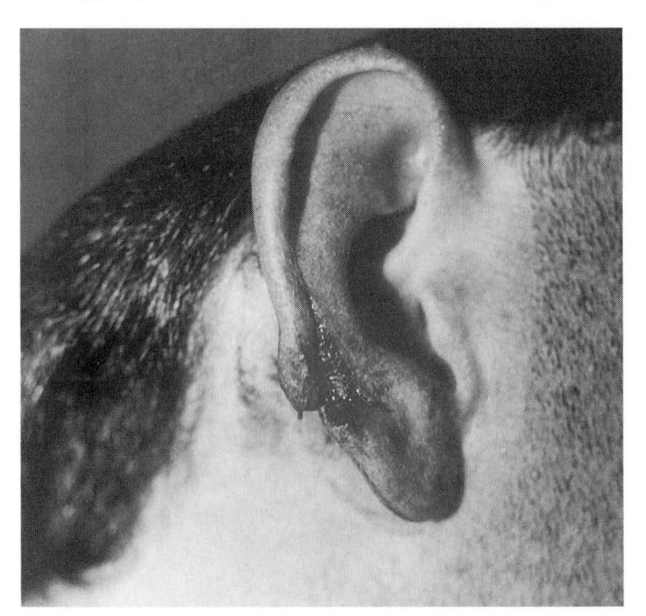

FIGURE 20-10 ■ Laceration of the external ear. This injury requires suturing to prevent permanent deformity of the ear.

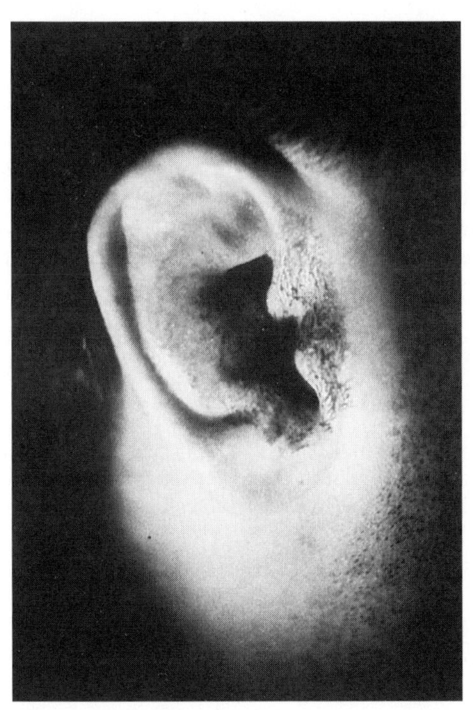

FIGURE 20-11 ■ Auricular hematoma, or "cauliflower ear." This condition is shown in its acute stage. If the hematoma is allowed to develop, the underlying cartilage is destroyed, resulting in permanent deformity of the external ear. Hearing acuity is affected secondary to the decreased ability to funnel sound waves into the middle ear.

further medical evaluation. Infection of the middle ear, otitis media, causes the membrane to appear distended secondary to the collection of fluids and pus. A collection of fluids may also be visible, otitis media with effusion. These substances may also occlude the membrane.

- **Periauricular area:** Carefully inspect the area surrounding the ear for signs of a basilar skull fracture, characterized by ecchymosis around the mastoid process, known as "**Battle's sign**."

Inspection of the nose

- **Alignment:** Inspect the nose for proper alignment and symmetry on each side of the sagittal plane. Asymmetry may be caused by a fracture or swelling. Any question regarding the presence of a deformity can be resolved by asking the patient to view his or her nose in a mirror to see if it looks normal.
- **Epistaxis:** Observe for bleeding from the nose. Bleeding from the nasal passage is common after trauma to the nasal bones and is usually the result of mucosal laceration. Light bleeding may indicate epistaxis from the anterior portion of the nose; moderate to heavy bleeding indicates posterior epistaxis.[9] Lacerations of the skin covering the nose are also common in patients with these injuries and may or may not have an associated fracture. Universal precautions are indicated.
- **Septum and mucosa:** View the nasal septum and its mucosal lining using an otoscope (see Inspection Findings 20-1) or penlight. On inspection, the septum appears symmetrical and straight; asymmetry or angulation of the nasal passage indicates a deviated septum. Bony fragments may also be seen within the nasal passage.
- **Eyes and face:** Inspect the area beneath the eyes for the presence of ecchymosis. After a nasal or skull fracture, blood follows the contour of the bone to rest beneath the eyes (periorbital ecchymosis), a clinical sign termed **raccoon eyes** (Fig. 20-12).

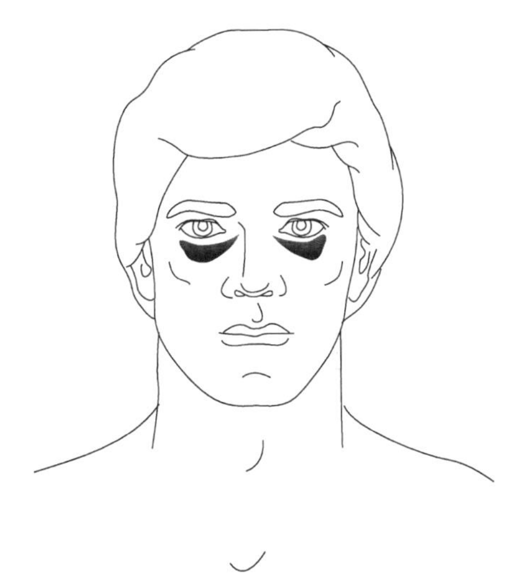

FIGURE 20-12 ■ Raccoon eyes. After a nasal fracture, hemorrhage follows the contour of the face and pools beneath the eyes. This condition can also result from a skull fracture.

Inspection Findings 20-1
Use of an Otoscope for Inspection of the Ear and Nose

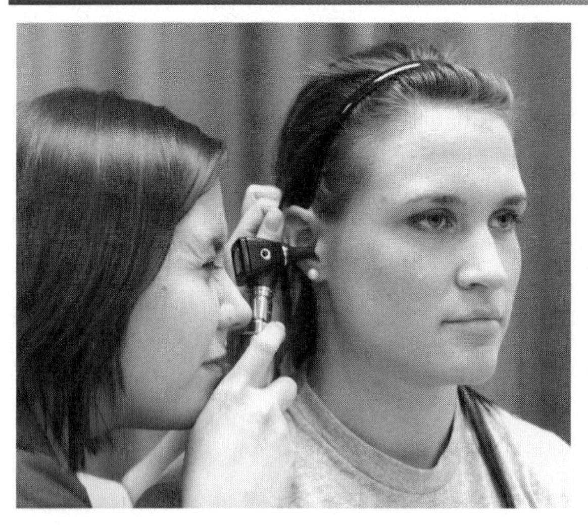

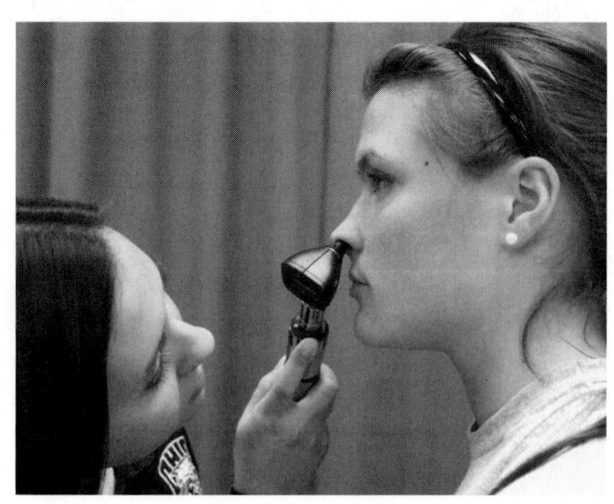

An otoscope with a speculum that fits snugly within the ear canal, without causing pain, is used to inspect the tympanic membrane. The speculum needs to be placed only slightly into the ear canal to view the structures. Visualization is improved when the pinna is pulled upward and backward (some clinicians prefer to pull the earlobe downward).

An otoscope is used to visualize the tympanic membrane and nasal passage.

Patient Position	Seated or standing
Position of Examiner	Position to easily access the patient's ear or nose.
Evaluative Procedure	Select and fit a speculum on the otoscope that will fit snugly into the opening. When inspecting the ear, open the auditory canal by gently pulling upward and backward on the pinna or downward on the earlobe. Look through the otoscope and insert it gently into the canal. Deep penetration is not necessary.
Positive Test	***Ear:*** Reddened and/or bulging tympanic membrane; fluid buildup behind the tympanic membrane; fluid in the ear canal; ruptured tympanic membrane ***Nose:*** Deviation or deformity of the nasal passage(s)
Implications	***Ear:*** Reddened and/or bulging tympanic membrane is indicative of middle ear infection (acute otitis media). Fluid behind the tympanic membrane (otitis media effusion) is not necessarily indicative of an infection. Fluid in the ear canal may represent otorrhea, or leakage of cerebrospinal fluid, and is associated with a skull fracture. A rupture tympanic membrane may result from a blow to the ear ***Nose:*** Fracture, deviated septum
Comments	Cerumen may obscure the tympanic membrane. To clear cerumen, gently flush the ear with hydrogen peroxide or warm water. Do not do this if a tympanic membrane rupture is suspected.
Evidence	Absent or inconclusive in the literature

Inspection of the throat

- **Respiration:** Observe the patient's breathing pattern for signs of respiratory distress (see Chapter 15). Even relatively minor blows to the throat can disrupt breathing. Any difficulty in breathing must be considered a medical emergency.
- **Thyroid and cricoid cartilage:** Inspect these cartilages for deformity. Swelling may appear rapidly and obliterate the borders of the thyroid cartilage. Any deformity in this structure must be treated as a medical emergency because of the potential jeopardy to the airway.[10]

Inspection of the face and jaw

- **Bleeding:** Facial and tongue lacerations are often accompanied by profuse bleeding. Although controlling bleeding must be addressed, the possibility of underlying trauma must not be overlooked (see the section on on-field management of facial lacerations).
- **Ecchymosis:** The presence of periorbital ecchymosis may be the result of fracture to the nasal bones, maxilla, or zygoma. In addition, it can occur without a fracture (e.g., black eye). Ecchymosis below the alveolar process and at the angle of the mandible is common after mandibular fracture.
- **Symmetry:** Inspection of the uninjured face usually reveals symmetry between the right and left halves. With facial pathology such as zygomatic fracture, TMJ injury, or mandibular fracture, this symmetry may be lost secondary to bony deformity or swelling. Inspection of the face also includes inspecting the patient's eye movements for equality. If the maxilla or zygoma is fractured, eye movement may be asymmetrical (see Chapter 19).
- **Muscle tone:** As the patient responds to your questions, the movements of his or her mouth, eyebrows, and forehead are inspected for symmetry. A unilateral paralysis of the facial muscles, Bell's palsy, is the result of traumatic or organic inhibition of the facial nerves or can be associated with a stroke.

Inspection of the oral cavity

- **Lips:** Because of the high potential for infection and scarring, any laceration extending across the vermillion border onto the lips requires a referral to a physician for further evaluation.
- **Teeth:** Although most types of tooth fractures are readily apparent during gross inspection, chipped teeth and fractures involving the root are more subtle. Using a penlight and dental mirror, inspect both the inner and outer sides of the tooth's surfaces for chipped crowns and other defects. Although most acute dental trauma only involves one tooth, trauma to the surrounding teeth must also be ruled out (Fig. 20-13).[11]

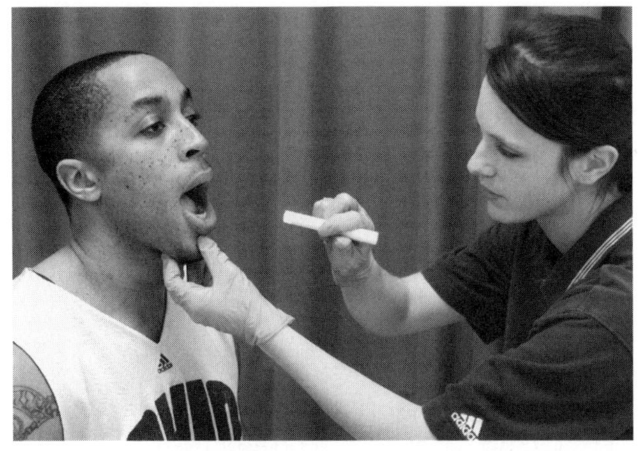

FIGURE 20-13 ■ Inspection of the oral cavity to rule out tooth fractures and to locate the source of bleeding.

- **Tongue:** The dorsal and ventral surfaces of the tongue are inspected for lacerations.
- **Lingual frenulum:** The integrity of the lingual frenulum is observed as the patient lifts the tongue (Fig. 20-14). This structure can become lacerated secondary to teeth fractures.
- **Gums:** The inner and outer border of the gums is inspected for lacerations, an abscess, or **gingivitis**. For conditions of insidious onset for patients with a history of smoking or smokeless tobacco use, inspect the gums and tongue for white or red lesions and nonhealing open wounds. Leukoplakia, precancerous cells, often form in the area of contact with smokeless tobacco.

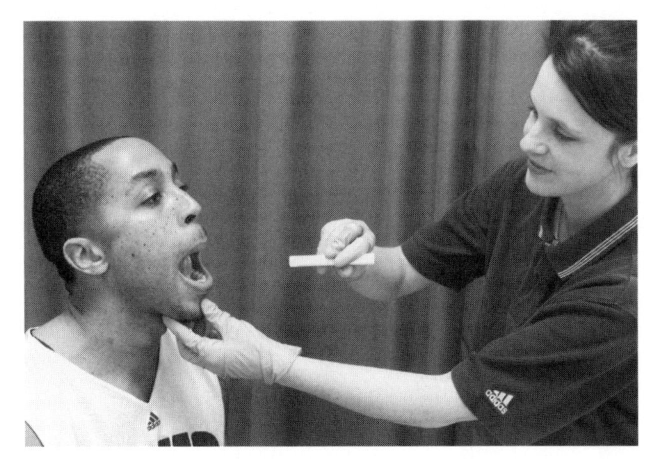

FIGURE 20-14 ■ Inspection of the lingual frenulum. The patient is asked to lift the tongue to the roof of the mouth.

Gingivitis Inflammation of the gums.

PALPATION

Because of the relatively subcutaneous location of the facial bones and mandible, these structures are easily palpated. Although the internal structures of the ears, nose, and throat cannot be palpated, the overlying and surrounding areas must be examined for tenderness and concurrent injury.

Palpation of the Anterior Structures

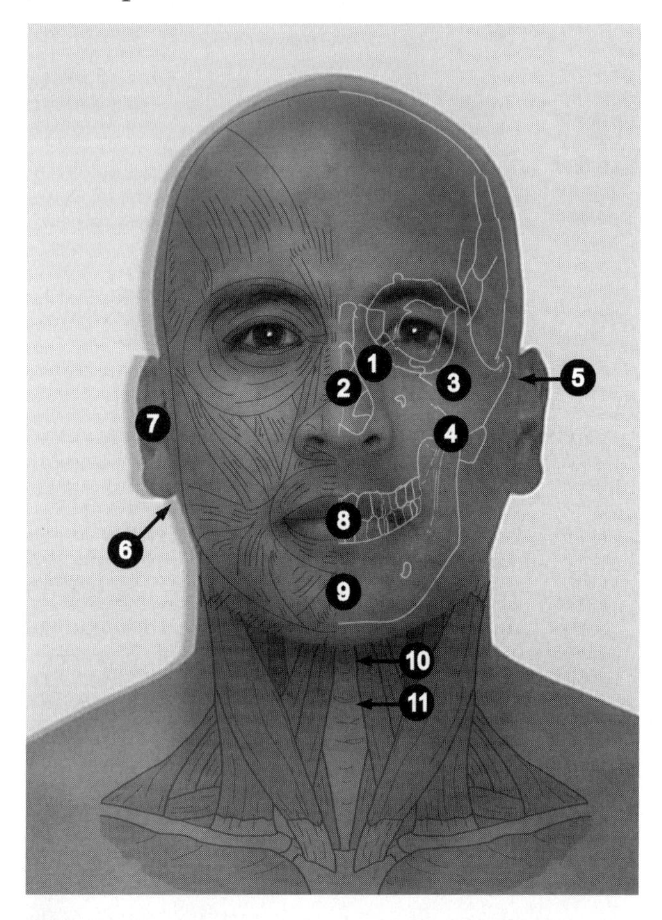

1 Nasal bone: Begin palpation of the nasal bone at the point that the zygomatic and maxillary bones merge beneath the medial portion of the orbit. Applying light yet firm pressure, continue to palpate medially to the base of the nasal bone and up to the bridge of the nose, noting painful areas or crepitus. Palpation of the nasal bones is not necessary if a fracture is visually apparent. From the upper boundaries of the nasal bone, proceed upward and laterally to palpate the frontal bone above the nose and eyes.

2 Nasal cartilage: From the bridge of the nose, continue palpating distal to the nasal cartilage at the tip of the nose. Normally, this structure should align with the center of the bridge.

3 Zygoma: Begin to palpate the face at the junction between the temporal and zygomatic bones, just anterior to the auditory canals and above the TMJ. Palpate anteriorly and medially along the zygomatic arches as they pass beneath the eyes and merge with the maxillary bones bilaterally.

4 Maxilla: From the crest of the zygomatic arch, palpate upward along the maxillary bones. The fused joint where the maxillary and nasal bones join is marked by a sudden slope. Palpation continues to the crest of the nasal bones. Palpate the remainder of the maxillary bone by moving inferiorly from the nose and outward along the upper margin of the teeth.

5 TMJ: Open the jaw to move the coronoid process from under the zygomatic arch. Although this structure is often not directly palpable, the area can be palpated for underlying tenderness.

Placing the tips of the index and middle fingers over the TMJ, note the presence of any clicking or crepitus as the mouth is opened and closed (Fig. 20-15). These conditions are pathological, indicating a disruption of the joint's normal biomechanics. As the mouth is opened wide, a small depression is normally felt within the joint as the mandibular head and neck slide forward. Swelling can fill this area.

Palpate the posterior aspect of the TMJ by placing the fifth finger in the opening of the external auditory meatus (Fig. 20-16). The bilateral movement of the TMJ normally is smooth and equal as the mouth is opened and closed. Any discrepancy in this motion may indicate TMJ dysfunction, a TMJ dislocation, or a mandibular fracture.

6 Periauricular area: To rule out the presence of a fracture, palpate the temporal bone surrounding the external ear and its mastoid process.

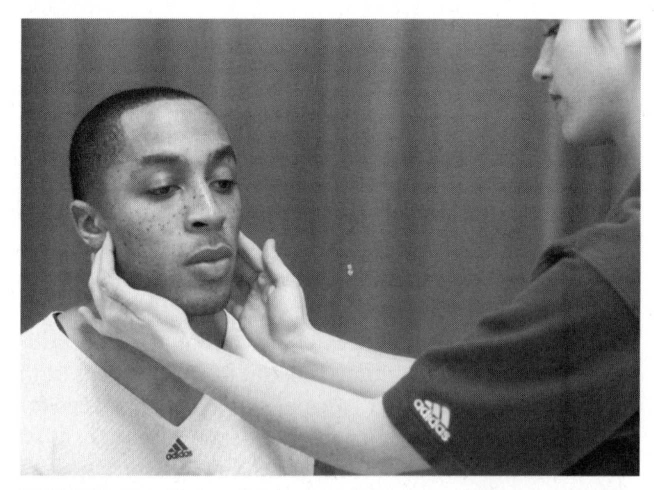

FIGURE 20-15 ■ External palpation of the external temporomandibular joint. The temporomandibular joint is palpated while the mouth is opened and closed. Asymmetry of movement and clicking or locking of the joint are noted.

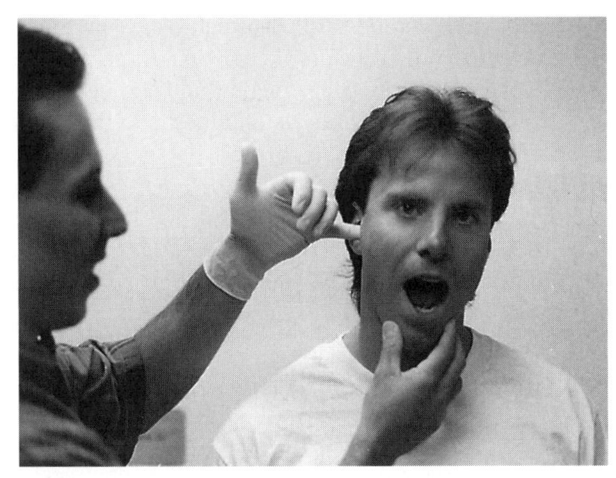

FIGURE 20-16 ■ Palpation of the internal temporomandibular joint. Wearing gloves, the examiner lightly places a finger in the outermost portion of the auditory canal to further palpate the mechanics of the temporomandibular joint as the mouth is opened and closed.

7 **External ear:** Palpate the auricle to determine tenderness and swelling. In cases of repeated trauma to the external ear, as commonly occurs in wrestlers, hard nodules may be felt within the auricle. Pain associated with a middle or inner ear infection is increased by tugging on the earlobe. Locate the lymph nodes just inferior and posterior to the ear. They can become enlarged secondary to infection.

8 **Teeth:** Palpate the teeth after an oral injury with caution. Gentle pressure is sufficient to check the integrity of the tooth's attachment to the alveolar processes (Fig. 20-17). An alternative is to have the patient use the tongue to apply this pressure. Any suspicion of a loosened tooth warrants consultation with a dentist. The procedure for the management of a lost tooth is covered in the related section on on-field management.

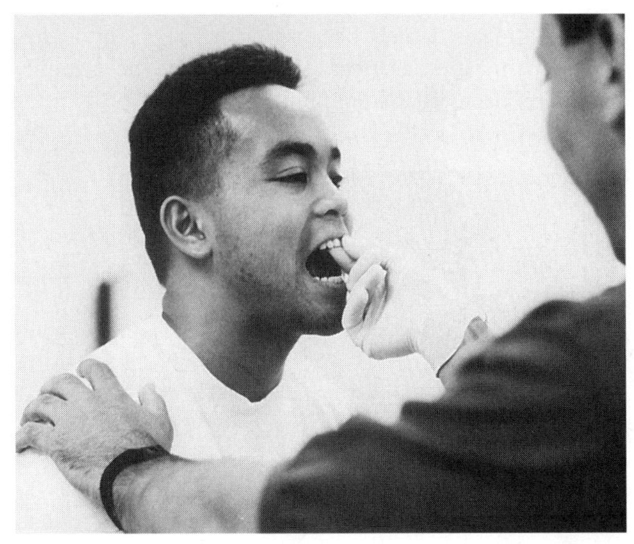

FIGURE 20-17 ■ Palpation of the teeth. Because of the possibility of exposure to bloodborne pathogens, gloves must be worn during this process.

9 **Mandible:** Begin the palpation of the chin at the mental protuberance (cleft of the chin). From here, progress posteriorly, palpating the lateral and posterior portion of the mandible and the lower alveolar processes. The mandibular ramus and the lateral border of the angle of the mandible become obscured by the masseter muscle.

10 **Hyoid bone:** Palpate the hyoid bone, located approximately one finger breadth superior to the thyroid cartilage. The integrity of the hyoid bone can be determined by gently grasping it between the thumb and index fingers. The bone glides downward as the patient swallows.

11 **Cartilages:** Begin the palpation of the cartilages at the sternal notch. Continue upward to find the series of depressions and hardened bands of the tracheal cartilage. Then proceed upward to find the cricoid cartilage and the thick body of the thyroid cartilage.

Palpation of the Lateral Structures

The four primary muscles of mastication are the temporalis, masseter, and medial and lateral pterygoid.

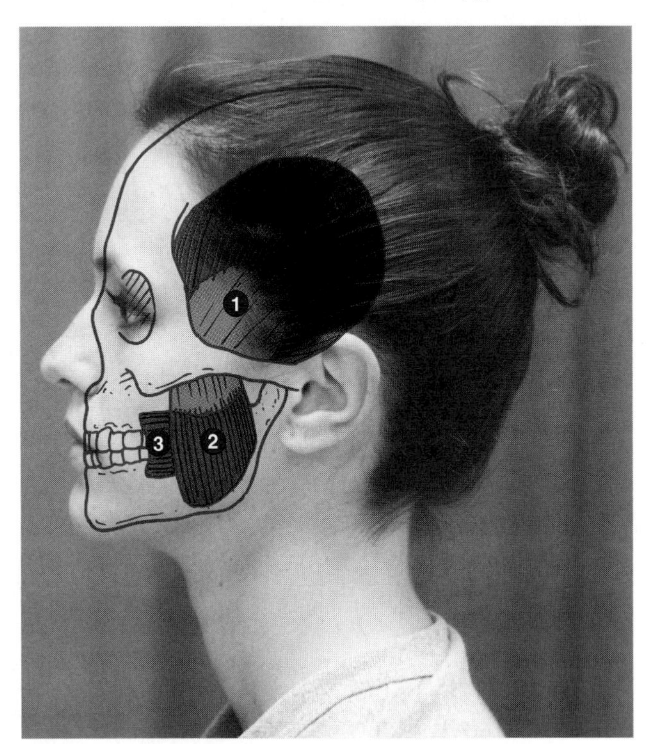

1 **Temporalis:** Palpate the belly of the temporalis superior to the ears. To make the muscle more prominent, ask the patient to clench the teeth.

2 **Masseter:** The masseter is palpable superior to the mandible, near its angle. Clenching the teeth activates this muscle and makes it easily palpable. The medial and lateral pterygoid muscles lie beneath the masseter muscle.

3 **Buccinator:** Located in the space between the maxilla and mandible, the buccinator in blowing (stabilizing the cheek) and is a secondary muscle of mastication. The muscle is located just lateral to the mouth on both sides and becomes prominent with puffing the cheeks.

Functional Assessment

The functional tests for the ear, nose, and throat provide information about the pathology and impairment of hearing, balance, smell, and swallowing.

Tests for the ear

- **Hearing:** Transitory hearing loss is to be expected immediately after a blow to the ear. Failure to regain normal hearing within 1 hour after injury is significant and warrants referral for further medical evaluation and visualization of the tympanic membrane.
- **Balance:** The patient is questioned regarding balance and dizziness, each of which may occur secondary to either ear or brain trauma. Neurologic balance assessment is discussed in Chapter 21.

Tests for the nose

- **Smell:** The olfactory senses may be obscured by epistaxis but should return after the bleeding has subsided. The loss of olfactory function is more commonly attributed to brain trauma than to trauma directly to the nose itself.

Tests for temporomandibular involvement

Functional testing for TMJ pathology involves having the patient slowly open and close the mouth. Normally, the mouth can open wide enough to insert two knuckles (Special Test 20-1).

To identify malocclusion, select a point, such as the junction between the two middle lower incisors, for use as a reference point (Fig. 20-18). Normally, the jaw moves smoothly and evenly with no interruption. After injury to the TMJ, mandible, or maxilla, opening and closing the jaw may demonstrate a lateral deviation and the bite may be maloccluded.

Use the same reference point to evaluate the distance and quality of lateral excursion of the jaw. Then this can be compared with the point between the incisors of the upper jaw by asking the patient to move the jaw right and left. The distance that the lower reference point moves relative to the upper reference point is measured with a ruler and compared bilaterally. Normally, the movement is bilaterally equal and completed in a smooth and pain-free manner.

The point in the range of motion (ROM) where tracking deviations occur can be indicative to the nature of the pathology. Lateral deviations opposite of the involved side that occur early in the ROM are often the result of muscle spasm, deviations in the midpoint are associated with muscle spasm, and deviations at the end of the ROM are caused by posterior capsulitis.[3]

Neurologic Testing

Loss of the associated special senses (hearing and smell) can indicate the presence of closed head trauma that has disrupted one or more cranial nerves. The evaluation of these conditions is described in Chapter 21. Decreased sensation in the upper cheek region may indicate involvement of the infraorbital nerve, such as entrapment associated with a blow-out fracture (Chapter 19).

Facial Pathologies and Related Special Tests

Pathology to the ear, nose, and throat is relatively uncommon in athletes, largely because of the use of protective mouthguards and headgear. Also, rules have been implemented to decrease the possibility of injury by prohibiting

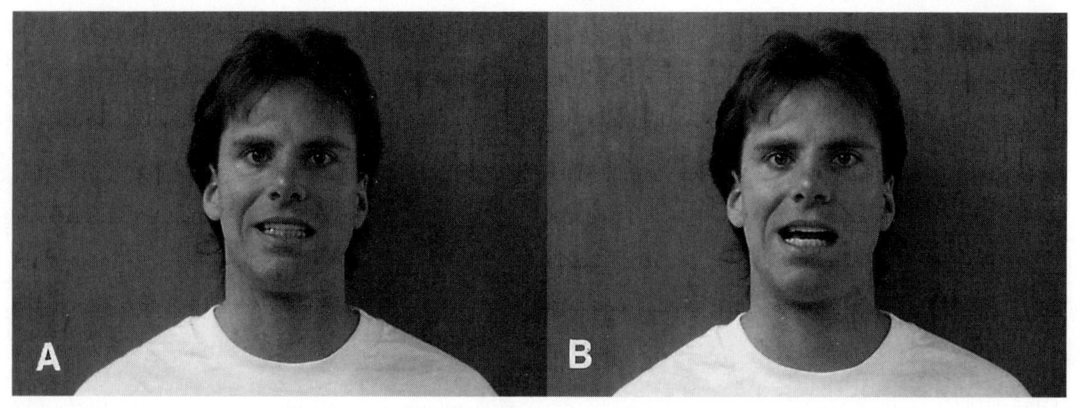

FIGURE 20-18 ■ Observation for malocclusion of the teeth. (A) Normally, the mandible travels in a straight line. (B) Trauma to the temporomandibular joint or a fracture of the mandible causes the jaw to track laterally and results in a malalignment of the teeth.

Special Test 20-1
Temporomandibular Joint Range of Motion

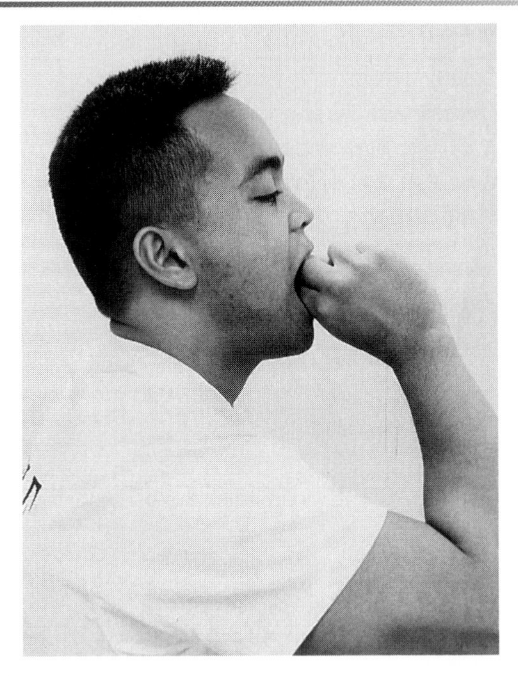

The temporomandibular joint should provide enough motion to allow two fingers to be inserted into the mouth.

Patient Position	Seated or standing
Position of Examiner	In front of the patient
Evaluative Procedure	The patient attempts to place as many flexed knuckles as possible between the upper and lower teeth.
Positive Test	The patient is unable to place a minimum of two knuckles within the mouth.
Implications	***Less than two fingers:*** TMJ hypomobility ***Three or more fingers:*** TMJ hypermobility
Evidence	Absent or inconclusive in the literature

TMJ = temporomandibular joint.

blows to the face and head. Although limited in number, injuries to this area can involve major trauma with the potential for long-term complications of impaired hearing, smell, and speech and undesirable esthetic changes. Laryngeal injury can be life threatening secondary to obstruction of the airway.

Ear Pathology

Most athletic-related ear injuries are the result of a single traumatic force or invading organisms and diseases. Although this trauma may be visible to the unaided eye, it may not be visible to untrained personnel. Thus, the decision to refer the patient to a physician is based on the complaints reported.

Auricular hematoma

Repeated episodes of blunt trauma or shearing forces to the external ear can result in an auricular hematoma,[12] also termed "cauliflower ear." Swelling within the skin of the outer ear develops within hours of the injury. Pooling of blood between the skin and the cartilage separates the two, depriving the cartilage of its source of nutrition. With time, the hematoma can scar, causing a deformed appearance to the external ear (see Fig. 20-11).[13]

The chief complaint is pain in the external and middle ear, accompanied by ecchymosis and swelling of the auricle. The external ear is inspected for open wounds and drainage from the middle ear. Palpation reveals increased tenderness and, initially, the "boggy" feel of swelling. Untreated cases with scarring appear smooth but feel

Examination Findings 20-1
Auricular Hematoma

Examination Segment	Clinical Findings
History	***Onset:*** Acute or chronic ***Pain characteristics:*** The external ear ***Other symptoms:*** Not applicable ***Mechanism:*** A single or repeated trauma to the external ear, resulting in a subcutaneous hematoma ***Predisposing conditions:*** Not applicable
Inspection	The external and possibly the middle ear appear violently red. Swelling secondary to a hematoma is visible.
Palpation	Palpation of an acute injury produces pain and confirms the presence of a hematoma. Palpation of a chronic injury may reveal hardened nodules within the ear.
Special Tests	Not applicable
Neurologic Screening	Impairment of cranial nerve VIII (acoustic nerve: hearing and balance)
Vascular Screening	Not applicable
Functional Assessment	Hearing and balance should be checked.
Imaging Techniques	Not applicable
Differential Diagnosis	Not applicable
Comments	Auricular hematomas require an immediate referral to a physician.

hardened on palpation (Examination Findings 20-1). The inner ear is also examined using an otoscope (see information on the tympanic membrane).[14]

In cases caused by a blow to the head, brain trauma also must be ruled out. A concurrent basilar skull fracture may result in ecchymosis at the mastoid process (Battle's sign). Patients suspected of having a concurrent skull fracture must be immediately referred to a physician for a definitive diagnosis.

Often, the physician elects to use a small needle to aspirate the hematoma, decreasing the amount of separation between the skin and the cartilage. If the fluid accumulation is actually within the cartilage, a more extreme excision and drainage is needed to fully clear the hematoma.[12] Chronic cauliflower ear may require surgical correction.[15] After this procedure is performed, or as a method of initial management of a patient with this condition, the ear may be casted with pieces of plaster casting material or gauze and **flexible collodion** to prevent further fluid accumulation.[12] None of these treatments has demonstrated effectiveness over another.[16] Prophylactic antibiotics are used to reduce the chance of infection following drainage.[12]

Flexible collodion A mixture of ether, alcohol, cellulose, and camphor that dries to form a firm, protective layer.

Tympanic membrane rupture

The mechanism of injury for a tympanic membrane rupture is a sudden change of air pressure on the tympanic membrane caused by blunt trauma or by a decreased ability to regulate inner ear pressure secondary to an infection. The use of hyperbaric oxygen chambers may increase the risk of tympanic membrane ruptures secondary to the high atmospheric pressures used in this procedure.[17] The membrane may also be ruptured through direct trauma, such as sticking a sharp object in the ear (Examination Findings 20-2).

An otoscope with a speculum that fits snugly within the ear canal, without causing pain, is used to inspect the tympanic membrane. The speculum needs to be placed only slightly into the ear canal to view the structures. Visualization is improved when the pinna is pulled upward and backward (some clinicians prefer to pull the earlobe downward).

Reddish-brown **cerumen** may be seen as the speculum enters the ear canal, possibly obscuring the view of the tympanic membrane. Any fluids in the canal are unusual and minimally indicate a rupture to the tympanic membrane

Examination Findings 20-2
Tympanic Membrane Rupture

Examination Segment	Clinical Findings
History	***Onset:*** Acute ***Pain characteristics:*** Pain, often excruciating, in the middle ear, radiating inward and outward ***Other symptoms:*** **Tinnitus** ***Mechanism:*** A mechanical pressure (e.g., a slap to the ear or a blocked sneeze) that causes the tympanic membrane to burst or a mechanical intrusion through the membrane (e.g., cleaning the ears with a ballpoint pen) ***Predisposing conditions:*** Upper respiratory infection, otitis media
Inspection	Blood or fluids may be observed leaking from the ear. Inspection with an otoscope reveals redness and the perforation may be visible.
Palpation	Not applicable
Special Tests	Hearing assessment
Neurologic Screening	Not applicable (in this case, hearing reduction is the result of a mechanical deficit)
Vascular Screening	Not applicable
Functional Assessment	There is a marked hearing loss in the involved ear. Valsalva maneuver may result in the audible escape of air from within the inner ear.
Imaging Techniques	Not applicable
Differential Diagnosis	Not applicable
Comments	The resulting pain and inflammatory response may result in transient dizziness. The ear must be kept dry and the patient referred to a physician.

secondary to otitis media. In a worst-case scenario, this is caused by a skull fracture. Disruption of the tympanic membrane warrants the referral for further examination by a physician.

The tympanic membrane's healing properties and process are different from those of other soft tissues. The defect tends to heal without first closing, resulting in a permanent fissure in the tympanic membrane.[18]

Otitis externa

Otitis externa is an infection of the external auditory meatus commonly termed "swimmer's ear" because of its prevalence in individuals who participate in water activities. The condition is usually caused by inadequate drying of the ear canal. The dark, damp environment encourages the growth of bacteria or fungus, resulting in the inflammation of the external auditory meatus. The presence of psoriasis, eczema, excessively oily skin, and open wounds within the ear can predispose an individual to otitis externa. Overcleaning of the external auditory canal may inadvertently remove a protective chemical layer, also predisposing a person to otitis externa. In addition, a narrow inner ear can predispose an individual to otitis externa by preventing adequate drying and encouraging the growth of bacteria.[19]

The chief complaint is one of constant pain and pressure, possibly accompanied by itching in the ear. The patient may complain of a hearing deficit and dizziness. The area is red, and a clear discharge from the middle ear may be present. The lymph nodes around the ear may be enlarged. In severe cases, the mastoid process may be enlarged and tender to the touch. Tugging on the earlobe usually increases pain.

A physician may prescribe acid-based drops mixed with antibiotics or corticosteroids (or both). A wick may be placed in the ear to maintain dryness. Patients, especially swimmers, should refrain from entering the water and keep their ears dry.

Otitis media

Upper respiratory infections and bacterial or viral invasion can cause an inflammation of the ear's mucous membranes,

Tinnitus Ringing in the ears.
Cerumen A reddish-brown wax formed in the auditory meatus.

blocking the eustachian tubes and increasing the pressure within the inner ear. Upper respiratory infections, airplane travel, and seasonal allergies may predispose an individual to acute otitis media, and the condition is particularly prevalent in young children. Another condition, otitis media with effusion, occurs when fluid collects in the middle ear but no bacterial or viral infection is present.[20] In addition to having a history of upper respiratory problems, other complaints include a feeling of the ear's being blocked and pressure and pain within the inner ear. Inspection with an otoscope reveals fluid buildup in the middle ear and an opaque, reddened, and bulging tympanic membrane. Otitis media may result in hearing loss in the affected ear. This hearing loss can be confirmed by striking a tuning fork and placing the stem on the center of the forehead (the **Weber test**); in the presence of otitis media, the patient hears the vibration louder in the affected ear. Otitis media may also lead to tympanic membrane rupture.

*** Practical Evidence**

A bulging tympanic membrane is highly suggestive of otitis media.

Oral antibiotics are usually prescribed for patients who are suffering from acute otitis media but are not warranted for otitis media with effusion. Antihistamine medications, commonly used to combat allergies, should not be used with acute otitis media or otitis media with effusion, as they may cause a longer duration of the middle ear effusion. Decongestants may help reduce nasal congestion, although neither antihistamines or decongestants are associated with a shorter duration of acute otitis media.[20]

Nasal Injuries

The nasal bones, the most commonly fractured bones of the face and skull and the third most common of all fractures, are fractured by direct blows to the nose.[22] Bleeding typically occurs immediately after the trauma but is usually easily controlled (see the section on on-field evaluation and management of nasal injuries). Athletes competing in contact or collision sports often have a history of nasal fractures. However, deformity of the nose should not be assumed to be preexisting.

Other than bleeding, the chief complaint is pain on and around the nose. On inspection, the nose may be visibly deformed, but the lack of a deformity does not conclusively rule out a nasal fracture. Swelling in and around the nose may obscure minor deformities, thus making palpation difficult. With time, ecchymosis develops and settles under the inferior aspect of the eyes ("raccoon eyes"). Palpation reveals tenderness at the fracture site and the surrounding areas. Crepitus may be identifiable at the fracture site as well (Examination Findings 20-3).

Using an otoscope or penlight inspect the internal nose for deviation of the septum. The patient should attempt to breathe through one nostril while holding the opposite one closed. The nostril should close during inhalation, and breathing should be unobstructed. The exhalation should be easy and unencumbered. Inspection of the nasal cavity may reveal a deviated septum or septal hematoma. Septal hematomas require immediate removal by a physician because of the associated risk of infection and subsequent necrosis of the articular cartilage, resulting in a saddle-nose deformity (Fig. 20-19).[22,23] If a nasal fracture, deviated septum or septal hematoma is suspected, the patient requires a physician referral.

Although radiographs are often used to identify the presence of a nasal fracture, their use has low reliability as a diagnostic tool and is discouraged.[22–24] Displaced nasal fractures or deviated septa require closed or open reduction for realignment. This procedure can be delayed to allow associated swelling to subside with no change in outcome.[23]

Throat Injury

Trauma to this area often results in respiratory distress and the inability to speak, leading to agitation of the patient. The insulting blow to the anterior throat, if it includes the **carotid sinus**, can result in the loss of consciousness. Pain is increased during swallowing or while taking deep, gasping breaths of air. Bruising over and around the larynx is common, and the usual palpable definition of the larynx is lost because of deformity or swelling. There may be a noticeable change in the patient's voice.[25] The inside of the mouth is examined with the use of a penlight to detect

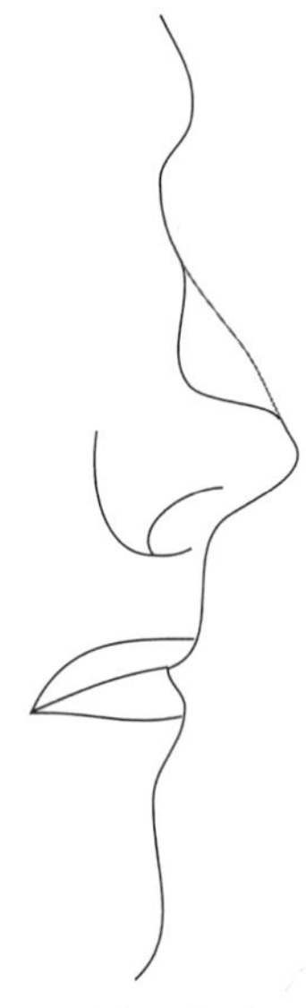

FIGURE 20-19 ■ Saddle-nose deformity. An untreated septal hematoma and its infection causing necrosis of the nasal cartilage can result in deformity of the nose.

Carotid sinus An area near the common carotid artery that, when stimulated, results in vasodilation and a lowering of the heart rate. When this occurs suddenly, unconsciousness may occur.

Examination Findings 20-3
Nasal Fractures

Examination Segment	Clinical Findings
History	***Onset:*** Acute ***Pain characteristics:*** The bridge of the nose and nasal cartilage, possibly radiating into the frontal and zygomatic bones ***Other symptoms:*** Bleeding normally accompanies nasal fractures. ***Mechanism:*** A direct blow to the nose ***Predisposing conditions:*** Not applicable
Inspection	The nose may be visibly malaligned and/or swollen. Ecchymosis may accumulate beneath one or both eyes ("raccoon eyes"). The internal nose requires inspection with an otoscope or penlight for the presence of a deviated septum or septal hematoma. Swelling may mask any deviation.
Palpation	Palpation of the traumatized area elicits pain. Crepitus may be felt over the fracture site.
Special Tests	None
Neurologic Screening	Not applicable
Vascular Screening	Not applicable
Functional Assessment	The sense of smell and breathing through the nose may be obstructed by bleeding or a deviated septum (or both).
Imaging Techniques	Radiographs may be obtained, but are not accurate in identifying the presence of a nasal fracture and their use is discouraged.[22] Optimal imaging is obtained from CT images and pathology to the orbit or other facial structures can concurrently be assessed.[23]
Differential Diagnosis	Epistaxis resulting from URI, sinus conditions, or other general medical state; nasal cartilage pathology; septal hematoma
Comments	Patients who have suffered a nasal fracture should also be screened for injury to the eyes and head.

CT = computed tomography; URI = upper respiratory infection.

the presence of bloody sputum, indicating an injury to the inside of the throat. Palpation may reveal a displaced cartilage and extreme tenderness or crepitus (Examination Findings 20-4). No attempt is made to correct any deviations because of the possibility of worsening the condition. Immediate referral to a physician or activation of the emergency action system is indicated because airway compromise may develop as swelling continues.

Facial Fractures

Protective facial equipment, such as a football helmet's facemask or a catcher's mask, is useful in deflecting many otherwise injurious forces. However, most equipment leaves at least a portion of the face exposed to potential injury. Also see Orbital Fractures, p. 825.

Mandibular fractures

Mandibular fractures, the second most common type of facial fracture, ranking behind nasal fractures, are the result of a high-velocity impact to the jaw.[26] The chief complaint of a mandibular fracture is pain in the jaw that is increased by opening and closing the mouth. Difficulty with or discrepancies in jaw movement may also be noted by the patient (Fig. 20-20). Crepitus may be felt during palpation of the fracture site. Mandibular fractures typically result in a malocclusion of the jaw and teeth, a fact that warrants referral to a physician (Examination Findings 20-5). The **tongue blade test** may be used to reinforce the suspicion of a mandibular fracture (Special Test 20-2).

Zygoma fractures

Direct blows to the cheek and inferior periorbital area may result in a fracture of the zygoma, especially at the arch. Examination findings reveal pain, discoloration, and possible depression of the zygomatic arch at the site of injury. Displaced fractures may result in malalignment of the eyes. Attempted eye movements may increase the pain or be performed with difficulty. Subconjunctival hematoma and periorbital swelling may be noted. Pain is elicited with palpation along the zygomatic arch and the lateral rim of the orbit. Occasionally, a step-off deformity is noted during palpation of the fracture site.[26] Definitive diagnosis of a zygomatic fracture is based on the findings of CT scans.

Maxillary fractures

Fractures of the maxillae tend to occur concurrently with nasal fractures. Pain is described through the midportion of the face. Deformity found on inspection is rare, but ecchymosis and swelling along the alveolar processes are common. Crepitus may be elicited at the fracture site.

LeFort fractures

The LeFort system is used to classify midface fractures. Because these fractures are normally the result of extremely high-impact forces (e.g., automobile accidents), their incidence in athletes is unusual. Figure 20-21 presents the LeFort classification system and identifies the bony segments involved. This type of fracture is so extensive that when the upper teeth are pulled forward, the fractured segment and the associated portion of the face are also displaced forward, roughly resembling the anterior drawer test in the knee. Sinus fluid may also be observed running from the nose.

Dental Conditions

Oral injury rates have been determined for both female and male intercollegiate athletes.[29,30] In female athletes, the injury rate ranges from 1.5% in softball players to 7.5% in basketball players; soccer, field hockey, and lacrosse

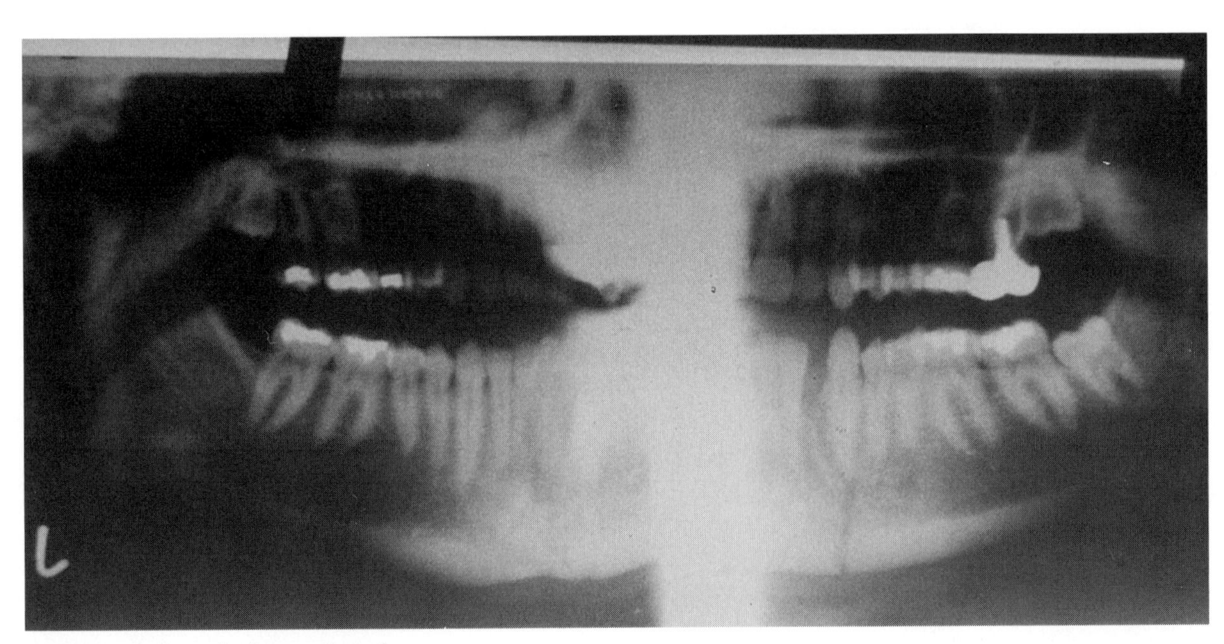

FIGURE 20-20 ■ Radiograph of a mandibular fracture.

Examination Findings 20-4
Throat Trauma

Examination Segment	Clinical Findings
History	***Onset:*** Acute ***Pain characteristics:*** Anterior neck, possibly radiating into the chest secondary to an obstructed airway ***Other symptoms:*** Difficulty breathing ***Mechanism:*** A crushing force to the anterior neck ***Predisposing conditions:*** Not applicable
Inspection	Bruising or other signs of trauma are present over the anterior throat. Swelling or deformity may be present. Bloody sputum in the mouth and throat. The patient may be coughing in an attempt to clear the airway. The patient's voice may be noticeably altered.
Palpation	Palpation produces tenderness. Crepitus is present. Displacement of the cartilage or fracture of the hyoid bone may be felt.
Special Tests	None
Neurologic Screening	Not applicable
Vascular Screening	Not applicable
Functional Assessment	The patient has difficulty breathing. There is an inability to speak or difficulty speaking (aphasia).
Imaging Techniques	
Differential Diagnosis	Fractured larynx, contusion
Comments	Absence of breathing requires activation of the emergency action system. Immediate referral to a physician is indicated. Ice packs may be applied to control the swelling, but care must be taken not to compress the traumatized tissues. The vital signs require continuous monitoring.

Examination Findings 20-5
Mandibular Fracture

Examination Segment	Clinical Findings
History	***Onset:*** Acute ***Pain characteristics:*** Ramus or mental protuberance of mandible ***Other symptoms:*** Not applicable ***Mechanism:*** Direct blow to the mandible on its anterior or lateral aspects ***Predisposing conditions:*** Not applicable
Inspection	Swelling or gross deformity may be seen over the fracture site. A step deformity between the teeth may be noted on the involved side. Malocclusion of the teeth may be noted or described by the patient. Intraoral and extraoral ecchymosis may be noted.
Palpation	Tenderness, crepitus, or bony deformity is present over the fracture site.
Joint and Muscle Function Assessment	***AROM:*** Pain is experienced when opening and closing the mouth, or this motion is prohibited secondary to pain. The mandible may track laterally or asymmetrically. ***MMT:*** See special tests. ***PROM:*** Not applicable
Joint Stability Tests	***Stress tests:*** The structures of the TMJ may be affected. However, the integrity of these structures should not be checked in the presence of a known fracture. ***Joint play:*** Not applicable
Special Tests	Tongue blade test
Neurologic Screening	Cranial nerves V or VII (or both) may be traumatized by the fracture (see Chapter 21).
Vascular Screening	Not applicable
Functional Assessment	Difficulty opening and closing the mouth Chewing food is limited by pain
Imaging Techniques	AP radiographs and/or CT scans are used to identify the presence, and shape, of fracture lines.
Differential Diagnosis	TMJ sprain, TMJ dislocation
Comments	Mandibular fractures may also be accompanied by a TMJ dislocation. Persons suspected of suffering a mandibular fracture or dislocation should be referred to a physician for further evaluation and treatment.

AP = anteroposterior; AROM = active range of motion; CT = computed tomography; MMT = manual muscle test; PROM = passive range of motion; TMJ = temporomandibular joint.

Special Test 20-2
Tongue Blade Test

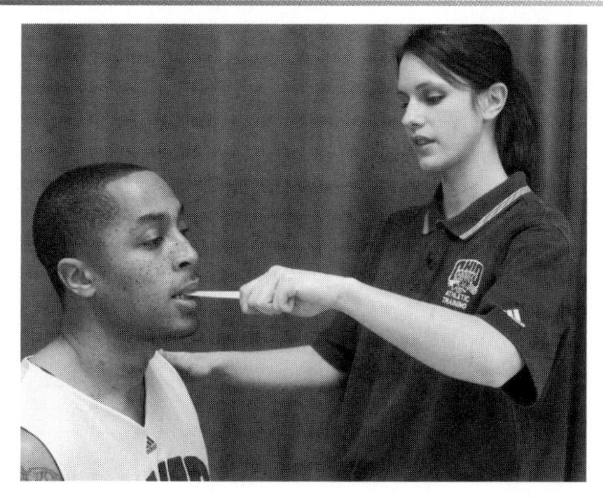

In the presence of a fractured mandible, the patient will not be able to bite down hard on the tongue depressor.

Patient Position	Seated
Position of Examiner	Standing in front of the patient
Evaluative Procedure	A tongue blade (tongue depressor) is placed in the patient's mouth. As the patient attempts to hold the tongue blade in place, the examiner rotates (twists) the blade.
Positive Test	The patient is unable to maintain a firm bite or pain is elicited.
Implications	Possible mandibular fracture
Evidence	Absent or inconclusive in the literature

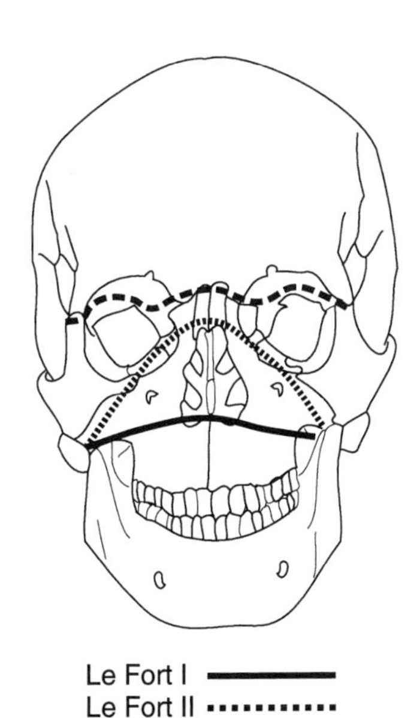

FIGURE 20-21 ■ Classification of LeFort fractures. Type I fractures involve only the maxillary bone; type II extend up into the nasal bone; type III cross the zygomatic bones and the orbit.

players also have high rates. The highest oral injury rates for male athletes occur in basketball players, followed by ice hockey, lacrosse, football, soccer, baseball, and volleyball players.

The preparticipation physical examination questionnaire should ascertain the presence of dental appliances such as crowns, caps, or implants. This dental work must be evaluated for loosening, fracture, or luxation along with the natural dental structures. The numeric system used by dentists in referencing the teeth is presented in Figure 20-22. With all dental injuries, the examiner must establish the presence of a suitable airway, rule out the presence of head injury and evaluate and manage concurrent lacerations.

Patients with oral injuries must be carefully evaluated to ensure prompt management to limit is physical deformity and disability. The time and mechanism of injury define the risk of associated injuries and influence the treatment.[7]

Tooth fractures

Tooth fractures, ranging from simple chips of the crown to full avulsions of the crown from its roots, are classified on a scale of I to IV (Fig. 20-23). Class I injuries, chip fractures, may be subtly noticed during eating, drinking, talking, or

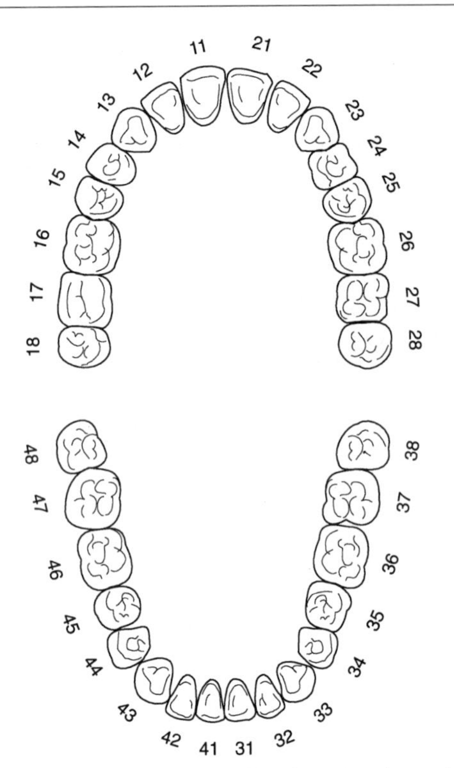

FIGURE 20-22 ■ Numbering system for referencing the teeth. The upper right teeth are numbered by 10s, the upper left by 20s, the lower left by 30s, and the lower right by 40s.

other activity in which the tongue is scraped across the teeth. These injuries may be self-evaluated when the patient looks in a mirror. Class II, III, and IV fractures are more easily recognized secondary to pain, sensitivity to extreme temperatures of food or drink, or obvious deformity. The degree of sensitivity depends on the extent of the fracture. Fractures into the enamel are usually minor irritations, but dental referral can be delayed.[7] Fractures involving the dentin and the pulp cavity are painful and sensitive to hot and cold temperatures. Fracture of the tooth's root generally require radiographic identification.[7]

Tooth luxations

A tooth luxation ranges from a tooth's being avulsed from the socket to its being driven into the bone (Fig. 20-24). A subtle tooth dislocation, one that is loosened in its socket, is not always visibly recognized. It may be discovered while the patient is chewing or applying pressure on it with the tongue. An **intruded tooth** is marked by its depression into the alveolar process relative to the contiguous teeth and to its match on the opposite side. An **extruded tooth** is partially withdrawn from the bone and may be tilted anteriorly or posteriorly or may be twisted. A **tooth avulsion** is marked by the intact tooth's being displaced from the alveolar process and may represent a medical emergency.[7]

Fracture of the tooth's root can also result in luxation (Fig. 20-25). A fracture of the cervical third of the tooth may be repaired or permanently secured using dental hardware. Fractures to the middle third typically result in the loss of the tooth. The best prognosis occurs when the fracture occurs in the apical third (root) because the tooth is not greatly displaced in its socket.

The teeth can be evaluated for loosening through gentle palpation. If uncertainty exists as to whether a tooth has been partially dislodged, the patient may be given a mirror to conduct a self-assessment. A loose tooth should be left in place so that it can be properly managed by a dentist.

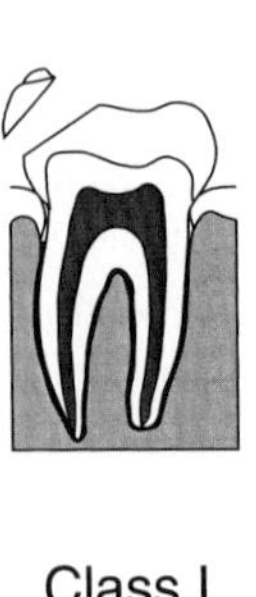

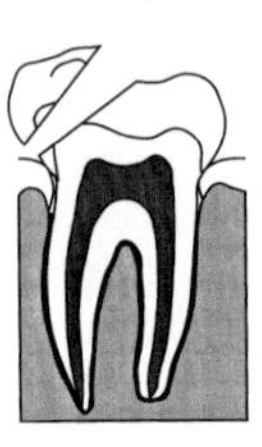

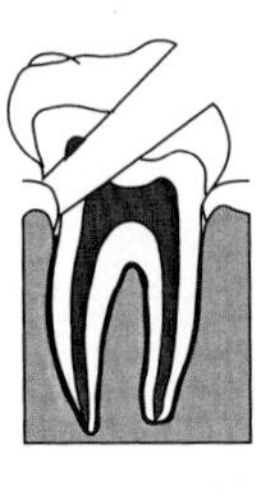

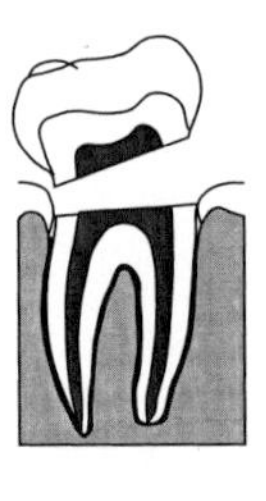

FIGURE 20-23 ■ Classification scheme for tooth fractures.

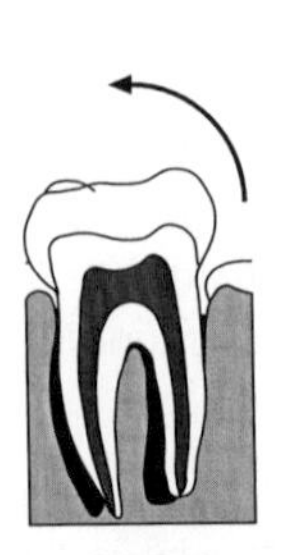

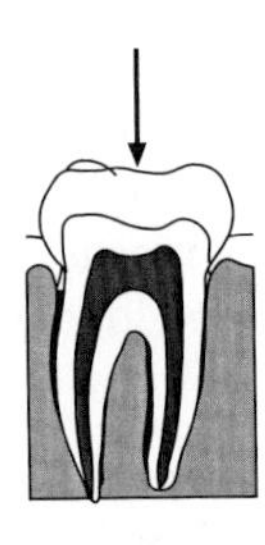

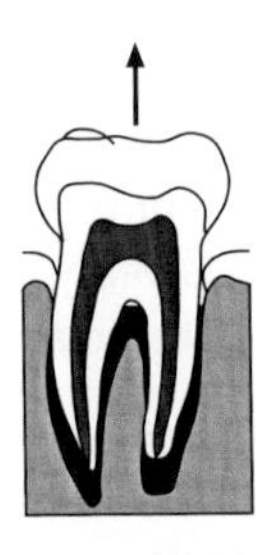

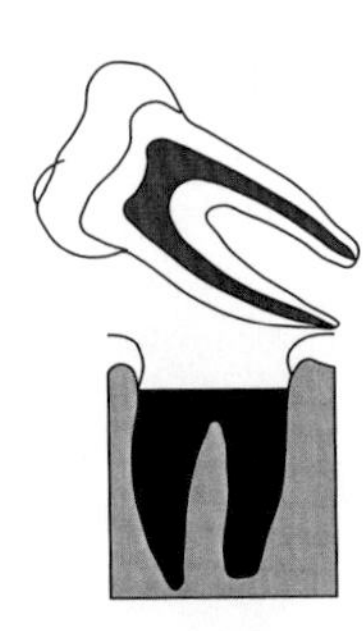

FIGURE 20-24 ■ Classification scheme for tooth luxations.

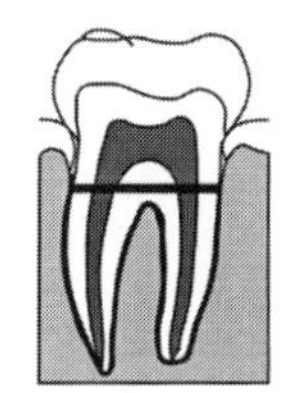
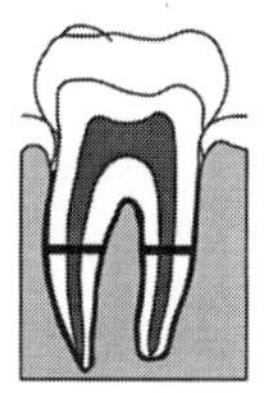
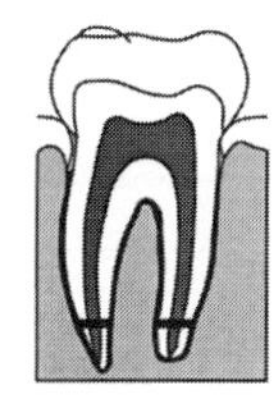

FIGURE 20-25 ■ Classification scheme for root fractures.

In the event of an avulsed tooth, the patient is keenly aware of the injury and concomitant injuries, such as a mandible fracture, should be suspected. Other types of tooth luxations result in pain, bleeding from the socket, and temperature hypersensitivity. After the condition is recognized, the patient must be properly managed to maximize the potential of saving the tooth. Management of the luxated tooth is found in the "On-Field Evaluation and Management of Injuries to the Face and Related Areas" section of this chapter.

Dental caries

Also known as cavities and tooth decay, dental caries is a disease of the teeth that results in damage to the hard structures. The primary cause of tooth decay is **plaque**, which adheres to the teeth. Bacteria within the plaque contain acids that begin to dissolve the tooth's enamel. High intakes of sugars and starches, consuming acid-rich food, and poor oral hygiene all contribute to the development of dental caries.

Most dental caries are initially painless and are only identified on radiographic examination. As the size of the decay enlarges and its depth into the tooth increases, the patient complains of the tooth's sensitivity to heat and cold. If the decay is allowed to progress, the defect will become visible to the unaided eye. In advanced cases, an abscess develops and the tooth's enamel and pulp are lost.

Temporomandibular Joint Dysfunction

TMJ dysfunction is a broad term that encompasses pain, decreased range of motion, audible noises, and decreased pain when opening and closing the mouth.[3] Although TMJ dysfunction often has an insidious onset, a prior history of injury to the TMJ including sprains, cartilage tears, subluxations, or dislocations may be identified.

Acutely, the TMJ is usually injured when a blow is received on the point of the chin or across the jaw. The initial complaint is jaw pain and possibly clicking at the joint. Muscle guarding resulting from either a physical or psychological nature increases tension in the lateral pterygoid muscle, pulling the articular disk posteriorly and stretching the joint capsule and its ligaments. TMJ derangements are classified as reducing or nonreducing.[3] Reducing derangements are characterized by "clicking" or "clunking" that represents the subluxation and reduction of the disk, usually at the midpoint of the ROM. Nonreducing derangements are characterized by the joint freezing and represents a torn portion of the disk presenting a mechanical block to motion. The nonreducing type often requires surgical correction. Intracapsular bleeding can result in joint ankylosis.[27]

On inspection, the mouth may open and close in an asymmetrical fashion, causing the lower jaw to deviate in one direction. The jaw may meet a mechanical block that limits the ROM. Palpation of the TMJ reveals localized tenderness and possibly crepitus or clicking at the joint. A stethoscope should be used to auscultate the TMJ during active ROM. Complaints of—or the presence of—audible crepitus alone are not indicative of TMJ dysfunction, these symptoms must be associated with other signs and symptoms of TMJ dysfunction (Examination Findings 20-6). Secondary symptoms including headache, earache, and dizziness may also be reported.[3]

Temporomandibular joint dislocation

Dislocations often result in an observable displacement of the mandible. However, subtle subluxations that spontaneously reduce may be less evident (Fig. 20-26). The mechanism of injury is a blow of sufficient force to move the mandible laterally, such as being punched. The rotation of the mandible causes the joint opposite the direction of displacement to anteriorly dislocate. The upper and lower teeth are malaligned, and movement of the jaw may be significantly impaired.

Blows to the point of the mandible, driving the bone toward the skull, may result in a fracture along the mandibular ramus or, on rare occasion, the temporal bone. Similar to TMJ dislocations, mandibular fractures result in malocclusion of the teeth, crepitus and deformity over the fracture site, and the inability to normally open and close the mouth.

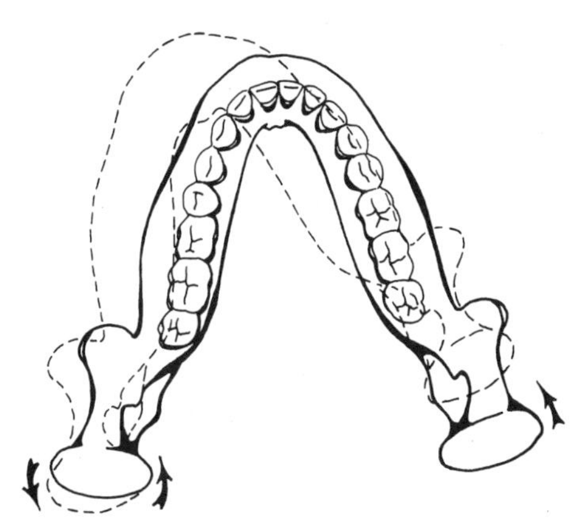

FIGURE 20-26 ■ Malocclusion of the jaw following a mandibular dislocation. Correlate this illustration with Figure 20-18B. (Courtesy of Perry, JF, Rohe DA, and Garcia AO: *The Kinesiology Workbook*, ed 2, Philadelphia: FA Davis, 1996.)

Plaque Food, mucus, and bacteria that collect and harden on the exposed portions of the teeth; it can harden into tartar.

Examination Findings 20-6
Temporomandibular Joint Dysfunction

Examination Segment	Clinical Findings
History	***Onset:*** Acute, insidious, or chronic ***Pain characteristics:*** Area of the TMJ ***Other symptoms:*** Clicking or locking of the joint Headache, ear ache, and dizziness may also be reported ***Mechanism:*** Trauma to the mandible or progressive joint degeneration ***Predisposing conditions:*** Laxity, disk degeneration, bruxing arthritis, missing or malaligned teeth, emotional stress
Inspection	Inspection of the joint may be unremarkable. Swelling may be located over the joint. Malocclusion of the jaw may be noted.
Palpation	Tenderness exists over the joint surfaces. Palpation of the external and internal structures may reveal clicking as the mouth is opened and closed.
Joint and Muscle Function Assessment	***AROM:*** Active range of motion may be decreased secondary to pain or mechanical blockage of the TMJ. Any lateral deviation in the motion indicates joint pathology. ***MMT:*** Clenching the teeth may cause pain. ***PROM:*** Not applicable
Joint Stability Tests	***Stress tests:*** Not applicable ***Joint play:*** Not applicable
Special Tests	None
Neurologic Screening	Not applicable, but TMJ dysfunction has been implicated in causing headaches, decreased strength, and other symptoms.
Vascular Screening	Within normal limits
Functional Assessment	Observe the jaw for true inferior and superior movement as the mouth is opened or closed.
Imaging Techniques	CT and MR images are obtained to identify joint structure and possible disk pathology.
Differential Diagnosis	Mandibular fracture
Comments	Individuals suffering from persistent TMJ pain should be referred to a physician for further evaluation. Instruct the patient not to eat hard foods (e.g., apples) that would cause pain during biting.

AROM = active range of motion; CT = computed tomography; MMT = manual muscle test; MR = magenetic resonance; PROM = passive range of motion; TMJ = temporomandibular joint.

On-Field Examination and Management of Injuries to the Face and Related Areas

Owing to the proximity of the maxillofacial area to the airway, the presence of an unencumbered airway must be established. The athlete may concurrently sustain a laceration and injury to the maxillofacial structures. After establishing the presence of an airway, the responder must control bleeding before proceeding with a complete on-field examination.[28] As with all open wounds, standard precautions for bloodborne pathogens must be implemented.

Lacerations

Lacerations may mask underlying injuries. After the bleeding is controlled, the area around the laceration is palpated for tenderness, being careful to delineate between tenderness from the insulting blow that caused the injury and any actual fractures that may have occurred.

The presence of any foreign particles or objects within the laceration must be determined before any subsequent treatment. An imbedded object must be left in place. The surrounding area can be cleaned and dressed until the object can be removed and the wound can be further managed by a physician.

Next, the extent of the wound must be determined. As a general rule, any facial laceration requires a referral to a physician for possible suturing or gluing to limit the extent and visibility of any scars. The sooner the referral occurs, the better it is, but the physician should see the patient within 24 hours after the injury.[26] If the bleeding can be controlled and the wound closed and dressed with a sterile bandage, the athlete may return to competition. The bandage covering the wound must be sufficient to protect other competitors from contact with the athlete's blood.

In the case of lacerations of the throat, the athlete is assessed for difficulty with breathing and transported by trained personnel who can aid the athlete on route to the hospital. If the laceration avulses a piece of the ear, nose, or tongue, the avulsed tissue is cleaned with sterile water, wrapped in sterile gauze, put on ice, and transported with the athlete to the medical facility for possible reimplantation. Microsurgical techniques may be able to salvage these parts, giving the athlete a better cosmetic repair and normal function.

Laryngeal Injuries

Laryngeal injuries present a difficult decision for the examiner because of their potential to become life threatening. Early signs of potentially catastrophic injury include progressive swelling (indicating bleeding), crepitation (indicating the presence of subcutaneous air), audible **stridor** (indicating a narrowing of the airway), and blood exiting the oral cavity.

The decision must be made to move the athlete to the sideline before transport or to transport the athlete directly from the field. In cases in which the athlete has trouble breathing, it is prudent to stabilize the athlete and transport him or her to a hospital using emergency medical personnel capable of managing an obstructed airway. The athlete may first be moved to the sideline if no signs of breathing difficulty are noted. Ice may be applied to the anterior throat, but care must be taken not to compress the underlying structures. The pressure applied could be enough to displace the injured area, causing obstruction of the airway.

Facial Fractures

The forces required to fracture the facial bones (i.e., the zygoma, frontal, maxillary, and mandible bones) are usually of considerable magnitude. The athlete is not only "down" from the injury but may also be stunned or rendered unconscious by head injury from the incident. In this case, the examination and on-field management of the head injury takes precedence (see Chapter 21).

LeFort fractures and other fractures around the nose and mouth can compromise the airway. In this case, maintaining an open airway is the highest treatment priority.[29] Athletes suffering stable facial fractures that do not jeopardize the airway can be carefully moved to the sidelines. Athletes with suspected facial fractures can be removed to the sideline for further evaluation and treatment. If the athlete has an obvious fracture, movement of the athlete's head and neck is restricted. As long as it does not increase the athlete's discomfort, a Philadelphia collar can be used to stabilize the jaw and prevent unwanted motion while the athlete is transported to a medical facility (Fig. 20-27).

Temporomandibular Joint Injuries

The TMJ may be injured along with the mandible from a blow to the jaw. If a fracture of the mandible is unlikely, the athlete can be carefully assisted to the sideline for a full assessment of the TMJ. Injuries that produce malocclusion warrant the removal of the athlete from participation immediately and referral to a physician or dentist. If the TMJ is dislocated, the athlete can be immobilized with a Philadelphia collar as long as it does not create further pain. This athlete also requires a referral for immediate treatment.

Nasal Fracture and Epistaxis

Nasal fractures are usually accompanied by epistaxis, which must be controlled before further evaluation or management of the injury occurs. Although squeezing the nostrils and tilting the head forward is an adequate form of

Stridor A harsh, high-pitched sound resembling blowing wind that is experienced during respiration.

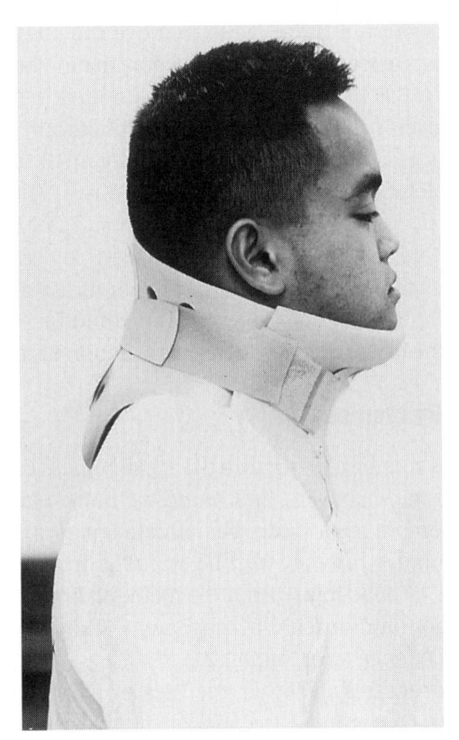

FIGURE 20-27 ■ Use of a Philadelphia collar for immobilizing a suspected mandibular fracture. Avoided applying too much pressure to the fracture site

management for nasal bleeding, this method may be prohibited secondary to pain arising from the fracture. Applying a cold pack to the nose and surrounding area also may stop the bleeding. The nose may be packed with rolled gauze or a tampon that has been cut into quarters. (These should be precut and kept in the athletic trainer's medical kit.) Another technique to control bleeding involves placing a rolled cotton gauze pad between the anterior upper lip and gum. The pressure from the lip required to hold the gauze in place applies pressure on the arteries that supply the anterior nasal mucosa, potentially stopping bleeding.[9]

The nose, nasal cartilage, and adjacent maxillary, zygomatic, and frontal bones are palpated for tenderness and crepitus. If the nose is obviously deformed, the athlete is discouraged from viewing the injury in a mirror or feeling the deformity because doing so may increase his or her anxiety or cause the onset of shock. Suspected nasal fractures may be packed with a small bag of ice to assist in controlling pain and limiting the amount of bleeding until the athlete is seen by a physician. Reduction of displaced fractures should be made 5 to 10 days after injury.[5]

Dental Injuries

An athlete suffering tooth trauma usually reports to the sidelines for evaluation. Because continued participation can result in a complete tooth avulsion, athletes suffering from any form of tooth injury other than a class I fracture must be removed from competition and evaluated by a dentist (see Fig. 20-23).

Table 20-3	Emergency Management of Dental Injuries

- Before reimplanting an avulsed tooth, rinse it with water or saline solution. Allow the athlete to hold the tooth in its socket by biting on gauze. Make sure that the tooth is reimplanted in its proper orientation.
- If the tooth is not reimplanted immediately, store it in a secure biocompatible storage environment such as an emergency tooth preserving system or in fresh whole milk in a plastic container with a tightly fitting top. Do not store it in water.[34]
- Do not attempt to clean, sterilize, or scrape the tooth in any way other than as noted above.
- Transport the athlete and the tooth to a dentist as quickly as possible.

Usually a fractured tooth is not a cause of immediate danger to the athlete unless the remaining portion is loose. If no loosening has occurred, the athlete can return to activity as long as a mouthpiece is used. However, follow up by a dentist must occur as soon as possible. The athlete should expect extreme discomfort, especially if the fracture penetrates the pulp cavity.

Every reasonable attempt must be made to find a tooth that has been luxated. The primary problem leading to failure of the tooth to survive involves the death of the periodontal ligament attached to the avulsed tooth. All treatment must focus on the survival of this ligament.[32,33] To improve the tooth's chances of survival, the emergency procedures listed in Table 20-3 are recommended.[31]

✱ Practical Evidence

With proper care, as recommended by the American Dental Association[30] and the American Association of **Endodontics**, it is estimated that 90% of all avulsed teeth can be permanently reimplanted.[31]

Current recommendations support the immediate reimplantation of an avulsed tooth.[34] If the tooth is visibly contaminated, wash it using cool tap water before reimplantation.

REFERENCES

1. Widmark, G, et al: Evaluation of TMJ surgery in cases not responding to conservative treatment. *Cranio*, 13:44, 1995.
2. Moss, RA, et al: Oral habits and TMJ dysfunction in facial pain and non-pain subjects. *J Oral Rehabil*, 22:79, 1995.
3. Sailors, ME: Evaluation of sports-related temporomandibular dysfunctions. *J Athl Train*, 31:346, 1996.
4. Puzas, JE, et al: Degradative pathways in tissues of the temporomandibular joint. Use of in vitro and in vivo models to characterize matrix metalloproteinase and cytokine activity. *Cells Tissues Organs*, 169:248, 2001.

Endodontics The field of dentistry specializing in the management of injuries and diseases affecting the pulp of a tooth.

5. Kucik, CJ, Clenney, T, and Phelan, J: Management of acute nasal fractures. *Am Fam Physician*, 70:1315, 2004.
6. Labuguen, RH: Initial evaluation of vertigo. *Am Fam Physician*, 73:244, 2006.
7. Douglass, AB, and Douglass, JM: Common dental emergencies. *Am Fam Physician*, 67:511, 2003.
8. Guler, N, et al: Temporomandibular internal derangement: correlation of MRI findings with clinical symptoms of pain and joint sounds in patients with bruxing behavior. *Dentomaxillofac Radiol*, 32:304, 2003.
9. Weir, JD: Effective management of epistaxis in athletes. *J Athl Train* 32:254, 1997.
10. Bechman, SM: Laryngeal fracture in a high school football player. *J Athl Train*, 28:217, 1993.
11. Beachy, G: Dental injuries in intermediate and high school athletes: A 15-year study at Punahou School. *J Athl Train*, 39:310, 2004.
12. Ghanem, T, Rasamny, JK, and Park, SS: Rethinking auricular trauma. *Laryngoscope*, 115:1251, 2005.
13. O'Donnell, BP, and Eliezri, YD: The surgical treatment of traumatic hematoma of the auricle. *Dermatol Surg*, 25:803, 1999.
14. Fincher, AL: Use of the otoscope in the evaluation of common injuries and illnesses of the ear. *J Athl Train*, 29:52, 1994.
15. Vogelin, E, et al: Surgical correction of cauliflower ear. *Br J Plast Surg*, 51:359, 1998.
16. Jones, SEM, and Mahendran, S: Interventions for acute auricular haematoma. *Cochrane Database of Systematic Reviews* 2004, Issue 2. Art. No.: CD004166. DOI: 10.1002/14651858.CD004166.pub2
17. Plafki, C, et al: Complications and side effects of hyperbaric oxygen therapy. *Aviat Space Environ Med*, 71:194, 2000.
18. Gladstone, HB, Jackler, RK, and Varav, K: Tympanic membrane wound healing. An overview. *Otolarynol Clin North Am*, 28:913, 1995.
19. Goodman, RA, et al: Infectious disease in competitive sports. *JAMA*, 271:862, 1994.
20. Ramakrishnan, K, Sparks, RA, and Berryhill, WE: Diagnosis and treatment of otitis media. *Am Fam Physician*, 76:1650, 2007.
21. Karma, PH, et al: Otoscopic diagnosis of middle ear effusion in acute and non-acute otitis media. I. The value of different otoscopic findings. *Int J Pediatr Otorhinolaryngol*, 17:37, 1989.
22. Mondin, V, Rinaldo, A, and Ferlito, A: Management of nasal bone fractures. *Am J Otolaryngol*, 26:181, 2005.
23. Kucik, CJ, Clenney, T, and Phelan, J. Management of acute nasal fractures. *Am Fam Physician*, 70:1315, 2004.
24. Logan, M, O'Driscoll, K, and Masterson, J: The utility of nasal bone radiographs in nasal trauma. *Clin Radiol*, 49:192, 1994.
25. Bechman, SM: Laryngeal fracture in a high school football player. *J Athl Train*, 28:217, 1993.
26. Matthews, B: Maxillofacial trauma from athletic endeavors. *J Athl Train*, 25:132, 1990.
27. Muhtaroğullari, M, Demiralp, B, and Ertan, A: Non-surgical treatment of sports-related temporomandibular joint disorders in basketball players. *Dent Traumatol*, 20:388, 2004.
28. Mihalik, JP, et al: Maxillofacial fractures and dental trauma in a high school soccer goal keeper: A case report. *J Athl Train*, 40:116, 2005.
29. Lephart, SM, and Fu, FH: Emergency treatment of athletic injuries. *Sports Dentistry*, 35:707, 1991.
30. Ad Hoc Committee on Treatment of the Avulsed Tooth: American Association of Endodontists: Recommended guidelines for the treatment of the avulsed tooth. *Dent Clin North Am*, 39:221, 1997.
31. Krasner, P: The athletic trainer's role in saving avulsed teeth. *J Athl Train*, 24:139, 1989.
32. Andreasen, JO, and Kristersson, L: The effect of limited drying or removal of the periodontal ligament. Periodontal healing after reimplantation of mature permanent incisors in monkeys. *Acta Odontol Scand*, 39:1, 1981.
33. Andreasen, JO: Relationship between cell damage in the periodontal ligament after reimplantation and subsequent development of root resorption. A time-related study in monkeys. *Acta Odontol Scand*, 39:15, 1981.
34. Flores, MT, et al: Guidelines for the management of traumatic dental injuries. II. Avulsion of permanent teeth. *Dental Trauma*, 23:130, 2007.

CHAPTER 21

Head and Cervical Spine Pathologies

The potential for catastrophic head or cervical spine injuries and their life-ending or altering consequences necessitates development of a clear plan for evaluation and management. Fortunately, the overall rate of injury to these body areas is relatively low.[1] However, when it does occur, the outcomes can be fatal or result in long-term physical and/or mental deficits.[2]

Most often the result of direct contact with another player, head injuries occur more frequently in college athletics than in high school and tend to be more frequent in women's than in men's sports.[3] Sports in which blows to the head are commonplace—football, baseball, and ice hockey—have rules mandating the use of protective headgear. The use of helmets has greatly reduced the number and severity of head injuries in football, but various styles and brands have differing levels of effectiveness.[3–6] Ironically, the football helmet has been implicated in increasing the number of injuries to the cervical spine.

Regular inspection of helmets is needed to ensure proper maintenance and continued protection. Athletes must be knowledgeable about the risks associated with participation in sports and be instructed in the proper techniques necessary to avoid serious head and cervical spine injuries.

This chapter is dedicated to the immediate and follow-up evaluation and management of athletes with head and cervical spine injuries. A well-organized procedure for the emergency management of head and cervical spine trauma is crucial to this process and must be rehearsed regularly by the medical staff to ensure appropriate care. Chapter 14 describes the anatomy of the cervical spine, evaluation of noncatastrophic cervical spine conditions, and injury to the brachial plexus.

Clinical Anatomy

With the exception of a small opening on the skull's base, through which the brain stem and spinal cord pass, the brain is almost fully encased in bone (Fig. 21-1). In adults, the cranial bones are rigidly fused by cranial sutures, making the skull a single structure. In infants and children, the sutures are more pliable because they are continually being remodeled during growth.

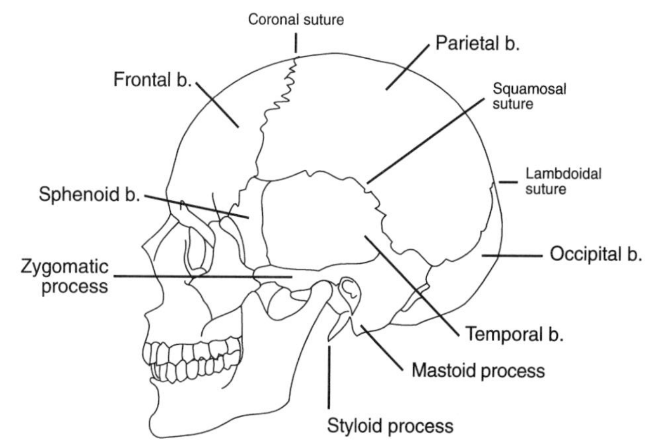

FIGURE 21-1 ■ Lateral view of the bones of the skull.

The skull's design allows for maximum protection of the brain. The density of the bone reduces the amount of physical shock transmitted inwardly. The rounded shape of the skull also has protective qualities. When an object strikes a rounded object, it tends to be deflected quickly. Consider, for example, two scenarios: dropping a brick on a tabletop and dropping a brick on a basketball. When the brick hits the tabletop, it stays there, transmitting its force into the table. When a brick is dropped onto a basketball, although some of the force is transmitted into the ball, the remaining force is dissipated as the brick deflects off the round surface. Lastly, the skin covering the skull increases the cranium's ability to protect the brain by absorbing and redirecting forces from the skull. The skin greatly increases the skull's strength, increasing its breaking force from 40 pounds per square inch to 420 to 490 pounds per square inch.[7]

The Brain

The brain is the most complex and least understood part of the human body. Its anatomy and function are presented in this chapter only as they relate to athletic injuries. Table 21-1 presents an encapsulated description of the major brain areas and their primary functions.

Table 21-1 Brain Function by Area

Area	Function
Cerebrum	Motor function Sensory information (e.g., touch, pain pressure, temperature) Special senses (vision, hearing, smell, taste) Cognition Memory
Cerebellum	Balance and coordination. Smooth, synergistic muscle control.
Diencephalon	Routing of afferent information to the appropriate cerebral areas Body temperature regulation Maintenance of the necessary water balance Emotional control (anger and fear)
Brain Stem	Heart rate regulation Respiratory rate regulation Control over the amount of peripheral blood flow

The cerebrum

The largest section of the brain, the cerebrum is composed of two **hemispheres** separated by the **longitudinal fissure**. Each hemisphere is divided into **frontal**, **parietal**, **temporal**, and occipital lobes, which are separated by sulci and fissures and are named for the overlying cranial bones (Fig. 21-2).

The cerebrum is responsible for controlling the body's primary **motor functions**, both gross muscle contraction and coordination of the muscle contractions in a specific sequence. **Sensory information**, including temperature, touch, pain, pressure, and proprioception, is processed in this region of the brain, along with the **special senses**: visual, auditory, olfactory, and taste. **Cognition**, including spatial relationships, behavior, memory, and association, also occurs in the cerebrum.

With a few exceptions, the cerebrum communicates contralaterally with the rest of the body. The right hemisphere controls the motor actions and interprets much of the sensory input of the body's left side, and vice versa.

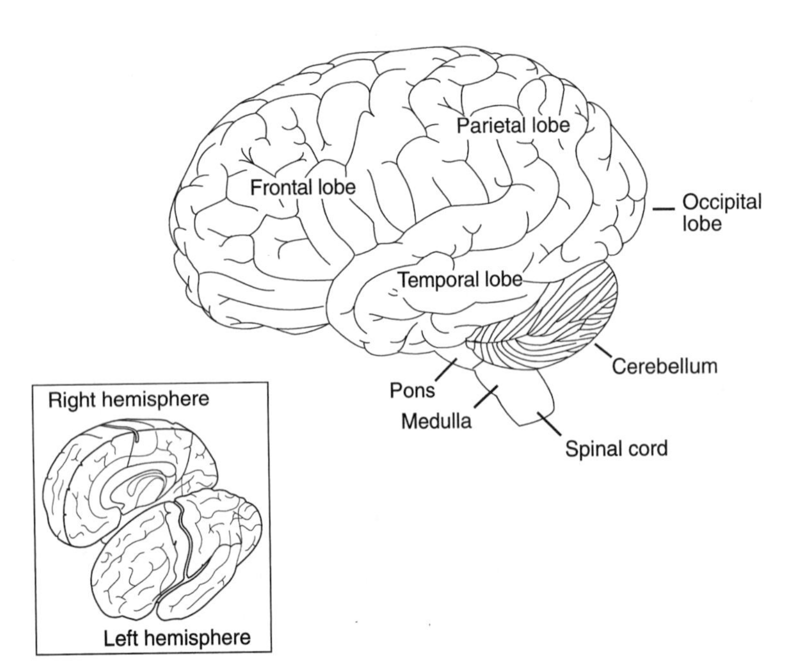

FIGURE 21-2 ■ Regions of the brain, with insert showing the cerebral hemispheres.

Clinically the same cross over occurs: motor impairment of the body's left side usually reflects damage to the brain's right hemisphere

The cerebellum

Designed to allow the quick processing of both incoming and outgoing information, the cerebellum provides the functions necessary to maintain **balance and coordination**. Visual, tactile, auditory, and proprioceptive information from the cerebrum is routed to the cerebellum for immediate processing. The outgoing information is relayed to the muscles via the cerebrum and descending pathways to properly orchestrate the necessary movements.

Fluid, synergistic motions, whether performing a back flip in gymnastics or lifting a cup of coffee, are initiated and controlled by the cerebellum. Facilitative impulses are relayed from the cerebellum to the contracting muscles, and an inhibitory stimulus is sent to the antagonistic muscles. Individuals who have suffered trauma to the cerebellum are recognizable by their uncoordinated, segmental, robot-like movements. Cerebellar injuries are relatively rare in athletes. However, severe blows to the posterior aspect of the skull or acceleration and deceleration mechanisms that cause rotation of the brain stem can injure the cerebellum.

The diencephalon

Formed by the **thalamus**, **hypothalamus**, and **epithalamus**, the **diencephalon** acts as a processing center for conscious and unconscious brain input. In its gatekeeping role, the thalamus monitors sensory information ascending the spinal cord, routing the specific types of information to the appropriate area of the brain. In addition to regulating some of the body's hormones, the hypothalamus is the center of the body's autonomic nervous system, regulating **sympathetic** and **parasympathetic nervous system** activity. Body temperature, water balance, gastrointestinal activity, hunger, and emotions are controlled by the hypothalamus.

The brain stem

Formed by the **medulla oblongata** (medulla) and the pons, the brain stem serves to relay information to and from the central nervous system (CNS) and controls the involuntary systems. Literally translating as "bridge," the **pons** serves to link the cerebellum to the brain stem and spinal cord, connecting the upper and lower portions of the CNS. In addition, receptors in the pons regulate the respiratory rate.

The medulla serves as the interface between the spinal cord and the rest of the brain. Involuntary functions of heart rate, respiration, blood vessel diameter (vasodilation and vasoconstriction), coughing, and vomiting are regulated by the **medullary centers**.

Sympathetic nervous system The part of the central nervous system that supplies the involuntary muscles.

Parasympathetic nervous system A series of specific effects controlled by the brain regulating smooth muscle contractions, slowing the heart rate, and constricting the pupil.

The Meninges

The brain and spinal cord are buffered from the bony surfaces of the cranium and spinal column by three meninges: the **dura mater**, **arachnoid mater**, and **pia mater**. The progressive densities of the meninges support and protect the brain and spinal cord. Arterial and venous blood supplies are provided through these structures, as are the production and introduction of the **cerebrospinal fluid** (CSF).

The dura mater

Literally translating as "hard mother," the dura mater is the outermost meningeal covering, also serving as the periosteum for the skull's inner layer. The **falx cerebri** is a fold in the dura mater in the longitudinal fissure between the two cerebral hemispheres. The void between the two cerebellar hemispheres is filled by another fold of the dura mater, the **falx cerebelli**.

Arteries in the dura mater, the **meningeal arteries**, primarily supply blood to the cranial bones. Blood supply to the dura mater is provided by fine branches from the meningeal arteries. At various points around the brain, the dura mater forms two layers. The space between these layers forms the **venous sinuses**, which serve as a drainage conduit to route used blood into the internal jugular veins in the neck.

The arachnoid mater

The name "arachnoid" is gained from this structure's resemblance to a cobweb ("arachne" is the Greek word for "spider"). Similar to a cobweb, the fibers forming the arachnoid are thin yet relatively resilient to trauma. The arachnoid mater is separated from the dura mater by the narrow **subdural space**. Beneath the arachnoid is a wider separation, the **subarachnoid space**, containing the CSF.

The pia mater

The innermost meningeal membrane, the pia mater, envelops the brain, forming its outer "skin." This delicate membrane derives its name from the Latin word for "tender"; therefore, the pia mater is the "tender mother." The pia mater follows the brain's contour, intruding into its fissures and sulci.

Cerebrospinal Fluid

Originating from the **choroid plexuses** deep within the brain and secreted by cells surrounding the cerebrum's blood vessels, CSF slowly circulates around the brain and spinal cord within the subarachnoid space. From the lateral ventricles, CSF is forced into the third and fourth ventricles by a pressure gradient. After it is in the fourth ventricle, a small proportion of the CSF enters the central canal of the spinal cord. The remaining fluid flows down the spinal cord on its posterior surface and returns to the brain on the anterior portion of the subarachnoid space.

Because of the presence of the subarachnoid space and its watery content, the CNS floats within the body. This arrangement serves as another buffer against external forces being transmitted to the CNS. Although beneficial in dissipating the high-velocity impacts associated with collision sports, this protective configuration is most useful in buffering more repetitious forces, such as those seen when running.

Blood Circulation in the Brain

When the body is at rest, the brain demands 20% of the body's oxygen uptake. For each degree (centigrade) the body's core temperature increases, the brain's need for oxygen increases by 7%. Blood supply to the brain is provided by the two **vertebral arteries** and the two **common carotid arteries**. Each common carotid artery diverges to form an **internal carotid artery** and an **external carotid artery**. The external carotid arteries continue upward to supply blood to the head and neck, with the exception of the brain. The internal carotid arteries move toward the center of the cranium to assist in supplying the brain with blood.

The two internal carotid arteries and the two vertebral arteries converge to form a collateral circulation network, the **circle of Willis** (Fig. 21-3). If one of the cranial arteries is obstructed, the design of the circle of Willis permits at least a partial supply of blood to the affected area.

Examination of Head and Cervical Spine Injuries

The ability to identify and properly manage patients with serious head and cervical spine injuries may affect whether the person lives, dies, or becomes permanently disabled.

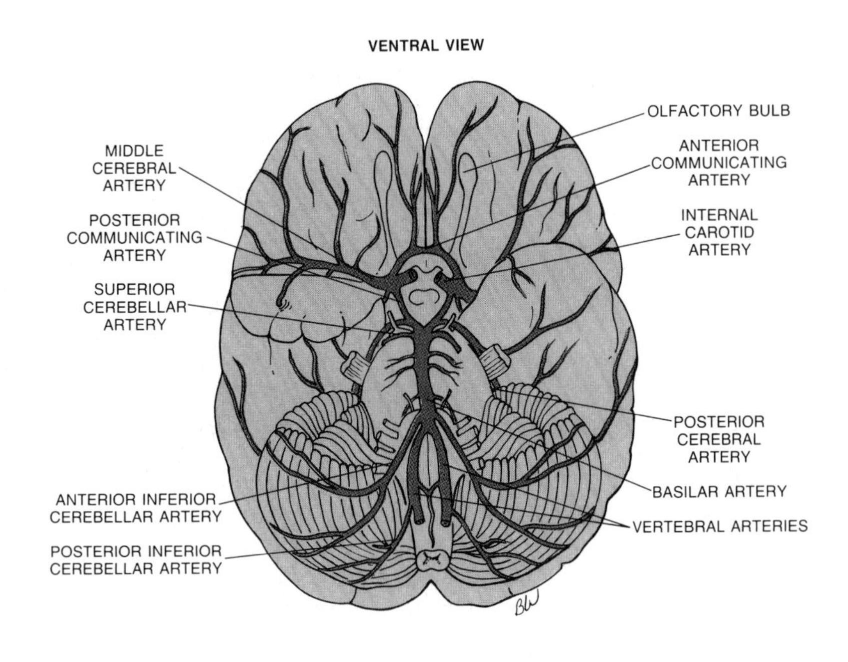

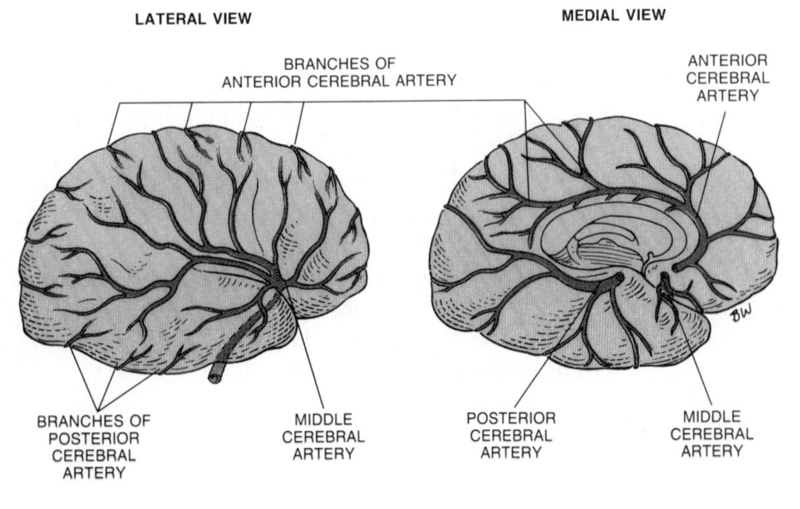

FIGURE 21-3 ■ Blood supply to the brain. The circle of Willis provides collateral circulation to the brain's regions (From Venes D (ed): *Taber's Cyclopedic Medical Dictionary*, ed 21, Beth Anne Willert, MS, medical illustrator. Philadelphia: FA Davis, 2009.)

Examination Map

EVALUATION OF ATHLETE'S POSITION

DETERMINATION OF CONSCIOUSNESS

Level of Consciousness

Primary Survey

Secondary Survey

HISTORY

Location of Symptoms
Cervical pain
Head pain

Mechanism of Injury
Coup
Contrecoup
Repeated subconcussive forces
Rotational/shear force
Cervical spine mechanism
- Flexion/axial loading
- Extension
- Lateral bending/rotation

Loss of consciousness
History of concussion
Weakness
Persistent symptoms

INSPECTION

Inspection of the Bony Structures
Position of the head
Cervical vertebrae
Mastoid process
Skull and scalp

Inspection of the Eyes
General
Nystagmus
Pupil size
Pupil reaction to light

Inspection of the Nose and Ears
Fluid escaping

PALPATION

Palpation of the Bony Structures
Spinous processes
Transverse processes
Skull

Palpation of Soft Tissue
Musculature
Throat

FUNCTIONAL ASSESSMENT

Neurocognitive Function
Behavior
Analytical skills
Information processing
Memory
- Test for retrograde amnesia
- Test for anterograde amnesia

Neuropsychological testing

Balance and Coordination
Romberg test
Tandem walk test
Balance Error Scoring System

Vital Signs
Respiration
Pulse
Blood pressure
Pulse pressure

NEUROLOGIC EXAMINATION

Cranial Nerve Function
Eyes
Face
Ears
Shoulder and neck

Spinal Nerve Root Evaluation
Upper quarter screen
Lower quarter screen

PATHOLOGIES AND SPECIAL TESTS

Head Trauma

Mild Traumatic Brain Injury
Standardized Assessment of Concussion
Concussion Rating Systems

Postconcussion Syndrome

Second Impact Syndrome

Intracranial Hemorrhage
Epidural hematoma
Subdural hematoma

Skull Fractures

Cervical Spine Trauma
Cervical Fracture/Dislocation
Transient Quadriplegia

Although some signs and symptoms of brain trauma are blatantly obvious, such as unconsciousness, some potentially catastrophic head injuries initially have few, if any, outward signs or symptoms. This section describes the signs and symptoms of brain and spine trauma, and the section that follows describes the on-field management of athletes with these conditions. Many of these evaluative procedures are performed on the field.

Evaluation Scenarios

Before discussing how to evaluate and manage athletes with head and cervical spine injuries, the possible scenarios under which an evaluation may have to be performed must be considered. The best-case scenario is one in which the athlete is conscious and responsive to stimuli. The worst-case scenario is that of a prone, unconscious athlete who is not breathing and has no pulse. In either case, the decisions made by the medical staff are critical in the optimal management of athletes with catastrophic conditions.

The basic premise of on-field management is: **All unconscious athletes must be managed as if a fracture or dislocation of the cervical spine exists until the presence of these injuries can be definitively ruled out.**

Ideally, athletes with head and cervical spine injuries are evaluated on the field by at least two responders. One responder must ensure stabilization and immobilization of the athlete's head and cervical spine by grasping the sides of the head or helmet and applying **in-line stabilization** on the cervical spine until significant pathology has been ruled out. A second responder performs the necessary palpation, sensory, and motor assessments (Fig. 21-4). One person acts as the leader and directs the actions of all others at the injury scene. In situations in which only one responder is present, other on-site personnel may be directed to assist in the management of the athlete's condition. Prior discussion and practice are necessary to ensure orderly and precise action by the support staff.

Evaluation of the Athlete's Position

The initial assessment of an on-field head and cervical spine injury may be complicated further by the position in which the athlete is found. A supine athlete is in the optimal position for subsequent evaluation and management. When athletes are in the sidelying or prone position, the evaluation is more difficult.

If, as determined according to the assessments described the next section, the athlete's vital signs are present, there is no need to move the athlete until a complete on-field evaluation is performed and the athlete's disposition is determined. However, when an athlete is prone or sidelying, the absence of vital signs takes precedence over the possibility of a spinal fracture. The athlete must be rolled into the supine position in the safest manner possible. These procedures are discussed in the "On-Field Management of Head and Cervical Spine Injuries" section of this chapter.

Determination of Consciousness

When an athlete is "down" on the field or court, the first priority is to establish the athlete's level of consciousness. A moving and speaking athlete demonstrates that the ABCs are present and functioning. Even under these circumstances, however, a cervical fracture must be suspected, and the athlete's vital signs require regular monitoring. At the scene of a possible head or cervical spine injury, the athlete's head is stabilized and immobilized by grasping the sides of the helmet or head and applying in-line stabilization on the cervical spine until pathology to the spine has been ruled out.

- **Level of consciousness:** While moving toward the scene of the injury, note whether the athlete is moving. At the scene, make an attempt to communicate with the athlete. If spoken communication fails, the athlete's responsiveness to painful stimuli is checked by applying pressure to the lumina of a fingernail or rubbing the sternum (Fig. 21-5). The use of ammonia inhalants is discouraged because of the possibility of the athlete's jerking the head and cervical spine when awakening.
- **Primary survey:** If the athlete is unconscious or unable to communicate, check the athlete's airway, breathing and circulation (ABCs) by looking, listening, and feeling for breathing (Fig. 21-6). The Emergency Action System should be activated if the athlete continues to remain unconscious. If breathing is absent, use a modified jaw thrust to open the airway. In the event that no carotid or radial pulse is found, send someone to summon advanced medical assistance and initiate emergency cardiac procedures including cardiopulmonary resuscitation and automated external defibrillator (AED) use. The "On-Field Management of Head and Cervical Spine Injuries" section of this chapter and Chapter 2 contain further discussion of this topic.
- **Secondary survey:** Although the suspicion of brain or cervical spine trauma takes precedence, do not overlook the possibility of other trauma to the body. Inspect the extremities and torso for bleeding or indications of fractures or dislocations.

The following components of an assessment of a head- or cervical spine–injured athlete assume a sideline evaluation is being conducted. A descriptive on-field management procedure is detailed later in this chapter.

FIGURE 21-4 ■ Head and cervical spine trauma is best managed by two responders. One stabilizes the head while the second conducts the examination.

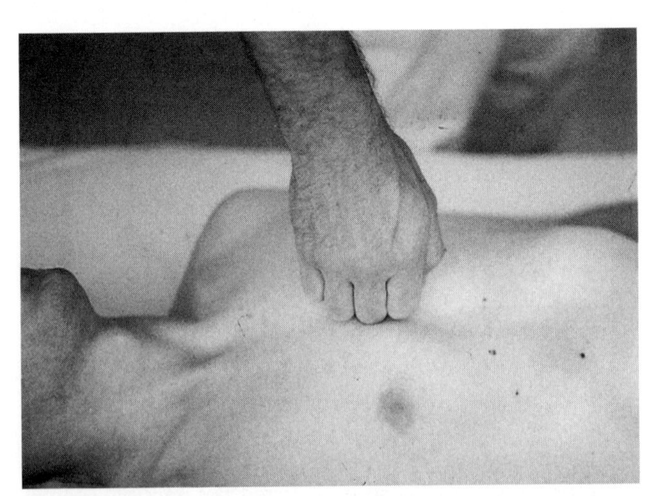

FIGURE 21-5 ■ Attempting to elicit a pain response from an unconscious patient. This test is performed by squeezing the patient's fingernail, pinching the patient, or applying pressure with a knuckle to the sternum.

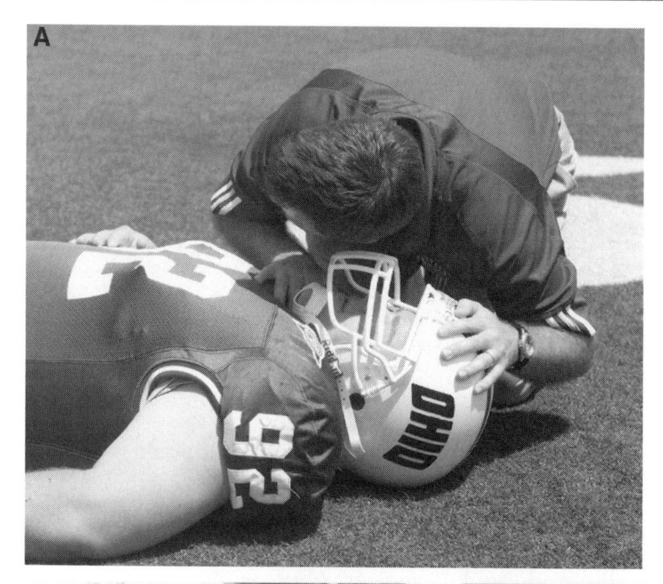

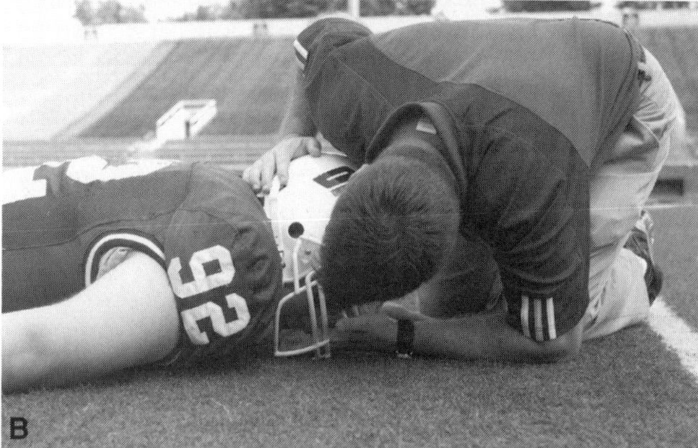

FIGURE 21-6 ■ Establishing the presence of an open airway, breathing, and circulation. (A) Supine athlete. (B) Prone athlete.

History

The history-taking process of an athlete with a head injury not only determines the injury mechanism but also assesses the athlete's level of brain function. Much of this portion of the evaluation is initially conducted when the athlete is on the field. Then this evaluation is repeated at regular intervals on the sidelines. In the event that the athlete becomes unconscious, proceed to the inspection phase of the evaluation while continuing to monitor the vital signs. Throughout the evaluation, the athlete must be questioned and observed for the presence of subtle signs and symptoms indicating a head injury (Table 21-2).

- **Location of symptoms:** Question the athlete about the location and type of pain or other symptoms experienced after the injury.
  - **Cervical pain:** The most significant finding during this portion of the examination is cervical pain or muscle spasm. The significance of this finding is magnified when it is accompanied by pain, numbness, or burning, which may or may not radiate into the extremities.

Table 21-2 Signs and Symptoms of a Head or Cervical Spine Injury to Note Throughout the Evaluation

Area	Signs and Symptoms
Brain	Amnesia (retrograde and anterograde)
	Confusion
	Disorientation
	Irritability
	Incoordination
	Dizziness
	Headache
Ocular	Blurred vision
	Photophobia
	Nystagmus
Ears	Tinnitus
	Dizziness
Stomach	Nausea
	Vomiting
Systemic	Unusually fatigued

  - **Head pain:** Diffuse headaches are a common complaint after brain trauma. Localized pain can indicate a contusion, skull fracture, or intracranial hemorrhage.
- **Mechanism of head injuries:** The type of and severity injury inflicted to the head and cervical spine depends on the nature of the force delivered (Fig. 21-7). This information may be obtained by someone who witnessed the injury if the athlete is unconscious or groggy.
  - **Coup:** A coup injury results when a relatively stationary skull is hit by an object traveling at a high velocity (e.g., being struck in the head with a baseball). This type of mechanism results in trauma on the side of the head that was struck.
  - **Contrecoup:** A contrecoup injury occurs when the skull is moving at a relatively high velocity and is suddenly stopped, such as when falling and striking the head on the floor. The fluid within the skull fails to decrease the brain's momentum proportional to that of the skull, causing the brain to strike the skull on the side opposite the impact. This mechanism includes forces that are transmitted up the length of the spinal column, such as when falling and landing on the buttocks.
  - **Repeated subconcussive forces:** Athletes receiving repeated nontraumatic blows to the head (e.g., in boxing or while heading a soccer ball) have a higher degree of degenerative changes within the CNS, including dementia.[8–10] A history of repeated concussions can result in cumulative neurologic and

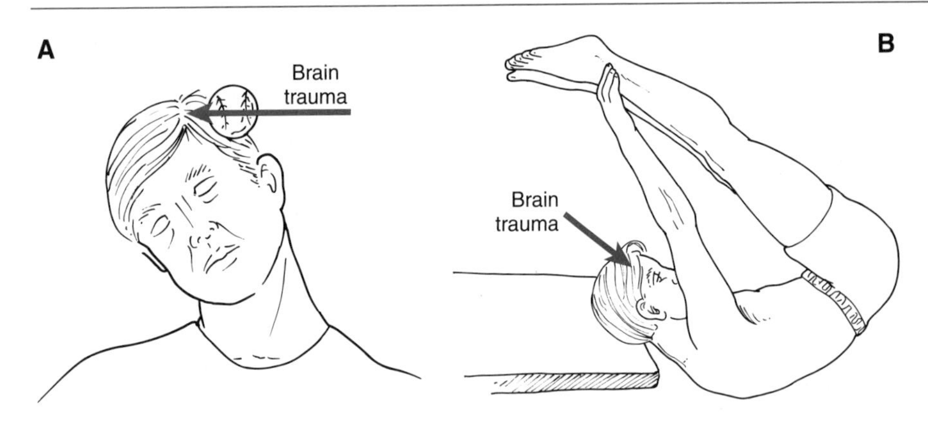

FIGURE 21-7 ■ Mechanisms of an athletic head injury. (A) Coup mechanism caused by a moving object's striking the head, resulting in brain trauma on the side of the impact. (B) Contrecoup mechanism caused by a moving head striking a stationary object. Trauma occurs to the brain on the opposite side of the impact as it rebounds off the skull.

cognitive deficits by disrupting electroencephalographic (EEG) activity.[9,11]

- **Rotational or shear forces:** Sudden twisting forces or acceleration and deceleration can disrupt neural activity and result in cerebral concussion symptoms.
- **Mechanism of cervical spine injuries:** Most of the forces directed toward the cervical spine are capable of being dissipated by the energy-absorbing properties of the cervical musculature and intervertebral disks.[12] The mechanisms of injury to the cervical spine involve flexion, extension, or lateral bending and may be accompanied by a rotational component.

Flexion of the cervical spine combined with an axial load applied to the crown of the head is the mechanism most likely to produce catastrophic injury.[12–16] As the crown of the head makes contact, the cervical spine and skull flexes. As soon as the cervical spine is flexed to approximately 30 degrees, the cervical spine's lordotic curve is lost (Fig. 21-8). In this position, the effectiveness of the cervical spine's energy-dissipating mechanism is rendered ineffective, thus transmitting forces directly to the cervical vertebrae, creating an axial load through the vertical axis of the segmented columns (Fig. 21-9).

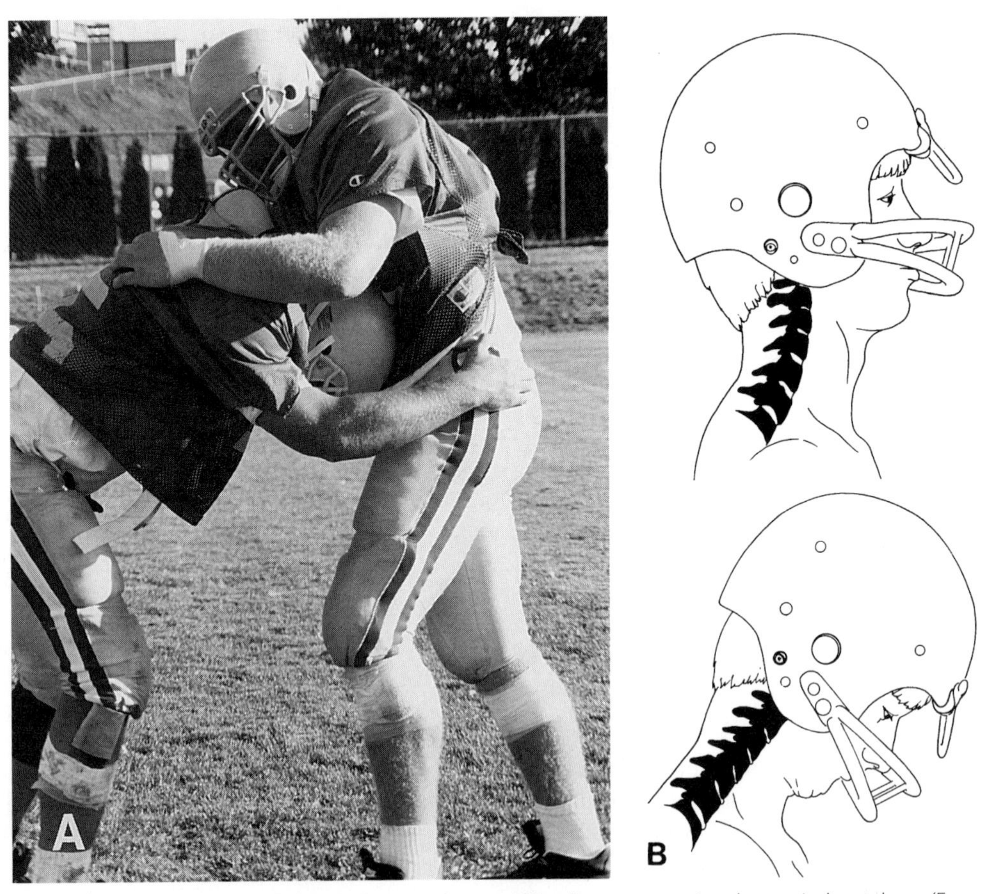

FIGURE 21-8 ■ Making contact with the crown of the helmet results in axial loading, compressing the cervical vertebrae. (From Torg, JS: The epidemiologic, biomechanical, and cinematographic analysis of football induced cervical spine trauma. *Athl Train J Natl Athl Train Assoc*, 25:147, 1990.)

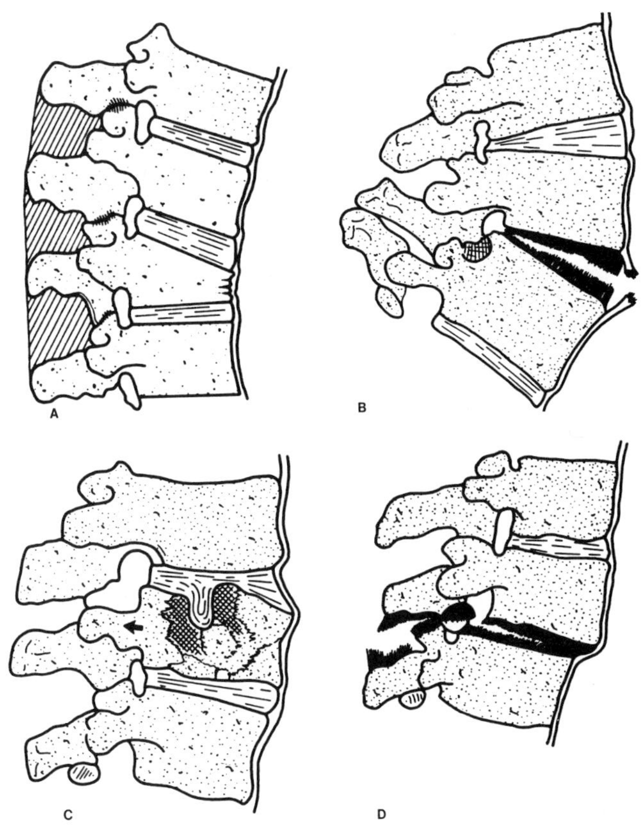

FIGURE 21-9 ■ Mechanisms of cervical spine injuries and the resulting trauma. (A) Flexion mechanism resulting in compression of the vertebral body. (B) Extension mechanism resulting in tearing of the anterior longitudinal ligament and intervertebral disk. (C) Compression mechanism resulting in a posterior burst of the bone. (D) Flexion and rotation injury resulting in a dislocation of the cervical vertebrae. (From Mueller, FO and Ryan, AJ: *Prevention of Athletic Injuries: The Role of the Sports Medicine Team*. Philadelphia: FA Davis, 1991.)

- **Loss of consciousness:** This portion of the history-taking process is closely related to the determination of the athlete's memory status. Record the responses given by the athlete immediately after the injury for future comparison. The athlete is questioned regarding a momentary loss of consciousness after the impact (e.g., "Did you black out?"). The athlete may also describe "seeing stars" at the time of the impact, which indicates transitory unconsciousness.

✱ Practical Evidence

Loss of consciousness is often thought to be the best predictor of the severity of the head injury and ensuing symptoms. Several studies suggest that the presence of amnesia is a more sensitive predictor of cognitive deficits and other symptoms.[17]

- **History of concussion:** A recent history of concussion increases the risk for subsequent concussions, increases the symptoms of the current condition delays recovery, and may predispose the individual to second impact syndrome.[17,18] The history of concussions must be readily available from the athlete's medical file.
- **Complaints of weakness:** A general malaise is to be expected after a cerebral concussion. Reports of muscular weakness in one or more extremities is a more serious finding, possibly indicating trauma to the brain, spinal cord, or one or more spinal nerve roots.
- **Persistent symptoms:** Difficulty concentrating, fatigue, and emotional instability are all symptoms that might linger after a concussive event. The presence of any of these symptoms precludes further athletic participation.

Inspection

If the athlete is wearing protective headgear at the onset of the inspection process, a decision must be made regarding whether and when to remove it. The helmet should not be removed if there is any lingering suspicion of a cervical spine fracture or dislocation. Much of the inspection and palpation process can be performed with the helmet still in place.

Inspection of the bony structures

- **Position of the head:** Observe the way in which the head is positioned. Normally the head should be upright in all planes. A laterally flexed and rotated skull that is accompanied by muscle spasm on the side opposite that of the tilt may indicate a dislocation of a cervical vertebra.
- **Cervical vertebrae:** Viewing the athlete from behind, observe the alignment of the spinous processes. A vertebra that is obviously malaligned (i.e., rotated or displaced anteriorly or posteriorly) can signify a vertebral dislocation.
- **Mastoid process:** Note any ecchymosis over the mastoid process, Battle's sign, which may indicate a basilar skull fracture. This finding would emerge several hours following the injury.
- **Skull and scalp:** Inspect the athlete's skull and scalp for the presence of bleeding, swelling, or other deformities.

Inspection of the eyes

- **General:** Note the general attitude of the athlete's eyes. A dazed, distant appearance may be attributed to mental confusion and disruption of cerebral function.
- **Nystagmus:** While observing both of the athlete's eyes simultaneously, look for the presence of involuntary cyclical movement, or nystagmus. This clinical sign, although it may normally occur, may indicate pressure on the eyes' motor nerves or disruption of the inner ear.
- **Pupil size:** Observe the equality of the pupils. A unilaterally dilated pupil, anisocoria, can be indicative of an intracranial hemorrhage's placing pressure on cranial nerve III, although some people may normally display unequal pupil sizes (Fig. 21-10). Although this condition is benign, its presence should be detected during the preparticipation physical examination and recorded in

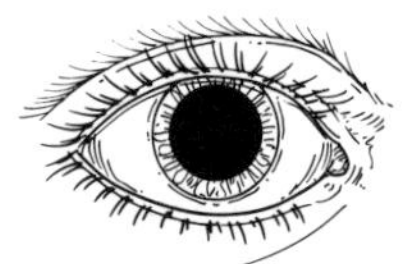
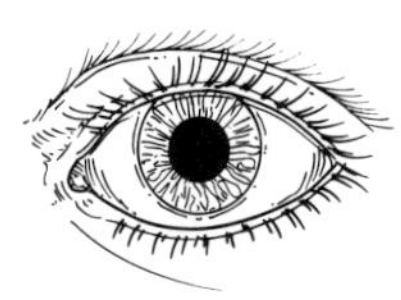

FIGURE 21-10 ■ Anisocoria, or unequal pupil size. This condition may result from pressure on the oculomotor nerve (cranial nerve III) or may be congenital.

the athlete's medical file to avoid confusion during the evaluation of a head injury.

- **Pupillary reaction to light:** Refer to Box 19–1 and see the "Neurologic Testing" section of this chapter for the process and implications of negative pupillary reaction tests.

Inspection of the nose and ears

Bleeding from the ears, even in the absence of CSF in the fluid, may indicate a skull fracture. Bleeding from the nose could represent either a nasal fracture or a skull fracture. Ecchymosis under the eyes, "raccoon eyes," can indicate a skull fracture or nasal fracture. Cerebrospinal fluid (CSF) may also leak from the ears and nose when a skull fracture is present and the dura is torn, opening the intracranial space to the nose or nasal tract.[19] The halo test is used to determine if CSF is present in fluids leaking from the nose or ears (Special Test 21-1).

PALPATION

Palpation should not be performed over areas of obvious deformity or suspected fracture, especially in the cervical spine and skull. Placing too much pressure on these structures may cause the bony fragment to displace, possibly resulting in catastrophic consequences. Refer to Chapter 14 for a detailed description of the palpation of the cervical spine.

Palpation of the Bony Structures

1 Spinous processes: Position the patient sitting and leaning slightly forward. Standing behind the athlete, palpate the spinous processes of C7, C6, and C5 (Fig. 21-11). At approximately the C5 level, the spinous processes become less defined. Continue to palpate the area over the spinous processes of C4 and C3, noting for tenderness or crepitus.

2 Transverse processes: Although the transverse processes of C1 are the only ones that are directly palpable (approximately two finger widths below the mastoid process), palpate the areas over the transverse processes of the remaining cervical vertebrae.

3 Skull: Begin the palpation of the skull at the inion, the occipital bone's posterior process. Continue to palpate anteriorly toward the face, palpating the temporal bones and their mastoid processes, and the sphenoid, zygomatic, parietal, and frontal bones (see Fig. 21-1). Palpation of the facial structures is described in Chapter 20.

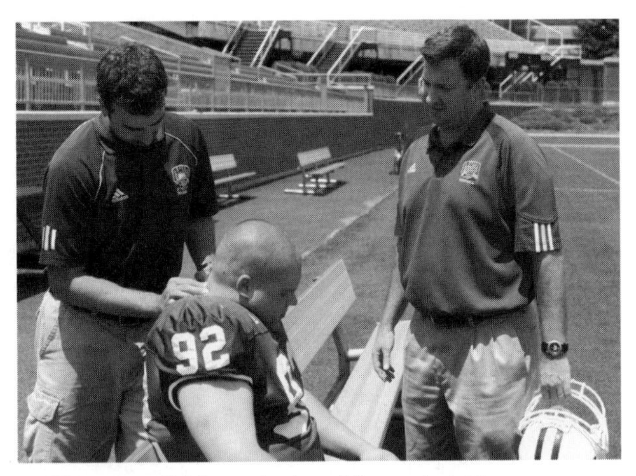

FIGURE 21-11 ■ Sideline palpation of the cervical spine.

Palpation of Soft Tissue

1 Musculature: To identify muscular spasm, palpate the trapezius and sternocleidomastoid muscles. In addition to the muscle's reaction to a strain, spasm may result from insult to a cervical nerve root or may reflect the body's protective response to a cervical fracture or dislocation.

2 Throat: Perform complete palpation of the anterior throat, if warranted, to rule out trauma to the larynx, trachea, or hyoid bone.

Functional Assessment

The goal of the functional testing of an athlete with a head or cervical spine injury is to assess the status of the CNS. This portion of the examination begins with assessment of the athlete's airway, breathing, circulation, and level of consciousness. This section of the chapter assumes that the patient is conscious and capable of responding to the functional tasks presented. The cervical spine must be assessed first to rule out bone or joint dysfunction.

*** Practical Evidence**

The examination of head injuries, the determination of the severity of the condition, and return-to-play decisions are largely based on self-reported symptoms. Many athletes may be unaware that symptoms are present or may understate the magnitude of symptoms for fear of being withheld from competition. For this reason quantifiable clinical measures such as computer-based neuropsychological tests, the Standardized Assessment of Concussion instrument, or other such tools should be used whenever possible, but should not be the sole basis for determining the patient's disposition.[17a]

Neurocognitive function

Trauma to the cerebrum can result in unusual communication between the patient and the examiner. This can

Special Test 21-1
Halo Test

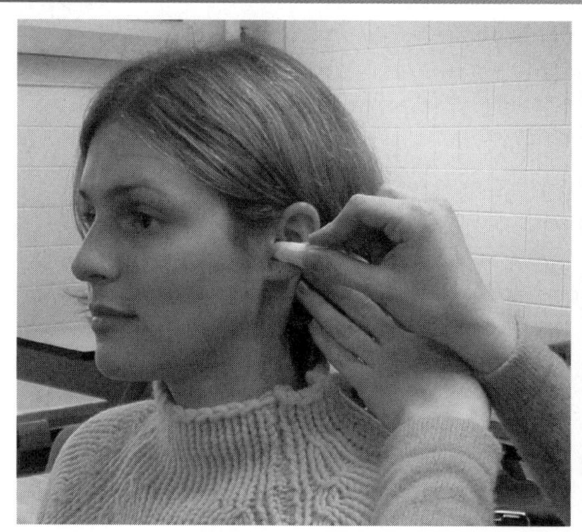

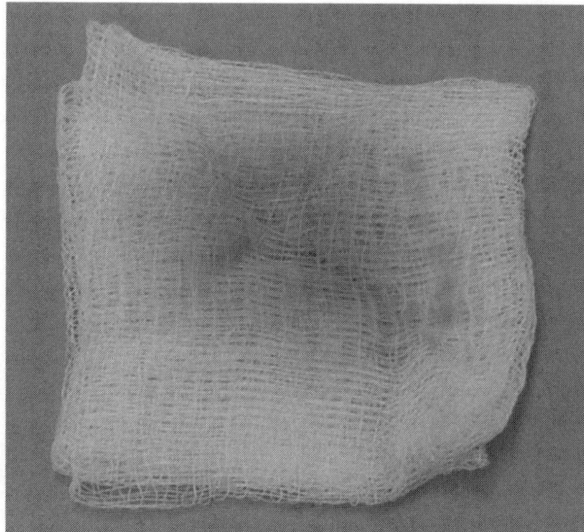

The halo test determines the presence of cerebrospinal fluid in any fluid escaping from the ears or nose.

Patient Position	Lying or sitting
Position of Examiner	Lateral to the patient's ear
Evaluative Procedure	Fold a piece of sterile gauze into a triangle. Using the point of the gauze, collect a sample of the fluid leaking from the ear or nose and allow it to be absorbed by the gauze.
Positive Test	A pale yellow "halo" will form around the sample on the gauze.
Implications	Cerebrospinal fluid (CSF) leakage, indicative of a skull fracture. The frontal bone and ethmoid bone are most commonly involved.[19]
Comments	CSF leakage from the intracranial space to the nose significantly increases the risk of infection.[19]
Evidence	Absent or inconclusive in the literature

manifest itself through inappropriate behavior, irrational thinking, and apparent mental disability or personality changes.

- **Behavior:** The individual's behavior, attitude, and demeanor may become altered after brain trauma. This may take the form of violent, irrational behavior; inappropriate behavior; and belligerence. After a head injury, the athlete may verbally or physically lash out at those attempting to assist.
- **Analytical skills:** The patient's analytical skills can be determined using **serial 7's**. The patient is asked to count backwards from 100 by 7's (e.g., 100, 93, 86, 79...).
- **Information processing:** The athlete's ability to process the information and assimilate facts should be noted. Confusion regarding relatively simple directions, such as "Sit on the bench," indicates profound cognitive dysfunction.

Memory. One of the most obvious dysfunctions after brain trauma is the loss of memory. The inability to recall events before the onset of the injury is termed **retrograde amnesia** (Special Test 21-2). When the athlete cannot remember events after the onset of injury, it is termed **anterograde amnesia** (Special Test 21-3) or posttraumatic amnesia (Fig. 21-12). Although significant retrograde amnesia is a cause for concern, fading or fogging memory identifies a progressive deterioration of cerebral function. The patient should be questioned regarding the sequence of events after the injury:

- How did you get to the sidelines?
- Who has spoken to you since?
- Do you remember my asking you those questions before?

Neuropsychological testing. Memory and cognitive testing provide a subjective assessment of the athlete's mental abilities. The use of objective neuropsychological

Special Test 21-2
Determination of Retrograde Amnesia

Patient Position	On-field: In the athlete's current position (see instructions regarding moving the athlete) Sideline: Standing, sitting, or lying down
Position of Examiner	In a position to hear the patient's response
Evaluative Procedure	The patient is asked a series of questions beginning with the time of the injury. Each successive question progresses backward in time, as described by the following set of questions: What happened? What play were you running? (or other applicable question regarding the patient's activity at the time of injury) Where are you? Who am I? Who are you playing? What quarter is it (or what time is it)? What did you have for a pregame meal (or what did you have to eat for lunch)? Who did you play last week?
Positive Test	The patient has difficulty remembering or cannot remember events occurring before the injury.
Implications	Retrograde amnesia, the severity of which is based on the relative amount of memory loss demonstrated by the inability to recall events Not remembering events from the day before is more significant than not remembering more recent events The same set of questions should be repeated to determine whether the memory is returning, deteriorating, or remaining the same. Further deterioration of the memory or acutely profound memory loss that does not return in a matter of minutes warrants the immediate termination of the evaluation and transportation to an emergency medical facility.
Comments	Try to ask questions that you know the answers to or can otherwise verify. Record the patient's responses. Retrograde and/or anterograde memory loss is a common deficit associated with concussion.[20]
Evidence	Absent or inconclusive in the literature

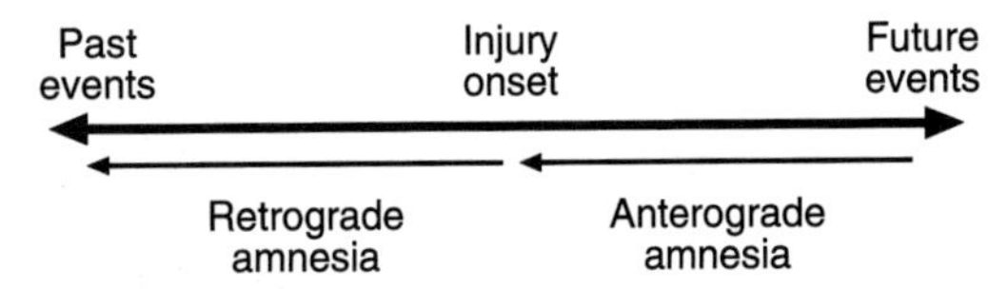

FIGURE 21-12 ■ Types of amnesia. Loss of memory from onset backward in time is known as retrograde amnesia. Loss of memory after the onset of an injury is anterograde amnesia.

tests and objective balance tests (see the information on the Balance Error Scoring System in the next section) objectively quantify the amount of dysfunction demonstrated by the athlete.[9,20–26] Neuropsychological testing can identify attention deficits and delayed memory function in athletes suffering mild traumatic brain injury.[9] Most cognitive deficits resolve within 7 to 14 days[27] although younger—high school aged—athletes tend to recover more quickly than older athletes.[17] Neurocognitive symptoms may persist after physical symptoms have resolved[28] and a history of multiple concussions further delays the recovery of neurologic function.[29]

Table 21-3 presents a description of the six most commonly used neuropsychological tests in sports medicine.[23] Although tests have shown statistical reliability, their weight in making return to play decisions is still being determined.[22,30]

Several computer-based programs are available for athletic neuropsychological testing. Measuring variables such as memory, reaction time, and information processing speed, the information obtained from these systems may be a valuable supplement to the return-to-play decision-making process.[17] Performance (scores) can be influenced by the patient's sex, sport(s) played, alertness at the time of testing, motivation, and other variables such as SAT scores.[31] Interestingly, a history of prior concussion does not appear to influence performance.[31]

Special Test 21-3
Determination of Anterograde Amnesia

Patient Position	Sitting or lying
Position of Examiner	In a position to hear the patient's response
Evaluative Procedure	The athlete is given a list of four unrelated items with instructions to memorize them, for example: Hubcap Film Dog tags Ivy The list is immediately repeated by the patient to ensure that it has been memorized. The patient is asked to repeat the list to the examiner every 5 minutes.
Positive Test	The inability to recite the list completely
Implications	Anterograde amnesia, possibly the result of intracranial bleeding or concussion
Comment	This test is usually performed after the test for retrograde amnesia.
Evidence	Absent or inconclusive in the literature

The return-to-play decision should be based on the patient's current score relative to the preinjury score. However, many computer-based neuropsychological tests have low to moderate test–retest reliability.[32]

Balance and coordination

After a head injury, the athlete's balance and coordination may be hindered secondary to trauma involving the cerebellum or the inner ear. A profound loss of muscular coordination, ataxia, may be obvious as the athlete attempts to perform even simple tasks. The **Romberg test** (Special Test 21-4) and **tandem walking** (Special Test 21-5) are used to determine cerebellar function by determining the level of balance and coordination.

After a head injury, an electronic balance system can be used to objectively determine the amount of balance disruption. In the absence of these devices, a quantifiable clinical test should be used. The **balance error scoring system** (BESS), a newer clinical test that has been developed to evaluate impairment of balance and coordination, is more applicable and sensitive to the athletic population (Special Test 21-6).[34,35] In this procedure, balance is first tested on a firm surface and then again with the patient standing on foam.

Baseline balance measurements should be obtained before the start of each season. During baseline testing, the patient should be well rested and free from any lower extremity musculoskeletal injury. After injury, the BESS can be administered on the sidelines or in the clinic with the results then compared with the baseline measures, but should be performed under the same conditions as the baseline.[38] For example, if baseline measures were obtained in a quiet room, postinjury testing should also be performed in a quiet room. If baseline information is not available, the patient's BESS score can be compared with recovery curves for the normal population.[23,34,35]

Vital signs

Techniques for determining the vital signs are described in Chapter 15, review of systems. The following are qualitative parameters that are relevant after a head or cervical spine injury.

- **Respiration:** In addition to the number of breaths per minute, the quality of the respirations are determined:

Type	Characteristics	Implications
Apneustic	Prolonged inspirations unrelieved by attempts to exhale	Trauma to the pons
Biot's	Periods of apnea followed by hyperapnea	Increased intracranial pressure
Cheyne-Stokes	Periods of **apnea** followed by breaths of increasing depth and frequency	Frontal lobe or brain stem trauma
Slow	Respiration consisting of fewer than 12 breaths per minute	CNS disruption
Thoracic	Respiration in which the diaphragm is inactive and breathing occurs only through expansion of the chest; normal abdominal movement is absent	Disruption of the phrenic nerve or its nerve roots

Apnea The temporary cessation of breathing.

Table 21-3 Neuropsychological Assessment Tests Used for Mild Head-Injured Athletes

Test and Publisher	Description
Trail Making Test A & B (Reitan Neuropsychological Laboratory, Tucson, AZ)	**Description:** The patient sequentially connects a series of numbers (Trail Making A) or series of alternating letters and numbers (Trail Making B). **Measurement:** The time required for successful completion **Assessment:** Visual conceptual, visuomotor tracking, general brain function
Wechsler Digit Span Test (WDST) (Psychological Corporation, San Antonio, TX)	**Description:** The patient is presented with a random list of single-digit numbers (0–9 with no repetition) and asked to repeat the list in the same order (Digits Forward) or reverse order (Digits Backwards). The first bout begins with 3 numbers and the next has 4 numbers, progressing up to 10. **Measurement:** The number of successful trials is recorded for each part. **Assessment:** Short-term memory, auditory attention, concentration
Stroop Color Word Test (Stoelting Co., Wood Dale, IL)	**Description:** Patients are presented with a list of 100 words (5 columns × 20 words each). The test itself consists of three trials, each 45 seconds in length. In the first trial, the patient is asked to read through the list as quickly as possible and read aloud the words "red," "green," and "blue," which are written in black ink. During the second trial, words are replaced with "XXXX" written in red, green, or blue ink, which the patient must identify the proper color. In the third trial, the words "red," "green," and "blue" are written in a color other than their own (e.g., "red" is written in blue ink and "blue" is written in green ink). The patient must identify the color the word is printed in, not the word itself. **Measurement:** Sum total of the number of correct responses in each subset **Assessment:** Cognitive processing speed, concentration ability to filter out distractions (inhibition)
Hopkins Verbal Learning Test (Johns Hopkins University, Baltimore, MD)	**Description:** The patient is read a list of 12 words grouped into 3 semantic categories of 4 words each 3 times. After each reading, the patient is asked to recall as many words as possible. After a 20-minute break, the patient is read a list of 24 words, 12 words from the original list, 6 words that are closely related, and 6 unrelated words. **Measurement:** The number of incorrect responses from the fourth trial subtracted from the total number of correct responses from the first three trials **Assessment:** Language function, short-term memory
Symbol Digit Modalities Test (Western Psychological Services, Los Angeles, CA)	**Description:** Patients are given 30 seconds to memorize a list of nine symbols and their corresponding symbols. In one version of the test, the patient is asked to repeat the symbols corresponding to a four-digit number. An alternate form has the patient write the number that corresponds to a specific symbol. **Measurement:** The number of correct responses divided by the total number of completed responses **Assessment:** Psychomotor speed, concentration, visual speed, and visual perception
Controlled Oral Word Association Test (COWAT) (Psychological Assessment Resources, Inc. Odessa, FL)	**Description:** The patient is given three word naming trials based on two groups of letters, "C–F–L" and "P–R–W." In the first session, the patient is then asked to say as many words as possible that begins with that letter of the alphabet, starting with the first letter within the first code group and then progressing to the subsequent letter. The second code group is used in the second session. Proper names, numbers, and different variations of the same word (e.g., "count," "counting," "counted") are not allowed. This is repeated for three trials. **Measurement:** The raw score based on the total number of acceptable words produced in the three trials. The publisher of the COWAT provides formulas that allow the score to be adjusted based on the patient's age, gender, and level of education. **Assessment:** Verbal fluency

Special Test 21-4
Romberg Test

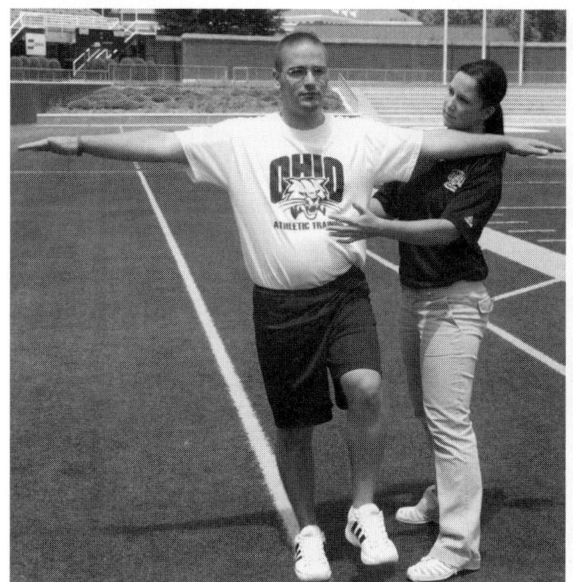

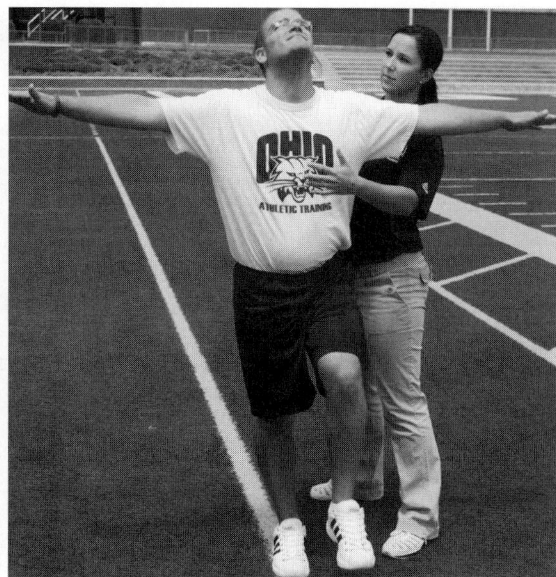

The Romberg test is used to determine the patient's balance and coordination.

Patient Position	Standing with the feet shoulder width apart
Position of Examiner	Standing lateral or posterior to the patient, ready to support the patient as needed
Evaluative Procedure	The patient shuts the eyes and abducts the arms to 90° with the elbows extended. The patient tilts the head backward and lifts one foot off the ground while attempting to maintain balance. If this portion of the examination is adequately completed, the patient is asked to touch the index finger to the nose (with the eyes remaining closed).
Positive Test	The patient displays gross unsteadiness.
Implications	Lack of balance and/or coordination indicating cerebellar or cranial nerve VIII dysfunction
Comments	Changes in balance as measured by clinical balance equipment are commonly associated with concussions.[33]
Evidence	Absent or inconclusive in the literature

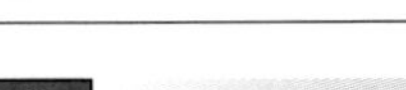
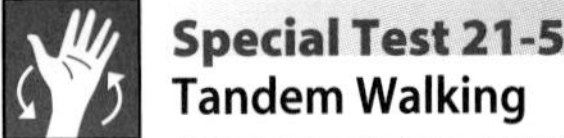

Special Test 21-5
Tandem Walking

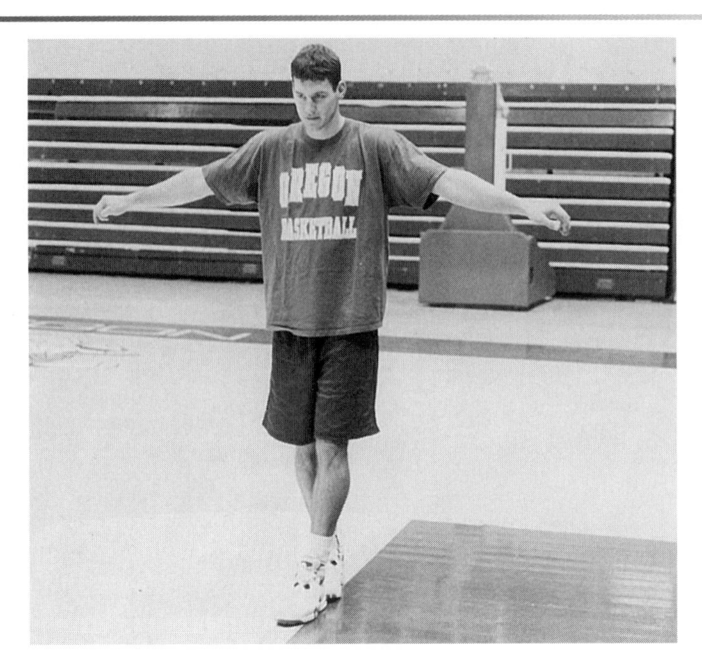

The tandem walk test determines the patient's balance.

Patient Position	Standing with the feet straddling a straight line (e.g., sideline)
Position of Examiner	Beside the patient ready to provide support
Evaluative Procedure	The patient walks heel-to-toe along the straight line for approximately 10 yards. The patient returns to the starting position by walking backward.
Positive Test	The patient is unable to maintain a steady balance.
Implications	Cerebral or inner ear dysfunction that inhibits balance
Evidence	Absent or inconclusive in the literature

- **Pulse:** The pulse rate and quality must be monitored at regular intervals until the possibility of brain or spinal injury has been ruled out. Pulse abnormalities attributed to these conditions include:

Type	Characteristics	Implication
Accelerated	Pulse >150 beats per minute (bpm) (>170 bpm usually has fatal results)	Pressure on the base of the brain; shock
Bounding	Pulse that quickly reaches a higher intensity than normal, then quickly disappears	Ventricular systole and reduced peripheral pressure
Deficit	Pulse in which the number of beats counted at the radial pulse is less than that counted over the heart itself	Cardiac arrhythmia
High Tension	Pulse in which the force of the beat is increased; an increased amount of pressure is required to inhibit the radial pulse	Cerebral trauma
Low Tension	Short, fast, faint pulse having a rapid decline	Heart failure; shock

- **Blood pressure:** Blood pressure readings should be taken concurrently or immediately after each pulse measurement. These measurements are recorded and repeated at regular intervals. Blood pressure is normally high after physical exertion. Blood pressure that does not decrease over time or continues to increase may be a sign of severe intracranial hemorrhage.
- **Pulse pressure:** To calculate the pulse pressure, the diastolic pressure is subtracted from the systolic pressure. The normal pulse pressure is approximately 40 mm Hg. A pulse pressure of greater than 50 mm Hg may indicate increased intracranial bleeding

Neurologic Assessment

Twelve pairs of cranial nerves (CNs), identified by Roman numerals (CN I to CN XII), arise from the brain and transmit both sensory and motor impulses (Table 21-4). The **ganglia** of the sensory component are located outside the CNS; the ganglia of the motor nerves are located within the CNS. Increased intracranial pressure results in

Table 21-4 Cranial Nerve Function

Number	Name	Type	Function
I	Olfactory	Sensory	Smell
II	Optic	Sensory	Vision
III	Oculomotor	Motor	Effect on pupillary reaction and size Elevation of upper eyelid Eye adduction and downward rolling
IV	Trochlear	Motor	Upward eye rolling
V	Trigeminal	Mixed	Motor: Muscles of mastication Sensation: Nose, forehead, temple, scalp, lips, tongue and lower jaw
VI	Abducens	Motor	Lateral eye movement
VII	Facial	Mixed	Motor: Muscles of expression Sensory: Taste
VIII	Vestibulocochlear	Sensory	Equilibrium Hearing
IX	Glossopharyngeal	Mixed	Motor: Pharyngeal muscles Sensory: Taste
X	Vagus	Mixed	Motor: Muscles of pharynx and larynx Sensory: Gag reflex
XI	Accessory	Motor	Trapezius and sternocleidomastoid muscles
XII	Hypoglossal	Motor	Tongue movement

Clinical Application

Function	Cranial Nerves	How Tested
Eye Assessment	II, III, IV, VI	Visual acuity, pupillary reaction, and tracking
Balance	VIII	Romberg test, BESS
Speaking/Hearing	VIII, IX, X, XII	Speaking to the patient; the patient speaking
Facial Expression	V, VII, XII	Smile, frown, stick out tongue
Smelling	I	Based on self-reported symptoms (often a "foul odor")
Shoulder Shrug	XI	Resist shoulder girdle raise

impairment of the motor component of the cranial nerves involved but leaves their sensory component intact.

Cranial nerve function

An assessment of the cranial nerves must be conducted immediately after the injury and repeated at 15- to 20-minute intervals until the severity of the head injury has been determined. Accumulation of blood within the cranium shifts the brain hemisphere, placing pressure on the cranial nerves, impairing their function. Information regarding the loss of many of these functions, such as vision, smell, and taste, is volunteered by the athlete. The following tests are ordered by the affected organ rather than by the cranial nerves themselves.

- **Eyes:** Vision (CN II) is assessed using a Snellen chart (see Fig. 19-5) or by reading an object of reasonable size for normal vision, such as the amount of time remaining on the scoreboard. With the use of a penlight, the **pupil's reaction to light** (CN III) is determined by covering one of the athlete's eyes and briefly shining the light into the opposite pupil. Normally, the pupil should constrict when the light strikes it and dilate when the light is removed. Using a penlight, finger, or other object held approximately 2 feet from the athlete's nose, the equality of **eye movement** (CNs III, IV, and VI) is determined by moving the object up, down, left, right, and, finally, inward toward the athlete's nose.

Ganglion (nerve) (pl. ganglia) A collection of nerve cell bodies housed in the central or peripheral nervous system.

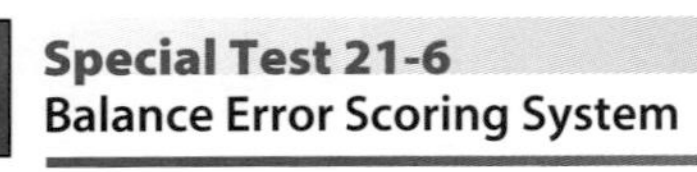

Special Test 21-6
Balance Error Scoring System

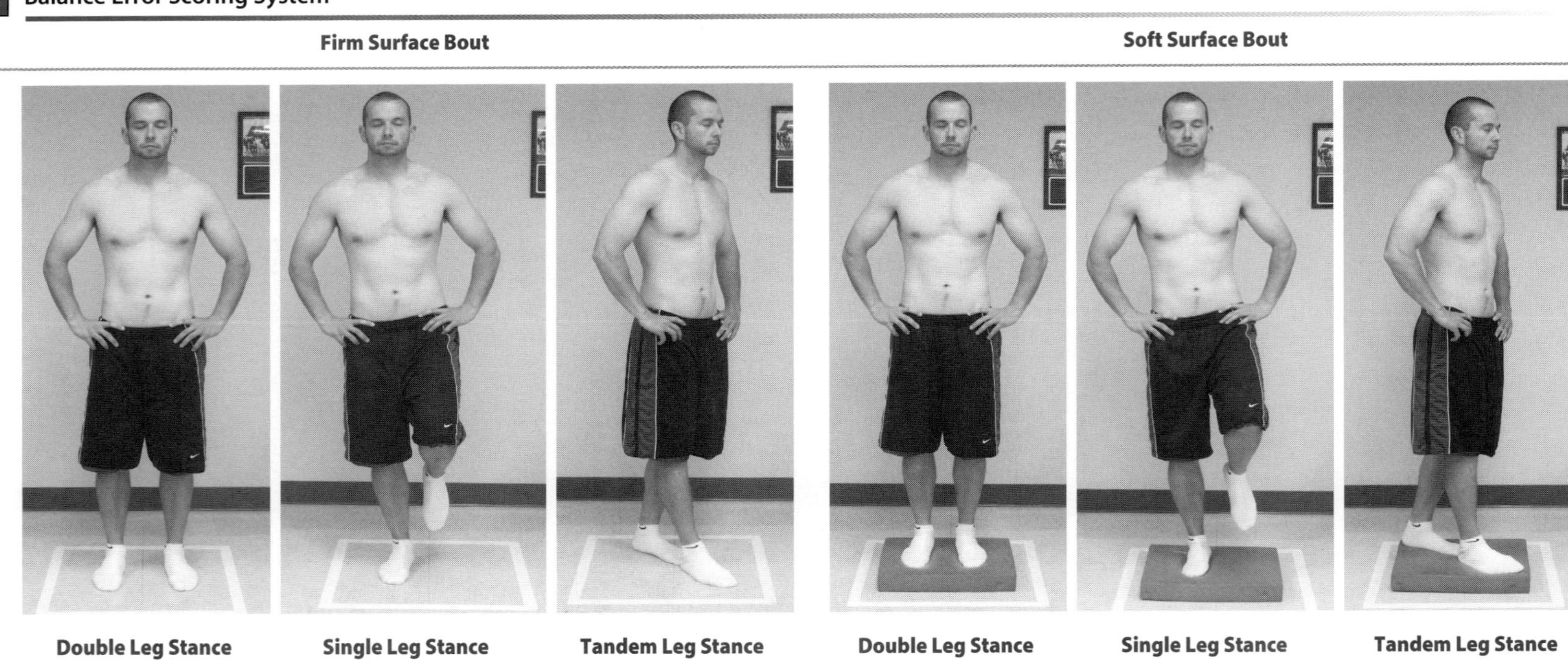

The balance error scoring system involves three different stances, each completed twice, once while standing on a firm surface and again while standing on a foam surface.

Patient Position	The patient is barefoot or wearing socks. The ankle must not be taped during the test. The patient assumes the following stances for each phase of the test: ***Phase 1:*** Double leg stance ***Phase 2:*** Single leg stance—standing on the nondominant leg. The non–weight-bearing hip is flexed to 20°–30° and the knee is flexed to 40°–50°. ***Phase 3:*** Tandem leg stance—The nondominant leg is placed behind the dominant leg and the patient stands in a heel–toe manner. The patient's hands are placed on the iliac crests. The eyes are closed during the test.
Position of Examiner	The examiner stands in front of the athlete. A stopwatch is required to time the trials. A second clinician acts as a spotter.
Evaluative Procedure	The first battery of tests is performed with the patient standing on a firm surface. The patient assumes the double leg stance and attempts to hold the position for 20 seconds. The test is repeated using the single leg stance and then the tandem leg stance. The second battery of tests is performed with the patient standing on a piece of medium density foam (60 kg/m^3) that is 45 cm × 45 cm and 13 cm thick. The trial is incomplete if the patient cannot hold the testing position for a minimum of 5 seconds.

Scoring	One point is scored for each of the following errors: Lifting hands off the iliac crest Opening the eyes Stepping, stumbling, or falling Moving the hip into more than 30° of flexion or abduction Lifting the foot or heel Remaining out of the testing position for more than 5 seconds If more than one error occurs simultaneously, only one error is recorded. Patients who are unable to hold the testing position for 5 seconds are assigned the score of 10.
Positive Test	Scores that are 25% above the patient's baseline or the norm[36] An increase in 3 BESS errors represents a clinically significant change. Performance on the BESS improves with repeated testing, a practice effect.[36,37]
Implications	Impaired cerebral function
Modification	Not applicable
Comments	To improve accuracy, BESS pretests and postinjury tests should be administered in the same environmental conditions (e.g., athletic training facility, sideline).[38] BESS scores correlate well with scores acquired from more sophisticated balance equipment.[34]
Evidence	***Intra-rater Reliability:*** Not Reliable — Very Reliable Poor / Moderate / Good 0 0.1 0.2 0.3 0.4 0.5 0.6 0.7 0.8 0.9 1.0

Diplopia experienced after the injury may indicate cerebral dysfunction; pressure on CN III, IV, or VI, causing spasm of the eye's extrinsic muscles; or a fracture of the eye's orbit. Diplopia that does not rapidly subside indicates the immediate need for advanced medical assistance.

- **Face:** The athlete is asked to raise the eyebrows and forehead, smile, and frown (CN VII); clench the jaw (CN V); swallow (CNs IX and X); and stick out the tongue (CN XII).
- **Ears:** The functions of CN VIII include hearing, in which any disruption should be apparent. Tinnitus demonstrates possible malfunctions of CN VIII. Balance and equilibrium can be assessed through the Romberg test.
- **Shoulders and neck:** If the presence of a cervical injury has been ruled out, strength assessment of the cervical spine musculature should be performed (see Manual Muscle Tests 14-1 to 14-4). Resisted shoulder shrugs are used to determine the integrity of CN XI.

Spinal nerve root evaluation

A complete neurologic evaluation is required when brain or spinal cord trauma is suspected. A complete upper and lower quarter neurologic screen is necessary to test for normal sensory, motor, and reflex functions (see Chapter 1). The neurologic tests to be performed while the athlete is still down are less nerve root-specific and are explained in the "On-Field Management of Head and Cervical Spine Injuries" section of this chapter.

Head and Cervical Spine Pathologies and Related Special Tests

Organized football has a fatality rate of three deaths per 100,000 participants.[39] Many of these fatalities are attributed to head or cervical spine trauma.[39] However, head and cervical spine trauma can—and does—occur in sports other than football. Therefore, emergency preparedness is not limited to the sport of football but, rather, should encompass all of an institution's or organization's athletic programs.

The ability to correctly identify and manage athletes with these conditions in a timely, safe, and efficient manner is a determining factor related to the successful management of a potentially catastrophic injury. Prudent decision making is necessary to determine the athlete's status and disposition. More so than any other type of injury described in this text, a consistent standardized plan of action must be implemented immediately in the management of these conditions.[40]

Head Trauma

Protective headgear has greatly reduced the number and severity of brain injuries in sports mandating their use. The incidence of skull fractures and skin lacerations in areas directly protected by the helmet has been virtually eliminated. The symptoms of head injuries may increase with time, so even athletes who have been released in apparently good health after a head injury need to be given information about signs and symptoms of head injuries. These instructions should also be communicated to the athlete's parents, roommate, or spouse (see "Home Instructions").

Traumatic brain injury

Traumatic brain injury (also referred to as a concussion), is characterized by immediate but transient posttraumatic impairment of brain function. Mental confusion, alteration of mental status, and amnesia are the hallmarks of concussion symptoms that may or may not also include the loss of consciousness.[1,17] Some brain cells are destroyed as a direct result of the concussive force, and other cells are placed at risk of further trauma secondary to changes in cerebral blood flow, increased intracranial pressure, and apnea.[41] After the trauma, a paradoxical period occurs that involves an increased demand for glucose to fuel cell metabolism along with a decrease in the blood flow needed to deliver these nutrients.[41] During this time, the risk for further brain trauma increases if the athlete is allowed to return to competition and suffers another head injury.[18]

Repeated head trauma may produce cumulative degenerative effects on brain function. Athletes with a history of multiple concussions can display the signs and symptoms of a current concussion in the absence of a recent history of head trauma.[29] In addition, a concussion may produce lingering effects, be magnified by subsequent concussions, or mask underlying brain trauma.

No anatomic or physiologic findings exist on which to base a diagnosis of a concussion or determine its severity. The diagnosis of a concussion is based on the duration of the loss of consciousness (if any) and neuropsychological findings.[41] In the absence of a loss of consciousness, the immediate signs of a concussion are based on the patient's behavior (Table 21-5).[17] Approximately 85% to 90 percent of slight to mild concussions are not reported until after the practice or game.[23] Other symptoms associated with concussions include dizziness, tinnitus, nausea, memory loss, and motor impairment, with the symptoms occurring along a continuum ranging from no disruption to total disruption (Table 21-6). Severe cases may also be marked by convulsions, vomiting, and loss of bowel and bladder control (Examination Findings 21-1). Delayed symptoms may include personality changes, fatigue, sleep disturbances,

Table 21-5 Behavioral Signs and Symptoms of Concussion

Sign	Behavior
Vacant Stare	Confused or blank facial expression
Delayed Verbal and Motor Responses	Slow to answer questions or follow instructions
Inability to Focus Attention	Easily distracted; unable to complete normal activities
Disorientation	Walking in the wrong direction; time, date, and place disorientation
Slurred or Incoherent Speech	Rambling, disjointed, incomprehensible statements
Gross Incoordination	Stumbling; inability to walk a straight line
Heightened Emotions	Appearing distraught, crying for no apparent reason, emotional responses that are out of proportion to the circumstances
Memory Deficits	As evidenced by the retrograde and anterograde memory tests

lethargy, depression, and difficulty performing activities of daily living.[41] Because concussion symptoms are multifaceted and vary from person to person, techniques that assess neurocognitive functioning, patient-described symptoms, and postural control must be used. Magnetic resonance imaging (MRI) may be used to identify other forms of traumatic brain injury, and computed tomography (CT) scans may be used to image intracranial bleeding or swelling.[41]

A postconcussion symptom scale (or postconcussion checklist) should be used to monitor the patient following mild traumatic brain injury (Table 21-7).[40] When compared to baseline (pre-injury) scores, these scales help to provide an objective assessment of changes in the patient's symptoms (Fig. 21-13). Most standardized symptoms scales demonstrate moderate to good statistical reliability.[42,43]

The **Standardized Assessment of Concussion Instrument** (SAC) has been developed specifically for athletes (Special Test 21-7).[41,44] The SAC protocol is a useful adjunct to neuropsychological and balance testing, but does not replace formal neurologic testing or medical evaluation.

The magnitude of severely brain injured individuals can be quantified using the **Glasgow coma scale** (Table 21-8). The normal score on this battery is 15. Patients scoring 11 or higher on this instrument have an excellent prognosis for recovery. Scores of 7 or less represent serious brain dysfunction.

Concussion rating systems. Several different rating scales are used to quantify the severity of concussions; however, their use is not recommended by all authorities. Quantifying concussion severity before all symptoms have

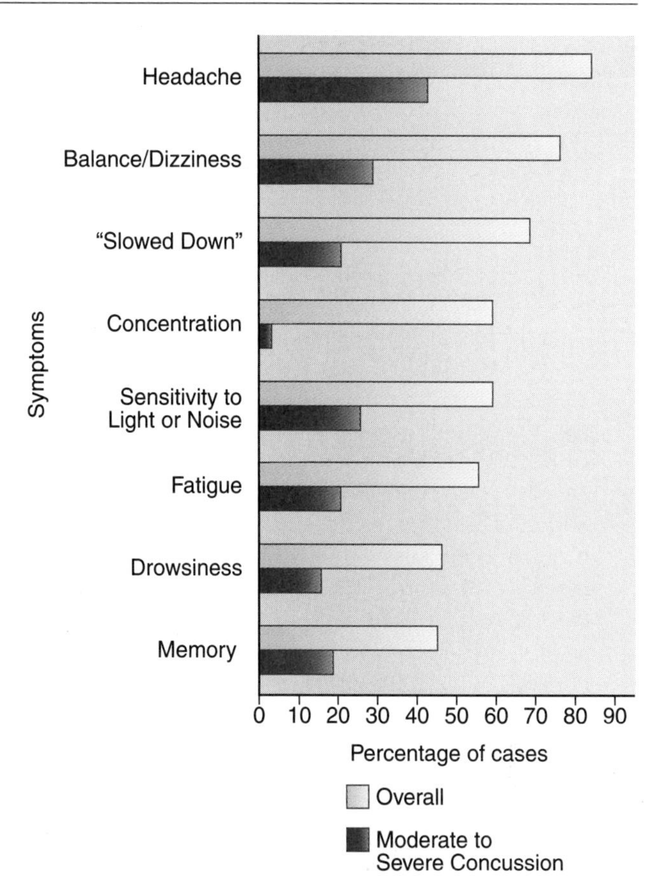

FIGURE 21-13 ■ Graph of cumulative effects associated with recurrent concussion in collegiate football players. (From Guskiewicz, KM, et al: Cumulative effects associated with recurrent concussion in collegiate football players. The NCAA concussion study. *JAMA*, 290:2549, 2003.)

cleared may provide inaccurate expectations of recovery.[45] Table 21-9 presents five of the commonly used classification systems for athletic-related head trauma.[46–48] There is disparity among these systems, with different emphases on loss of consciousness and postconcussion symptoms. In one system, an athlete may be classified as having a grade III concussion, yet in another system this same person may only have a grade I concussion.[23] Likewise, the systems are considered to be overly conservative for the athletic population.[23]

These systems are presented as a framework of the different classification schemes that are used with an athletic population. Institutions should use these systems as the basis for their own standard operating procedures. To determine the extent of the injury, the findings of a cerebral concussion evaluation should be compared with the dysfunction guide in Table 21-6.

*** Practical Evidence**

Loss of consciousness, amnesia lasting longer than 15 minutes, or any worsening of the symptoms presented in Table 21-6 warrant a physician referral.[50]

Table 21-6 Dysfunction Guide for Evaluating the Extent of Cerebral Concussions

Function	Slight	Severe	Comments
Consciousness	No loss of consciousness	Unconscious for 10 seconds to 1 minute or altered consciousness for less than 2 minutes	Institutional standard operating procedures should identify the minimum duration of unconsciousness required to activate emergency medical services.
Memory	The patient is initially unable to remember the immediate events leading to the trauma	Retrograde amnesia: Inability to remember events before the mechanism of injury Anterograde amnesia: Inability to remember events after the injury	Transitory loss of memory of the injurious contact is to be expected and often associated with a brief loss of consciousness ("seeing stars" or "blacking out").
Cognitive Function	Slight transient mental confusion ("What happened?")	Disorientation to person, place, or time Demonstration of violent, aggressive, and otherwise inappropriate behavior or language Inability to process information "normally"	These traits may be expected immediately after the injury. Their continued presence is correlated with the severity of the injury.
Balance and Coordination	Slight unsteadiness or unsteadiness that rapidly subsides	Profound disruption of balance and coordination; inability to walk without assistance and difficulty performing basic manual skills	These functions are based not only on the results of Romberg's test and the heel-toe walk but also on general observation.
Tinnitus	None or transitory	Prolonged tinnitus or tinnitus worsening over time	Ringing in the ears may be described immediately after the blow but should subside with time.
Pupil Size	Equal; both pupils responsive to light	Dilated pupil that is unresponsive to light	Pupillary change indicates increased intracranial pressure on CN III, indicative of intracranial bleeding. Unequal pupil size (anisocoria) may be normally present.
Nystagmus	Absent	Present	Nystagmus indicates increased intracranial pressure or inner ear dysfunction. This may be a normal finding.
Vision	Normal or initially blurred, which quickly subsides	Persistent blurred or double vision	The athlete's normal vision should be taken into account (i.e., if the athlete wears glasses).
Nausea	None or slight	Vomiting	Cumulative effect
Pulse	Within normal limits, possible decreasing with rest	Abnormally increasing or decreasing	Abnormal changes in pulse indicate intracranial hemorrhage.
Blood Pressure	Within normal limits	Rapidly rising or falling	Rapid blood pressure changes suggest intracranial hematoma.
Respirations	Normal	Abnormal	See "Functional Testing" section of this chapter.

CN = cranial nerve.

Examination Findings 21-1
Concussion

Examination Segment	Clinical Findings
History	***Onset:*** Acute ***Chief complaints:*** Headache, ringing in the ears, blurred vision, dizziness, unconsciousness (see Tables 21-2 and 21-4) ***Mechanism:*** Blow to the skull or spinal column transmitting an injurious force to the brain ***Predisposing conditions:*** A recent history of a cerebral concussion or a past history of repeated subconcussive forces to the head
Inspection	***Eyes:*** Generally may appear glazed or dazed. Pupil sizes should be equal; a unilaterally dilated pupil may indicate pressure on CN III. Nystagmus may indicate pressure on the CNs or dysfunction within the inner ear. ***Nose and ears:*** Any fluid draining from the nose and ears is checked for the presence of CSF. ***General:*** Severe concussions may result in convulsions. The entire skull requires inspection for secondary bleeding or contusions. The area over the mastoid process and the area beneath the eyes are checked for ecchymosis, indicating a skull fracture.
Palpation	If the patient was not wearing a helmet at the time of injury, palpate the skull to determine areas of point tenderness, possibly indicating the presence of a skull fracture.
Functional Tests	***Memory:*** Transient retrograde amnesia of the events leading up to the injury is possible. An increased scope of memory loss may indicate a severe concussion. The presence of anterograde amnesia warrants immediate referral to a physician. ***Cognitive function:*** The patient may display confused, violent, or aggressive behavior and may have diminished analytical function. ***Balance and coordination:*** These functions are diminished immediately after the injury but should return rapidly. Romberg's test and heel–toe walk (balance and coordination) ***Eyes:*** Blurred vision and unequal pupil size are present. ***Motor function:*** Partial and transitory motor loss may occur secondary to trauma to the motor and premotor cortexes. ***Vital signs:*** Monitor pulse, blood pressure, and respiration.
Special Tests	Halo test
Neurologic Screening	Retrograde amnesia test and anterograde amnesia test repeated at regular intervals. Balance Error Scoring System Cerebral function tests (e.g., 100 minus 7) Standardized Assessment of Concussion score Glasgow coma scale (used with profoundly head-injured patients) CN assessment Sensory testing Motor testing
Vascular Screening	Within normal limits
Imaging Techniques	MRI or CT scans are used to rule out intracranial hemorrhage, but these findings are not directly useful in making return-to-play decisions.[17]
Differential Diagnosis	Intracranial hemorrhage, second impact syndrome, heat illness, drug overdose or interaction
Comments	The possibility of a cervical spine fracture must be assumed until such an injury can be ruled out. When the severity of the injury is in doubt, refer the patient to a physician for further evaluation. Athletes who are unconscious for a measurable period of time must be cleared by a physician before returning to competition. An athlete with a history of multiple head trauma or having symptoms after little or no physical trauma should always be referred for further assessment by a physician (see "Postconcussion Syndrome and Second Impact Syndrome" section).

CN = cranial nerve; CT = computed tomography; CSF = cerebrospinal fluid; MRI = magnetic resonance imaging.

Table 21-7 Postconcussion Symptom Scale

Symptom	Preseason Baseline	Time of Injury	2 to 3 Hours Postinjury
Headache	0	2	4
Nausea	0	3	2
Vomiting	0	0	2
Dizziness	0	4	2
Poor Balance	0	4	2
Sensitivity to Noise	0	1	2
Ringing in the Ears	0	5	1
Sensitivity to Light	0	3	3
Blurred Vision	1	3	2
Poor Concentration	0	2	3
Memory Problems	0	2	2
Drowsiness	0	4	4
Fatigue	1	5	4
Sadness/Depression	1	5	4
Irritability	0	4	5
Neck Pain	0	0	0
TOTAL SCORE	3	47	42

Each symptom is graded on a scale of 0 (none) to 6 (severe). Columns are summed to demonstrate the patient's current state.

Table 21-8 The Glasgow Coma Scale

Response	Points	Action
Eye Opening		
Spontaneously	4	Reticular system is intact; patient may not be aware
To verbal command	3	Opens eyes when told to do so
To pain	2	Opens eyes in response to pain
None	1	Does not open eyes to any stimuli
Verbal		
Oriented, converses	5	Relatively intact CNS; aware of self and surroundings
Disoriented, converses	4	Well articulated, organized, but disoriented
Inappropriate words	3	Random, exclamatory words
Incomprehensible	2	No recognizable words
No response	1	No audible sounds or intubated
Motor		
Obeys verbal commands	6	Readily moves limbs when told to
Localizes painful stimuli	5	Moves limb in an effort to avoid pain
Flexion withdrawal	4	Pulls away from pain with a flexion motion
Abnormal flexion	3	Exhibits decorticate rigidity
Extension	2	Exhibits decerebrate rigidity
No response	1	Demonstrates dypotonicity, flaccid: Suggests loss of medullary function or spinal cord injury

CNS = central nervous system.

Special Test 21-7
Standardized Assessment of Concussion

Orientation (1 point each)

	Correct
Month	☐
Date	☐
Day of week	☐
Year	☐
Time (within 1 hour)	☐
Score	____/5

Delayed Recall (1 point each)

	Correct
Word 1	☐
Word 2	☐
Word 3	☐
Word 4	☐
Word 5	☐
Score	___/5

Immediate Memory (1 point for each correct response)

	Trial 1	Trial 2	Trial 3
Word 1	☐	☐	☐
Word 2	☐	☐	☐
Word 3	☐	☐	☐
Word 4	☐	☐	☐
Word 5	☐	☐	☐
Score	☐	☐	___/15

Summary of Total Scores

Orientation	___/5
Immediate memory	___/15
Concentration	___/5
Delayed recall	___/5
TOTAL SCORE	___/30

Concentration
Reverse Digits (1 point each for each string length)

		Correct
3–8–2	5–1–8	☐
2–7–9–3	2–1–6–8	☐
5–1–8–6–9	9–4–1–7–5	☐
6–9–7–3–5–1	4–2–8–9–3–7	☐

Months of the Year in Reverse Order (1point for sequence correct)

	Correct
Dec–Nov–Oct–Sept–Aug–July	
June–May–Apr–Mar–Feb–Jan	☐
Score	___/5

The following are performed between the Immediate Memory and Delayed Recall portions of the SAC, along with tests for memory, cerebral function, and strength.

Neurologic Screening
- Recollection of the injury
- Strength:
- Sensation:
- Coordination

Exertional Maneuvers (when appropriate)
- 1 40-yard sprint
- 5 sit-ups
- 5 push-ups
- 5 knee bends

Procedures

(Administration time is approximately 5 minutes): Proper training is required for appropriate use.

Orientation	Patient is asked to identify the current place in time and receives 1 point for each correct response.
Immediate Memory	The patient is asked to memorize a list of 5 random words. The list of words is repeated 3 times in succession, with 1 point being awarded for each correct response for a maximum total of 15 points. This list of words will be used for the delayed memory testing, but do not inform the patient as such.
Neurologic Screening	The patient is evaluated for loss of consciousness, amnesia, etc.
Concentration	***Reverse digits:*** The patient is given a sequence of numbers and asked to repeat them in reverse order (i.e., 2–8–3 would be recited as 3–8–2). If the patient correctly responds on the first attempt, progress to the next string length. If the patient incorrectly responds on the first attempt, use a second set of digits for the second attempt. If the patient incorrectly responds on the second attempt, move on to months of the year. ***Months of year:*** The patient is asked to recite the months of the year in reverse order.
Delayed Recall	Approximately 5 minutes after the "Immediate Memory" test, the patient is asked to recall the list of words that were used for the immediate memory test. One point is awarded for each correct response.
Total	The scores for each of the four sections are totaled to yield an overall index of impairment. A decrease from baseline of 2 points is clinically significant.[36]
Comments	Normal females score higher on the SAC than males.
Evidence	Absent or inconclusive in the literature

Table 21-9 Concussion Rating Systems

Rating System	Signs and Symptoms		
	Grade I	**Grade II**	**Grade III**
American Academy of Neurology[46]	No loss of consciousness Transient confusion Concussion symptoms resolve in less than 15 minutes	No loss of consciousness Transient confusion Concussion symptoms or mental status abnormalities on examination resolve in more than 15 minutes	Any loss of consciousness either brief (seconds) or prolonged (minutes)
American College of Sports Medicine Guidelines[46]	None or transient retrograde amnesia None to slight mental confusion No loss of coordination Transient dizziness Rapid recovery	Retrograde amnesia; memory may return slight to moderate mental confusion Moderate dizziness Transitory tinnitus Slow recovery	Sustained retrograde amnesia; anterograde is possible with intracranial hemorrhage Severe mental confusion Profound loss of coordination Obvious motor impairment Prolonged tinnitus Delayed recovery
Cantu Concussion Rating Guidelines[49]	No loss of consciousness Concussion symptoms resolving in less than 15 minutes Posttraumatic amnesia for less than 30 minutes	Loss of consciousness for less than 5 minutes Posttraumatic amnesia for more than 30 minutes but less than 24 hours	Loss of consciousness for more than 5 minutes Posttraumatic amnesia for more than 24 hours
Colorado Medical Society Concussion Rating Guidelines[48]	No loss of consciousness Transient confusion No amnesia	No loss of consciousness Transient confusion Amnesia	Loss of consciousness
Prague Group[45]	Simple Injury resolves over 7–10 days	Complex Persistent symptoms, specific, specific sequelae, prolonged loss of consciousness (>1 minute) or prolonged cognitive impairment	

Return-to-play criteria. Determining the time for the safe return to play after a head injury is a medical challenge. Some severe head injuries may not produce significant signs or symptoms for some time after the actual trauma. This fact alone suggests that it is better to err on the side of caution when making return-to-play decisions. The *National Collegiate Athletic Association's Sports Medicine Handbook* recommends that athletes who have been rendered unconscious should not be returned to activity that day and should not return to activity while displaying postconcussion symptoms, including a headache.[51]

An athlete who sustains a mild concussion may be allowed to return to participation after all the signs and symptoms have cleared and remain clear with exertional activity. Athletes sustaining a moderate or severe concussion should not return to competition for several days, weeks, or months after the injury. Table 21-10 presents the recommended time to return to competition after cerebral concussions, assuming that all of the athlete's symptoms have cleared.[52] This table clearly illustrates the inherent risk of early concussion grading.

Using concussion grading immediately following the injury may not provide sufficient return-to-play guidelines. The Zurich group recommends the following process[17a]:

1. No activity, complete rest. Once asymptomatic, proceed to next activity level.
2. Light aerobic exercise such as walking or stationary cycling, no resistance training.
3. Sport-specific exercise (e.g., skating in hockey, running in soccer), progressive addition of resistance training at steps 3 or 4
4. Non-contact training drills
5. Full contact training after medical clearance.
6. Game participation

Athletes move to the next level if they are asymptomatic at that level and no post-activity symptoms occur. If symptoms recur during or after activity, the athlete drops back to the previous level. Treatment of concussions may also require "cognitive rest" such as avoiding studying or attending classes.

Table 21-10 Guidelines for Returning to Play After a Cerebral Concussion

Grade	1st Concussion	2nd Concussion	3rd Concussion
Grade 1 (mild)	May return to play if asymptomatic.	Return to play in 2 weeks if the athlete is asymptomatic during the previous week.	Terminate season; may return to play the following season if asymptomatic.
Grade 2 (moderate)	Return to play after being asymptomatic for 1 week.	Out a minimum of 1 month; may return to play then if asymptomatic for 1 week; consider terminating season.	Terminate season; may return to play the following season if asymptomatic.
Grade 3 (severe)	Out a minimum of 1 month; may then return to play if asymptomatic for 1 week.	Terminate season; may return to play the following season if asymptomatic. Consider terminating Career.	Terminate career in contact sports.

External provocation tests can be used to determine if exercise will cause the symptoms to return.[46] The athlete performs exercises (e.g., a 40-yard sprint, 5 push-ups, 5 sit-ups) and is then evaluated for the presence or reoccurrence of concussion symptoms. The athlete should be withheld from competition if symptoms are present or if he or she is unable to complete the exercises.

Returning an athlete who has sustained a head injury to competition is ultimately a physician's decision. Prematurely returning an athlete to competition can increase the effects of postconcussion syndrome, increase the risk of subsequent concussions, and predispose the individual to second impact syndrome.[11] There is universal agreement, however, that the athlete should not be returned to practice or competition while experiencing any concussion symptoms or be returned to competition on the same day in which consciousness was lost. After a grade I or grade II concussion, the athlete should be returned to activity under controlled conditions, progressively working toward unrestricted participation.[23]

*** Practical Evidence**

In contact sports such as football, an athlete who sustains a "mild" head injury has three to four times the risk of sustaining another head injury.[29,53]

Postconcussion syndrome

Athletes suffering a cerebral concussion may describe a number of cognitive impairments for some time after the injury.[52] The extended duration of these symptoms is thought to be related to altered neurotransmitter function.[54] Postconcussion syndrome, residual concussion symptoms that persist for more than 3 months after the injury represent disruption of the brain, especially the upper brain stem, frontal lobe, and temporal lobe.[55]

Postconcussion syndrome is characterized by decreased attention span, trouble concentrating, impaired memory, and irritability over both the short and long term (Table 21-11).[56] Exercise may cause headaches, dizziness, and premature fatigue.[54] Long-term consequences of postconcussion syndrome are balance disruptions, decreased cognitive performance, and emotional depression.[17,57] With time, social interaction, academic performance, and job performance are significantly impaired.[17] These symptoms may predispose the individual to second impact syndrome and may require that the patient be further evaluated by a neurosurgeon. Cognitive rest, possibly including school work and exertion during ADLs may also be indicated.[45] The athlete should not be returned to competition until postconcussion syndromes have ceased. CT scans and neuropsychologic tests must show negative findings.

Second impact syndrome

A rare but possible consequence of returning an athlete to competition too soon after a concussion is an increased risk of second impact syndrome, the result of a second concussion occurring while the individual is still symptomatic from

Table 21-11 Early and Late Signs and Symptoms of Postconcussion Syndrome

Early	Late
Disorientation	Lack of concentration
Confusion	Poor memory
Headache	Irritability
Dizziness	Depression
Blurred vision	Anxiety
Nausea	Fatigue
Drowsiness	Headache
Sleep disturbance	Sleep disturbance

an earlier concussion. The second trauma, often a minor blow or contrecoup mechanism, increases cerebrovascular congestion, or a loss of cerebrovascular autoregulation, leading to brain edema and increased intracranial pressure.[17]

The second trauma is thought to disrupt the autoregulation of the brain's blood supply, resulting in vasodilation and the subsequent engorgement of the intracranial vasculature.[58] The increased blood flow and vascular expanse increase the intracranial pressure and quickly disrupt the normal function of the brain stem. Outward signs of spinal and cranial nerve involvement occur within 2 minutes of the trauma.

Initially the athlete may display the signs and symptoms of a grade I concussion but quickly collapses in a semicomatose state. Pressure on the cranial nerves results in rapidly dilating pupils that are unresponsive to light and the loss of eye motion.[54] As the pressure continues to build, the athlete displays signs of respiratory distress secondary to disruption of phrenic nerve activity.

Intervention must be swift and concise. The physician, paramedic, or other qualified personnel should intubate the athlete and may induce hyperventilation to facilitate vasoconstriction secondary to decreased carbon dioxide in the bloodstream. Even in the best-case scenarios, second impact syndrome has a 50% mortality rate. This severity emphasizes the importance of preventing this occurrence by prohibiting athletes from returning to athletic competition until all symptoms of a cerebral concussion have subsided and a physician has cleared the athlete's return to activity.

Intracranial hemorrhage

Rupture of the blood vessels supplying the brain results in an intracranial hematoma, named relative to the meninges (Fig. 21-14). Intracranial hematoma may also develop after disruption of the sinus separating the two brain hemispheres. Subsequent hematoma formation within the enclosed space (the cranium) places pressure on the brain and may have catastrophic results (see Table 21-2). The length of time until the onset of symptoms varies, depending on the type of bleeding involved (arterial or venous) and the location relative to the dura mater (above or below it).

Epidural hematoma. Arterial bleeding between the dura mater and the skull results in the rapid formation of an epidural hematoma, with the onset of symptoms occurring within hours after the initial injury. The mechanism of this injury is that of a concussion, a blow to the head that jars the brain. Because of the concussive mechanism, the athlete may be briefly unconscious and may show the signs and symptoms of mild concussion, although these are not prerequisite symptoms. These symptoms quickly subside, and the athlete progresses through a very **lucid** period (Table 21-12).

As the size of the hematoma increases, the athlete's condition deteriorates at a rate proportional to the amount of intracranial bleeding. The individual becomes disoriented, displays abnormal behavior, and complains of or displays drowsiness. A headache of increasing intensity may be reported, indicating pressure on the periosteum of the skull or an insult to the dura mater. Continued expansion of the hematoma results in outward symptoms via the cranial nerves; a unilaterally dilated pupil is the most common sign.

Subdural hematoma. Hematoma formation between the brain and dura mater usually involves venous bleeding. This type of injury accounts for the majority of deaths resulting from athletic-related head trauma.[59] Because venous bleeding occurs at a lower pressure than arterial bleeding and because the blood collects within the fissures and sulci, the symptoms occur hours, days, or even weeks after the initial trauma. Whereas acute subdural hematomas become symptomatic within 48 hours, chronic hematomas may not manifest symptoms until 30 days after the trauma.[60]

Subdural hematomas are classified as simple or complex. No direct cerebral damage is associated with a simple subdural hematoma. Complex subdural hematomas are

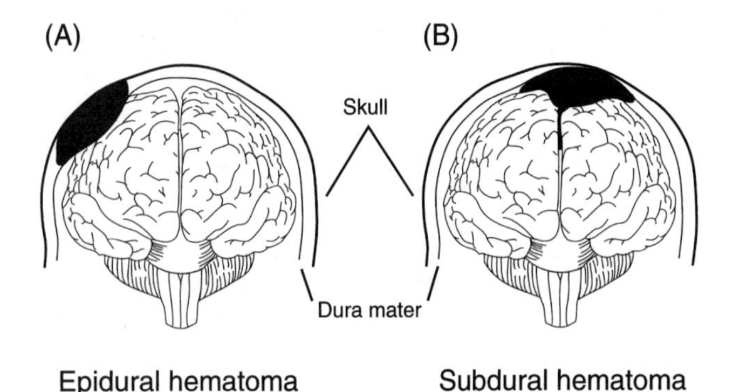

FIGURE 21-14 ■ Intracranial hemorrhage. (A) Epidural hematoma, arterial bleeding between the skull and dura mater. (B) Subdural hematoma, venous bleeding between the dura mater and brain. The meningeal spaces have been enlarged for clarity.

Table 21-12	Progression of Symptoms Associated with an Epidural Hematoma
Patient is unconscious or has other signs of a concussion (these are not prerequisite findings).	
The patient has a period of very lucid consciousness, perhaps eliminating the suspicion of a serious concussion.	
Patient appears to become disoriented, confused, and drowsy.	
Complaints of a headache that increase in intensity with time	
Signs and signals of cranial nerve disruption	
Onset of coma	
If untreated, death or permanent brain damage occurs.	

Lucid Mentally clear.

characterized by contusions of the brain's surface and associated cerebral swelling.

Initially after the injury, the individual is very lucid, even to the point of not displaying any of the signs or symptoms of a cerebral concussion. However, as blood accumulates within the brain, the patient begins to develop headaches, accompanied by a clouding of consciousness.[61] Further hematoma formation results in the impairment of cognitive, behavioral, and motor ability, and signs of cranial nerve dysfunction may be observed. The potentially long duration between the trauma and the onset of symptoms illustrates the need for home instructions identifying the latent signs and symptoms of head injuries.

Skull fractures

The prevalence of skull fractures is much higher in athletes who are not wearing headgear than in those who are. However, skull fractures can still occur in a head that is protected, especially in the bones around the helmet's periphery. Skull fractures are typically classified as **linear, comminuted,** or **depressed** (Fig. 21-15).

Linear fractures, referred to as hairline fractures in long bones, are caused by a blunt impact to the cranium. The subsequent swelling causes the loss of the skull's rounded contour in the traumatized area. Comminuted skull fractures result in fragmentation of the skull. A slight depression is felt during gentle palpation of the fractured area. If the blunt force is of enough intensity or fails to become deflected by the round shape of the skull, a depressed fracture can occur. The skull's indentation is obvious on gross inspection. Additional concern is focused around the possibility of the fractured pieces of bone lacerating the meninges and brain.

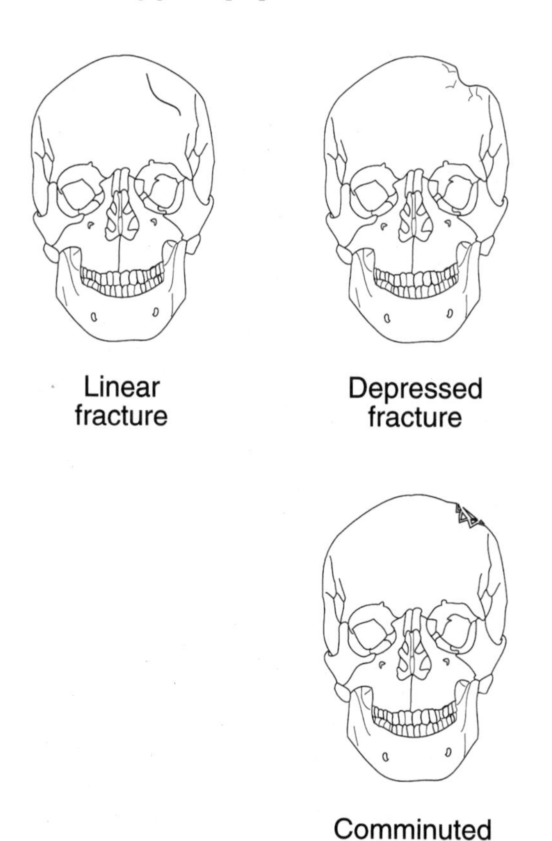

FIGURE 21-15 ■ Types of skull fractures: linear, depressed, and comminuted.

Although depressed skull fractures are often obvious during inspection, linear and comminuted fractures are less evident. The traumatic impact often results in a laceration of the overlying skin. Although the bleeding must be controlled, no material or object should be inserted into the laceration or possible fracture site. Fractures of the ethmoid or temporal bones may result in the leakage of CSF from the nose or ears or in bleeding from the ears (see Special Test 21-1). With time, ecchymosis may accumulate beneath the eyes and over the mastoid process (Battle's sign; Examination Findings 21-2). In addition to these symptoms, the patient may also describe the signs and symptoms of a concussion caused by the blow to the skull.

*** Practical Evidence**

After a blow to the head, and one or more episodes of vomiting, the probability of a skull fracture triples in adults and more than doubles in children.[62]

Cervical Spinal Cord Trauma

The advent of protective football helmets made the head an attractive weapon for blockers, tacklers, and ball carriers. The resulting axial load on the cervical spine caused a high rate of cervical fractures and dislocations, many producing catastrophic results. During the 1976 season, the National Collegiate Athletic Association (NCAA) and the National Federation of State High School Associations (NFHSA) adopted rules outlawing contact with opposing players using the top (crown) of the helmet ("spearing"), a rule change that drastically reduced the incidence of cervical injury in football players.[6,12] Despite this ruling, reviews of game films estimate that spearing still occurs in 19% of football plays, most of which go unpenalized.[16]

Spinal cord function is inhibited by one of two mechanisms: (1) impingement or laceration secondary to bony displacement and (2) compression secondary to hemorrhage, edema, and ischemia of the cord.[63] Although the effects of pressure placed on the spinal cord, with no death of its cells, are often transitory and reversible, actual trauma to the spinal cord itself is rarely reversible and results in permanent disability.

Not all athletes suffering from bony cervical trauma remain on the field. In fact, an athlete who has suffered a cervical fracture or dislocation may walk off under his or her own power. With this in mind, any complaints of pain in the cervical spine, with or without symptoms radiating into the extremities, should always be thought of as a catastrophic injury until otherwise ruled out. Torg[64] has

Examination Findings 21-2
Skull Fractures

Examination Segment	Clinical Findings
History	***Onset:*** Acute ***Pain characteristics:*** Pain over the point of impact; a headache may be described secondary to the trauma. ***Other symptoms:*** The patient may report vomiting.[62] ***Mechanism:*** Blunt trauma to the head; either the skull's being struck by a moving object or the skull's striking a stationary object ***Predisposing conditions:*** Not applicable
Inspection	Bleeding may occur secondary to the blow. Ecchymosis under the eyes ("raccoon eyes") and over the mastoid process (Battle's sign) may be noted. The rounded contour of the skull over the impacted area may be lost.
Palpation	Crepitus may be felt over the fracture site. Palpation should not be performed over areas of obvious fracture.
Special Tests	Halo test
Neurologic Screening	Same as for evaluation of a cerebral concussion: Cranial nerve assessment, sensory testing, and motor testing
Vascular Screening	Within normal limits, unless associated shock symptoms
Functional Assessment	General unwillingness to move
Imaging Techniques	Computed tomography
Differential Diagnosis	Traumatic brain injury
Comments	The presence of a cervical fracture or dislocation must be ruled out. No object should be inserted into the site of a skull laceration (e.g., cleaning the wound, removing deeply impaled objects). Traumatic brain injury may also be associated with this injury. Athletes suspected of suffering from a skull fracture should be immediately referred to a physician.

categorized risk groups, based on underlying trauma, as to their conditions predisposing the athlete to further cervical trauma (Table 21-13).

Trauma to the spinal cord above the C4 level has a high probability of death secondary to disruption of the function of the brain stem or the phrenic nerve. Trauma to the spinal cord anywhere along its length can result in the permanent loss of function of the nerves distal to the traumatized area.

The anatomy of the cervical spine is covered in Chapter 14. Before proceeding with this portion of the chapter, readers should take a moment to refresh their memory as to the important structures and anatomical relationships of this body area. Likewise, Chapter 14 also discusses injuries to the brachial plexus.

Cervical fracture or dislocation

The signs and symptoms of a cervical fracture and those of a dislocation are quite similar. Often these two conditions occur concurrently (Fig. 21-16). Cervical fractures alone do not cause spinal cord trauma. Rather, spinal cord trauma secondary to vertebral fractures results when a bony fragment lacerates the cord; swelling compresses the cord; ischemia affects the cord's cells; or the vertebra shifts, narrowing the spinal canal.

Cervical dislocations represent a much more serious direct threat to the spinal cord. Most often affecting the lower cervical vertebrae (C4–C6) when the cervical spine is forced into flexion and rotation, the superior articular facet passes over the inferior facet. The resulting dislocation decreases the diameter of the spinal canal, often compressing the cord.

The signs and symptoms of a stretch or pinch of the brachial plexus can mimic many of those of a spinal cord injury. The primary differences are found in the relatively rapid fading of symptoms associated with brachial plexus trauma and the fact that the symptoms most often occur unilaterally.

Table 21-13 Risk Factors of Predisposing Conditions Resulting in Permanent Disability

Minimal Risk	Moderate Risk	Extreme Risk
Asymptomatic bone spurs	Acute lateral disk herniation	Acute large central disk
Brachial plexus neurapraxia	Cervical radiculopathy–radial spur	Herniation
Certain healed facet fractures	Facet fractures	Cervical cord anomaly
Healed disk herniation	Lateral mass fractures	Occipitocervical dislocation
Healed lamina fracture	Nondisplaced healed ring of C1 fracture	Odontoid fracture
Healed spinous process fracture	Nondisplaced odontoid fractures	Ruptured C1–C2 transverse ligament
		Stenosis of the cervical canal
		Total ligamentous disruption of the lower cervical spine
		Unstable fracture or dislocation
		Unstable **Jefferson's fracture**

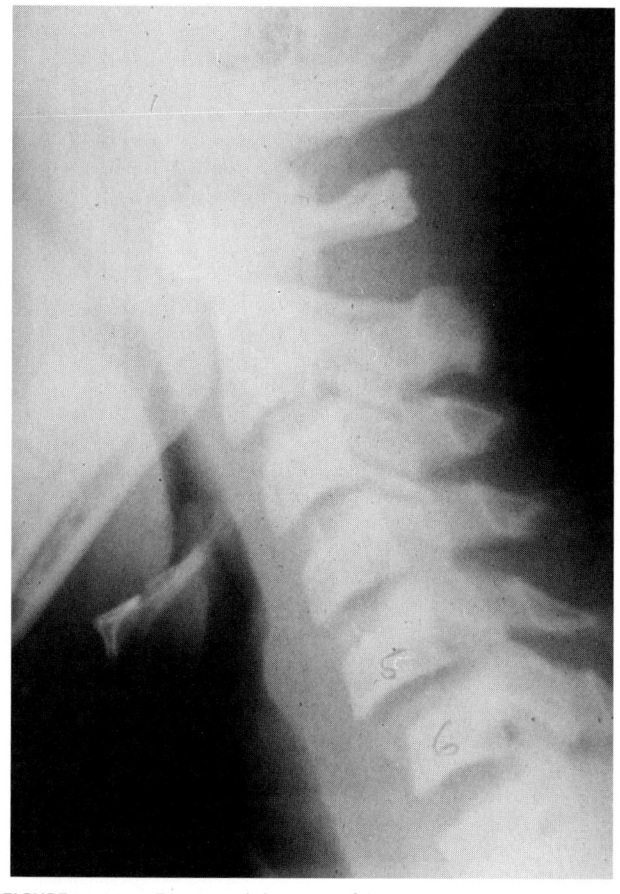

FIGURE 21-16 ■ Fracture–dislocation of the C6 vertebra. Note the posterior displacement of the vertebral body relative to C5 and the fracture of the C6 spinous process.

Jefferson's fracture A fracture of a circular bone in two places; similar to breaking a doughnut in half.

Trauma to the cervical spine itself is identified by pain along its posterior and lateral structures and possible spasm of the surrounding muscles. If there is associated damage to the spinal cord or if displaced bone or swelling is compressing the cord, symptoms are referred to the involved nerve distributions and in those nerves located distal to the site of the insult. Typically, these symptoms involve pain, burning, or numbness radiating into the extremities (Examination Findings 21-3). Fractures of the vertebral body may produce little or no symptoms unless the cervical spine and head are positioned in a manner that places a load on the involved body.

Other than the actual physical trauma, the spinal cord tissue is further damaged by ischemia. Pharmacologically, the use of ganglioside (GM-1), methylprednisolone, and other medications has shown promise in limiting spinal cord trauma.[67,68] The strategy of medically increasing the patient's mean arterial blood pressure above 85 mm Hg has also been demonstrated to assist in reducing the long-term effects of spinal cord trauma.[69]

Transient quadriplegia

Blows to the head that force the cervical spine into hyperextension, hyperflexion, or produce an axial load may result in transient quadriplegia, a body-wide state of decreased or absent sensory and motor function.[65,70,71] This results from neurapraxia of the cervical spinal cord and is predisposed by stenosis of the spinal foramen (especially at the C3–C4 level), congenital fusion of the cervical canal, abnormalities of the posterior arch, or cervical instability.[65] The risk of transient quadriplegia is increased when the ratio between the diameter of the spinal canal and the diameter of the vertebral body is 0.80 or less.[65,72] The narrowing of the spinal canal predisposes the spinal cord to compressive and contusive forces, a condition referred to as spear tackler's spine.[65]

Examination Findings 21-3
Cervical Fracture or Dislocation

Examination Segment	Clinical Findings
History	***Onset:*** Acute ***Pain characteristics:*** Pain in the cervical spine Chest pain ***Other symptoms:*** Numbness, weakness, or paresthesia radiating into the extremities Cervical muscle spasm Loss of bladder or bowel control ***Mechanism:*** Fractures most commonly secondary to an axial load placed on the cervical vertebrae. Dislocations most commonly resulting from hyperflexion or hyperextension and rotation of the cervical spine. ***Predisposing conditions:*** Increased risk of cervical fracture if the normal lordotic curve of the cervical spine is decreased.[65]
Inspection	Malalignment of the cervical spine spinous processes may be observed. The head may be abnormally tilted and rotated. Unilateral cervical dislocations result in the head's tilting toward the site of the dislocation. The muscles on the side opposite the dislocation (tilt) are in spasm. Those muscles on the side of the dislocation are flaccid. Swelling may be present over the ligamentum nuchae.
Palpation	Tenderness, crepitus, or swelling may be present over the cervical spine Unilateral or bilateral muscle spasm may be present.
Joint and Muscle Function Assessment	ROM testing should not be performed if numbness, weakness, or paresthesia radiating into the extremities or bowel and bladder signs are present.
Joint Stability Tests	***Stress tests:*** Not performed acutely ***Joint play:*** Not performed acutely
Special Tests	Not applicable in acute conditions in which a fracture or dislocation is suspected
Neurologic Screening	Upper quarter and lower quarter neurologic screens
Vascular Screening	Within normal limits
Functional Assessment	Within normal limits
Imaging Techniques	Radiographs, MRI, CT scans[66]
Differential Diagnosis	Brachial plexus neuropathy, intervertebral disk injury, cervical vertebra sprain, strain of the cervical musculature.
Comments	Athletes suspected of suffering a spinal cord injury should be immediately stabilized and transported Trauma to the brain stem or phrenic nerve may result in cardiac arrest.

CT = computed tomography; MRI = magnetic resonance imaging; ROM = range of motion.

Initially, the signs and symptoms of transient quadriplegia resemble those of a catastrophic cervical injury. Symptoms range from sensory dysfunction to burning pain, numbness, or paresthesia in the upper and lower extremities. Likewise, upper and lower extremity motor function is inhibited, ranging from muscular weakness to complete paralysis. However, these symptoms clear within 15 minutes to 48 hours. Pain within the cervical spine is limited to burning paresthesia.[65]

The definitive diagnosis of transient quadriplegia is made through imaging and electrophysiologic testing. Radiographic examination is used to rule out fractures or congenital abnormalities of the cervical spine, and CT scans are used to gain a better definition of the cervical bony anatomy. The integrity of the spinal cord and its roots is determined through the use of MRI scans, **electromyelograms**, and nerve conduction velocity testing.

Return-to-play criteria

Athletes must not be returned to competition while neurologic symptoms including pain, motor weakness, paresthesia, or numbness are present. The cervical spine must demonstrate a preinjury level of strength and range of motion. Clinical and radiographic examination should reveal no evidence of spinal stenosis, disc injury, or vertebral instability, and the cervical spine should have its normal lordotic curvature.

On-Field Examination and Management of Head and Cervical Spine Injuries

The decisions made during a crisis situation are key to the proper management of head and cervical spine trauma. It is the medical staff's responsibility to have a preplanned course of action that has been discussed and approved by the athletic training staff, physician, emergency medical service (EMS), and administration (see Chapter 2). Before the start of each season, these procedures must be reviewed by the involved parties, with each understanding not only his or her own roles but also those of the others. Further, the techniques discussed in this text must be reviewed and rehearsed until each member is comfortable performing the techniques described. The procedures described in this section assume that more than one responder knowledgeable of the plan is present.

Because of the importance of not unnecessarily moving an athlete with a spinal injury and the potentially catastrophic ramifications of doing so, athletic trainers should conduct meetings with each team, instructing the athletes not to help injured players to their feet. In too many instances, these well-intentioned actions have resulted in an athlete's death or permanent paralysis.

This section assumes that the responder has a minimum of emergency cardiac care (ECC) certification which includes cardiopulmonary resuscitation and use of automatic external defibrillator. The procedures discussed in this section are not intended to supersede formal ECC training. Refer to Chapter 2 for more information on emergency preparedness.

Equipment Considerations

When, where, and how to remove a helmet after a spinal injury is a debatable issue.[73–75] The consensus opinion is the football helmet should not be removed during the prehospital care of a patient with a spinal injury.[76] The movement associated with removing the helmet places the spinal cord at too great of a risk for further injury, especially when the following are considered:

- The airway is still accessible by removing the face mask.[73]
- A cervical collar can be applied to the cervical spine while the helmet is still in place, although shoulder pads may make this difficult.
- The skull can be adequately secured to the spine board.
- Football helmets are radiographic translucent (Fig. 21-17). In most cases a definitive diagnosis can be made before removal.[66]
- Removing the helmet without removing the shoulder pads results in the cervical spine's being placed in extension.[74]

In cases of improperly fitting helmets, the inability to remove the face mask, the inability to access the airway, or other extraordinary circumstances, the helmet and shoulder pads must be removed. These procedures are described in the following sections.

The strongest argument in support of removing the helmet and shoulder pads involves the necessity, or the potential necessity, of **defibrillating** the athlete.[74] Proper protocol for the use of an AED requires that the athlete's chest be completely exposed and dry (Fig. 21-18). The contact points for the defibrillator pads are over the apex of the heart and inferior to the right clavicle. If these pads were to come into contact with wet shoulder pads, the defibrillator's current could arc, an event that would not only decrease the defibrillator's effectiveness but could also defibrillate the operator.

This section first discusses making the airway and chest accessible for CPR or the physical examination of these areas. Regardless of the athlete's condition, the helmet or shoulder pads must be removed at some point, whether on the field or in the hospital, and safely doing so is not an easy task. These techniques must be practiced and rehearsed before actually performing them on stricken athletes

---

Electromyelogram The recording of the electrical activity within a muscle.

Defibrillation (defibrillating) The process of restoring a normal heartbeat.

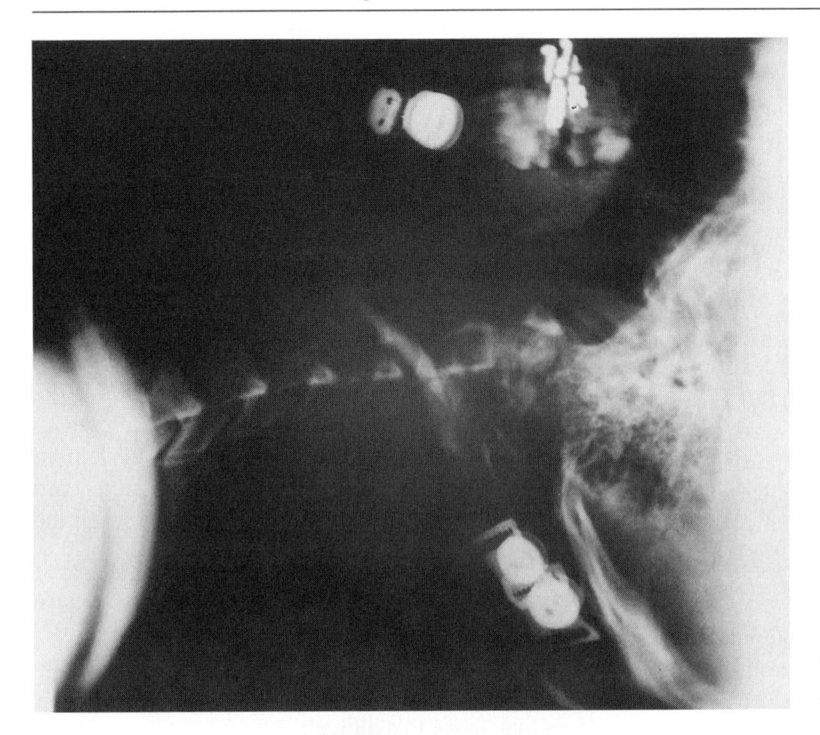

FIGURE 21-17 ■ Radiograph of the cervical spine through a helmet. Note the metal snaps for the chin strap.

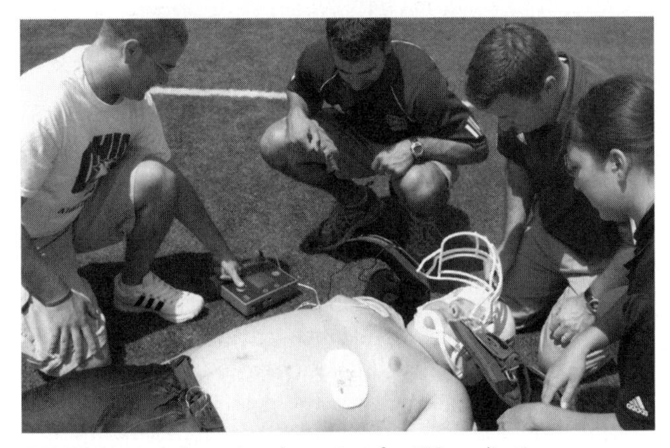

FIGURE 21-18 ■ Preparing the patient for AED application.

requiring assistance. Often it is necessary to assist hospital personnel with this procedure because they may be unfamiliar with the sports equipment.

Face mask removal

An alternative to removing the athlete's helmet is to remove the face mask. which is commonly held in place by four plastic clips (Fig. 21-19).[73] The face mask should be removed if spinal cord injury is suspected, if there is any possibility that rescue breathing or CPR be administered, or if the patient will be transported on a spineboard.[76]

*** Practical Evidence**

The fastest method of face mask removal that imposes the least amount of movement is a cordless electric screwdriver. Because the screwdriver is not 100% reliable in removing screws, an alternative tool to cut the clips should always be available.[77–79]

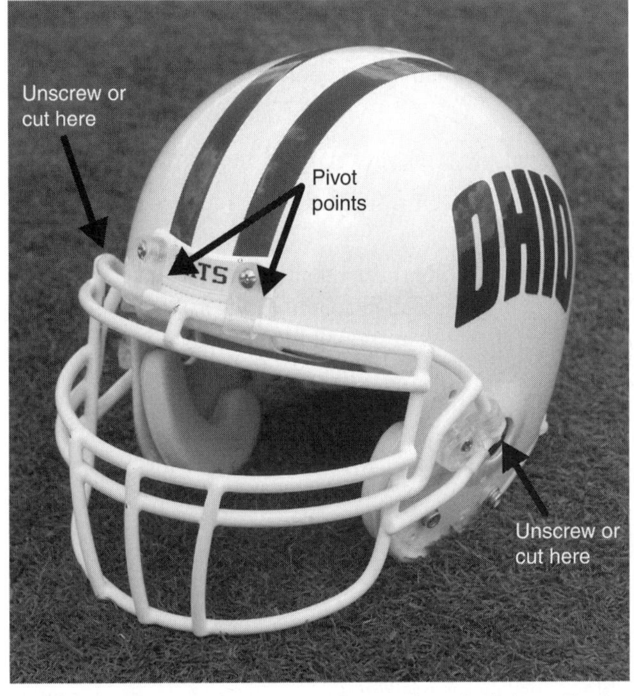

FIGURE 21-19 ■ Clips attaching the face mask to the helmet. The lateral clips are cut or unscrewed, but the superior ones remain in place as pivot hinges for the face mask.

Unfastening the two lower clips allows the face mask to swing away from the athlete's face, making the mouth and nose accessible for assisted ventilation (Fig. 21-20). A scalpel, box opener, or other type of razor knife can be used to cut the clips, but these methods have the risk of cutting the athlete or the athletic trainer. Also, because the plastic hardens with age, older clips become harder to cut. Other

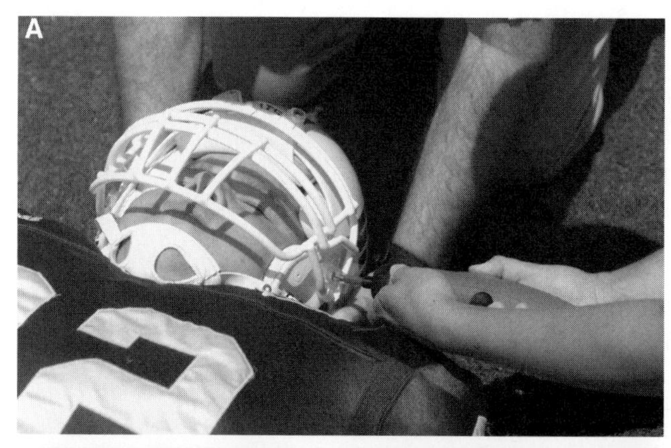

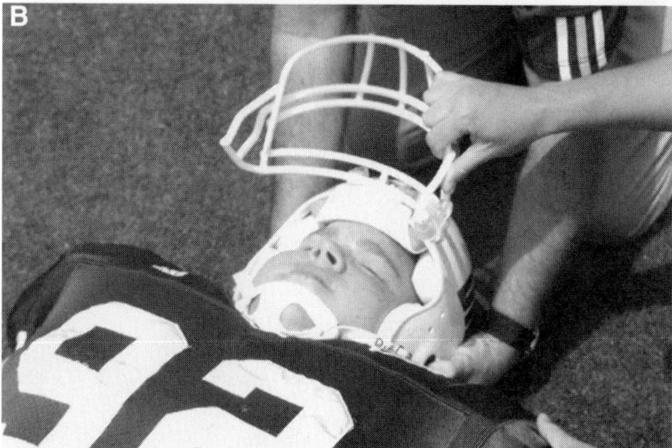

FIGURE 21-20 ■ Using an electric screwdriver to remove the screws attaching the face mask to the helmet and exposing the athlete's airway. Because of the possibility of damage or rusting of the screw or bolt, a cutting-type face mask removal tool should always be available.[76]

methods of removing the face mask include unscrewing the bolts that attach the clips to the helmet or using a specifically designed cutting instrument.

Regardless of the method used to remove the face mask, this procedure requires two people. In-line stabilization of the head and cervical spine must be maintained, and the cervical spine must be guarded against any movement that may occur during this process, especially avoiding hyperflexion of the cervical spine.

Chest exposure

Auscultation of heart sounds, external cardiac compression during CPR and use of an AED require that the athlete's sternum be exposed. First the athlete's shirt is cut to expose the shoulder pads and, if the shirt is particularly tight fitting, it is cut along the anterior portion of the sleeves. Next, the clinician cuts or unfastens the rib straps on the sternal portion of the pads and cuts the laces holding together the anterior portion of the pad. The halves are spread to expose the sternum (Fig. 21-21).

Helmet removal

In cases necessitating the removal of the helmet (e.g., improperly fitting helmet, inability to secure the head to the spineboard with the helmet on), two people are necessary to perform the process in a manner that minimizes the amount of cervical spine motion (Fig. 21-22). A semirigid collar can be fitted to the cervical spine before removing the helmet if the relationship of the helmet, shoulder pads, and surface provides sufficient room to do this with a minimum of movement; this may also require removing the shoulder pads (see the section on spine boarding the athlete).

While maintaining in-line stabilization, the other responder cuts the chin strap or straps. A flat instrument, such as the handle of a pair of scissors, is slid between the cheek pad and the helmet. A twist of this instrument causes the pad to unsnap and separate from the helmet. The pad is removed, and the procedure is repeated on the opposite side. The person who has been applying the in-line stabilization now slips a finger in each ear hole and spreads the helmet. As the helmet is slowly slid off the head, the second responder reaches behind the neck to support the cervical spine and provide a firm grip on the head.

Shoulder pad removal

The shoulder pads are removed only when the athlete's life is in jeopardy or such a state is imminent.[76] This decision warrants that the immediate threat to the athlete's life outweigh the possibility of spinal cord injury that may result from moving the athlete. This decision should be made by a physician, if one is present. Otherwise, the decision is made by the attending athletic trainer, emergency medical technician, or paramedic.

This procedure is most safely performed after the cervical spine has been stabilized by a hard or firm collar and the helmet removed. The responder begins this procedure by performing the steps described in the section on exposing the chest. After the anterior and axillary shoulder straps have been cut, the two halves of the shoulder pads may be widened. While one person continues to support the athlete's head, the shoulder pads are slid off the shoulders and over the head (Fig. 21-23).

Initial Inspection

The initial inspection encompasses contingencies that must be noted on arrival at the accident scene. These factors provide clues to the severity of the injury and insight regarding the proper on-field management of the patient.

- **Encumbering circumstances:** Encumbering circumstances are factors that make the worst-case scenarios even more difficult to handle. Examples of these include a diver who is still in the water, a football player who is lying on top of another player, a gymnast in a soft landing pit, or a hockey player whose head and neck are still against the boards.
- **Movement:** Any movement by the athlete must be noted. Unconscious athletes may be lying perfectly still or may have a seizure. Likewise, conscious athletes may lie still out of fear or grogginess.

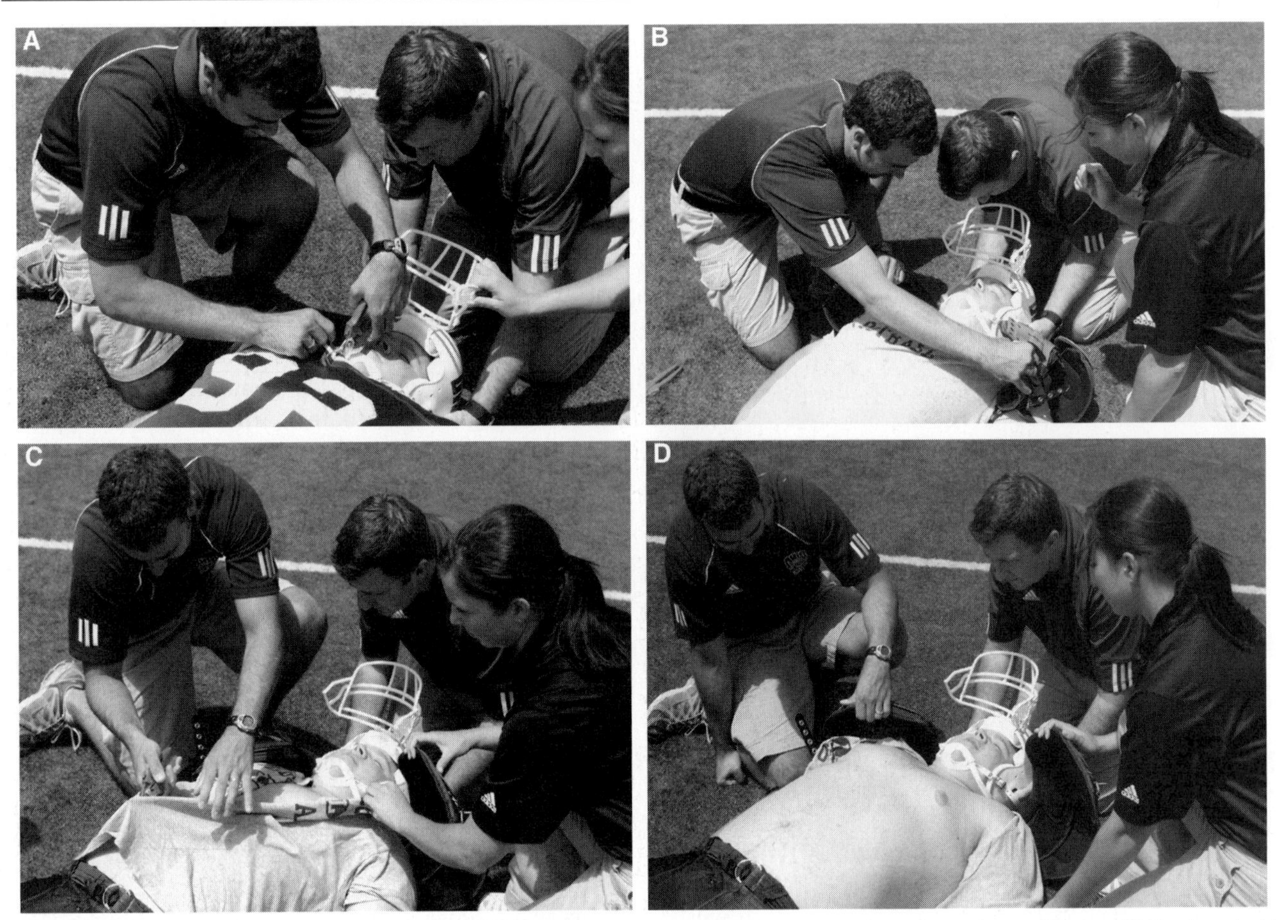

FIGURE 21-21 ■ Exposing the athlete's sternum so that cardiopulmonary resuscitation can be performed. (A) The jersey is cut. (B) The laces holding the shoulder pads together are cut and the halves of the shoulder pads are spread. (C) The underlying t-shirt is cut. (D) The shoulder pads and shirts are moved back to expose the athlete's chest. See also Figure 21-18 for the placement of AED electrodes.

- **Position:** Ideally, the athlete should be supine. Athletes who are sidelying or prone eventually must be rolled, but these initial assessments must be made before the decision to move the athlete is made.
- **Posture:** The alignment of the athlete's arms, legs, and cervical spine relative to the trunk is noted (Inspection Findings 21-1). Splayed extremities must be aligned with the rest of the body if spine boarding or rolling the athlete is required. Male athletes who are suffering from a lesion of the spinal cord at the thoracic or cervical level may also demonstrate **priapism**.

Initial Action

After arriving at the scene, the responder's actions within the first 3 or 4 minutes strongly determine whether the athlete lives, dies, or becomes permanently disabled. Despite this urgency, the responder must not rush through these processes but must perform each with care and diligence.

- **Stabilize the cervical spine:** One responder must immediately assume control of the head by applying in-line stabilization. If the athlete is wearing a helmet, in-line stabilization is achieved by firmly grasping the sides of the helmet in the area of the ear holes and applying firm stabilization along the vertical axis of the cervical spine (Fig. 21-24). If the athlete is not wearing a helmet, stabilization is applied by grasping the skull beneath the occipital bone and mandible on each side, being careful not to alter the position of the spine and especially avoiding flexion.

  From this point until the situation resolves, either by the determination that no cervical spine injury exists or by the athlete's placement on a spine board, the person at the head maintains the in-line stabilization and directs the other individuals providing assistance. Movement of the spinal column may result in a fragmented or displaced piece of bone's lacerating the spinal cord and causing death or permanent disability.
- **Clear airway:** Remove the athlete's mouthpiece. In addition, inspect the mouth for other objects that may become lodged in the athlete's airway.
- **Determine the level of consciousness:** In cases in which the athlete is not obviously responsive, the level of consciousness can be determined by calling the

Priapism Spontaneous penile erection.

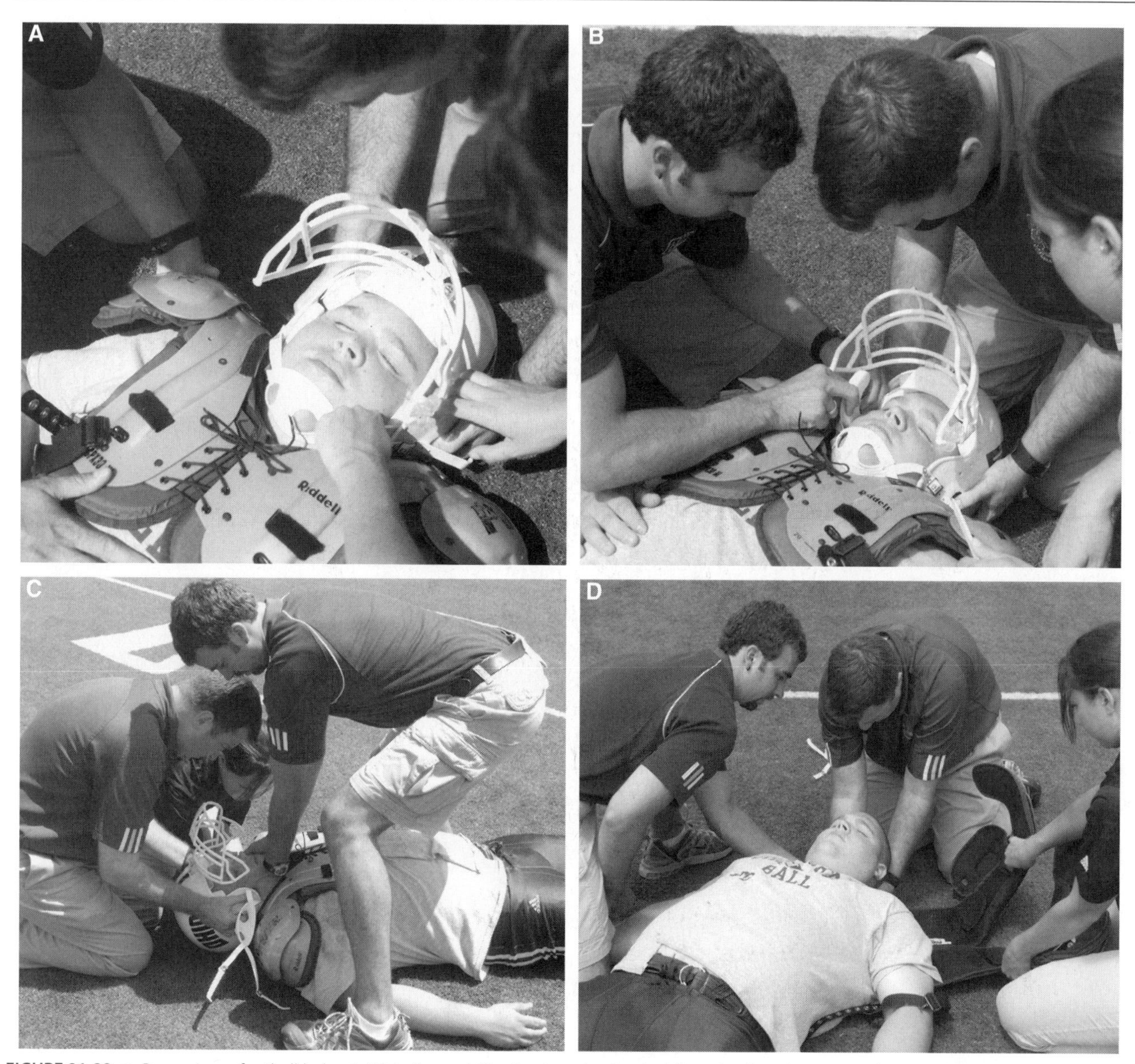

FIGURE 21-22 ■ Removing a football helmet. (A) In-line stabilization is maintained while a cheek pad is removed using a blunt object. (B) The opposite cheek guards is removed. (C) The chin strap is uncut or unsnapped. (D) Secondary stabilization is applied to the cervical spine as the helmet is spread and slid off the athlete's head.

athlete's name and asking, "CAN YOU HEAR ME?" If this verbal stimulus fails to evoke a motor response, the athlete's response to a painful stimulus can be determined by applying pressure to the bed of a fingernail (see Fig. 21-5). Failure to evoke a response through either of these methods indicates that the athlete is unconscious. At this time, the athlete's ABCs should be reevaluated.

- **Secondary screen:** The torso and extremities are observed for any signs of additional trauma such as a fracture, joint dislocation, or bleeding. Of these pathologies, controlling bleeding takes the highest priority because of the need to preserve the athlete's blood pressure.

Management of the unconscious athlete

Figure 21-25 presents a flowchart describing the management of an unconscious athlete. Sustained unconsciousness (based on the institution's standard operating procedures) warrants the activation of the emergency medical system. If the athlete regains consciousness, follow the procedures described in the "Management of the Conscious Athlete" section. The athlete's cervical spine continues to be stabilized using in-line stabilization during these procedures.

- **Airway:** Permanent brain damage can occur within 4 minutes after oxygen deprivation. Establish that the athlete has an open airway by looking, listening, and feeling for breaths (see Fig. 21-6). Occlusion of the

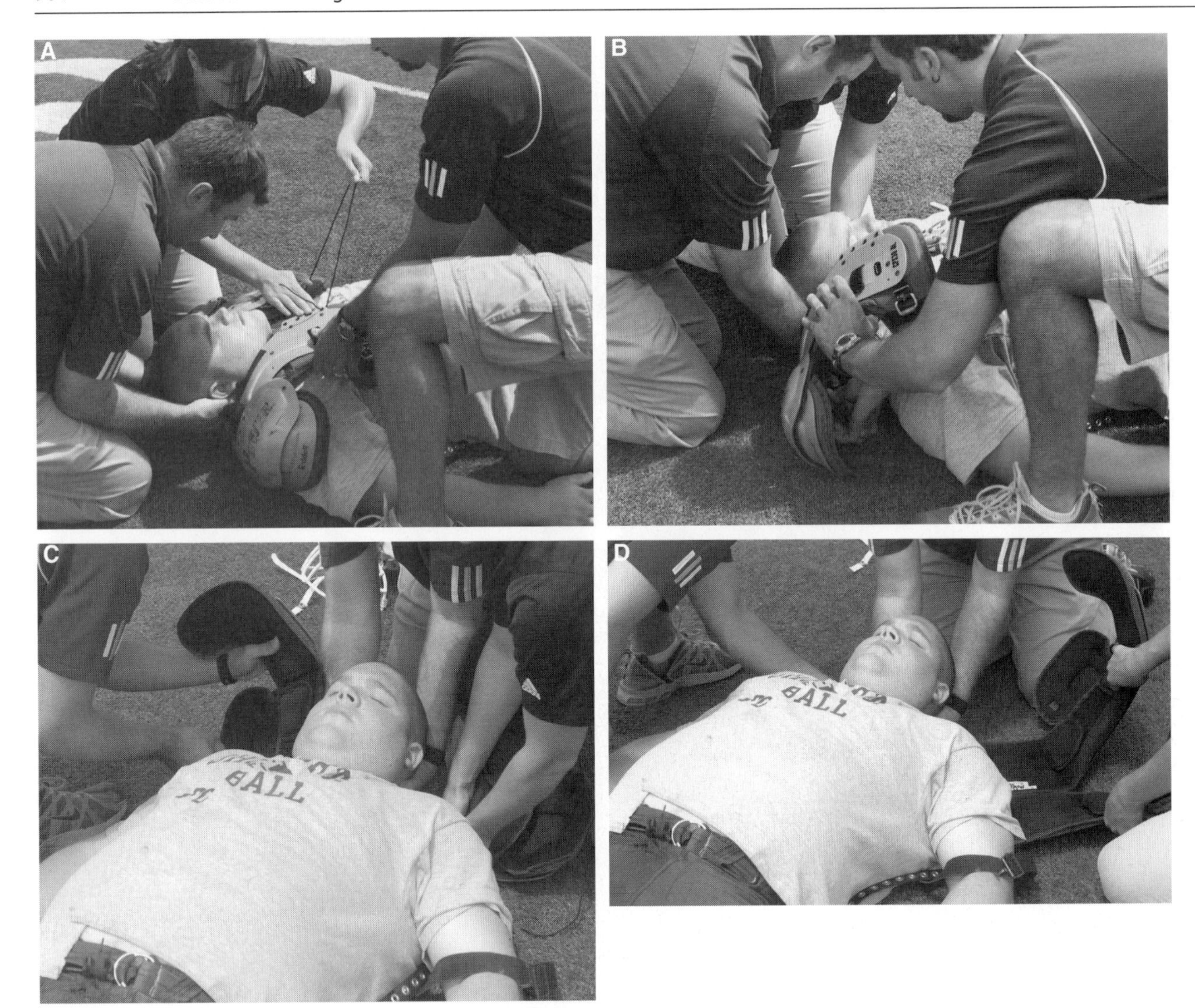

FIGURE 21-23 ■ Removing the shoulder pads. After removing the athlete's jersey and unsnapping or cutting the axial straps: (A) The sternal laces holding the pads together are cut or untied. (B) The shoulder pad is spread. (C) The one half of the shoulder pads are slid from under the athlete. (D) The shoulder pads are pulled from under the athlete. Note that in-line cervical stabilization is maintained throughout this procedure.

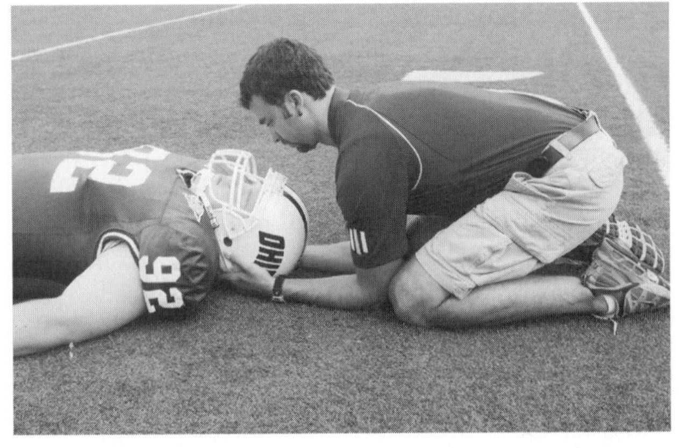

FIGURE 21-24 ■ Applying in-line stabilization to the cervical spine.

airway can occur secondary to intrinsic blockage (crushing or swelling of the larynx or trachea), extrinsic blockage (external hematoma), foreign body blockage (mouthpiece, gum), or central blockage (flaccid tongue) of the airway. Foreign bodies must be manually dislodged from the athlete's airway; tongue forceps can be used for this purpose or to grasp the tongue and remove it from the airway. Complete obstruction of the airway owing to intrinsic and extrinsic blockage may require use of nasopharyngeal airway or an emergency **tracheotomy**, a technique that must be performed only by trained personnel.

Tracheotomy A method of delivering air to the lungs by incising the skin and trachea and inserting a tube to form an airway; an emergency technique used only when the athlete's life is threatened by an immovable obstruction to the upper airway. Training is required to perform this technique properly.

Inspection Findings 21-1
Postures Assumed After Spinal Cord Injury

Decerebrate Posture

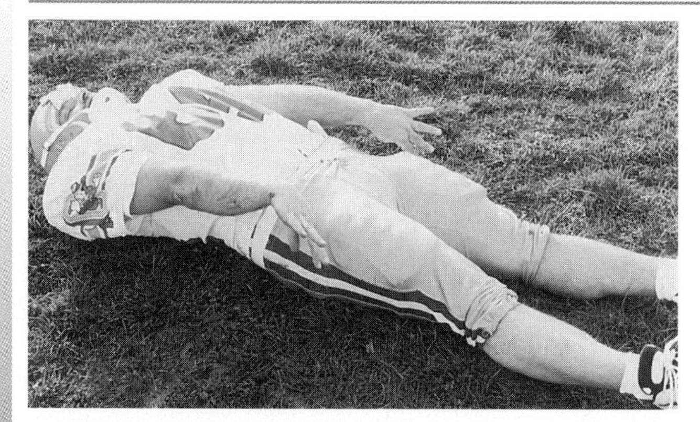

Description	Extension of the extremities and retraction of the head
Pathology	Lesion of the brain stem; also possible secondary to heat stroke

Decorticate Posture

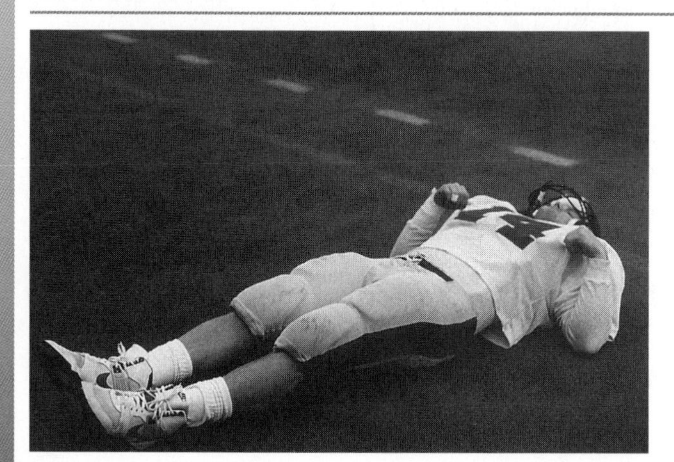

Description	Flexion of the elbows and wrists, clenched fists, and extension of the lower extremity
Pathology	Lesion above the brain stem

Flexion Contracture

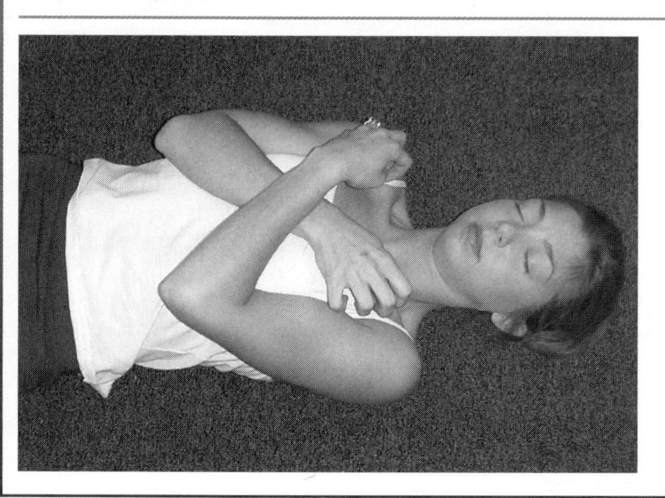

Description	Arms flexed across the chest
Pathology	Spinal cord lesion at the C5–C6 level

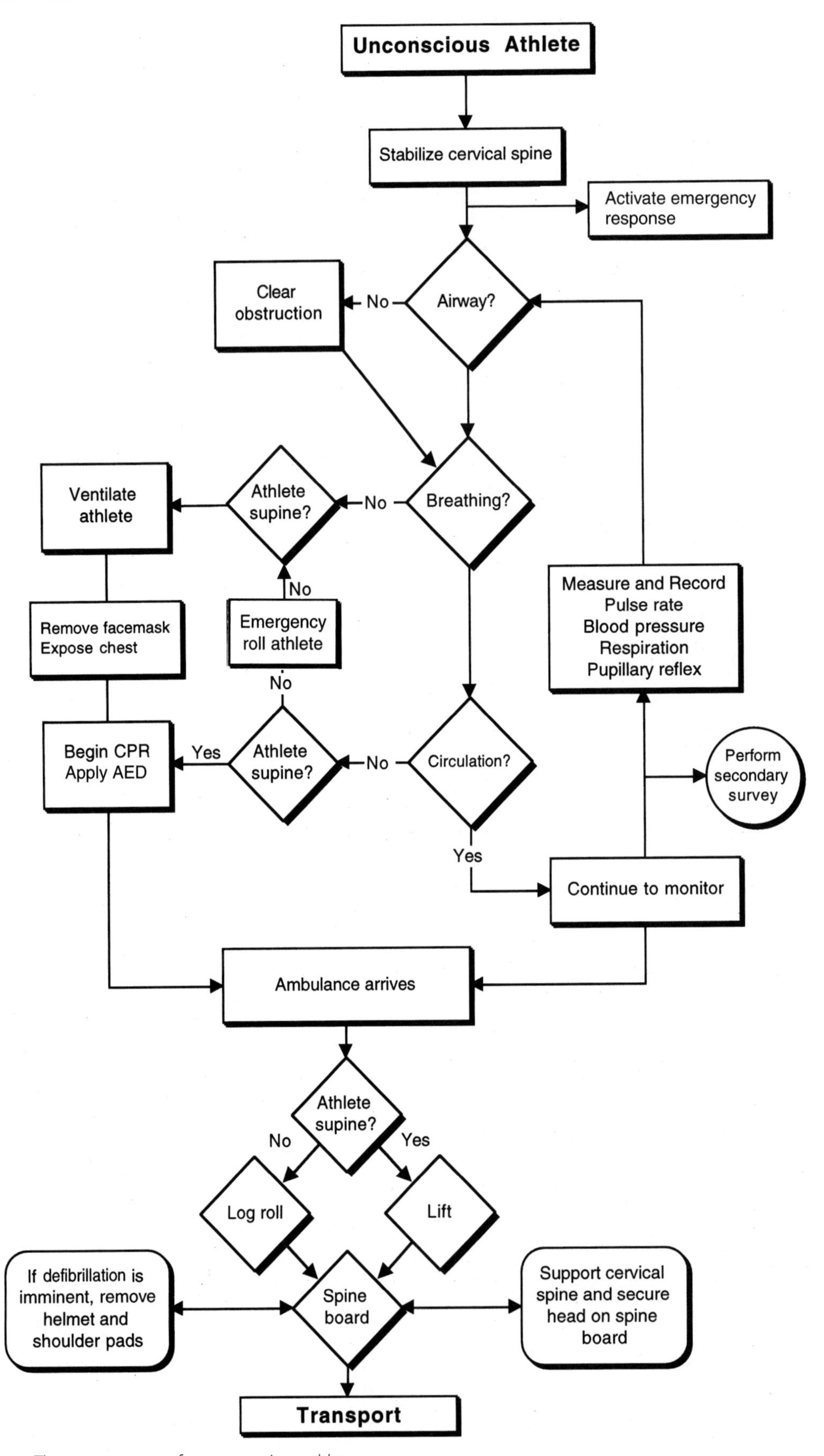

FIGURE 21-25 ■ The management of an unconscious athlete.

- **Breathing:** Breathing is determined by looking, listening, and feeling for signs of breathing. The absence of breathing or a respiratory rate of fewer than 10 or greater than 30 breaths per minute requires assisted ventilation:
- **Emergency roll:** Emergency rolls differ from standard spine boarding techniques and are used only in cases in which the athlete does not have a pulse or is not breathing. Bystanders must be recruited to quickly roll the athlete to the supine position, foregoing the immediate use of a spine board. Although this is done rapidly, in-line stabilization must be maintained with continued stabilization of the cervical spine. At this time, the chest must be exposed so that proper chest compressions and AED procedures can be initiated.
- **Removal of the face mask:** The face mask is removed to access the athlete's mouth and nose.
- **Jaw thrust:** A jaw thrust maneuver to open the airway is used rather than the head-tilt method.
- **Ventilation:** The responder gives two quick breaths to ventilate the athlete. The use of a one-way mask or bag valve mask is recommended. An oral–pharyngeal airway may be inserted by personnel who have been trained in this procedure.
- **Circulation:** Ideally, the carotid pulse is used to determine that the heart is beating. If the athlete's cervical spine is inaccessible, either because of equipment or the athlete's position on the ground, the pulse can be identified over the radial, ulnar, or femoral or popliteal arteries. If the athlete is not breathing but has a heartbeat, then **rescue breathing** is initiated. If the athlete does not have a pulse, then **CPR** is begun and an AED is used.

Management of the unconscious but breathing athlete

This section assumes that the athlete has an open airway and the cardiopulmonary system is functioning normally. Although these findings initially appear to be normal, they require continuous monitoring because the worst-case scenario involves the athlete's progressing to cardiac arrest. Lesions in the C1 region of the spinal cord alter brain stem function and result in almost immediate cardiac arrest. C2 to C4 lesions or subsequent hemorrhage and hematoma formation at these levels can interrupt the phrenic nerve, possibly resulting in a delayed onset of respiratory arrest.

- **Cervical spine evaluation:** Gently palpate the cervical spine for signs of gross bony deformity or swelling. The absence of these signs, however, does not rule out the possibility of cervical spine injury.
- **Blood pressure:** The athlete's blood pressure is monitored and recorded so that any change over time may be identified. If a blood pressure cuff is not immediately available, the athlete's blood pressure can be estimated based on where the pulses can be palpated[80]:

Palpable Pulse	Minimum Systolic Blood Pressure, mm Hg
Carotid artery	60
Femoral artery	70
Radial artery	90

- **Pupil responsiveness:** The athlete's eyelids are opened to observe for pupillary response. The act of opening the eyelids alone should cause the pupils to constrict. The absence of pupillary response indicates that the brain is not receiving oxygen or that substantial brain trauma has occurred.
- **Continuation of monitoring:** The athlete's respirations, blood pressure, pupillary reflex, and pulse are monitored and recorded every 5 minutes. Decreased respiration, increased blood pressure, and decreased heart rate are signs of an expanding intracranial lesion.

Management of the conscious athlete

The on-field management described in this section assumes that the athlete has been determined to be conscious, in-line stabilization has been applied to the athlete's cervical spine, the athlete's mouthpiece has been removed, and the presence of an open airway has been established.

As long as the athlete displays stable vital signs, no attempts should be made to move the athlete until the possibility of a spinal fracture has been ruled out or the athlete is stabilized with a spine board and cervical collar. The athlete may express the desire to move or may attempt to do so. Either through verbal commands or gentle restraint, the athlete should not be allowed to move until the possibility of a fracture has been ruled out.

History

Question the athlete regarding any loss of consciousness, the mechanism of the injury, and any areas of pain or paresthesia in the cervical spine or radiating into the extremities. Any significant findings of pain or numbness radiating into the extremities or cervical pain warrant the immediate spine boarding of the athlete and transport to the hospital.

- **Loss of consciousness:** Determine if the athlete lost consciousness, even for a brief period of time. A transitory loss of consciousness may be described as "blacking out" or "seeing stars."
- **Mechanism of injury:** Identify how the injurious force was delivered. A direct blow to the head can result in either brain or cervical spine trauma. If this mechanism forces the cervical spine into flexion or extension, cervical spine trauma should be suspected. If the athlete cannot recall the onset of injury, bystanders or witnesses may be able to describe it.
- **Symptoms:** Question the athlete regarding the symptoms that indicate spinal pathology. Positive findings

for any of the following support the assumption that a spinal cord or cervical vertebral injury is present:

- Pain in the cervical spine
- Numbness, tingling, or burning pain radiating through the upper or lower extremities
- Sensation of weakness in the cervical spine, upper extremities, or lower extremities
- Burning or aching in the chest secondary to cardiac inhibition

Inspection

This inspection process supplements the information gained during the observations made on the way to the scene and may be conducted concurrently with the previously described segments of the examination. If the athlete is supine, the inspection of the posterior cervical structures can be delayed until the athlete is moved to the sidelines or omitted if the athlete is being transported to the hospital.

- **Cervical vertebrae:** Observe the cervical vertebrae spinous processes, if visible. They should display a normal alignment.
- **Cervical musculature:** Observe for the presence of muscle spasm indicating a cervical fracture, a dislocation, or a strain of the cervical muscles.

Palpation

Palpation is conducted to confirm any visual findings of malalignment and identify underlying pathology. Too much pressure during palpation must be avoided to prevent the possible displacement of a bony fragment. If the athlete is supine, palpation can be performed by reaching beneath the athlete. Certain pieces of equipment, such as cervical collars, can prohibit palpation while the athlete is either prone or supine.

- **Cervical spine:** Palpate the area over the spinous and transverse processes for signs of vertebral malalignment, crepitus, or tenderness. Any of these signs signifies the possibility of a cervical fracture or dislocation.
- **Cervical musculature:** Palpate the cervical musculature for signs of spasm in the upper portion of the trapezius, levator scapulae, or sternocleidomastoid muscles. Unilateral spasm is an indication of a cervical vertebral dislocation, especially when the skull is rotated and tilted toward the opposite side.

Neurologic Testing

- **Sensory testing:** Although formal dermatome testing may be conducted while the athlete is on the field, the essential finding is that of normal and bilaterally equal sensation in the upper and lower extremities. Sensation may be compared by stroking along the following body areas:

Upper Extremity		Lower Extremity	
Area	Dermatome	Area	Dermatomes
Superior shoulder	C4	Lateral thigh	L1, L2, L3
Lateral humerus	C5	Lateral lower leg and foot	L5, S1
Lateral forearm	C6	Medial lower leg and foot	L4
Middle finger	C7		
Medial forearm	C8		
Medial humerus	T1		

- **Motor testing:** If no other signs and symptoms of cervical vertebral involvement exist, the athlete's ability to perform active motion of the upper and lower extremities and resisted movements of the upper extremity may be assessed.
- **Active motion:** Active movements are first performed on the small joints because motion of the large joints (e.g., knees and hips) may result in a significant shift of the body. Begin by asking the athlete to wiggle the toes and fingers, progressing to movement of the ankles, wrists, knees, elbows, hips, and shoulders. Each of these motions should be performed smoothly and appear bilaterally equal.

Removing the Athlete from the Field

Each on-field incident ends with the decision of how to remove the athlete from the field. The extremes of the possible scenarios range from the athlete walking off the field without assistance to rolling and placing the athlete on a spine board. Cases that lie between these extremes require that the medical staff make a decision about the best method to safely remove the athlete.

Any suspected cervical spine trauma mandates that the athlete be placed on a spine board and transported to a hospital via an ambulance squad. The use of stretchers without a spine board is to be avoided in these cases. In addition, if any doubt exists, the most conservative form of management should be chosen.

Walking the athlete off the field

Removing athletes from the field under their own power is not as straightforward as standing the athlete up and having him or her walk off the field. After a head injury, the sudden change from a lying to a standing position may make the blood pressure drop suddenly, causing the athlete to faint or become unsteady.

The athlete's body should be allowed to gradually adjust to the change in positions, using a three-step process. First, the athlete is brought to a sitting position with the knees bent. The athletic trainer is positioned behind the athlete, providing support and being ready to assist the athlete if dizziness occurs. This position is maintained until the athlete feels comfortable with the position. The athlete then kneels forward on one knee and again waits, to ensure that dizziness does not occur. Finally, the athlete is brought to the standing position, with assistance being provided on either side. If the symptoms increase in any of these positions, the athlete should be transported in a supine or sitting position.

Using a spine board

In-line stabilization is maintained throughout these procedures until the athlete's skull is securely affixed to the spine board. These procedures should be discussed and practiced with the emergency medical squad.

Cervical spine stabilization. If possible, the cervical spine should be stabilized using a semirigid collar, such as a Philadelphia collar prior to spineboarding (see Fig. 20-27). These devices are most easily applied when the athlete is not wearing shoulder pads or a helmet. Other types of collars, such as a vacuum splint cervical immobilizer, can be used for stabilization when the helmet and shoulder pads are still in place.[81]

After the two halves of the collar are separated, the posterior shell is compressed and slid behind the cervical spine, taking care to prevent spinal movement. This section should fit snugly beneath the athlete's occipital and mastoid processes. The anterior shell is fitted so that it envelops the chin. Most models have an opening on the sternal pad that allows access to the trachea in case a tracheotomy must be performed.

The supine athlete. When spine boarding spinal injury the six-plus person lift is recommended.[76] In this case, one person applies in-line stabilization (referred to as the leader) and an appropriate number of people controlling the athlete's torso and legs, while another person manipulates the spine board (Fig. 21-26). The leader maintains in-line stabilization throughout the lift and subsequent stabilization of the athlete on the spine board and is responsible for instructing and guiding the remaining personnel in the sequence to be performed.

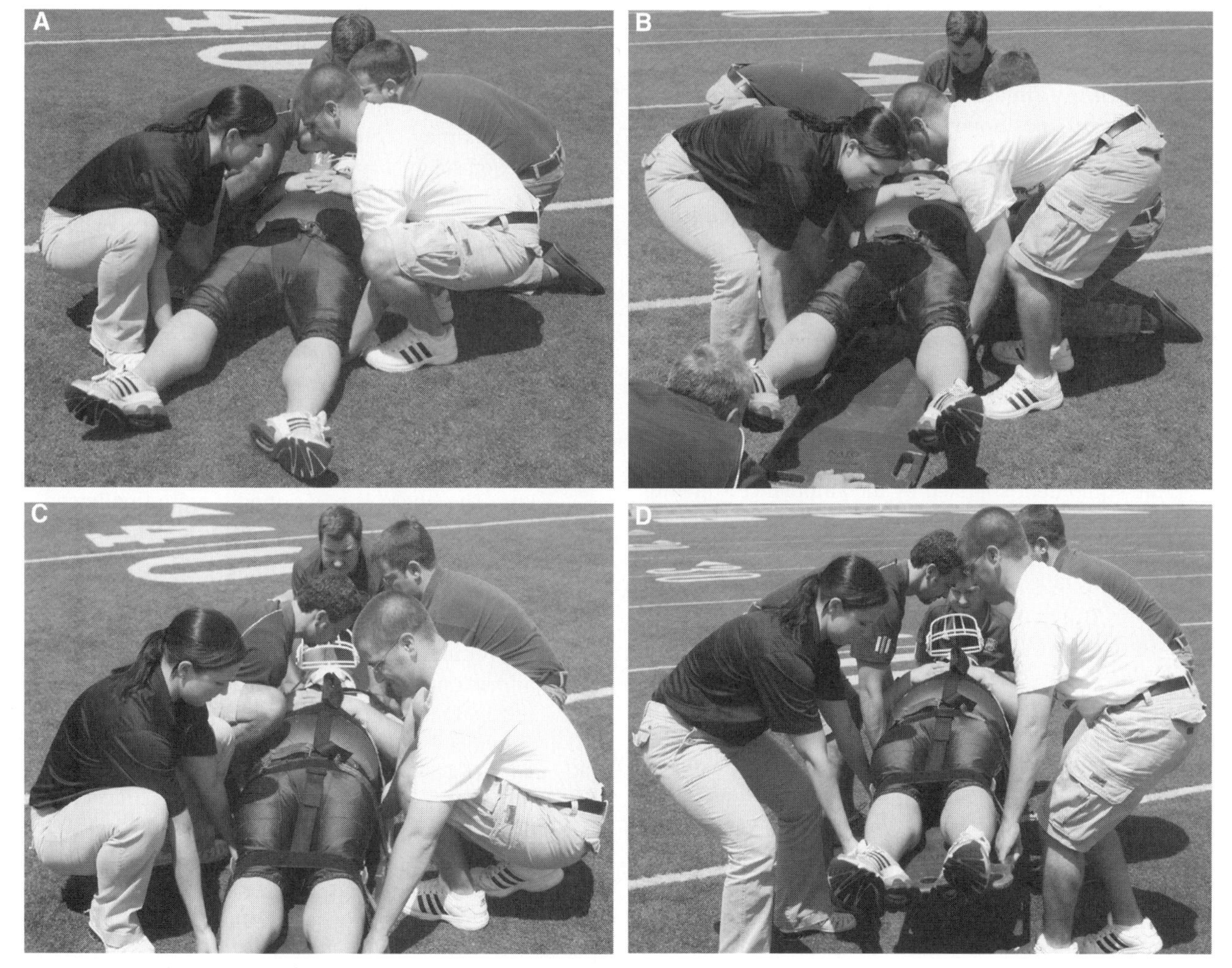

FIGURE 21-26 ■ The six-person lift for spine boarding a supine athlete; see text for details.

The process of using a spine board for an athlete who is supine involves lifting the athlete, sliding the board under the person, then placing the athlete on the board.

1. **Align the athlete:** Before the athlete is placed on the board, the extremities must be aligned with the body. If possible, cross the athlete's arms across the chest.
2. **Position the personnel:** Depending on the height and weight of the athlete, at least one person should be positioned on each side of the chest, pelvis, and legs. Larger people will require more rescuers.
3. **Lift the athlete:** On the leader's command, the athlete is lifted 4 to 6 inches. The following command is used: "On the count of three, we will lift the athlete until I say 'stop.' Start and stop on my command. Ready? One, two, three, lift." The personnel positioned at the torso and legs are responsible for maintaining axial alignment of the spinal column by staying with the leader's pace.
4. **Slide the spine board:** With the board on the ground, slide the spine board from the athlete's feet toward the head. The final position should place the board under the athlete so that the top of the spine board is matched with the athlete's head.
5. **Return the athlete:** After the leader is satisfied with the board's position relative to the athlete, he or she gives the command, "On the count of three, we lower the athlete to the board. Start and stop on my command. Ready? One, two, three, lower." Again, it is the torso personnel who are responsible for meeting the pace of the leader. Minor adjustments may be needed after the athlete is positioned on the board.
6. **Secure the athlete:** After the athlete is properly positioned on the spine board, the torso is secured, using the strapping techniques applicable to the equipment being used. The cervical spine must be secured, using the equipment supplied by the ambulance squad or using commercially available equipment (Fig. 21-27). If the helmet is left on, the head may be secured to the board by tape.

The prone athlete. Athletes in the prone position who are breathing but unconscious may be rolled onto the spine board in a safer and more orderly manner than that described in the section on the on-field management of an unconscious athlete who is not breathing. The basic procedures are the same as those described for spine boarding an athlete in the supine position, but the athlete must be rolled 180 degrees rather than 90 degrees (Fig. 21-28). The person who is providing in-line stabilization to the cervical spine is again the operation's leader. A minimum of three additional people is necessary for this procedure to be safely performed. A fourth additional person is recommended to manipulate the spine board.

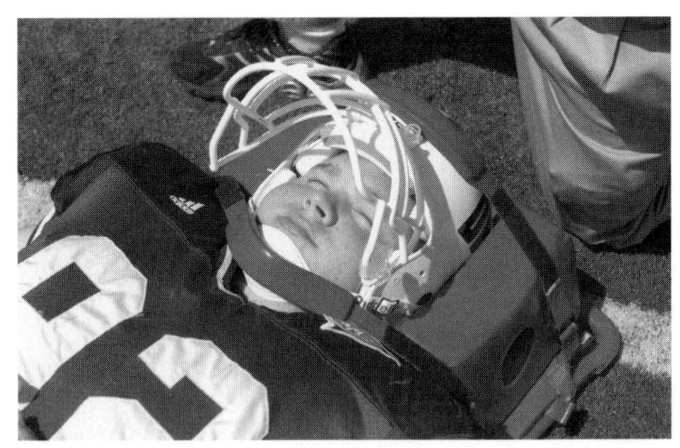

FIGURE 21-27 ■ The spineboarding process is completed by immobilizing the patient's head.

1. **Align the athlete:** Before the athlete is placed on the board, the extremities are aligned with the body. The arm on the side toward which the athlete is to be rolled is abducted to 180 degrees. In Figure 21-28, the right arm is fully abducted prior to rolling.
2. **Position the personnel:** When the minimum of three personnel is used at the torso, one is positioned at the shoulders, one at the hips, and one along the legs. The hands should be spaced along the athlete, gripping underneath the athlete. Tall, heavy, or large individuals may require more personnel in order to be moved safely.
3. **Roll to the side:** On the leader's instructions, the athlete is rolled 90 degrees. The command is given: "On the count of three, we will roll the athlete toward the board. Start and stop on my command. Ready? One, two, three, roll." The personnel used at the torso are responsible for maintaining axial alignment of the spinal column by staying with the leader's pace.
4. **Slide the spine board:** If a single person is given the responsibility of manipulating the spine board, it should be slid so that it is resting against the athlete. The board is positioned longitudinally so that the head of the spine board is matched with the athlete's head.
5. **Placement:** After the leader is satisfied with the board's position relative to the athlete, he or she gives the command: "On the count of three, we will roll the athlete on the board. Start and stop on my command. Ready? One, two, three, roll." The torso personnel are responsible for meeting the pace of the leader. Minor adjustments may be needed after the athlete is positioned on the board.
6. **Secure the athlete:** The athlete is secured on the spine board as described in the previous section.

Home Instructions

Because of the delayed onset of symptoms associated with intracranial hemorrhage, there is always the potential for a more serious condition to develop. The attending physician,

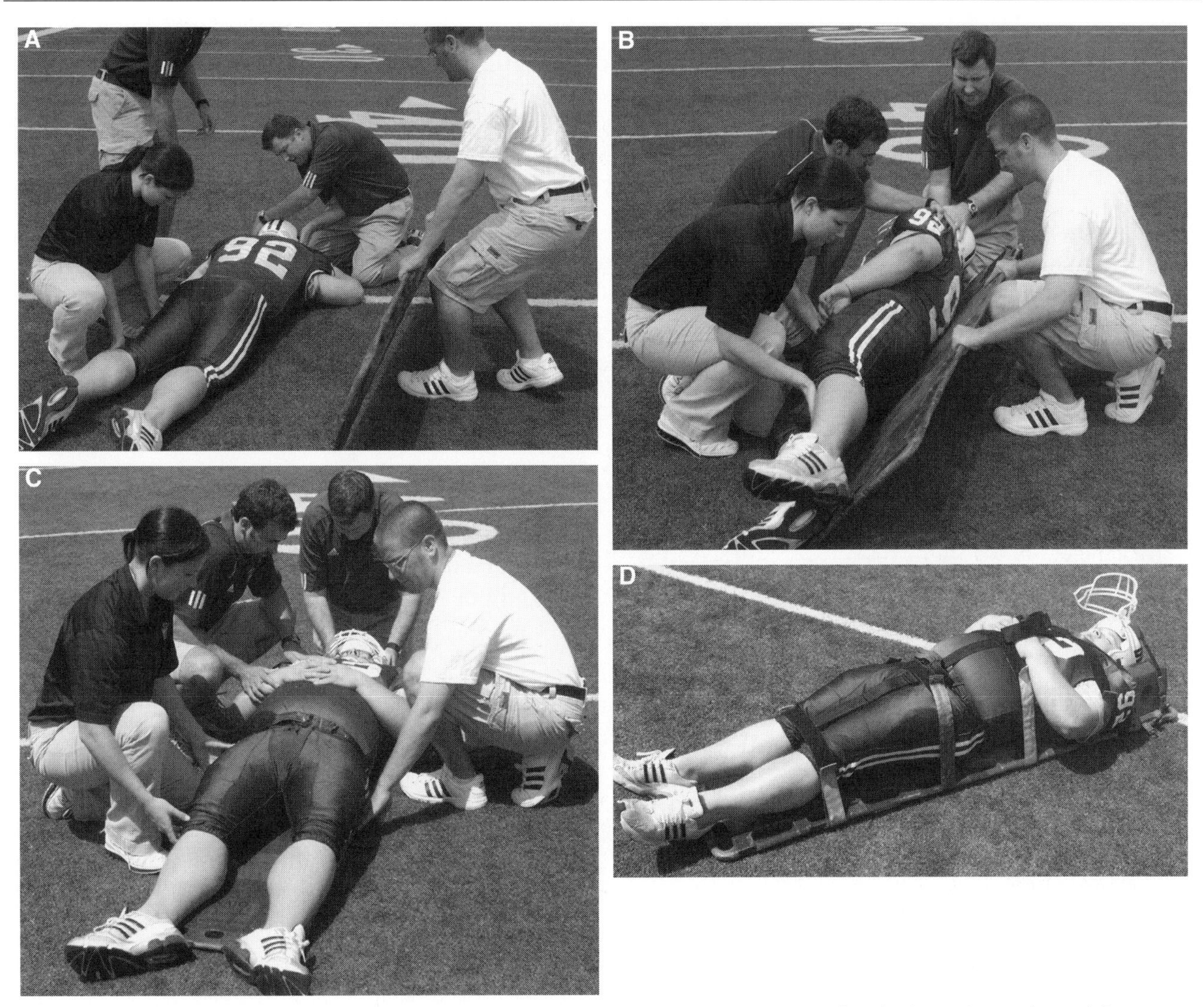

FIGURE 21-28 ■ Spine boarding a prone athlete; see text for details. Note the cross-armed position of the leader applying in-line stabilization.

in some cases, may elect to admit the athlete to the hospital for observation. In other cases, the athlete is allowed to return home.

Inform the athlete's parents or roommates of the delayed progression of the signs and symptoms of head injuries and alert them to the appropriate course of action. A good method of doing this is through the use of a business card-sized instruction booklet. A list of emergency numbers (e.g., athletic trainer, physician, emergency room) is printed on the front cover. The card then opens to display a list of signs and symptoms to alert the individual to a deteriorating condition (Fig. 21-29).

Behavioral changes, forgetfulness, confusion, anger, aggression, and malaise are the most outward signs. In addition, the athlete may describe nausea, vomiting, a headache with increasing severity, and a loss of appetite. Although these symptoms may be caused by other conditions, their presence after a head injury may be cause for concern. The onset of any of the other signs and symptoms of a cerebral injury may also indicate a severe head injury (see Tables 21-5 and 21-6).

Permission to take aspirin or other pain-relieving medication must be given by the physician. Many of these medications, as well as alcoholic drinks, inhibit the clotting mechanism, potentially increasing the rate of intracranial bleeding. Analgesic medications may also mask underlying symptoms, thus delaying their recognition.

Prohibiting sleep after a concussion is largely founded in fiction rather than fact. Although it is necessary to keep the athlete conscious immediately after the injury, sleep should—and must—be permitted at night. The athlete's parents or roommate can be asked to check on the athlete at regular intervals. If enough doubt surrounds the athlete's condition to prohibit sleep, the physician will admit the athlete to the hospital for observation. The medical staff or emergency room personnel should be contacted immediately if any of the latent signs or symptoms of intracranial hemorrhage are manifested.

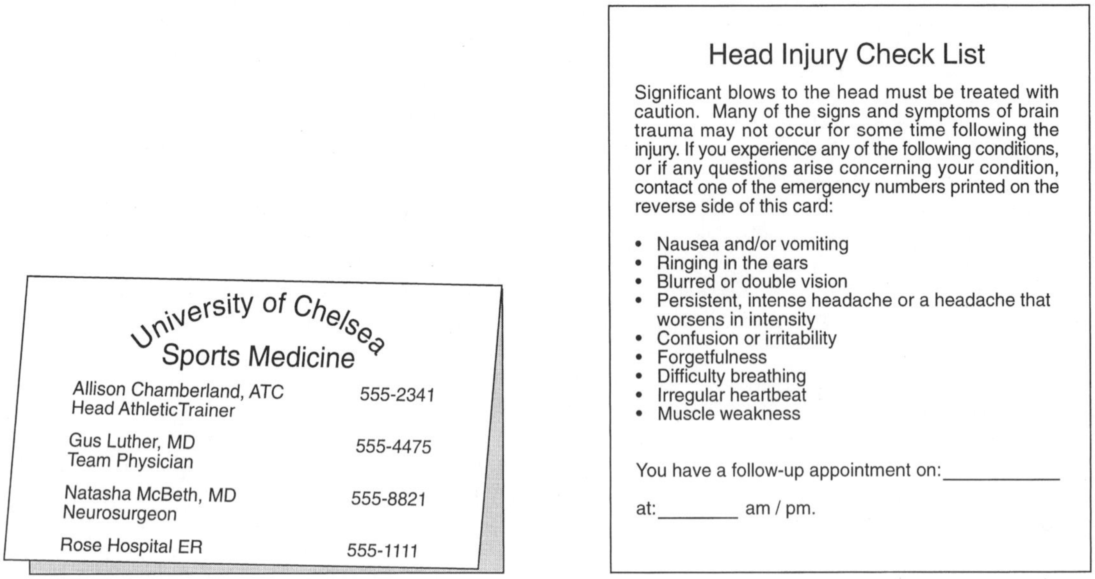

University of Chelsea
Sports Medicine

Allison Chamberland, ATC 555-2341
Head AthleticTrainer

Gus Luther, MD 555-4475
Team Physician

Natasha McBeth, MD 555-8821
Neurosurgeon

Rose Hospital ER 555-1111

Head Injury Check List

Significant blows to the head must be treated with caution. Many of the signs and symptoms of brain trauma may not occur for some time following the injury. If you experience any of the following conditions, or if any questions arise concerning your condition, contact one of the emergency numbers printed on the reverse side of this card:

- Nausea and/or vomiting
- Ringing in the ears
- Blurred or double vision
- Persistent, intense headache or a headache that worsens in intensity
- Confusion or irritability
- Forgetfulness
- Difficulty breathing
- Irregular heartbeat
- Muscle weakness

You have a follow-up appointment on:___________

at:________ am / pm.

FIGURE 21-29 ■ Business card method of communicating home instructions to a head-injured athlete.

REFERENCES

1. Tommasone, BA, and Valovich McLeod, T: Contact sport concussion incidence. *J Athl Train,* 41:470, 2006.
2. Boden, BP, et al: Catastrophic head injuries in high school and college football players. *Am J Sports Med,* 35:1075, 2007.
3. Gessel, LM, et al: Concussions among United States high school and college athletes. *J Athl Train,* 42:495, 2007.
4. Zemper, ED: Cerebral concussion rates in various brands of football helmets. *Athl Train J Natl Athl Train Assoc,* 24:133, 1989.
5. Zemper, ED: Analysis of cerebral concussion frequency with the most commonly used models of football helmets. *J Athl Train,* 29:44, 1994.
6. Heck, JF, et al: National Athletic Trainers' Association position statement: Head-down contact and spearing in tackle football. *J Athl Train,* 39:101, 2004.
7. Nelson, WE: Athletic head injuries. *Athl Train J Nl Athl Train Assoc,* 19:95, 1984.
8. Tysvaer, AT, and Lochen, EA: Soccer injuries to the brain. A neuropsychologic study of former soccer players. *Am J Sports Med,* 19:56, 1991.
9. Killam, C, Cautin, RL, and Santucci, AC: Assessing the enduring residual neuropsychological effects of head trauma in college athletes who participate in contact sports. *Arch Clin Neuropsych,* 20:599, 2005.
10. Spear, J: Are professional footballers at risk of developing dementia? *Int J Geriatric Psych,* 10:1011, 1995.
11. Sports-related recurrent brain injuries: United States. *Morb Mortal Wkly Rep,* 14:224, 1997.
12. Torg, JS: Epidemiology, biomechanics, and prevention of cervical spine trauma resulting from athletics and recreational activities. *Oper Techn Sports Med,* 1:159, 1993.
13. Torg, JS: The epidemiologic, biomechanical, and cinematographic analysis of football induced cervical spine trauma. *Athl Train J Nl Athl Train Assoc,* 25:147, 1990.
14. Otis, JS, Burstein, AH, and Torg, JS: Mechanisms and pathomechanics of athletic injuries to the cervical spine. In Torg, JS (ed): *Athletic Injuries to the Head, Neck, and Face* (ed 2). St Louis, Mosby-Year Book, 1991, p 438.
15. Torg, JS, et al: The epidemiologic, pathologic, biomechanical, and cinematographic analysis of football-induced cervical spine trauma. *Am J Sports Med,* 18:50, 1990.
16. Heck, JF: The incidence of spearing by high school football carriers and their tacklers. *J Athl Train,* 27:120, 1992.
17. Theye, F, and Mueller, KA: "Heads up": Concussions in high school sports. *Clin Med Res,* 2:165, 2004.

17a. McCrory P, Meeuswisse W, Johnson K, et al: Consensus statement on concussion in sport. 3rd International conference on concussion in sport held in Zurich, November 2008. *Clin J Sport Med,* 19:185, 2009.

18. Guskiewicz, KM, et al: Epidemiology of concussions in collegiate and high school football players. *Am J Sports Med,* 28:643, 2000.
19. Abuabara, A: Cerebrospinal fluid rhinorrhea: Diagnosis and management. *Med Oral Patol Oral Cir Bucal,* 12:E397, 2007.
20. Miller, JR, et al: Comparison of preseason, midseason, and postseason neurocognitive scores in uninjured collegiate football players. *Am J Sports Med,* 35:1284, 2007.
21. Oliaro, SM, Guskiewicz, KM, and Prentice, WE: Establishment of normative data on cognitive tests for comparison with athletes sustaining mild head injury. *J Athl Train,* 33:36, 1998.
22. Onate, JA, et al: A comparison of sideline versus clinical cognitive test performance in collegiate athletes. *J Athl Train,* 35:155, 2000.
23. Guskiewicz, KM: Concussion in sport: The grading system dilemma. *Athl Ther Today,* 6:18, 2001.
24. Bohnen, N, Twinjstra, A, and Jolles, J: Performance in the Stroop color word test in relationship to the persistence of symptoms following mild head injury. *Acta Neurol Scand,* 85:116, 1992.

25. Hinton-Bayre, AD, Geffen, G, and McFarland, K: Mild head injury and speed of information processing: A prospective study of professional rugby league players. *J Clin Exp Neuropsychol,* 19:275, 1997.
26. Iverson, G, Franzen, M, and Lovell, M: Normative comparisons for the controlled oral word association test following acute traumatic brain injury. *J Clin Exp Neuropsychol,* 13:437, 1999.
27. McClincy, MP, et al: Recovery from sports concussion in high school and college athletes. *Brain Injury,* 20:33, 2006.
28. Broglio, SP, Macciocchi, SN, and Ferrara, MS: Neurocognitive performance of concussed athletes when symptom free. *J Athl Train,* 42:504, 2007.
29. Guskiewicz, KM, et al: Cumulative effects associated with recurrent concussion in collegiate football players. The NCAA concussion study. *JAMA,* 290:2549, 2003.
30. Randolph, C, McCrea, M, and Barr, WB: Is neuropsychological testing useful in the management of sport-related concussion? *J Athl Train,* 40:139, 2005.
31. Brown, CN, Guskiewicz, KM, and Bleiberg, J: Athlete characteristics and outcome scores for computerized neuropsychological assessment: A preliminary analysis. *J Athl Train,* 42:515, 2007.
32. Broglio, SP, et al: Test-retest reliability of computerized concussion assessment programs. *J Athl Train,* 42:509, 2007.
33. Broglio, SP, Macciocchi, SN, and Ferrara, MS: Sensitivity of the concussion assessment battery. *Neurosurgery,* 60:1050, 2007.
34. Riemann, BL, and Guskiewicz, KM: Effects of mild head injury on postural stability as measured through clinical balance testing. *J Athl Train,* 35:19, 2000.
35. Balance Error Scoring System (BESS) *User's Manual.* University of North Carolina, Chapel Hill, NC, Sports Medicine Research Laboratory.
36. Valovich, TCV, et al: Psychometric and measurement properties of concussion assessment tools in youth sports. *J Athl Train,* 41:399, 2006.
37. Valovich, TC, Perrin, DH, and Gansneder, BM: Repeat administration elicits practice effect with the Balance Error Scoring System but not with the Standardized Assessment of Concussion in high school athletes. *J Athl Train,* 38:51, 2003.
38. Onate, JA, Beck, BC, and Van Lunen, BL: On-field testing environment and Balance Error Scoring System Performance during preseason screening of healthy collegiate baseball players. *J Athl Train,* 42:446, 2007.
39. Mueller, FO, and Colgates, B: Annual survey of football injury research 1931–2007. National Center for Catastrophic Sport Injury Research. Retrieved from http://www.unc.edu/depts/nccsi/SurveyofFootballInjuries.htm. (Accessed: October 22, 2008).
40. Oliaro, S, Anderson, S, and Hooker, D: Management of cerebral concussion in sports: The athletic trainer's perspective. *J Athl Train,* 36:257, 2001.
41. AOSSM Concussion Group: Concussions in sports. Rosemont, IL, American Orthopaedic Society for Sports Medicine, 1999. Retrieved from http://www.intelli.com/vhosts/aossm-isite/databases/Concussion.doc. (Accessed November 19, 2008).
42. Lovell, MR, et al: Measurement of symptoms following sports-related concussion: Reliability and normative data for the post-concussion scale. *Appl Neuropsych,* 13:166, 2006.
43. Piland, SG, et al: Structural validity of self-report concussion-related symptom scale. *Med Sci Sport Exer,* 38:27, 2006.
44. McCrea, M, et al: Standardized assessment of concussion in football players. *Neurology,* 48:586, 1997.
45. McCrory P, et al: Summary and agreement statement of the 2nd International Conference on Concussion in Sport, Prague 2004. *Clin J Sport Med,* 15:48, 2005.
46. Practice parameter: The management of concussion in sports (summary statement). *Neurology,* 48:581, 1997.
47. Cantu, RC, and Micheli, LJ (eds): *American College of Sports Medicine Guidelines for the Team Physician.* Philadelphia: Lea & Febiger, 1991, p 93.
48. Colorado Medical Society: *Report of the Sports Medicine Committee: Guidelines for the Management of Concussion in Sports* (revised). Paper presented at the Colorado Medical Society, Denver, CO, 1991.
49. LeBlanc, KE: Concussions in sports: Guidelines for return to competition. *Am Fam Physician,* 50:801, 1994.
50. Guskiewicz, KM, et al: National Athletic Trainers' Association position statement: Management of sport-related concussion. *J Athl Train,* 39:280, 2004.
51. NCAA Guideline 2i: Concussion or mild traumatic brain injury (mTBI) in the athlete. In Klossner, D (ed): *NCAA Sports Medicine Handbook.* Indianapolis, IN, National Collegiate Athletic Association, 2007, p 46.
52. Cantu, RC: Criteria for return to competition after a closed head injury. In Torg, JS (ed): *Athletic Injuries to the Head, Neck, and Face* (ed 2). St Louis, Mosby-Year Book, 1991, p 326.
53. Gerberich, SG, et al: Concussion incidences and severity in secondary school varsity football players. *Am J Public Health,* 73:1370, 1983.
54. Cantu, RC: Head and spine injuries in youth sports. The young athlete. *Clin Sports Med,* 14:517, 1995.
55. Bigler, ED: Neuropsychology and clinical neuroscience of persistent post-concussive syndrome. *J Int Neuropsychol Soc,* 14:1, 2008.
56. Erlanger, DM, et al: Neuropsychology of sports-related head injury. Dementia pugilistica to post concussion syndrome. *Clin Neuropsychol,* 13:193, 1999.
57. Geurts, AC, Knoop, JA, and van Limbeek, J: Is postural control associated with mental functioning in the persistent postconcussion syndrome? *Arch Phys Med Rehabil,* 80:144, 1999.
58. Sanders, RI, and Harbaugh, RE: The second impact in catastrophic contact: Sports head trauma. *JAMA,* 252:538, 1984.
59. Muller, FO: Fatalities from head and cervical spine injuries occurring in tackle football: 50 years' experience. *Clin Sports Med,* 17:169, 1998.
60. White, RJ: Subarachnoid hemorrhage: The lethal intracranial explosion. *Emerg Med Clin North Am,* May:74, 1994.
61. Logan, SM, Bell, GW, and Leonard, JC: Acute subdural hematoma in a high school football player after 2 unreported episodes of head trauma: A case report. *J Athl Train,* 36:433, 2001.
62. Nee, PA, et al: Significance of vomiting after head injury. *J Neurol Neurosurg Psychiatry,* 66:470, 1999.
63. Bailes, JE: Management of cervical spine sports injuries. *Athl Train J Natl Athl Train Assoc,* 25:156, 1990.
64. Torg, JS: Criteria for return to collision activities after cervical spine injury. *Oper Techn Sports Med,* 1:236, 1993.
65. Torg, JS, et al: Spear tackler's spine: An entity precluding participation in tackle football and collision activities that expose the cervical spine to axial energy inputs. *Am J Sports Med,* 21:640, 1993.

66. Waninger, KN: Management of the helmeted athlete with suspected cervical spine injury. *Am J Sports Med,* 32:1331, 2004.
67. Geisler, FH: Clinical trials of pharmacotherapy for spinal cord injury. *Ann NY Acad Sci,* 845:374,1998.
68. Seidl, EC: Promising pharmacological agents in the management of acute spinal cord injury. *Crit Care Nurs Q,* 22:44, 1999.
69. Vale, FL, et al: Combined medical and surgical treatment after acute spinal cord injury: Results of a prospective pilot study to assess the merits of aggressive medical resuscitation and blood pressure management. *J Neurosurg,* 87:239, 1997.
70. Scher, AT: Spinal cord concussion in rugby players. *Am J Sports Med,* 18:50, 1990.
71. Torg, JS: Cervical spine stenosis with cord neurapraxia and transient quadriplegia. *Athl Train J Nl Athl Train Assoc,* 25:156, 1990.
72. Torg, JS, et al: The relationship of developmental narrowing of the cervical spinal canal to reversible and irreversible injury of the cervical spinal cord in football players. *J Bone Joint Surg,* 78(A):1308, 1996.
73. Gale, SD, Decoster, LC, and Swartz, EE. The combined tool approach for face mask removal during on-field conditions. *J Athl Train,* 43:14, 2008.
74. Feld, F: Management of the critically injured football players. *J Athl Train,* 28:206, 1993.
75. NCAA Guideline 4e: Guidelines for helmet fitting and removal in athletics. In Klossner D (ed): *NCAA Sports Medicine Handbook.* Indianapolis, IN, National Collegiate Athletic Association, 2007, p 89.
76. Kleiner, DM, et al: Prehospital care of the spine-injured athlete. A document from the inter-association task force for appropriate care of the spine-injured athlete. National Athletic Trainers' Association, Dallas, TX. 2001.
77. Decoster, LC, Shirley, CP, and Swartz, EE: Football face-mask removal with a cordless screwdriver on helmets used for at least one season of play. *J Athl Train,* 40:169, 2005.
78. Swartz, EE, et al: The influence of various factors on high school football helmet face mask removal: A retrospective, cross-sectional analysis. *J Athl Train,* 42:11, 2007.
79. Swartz, EE, et al: Football equipment design affects face mask removal efficiency. *Am J Sports Med,* 33:1, 2005.
80. Caroline, N: *Emergency Care in the Streets* (ed 3). Boston, Little, Brown, 25:147, 1990.
81. Ransone, J, Kersey, R, and Walsh, K: The efficacy of rapid form cervical vacuum immobilizer in the cervical spine immobilization of the equipped football player. *J Athl Train,* 35:65, 2000.

CHAPTER 22

Environment-Related Conditions

The onset of environment-related injury or illness is not limited to temperature extremes or outdoor activities. The harmful gain or loss of heat to and from the external environment can occur during any physical activity. The body has the ability to adapt to exercise in most of the environmental extremes seen in athletics. Except for accidental exposure to very hot or very cold temperatures, environmentally related injuries or illnesses are completely preventable.

Clinical Anatomy and Physiology

Regulation of the body's core temperature occurs in the hypothalamus and other brain centers. Normally, the skin temperature is higher than that of the surrounding environment. The body's core temperature is greater than that of the skin and extremities. In this chapter, the term "core temperature" is used to describe the actual temperature within the viscera.

Just as a furnace receives input from a thermostat, the hypothalamus receives input from thermoreceptors located in the skin, spinal cord, abdomen, and brain. In response to changes in the core temperature, the hypothalamus directs blood toward or away from the skin, regulating the amount of cooling. Increasing blood flow to the skin decreases the core temperature. Conversely, decreasing blood flow to the skin increases the core temperature. Core temperature is controlled by increasing mechanical and chemical heat production when the core temperature drops too low or increasing sweating when the core temperature rises too high (Fig. 22-1).

Heat Transfer

Heat exchange to and from the body occurs through radiation, conduction, convection, and evaporation. Each of these mechanisms relies on a temperature gradient between the body and the surrounding environment. The greater this difference, the greater the magnitude and rate of the exchange to and from the body.

Radiation

All objects emit heat in the form of infrared radiation. Normally, this exchange occurs in the form of the body's losing heat into the environment. However, when the body is placed in an exceedingly warm environment, such as a hot, humid day, sitting in a sauna, or practicing in a wrestling room, the body gains heat through radiation.

Conduction and convection

The body can gain or lose heat when it is in contact with an object that has a temperature warmer or cooler than itself. Because the air contains molecules, the body can exchange heat directly with the atmosphere via **conduction**. The use of a hot pack or ice pack are examples of the body's gaining or losing heat through conduction. The efficiency of conduction in still, standing air is quite poor. Circulating the air across the body enhances the cooling

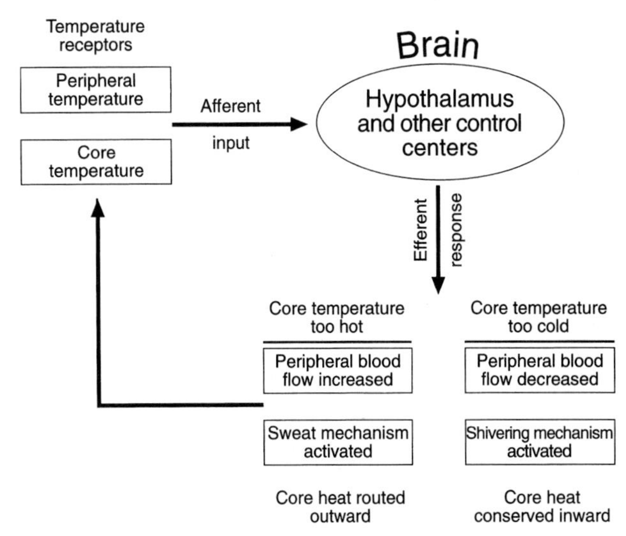

FIGURE 22-1 ■ The body's thermoregulatory system. Thermoreceptors in the extremities, skin, and within the viscera monitor the body's temperature. High temperatures result in increased peripheral blood flow and activate the sweating mechanism to route the heat away from the core. Cold core temperatures activate a mechanism that conserves the core temperature.

Examination Map

HISTORY

Past Medical History

Weight loss

Recent history of illness

Sickle cell trait

Inadequate nutrition

Prior environmental illness or injury

History of the Present Condition

Mechanism of injury

Environmental conditions

Thirst

Conditioning level

Body build

Drug and alcohol use

INSPECTION

Skin color

Muscle tone

Pupils

PALPATION

Skin temperature

REVIEW OF SYSTEMS

Cardiovascular
- Pulse
- Blood pressure
- Core temperature

Respiration

Neurologic

Genitourinary
- Urine specific gravity

PATHOLOGIES AND SPECIAL TESTS

Heat Illness

Heat cramps

Heat syncope

Heat exhaustion

Heat stroke

Exertional hyponatremia

Cold Injuries

Hypothermia

Frostbite

process via **convection**. The use of a room fan is an example of convective cooling.

Conduction and convection most commonly occur between the skin and the air. During swimming, water is the environmental medium through which most heat is lost. This explains why the temperature of competitive swimming pools is kept relatively low.

Evaporation

The evaporation of water from the skin carries heat with it, cooling the skin and subsequently lowering the core temperature. During physical exertion, the body depends primarily on evaporation for heat loss. In response to exercise, the body's perspiration rate increases, covering the body with fluids to be evaporated, thus removing heat.

Other mechanisms

Heat is lost from the body through several other mechanisms, many of which are inconsequential (or impractical) during physical exercise. Respiration is the most common and applicable of these methods. As air passes into the lungs, it travels through warm, moist passages, humidifying it. During expiration, water and heat are lost. Elimination through urination, defecation, or vomiting also transfers heat from the body. However, these mechanisms cause dehydration.

Blood Flow and Heat Exchange

To maintain its core temperature during exercise, the body must balance the amount of heat gained and heat lost. The body responds to a hot, humid environment by increasing the blood flow to the extremities and subcutaneous vessels. The vessels in the skin dilate, allowing more blood to carry heat away from the core to be released into the environment.

The proportion of heat lost via radiation, conduction, convection, and evaporation depends on the intensity of exercise, **relative humidity**, and **ambient** temperature.[1] Heat lost via conduction, convection, and radiation decreases as the ambient temperature increases. Increased humidity decreases the effectiveness of the sweating mechanism.

The total volume of the body's blood vessels is approximately four times greater than that of the heart's pumping capacity. The body compensates for this disparity by routing more blood to the areas having a higher oxygen demand and decreasing the supply to areas with a lesser demand. The brain has the highest priority for oxygen.

During exercise, a worsening cycle occurs when the body's core temperature begins to increase above normal. Increased core temperature caused by exercise increases systemic metabolism. This, in turn, further increases the core temperature. For every 1% of body weight lost through sweating, there is a 0.49°F to 0.65°F (0.27°C to 0.37°C) increase in core temperature. The heart rate also increases 3 to 5 beats per minute.[1] As the core temperature rises above 104.0°F (40.07°C), a linear relationship between the core temperature and metabolic demands develops (Fig. 22-2).[2] After the body's internal temperature reaches 107.6°F (42.0°C), the cardiovascular system can no longer meet the metabolic oxygen demand necessary to sustain life.

The brain is constantly monitoring the oxygen requirements of the exercising muscles, internal organs, and brain, making the adjustments necessary to maintain

Relative humidity The ratio between the amount of water vapor in the air and the actual amount of water the air could potentially hold based on the current temperature.

Ambient Pertaining to the local environment.

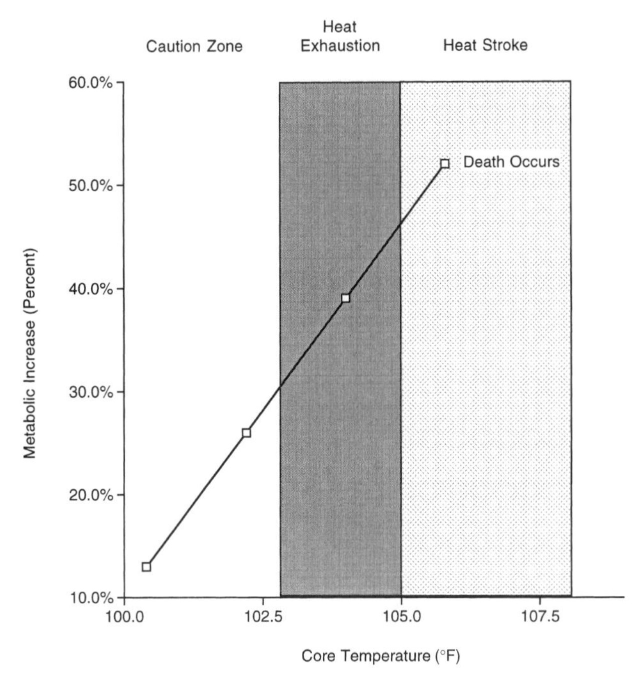

FIGURE 22-2 ■ Linear relationship between core temperature and metabolism.

the viability of each while also keeping the core temperature within acceptable limits. Blood flow to the working muscles is increased, decreasing the supply of oxygen available to the other areas of the body. When this exertion occurs in a hot or humid environment, blood flow to the cutaneous vessels is increased to cool the core temperature. This rerouted blood draws more blood from the viscera and the brain, causing the core temperature to increase. Increased metabolism associated with the temperature rise and the exercising muscles further increases the core temperature.

Sweating Mechanism

Sweating reduces the body's internal temperature by carrying heat outward, where it can evaporate into the atmosphere. This process is inherently efficient because water conducts heat 25 times more rapidly than air.[3] Unfortunately, the sweating process is also self-depleting.

Sweat is not pure water. When sweat leaves the body, it also carries electrolytes, namely sodium (salt) and potassium, with it. The body's ability to efficiently sustain prolonged activity is directly related to the replacement of both water and electrolytes. When water is not replaced, the efficiency of the cooling mechanism is impaired. The plasma volume is reduced, decreasing blood pressure, causing the heart to work harder to deliver blood to the areas requiring it. When the electrolytes are not replaced, metabolic efficiency is hindered by depriving the body of essential substances required for normal physiologic function. The combined effects of increased core temperature and dehydration significantly alter cardiovascular function more so than either dehydration or increased temperature alone.[4]

The total amount of sweat lost is based on the sweating rate, calculated as[1]:

$$\text{Sweat rate} = \frac{\text{(pre-exercise body weight} - \text{post-exercise body weight} + \text{fluid intake} - \text{urine volume)}}{\text{Time in hours}}$$

Replenishing water before, during, and after exercise keeps the net fluid loss to a minimum, increases the efficiency of the sweating mechanism, and assists in preventing dehydration.

Heat Conservation

Just as excessive heat gain is harmful to the body, so is excessive loss of heat. The body conserves heat by reversing the process used to cool the body. Blood is routed away from the superficial vessels and the skin, maintaining the core temperature. When the temperature drops below 86°F (30°C), muscle tone increases and, eventually, shivering begins. The increased metabolism associated with these muscle contractions serves as a source of heat to rewarm the core. Chronic or prolonged exposure to a cold environment results in chemical thermogenesis, a process in which epinephrine is secreted into the bloodstream, increasing the metabolism of nonmuscular cells.[5]

Ambient Temperature Influence

The ambient temperature, humidity, wind velocity, and radiant heat all influence the risk of environmental illness.[6] The term "heat illness" is probably a misnomer because its onset is more directly related to the relative humidity (RH) than to the actual temperature of the air. Until the ambient air temperature exceeds 95°F (35°C) or the relative humidity reaches 75%, sweating and evaporation account for most of the heat loss.[7] The percentage at which relative humidity raises the risk of heat illness is decreased by 10% for every 5°F increase in air temperature (i.e., at 70°F the humidity danger zone is 80% RH; at 90°F, the danger zone is 40% RH). After the relative humidity reaches 100% and the air temperature reaches that of the skin, the body can no longer lose heat into the environment. The resulting core temperature can increase to fatally high levels.

Acclimatization

Physiologic systems can adapt to exercise in hot, humid environments through improved efficiency of the metabolic and cooling processes. "Acclimation" is used to describe physiologic changes that occur in a controlled environment. "Acclimatization" describes the physical adaptations that occur in a natural environment.[6] Acclimatization is achieved by gradually exposing the exercising athlete to the environmental condition over a period of several days to weeks, depending on the magnitude of the environmental change.

The process of making the body more efficient involves the modification of four components[3]:

1. Increased glycogen stores increase the amount of **adenosine triphosphate** (ATP) available to skeletal and cardiac muscle and provide an immediate source of energy.
2. The heart's efficiency is improved by increasing cardiac output and stroke volume, allowing the heart to deliver more blood to the working muscles at a lower pulse rate. The improved efficiency of cardiac and skeletal muscle contraction results in decreased metabolic heat production.
3. The body's sweat threshold temperature is lowered and the volume of sweat is increased, enhancing the rapid removal of heat from the body and preventing the core temperature from reaching the danger zone.
4. Improved renal function results in a decreased level of salt being lost in the sweat, which, through osmotic properties, retains extracellular fluid (ECF) and plasma volume.

Clinical Examination of Environmental Conditions

The evaluative process of patients with environmental injuries and illnesses requires knowledge of the symptoms and information about the environmental conditions and other factors that may predispose the individual to these injuries. Because of the relatively straightforward evaluation of patients with these conditions, the format of the evaluative process has been altered from those presented in previous chapters.

*** Practical Evidence**

Adolescents are at greater risk of heat illness than adults because they (1) begin practice sessions underhydrated, (2) drink insufficient amounts during exercise, (3) require a longer time needed to acclimatize to hot conditions, and (4) have a greater body area to body mass ratio.[8,9]

History

Past medical history

- **Weight loss:** Recent weight loss can increase the risk of environmental illness, especially when it is caused by water loss. The use of weight charts can identify individuals who are predisposed to heat illness secondary to water loss (see "Prevention of Heat Illnesses").
- **Recent history of illness:** Vomiting or diarrhea increases the amount of water and electrolytes lost from the body. Other illnesses increase the body's metabolic demands and decrease the body's resistance to stress by increasing the core temperature.
- **Sickle cell trait:** Affecting primarily African Americans, the presence of **sickle cell trait** can result in **exertional sickling,** a heat and/or altitude-related condition that must be differentiated from heat exhaustion or heat stroke. Sickling of red blood cells can result in a blockage of the blood vessels, leading to potentially fatal **ischemic rhabdomyolysis.**[10]
- **Nutrition:** Dieting or poor nutritional habits may increase the risk of environmental illness. Decreased intake of fluids and electrolytes decrease the plasma volume and may inhibit the metabolism necessary for athletic activity. High-protein diets may decrease the body's ability to cope with cold environments.
- **History of environmental illness:** Previous heat-related illnesses predispose the individual to repeat episodes.

History of the present condition

- **Environmental conditions:** The magnitude of environmental extremes decreases the duration of exposure required for the onset of symptoms. Heat exposure is compounded by humidity, and cold exposure is compounded by wind. These conditions, discussed in the "Environmental Pathologies and Related Special Tests" section, must be determined before competition or practice and influence whether or not the activity will be held or modified.
- **Thirst:** The thirst response is triggered when the patient's body weight is decreased 1% to 2% by fluid loss.[6] Some systemic conditions may also alter the thirst response. Diets, especially those rich in salty and fried foods, may also increase the thirst response. Note that electrolyte depletion alone does not trigger the thirst response.
- **Conditioning level:** People who are poorly conditioned or are not acclimatized are susceptible to heat illness. Proper conditioning assists in adapting to both hot and cold environments.[11]
- **Body build:** Large muscle mass is a predisposition to heat illness secondary to increased metabolism.
- **Drug and alcohol use:** Certain medications, including amphetamines, antihistamines, laxatives, diet pills, tricyclic antidepressants, and diuretics, predispose an individual to heat illness.[8]
- **Other complaints:** Heat illness may cause the person to become confused and aggressive and have headaches. Individuals suffering from cold injuries express a desire to warm up or, in extreme cases, to sleep.

Inspection

- **Skin:** The color of the skin can provide evidence of the underlying condition. Minor heat-related conditions cause the skin to become pale. Heat stroke, a medical

---

Adenosine triphosphate (ATP) An energy-yielding enzyme used during muscular contractions.

Sickle cell trait Carrying one sickle gene, associated with sickle cell anemia.

emergency, often results in dark or red skin. In the majority of athletic-related heat illness, the athlete sweats profusely. Cold injury causes the skin to have a waxy appearance that is red in minor cases or pale in more severe cases.

- **Muscle tone:** As the core temperature increases, the muscle tone decreases to reduce the amount of metabolic heat produced and assist in routing the heat outward to the skin. The exception to this is heat cramps. The body responds to a cold environment by increasing muscle tone by shivering.
- **Pupils:** Exposure to extreme heat or cold causes pupillary dilation and decreased responsiveness to light, an indication of decreased brain function.

Palpation

- **Skin temperature:** During heat exhaustion, the skin often feels cool and clammy to the touch. During heat stroke, the skin feels hot. Cold exposure results in decreased skin temperature.

Review of Systems

Also refer to Review of Systems, p. 575 in Chapter 15.

- **Cardiovascular**
  - **Pulse:** Heat illnesses result in tachycardia in response to meet the body's demand for oxygen. Cooling of the core temperature causes the heart rate to become slow and the pulse to weaken.
  - **Blood pressure:** During heat exhaustion and hypothermia, the blood pressure decreases and may result in syncope. Heat stroke causes an increase in the blood pressure.
  - **Core temperature:** A core temperature greater than 104°F (40°C) is indicative of heat stroke and requires the immediate cooling of the patient and activation of the emergency action plan. Cardiorespiratory changes begin to occur once the core temperature falls to 94°F (34.4°C) and below.
- **Respiration:** Paralleling the findings of the heart rate, heat exposure increases the respiratory rate; cold exposure causes it to slow.
- **Neurologic:** Prolonged increases or decreases of the intracranial temperature result in an altered cognitive function. Increased temperature results in dizziness, confusion, violent behavior, and unconsciousness. Cooling of the brain causes the individual to become drowsy, eventually drifting into unconsciousness.
- **Genitourinary:** Urine specific gravity (USG) of greater than 1.020 may indicate dehydration. Heat cramps are likely to occur when USG is greater than 1.016. A USG of less than 1.010 is considered adequate hydration.[1,6] Refractometry is more accurate and more reliable than urine reagent strips in assessing USG.[12]

*** Practical Evidence**

To assess core temperature accurately, rectal temperature must be used. Oral, axillary, aural, temporal, and forehead temperatures give invalid results and could mistakenly minimize the severity of a heat illness.[13]

Environmental Pathologies and Related Special Tests

The delineation between heat and cold pathologies is obvious. What is more difficult, however, is the delineation between the various types and severity of heat and cold injuries and illnesses. The importance of preventing environmental injuries is emphasized throughout this chapter. Illnesses from exposure to hot or cold environments are preventable, unlike the relatively unpreventable nature of most of the other injuries described in this text.

Heat Illnesses

The effects of participating in a hot, humid environment, collectively referred to as **hyperthermia,** range from the relatively minor symptoms associated with heat cramps and heat exhaustion to the potentially fatal effects of heat stroke. These are not always progressive conditions. A person may collapse from heat stroke without first displaying the signs and symptoms of the less serious conditions. A comparison of the signs and symptoms of heat cramps, heat syncope, heat exhaustion, and heat stroke is presented in Examination Findings 22-1.[14]

*** Practical Evidence**

Body mass index (BMI) is a significant predictor for the onset of exertional heat illness. A study of military recruits indicated that individuals having a BMI greater than 22 kg/m^2 were eight times more likely to sustain a heat-related illness than recruits with a BMI less than 22 kg/m^2.[11]

The onset of heat-related illnesses is directly associated with the environment and based on the relationship between air temperature and humidity. The onset of heat illness is not limited to the summer or outdoor activities. Hot, humid gymnasiums, wrestling rooms, or even swimming pools can be the sites of heat illness. Certain individuals may be predisposed to acquiring heat-related illnesses (Table 22-1). Despite the varying times and locations in which heat illness can occur, they are all preventable through adequate rehydration and conditioning.

Exercising in high heat and humidity conditions may result in a **heat rash** (also known as prickly heat). The rash tends to occur in areas covered with occlusive clothing (neck, trunk, axilla, groin) and is instantly and intensely itchy.[8]

Examination Findings 22-1
Heat Illness

Evaluative Finding	Heat Cramps	Heat Syncope	Heat Exhaustion	Heat Stroke
Hydration Status	Dehydrated	Dehydrated	Dehydrated	Dehydrated
Core Temperature*	WNL**	WNL	102°F–104°F (38.9°C–40°C)	Greater than 104°F (40°C)
Skin Color and Temperature	WNL	Pale	Cool/clammy Pale	Hot Red
Sweating	Moderate to profuse	WNL	Profuse	Slight to profuse The skin may be wet or dry
Pulse	WNL	Decreased	Rapid and weak	Increased
Blood Pressure	WNL	A sudden, imperceptible drop in blood pressure, which rapidly returns to normal	Low	High
Respiration	WNL	WNL	Hyperventilation	Rapid hyperventillation
Mental State	WNL Possible fatigue	Fatigue Dizziness Fainting	Dizziness Fatigue Slight confusion	Dizziness Drowsiness confusion/disorientation Emotional instability Violent behavior
Neuromuscular Changes	Cramping in one or more muscles		Muscle cramps Weakness	Weakness Decerebrate posture
Gastrointestinal and Urinary Changes			Intestinal cramping Nausea Vomiting Diarrhea Decreased urinary output	Nausea Vomiting Diarrhea
Central Nervous System			Syncope Headache	Headache Unconsciousness Seizures Coma
Other Findings	Thirst	"Tunnel vision" may be reported.	Thirst Loss of appetite (anorexia) Chills	Dilated pupils

WNL = within normal limits.
*As determined by the rectal temperature.
**Within normal limits for an exercising athlete.

Heat cramps

Heat cramps are easily recognized by the painful spasm or cramping of skeletal muscle, most often affecting the lower extremity muscles, and are most apt to occur during the first 3 weeks of practice in high heat and/or humidity.[15] The underlying cause of heat cramps is debatable, but dehydration and loss of electrolytes secondary to excessive sweating, neuromuscular fatigue,[7,14] sodium depletion,[6] or a spinal

Table 22-1 Conditions Predisposing to Heat Illness

Predisposing Condition	Rationale
Large Body Mass	Large muscle mass increases the body's heat production. Large layers of adipose tissue decrease the heat exchange mechanism.
Age	The heat exchange mechanism of the young and old does not efficiently remove heat.
Conditioning Level	Individuals who are poorly conditioned or conditioned athletes who are not acclimated to the environment produce increased levels of metabolic heat and are less efficient at dissipating the heat.
Poor Hydration	Internal fluids are required for maximum efficiency of the heat transfer mechanism. Illnesses, especially those involving vomiting or diarrhea, dehydrate the body. Lack of hydration before, during, and after exercise.
History of Heat Illness	A history of heat-related illness can indicate a chronically inadequate level of hydration or nutrition. An athlete with a recent history of heat-related illness may not have sufficient time to rehydrate.
Medications and Other Substances	Diuretic and laxative medications and alcohol promote fluid loss via urination and defecation. Creatine and anabolic steroids increase muscle mass and tend to increase the level of intramuscular fluids. Antihistamines, decongestants (pseudoephedrine), and amphetamines increase metabolism, cause vasoconstriction, or otherwise increase the risk of heat illness.

neural mechanism[16] are most often implicated. Unconditioned individuals or otherwise conditioned athletes who are not acclimatized to participating in a hot, humid environment are most susceptible to heat cramps. These environmental conditions increase the person's sweating rate and volume, rapidly depleting the body of electrolytes. There have, however, been reports of "heat cramps" in cool conditions.[17] Sodium loss through sweating—often over several days—is compounded by inadequate intake of dietary salts and/or ingesting hypotonic fluids.[17] The decreased plasma sodium chloride (NaCl) concentrations alters the sodium-potassium pump and changes action potential changes across the cell membrane.[6] The compacted interstitial volume results in the mechanical deformation of individual motor nerves and an increase in neurotransmitter levels, causing these sites to become easily excited. When combined with other ionic changes, random, uncontrolled muscle contractions (cramps or spasms) may result.[6,17]

Heat cramps can be differentiated from exercise-induced cramps by the location of the muscle spasm. Exercise induced cramps tend to involve the entire muscle or muscle group. Heat cramps tend to affect individual muscle bundles.[6]

Heat syncope

A fainting spell caused by hot, humid environments, heat syncope is sometimes included as a symptom of heat exhaustion.[16] Unlike fainting caused by heat exhaustion, the patient with heat syncope does not have an abnormally elevated core temperature and is normally hydrated.[3] When a person is exposed to high environmental temperatures, vascular shunting routes the blood outward to the skin and extremities to lower the core temperature. A sudden shift in blood flow causes cardiac filling pressure and stroke volume to decline rapidly, decreasing cardiac output and blood pressure and depriving the brain of oxygen. The onset of syncope is also associated with dehydration, decreased or inhibited venous return, decreased cardiac output, and cerebral ischemia.[14] Syncope can also have a metabolic, neurologic, or cardiovascular origin or can be the result of a drug reaction. These issues are discussed in Chapter 15.

Heat exhaustion

Heat exhaustion is characterized by sudden, extreme fatigue as the body attempts to supply blood to the brain, exercising muscles, and skin. Unlike in heat stroke, the hypothalamus continues to function properly with heat exhaustion.

The physiologic effects of heat exhaustion can be traced to water and electrolytes lost through sweating.[6] When these events are accompanied by profuse sweating and when fluids and electrolytes are not replaced, the body's volume of circulating fluid is depleted.

Heat exhaustion is classified according to its onset: water depletion or electrolyte depletion. Sweating, vomiting, diarrhea, and excessive urination without substantial rehydration cause a net water loss from the body, all predisposing conditions for heat stroke. Water depletion heat exhaustion has a rapid onset and, if untreated, can progress to heat stroke.[6]

Excessive loss of electrolytes from the body causes a loss of ECF, reducing the plasma volume and subsequently reducing cardiac output and decreasing blood pressure. Severe cases of salt and electrolyte depletion result in peripheral vascular collapse, presenting the signs and symptoms of traumatic shock. Electrolyte depletion heat stroke tends to occur after several days of exercising in a hot environment.[6]

The presence or absence of thirst is a way of determining whether a heat illness is caused by water deprivation or salt deprivation. People who are water depleted describe thirst. Salt-depleted individuals have no such craving. Heat exhaustion caused by salt depletion is not resolved by the ingestion of plain water. Most athletic-related cases of heat exhaustion are caused by water depletion, but the two can occur in conjunction with each other.

Individuals suffering from heat exhaustion have a rectal temperature less than 104°F (40°C) and present with profuse sweating, causing the skin to feel cool and clammy. In response to cardiovascular demands, pulse and respiration are rapid, but the loss of fluids causes the pulse to feel weak and reduces the blood pressure. The individual may complain of a headache and appear to be fatigued and confused.

Heat stroke

A medical emergency, heat stroke represents the failure and subsequent shutdown of the body's thermoregulatory system. Heat stroke occurs when the body is unable to shed its excess heat into the environment, causing the core temperature to rise above 104°F (40°C). After this shutdown, the core temperature continues to increase, placing the cells of the internal organs and, most importantly, the brain, at risk. The body attempts to maintain arterial blood pressure at the expense of thermoregulation and blood flow to the skin, which is needed for cooling.[6] Subsequently, all of the body's systems begin to fail. If untreated, death can occur from heat stroke within 20 minutes.

Heat stroke is classified as classic or exertional. **Classic heat stroke** most often affects infants and the elderly, occurring during a period when they are exposed to a hot environment and unable to rehydrate or cool themselves. Classic heat stroke, which is not generally associated with physical exertion, is characterized by the absence of sweat, a potentially fatal misconception when applied to athletes. The lack of sweating is often, and incorrectly, correlated with exertional heat stroke, which most commonly affects athletes.

Exertional heat stroke occurs within a matter of hours during exercise in a hot and humid environment. In this scenario, profuse sweating occurs and fluids are not replaced, depleting the body of water and electrolytes. Most athletes suffering from exertional heat stroke are sweating. Using the definition of classic heat stroke, athletes suffering from exertional heat stroke may be misevaluated because of the presence of sweating. However, exertional heat stroke may occur without significant dehydration.[6]

The athlete's probability of survival is directly related to the quick identification of heat stroke and the immediate initiation of treatment. The only practical difference between heat stroke and heat exhaustion that can be determined on the field is the athlete's mental state. Violent behavior followed by unconsciousness is a characteristic trait of heat stroke. The athlete's skin may feel hot compared with the expected finding of heat exhaustion, in which the skin tends to feel damp and cool. As brain function diminishes, the pupils become fixed and dilated and the athlete may assume a decerebrate posture (see p. 905). The attempt to maintain blood pressure may account for the incidence of liver and kidney failure associated with heat illnesses.

Exertional hyponatremia

Exertional hyponatremia occurs when the person's serum-sodium level drops below 130 to 135 mmol/L and is triggered by excessive fluid consumption coupled by inappropriate fluid retention ("water intoxication") or inadequate water and sodium replacement.[14,19] In other words, consuming too much or too little fluid and sodium can lead to the onset of exertional hyponatremia. The intravascular and extracellular fluids have a lower sodium density that the intracellular fluids, causing water to diffuse into the cells. As the water content within the cell walls increase, the size of the cells increase, resulting in neurologic and physiologic dysfunction.[14] Untreated, exertional hyponatremia can result in death.

The initial signs and symptoms of exertional hyponatremia often first affect the central nervous system (Examination Findings 22-2). The patient demonstrates an altered mental/cognitive state including lethargy and disorientation. Outwardly, vomiting and swelling of the extremities may be noted. Pulmonary and cerebral edema leads to seizures, unconsciousness, and, if untreated, death.[14] The patient's core temperature is less that 104°F (40°C), differentiating the condition from heat stroke.

Patients suspected of suffering exertional hyponatremia must be immediately transported for emergency medical intervention. Do not administer fluids until the patient is examined by a physician.[14]

Prevention of Heat Illness

Table 22-2 lists steps to reduce the incidence of athletic heat illnesses and the rationale for doing so. Environmental heat conditions need to be determined before and during outdoor athletic competition. Traditionally, this has been done with the use of a sling psychrometer, a device that determines relative humidity through the temperatures derived from a dry thermometer and a wet one. The wet bulb globe temperature alone is often sufficient information to indicate the need to modify the activity. Practice should be suspended when the wet bulb temperature exceeds 82°F (27.8°C).[20] The temperature and humidity can also be obtained from local radio stations or dial-in weather services, but these reports may not accurately depict local weather conditions. High temperature and humidity require that the activity be modified accordingly (Table 22-3).

The **WBGT Index** is another method of measuring environmental conditions. By factoring the ambient air temperature, humidity, and radiant heat conditions and comparing them to a chart, the intensity, duration, and required length of rest periods can be determined.[15]

In regions where the temperature is normally hot and humid, practices should be regularly scheduled to avoid environmental extremes. However, in many regions, the summer months may be predominated by these conditions.[21] Altering the duration and intensity of the activity is also useful in preventing hyperthermia. Longer events performed at a slower pace have less risk of heat illness than do shorter, more intense activities held in the same environmental conditions.[22]

Examination Findings 22-2
Exertional Hyponatremia

Examination Segment	Clinical Findings
History	***Onset:*** Acute ***Pain characteristics:*** Not applicable ***Other symptoms:*** Not applicable ***Mechanism:*** Not applicable ***Predisposing conditions:*** Exercise of greater than 4 hours coupled with high fluid and sodium intake or inadequate replacement of sodium NSAID use[18]
Inspection	Swelling of the feet, hands, and extremities
Palpation	Not applicable
Review of Systems	***Cardiovascular:*** Pulmonary edema ***CNS:*** Headaches that worsen with time Altered consciousness Cerebral edema Coma Seizures ***Mental state:*** Confusion/disorientation ***Core temperature:*** Less than 104°F (40°C) ***Gastrointestinal:*** Nausea Vomiting
Functional Assessment	The patient is disoriented and lethargic before becoming unconsciousness.
Laboratory Tests	Low blood-sodium level
Differential Diagnosis	Heat stroke, heat exhaustion, ischemic rhabdomyolysis

Table 22-2 Prevention of Heat Illness

Technique	Rationale
Acclimation	Improves the efficiency of muscle contraction, improves the efficiency of the cardiovascular system, lowers sweat threshold, and improves kidney function.
Proper Nutrition and Hydration	Provides the body with the fluids and electrolytes to maintain homeostasis during exercise.
Avoidance of Environmental Extremes	When practical, exercise in less hot or humid environments to maximize heat transfer from the body.
Wearing Appropriate Clothing	Allows evaporation of perspiration to promote heat loss from the body when appropriate clothing is worn; therefore, full pads practices should not be conducted in extreme heat or humidity
Rest Periods	Allows recovery and rehydration for athletes; includes activities such as cooling off in a cool area, consuming fluids, and allowing clothing changes during breaks

During two-a-day practices, the proportion of body weight lost because of dehydration can be calculated through the use of weight charts (Fig. 22-3). Athletes record their weight before and after each practice, with the percentage of body weight lost determining the risk of complications caused by the heat. Athletes who lose 3% of their weight from the start of one practice to the start of the next require continuous monitoring during practice. In addition, they are required to consume water frequently. Athletes displaying a 5% weight loss should be prohibited from practice. Those having a 7% drop in weight are in extreme danger and should be withheld from participation until the weight loss is reduced to 3% (see the following section on rehydration).

Sports gear made of substances that completely isolate the body from the external environment, such as neoprene™ or rubber, creates an environment with a temperature equal to or greater than the core temperature. Subsequent sweating raises the relative humidity within the suit to levels nearing 100%, actually predisposing the athlete to heat illness.

Athletes should report to practice physically fit and acclimated to the environment in which they will be competing.

Table 22-3 Guidelines for Modification of Athletic Competition in Hot or Humid Environments

Dry Bulb Temperature (°F)	Wet Bulb Temperature (°F)	Humidity (%)	Consequences
80–90	68	<70	No extraordinary precautions are required for athletes not predisposed to heat illness. Athletes who are predisposed (e.g., unconditioned, unacclimated, or losing more than 3% of body weight from water loss) require close observation.
80–90 90–100	69–79 <70	>70	Regular rest breaks are necessary.
			Loose, breathable clothing should be worn, and wet uniforms require regular changing.
90–100 >100	>80	>70	Practice should be shortened and modified. The use of protective equipment covering the body should be curtailed.
	>82		Practice should be canceled.

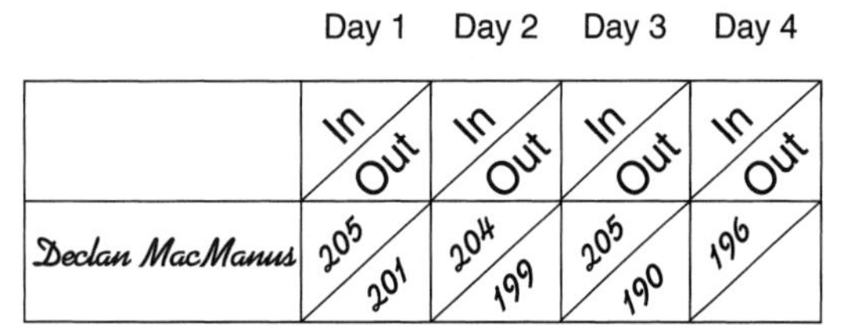

FIGURE 22-3 ■ Weight chart. Each athlete weighs "in" before practice and weighs "out" afterward. In the example, the athlete should have been restricted from practice on day 4 because of a 5% loss of body weight.

Athletes who have trained in a cool, dry environment are still predisposed to heat illness when moving to hot, humid areas.

Rehydration

Most heat-related illness can be prevented by keeping athletes properly hydrated before, during, and after the activity (Table 22-4).[1] The goal of any rehydration strategy is to match the amount of fluids and sodium ingested during activity to the fluids and sodium lost during activity. In many cases it is impractical to precisely match fluid intake with fluid loss with causing bloating and gastrointestinal upset (which would further dehydrate the body). Although the emphasis on maintaining this balance occurs during activity, pre- and post-activity strategies are also important.[17]

Proper hydration assists in heat dissipation by increasing blood flow to the skin and increasing the sweating rate, keeping the core temperature relatively low. Maintaining a proper fluid balance maintains the central blood volume that sustains cardiac output and prevents plasma **hypertonicity**.[6]

The goal of pre-exercise hydration is to preload the body with fluid stores. During activity, the goal of hydration is to prevent the athlete from losing more than 2% of the body weight through water loss. Athletes are encouraged to drink beyond their thirst level at a rate of approximately 7 to 10 fluid ounces every 10 to 20 minutes. After activity, athletes must be encouraged to consume fluids at a rate that is approximately 25% to 50% beyond that lost through sweating and urination. Ideally, water, carbohydrates, and electrolytes should be replenished within 2 hours after the activity.[1]

Table 22-4 Rehydration Strategies

Strategy	Comments
Pre-exercise Hydration	At 2–3 hours before competition: Consume 500–600 mL (17–20 fl oz.) of water or sports drink. At 10–20 minutes before competition: Consume 200–300 mL (7–10 fl oz.) of water or sports drink.
Hydration Maintenance	Every 10–20 minutes: Consume 200–300 mL (7–10 fl oz.) of water or sports drink. Prevent the athlete from losing more than 2% of body weight through water loss.
Post-exercise Hydration	Within 2 hours: Replace water, carbohydrates, and electrolytes lost during activity.

*** Practical Evidence**

The use of carbohydrate drinks before exercise can assist in increasing glycogen stores. A combination of water and a sports drink having a sodium concentration of up to 1150 mg per liter is effective in reducing the onset of heat-related illnesses.[17]

Simply ingesting fluids does not necessarily mean that the athlete will be rehydrated. Factors including the type, amount (volume), and **osmolality** of the fluid affect the body's ability to absorb—and therefore use—the fluid. After exiting the

---

Hypertonic (hypertonicity) Having an increased osmotic pressure relative to the body's other fluids.

Osmolality A substance's concentration in a fluid affecting its tendency to cross a membrane (osmosis).

stomach, fluids are absorbed in the small intestine. The volume of the fluid must be large enough to trigger gastric emptying.[6] Often, the volume and osmolality of water consumption after exercise is not sufficient to rehydrate the body. Plain water, especially in small amounts, decreases osmolality, which limits the thirst response and increases urinary output. Including carbohydrates in the fluid increases the rate of intestinal absorption; the addition of a small amount of sodium may increase the thirst response.[6]

For maximum benefit, these drinks should contain a 6% concentration of carbohydrates. Carbohydrate concentrations above 8% can reduce gastric emptying and slow the absorption of fluids from the intestines.[1,23]

On-Field Examination and Management of Heat Illnesses

The management of patients with all types of heat illnesses requires rehydrating with cool water (the exception to this is exertional hyponatremia). Electrolytes, especially salt, often need to be replaced, but the use of salt tablets should be avoided because of their potentially counterproductive effects.[7] Dehydration, the root cause of many forms of heat illness, presents with a common set of symptoms (Table 22-5).[1]

Salt tablets delay gastric emptying and, if insufficient water is provided, fluids may be drawn from the extracellular space, causing further dehydration. In addition, salt tablets are often poorly tolerated, irritating the stomach lining and possibly resulting in nausea and vomiting, especially if administered without plentiful fluids. The use of commercial electrolyte drinks before, during, and after competition may be an effective method of reducing heat illnesses. However, drinking water should not be neglected.

Heat Cramps

Heat cramps are managed by controlling the symptoms and replacing fluids and electrolytes. While the athlete is on the field, the cramping muscle or muscles should be stretched

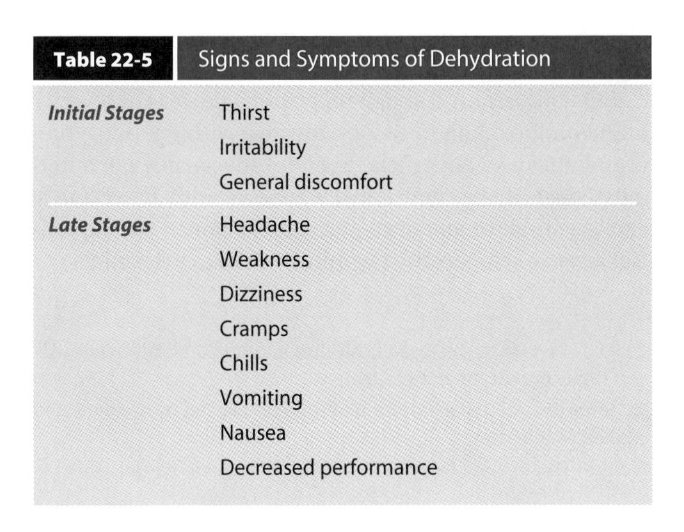

Table 22-5	Signs and Symptoms of Dehydration
Initial Stages	Thirst
	Irritability
	General discomfort
Late Stages	Headache
	Weakness
	Dizziness
	Cramps
	Chills
	Vomiting
	Nausea
	Decreased performance

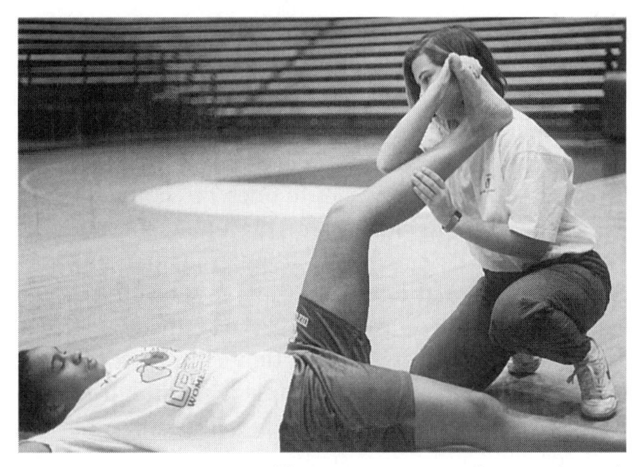

FIGURE 22-4 ■ Treatment of heat cramp spasms by stretching the involved muscle group.

until the spasm subsides (Fig. 22-4). After the athlete is returned to the sidelines, ice packs are applied to the involved area and the athlete's fluids and electrolytes are replenished. At the first sign of muscle twitching the athlete should be encouraged to drink 16 to 20 ounces of a sports electrolyte drink to which 3 grams of salt has been added. Salt tablets containing 1 gram of NaCl per tablet may be administered with a plentiful amount of water. More severe cases of heat cramps or heat cramps that are associated with heat exhaustion may require the intravenous administration of fluids and sodium.[17]

Heat Exhaustion and Heat Stroke

The treatment goals for athletes suffering from heat exhaustion or heat stroke are to reduce the core temperature and replace fluids and electrolytes. In each case, first aid cooling must be initiated by moving the athlete from the hot environment to a shaded area or indoors; removing excess clothing; elevating the legs; and cooling the body through the use of ice packs, cold water immersion, or fan-sprayed mist.

Patients with heat exhaustion can usually be adequately managed by applying ice packs to the superficial arteries located at the lateral neck, axilla, groin, and popliteal fossa (Fig. 22-5). A fan-sprayed mist has been used not only to

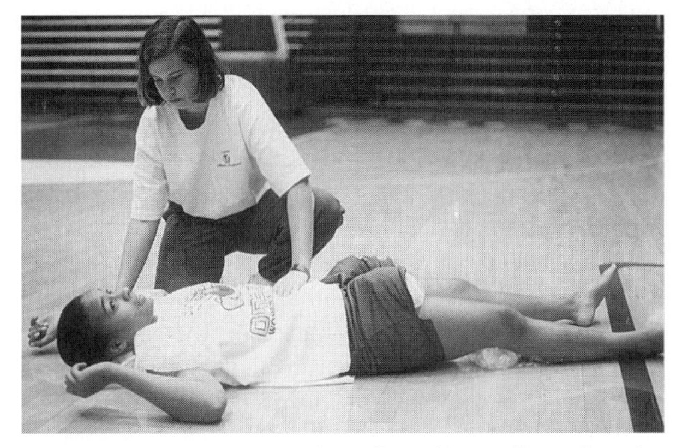

FIGURE 22-5 ■ Emergency cooling of an athlete suffering from heat illness. Packing the areas in which arteries are relatively subcutaneous (e.g., the popliteal fossa, femoral triangle, axilla, and neck) serves to cool the core temperature.

treat but also to prevent heat illnesses. These devices, often seen on football sidelines, spray a cool mist on the athlete to reduce the core temperature. However, their efficacy is questionable.[6] A cold shower is also an efficient method of reducing the core temperature, but the athlete should not be permitted to enter the shower unescorted.

If heat stroke is suspected, the emergency medical system should be activated. Although ice packs may be used, the ideal method of management of someone with heat stroke involves immersing the individual in 8 to 10 inches of cold water with a temperature at or below 55°F (12.8°C).[20] A shallow animal watering trough or child's swimming pool filled with water and ice can be used for this purpose, but the use of deep whirlpools should be avoided because of the inherent risk of drowning. To prevent overcooling, the patient is removed from the cooling tub when the core temperature decreases to 102°F (38.9°C).

If the athlete is conscious and cooperative, copious amounts of fluids are administered. In extreme cases of heat stroke, the physician orders **Ringer's lactate** to be administered intravenously. If the athlete's symptoms do not subside or if heat stroke is suspected, he or she must be immediately transported to the hospital because of the potentially fatal consequences.

Cold Injuries

Athletes who are competing outdoors in cold, damp environments are most predisposed to hypothermia. Indoor activities, except under the most unusual circumstances, do not normally predispose the athlete to cold injury. An exception to this is prolonged activity in a very cold swimming pool.

Hypothermia

Systemic cooling of the body, hypothermia, results from exposure to cold, damp air or immersion in cold water. The onset of hypothermia is not limited to subfreezing conditions. The body's core temperature begins to decrease when the ambient temperature is less than the body temperature and influenced by other environmental conditions such as wind and water. Clothing that has become wet from rain, snow, perspiration, or other means conducts heat away from the core, increasing the risk of hypothermia.

After the core temperature drops below 95°F (35°C), shivering, the first sign of hypothermia, appears, providing a short-term source of heat by increasing the body's metabolism. Impairment of the body's regulatory systems occurs when the core temperature drops below 94°F (34.4°C), predisposing the individual to cardiac irregularities and impairing the heart's responsiveness to treatment. A decreased cardiac stroke volume and an increased blood viscosity reduce the amount of blood reaching the brain, resulting in impaired mental function.

Cooling of the brain stem depresses the respiratory rate, resulting in body-wide anoxia. Systemic metabolism decreases, resulting in decreased metabolic heat production and further lowering of the core temperature. As the temperature continues to decrease, kidney function is impaired, disrupting the body's electrolyte balance.

A core temperature between 90°F and 94°F (32.2 and 34.4°C) is classified as mild hypothermia. Initially, the athlete complains of feeling cold, and the shivering response is initiated. Interest in the activity at hand wanes and is replaced by the desire to warm up. Signs of motor and mental impairment are indicated by decreased athletic performance. Severe hypothermia, a potentially fatal condition, results when the core temperature drops below 90°F (32.2°C). The athlete's desire to warm up is overridden by the desire to sleep, causing the athlete to appear uncoordinated and have slurred speech. An examination of the vital signs reveals decreased heart rate, respiration, and blood pressure (Examination Findings 22-3).

Frostbite

Unlike hypothermia, frostbite occurs only when the body is exposed to subfreezing temperatures. In response to this environment, the body protects the integrity of the core temperature at the expense of blood flow to the extremities, with the toes and fingers being the most vulnerable sites. During competition, the nose and cheeks are often uncovered, increasing the possibility of frostbite at these areas. The freezing of the ECF results in hypertonicity, dehydrating the cells by drawing the fluids out from the cell membrane via osmosis, an event that is more damaging than the actual extracellular ice formation. However, ice forming within the cell results in the permanent disruption of the cell membrane.

The magnitude and rate of nerve transmission is reduced when the nerves are cooled. This interruption makes the athlete initially unaware of the potential damage to the skin. As the freezing progresses, the athlete experiences a cold, burning sensation that suddenly ceases and is replaced by a sensation of comfortable warmth, a warning sign of severe frostbite.

Frostbite occurs through progressing degrees of severity, based on the depth of tissues affected, with one stage preceding the next. Superficial frostbite affects only the outermost layer of skin and initially appears with **hyperemia** and the development of edema within 3 hours. The superficial layer of skin **sloughs** within 1 week after the injury.

Ringer's lactate A salt-based solution administered intravenously as a replacement for lost electrolytes.

Hyperemia A red discoloration of the skin caused by an increased capillary blood flow.

Slough The peeling away of dead skin from living tissue.

Examination Findings 22-3
Hypothermia

Examination Segment	Clinical Findings
Onset	Gradual
Predisposing Factors	Prolonged exposure to a cold, damp or windy environment
Pupils	Dilated in severe hypothermia
Pulse	Slow and weak
Blood Pressure	Hypotension
Respiration	Shallow and irregular
Muscular Function	***Slight:*** Shivering ***Mild:*** Motor impairment ***Severe:*** Extreme motor impairment followed by muscle rigidity
Mental Status	***Slight:*** The athlete's mental focus begins to drift from the task at hand ***Mild:*** Desire to warm up ***Severe:*** Desire to sleep

Deep frostbite initially presents with the same signs and symptoms of superficial frostbite. However, destruction of the skin's full thickness occurs. Blisters appear in 1 to 7 days. This tissue sloughs to expose a hard, black layer of tissue. Disruption of the blood supply to the affected body part and distal structures creates an environment that encourages the development of **gangrene**. The most severe cases of frostbite involve the total destruction of the tissues in the area, including bone.

Prevention of Cold Injuries

Common sense is the guide in preventing cold injuries. Environmental conditions are a combination of ambient air temperature and wind. Wind chill can quickly lower the air temperature equivalent to dangerously low levels capable of freezing the skin in a matter of minutes or even seconds (Table 22-6). In extremely cold temperatures, the person's skin should be covered as completely as possible and practical for the sport. Multiple layers of clothing provide better insulation from the external environment than a single layer (Table 22-7).

Diet may be a factor contributing to the onset or prevention of hypothermia. Individuals who face prolonged exposure to subfreezing environments should avoid high-protein diets. Compared with diets high in carbohydrates or fats, those that are high in protein increase an individual's metabolic water requirements, thus decreasing their tolerance to cold.

Gangrene The death of bony or soft tissue resulting from a decrease in, or loss of, blood supply to a body area.

On-Field Examination and Management of Cold Injuries

As with heat injuries, the management of patients with cold injuries involves removing the athlete from the insulting environment. In this case, the athlete must be placed in a warm, dry environment, allowing the body to return to its normal temperature.

Hypothermia

After the athlete has been placed in a warm environment, the wet clothing is removed and the body is dried. Then the athlete is dressed in dry clothing or wrapped in a blanket.

Techniques to rapidly rewarm the body, such as immersion in a hot bath, must be avoided. Rapid rewarming dilates the peripheral vessels, causing lactic acid to be routed to the core. This leads to rebound hypothermia, which can cause a further decrease in core temperature secondary to hypotension and ventricular fibrillation. Athletes should not be allowed to sleep. Doing so decreases metabolism and delays rewarming of the core temperature. Warm drinks are not effective in raising the core temperature, and the use of alcoholic drinks must be avoided because of their depressant effects. The core may be quickly and safely rewarmed by having the athlete breathe in the mist of a humidifier or other source of hot,

Table 22-6 Calculation of the Wind Chill Factor

Wind Speed, MPH	Actual Thermometer Reading (°F)											
	50	40	30	20	10	0	−10	−20	−30	−40	−50	−60
	Wind Chill Factor (°F)											
Calm	50	40	30	20	10	0	−10	−20	−30	−40	−50	−60
5	48	37	27	16	6	−5	−15	−26	−36	−47	−57	−68
10	40	28	16	4	−9	−24	−33	−46	−58	−70	−83	−95
15	36	22	9	−5	−18	−32	−45	−58	−72	−85	−99	−112
20	32	18	4	−10	−25	−39	−53	−67	−82	−96	−110	−124
25	30	16	0	−15	−29	−44	−59	−74	−88	−104	−118	−133
30	28	13	−2	−18	−33	−48	−63	−79	−94	−109	−125	−140
35	27	11	−4	−20	−35	−51	−67	−82	−98	−113	−129	−145
40	26	10	−6	−21	−37	−53	−69	−85	−100	−116	−132	−148
	Little danger				Moderate danger			Extreme danger				
					Skin freezes within 1 min			Skin freezes rapidly (< 1 min)				

moist air.[24] Blankets, clothing, and so on can also be used to gently warm the individual.

Frostbite

Initially, frostbite can be limited by the athlete keeping the affected body part moving, increasing the amount of metabolic heat production. When the athlete is still in the cold environment, frostbite of the fingers can be treated by the person tucking the fingers in the axilla or crotch. Once out of the environment, mild frostbite can be treated by immersing the body part in a warm (104°F to 110°F; 40°C to 43.3°C) bath. The affected area should never be rubbed and snow should not be applied.

Frostbite that affects more than the superficial skin should not be thawed if the risk of refreezing exists. After the frozen part thaws, the athlete must not be allowed to walk on or use the affected part. If the athlete is still in the cold environment, steps must be taken to prevent hypothermia. Athletes suspected of suffering from frostbite must be immediately referred to a hospital so that a definitive diagnosis may be made and proper treatment initiated.

Table 22-7 National Collegiate Athletic Association's Recommended Guidelines for Reducing Cold Stress[23]

Guideline	Comments
Layer Clothing	Wearing several thin layers of clothing is best to retain body heat; layers may be added or removed as needed.
Cover the Head	As much as 50% of the body's heat is lost through the head.
Protect the Hands	The use of mittens rather than gloves is recommended to protect the fingers from frostbite.
Stay Dry	Water increases the rate of heat loss from the body. Rather than wearing clothes made of cotton, wearing those made of polypropylene, wool, or other material that wicks moisture away from the skin is recommended.
Stay Hydrated	Fluids are needed to maintain the body'score temperature and are as important in preventing cold injuries as heat injuries.
Maintain Energy Level	A negative energy balance increases the risk of hypothermia. Proper eating and consuming "energy snacks" and sports drinks helps maintain a positive energy balance.
Warm Up Thoroughly	A thorough warm-up is required before competition to elevate the core temperature.
Warm Incoming Air	The use of a scarf or mask across the mouth warms incoming air.
Avoid Alcohol, Nicotine, and Other Drugs	These agents cause vasoconstriction or vasodilation of the superficial blood vessels, hindering regulation of the core temperature.
Never Train Alone	An injury that prevents the athlete from walking may be catastrophic in cold climates.

REFERENCES

1. Casa, DJ, et al: National Athletic Trainers' Association Position Statement: Fluid replacement for athletes. *J Athl Train,* 35: 212, 2000.
2. Sheehy, SB: Environmental emergencies. In Sheehy, SB (ed): *Mosby's Manual of Emergency Care* (ed 3). St Louis, CV Mosby, 1990, p 300.
3. Davidson, M: Heat illness in athletics. *Athl Train J Nl Athl Train Assoc,* 20:96, 1985.
4. Gonzalez-Alonso, J: Separate and combined influences of dehydration and hyperthermia on cardiovascular response to exercise. *Int J Sports Med,* 2(S):111, 1998.
5. Nimmo, M: Exercise in the cold. *J Sports Sci,* 22:898, 2004.
6. Casa, DJ: Exercise in the heat. II. Critical concepts in rehydration, exertional heat illness, and maximizing performance. *J Athl Train,* 34:253, 1999.
7. Birrer, RB: Heat stroke. Don't wait for the classic signs. *Emerg Med Clin North Am,* July:43, 1994.
8. Howe, AS, and Boden, BP: Heat-related illnesses in athletes. *Am J Sports Med,* 35:1384, 2007.
9. Bergeron, MF, et al: Youth football: Heat stress and injury risk. *Med Sci Sports Exerc,* 37:1421, 2005.
10. Eichner, ER : Sickle cell trait. *J Sport Rehabil,* 16:197, 2007.
11. Cleary, M: Predisposing risk factors on susceptibility to exertional heat illness: Clinical decision-making considerations. *J Sport Rehabil,* 16:204, 2007.
12. Stuempfle, JG, and McCaw, ST: Ground reaction forces among gymnasts and recreational athletes in drop landings. *J Athl Train,* 38:315, 2003.
13. Casa, DJ, et al: Validity of devices that assess body temperature during outdoor exercise in heat. *J Athl Train,* 42:333, 2007.
14. Binkley, HM, et al: National Athletic Trainers' Association position statement: Exertional heat illnesses. *J Athl Train,* 37: 329, 2002.
15. Cooper, ER, Ferrara, MS, and Broglio, SP: Exertional heat illness and environmental conditions during a single football season in the Southeast. *J Athl Train,* 41:332, 2006.
16. Noakes, TD: Fluid and electrolyte disturbances in heat illness. *Int J Sports Med,* 2(S):146, 1998.
17. Bergeron, MF: Exertional heat cramps: Recovery and return to play. *J Sport Rehabil,* 16:190, 2007.
18. Wharam, PC, et al: NSAID use increases the risk of developing hyponatremia during an Ironman triathlon. *Med Sci Sports Exerc,* 38:618, 2006.
19. Siegel, AJ: Exercise-associated hyponatremia: Role of cytokines. *Am J Med,* 119(7 Suppl 1):S74, 2006.
20. American College of Sports Medicine: Position stand on prevention of thermal injuries during distance running. *Med Sci Sports Exerc,* 16:ix, 1984.
21. Francis, K, Feinstein, R, and Brasher, J: Optimal practice times for the reduction of the risk of heat illness during fall football practice in the southeastern United States. *Athletic Training: J Athl Train,* 26:76, 1991.
22. Noakes, TD, et al: Metabolic rate, not percent dehydration, predicts rectal temperatures in marathon runners. *Med Sci Sports Exerc,* 23:443, 1991.
23. National Collegiate Athletics Association: Sports Medicine Handbook 2008-09 (ed 20). Retrieved from http://www.ncaa.org/wps/ncaa?ContentID=1446. (Accessed October 22, 2008).
24. Bowman, WD: Outdoor emergency care: Comprehensive *First Aid of Nonurban Settings.* Lakewood, CO, National Ski Patrol System, 1988, p 291.

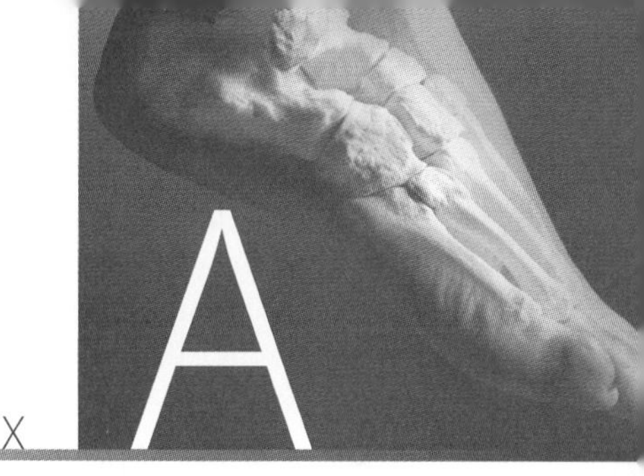

APPENDIX A

Reflex Testing

Deep tendon reflexes are elicited with a threshold response after a quick stretch of the muscle tendon that causes a reflexive muscular contraction. The procedure involves tapping the tendon with a reflex hammer with enough force to elicit the response. Practice is required to develop the right touch to elicit a reflex response. The amount of pressure required to elicit a response varies from reflex to reflex and from person to person.

Obtaining a reflex response is facilitated by having the patient slightly tense an unrelated muscle during the reflex test (Fig. A1). If the patient is anxious, instruct him or her to close the eyes so that he or she will not anticipate the test.

Reflexes must be checked bilaterally with each limb held at approximately the same position with equal amounts of muscular tension. The reflex can be graded on a four-point scale:

Grade	Response
0	No reflex elicited
1+	Hyporeflexia: Reflex elicited with reinforcement (precontracting the muscle)
2+	Normal response
3+	Hyperreflexia (brisk)
4+	Hyperactive with clonus

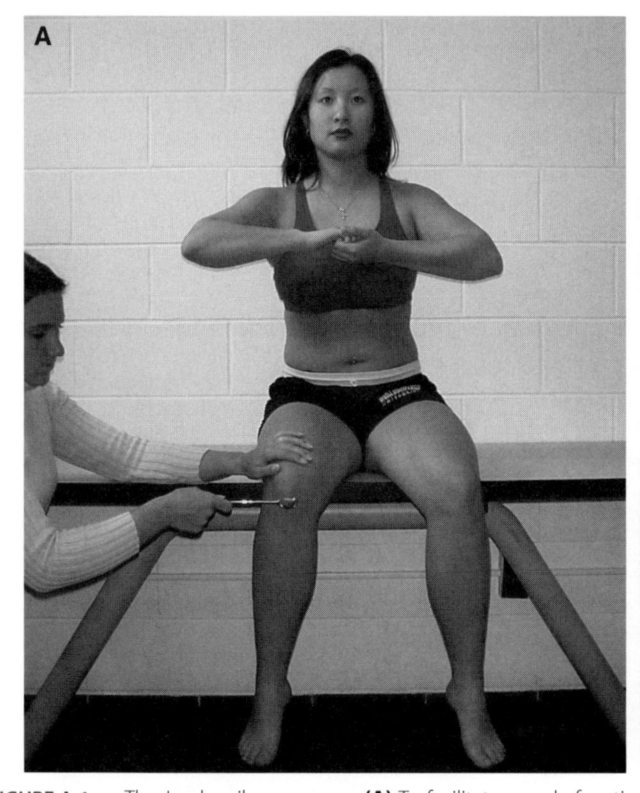

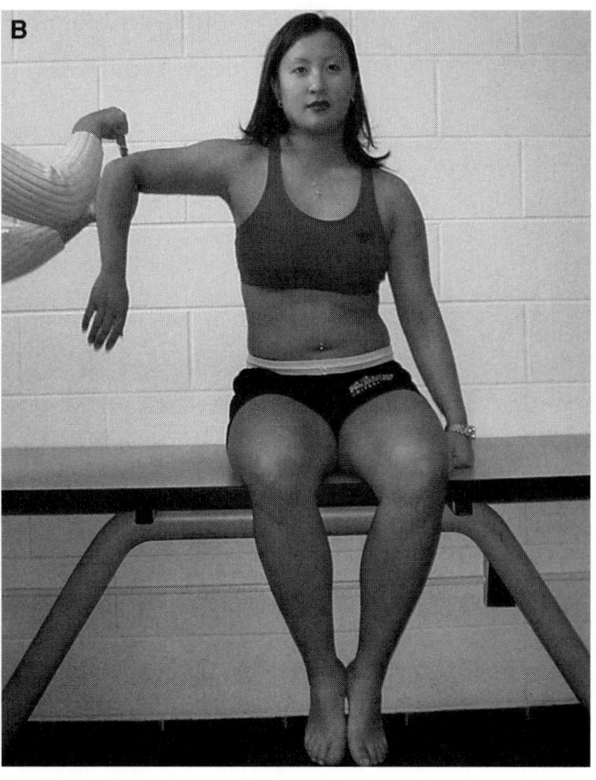

FIGURE A-1 ■ The Jendrassik maneuvers. **(A)** To facilitate muscle function during lower extremity reflex testing, have the patient attempt to pull the hands apart as shown. **(B)** Muscle facilitation during upper extremity reflex testing. The patient presses the medial aspects of the feet against each other.

All of the reflexes in the extremity being tested should be assessed and compared to the same reflex in the opposite extremity. For example, in a patient who exhibits poor muscle tone, a reflex that must be elicited with reinforcement might be assessed as abnormal. However, further assessment would reveal that all of the remaining reflexes are also grade 1. Therefore, this is the baseline assessment naturally found in this individual.

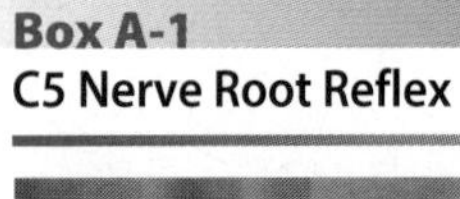

Box A-1
C5 Nerve Root Reflex

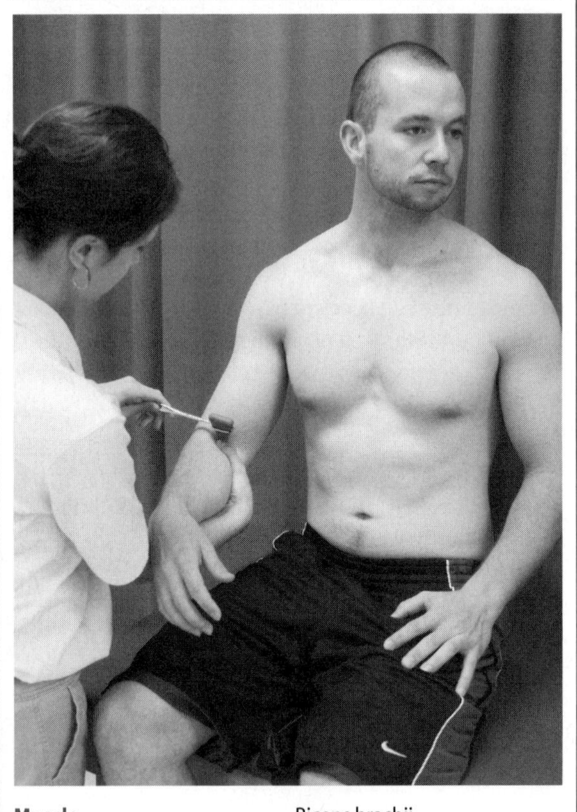

Muscle	Biceps brachii
Patient Position	Seated looking away from the tested side
Position of Examiner	Standing to the side of the patient, cradling the forearm with the thumb placed over the tendon
Evaluative Procedure	The thumb is tapped with the reflex hammer.
Innervation	Musculocutaneous nerve
Nerve Root	C5, C6

Box A-2
C6 Nerve Root Reflex

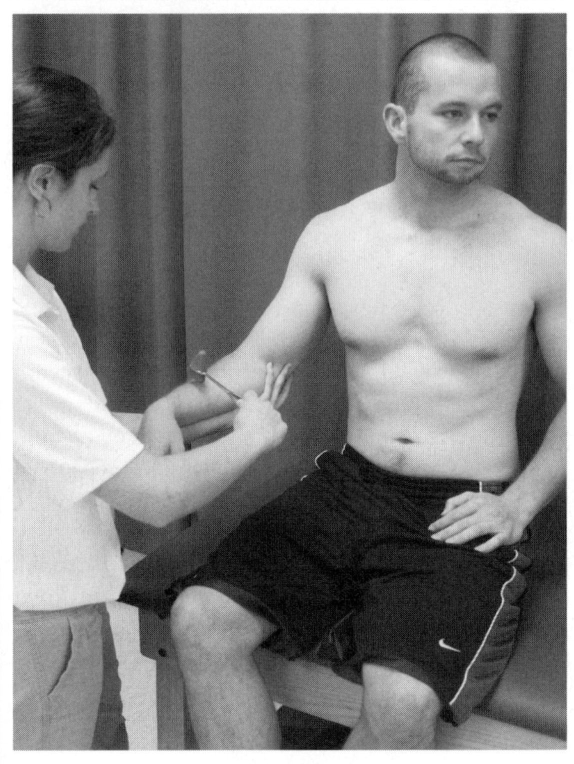

Muscle	Brachioradialis
Patient Position	Seated looking away from the tested side The elbow is passively flexed to between 60° and 90°
Position of Examiner	Cradling the patient's arm
Evaluative Procedure	The distal portion of the brachioradialis tendon is tapped with the reflex hammer. The proximal tendon may also be used.
Innervation	Radial nerve
Nerve Roots	C5, C6

Box A-3

C7 Nerve Root Reflex

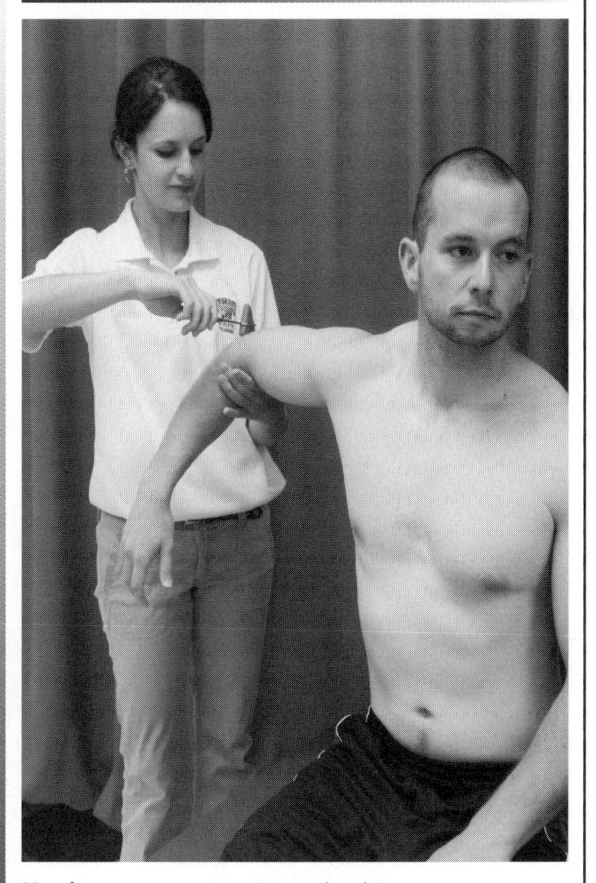

Muscle	Triceps brachii
Patient Position	Seated looking away from the tested side
Position of Examiner	Supporting the patient's shoulder abducted to 90° and the elbow flexed to 90°
Evaluative Procedure	The distal triceps brachii tendon is tapped with the reflex hammer.
Innervation	Radial nerve
Nerve Roots	(C6), C7, C8

Box A-4

L4 Nerve Root Reflex

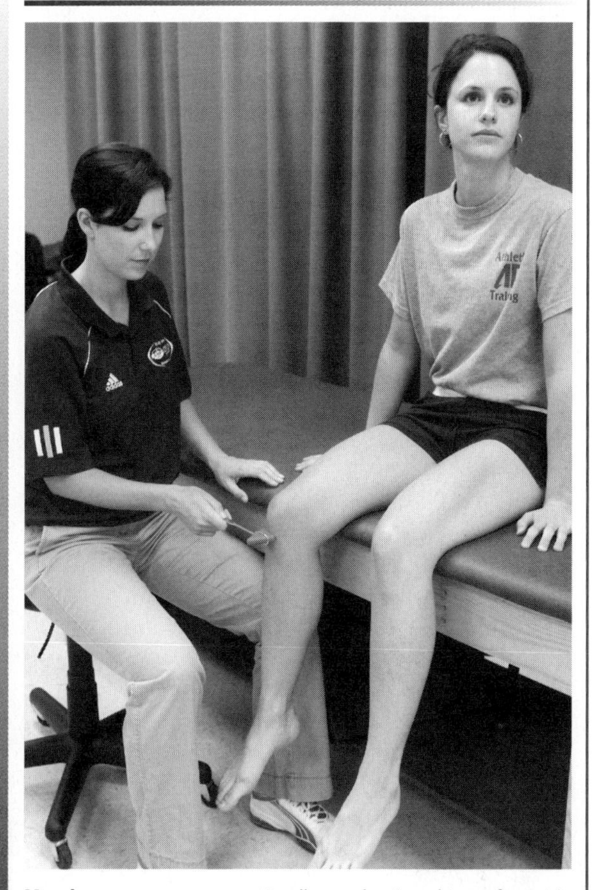

Muscle	Patellar tendon (quadriceps femoris)
Patient Position	Sitting with the knees flexed over the end of the table looking away from the tested side
Position of Examiner	Standing or seated to the side of the patient
Evaluative Procedure	The patellar tendon is tapped with the reflex hammer.
Innervation	Femoral nerve
Nerve Roots	(L2), L3, L4

Box A-5
L5 Nerve Root Reflex

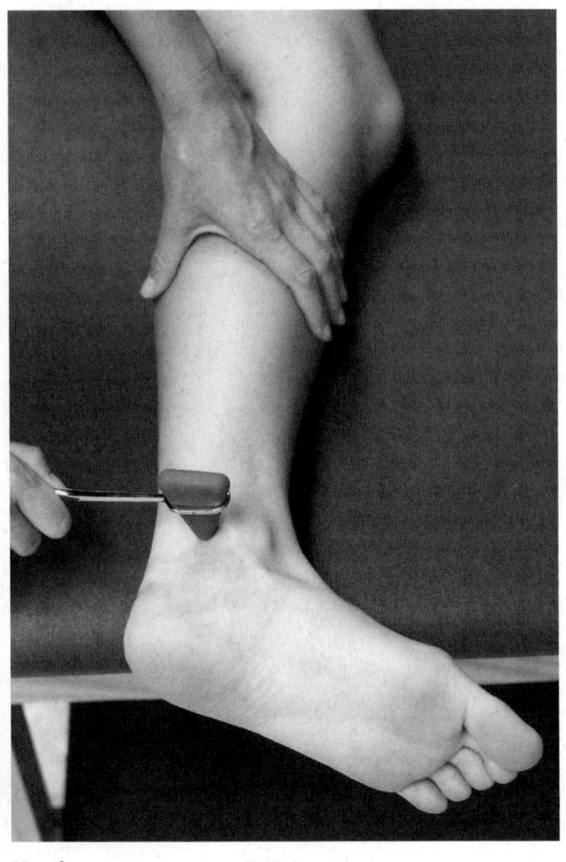

Muscle	Tibialis posterior
Patient Position	Sidelying on test side The test foot is off the edge of the table.
Position of Examiner	Standing or seated to the side of the patient
Evaluative Procedure	The tibialis posterior tendon is tapped with the reflex hammer posteriorly and just proximal to the medial malleolus.
Innervation	Tibial nerve
Nerve Roots	L5, (L4, S1)

Box A-6
L5 Nerve Root Reflex

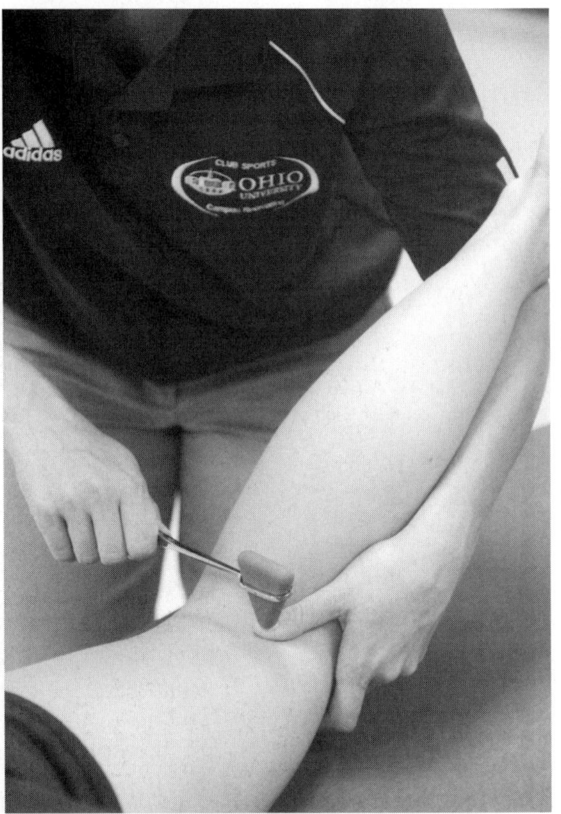

Muscle	Medial hamstrings (semitendinosus)
Patient Position	Supine with the knee slightly flexed looking away from the tested side
Position of Examiner	Standing or seated to the side of the patient. The thumb or finger is placed over the semitendinosus tendon immediately superior to the medial joint line.
Evaluative Procedure	The finger is tapped with the reflex hammer.
Innervation	Tibial nerve
Nerve Roots	L5, S1, (S2)

Box A-7
S1 Nerve Root Reflex

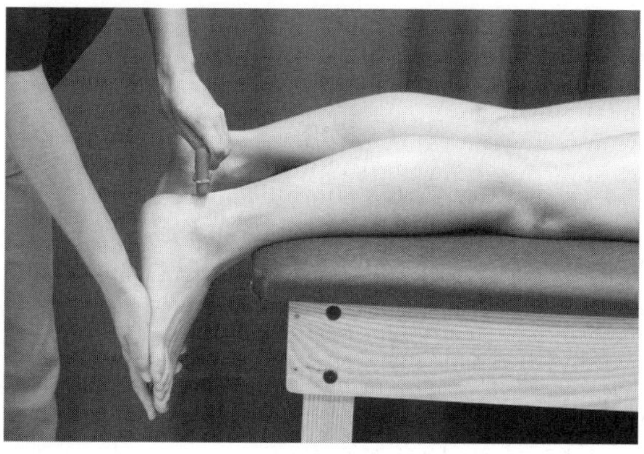

Muscle	Achilles tendon (triceps surae muscle group)
Patient Position	Prone with the feet off the edge of the table.
Position of Examiner	Seated or standing next to the patient, supporting the foot in its neutral position
Evaluative Procedure	The Achilles tendon is tapped with a reflex hammer.
Innervation	Tibial
Nerve Roots	S1, S2

Box A-8
S2 Nerve Root Reflex

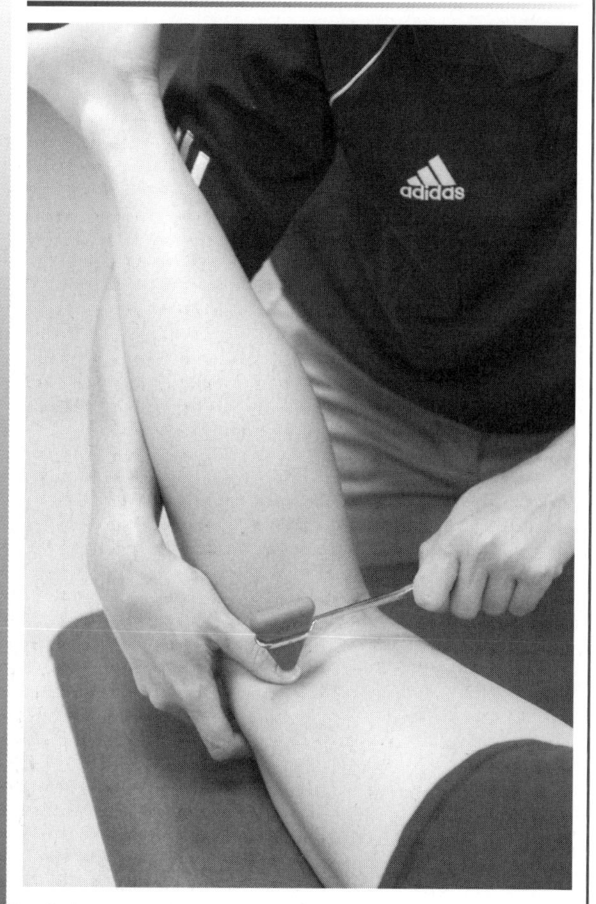

Muscle	Biceps femoris
Patient Position	Prone with the knee flexed to approximately 20°
Position of Examiner	Standing next to the patient The thumb is placed over the biceps femoris tendon just proximal to the joint line
Evaluative Procedure	The thumb is tapped with a reflex hammer.
Innervation	Tibial, common peroneal
Nerve Roots	L5, S1, S2, (S3)

APPENDIX B

Lower Extremity Functional Testing

Functional testing involves the application of controlled forces replicating the stresses that will be experienced during activity. The individual components of lower extremity function, including joint stability, range of motion, strength, and balance, are assessed during the evaluation of injury. The application of sport-specific functional tests assesses the patient's neuromuscular and proprioceptive status. Functional testing also challenges the athlete psychologically, requiring confidence that the limb can function under the stresses that will be placed on it during sports.

An athlete's functional status can be evaluated by using running, sprinting, and agility drills that emphasize quick starts, cutting, and stops. Actual sport skills such as backpedaling, cross-over steps, jumping, and so on may also be used. In addition, specific tests have been developed so that the injured leg's function can be assessed clinically. Although these tests may be sensitive in some patients, subjective complaints of difficulty with pivoting, cutting, and twisting may be the most sensitive determination of the ability to function. Patients who display gross joint laxity or muscle weakness should not perform these tests.

This appendix describes four common tests used for determining the functional ability of the patient with a lower extremity injury. These tests may be performed as a single set of one repetition on each limb or recorded as the average of three repetitions for each extremity. Positive tests indicate the presence of functional limitations that may suggest the inability to pivot, cut, and twist during activity.

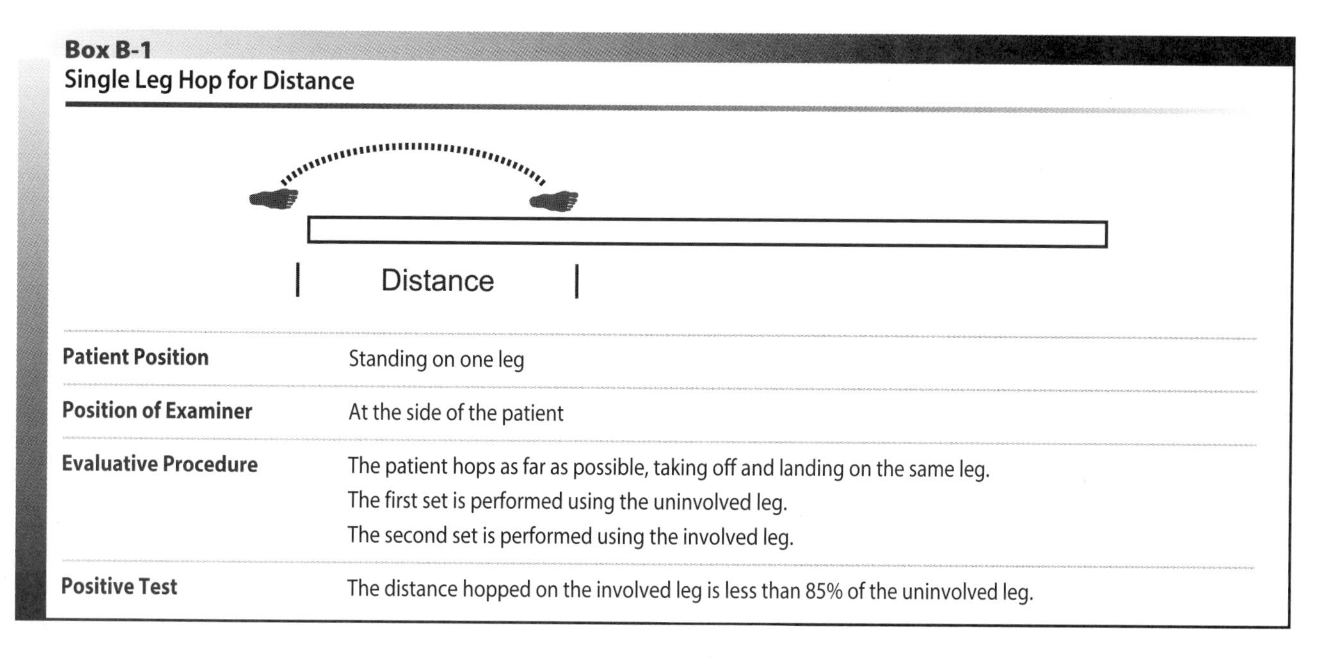

Box B-1
Single Leg Hop for Distance

Patient Position	Standing on one leg
Position of Examiner	At the side of the patient
Evaluative Procedure	The patient hops as far as possible, taking off and landing on the same leg. The first set is performed using the uninvolved leg. The second set is performed using the involved leg.
Positive Test	The distance hopped on the involved leg is less than 85% of the uninvolved leg.

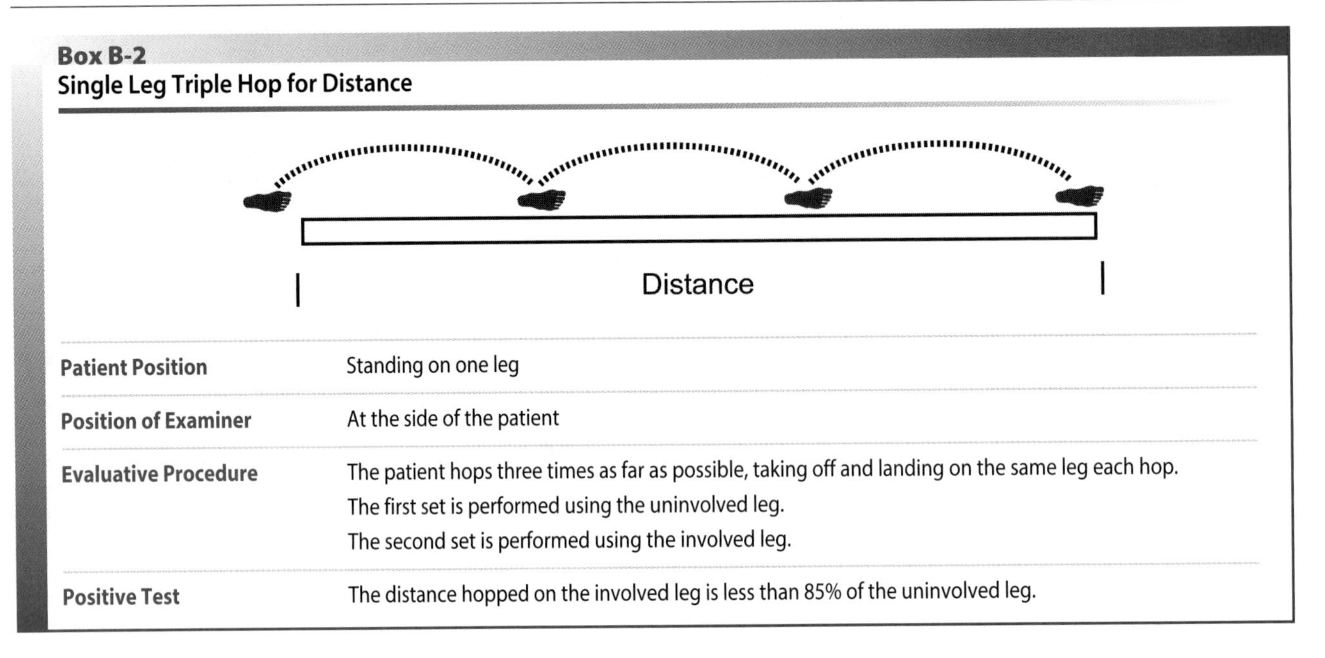

Box B-2

Single Leg Triple Hop for Distance

Patient Position	Standing on one leg
Position of Examiner	At the side of the patient
Evaluative Procedure	The patient hops three times as far as possible, taking off and landing on the same leg each hop. The first set is performed using the uninvolved leg. The second set is performed using the involved leg.
Positive Test	The distance hopped on the involved leg is less than 85% of the uninvolved leg.

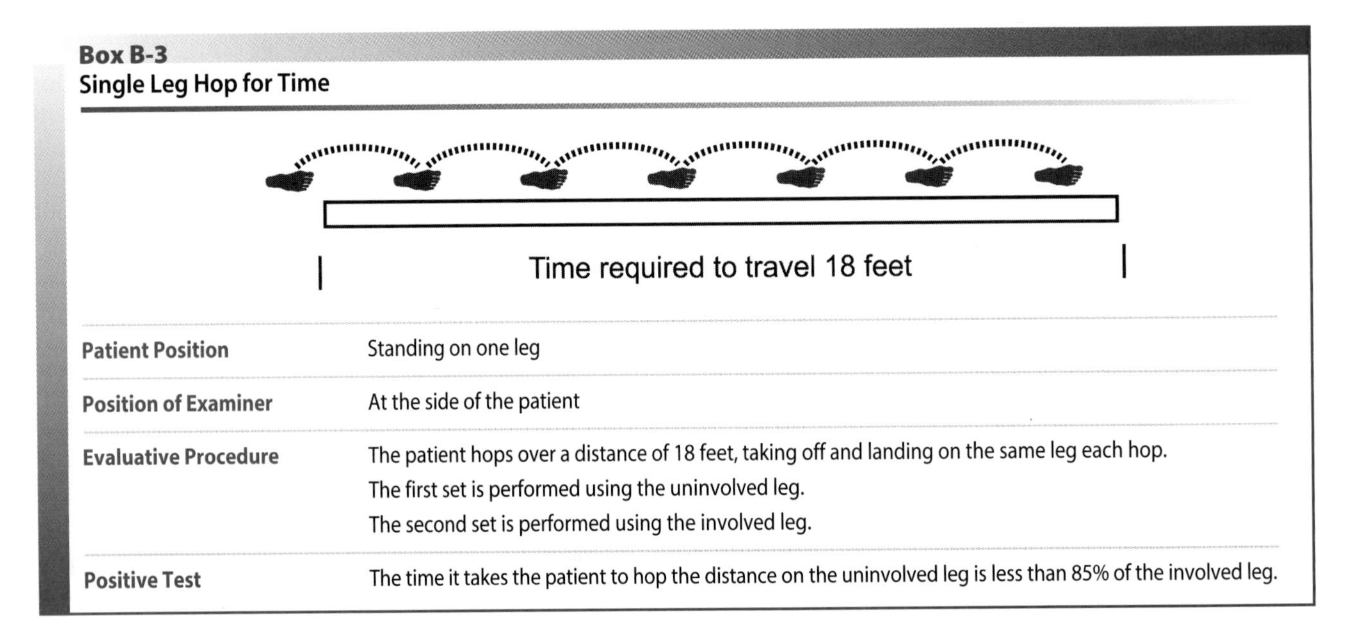

Box B-3

Single Leg Hop for Time

Patient Position	Standing on one leg
Position of Examiner	At the side of the patient
Evaluative Procedure	The patient hops over a distance of 18 feet, taking off and landing on the same leg each hop. The first set is performed using the uninvolved leg. The second set is performed using the involved leg.
Positive Test	The time it takes the patient to hop the distance on the uninvolved leg is less than 85% of the involved leg.

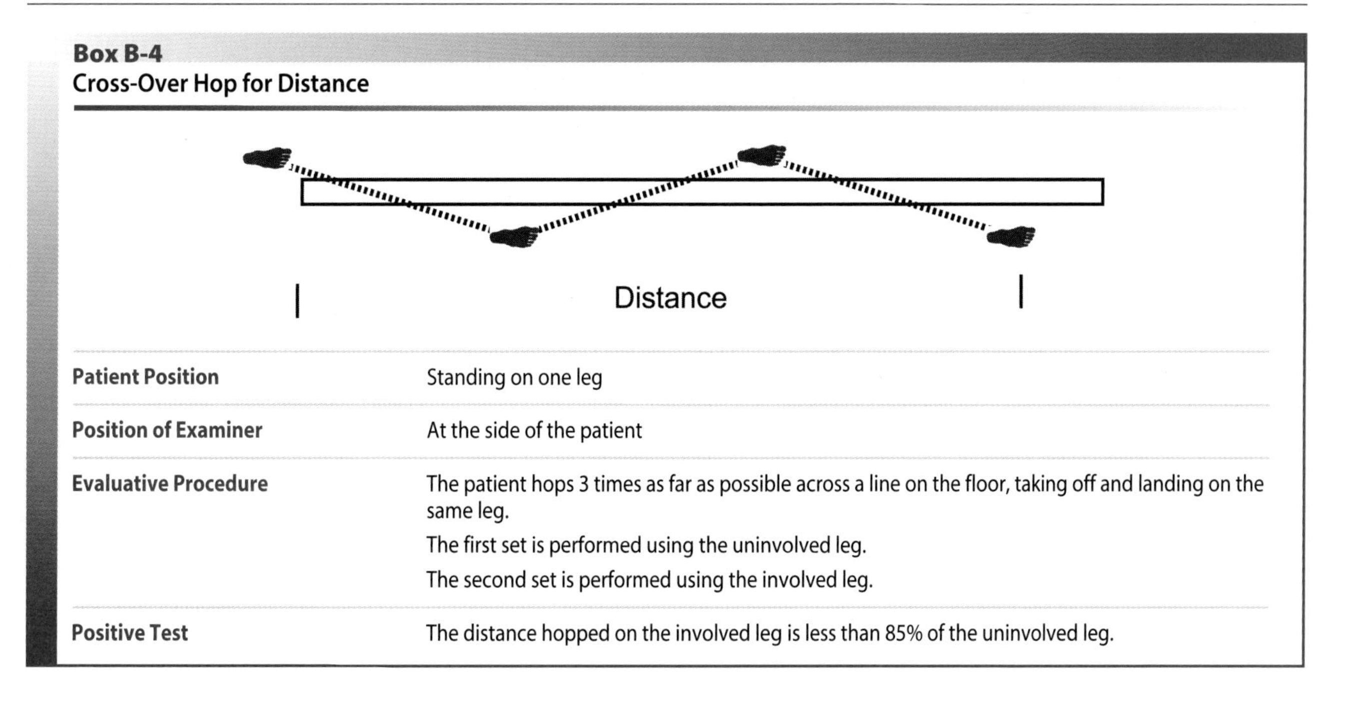

Box B-4
Cross-Over Hop for Distance

Patient Position	Standing on one leg
Position of Examiner	At the side of the patient
Evaluative Procedure	The patient hops 3 times as far as possible across a line on the floor, taking off and landing on the same leg. The first set is performed using the uninvolved leg. The second set is performed using the involved leg.
Positive Test	The distance hopped on the involved leg is less than 85% of the uninvolved leg.

Index

Note: Page numbers followed by f refer to figures; page numbers followed by t refer to tables; page numbers followed by b refer to boxes.

A

D

E

G

H

I

J

M

N

O

P

Q

U